REHABILITATION MEDICINE

REHABILITATION MEDICINE

Editor

JOSEPH GOODGOLD, M.D.

The Howard A. Rusk Professor and Chairman,
Department of Rehabilitation Medicine,
New York University School of Medicine,
Director of Rehabilitation Medicine Services,
New York University Medical Center,
New York, New York

with **670** *illustrations*

The C. V. Mosby Company

ST. LOUIS • WASHINGTON, D.C. • TORONTO   1988

MOSBY

A TRADITION OF PUBLISHING EXCELLENCE

Editor: Eugenia A. Klein
Developmental editor: Kathryn H. Falk
Assistant editor: Ellen Baker Geisel
Project manager: Patricia Tannian
Design: Gail Morey Hudson

The C.V. Mosby Company
11830 Westline Industrial Drive, St. Louis, Missouri 63146

Library of Congress Cataloging-in-Publication Data

Rehabilitation medicine/editor, Joseph Goodgold.
        p.   cm.
     Includes bibliographies and index.
     ISBN 0-8016-1838-X
     1. Medicine, Physical.   I. Goodgold, Joseph, 1920-
     [DNLM: 1. Rehabilitation.   WB 320 R3436]
RM700.R43   1988
617--dc19
DNLM/DLC
for Library of Congress   88-12756
                                                                        CIP

GW/MV/MV   9 8 7 6 5 4 3 2 1

Contributors

JUNG H. AHN, M.D.

Assistant Professor of Clinical Rehabilitation Medicine,
Project Director, Department of Rehabilitation Medicine, New
York University School of Medicine, New York Regional
Spinal Cord Injury System, New York, New York

JUSTIN ALEXANDER, Ph.D.

Coordinator, Comprehensive Rehabilitation Center, Veterans
Administration Hospital, Tampa, Florida

FRANCES SOMMER ANDERSON, Ph.D.

Formerly Senior Clinical Psychologist, Formerly Director,
Psychology Intern Training, Department of Psychology, Rusk
Institute of Rehabilitation Medicine, New York University
Medical Center, New York, New York

MERRILL P. ANDERSON, Ph.D.

Assistant Professor, Department of Medicine, Baylor College of
Medicine, Houston, Texas

PAUL BACH-Y-RITA, M.D.

Professor and Chairman, Department of Rehabilitation
Medicine, University of Wisconsin, Madison, Wisconsin

R. JAMES BARNARD, Ph.D.

Professor of Kinesiology, Department of Kinesiology, University
of California–Los Angeles, Los Angeles, California; Director of
Research, Nathan Pritikin Research Foundation,
Santa Monica, California

YEHUDA BEN-YISHAY, Ph.D.

Associate Professor of Clinical Rehabilitation, Co-Director,
Head Trauma Program, Rusk Institute of Rehabilitation
Medicine, New York University Medical Center,
New York, New York

EDWARD H. BERGOFSKY, M.D.

Professor of Medicine, Pulmonary-Critical Care Division, State
University of New York at Stony Brook, Stony Brook,
New York

BARBARA Z. BERK, M.D.

Fellow in Geriatrics, Teaching Assistant, Medicine, New York
University Medical Center, New York, New York

DORIS BERRYMAN, Ph.D.

Department of Recreation, Leisure, Physical Education and
Sport, New York University, New York, New York

JOSEPH BRUDNY, M.D.

Clinical Associate Professor, Department of Rehabilitation
Medicine, New York University School of Medicine,
New York, New York

SOPHIA CHIOTELIS, O.T.R., M.A.

Director, Occupational Therapy, Rusk Institute of Rehabilitation
Medicine, New York University Medical Center, New York,
New York

CHARLES D. CICCONE, Ph.D., P.T.

Assistant Professor, Division of Physical Therapy, Ithaca
College, Ithaca, New York

STEPHEN R. COLEN, M.D.

Assistant Professor of Surgery, New York University Medical
Center, Institute of Reconstruction Plastic Surgery, New York,
New York

RONALD W. CONLEY, Ph.D.

Department of Health and Human Services, Washington, D.C.

LEONARD DILLER, Ph.D.

Professor of Clinical Rehabilitation Medicine, Department of Rehabilitation Medicine, New York University Medical Center, New York, New York

PATRICIA DVONCH, Ph.D.

Formerly Associate Professor and Chairperson, Department of Rehabilitation Counseling, New York University, New York, New York

ARTHUR EBERSTEIN, Ph.D.

Professor and Director of Research, Department of Rehabilitation Medicine, New York University Medical Center, New York, New York

ANDREW EISEN, M.D., F.R.C.P. (C)

Professor, Department of Neurology, Associate Dean of Medicine, University of British Columbia; Head, Neuromuscular Diseases Unit, The Vancouver General Hospital, University of British Columbia, Vancouver, British Columbia

GORDON L. ENGLER, M.D.

Clinical Professor of Orthopedic Surgery, Director of Scoliosis and Spinal Deformities, New York University Medical Center, Department of Orthopaedic Surgery, New York, New York

SAUL H. FISHER, M.D.

Clinical Professor of Psychiatry, Department of Psychiatry, New York University School of Medicine, New York, New York

WILLIAM M. FOWLER, Jr., M.D.

Professor, Department of Physical Medicine and Rehabilitation, University of California School of Medicine, Davis, California

MICHAEL L. FREEDMAN, M.D.

Diane and Arthur Belfer Professor of Geriatric Medicine, Director, Division of Geriatrics, Department of Medicine, New York University Medical Center, New York, New York

SANFORD J. FRIEDMAN, M.D., F.A.C.C.

Instructor, Department of Medicine, Mount Sinai Hospital, New York, New York

LAWRENCE W. FRIEDMANN, M.D., F.A.C.A., F.I.C.A.

Chairman, Department of Physical Medicine and Rehabilitation, Nassau County Medical Center; Professor, Department of Rehabilitation Medicine, State University of New York at Stony Brook, Stony Brook, New York

MARTIN GRABOIS, M.D.

Professor and Chairman, Department of Physical Medicine, Baylor College of Medicine; Director, Pain Management Program, The Methodist Hospital, Houston, Texas

JACOB J. GRAHAM, M.D.

Attending Orthopaedic Surgeon, Chief, Scoliosis Service, Orthopaedic Institute, Hospital for Joint Diseases; Associate Clinical Professor, Orthopaedic Surgery, Mount Sinai School of Medicine; Assistant Clinical Professor, Orthopaedic Surgery, New York University School of Medicine, New York, New York

BRUCE B. GRYNBAUM, M.D.

Professor and Vice Chairman, Department of Rehabilitation Medicine, New York University Medical Center, New York, New York

STEPHEN L. GUMPORT, M.D.

Professor of Surgery, Director, Cancer Rehabilitation Service, Rusk Institute of Rehabilitation Medicine, New York University Medical Center, New York, New York

LAURO S. HALSTEAD, M.D.

Director, Post Polio Program, Professor, National Rehabilitation Hospital, Department of Medicine, Georgetown University Medical School, Washington, D.C.

ADAM N. HUREWITZ, M.D.

Research Assistant Professor of Medicine, Department of Medicine, State University of New York at Stony Brook, Stony Brook, New York

STEPHEN INKELES, M.D., M.P.H.

Director of Clinical Nutrition, Pritikin Longevity Center, Santa Monica, California; Clinical Instructor, Division of Clinical Nutrition, Department of Medicine, University of California–Los Angeles, Los Angeles, California

MASAYOSHI ITOH, M.D., M.P.H.

Associate Professor of Clinical Rehabilitation Medicine, Goldwater Memorial Hospital, Department of Rehabilitation Medicine, New York University School of Medicine, New York, New York

SARAN JONAS, M.D.

Professor of Clinical Neurology, Acting Chairman, Department of Neurology, New York University Medical Center, New York, New York

THOMAS KANTOR, M.D.

Professor of Clinical Medicine, Department of Medicine, New York University School of Medicine, New York, New York

ESIN KAPLAN, M.D.

Clinical Assistant Professor of Rehabilitation Medicine, Rusk Institute of Rehabilitation Medicine, New York University Medical Center, New York, New York

PAUL KAPLAN, M.D.

Chairman, Department of Physical Medicine and Rehabilitation, University of Missouri at Columbia, Columbia, Missouri

LAWRENCE I. KAPLAN, M.D.

Director, Department of Rehabilitation Medicine, Mount Sinai Services, City Hospital Center at Elmhurst, Elmhurst, New York

PATRICIA KERMAN-LERNER, M.A.

Chief, Speech Pathology and Audiology Service, Department of Rehabilitation Medicine, Goldwater Memorial Hospital, New York University Medical Center; Assistant Professor of Speech, New York University, New York, New York

HANS KRAUS, M.D.

Formerly Associate Professor, Department of Physical Medicine and Rehabilitation, New York University, New York, New York

SANTOSH LAL, M.D.

Assistant Professor of Physical Medicine and Rehabilitation, Northwestern University; Attending Physician, Rehabilitation Institute of Chicago, Chicago, Illinois

VALERY F. LANYI, M.D.

Clinical Associate Professor, Department of Rehabilitation Medicine, New York University Medical Center, New York, New York

MATHEW LEE, M.D., M.P.H.

Professor of Clinical Rehabilitation Medicine, Department of Rehabilitation Medicine, Goldwater Memorial Hospital, New York University School of Medicine, New York, New York

CLAUDETTE LeFEBVRE, Ph.D.

Department of Recreation, Leisure, Physical Education and Sport, New York University, New York, New York

HANS RICHARD LEHNEIS, Ph.D., C.P.O.

Director, Orthotics and Prosthetics, Department of Rehabilitation Medicine, New York University Medical Center, New York, New York

RALPH LUSSKIN, M.D.

Professor of Clinical Orthopedic Surgery, Department of Orthopedic Surgery, New York University School of Medicine, New York, New York

DONG M. MA, M.D.

Assistant Professor of Rehabilitation Medicine, Co-Director of EMG Laboratories, Rusk Institute of Rehabilitation Medicine, New York University Medical Center, New York, New York

ROBERT L. MAGNUSON, M.D.

Medical Director of Rehabilitation, Paradise Valley Hospital, National City, California

COLIN A. McLAURIN, Sc.D.

Director, Rehabilitation Engineering Center, University of Virginia, Charlottesville, Virginia

MARIAN T. MIGNANO, R.N., B.S.N., M.P.S.

Assistant Administrator and Director of Nursing, Rusk Institute of Rehabilitation Medicine, New York University Medical Center, New York, New York

JEFFREY MINKOFF, M.D.

Clinical Associate Professor, Director of Sports Fellowships, New York University; Associate Attending in Orthopedics, Lenox Hill Hospital; Associate Attending in Orthopedics, Hospital for Joint Diseases, New York, New York

PABLO MORALES, M.D.

Professor and Chairman, Department of Urology, New York University Medical Center, New York, New York

SANJEEV D. NANDEDKAR, Ph.D.

Medical Research Assistant Professor, Duke University Medical Center, Durham, North Carolina

MARY LYNN NEWPORT, M.D.

Senior Resident, Hospital for Joint Diseases/Orthopedic Institute, New York, New York

JOHN H. NOBLE, Jr., M.D.

Professor of Social Work and Rehabilitation Medicine, State University of New York at Buffalo, Buffalo, New York

JOACHIM L. OPITZ, M.D.

Consultant, Department of Physical Medicine and Rehabilitation, Mayo Clinic and Mayo Foundation; Associate Professor of Physical Medicine and Rehabilitation, Mayo Medical School, Rochester, Minnesota

HORACIO D. PINEDA, M.D.

Clinical Assistant Professor of Rehabilitation Medicine, Department of Physical Medicine and Rehabilitation, New York University Medical Center, New York, New York

ROBERT PRITIKIN, M.S., M.B.A.

President, Nathan Pritikin Research Foundation; Director, Pritikin Programs, Santa Monica, California

EDWARD S. RACHLIN, M.D., F.A.C.S.

Assistant Professor of Clinical Orthopedics, Department of Orthopedic Surgery, Rutgers University, New Brunswick, New Jersey; Associate Professor of Physical Medicine and Rehabilitation, Albert Einstein College of Medicine, New York, New York

MONROE B. ROSENTHAL, M.D.

Medical Director, Pritikin Programs, Santa Monica, California

MAURICE V. RUSSELL, M.S.W., Ed.D., A.C.S.W.

Professor and Director, Department of Social Service, New York University Medical Center, Department of Rehabilitation Medicine, New York, New York

ANN H. SCHUTT, M.D.

Consultant, Department of Physical Medicine and Rehabilitation, Mayo Clinic and Mayo Foundation; Associate Professor of Physical Medicine and Rehabilitation, Mayo Medical School, Rochester, Minnesota

BHAGWAN T. SHAHANI, M.D.

Professor of Neurology, Director of EMG Lab, Harvard Medical School, Boston, Massachusetts

ROY J. SHEPHARD, M.D., Ph.D.

Director, School of Physical and Health Education, University of Toronto, Toronto, Ontario, Canada

ORRIN SHERMAN, M.D.

Clinical Instructor, Orthopedics, New York University; Adjunct Attending in Orthopedics, Hospital for Joint Diseases, New York, New York

DAVID G. SIMONS, M.D.

Clinical Professor, Physical Medicine and Rehabilitation, Department of Physical Medicine and Rehabilitation, California College of Medicine, University of California–Irvine, Irvine, California

JIRI C. SIPAJLO, M.A.

Adjunct Assistant Professor of Driver Education and Safety, The Center for Safety, School of Education, New York University, New York, New York

CYNTHIA L. SMITH, M.D.

Assistant Attending Physician, Department of Physical Medicine and Rehabilitation; Medical Director, Preschool Education Department, Rusk Institute of Rehabilitation Medicine; Instructor of Rehabilitation Medicine, New York University Medical Center, New York, New York

JEROME STENEHJEM, M.D.

Medical Director of Rehabilitation, Scripps Memorial Hospital, Encinitas, California

RICHARD SULLIVAN, M.D.

Associate Professor and Acting Chairman, Department of Rehabilitation Medicine, New Jersey Medical School; Medical Director, Kessler Institute for Rehabilitation, West Orange, New Jersey

ROBERT SURY, M.D.

Clinical Instructor, Department of Rehabilitation Medicine, New York University Medical Center, New York, New York

SAMUEL S. SVERDLIK, M.D.

Director of Rehabilitation Medicine, St. Vincent's Hospital Center and Medical Center of New York City, New York, New York

HOWARD G. THISTLE, M.D.

Associate Professor of Clinical Rehabilitation Medicine; Associate Attending, University Hospital and Rusk Institute of Rehabilitation Medicine, Department of Rehabilitation Medicine, New York University, New York, New York

NICHOLAS A. TZIMAS, M.D.

Clinical Professor of Orthopaedic Surgery, New York University Medical Center, New York, New York

GAVRIL URSU, M.D.

Clinical Assistant Professor of Rehabilitation Medicine, New York University Medical Center; Clinical Assistant Attending, Department of Rehabilitation Medicine, Bellevue Hospital Center; Chief, Department of Physical Medicine and Rehabilitation, Rehabilitation Division, Peninsula Hospital Center, New York, New York

STANLEY F. WAINAPEL, M.D.

Associate Director, Department of Rehabilitation Medicine, St. Luike's–Roosevelt Hospital Center; Associate Professor of Clinical Rehabilitation Medicine, Columbia University College of Physicians and Surgeons, New York, New York

THEODORE WAUGH, M.D.

New York University Medical Center, Department of Orthopaedic Surgery, New York, New York

NANETTE KASS WENGER, M.D.

Professor of Medicine (Cardiology), Emory University School of Medicine; Director, Cardiac Clinics, Grady Memorial Hospital, Atlanta, Georgia

MURIEL ZIMMERMAN, O.T.R., M.A.

Associate Director, Occupational Therapy, Rusk Institute of Rehabilitation Medicine, New York University Medical Center, New York, New York

JOSEPH D. ZUCKERMAN, M.D.

Director, Geriatric Trauma Program, Hospital for Joint Diseases/Orthopaedic Institute; Assistant Professor of Orthopaedic Surgery, New York University School of Medicine, New York, New York

Dedication

This book is dedicated to Howard A. Rusk, Distinguished University Professor at New York University, as a mark of honor and gratitude for his unique leadership and foresight in the organization and development of rehabilitation medicine as a special discipline.

Dr. Rusk's roots were firmly entrenched in internal medicine (he holds the fourth certificate issued to its diplomates by the American Board of Internal Medicine), but his vision transcended a disease-oriented perspective to embrace what he called the fourth phase of medicine. This approach dictated the incorporation of social, economic, educational, vocational, and behavioral intervention as part of an integrated treatment regimen. Dr. Rusk's innovative ideas were disquieting to some of his colleagues, especially those in academic environments that favored an almost exclusive concern with basic and investigative medicine. On occasion the road to recognition of the importance and necessity for rehabilitative intervention has been rocky, but Dr. Rusk's message is now fully vitalized. Private and government social agencies are dedicated to his approach, and the growth of departments of rehabilitation medicine in every kind of care center, as well as the organization of academic departments in many medical schools, is evidence of its maturation.

This manuscript is also dedicated to my family, who showed remarkable forbearance with my eternal absorption with writing chores coupled with some neglect of their needs and interests. I therefore deeply thank those who were most affected. These include four women—Mildred, Ellen, Shelley, and Vanessa—and four men—Christopher, Justin, Spencer, and Benjamin.

Joseph Goodgold

Preface

In 1958, Howard A. Rusk, M.D., joined with The C.V. Mosby Company to publish the first edition of a text that bore the same title as this volume. His was the first comprehensive textbook to address the relatively new specialty of physical medicine and rehabilitation. For many years it deservedly enjoyed national and international popularity as *the* definitive source of information and the documentary vehicle for training of the medical and allied health professionals in the field. The last edition of the Rusk publication appeared in 1977.

The title *Rehabilitation Medicine* has been retained as a matter of tradition and historical continuity, but this book is entirely new. Its contents do not solely reflect the concepts and modus operandi of the Rusk Institute of Rehabilitation Medicine at New York University; the roster of collaborating authors has been drawn from throughout the United States and Canada to maximize the level of expertise of the contents. We have tried to avoid the presentation of singular viewpoints as dogma; instead many topics have been considered in expanded depth by experts who have quite different perspectives and opinions concerning the same subject. This is especially so in regard to therapeutics. For example, Doctors Simons, Grabois, and Kraus present distinctive discussions of pain. Cardiac rehabilitation is presented in varied and multiple discourses by Pritikin of California, Friedman of Mount Sinai in New York, Shepard of Toronto, and Wenger of Emory University in Georgia. Rehabilitation medicine is now firmly established as a comprehensive system of medical care that requires the integrated effort of many health care professionals. Therefore information dealing with the activities of allied health professionals and the participatory spectrum of other medical disciplines, such as neurology, neurosurgery, pediatrics, and orthopedics, represents a considerable part of the text.

I express my deep appreciation to the many colleagues and friends who have so generously and diligently given of their time and effort to contribute chapters to this volume. I also acknowledge the invaluable assistance of my secretarial staff, especially the indefatigable Linda Moy, and of the exceptionally capable and cooperative editors Eugenia Klein and Kathy Falk of The C.V. Mosby Company.

Joseph Goodgold

Contents

PART I | PATIENT EVALUATION

CHAPTER 1 | Evaluation

BRUCE B. GRYNBAUM AND ROBERT SURY

This chapter provides an overview of the process of evaluating patients in rehabilitation programs. Other chapters examine specific aspects of the evaluation process in greater detail and are referred to as appropriate. For example, discussion of such laboratory procedures as electromyography and pulmonary function testing are not covered here but are discussed in depth in later chapters.

The evaluation of a potential candidate for admission to a rehabilitation center requires a two-pronged approach:

1. The underlying disease process must be diagnosed by obtaining a precise history and performing a careful physical examination. In addition, specific laboratory procedures should be performed to confirm the diagnostic conclusions.
2. Rehabilitation medicine requires an extension of this basic diagnostic examination to determine the level of functional capacity that remains after stabilization of any disabling disease. In addition, the potential for recovering capabilities must be assessed as precisely as possible. Since rehabilitation medicine deals with the whole, integrated human as a patient, behavioral disturbances, educational and vocational issues, and social service factors, including the family and its environment, become essential components of current therapy and of plans for future care.

The multidisciplinary nature of the rehabilitation process begins at the initial evaluation and continues throughout the progressive care plan for the patient. The medical aspects are the province of the physician-physiatrist, who is frequently joined by consultative colleagues from other disciplines, usually neurology, neurosurgery, orthopedics, urology, plastic surgery, psychiatry, and pediatrics. The allied health professions that are essential parts of rehabilitation medicine include physical therapy, occupational therapy, rehabilitation nursing, psychology (behavioral science), social service, vocational services, speech pathology, recreational therapy, and orthotics and prosthetics.

ADMISSION TO THE REHABILITATION PROGRAM

Providing services for patients requiring less serious rehabilitation in an ambulatory, private practice setting is relatively simple, depending on the goals established by the attendant physician and the patient. It should be noted that the guidelines imposed by government agencies and third party insurance carriers are a critical determinant of fiscal feasibility and coverage under these circumstances, as well as in more structured programs. Providing care in a comprehensive rehabilitation center is considerably more complicated, depending on the rules and regulations of federal and local governments and third party carriers, the criteria of the institution itself, and the diagnostic process used by the facility.

Frequently the decision to admit must be made without the benefit of direct examination of the patient because referral is made from a distant facility or in response to pressure to discharge the patient because of diagnostic related group (DRG) regulations. In the latter instance it is not unusual for the referring institution to understate the significance of organic mental changes, serious behavioral manifestations, incontinence, feeding difficulties, and even some profound medical complications. All of these unidentified problems contribute to the ultimate success or failure of rehabilitation services and may even represent complete impediments to a successful outcome. Because of the frequent understatement of these sorts of problems, some rehabilitation centers schedule preadmission evaluation conferences or send a team out to the referring facility when possible. In Rusk Institute a full-time member of our team, usually a rehabilitation nurse, carefully screens the applications and makes investigative field trips. We have found that a more reliable and realistic appraisal may be obtained by such communication with the hospital staff (nurses and physical therapists) who have had direct responsibility for the patient.

HISTORY

The method of obtaining the patient's history in rehabilitation medicine differs from that used in other specialties. The elicitation of signs and symptoms may be the same, but the approach differs in its emphasis on functional capacities. The data obtained are organized in a standard format:

1. Basic vital statistics
2. Informant. The history may be obtained from the patient or from friends. When an interpreter is required, medically trained professional translators are most effective.
3. Chief complaint(s). The chief complaints are the main reasons the patient seeks the physician's assistance. They should be carefully listed and defined.
4. Present illness. The patient's symptoms are described in this section. In rehabilitation medicine, information should be elicited regarding the present illness and how it interferes with the patient's social life and ability to work and to perform normal daily activities.
5. Past medical history. Knowledge of the patient's lifelong health and specifically the patient's functional ability before the present illness is essential for setting rehabilitation goals. Family history also may be important, for example, in congenital neuromuscular diseases.
6. Review of systems. The review of systems in rehabilitation medicine emphasizes the cardiovascular, respiratory, neurologic, and musculoskeletal components. The patient's capacity for training depends on the status of these body functions.
7. Social history. The social history should include where and with whom the patient was living before admission and should address the issue of the patient's and family's plans following discharge. Is the housing accessible to the patient? Is the family capable of providing care at home, or will the patient require institutional placement should treatment result in inadequate functional improvements? The patient's standard of living, diet, and use of tobacco, alcohol, and illicit drugs should be noted and recorded.
8. Vocational history. Where the patient works, the extent of the patient's education, and other job skills help determine if the patient can return to the previous employment or will need vocational placement and retraining.

In addition to the diagnosis, the physiatrist is interested in the impact of disability on the patient's present and future way of life, the influence of surroundings, transportation problems, and whether the patient will have access to home, workplace, shopping, and restaurants. The patient's functional abilities will be influenced by family support, living conditions, educational level, employment, and future income.

PHYSICAL EXAMINATION

Although the format for the history and physical examination follows the pattern used in clinical medical practice, both rehabilitation medicine and other clinical disciplines are attempting to make the process more systematic and useful. The best-known example in the past 30 years is the method proposed by Weed[15] and identified as the problem-oriented patient record. These records identify the patient's medical problems by a numerical system based on priority and importance. With this system, further workup is planned and a treatment and education program for the patient and family is developed. The plan reflects the patient's responses and is continually updated. This approach to identifying patient problems and organizing therapeutic programs appears more rational, systematic, and amenable to evaluation of outcomes by statistical means and computer data management. The disadvantages of Weed's system are that it is time consuming and detracts from direct patient care. The system works best for patients with multiple medical problems but is probably not necessary for most patients.

During the physical examination, emphasis is placed on specific observations and on determination of functional capacity. The examination is outlined as follows:

1. Neurologic evaluation
   a. Mental status
   b. Motor system
   c. Sensory status
   d. Reflexes
   e. Vision
   f. Hearing
   g. Swallowing
   h. Speech and language
   i. Gait and mobility
2. Musculoskeletal, soft tissue, and joint evaluation
3. Cardiac and pulmonary status
4. Skin
5. Bladder and bowel function
6. Pain
7. Functional assessment
   a. PULSES Profile
   b. Barthel Index
   c. Glasgow Scale
   d. Ranchos Scale

Table 1-1. Glasgow Coma Scale

	Examiner's test	Patient's response	Assigned score*
Eye opening	Spontaneous	Opens eyes on own	E4
	Speech	Opens eyes when asked to in a loud voice	3
	Pain	Opens eyes when pinched	2
	Pain	Does not open eyes	1
Best motor response	Commands	Follows simple commands	M6
	Pain	Pulls examiner's hand away when pinched	5
	Pain	Pulls a part of body away when examiner pinches him	4
	Pain	Flexes body inappropriately to pain (decorticate posturing)	3
	Pain	Body becomes rigid in an extended position when examiner pinches victim (decerebrate posturing)	2
	Pain	Has no motor response to pinch	1
Verbal response (talking)	Speech	Carries on a conversation correctly and tells examiner where he is, who he is, and the month and year	V5
	Speech	Seems confused or disoriented	4
	Speech	Talks so examiner can understand victim but makes no sense	3
	Speech	Makes sounds that examiner can't understand	2
	Speech	Makes no noise	1

From Bond, RM: Standardized methods of assessing and predicting outcome. In Rosenthal, M, editor: Rehabilitation of the head injured adult, Philadelphia, 1983, FA Davis Co.
*Coma score (E + M + V) = 3 to 15.

Neurologic evaluation
Mental status

The following are evaluated in an attempt to ascertain the patient's mental status:
1. Orientation to time, place, and person
2. Memory
3. Attention span
4. Ability to perform calculations
5. Abstract thinking
6. Behavior
7. Ability to follow commands
8. Judgment
9. Insight
10. Mood

This information serves as a basis for evaluating the patient's mental ability to successfully complete the rehabilitation process.

Cognitive impairment is a serious obstacle, but it is not a complete deterrent to use of the rehabilitation process. The severity of impairment can be measured by the Glasgow Coma Scale (Table 1-1)[14]. In attempting to establish current status and to gauge improvement or deterioration, the scale evaluates three areas: eye opening, best motor responses, and verbal response. Each area is scored separately, and the scores are totaled to give a value of 3 to 15 points. Of patients with scores of 8 or less, 90% are in comas, whereas none of those with scores of 9 or more are comatose.[3]

It is difficult to predict the rehabilitative outcome based solely on the Glasgow Coma Scale because it measures only responses, not underlying disease. Patients whose coma is the result of reversible biochemical alterations, infections, or traumatic conditions often make much greater progress than do patients with hypoxia or anoxia caused by cerebrovascular disease or cardiac arrest.

Motor system

Inspection of the muscles may reveal atrophy, tumor, or spontaneous motor activity, such as faciculations or tremors. Palpation can reveal tenderness, masses (for example, nodules), and increased or decreased tonus. For instance, there is often a characteristic rubbery consistency or doughiness of the gastrocnemius muscle in patients with Duchenne's muscular dystrophy.

Changes in muscle tone, such as increases in spasticity or rigidity or decreases in hypotonia or flaccidity, should be evaluated. In upper motor neuron lesions spasticity may be especially prominent in the flexors of the arm and the extensors of the leg. In addition, increased resistance to passive stretching is followed by a rapid decrease in resistance, producing the "clasp-knife" reaction.

Extrapyramidal motor system disease produces a rigidity that is usually more pronounced in the limb flexors. This increased resistance on passive motion shows a uniform quality throughout the range of motion and has been compared to bending a lead pipe. A special type of rigidity, the "cogwheel" phenomenon, is described as intermittent, step-like, increased muscle tone on passive movement of the limb.

Hypotonia and flaccidity are characteristics of lower motor neuron lesions. Depending on the site of the lesion, individual rather than groups of muscles may be affected, unlike the case in upper motor neuron lesions. Hypotonia and flaccidity are associated with marked atrophy of the muscles.

To evaluate muscle strength, careful observation, positioning, and palpation are essential. An example of the importance of positioning is the handgrasp test. In complete radial nerve palsy the wrist is dropped. If the ability and strength of the patient's handgrasping are tested in this position, the grasp is weak, even though the ulnar and median innervated muscles are intact. However, when the wrist is placed in extension, which is a stabilizing position for grasp, the force of fist formation approaches normal.

The patient should be asked to move the joint through its complete range of motion. Careful evaluation is necessary to detect the substitution of a functioning muscle for one that is paralyzed. For example, in complete ulnar nerve palsy, the extensor digitorum simulates the action of the dorsal interossei in performing abduction of the fingers.

Individual muscle strength can be graded on a basis of 0 to 5 (Figure 1-1). This manual testing procedure is especially useful in peripheral nerve lesions. The most important part of the functional assessment of the patient's muscle strength is the ability to move against gravity in the upper extremity actions in activities of daily living (ADLs). In the lower extremities, the keystone is the patient's ability to ambulate "normally." For example, quadriceps function cannot be fully evaluated by checking resistance to extension of the leg at the knee; the patient's ability to walk up stairs carrying full body weight is a more critical test.

Sensory status

A thorough examination includes assessment of pain, heat, cold, vibratory and position sensation, touch, and discriminative sensory function, such as two-point discrimination. The findings can be reported as *anesthesia,* which refers to a complete loss of all sensation, or *hypesthesia,* a diminution of sensation. *Paresthesia* refers to feelings of burning, tingling, or "pins and needles" that arise spontaneously. *Dysthesia* is the unpleasant or painful sensations induced by a stimulus that is ordinarily painless. *Hyperesthesia* is the term for an increases sensitivity to various stimuli. Location, precipitating factors, relief, and other factors should all be identified. In suspected spinal cord lesions, sensory testing should be carried out to determine the level of the injury. Patients with transverse myelitis, spinal cord injuries, or dissociated sensory syndromes (loss of pain and thermal sense with preservation of the sense of touch), as seen in syringomyelia, should be evaluated to determine the level of lesion. Table 1-2 presents the Frankel classification[5] of neurologic deficit after spinal cord injury.

Table 1-2. Frankel classification of neurologic deficit after spinal cord injury

Grade	Description
A	Complete: no motor or sensory function below level of lesion
B	Sensory only: complete motor paralysis below level of lesion with some preservation of sensory function; includes sacral sparing
C	Motor useless: some motor power present below level of lesion, but it is of no practical use
D	Motor useful: useful motor power below level of lesion; these patients can move lower limbs and many can walk, with or without aids
E	Recovery: free of neurologic symptoms, that is, no weakness, sensory loss, or sphincter disturbance; abnormal reflexes may be present

From Frankel, HL, et al: Paraplegia 7:179, 1969.

This system is based on the presence or absence of sensation or motor function below the level of the lesion.

In determining the distribution of sensory abnormalities, it is important to define the presence of peripheral nerve, plexus, or spinal root patterns. Figure 1-2 can be a helpful reference.

If a patient complains of uncomfortable dysesthesias, for example, burning on the lateral thigh in the distribution of the lateral cutaneous femoral nerve, the injury is most likely a peripheral neuropathy, meralgia paresthetica. However, if the patient's symptoms are in the back and radiate down the lateral thigh and anterior foreleg, lower lumbar radiculopathy is a more consistent possibility.

Reflexes

The reflexes that should be evaluated include those of the biceps, triceps, and supinator muscles, knee and ankle jerks, and superficial abdominal and bulbocavernosus reflexes. They are tabulated with their segmented levels in Table 1-3. The reflex response can be hyperactive, absent, hypoactive, or normal.

In upper motor neuron lesions, the tendon reflexes are frequently hyperactive. Such hyperactivity can be associated with other abnormal reflexes such as Babinski's or Hoffmann's sign. In Babinski's sign, the great toe extends with the small toes fanned when the outer edge of the sole of the foot is stroked with a blunt instrument. The stimulus should not be painful. Hoffmann's sign is the flexion and abduction of the thumb in response to sharp flexion of the terminal phalanx of the middle digit.

The hyperreflexic state may also produce clonus, which is a series of rhythmic involuntary muscle contractions initiated by stretching. Clonus is termed *unsustained* if it stops after a few contractions despite continued stretching and

Text continued on p. 11.

MUSCLE EXAMINATION

Patient's Name_____Chart No._____

Date of Birth_____Name of Institution_____

Date of Onset_____Attending Physician_____M. D.

Diagnosis:

LEFT								RIGHT			
					Examiner's Initials						
					Date						
				NECK	Flexors	Sternocleidomastoid					
						Extensor group					
				TRUNK	Flexors	Rectus abdominis					
					Rt. ext. obl. / Lt. int. obl. } Rotators {	Lt. ext. obl. / Rt. int. obl.					
					Extensors	Thoracic group / Lumbar group					
					Pelvic elev.	Quadratus lumb.					
				HIP	Flexors	Iliopsoas					
					Extensors	Gluteus maximus					
					Abductors	Gluteus medius					
					Adductor group						
					External rotator group						
					Internal rotator group						
					Sartorius						
					Tensor fasciae latae						
				KNEE	Flexors	Biceps femoris / Inner hamstrings					
					Extensors	Quadriceps					
				ANKLE	Plantar flexors	Gastrocnemius / Soleus					
				FOOT	Invertors	Tibialis anterior / Tibialis posterior					
					Evertors	Peroneus brevis / Peroneus longus					
				TOES	M. P. flexors	Lumbricales					
					I. P. flexors (1st)	Flex. digit. br.					
					I. P. flexors (2nd)	Flex. digit. l.					
					M. P. extensors	Ext. digit. l. / Ext. digit. br.					
				HALLUX	M. P. flexor	Flex. hall. br.					
					I. P. flexor	Flex. hall. l.					
					M. P. extensor	Ext. hall. br.					
					I. P. extensor	Ext. hall. l.					

Measurements:

Cannot walk	Date	Speech	
Stands	Date	Swallowing	
Walks unaided	Date	Diaphragm	
Walks with apparatus	Date	Intercostals	

KEY

5 N Normal Complete range of motion against gravity with full resistance.
4 G Good* Complete range of motion against gravity with some resistance.
3 F Fair* Complete range of motion against gravity.
2 P Poor* Complete range of motion with gravity eliminated.
1 T Trace Evidence of slight contractility. No joint motion.
0 0 Zero No evidence of contractility.

S or SS Spasm or severe spasm.
C or CC Contracture or severe contracture.
* Muscle spasm or contracture may limit range of motion. A question mark should be placed after the grading of a movement that is incomplete from this cause.

Figure 1-1. Chart for recording muscle strength. (Reproduced with permission of the Department of Physical Therapy, Rusk Institute of Rehabilitation Medicine, New York University Medical Center.) *Continued.*

LEFT   RIGHT

				Examiner's Initials						
				Date						
				SCAPULA	Abductor	Serratus anterior				
					Elevator	Upper trapezius				
					Depressor	Lower trapezius				
					Adductors	{ Middle trapezius / Rhomboids				
				SHOULDER	Flexor	Anterior deltoid				
					Extensors	{ Latissimus dorsi / Teres major				
					Abductor	Middle deltoid				
					Horiz. abd.	Posterior deltoid				
					Horiz. add.	Pectoralis major				
					External rotator group					
					Internal rotator group					
				ELBOW	Flexors	{ Biceps brachii / Brachioradialis				
					Extensor	Triceps				
				FOREARM	Supinator group					
					Pronator group					
				WRIST	Flexors	{ Flex. carpi rad. / Flex. carpi uln.				
					Extensors	{ Ext. carpi rad. l. & br. / Ext. carpi uln.				
				FINGERS	M. P. flexors	Lumbricales				
					I. P. flexors (1st)	Flex. digit. sub.				
					I. P. flexors (2nd)	Flex. digit. prof.				
					M. P. extensor	Ext. digit. com.				
					Adductors	Palmar interossei				
					Abductors	Dorsal interossei				
					Abductor digiti quinti					
					Opponens digiti quinti					
				THUMB	M. P. flexor	Flex. poll. br.				
					I. P. flexor	Flex. poll. l.				
					M. P. extensor	Ext. poll. br.				
					I. P. extensor	Ext. poll. l.				
					Abductors	{ Abd. poll. br. / Abd. poll. l.				
					Adductor pollicis					
					Opponens pollicis					
				FACE:						

Additional data:

Figure 1-1, cont'd. Chart for recording muscle strength. (Reproduced with permission of the Department of Physical Therapy, Rusk Institute of Rehabilitation Medicine, New York University Medical Center.)

PERIPHERAL DISTRIBUTION   SEGMENTAL OR RADICULAR DISTRIBUTION

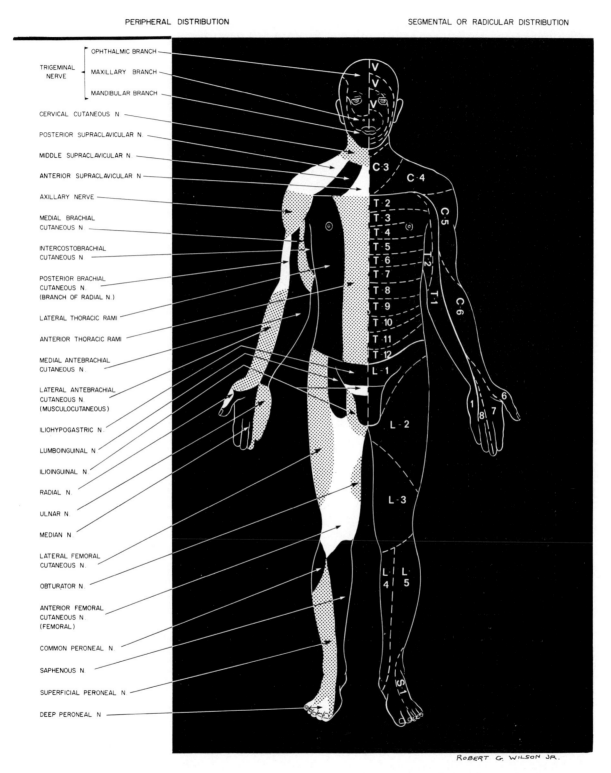

Figure 1-2. Distribution of the sensory spinal roots and the cutaneous fields of the peripheral nerves. *Continued.*

SEGMENTAL OR RADICULAR DISTRIBUTION

PERIPHERAL DISTRIBUTION

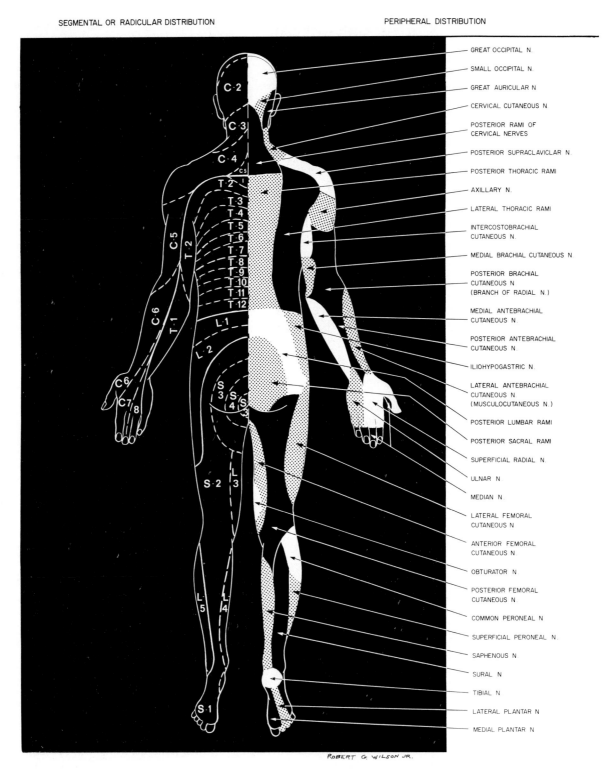

Figure 1-2, cont'd. Distribution of the sensory spinal roots and the cutaneous fields of the peripheral nerves.

Table 1-3. Muscle stretch reflexes

Reflex	Segmental level
Biceps	C5 and C6
Brachioradialis	C5 and C6
Triceps	C7 and C8
Abdominal	T8 to T12
Cremaster	L1 and L2
Knee	L3 and L4
Ankle	S1 and S2
Bulbocavernosus	S3 and S4
Superficial anal	S5 and coccygeal

sustained if the rhythmic contractions continue as long as the stretch is applied.

Absent or hypoactive reflexes are seen in lower motor neuron lesions. When the reflex responses are equal bilaterally, they must be carefully evaluated. If this bilaterality is the only observation, it probably is not pathologically significant and represents an individual variant. With other significant physical findings, however, bilateral lesions must be carefully excluded.

Vision

The fundus of the eye can be directly examined with an ophthalmoscope and tested by investigating visual acuity and visual fields. The oculomotor (III), trochlear (IV), and abducens (VI) nerves can be evaluated by the pupillary reflex and tests of extraocular muscle function.

Nystagmus is an involuntary rhythmic motion of the eyes seen in disorders of the brainstem or the vestibular portion of the auditory nerve, cerebellar disease, drug intoxications, or visual loss from birth or infancy. Nystagmus is termed "left" or "right," depending on the direction in which the eyes move most quickly. For example, eyes that drift slowly to the right and are corrected by a rapid return to the original position are said to have nystagmus to the left.

Hearing

Auditory function can be grossly tested by observing the patient's ability to hear a spoken word or a whisper. For more precise examination, audiometric instrumentation systems are required.

Swallowing

Swallowing disorders are a common ocurrence in patients undergoing rehabilitation, and many causes exist for dysphagia. For our purposes, they may be functionally classified, based on the type of food the patient is able to swallow. Our center uses the series of Dysphagia Diet Levels, which are based on ease of oral manipulation (see box). For instance, stroke patients with dysphagia often aspirate thin

---

DYSPHAGIA DIET LEVELS

1. Dysphagia NPO: single items ordered by occupational therapist with physician approval for trial feeding purposes; no other items by mouth.
2. Dysphagia Pureed: no liquids unless specified by physician's order; smooth, moist, blenderized foods only.
3. Dysphagia Mechanical Soft: no liquids unless specified by physician's order; pureed foods, minced and soft foods that require little chewing and are easy to control in the mouth are the only items included.
4. Thick Liquids: thickened liquids (for example, thickened cream soup) are easier to control in the mouth than thin liquids (for example, apple juice). They should be introduced gradually under supervision in conjunction with Dysphagia Pureed or Dysphagia Mechanical Soft Diet.
5. Medium Liquids: includes eggnogs, milkshakes, regular cream soups, and nectar; used as a transition from thick liquids to thin liquids.
6. Thin Liquids: includes clear liquids, gelatin, and milk and should not be ordered until thick liquids are tolerated. Thin liquids should be introduced gradually under supervision in conjunction with Dysphagia Pureed or Dysphagia Mechanical Soft Diet.

From New York University Medical Center Diet Manual.

---

liquids but may be able to tolerate thick fluids or solid food. Swallowing disorders are most effectively evaluated with video fluoroscopy.

Speech and language

There are three main categories of speech and language disorders:

1. Aphasia and dysphasia are cerebral disturbances that encompass loss of production or comprehension of spoken or written language.
2. Anarthria and dysarthria are defects in articulation but with intact mental functions. These motor disorders of the muscles of articulation can be the result of impairment of the upper or lower motor neurons. In bilateral upper motor neuron lesions (pseudobulbar and bulbar palsy), speech has a forced quality or may be absent. In lower motor neuron lesions, which cause bilateral paralysis of the palate, speech has a nasal quality. Ataxic dysarthria is seen in cerebellar lesions; speech is slow with breaks caused by the unnatural separation of the syllables of words (scanning). This is best demonstrated when the patient is asked to say "liquid electricity" or "Methodist Episcopal."
3. Aphonia or dysphonia is a loss or impairment of voice function caused by a disorder of the larynx or its innervation. With bilateral vocal cord paresis the patient can speak only in whispers, and inspiratory stri-

dor may be present. If one vocal cord is paralyzed, speech becomes hoarse and rasping.

Gait and mobility

Impairment of gait is seen in a wide variety of neurologic and orthopedic conditions. Observation of the patient's walk begins when he or she first enters the examining room, when gait is apt to be most natural and any need for assistance can be noted. If the patient is nonambulatory and uses a wheelchair for mobility, the extent of independence should be determined: Can the patient propel the wheelchair independently and transfer safely from it? How much assistance is needed? Gait laboratories are found in a number of facilities, but their real clinical value is yet to be fully established.

Musculoskeletal, soft tissue, and joint evaluation

The physical evaluation should include inspection, palpation, and measurement of pasive and active range of motion, as well as evaluation of muscle strength. Inspection should begin as soon as the patient enters the examining room. The right and left sides of the body should be compared for asymmetry, postural attitudes, scars, edema, atrophy, masses, or skin changes.

Palpation of muscles, bones, and joints is performed to detect both local and general spasm, masses, swelling, or tenderness. Passive and active range of motion can be evaluated with a goniometer, which measures the angular joint range of motion. Accurate assessment of joint range of motion documents not only the patient's disability but also the effectiveness of the treatment program. The ranges may be recorded on the forms shown in Figures 1-3 to 1-5.

Means other than goniometry may be used to evaluate range of motion. For example, to evaluate internal rotation of the shoulder, the patient can be asked to place his hand behind his back and to reach as far up superiorly as possible. The two sides can be compared and any difference recorded in centimeters. Finger flexion can be measured by noting the distance from fingertips to the palm of the hand. The range of back flexion can be measured as the distance from the fingertips to the floor when the patient bends forward without flexing his knees. Arthritis is such a common disability that a functional classification is extremely useful in diagnosis and evaluation of therapy. Table 1-4 shows the classification proposed by the American Rheumatism Association.[13]

Cardiac and pulmonary status

The essential features of cardiac and pulmonary disease are covered in detail in Chapters 17 and 27.

Skin

Decubitus ulcers are a major concern in patients with sensory loss, debilitation, or coma (see Chapter 11). The scope of the problem is highlighted by studies showing

Table 1-4. Functional criteria of the American Rheumatism Association

Level	Criteria
1	Patient performs all usual activities without handicaps
2	Patient performs normal activities adequately despite occasional discomfort in one or more joints
3	Patient is limited to few or no activities, but performs usual occupation and self-care
4	Patient is largely or wholly incapacitated, is bedridden or confined to a wheelchair, and has little or no self-care skills

From Steinbrocker, O, Traeger, CH, and Batterman, RL: JAMA 140:659, 1949.

Table 1-5. Spinal cord injury classification of decubitus ulcers

Grade	Criteria
I	Limited to superficial epidermal and dermal layers
II	Involving the epidermal and dermal layers and extending into the adipose tissue
III	Extending through superficial structures down to and including muscle
IV	Destruction of all soft tissue structures down to bone; there is communication with either bone or joint structures or both tissues may be affected

that the average nursing time required for patients with decubiti is 50% more than for equally ill patients without ulcers.[2]

These lesions may appear anywhere on the body but are more likely to form over bony prominences. The most common sites are over the ischial, sacral, and trochanteric prominences.[1] Decubitus ulcers can be classified according to a system recommended by the National Spinal Cord Injury Data Collection System (Table 1-5).[12]

Bladder and bowel function

Patients with complaints of urinary incontinence or retention should undergo more extensive urologic evaluation. For patients with a neurogenic bladder who use intermittent catheterizations, the frequency of catheterization, amount of residual urine, technique in performing the catheterization, and frequency of urinary tract infections should be noted. In patients using indwelling Foley catheters, the frequency of catheter replacement and of urinary tract infections should also be recorded. Cystometric studies help de-

Text continued on p. 19.

NEW YORK UNIVERSITY MEDICAL CENTER
INSTITUTE OF REHABILITATION MEDICINE
DEPARTMENT OF PHYSICAL THERAPY

NAME _____ AGE _____

DISABILITY _____ DIAGNOSIS _____ **IN ____ OUT ____**

RANGE OF MOTION TEST FOR UPPER EXTREMITY

1. Anatomical position is starting position. Range is measured with cauda as 0°, cranium as 180°. Rotating motions are from the midsagittal plane as 0° to lateral plane as 180°.

2. All ranges are expressed as passive range of motion. Check muscle chart attached for limitations caused by tightness, weakness, spasm, or contracture.

3. The scale is divided into units of 10°. Range of motion is recorded by filling in area of range

directly on attached sketch with date and examiner's initial.

4. Use of same sheet for subsequent tests is recorded in same color and dated accordingly.

5. Retrogression is marked by diagonal lines over area of previous test and dated.

6. If position is other than in sketch, indicate S for supine, P for prone.

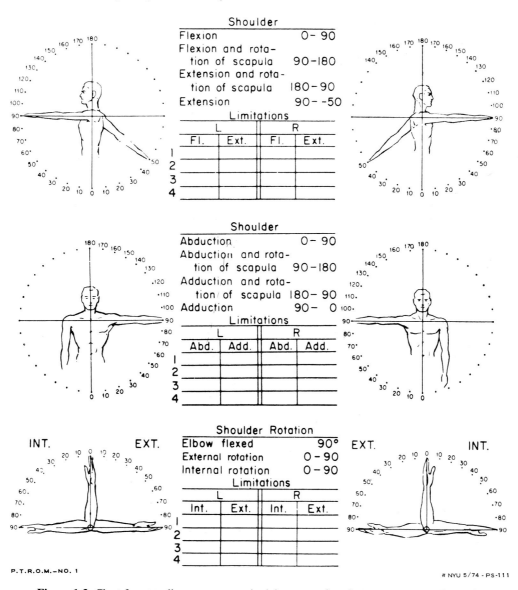

P.T.R.O.M.—NO. 1

\# NYU 5/74 - PS-111

Figure 1-3. Chart for recording upper extremity joint range of motion measurements. (Reproduced with permission of the Department of Physical Therapy, Rusk Institute Rehabilitation Medicine, New York University Medical Center.) *Continued.*

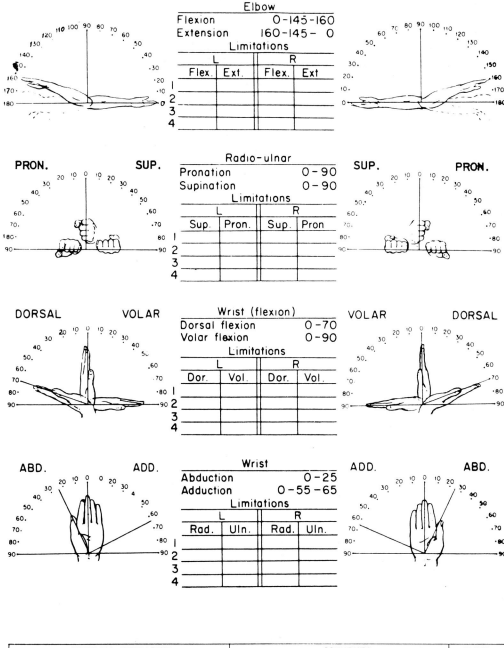

PHYSICAL THERAPIST	COMMENTS	DATE
1.	1.	
2.	2.	
3.	3.	
4.	4.	

Figure 1-3, cont'd. Chart for recording upper extremity joint range of motion measurements. (Reproduced with permission of the Department of Physical Therapy, Rusk Institute Rehabilitation Medicine, New York University Medical Center.)

NEW YORK UNIVERSITY MEDICAL CENTER
INSTITUTE OF REHABILITATION MEDICINE
DEPARTMENT OF PHYSICAL THERAPY

NAME _____ AGE _____

DISABILITY _____ DIAGNOSIS _____ IN ___ OUT ___

RANGE OF MOTION TEST FOR FINGER AND TOES

1. Anatomical position is starting position. Range is measured with cauda as 0°, cranium as 180°. Rotating motions are from the midsagittal plane as 0° to lateral plane as 180°.

2. All ranges are expressed as passive range of motion. Check muscle chart attached for limitations caused by tightness, weakness, spasm, or contracture.

3. The scale is divided into units of 10°. Range of motion is recorded by filling in area of range

directly on attached sketch with date and examiner's initial.

4. Use of same sheet for subsequent tests is recorded in same color and dated accordingly.

5. Retrogression is marked by diagonal lines over area of previous test and dated.

6. If position is other than in sketch, indicate S for supine, P for prone.

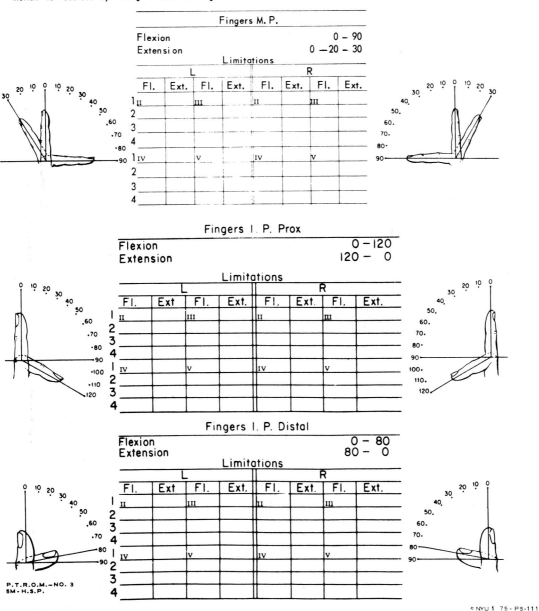

P.T.R.O.M.—NO. 3
5M-H.S.P.

✎ NYU 1 75 - PS-111

Figure 1-4. Chart for recording joint range of motion measurements for finger and toes. (Reproduced with permission of the Department of Physical Therapy, Rusk Institute of Rehabilitation Medicine, New York University Medical Center.) *Continued.*

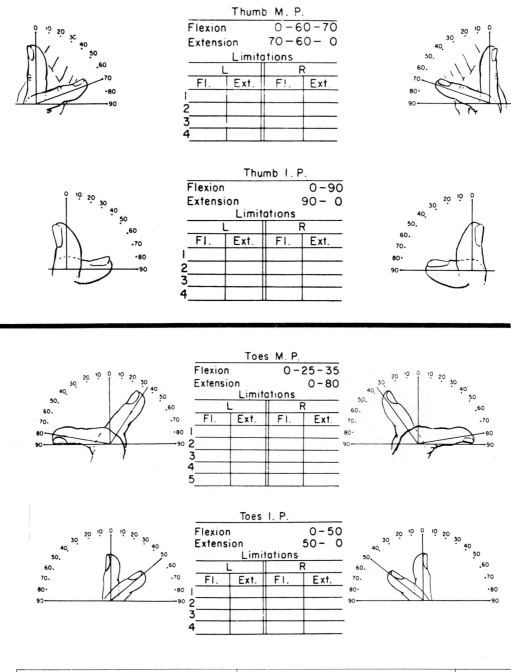

Figure 1-4, cont'd. Chart for recording joint range of motion measurements for finger and toes. (Reproduced with permission of the Department of Physical Therapy, Rusk Institute of Rehabilitation Medicine, New York University Medical Center.)

NEW YORK UNIVERSITY MEDICAL CENTER
INSTITUTE OF REHABILITATION MEDICINE
DEPARTMENT OF PHYSICAL THERAPY

NAME _____ AGE _____

DISABILITY _____ DIAGNOSIS _____ IN ___ OUT ___

RANGE OF MOTION TEST FOR LOWER EXTREMITY

1. Anatomical position is starting position. Range is measured with cauda as 0°, cranium as 180°. Rotating motions are from the midsagittal plane as 0° to lateral plane as 180°.

2. All ranges are expressed as passive range of motion. Check muscle chart attached for limitations caused by tightness, weakness, spasm, or contracture.

3. The scale is divided into units of 10°. Range of motion is recorded by filling in area of range

directly on attached sketch with date and examiner's initial.

4. Use of same sheet for subsequent tests is recorded in same color and dated accordingly.

5. Retrogression is marked by diagonal lines over area of previous test and dated.

6. If position is other than in sketch, indicate S for supine, P for prone.

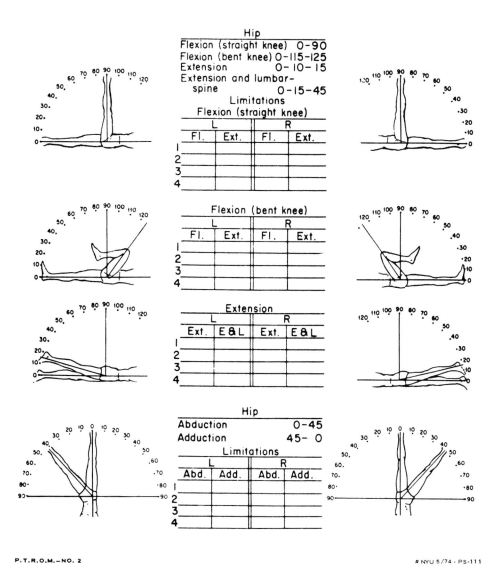

P.T.R.O.M.—NO. 2   # NYU 5/74 - PS-111

Figure 1-5. Chart for recording lower extremity joint range of motion measurements. (Reproduced with permission of the Department of Physical Therapy, Rusk Institute of Rehabilitation Medicine, New York University Medical Center.) *Continued.*

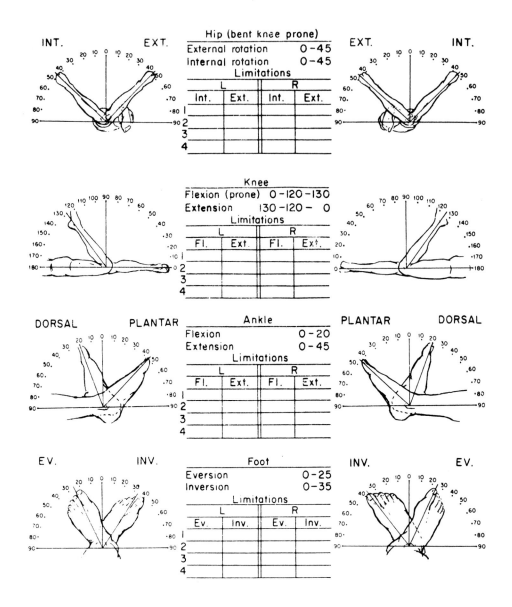

PHYSICAL THERAPIST	COMMENTS	DATE
1.	1.	
2.	2.	
3.	3.	
4.	4.	

Figure 1-5, cont'd. Chart for recording lower extremity joint range of motion measurements. (Reproduced with permission of the Department of Physical Therapy, Rusk Institute of Rehabilitation Medicine, New York University Medical Center.)

fine the presence of detrusor hyperreflexia and areflexia and sphincter dyssynergia.

The exact status of a bowel problem, which is most often neurogenic in etiology, must be carefully evaluated by determining the frequency of bowel movement, presence of bleeding, and type of stimulation, for instance, suppository or digital. At the time of admission, it is common for patients to have gastrointestinal tract dysfunction and, especially, to be severely constipated or even impacted.

Pain

Pain is a prime symptom prompting patients to seek medical care. It can be analyzed according to the following:
1. Quality. Is the pain sharp and knifelike, boring, heavy, burning, or throbbing?
2. Location. What is the exact site of the complaint? Does it radiate?
3. Temporal characteristics. How long does the pain last? When does it occur? When does it stop?
4. Provocative factors. What aggravates the pain? Motion? Posture? Weight bearing? Coughing?
5. Palliative factors. What relieves the pain? Medications? Physical therapy? Heat? Cold? Position changes?

The topic of pain is discussed in greater detail in Chapter 43.

Functional assessment

The goal of rehabilitation medicine is to restore patients to optimal functioning. The patient's performance is a dynamic process and must be repeatedly assessed and documented if progress is to be reliably monitored. Formalized assessment produces objective and explicit documentation of functional improvement, whereas most information provided in informal narrative form is of limited use because it is incomplete, does not use standard terminology, and is unsuitable for statistical analysis.

Four commonly used functional assessment scales are the following:
1. For overall disability evaluation
    a. PULSES Profile
    b. Barthel Index
2. For assessment of brain injury
    a. Glasgow Outcome Scale
    b. Rancho Los Amigos Levels of Cognitive Recovery (Ranchos Scale)

The *PULSES Profile*, developed by Moskowitz and McCann[11] in 1957, provides an overall functional profile of an individual. Six subcategories are measured:
1. Overall physical condition *(P)*
2. Upper extremity function *(U)*
3. Lower extremity function *(L)*
4. Sensory function (related to speech, vision, and hearing) *(S)*

5. Excretory function, or bowel and bladder control *(E)*
6. Mental and social status *(S)*

Within each of these subcategories the patient is rated from 1, essentially normal, to 4, severely disabled and dependent.

Two disadvantages that weakened the original PULSES Profile were that subscores from each of the six parts were not summed to give a total and that assignment of levels of achievement in each part was not correlated with the amount of assistance needed. These deficiencies were rectified by Granger[7] in 1975 in the adapted PULSES Profile. Its major differences from the original instrument are listed in the box on p. 20.

The original PULSES instrument allowed a global score of 6 (fully independent) to 24 (totally dependent). The adapted version correlates a score of 12 or more with severe disability.[6] However, since various combinations yield these total scores, PULSES lacks a degree of specificity.

The *Barthel Index,* developed in 1965 by Barthel and Mahoney, consists of 10 activities of daily living (ADLs) variables in which the patient receives a score[10] (see box on pp. 21 and 22). A score of 60 or less indicates severe disability.[6] However, a score of 100 shows only that a patient does not need an attendant, not necessarily that he is able to live completely alone.

Among the skills not measured by the Barthel Index are the patient's ability to cook or keep house. In addition, functional impairment related to general health status, communication skills, and psychosocial problems goes unnoted. For example, in the evaluation of stroke patients, the Barthel Index fails to measure changes in speech or cognitive function.

The *Glasgow Outcome Scale* was developed by Jennett and Bond to aid in the evaluation of brain damage and its prognosis (Table 1-6). The five categories measured by this scale tend to be so broad that important functional gains the patient makes while remaining at the same level of recovery are ignored. This disadvantage is particularly unfortunate in the light of evidence, gained through large-scale studies of head-injured patients, indicating that the greater part of recovery is achieved between 3 and 6 months after injury (Figure 1-6).[4]

The Ranchos Scale[8] is an eight-part scale developed to track recovery of head-injured patients and assess the appropriateness of the rehabilitation program (Table 1-7). It can be divided into three broad stages of recovery. In stages II and III, patients begin to respond to external stimuli. During stages IV, V, and VI, patients are alert but disoriented and have difficulty processing information. Patients in stages VII and VIII are capable of independent behavior at least in a familiar environment. The disadvantage in using this scale is its failure to take into account the patient's premorbid functional level or physical disabilities not related to the head injury that may impair function.

Text continued on p. 25.

THE PULSES PROFILE

P—Physical condition: includes diseases of the viscera (cardiovascular, gastrointestinal, urologic, and endocrine) and neurologic disorders

1. Medical problems sufficiently stable that medical or nursing monitoring is not required more often than at 3-month intervals
2. Medical or nursing monitoring is needed more often than at 3-month intervals but not each week
3. Medical problems are sufficiently unstable as to require intensive medical or nursing attention at least weekly
4. Medical problems require intensive medical or nursing attention at least daily (excluding personal care assistance only)

U—Upper limb functions: self-care activities (drink and feed self; dress upper and lower body; apply brace or prosthesis; groom self; wash; perineal care) dependent mainly on upper limb function

1. Independent in self-care without impairment of upper limbs
2. Independent in self-care with some impairment of upper limbs
3. Dependent on assistance or supervision in self-care with or without impairment of upper limbs
4. Dependent totally in self-care with marked impairment of upper limbs

L—Lower limb functions: mobility (transfer from chair, toilet, tub, or shower; walk; climb stairs; utilize wheelchair) dependent mainly on lower limb function

1. Independent in mobility without impairment of lower limbs
2. Independent in mobility with some impairment in lower limbs, such as needing ambulatory aids, a brace, or prosthesis; or else fully independent in a wheelchair without significant architectural or environmental barriers
3. Dependent on assistance or supervision in mobility with or without impairment of lower limbs; partly dependent in a wheelchair (or there are significant architectural or environmental barriers)
4. Dependent totally in mobility with marked impairment of lower limbs

S—Sensory components: relating to communications (speech and hearing) and vision:

1. Independent in communication and vision without impairment
2. Independent in communication and vision with some impairment, such as mild dysarthria, mild aphasia, or need for eyeglasses, hearing aid, or regular eye medication
3. Dependent on assistance, an interpreter, or supervision in communication or vision
4. Dependent totally in communication or vision

E—Excretory functions (bladder and bowel)

1. Complete voluntary control of bladder and bowel sphincters
2. Control of sphincters allowing normal social activities despite urgency or need for catheter, appliance, suppositories, etc.; able to care for needs without assistance
3. Dependent on assistance in sphincter management or else has occasional accidents
4. Frequent wetting or soiling from incontinence of bladder or bowel sphincters

S—Situational factors: intellectual and emotional adaptability, support from family unit, financial ability, and social interaction

1. Able to fulfill usual roles and perform customary tasks
2. Must make some modification in usual roles and performance of customary tasks
3. Dependent on assistance, supervision, or encouragement from a public or private agency as a result of any of the above considerations
4. Dependent on long-term institutional care (for example, chronic hospitalization or nursing home), excluding time-limited hospital for specific evaluation, treatment, or active rehabilitation

PULSES total: best score is 6, worst is 24.

Note: This adapted version of PULSES differs from the original in the following ways: (1) by relating levels 1 and 2 to function without assistance from another person and levels 3 and 4 to function with assistance from another person; (2) by relating section *U* to self-care activities, as well as to upper limb function; (3) by relating section *L* to mobility activities, as well as to lower limb function; (4) by relating the second *S* section to intellectual and emotional adaptability, support from the family unit, financial ability, social interaction, and type of supportive environment; and (5) by summing the scores to yield a global score.

Modified from Granger, CV, et al: Stroke 6:34, 1975. From Moskowitz, E, and McCann, CB: J Chron Dis 5:342, 1957.

THE BARTHEL INDEX

The Barthel Index is a measure of a person's ability to function independently and provides a score of the degree of severity. Originally called the Maryland Disability Index, the scale was used in three chronic disease hospitals in Maryland to standardize scoring instruments for measuring the degree of disability of clients with neuromuscular or musculoskeletal disorders. The Index primarily measures self-care and mobility. The values for each item are based on the time and amount of assistance needed by the patient in performing an activity. Items are weighted according to importance. For example, continence is weighted heavily as the incontinent client is seen as socially unacceptable to many persons in the environment.

Some environmental conditions effect scoring on the Barthel Index. If there are special environmental requirements (for instance wide doors in the patient's house), the score is lowered when these special needs are not met. Items are rated 0 or 5; 0, 5, or 10; or 0, 5, 10 or 15 depending on the item. The higher the score, the higher the degree of independence. A score of zero indicates complete dependence. The items are listed below with the possible scores in parentheses. The scores can only be any number presented here.

1. Feeding (10)
   10 = Independent. The patient can feed himself from a tray or table when someone puts the food within his reach. He must be able to put on an assistive device, if this is needed, cut up food, use salt and pepper, spread butter, etc. He must accomplish this in a reasonable time.
   5 = Some help is necessary (for instance, with cutting up food, as listed above.)
2. Moving from wheelchair to bed and returning (15)
   15 = Independent in all phases of this activity. Patient can safely approach the bed in his wheelchair, lock brakes, lift footrests, move safely to bed, lie down, come to a sitting position on the side of the bed, change the position of the wheelchair, if necessary, to transfer back into it safely, and return to the wheelchair.
   10 = Either some minimal help is needed in some step of this activity or the patient needs to be reminded or supervised for safety of one or more parts of this activity.
   5 = Patient can come to a sitting position without the help of a second person but needs a great deal of help to be lifted out of bed.
3. Personal toilet (5)
   5 = Patient can wash hands and face, comb hair, clean teeth, and shave. He may use any kind of razor but must put in blade or plug in razor without help, as well as get it from drawer or cabinet. Female patients must put on own make-up, if used, but need not braid or style hair.
4. Getting on and off toilet (10)
   10 = Patient is able to get on and off toilet, fasten and unfasten clothes, prevent soiling of clothes, and use toilet paper without help. He may use a wall bar or other stable object for support if needed. If it is necessary to use a bedpan instead of a toilet, he must be able to place it on a chair, empty it, and clean it.
   5 = Patient needs help because of imbalance or in handling clothes or in using toilet paper.
5. Bathing self (5)
   5 = Patient may use a bathtub or shower or take a complete sponge bath. He must be able to do all the steps involved in whichever method is employed without another person being present.
6. Walking on a level surface (15)
   15 = Patient can walk at least 50 yards without help or supervision. He may wear braces or prostheses and use crutches, canes, or a walkerette but not a rolling walker. He must be able to lock and unlock braces if used, assume the standing position and sit down, get the necessary mechanical aids into position for use, and dispose of them when he sits. (Putting on and taking off braces is scored under dressing.)
   10 = Patient needs help or supervision in any of the above but can walk at least 50 yards with a little help.
6a. Propelling a wheelchair (if appropriate) (5)
   5 = A patient cannot ambulate but can propel a wheelchair independently. He must be able to go around corners, turn around, and maneuver the chair to a table, bed, and toilet. He must be able to push a chair at least 50 yards. Do not score this item if the patient gets score for walking.
7. Ascending and descending stairs (10)
   10 = Patient is able to go up and down a flight of stairs safely without help or supervision. He may and should use handrails, canes, or crutches when needed. He must be able to carry canes or crutches as he ascends or descends stairs.
   5 = Patient needs help with or supervision of any one of the above items.
8. Dressing and undressing (10)
   10 = Patient is able to put on and remove and fasten all clothing, and tie shoelaces (unless it is necessary to use adaptations for this). The activity includes putting on and removing and fastening corset or braces when these are prescribed. Such special clothing as suspenders, loafer shoes, or dresses that open down the front may be used when necessary.
   5 = Patient needs help in putting on and removing or fastening any clothing. He must do at least half the work himself. He must accomplish this in a reasonable time.
   Women need not be scored on use of a brassiere or girdle unless these are prescribed garments.

Continued.

THE BARTHEL INDEX—cont'd

9. Continence of bowels (10)

    10 = Patient is able to control his bowels and have no accidents. He can use a suppository or take an enema when necessary (as for spinal cord injury patients who have had bowel training).

    5 = Patient needs help in using a suppository or taking an enema or has occasional accidents.

10. Controlling bladder (10)

    10 = Patient is able to control his bladder day and night. Spinal cord injury patients who wear an external device and leg-bag must put them on independently, clean and empty bag, and stay dry day and night.

    5 = Patient has occasional accidents or cannot wait for the bedpan or get to the toilet in time or needs help with an external device.

There have been variations on these items and of the entire scale. However, only the basic scale is presented here.

The scores are broken down into severity categories as follows (Urban Institute 1976):

0-20	Totally dependent
21-61	Severely dependent
62-90	Moderately dependent
91-99	Slightly dependent
100	Independent

The system is simple and easy to use and provides a rough index of severity. However, the system was designed for, and hence can only be used with, the physically handicapped. It is not designed to be used for eligibility determination or any other strict standard for a program. Rather, it is a quick reference that can be used to help indicate general patterns in improved client functioning in activities of daily living and mobility.

From Mahoney, FI, and Barthel, DW: Md St J Ed 14:61, 1965.

Table 1-6. The Glasgow Outcome Scale in its original form and in extended and contracted forms

Extended scale		Original scale	Contracted scales			
Dead		Dead	Dead	Dead or vegetative	Dead or vegetative	Dead
Vegetative		Vegetative	Dependent			Survivors
Degree of disability:	5	Severely disabled	Dependent	Severely disabled	Conscious	Survivors
	4	Severely disabled	Dependent	Severely disabled	Conscious	Survivors
	3	Moderately disabled	Independent	Independent	Conscious	Survivors
	2	Moderately disabled	Independent	Independent	Conscious	Survivors
	1	Good recovery	Independent	Independent	Conscious	Survivors
	0	Good recovery	Independent	Independent	Conscious	Survivors
Total categories	8	5	3		2	

Reproduced with permission from Bond, RM: Standardized methods of assessing and predicting outcome. In Rosenthal, M, editor: Rehabilitation of the head injured adult, Philadelphia, 1983, FA Davis Co.

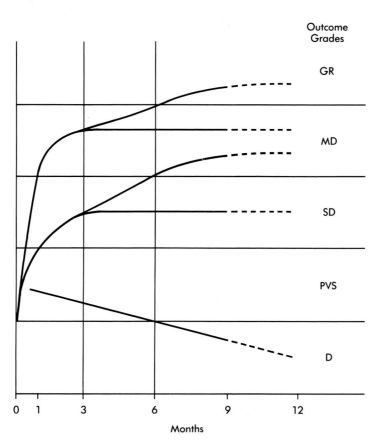

Figure 1-6. Outcome of severe head injury as measured by the Glasgow Outcome Scale. (From Bond, MR, and Brooks, DN: Scand J Rehabil Med 8:131, 1976.)

Table 1-7. Ranchos Los Amigos levels of cognitive recovery

Level		Description
I	No response	Patient appears to be in a deep sleep and is unresponsive to any stimuli presented to him.
II	Generalized response	Patient reacts inconsistently and nonpurposefully to stimuli in a nonspecific manner. Responses are limited in nature and are often the same regardless of stimulus presented. Responses may be physiological changes, gross body movements, and vocalization. Responses are likely to be delayed. The earliest response is to deep pain.
III	Localized response	Patient reacts specifically but inconsistently to stimuli. Responses are directly related to the type of stimulus presented as in turning the head toward a sound or focusing on a presented object. The patient may withdraw an extremity and vocalize when presented with a painful stimulus. He may follow simple commands in an inconsistent, delayed manner, such as closing his eyes or squeezing or extending an extremity. Once external stimuli are removed, he may lie quietly. He may also show a vague awareness of self and body by responding to discomfort, for instance, by pulling at a nasogastric tube or catheter or resisting restraints. He may show a bias toward responding to some persons, especially family and friends, but not to others.
IV	Confused-agitated	Patient is in a heightened state of activity with severely decreased ability to process information. He is detached from the present and responds primarily to his own internal confusion. Behavior is frequently bizarre and nonpurposeful, relative to his immediate environment. He may cry out or scream in disproportion to stimuli even after its removal, may show aggressive behavior, or attempt to remove restraints or tube or to crawl out of bed in a purposeful manner. He does not discriminate among persons or objects and is unable to cooperate directly with treatment efforts. Verbalization is frequently incoherent or inappropriate to the environment. Confabulation may be present; he may be hostile. Gross attention to environment is brief and selective attention often nonexistent. Being unaware of present events, patient lacks short-term recall and may be reacting to past events. He is unable to perform self-care activities without maximum assistance. If not disabled physically, he may perform automatic motor activities, such as sitting, reaching, and ambulating, as part of his agitated state but not necessarily as a purposeful act or on request.
V	Confused-inappropriate	Patient appears alert and is able to respond to simple commands fairly consistently. However, with increased complexity of commands or lack of any external structure, responses are nonpurposeful, random, or at best, fragmented toward any desired goal. He may show agitated behavior, not on an internal basis, as in level IV, but rather as a result of external stimuli and usually out of proportion to the stimulus. He has gross attention to the environment, is highly distractible, and lacks ability to focus attention to a specific task without frequent redirection. With structure, he may be able to converse on an automatic social level for short periods of time. Verbalization is often inappropriate; confabulation may be triggered by present events. Memory is severely impaired, with confusion of past and present in reaction to ongoing activity. Patient lacks initiation of functional tasks and often shows inappropriate use of objects without external direction. He may be able to perform previously learned tasks when structured for him but is unable to learn new information. He responds best to self, body, comfort, and, often, family members. The patient can usually perform self-care activities with assistance and may accomplish feeding with supervision. Management on the unit is often a problem if the patient is physically mobile, as he may wander off either randomly or with the vague intention of "going home."
VI	Confused-appropriate	Patient shows goal-directed behavior but is dependent on external input for a reaction. Response to discomfort is appropriate and he is able to tolerate unpleasant stimuli, for example, a nasogastric tube when the need for one is explained. He follows simple directions consistently and shows carryover for tasks he has relearned, for example, self-care. He needs at least supervision for old learning and needs at least maximal assistance for new learning with little or no carryover. Responses may be incorrect because of memory problems but are appropriate to the situation. They may range from delayed to immediate responses, and the patient shows decreased ability to process information with little or no anticipation or prediction of events. Earlier memories show more depth and detail than do more recent ones. The patient may show a beginning awareness of his situation by realizing he does not know an answer. He no longer wanders and is oriented (though inconsistently) to time and place. Selective attention to tasks may be impaired, especially with difficult tasks and in unstructured settings, but is functional for common daily activities. He may vaguely recognize some staff and be increasingly aware of self, family, and basic needs.

Table 1-7, cont'd. Ranchos Los Amigos levels of cognitive recovery

Level		Description
VII	Automatic-appropriate	Patient acts appropriately and is oriented within both hospital and home settings, goes through daily routine automatically but robotlike with minimal to no confusion, and has poor recall of what he has been doing. He shows increased awareness of self, body, family, food, people, and interaction in the environment. He is superficially aware of, but lacks insight into, his condition; the patient's judgment and problem solving abilities are decreased, and he does not plan realistically for his future. He shows carryover for new learning at a decreased rate and requires at least minimal supervision for learning and safety purposes. He is independent in self-care activities but must be supervised in home and community skills for safety. With structure, he is able to initiate tasks or social and recreational activities in which he now takes interest. His judgment remains impaired. Prevocational evaluation and counseling may be indicated.
VIII	Purposeful-appropriate	Patient is alert and oriented, is able to recall and integrate past and recent events, and is aware of and responsive to his culture. He shows carryover for new learning if acceptable to him and his life role, and he needs no supervision once activities are learned. Within his physical capabilities, he is independent in home and community skills. Vocational rehabilitation to determine the patient's ability to return to society as a contributor, perhaps in a new capacity, is indicated. He may continue to show decreases relative to premorbid abilities in quality and rate of processing, abstract reasoning, tolerance for stress, and judgment in emergencies or unusual circumstances. His social, emotional, and intellectual capacities may continue to be at a decreased level for him but still functional within society.

CONCLUSION

A precise, systematic record of the patient's total status on admission, derived from a complete history, physical examination, supportive laboratory studies, and specific evaluations by allied health professionals, is of critical importance. Functional tests are a basic component of the process. This chapter presents some of the less complicated testing approaches and reveals that a single perfect method is not yet available.

The initial evaluation process establishes a baseline status against which improvement, stasis, or regression can be measured. Regularly scheduled and carefully designed re-evaluation of every aspect of the patient's response to the rehabilitation program is equally important. Together these aspects allow the practitioner to define the current and ultimate state of functional capacity.

Formal quantifiable evaluation is also gaining a prominent position in the financing of the health services. The extension of the DRG-based renumeration criteria for health care services beyond the Medicare patient to everyone seems inevitable in the light of government policies. While the baseline for application to rehabilitative treatment has presented problems sufficient enough to defer implementation until recently, a strong movement exists to quantify functional outcomes as an appropriate instrument of mensuration. Under these circumstances, evaluation systems take on a full measure of significance.

REFERENCES

1. Agris, J, and Spira, M: Pressure ulcers: prevention and treatment, Ciba Foundation Symposium 31, Amsterdam, 1979, Elsevier–Excerpta Medica–North Holland.

2. Bliss, MR, McLaven, R, and Anton-Smith, AN: Preventing pressure sores in a hospital: controlled trial of large ripple mattress, Br Med J 1:394, 1967.

3. Bond, M: Standardized methods of assessing and predicting outcome. In Rosenthal, M, editor: Rehabilitation of the head injured adult, Philadelphia, 1983, FA Davis Co.

4. Bond, MR, and Brook, DN: Understanding the process of recovery as a basis for the investigation of rehabilitation for the brain injured, Scand J Rehab Med 8:127, 1976.

5. Frankel, HL, et al: The value of postural reduction in the initial management of closed injuries of spine with paraplegia and tetraplegia: comprehensive management and research, Paraplegia 7:179, 1969.

6. Granger, CV, Albrecht, GL, and Hamilton, BB: Outcome of comprehensive medical rehabilitation: measurement by Pulses profile and the Barthel Index, Arch Phys Med Rehabil 60:145, 1979.

7. Granger, CV, et al: Measurement of outcomes of care for stroke patients, Stroke 6:34, 1975.

8. Hagen, C: Language disorders secondary to closed head injury: diagnosis and treatment, Top Language Disorders 1:73, 1981.

9. Jannett, B, and Bond, MR: Assessment of outcome after severe brain damage, Lancet 1:480, 1975.

10. Mahoney, FI, and Barthel, DW: Functional evaluations: Barthel Index, Md State J Med 14:61, 1965.

11. Moskowitz, E, and McCann, CB: Classification of disability in the chronically ill and aging, J Chron Dis 5:342, 1957.

12. Stass, W, and LaManta, J: Decubitus ulcers. In Ruskin, A, editor: Current therapy in physiatry, physical medicine and rehabilitation, Philadelphia, 1984, WB Saunders Co.

13. Steinbrocker, O, Traeger, CH, and Batterman, RL: Therapeutic criteria in rheumatoid arthritis, JAMA 140:659, 1949.

14. Teasdale, G, and Jennett, B: Assessment of coma and impaired consciousness, Lancet 2:81, 1974.

15. Weed, LL: Medical records that guide and teach, N Engl J Med 278:593, 1968.

CHAPTER 2

The somatosensory evoked potential

RECORDING TECHNIQUES AND APPLICATIONS

ANDREW EISEN

Evoked potentials were first recorded in animals about 100 years ago.[25] However, human "hardcopy," short-latency somatosensory evoked potentials (SEPs) were not available until the late 1940s when Dawson[14] presented his averager to the Physiological Society of London, opening avenues for recording potentials of less than 10 μV. In those early days the SEP was superseded in clinical applicability by the simpler to record visual and auditory brainstem evoked potentials. However, over the last 10 to 15 years the situation has changed dramatically as our understanding of the basis, clinical uses, and limitations of SEPs has made rapid strides. The story is nevertheless incomplete. Several aspects of SEPs are poorly understood or controversial, partially because of the variety of stimulating and recording techniques used to elicit these potentials. The lack of uniformity in technique should not discourage research, however, since it indicates that, when fully understood, this test will have the flexibility to allow for appropriate, even ideal, test design for specific clinical problems.

This chapter reviews current concepts of the physiologic basis for SEPs, describes the different techniques available to elicit and record them, and addresses the problem of test design in the clinical setting.

EARLY LATENCY SENSORY EVOKED POTENTIAL COMPONENTS: THEIR NEURAL GENERATION

Until recently, the different early latency peaks of SEPs were considered to reflect sequential activation of neuronal generators (synapses in relay nuclei) excited by the ascending volley.[8,17,18] The acceptance of this concept formed a logical basis for concluding that missing or abnormal components were indicative of disease. Considerable effort was directed to proving that a given early latency peak is gen-

erated by a specific neuronal generator. Evidence favoring this view was based on animal experiments and human correlative studies.[25] However, there is increasing evidence that nonneuronal factors play an important role in the generation of some early latency SEP components, especially far-field potentials recorded using referential montages.

In the *bipolar cephalic montage* both recording electrodes are placed on the scalp. Mainly near-field potentials are recorded with this technique. They are characteristically negative (upgoing) at electrode G1 and are relatively large in amplitude when G1 is near the source, but the amplitude falls abruptly as G1 is moved away from the generator. The terms "active" and "inactive" are unsatisfactory in the context of bipolar scalp derivations. A frontal reference (G2), for example, is active, causing cancellation of potential differences having equal and opposite polarity to those recorded at G1 and eliminating most far-field potentials.*

Bipolar cephalic montages are relatively "noise" free, since they are devoid of respiratory and ECG interference. This means that only a few epochs need averaging; often 100 to 200 are sufficient. Thus this technique is ideal in the clinical setting.

Noncephalic recording of SEPs implies that G2 is placed away from the scalp. The opposite mastoid, earlobe, shoulder, arm, hand, and knee have all been chosen sites. Referential montages allow recording of both far- and near-

---

*The recording electrode close to the source of activity or generator recorded is referred to as the active exploring input terminal 1 or grid 1. The other electrode is the reference terminal 2 or grid 2 electrode. In somatosensory evoked recording the terms "terminal 1" and "terminal 2" or "grid 1" and "grid 2" are preferred because both electrodes are active, often equally so. By convention a potential difference that is negative at the input terminal 1 relative to the input terminal 2 causes an upward deflection.

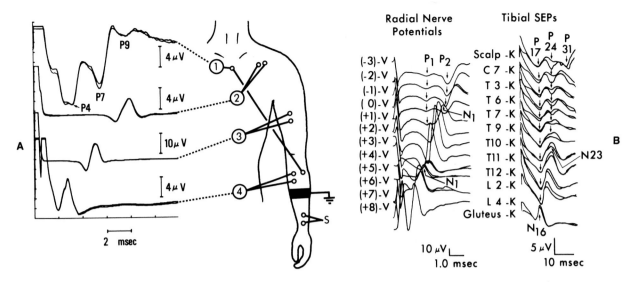

Figure 2-1. Peripheral nerve models of far-field potentials. **A,** Recording between sternum and forearm, three far fields are identified: P4, P7, and P9. They arise where volume conductor changes abruptly at elbow region (possibly insertion of brachialis muscle), mid–upper arm (possibly insertion of deltoid muscle), and region where brachial plexus is formed. **B,** *left,* Referential recording radial nerve (G1) against finger 5 (G2). Two far fields are recognized, one where wrist joins arm (P1) and another where finger joins hand (P2). Both are regions where marked change of volume conductor occurs. *Right,* For comparison, far fields recorded from scalp. Tibial nerve was stimulated. Recording montage Cz-knee.

field potentials. However, they do so at the cost of respiratory and ECG interference, and many epochs need to be averaged for the recognition of SEPs. Far-field potentials are small in amplitude and recordable diffusely over the scalp. They are usually positive (downgoing) and monophasic at G1, reflecting a moving front approaching the recording electrode. However, Kimura and co-workers[58] recently showed that under some circumstances far-field potentials may be of either polarity and biphasic. Their small amplitude is a limitation in clinical practice. Even with the extensive averaging that is invariably required to record most far-field potentials, they are not always successfully recorded in normal subjects.

Peripheral nerve models using referential recording have cast doubt that fixed neuronal generators (synapses in relay nuclei) are responsible for all far-field SEPs. Why, for instance, should stationary far-field peaks, such as P9, P11, P13, and P14 evoked by median nerve stimulation, which arise in a moving source, be recordable before they actually reach the GI electrode? The explanation lies in the surrounding volume conductor.[43,57-60] Whenever this changes abruptly in its electrophysical characteristics, a far-field potential emerges (Figure 2-1). For example, in a peripheral nerve model, in which a mixed nerve action potential is recorded between electrodes placed over the forearm and sternum, far-field potentials occur where the arm joins the forearm, the upper arm joins the shoulder, and the shoulder

joins the neck.[35] At these sites there is muscle insertion and the surrounding volume conductor changes dramatically. In addition, the junctions of the cervical cord and medulla, medulla and pons, pons and diencephalon, and diencephalon and thalamus are sites of considerable physical change in the volume conductor. The variation in the ease with which far-field potentials can be elicited could be explained by different degrees of change of the volume conductor in different individuals at these critical anatomic regions.

It is clear from the preceding that the origin of far-field SEPs is complex and the result of a variety of interacting factors, including fixed neural generators (synapses in relay nuclei), changes in the resistance or impedance of the volume conductor, and possibly sites of axonal branching and anatomic orientation of the traveling impulse.[35,43,57-60] Caution is therefore warranted before concluding that absence or alteration of a far-field potential reflects disease at a specific anatomic site.

Figure 2-2 shows the different short-latency SEP components recordable and the approximate anatomic structures they reflect. Of the far-field potentials, it seems likely that relay nuclei can be implicated only in the generation of P13/P27. The others are probably the result of physical alteration of the surrounding volume conductor as explained previously. The near-field components N17/N35 and N19/N37 are neurally generated, but it is likely that they reflect multiple and even independent thalamocortical projections.[32]

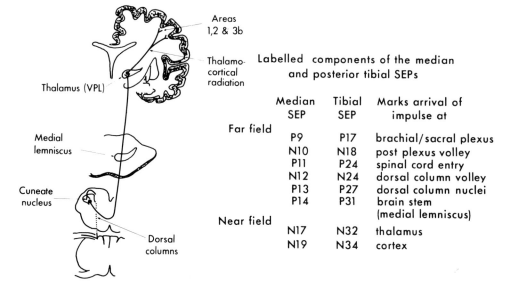

Labelled components of the median and posterior tibial SEPs

	Median SEP	Tibial SEP	Marks arrival of impulse at
Far field	P9	P17	brachial/sacral plexus
	N10	N18	post plexus volley
	P11	P24	spinal cord entry
	N12	N24	dorsal column volley
	P13	P27	dorsal column nuclei
	P14	P31	brain stem (medial lemniscus)
Near field	N17	N32	thalamus
	N19	N34	cortex

Figure 2-2. Somatosensory pathway. Most of labeled far-field potentials are not neuronally generated but reflect sites where there is abrupt change in electrophysical characteristics of surrounding volume conductor. Near-field potentials are neurally generated.

STIMULATION PROCEDURES

An electrical stimulation that is effective for eliciting an SEP has several important characteristics, including intensity, frequency, and site—for example, whether stimulation is of mixed or cutaneous nerve and of dermatomal or motor points. Electrical stimulation is preferred for routine use because it induces a synchronous volley and a most consistently recordable SEP. Other types of more natural stimulation (touch, vibration, stretch, and movement) are physiologic and of interest but usually require special equipment such as a torque motor.

Optimal intensity is different when stimulating a cutaneous nerve and when stimulating a mixed nerve. For mixed nerve stimulation the intensity need only be sufficient to induce a small visible muscle twitch. This is usually between 2 and 5 mA for the median or ulnar nerves and 3 to 12 mA for the tibial or peroneal nerves. These intensities evoke a mixed nerve action potential between 30% to 50% maximum amplitude, which is sufficient to elicit a maximum SEP. Low stimulus intensities preferentially excite the Ia muscle afferents. The afferents are predominantly if not entirely responsible for initiating the volley giving rise to the SEP. Recording a peripheral mixed nerve action potential at the same time as the SEP is good practice. It helps ensure that the stimulus applied is adequate and acts as a monitor of peripheral nerve normality. Conclusions regarding an abnormal SEP cannot be made without knowledge of the integrity of the peripheral component. The nerve action potential may be recorded at the elbow (with arm stimulation) rather than over Erb's point. Recording the brachial plexus potential is popular, but it can be difficult to obtain with surface electrodes, especially when the mixed ulnar nerve or cutaneous nerve stimulation is excited or when stimulation is carried out in thick-necked subjects.

The stimulus intensity required for cutaneous nerve stimulation should be at least three times the threshold (usually between 6 and 15 mA). This is best judged by the amplitude of the sensory nerve action potential, which should be maximal. Virtually any cutaneous nerve can be stimulated. If the nerve is anatomically deep, needle electrodes should be employed. Some of the cutaneous nerves more commonly used for eliciting SEPs are referred subsequently. When a specific site is correctly stimulated, sensation is perceived in the distribution of the cutaneous nerve and in conjunction a normal sensory nerve action potential is recorded.

Stimulation rate is also important. The early latency SEP components do not attenuate significantly below rates of 15 stimuli per second. This is obviously too fast for comfort, whereas rates between 2 and 5 stimuli per second are usually well tolerated. There is usually no need for random stimulation, but if electrocardiographic (ECG) artifacts are troublesome, random stimulation can help. Stimulating at a rate that is nonharmonic with the pulse or triggering the stimulus off a fixed component of the cardiac cycle also helps overcome ECG interference. As discussed below, stimulation rates considerably slower than 1 per second are required to elicit long-latency SEP components. Also, in disease the peripheral and central nervous systems may be unable to transmit trains of impulses at usual rates. In this situation slow stimulation rates may be able to elicit a potential that would not be evoked at faster rates.

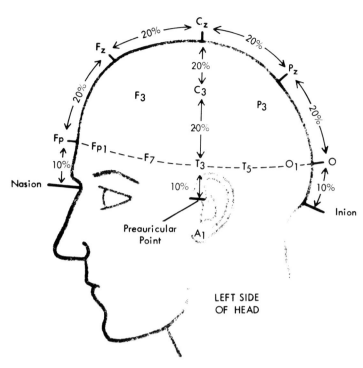

Figure 2-3. International 10-20 system depicted divides skull sagittally, coronally, and horizontally into 10% and 20% intervals marked from points indicated. For SEP recordings electrode placement is 1 cm posterior to C3 or C4 position and referred to as C3′ or C4′. (From Harner, PF, and Sannit, T: A review of the international ten-twenty system of electrode placement, Quincy, Mass, 1974, Grass Instrument Co.)

RECORDING SENSORY EVOKED POTENTIALS

Recording electrodes may be of either the surface or the scalp needle variety. The latter are less popular, although their higher impedance and the theoretic risk of infection should not be of concern. They are easily and rapidly inserted and are not uncomfortable. They obviate the need to abrade the scalp and apply substances for reducing impedance and securing electrodes to the scalp. Recording montages can be either cephalic bipolar, in which both electrodes are placed on the head, or referential, in which G2 is placed off the head (see previous discussion). Cephalic bipolar montages are preferred for routine clinical use because unwanted physiologic noise is limited to muscle electromyography (EMG), which is usually not a problem if the subject is encouraged to relax. Therefore the test should be carried out in an environment that produces relaxation. The subject should lie comfortably on a bed in a semidarkened room and should be encouraged to doze or even fall asleep. The ambient temperature should be maintained between 20° and 22° C (68° and 72° F). The subject should be covered with a blanket. Even anxious patients seldom need a sedative if the nature of the test is carefully explained.

SEPs should not be elicited with the patient sitting up, since this position makes cervical and lumbar spinal SEPs difficult or impossible to record. However, the sitting pos-

ture is used in some laboratories, because it is the preferred position for recording visual and auditory brainstem evoked potentials and thus can be used for multimodality studies.

As explained previously, cephalic-bipolar recordings cause cancellation of most small-amplitude far-field potentials. Because this is also true of montages connecting the neck (second or seventh cervical spinous process) to the cortex (C3, C4, Cz, and so on), they should be avoided.

There is no fixed rule as to the number of channels that should be recorded simultaneously. Four channels are commonly used, including a peripheral nerve potential, a spinal potential, and bipolar-cephalic and noncephalic potentials. The latency differences between these peripheral, spinal, and cortical potentials gives conduction times that are purely peripheral, central, and overlapping.[28] Useful as this may be, the derived measurements of conduction times do reflect central transit between any two specific sites.

The actual number of channels used should logically be determined by the purpose at hand. For example, in field distribution studies as many as 16 channels may be useful. On the other hand, one channel suffices if the SEP is being used to measure peripheral conduction velocities. Electrode placement is based on the international 10-20 system (Figure 2-3). For routine clinical work the G1 electrode for arm- and leg-elicited SEPs is placed, respectively, at C3 or C4

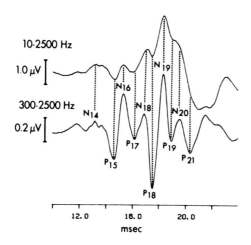

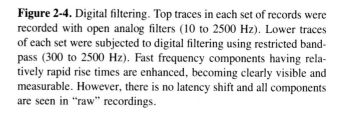

Figure 2-4. Digital filtering. Top traces in each set of records were recorded with open analog filters (10 to 2500 Hz). Lower traces of each set were subjected to digital filtering using restricted band-pass (300 to 2500 Hz). Fast frequency components having relatively rapid rise times are enhanced, becoming clearly visible and measurable. However, there is no latency shift and all components are seen in "raw" recordings.

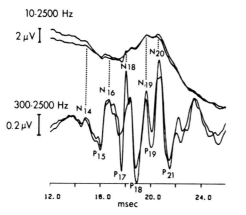

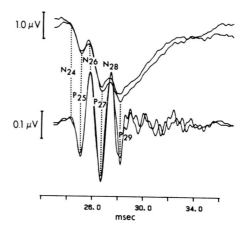

contralateral to the side of stimulation (arm recordings) or at Cz (leg recordings). The G2 electrode is placed at Fpz. An alternative G2 site for leg SEPs is at C3 or C4 contralateral to the side of stimulation. This site makes the onset of the SEP easier to identify and permits use of a common electrode for arm and leg recordings. For the arm it is the G1 electrode and, for the leg, the G2 electrode.

For noncephalic recording the G2 electrode can be placed anywhere, off the head, where it is more, but not entirely, inactive. Its placement is a matter of choice, since nothing indicates that a particular site for G2 makes far-field potentials easier to record. All noncephalic recordings pick up ECG and respiratory artifacts. This and the small amplitude of the potentials make recording difficult and require averaging of a large number of sweeps.

FILTERING

Both near- and far-field components of the SEP are composed of high- and low-frequency elements. Ideal filtering should include them while excluding frequencies that make up unwanted noise. Unfortunately, this is not possible. A relatively open bandpass (200 Hz to 2 kHz) required to include all SEP components also permits passage of most physiologic interference (EEG, ECG, EMG, and respiration). Automated rejection is useful in this regard, but even so the resulting SEP may have a poor morphology and components may be difficult to recognize or measure. Restrictive filtering, on the other hand, attenuates or obliterates either the high- or low-frequency components depending on the settings chosen. Thus there is no "correct" filter setting; the choice depends on the task at hand. Generally a relatively broad bandpass (10 to 2500 Hz) allows visualization of all the SEP components, although it produces a somewhat "noisy" record. However, if interest is limited to N20 (median nerve) or P40 (tibial nerve), a narrower bandpass of 0.5 Hz to 0.5 or 1 kHz gives a much smoother recording.

Restrictive filtering, for example, between 300 and 2000 Hz, dramatically enhances high-frequency, small-amplitude components but virtually abolishes the slow wave "N20" envelope.[32,67] Digital restrictive filtering is preferred to analog.[32,68] It can be designed for zero phase shift, is unlimited in range, and can be performed at any time. New, artificially induced components that are at times created with analog filtering are not a problem in the digital technique (Figure 2-4).

SIGNAL AVERAGING

Signal to noise ratio (SNR) improves by the square root of the number of sweeps that are averaged. Thus, if 100 sweeps are averaged, the mean amplitude of remaining random noise is reduced by a factor of 10 compared with a single sweep. However, improvement of SNR through averaging is not infinite. Too much averaging may be counterproductive because of "jitter" in the latency of the response. This particularly applies to long-latency components of the SEP (see below). In addition, some of the background noise may not be random; alpha rhythm and EMG activity are examples. These "grow" at the same rate as the rest of the signal and can cause confusion. It is better to average fewer responses (100 is often sufficient), but the procedure should be repeated several times to clearly identify time-locked components. Such duplicate runs are mandatory for even routine work; for the smaller-amplitude, more difficult to recognize components, three or four sets of averaging are recommended.

MEASURING EARLY LATENCY SENSORY EVOKED POTENTIAL COMPONENTS

Several characteristics of SEPs can be measured, including latency and interpeak conduction times and amplitude and morphology of the waveform. Latency is the most easily measured, but a normal latency SEP cannot be equated with a normal SEP. Indeed, focal central demyelination and axonal degeneration, like their peripheral nervous system counterparts, are liable to result in conduction block and amplitude reduction before or in the absence of conduction slowing. Latency or interpeak conduction times should be considered abnormal only when they exceed 3 standard deviations for a given component or conduction segment. Side-to-side comparison is often a more sensitive measure of subtle abnormality. For example, the side-to-side difference of the median N20 latency is less than 2 msec.[35]

Amplitude, in absolute terms, is too variable to use as a measure of abnormality, but a side-to-side difference in excess of 50% is abnormal. For arm SEPs the peak-to-peak amplitude between the N20 negativity and the P30 positivity is sufficiently consistent for comparison. For leg SEPs P40 is easily measured. In normal individuals side-to-side differences are less than 10%.

Morphology is the most sensitive characteristic of an SEP. Abnormal morphology invariably accompanies latency prolongation or amplitude reduction and frequently occurs before or in the absence of these changes. However, morphology is difficult to quantitate. An SEP's morphology should not be considered abnormal based simply on visual inspection, since abnormalities may easily be confused with a "noisy" but otherwise normal recording.

Computer-assisted methods that allow proper quantitative measurement of SEP morphology are now being developed. For example, a fast Fourier transform can be used to measure

the spectral energy of the median N20 and tibial P40 SEP components.[72,83] The log of the SEP spectral energy between 380 and 1000 Hz is measured and linearly scaled to a range of numbers between 0 (minimum) and 5 (maximum) morphologic distortion. The upper normal limit is 3, representing the normal mean + 3 SD.[72,83] This approach, which can only look at the spectral energy over a sizable time frame, for example, 20 msec, has recently become sophisticated enough that a true point by point analysis of the SEP's spectral energy can be accomplished in the time domain (Figure 2-4).[45] Another approach is to employ a dynamic time-warping algorithm. This was originally used in voice pattern recognition. In essence an unknown SEP is matched to a standard wave. Manipulation is required and is achieved by "shifting," "elongation," or "contraction" of the unknown SEP. The amount of manipulation is assigned a cost function, which normally does not exceed 2.5 determined in arbitrary units.[30] Warping of a normal SEP and of one recorded from a patient with multiple sclerosis is shown in Figure 2-5.

LONG LATENCY SENSORY EVOKED POTENTIAL COMPONENTS

The SEP has a total duration of 4 to 500 msec. When it is elicited by median nerve stimulation at the wrist, four or five components follow N20.[1,47] These have rarely been systematically analyzed but warrant exploration because of potential application in diffuse and deeply situated brain diseases.

Davis[12,13] first drew attention to "immediate positive responses" to sounds and other stimuli in humans. He described the "on-effect" of applying loud and faint 250 to 2000 cycle tones to the ongoing electroencephalogram (EEG) in an awake subject. The response, now equated with the vertex (V) response, was recorded by superimposition without the aid of computer averaging.

The following characterize the V potential (Figure 2-6):

1. It is of largest amplitude over the vertex where it appears as a triphasic positive-negative-positive potential. Peak-to-peak amplitude attains 40 μV. Onset latency is about 100 msec, and duration is between 200 and 300 msec.

2. It is nonspecific in terms of elicitation, being equally evoked by visual, auditory, and somatic stimuli.[1,2,12,13,47]

3. It may be less stable than short-latency evoked potential components, and its recovery cycle is possibly susceptible to the subject's mental state. However, ongoing thought processes do not appear to have a significant effect on latency or amplitude, and no attempt to control these characteristics has been made in previously reported studies. Even psychiatric illness may not influence the V potential.

4. The recovery cycle of the V potential is slow and is

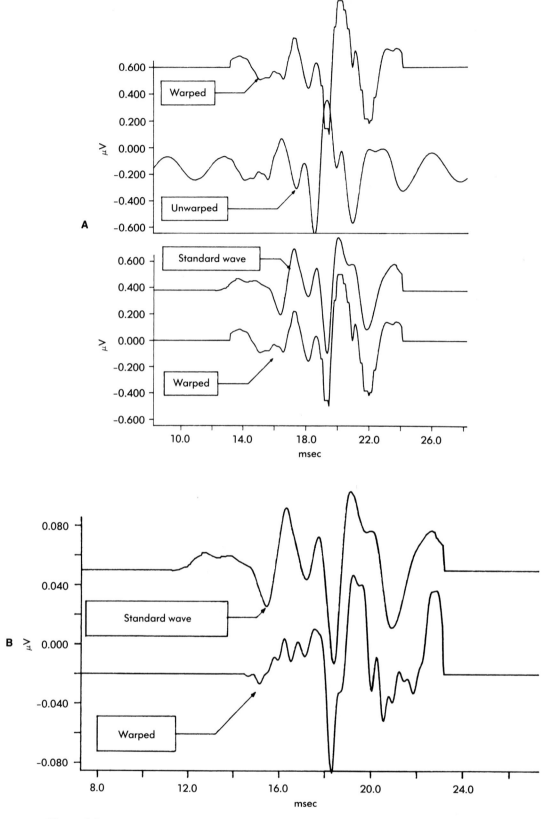

Figure 2-5. Dynamic time warping as means of morphologic measurement of SEP. **A,** Normal SEP has been warped to standard wave derived from 25 normal subjects. Warping required minimal adjustments, and cost factor incurred is small (2.4). **B,** Warping of SEP from patient with multiple sclerosis. Considerable manipulation was required in attempt to match to standard wave. Cost factor measured 13.7.

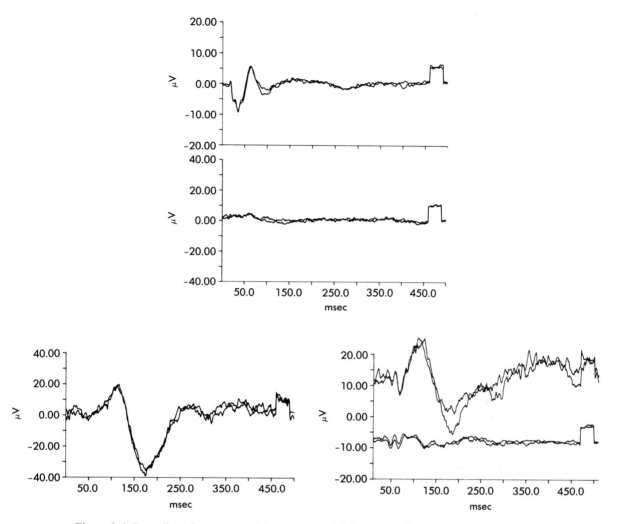

Figure 2-6. Recording of vertex potentials. Top traces: Median nerve stimulation. Montage channel 1 was C3-Fz; channel 2 was Cz-mastoid. Stimulus was applied at 1.5 Hz 100 averages. Early latency components (N20) are seen (channel 1) but no vertex potential (channel 2). Lower left traces: Typical normal vertex potential. Stimulus to median nerve at rate of 0.05 Hz. Only 10 epochs were averaged recorded from Cz-mastoid. Lower right traces: Channel 1, stimulus to tibial nerve at 0.05 Hz, 10 epochs recorded from Cz-mastoid. Large vertex potential is seen. Channel 2 is same as channel 1 at stimulus rate of 1.5 Hz, with 100 epochs recorded. Only early latency components (P40) are seen.

incomplete even after several minutes. The underlying determinants for the slow recovery cycle of the V potential are poorly understood but imply one or more of the following mechanisms: habituation, adaptation, fatigue, inhibition, and distraction. From a practical viewpoint the stimulus repetition rate should not exceed 0.02 to 0.03 Hz.[1,4,47]

Recordings using depth electrodes in human subjects clearly indicate that the V potential originates from deeply situated subcortical structures.[47] Exact localizing of the origin awaits further investigation. There is some evidence from depth electrode studies that the V potential as recorded over the scalp may be composed of a truly bilaterally synchronous evoked potential (the V potential) and a unilateral

(contralateral) evoked potential possibly reflecting late activity within the primary somatosensory cortex or its equivalent. Goff and co-workers[47] refer to the latter as the somatic late potential (SLP). When only surface recordings are used, it is impossible to separate the two because of superimposition and cancellation.

Several aspects of the V potential are clinically appealing. Slow stimulation rates are more comfortable and physiologic. In agitated patients, recording an easily measurable response after only one or two stimuli given a minute apart may be the only satisfactory way of eliciting any evoked potential. Similarly, single stimulus SEPs are appealing in the operating room where it is important to have a measure of changes at relatively short intervals (Figure 2-7). Slow

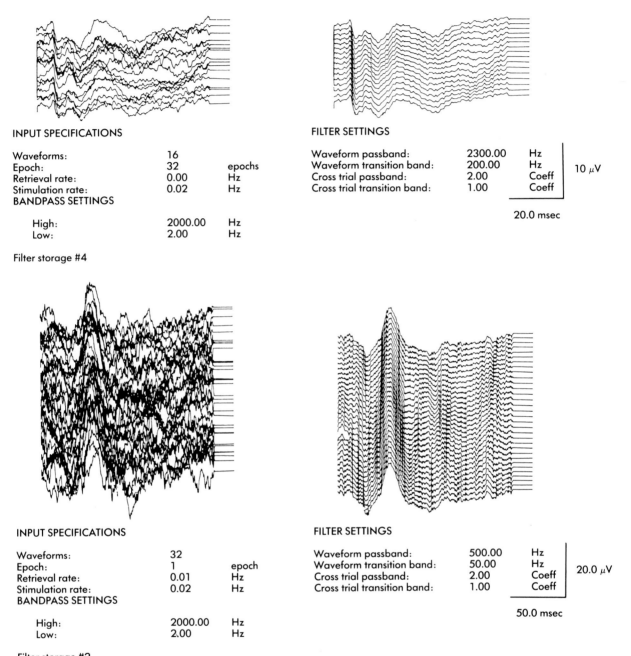

INPUT SPECIFICATIONS

Waveforms:	16	
Epoch:	32	epochs
Retrieval rate:	0.00	Hz
Stimulation rate:	0.02	Hz
BANDPASS SETTINGS		
High:	2000.00	Hz
Low:	2.00	Hz

Filter storage #4

FILTER SETTINGS

Waveform passband:	2300.00	Hz
Waveform transition band:	200.00	Hz
Cross trial passband:	2.00	Coeff
Cross trial transition band:	1.00	Coeff

10 μV

20.0 msec

INPUT SPECIFICATIONS

Waveforms:	32	
Epoch:	1	epoch
Retrieval rate:	0.01	Hz
Stimulation rate:	0.02	Hz
BANDPASS SETTINGS		
High:	2000.00	Hz
Low:	2.00	Hz

Filter storage #2

FILTER SETTINGS

Waveform passband:	500.00	Hz
Waveform transition band:	50.00	Hz
Cross trial passband:	2.00	Coeff
Cross trial transition band:	1.00	Coeff

20.0 μV

50.0 msec

Figure 2-7. Two-dimensional filtering used to enable recording of "single stimulus" SEPs. Bottom traces show vertex potentials. *Left:* Raw data from 32 vertex potentials, each a single sweep. *Right:* Effect of filtering. Potentials are clearly seen and measurable, even though each is only a single sweep. Top traces are early latency median SEPs. Each trace is average of only 32 epochs. Filtering allows easy measurement.

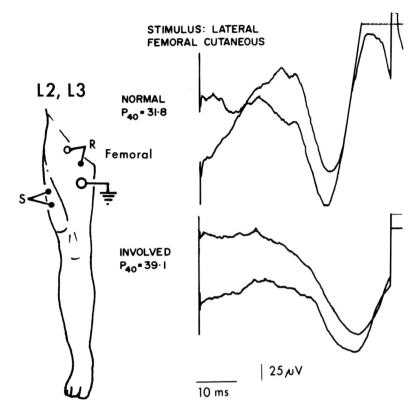

Figure 2-8. Use of SEPs for indirect evaluation of conduction through peripheral nerve (lateral femoral cutaneous). There is latency difference of 7.3 msec between diseased (lower SEPs) and normal (upper SEPs) recorded from Cz-Fz. Stimulation site S and peripheral nerve recording site R are indicated. Patient, a diabetic, had clinical picture of meralgia paresthetica.

stimulation rates do not preclude analysis of early latency components, which also are enhanced when elicited by stimuli applied at 1 per 30 to 40 seconds.

CLINICAL APPLICATION OF SENSORY EVOKED POTENTIALS

Interpretation of SEPs must take into consideration the clinical problem at hand. So doing allows appropriate "test design," a situation akin to the problem-solving approach used to advantage in EMG as a whole. The type of SEP most likely to give useful information must always be considered. For example, if the clinical problem is a lower trunk plexopathy, an ulnar, not a median, evoked SEP is the logical approach. In suspected spinal cord disease, which is virtually always symmetric, bilateral simultaneous stimulation of leg nerves or paraspinal elicited SEPs should be considered. The size of the SEP is proportional to the number of axons stimulated, and bilateral stimulation may allow recognition and measurement of a potential not possible with unilateral stimulation. In multiple sclerosis, leg SEPs, which incorporate conduction through the spinal cord as well as the cortex, are more useful than arm SEPs. Situations in which recording an SEP is inappropriate must also be rec-

ognized.[26] Most structural brain diseases are visualized and far better localized by CT scanning or magnetic resonance imaging. However, in the case of nonvisible lesions (toxic, infectious, or posttraumatic encephalopathies) there appears to be a place for recording long latency SEPs, which are possibly more useful than measurement of "central conduction times."[70]

Peripheral nerve disease
Peripheral nerves

The indications for using SEPs to evaluate peripheral nerves are several[24]:

1. To measure conduction through cutaneous nerves that are inaccessible for anatomic reasons and for which conventional conduction techniques are difficult or impossible. For example, the lateral femoral cutaneous, saphenous, and medial and lateral antebrachial nerves are all difficult to record. However, they are easily stimulated and doing so elicits a sizable SEP (Figure 2-8).
2. To verify axonal continuity after nerve injury. This is possible for some time before a peripheral sensory nerve action potential can be elicited.

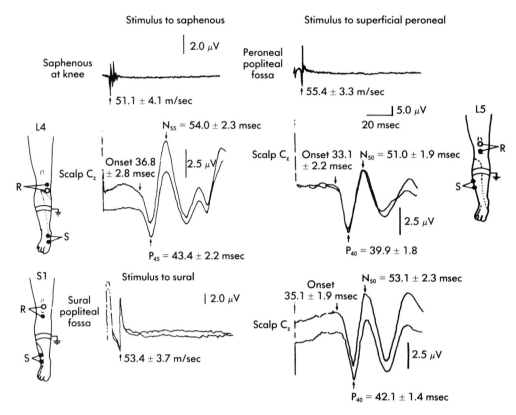

Stimulus to saphenous

Stimulus to superficial peroneal

Saphenous at knee

2.0 μV

Peroneal popliteal fossa

51.1 ± 4.1 m/sec

55.4 ± 3.3 m/sec

L4

5.0 μV
20 msec

L5

$N_{55} = 54.0 \pm 2.3$ msec

Scalp C$_z$

Onset 36.8 ± 2.8 msec

2.5 μV

Scalp C$_z$

Onset 33.1 ± 2.2 msec

$N_{50} = 51.0 \pm 1.9$ msec

R

S

$P_{45} = 43.4 \pm 2.2$ msec

2.5 μV

$P_{40} = 39.9 \pm 1.8$

S1

Stimulus to sural

$N_{50} = 53.1 \pm 2.3$ msec

Sural popliteal fossa

2.0 μV

Onset 35.1 ± 1.9 msec

R

Scalp C$_z$

S

53.4 ± 3.7 m/sec

Scalp C$_z$

2.5 μV

$P_{40} = 42.1 \pm 1.4$ msec

Figure 2-9. SEP can help assess conduction in neuropathies. **A,** Normal SEPs elicited by median nerve stimulation at wrist and elbow. Velocity calculated from latency differences is fast (75.8 m/sec). It reflects conduction through Ia afferents. **B,** Charcot-Marie-Tooth neuropathy. Lower trace is attempt to record near-nerve sural action potential. No response was seen after 2000 sweeps. SEP *(top traces)* is grossly slowed but easily recordable. Sural nerve biopsy showed few remaining myelinated axons. **C,** Ulnar neuropathy. Sensory nerve action potential *(lower trace)* is small and very dispersed. Stimulation of ulnar nerve at wrist elicited easily recorded SEP prolonged in latency.

3. As a means of measuring sensory conduction in neuropathies when sensory nerve action potentials cannot be recorded, as for example in Friedreich's ataxia, Charcot-Marie-Tooth neuropathy, or severe acquired chronic demyelinating neuropathies (Figure 2-9). In neuropathies, recording SEPs has the additional advantage of incorporating the otherwise inaccessible proximal segments of sensory nerve. This is of particular relevance in Guillain-Barré syndrome in which prolonged latency SEPs may be the sole or earliest conduction abnormality.[33,61]

It is possible to record an SEP in the absence of a sensory nerve action potential because the incoming peripheral volley is amplified within the central nervous system.[29] This central nervous system amplification explains the discrepancy between significant electrophysiologic abnormality and minimal clinical deficit encountered in some neurologic diseases.

When SEPs are used to study peripheral nerve disease, it is assumed that the central nervous system is intact. This may not be easy to establish. In some diseases, such as, central-peripheral axonopathies, diabetes, Charcot-Marie-Tooth disease, and some forms of acquired postinfectious polyradiculoneuropathy, there is both central and peripheral involvement.[24,25,93]

Use of SEPs to evaluate peripheral nerve disease requires only that continuity in conduction be documented, which allows a conduction time to be measured or velocity calculated. A single scalp recording channel is therefore perfectly valid and even desirable. There is neither need nor value in recording far-field potentials. The relevant ones, those generated distal to spinal cord entry, are not universally recordable and are even more difficult to evoke with cutaneous nerve stimulation. They are usually unrecordable in peripheral nerve disease. The best components to record are the median N19 or tibial P40 or their equivalents using a cephalic-bipolar montage (C3 or C4 against Fz for arm SEPs and Cz against Fz for leg SEPs). Because only the "slow" wave N19/P40 envelope is of interest, restrictive bandpass (0.5 Hz to 200 or 500 Hz), which smooths out unwanted fast frequency components, should be used. In some peripheral nerve diseases, routine stimulation rates of 1 to 4 per second elicit little or no response because the diseased or injured nerve is incapable of transmitting impulses at usual rates. Therefore, before concluding that an SEP is absent, one must try to elicit it using slow stimulation rates (0.03 to 0.05 Hz).

Plexopathies

SEPs are useful in documenting and localizing plexopathies. Mixed nerve, cutaneous nerve, and motor point stimulation are all suitable and have a role in eliciting the SEP. The choice depends on the part of the plexus involved (Table 2-1). In traumatic plexopathies the overriding question is whether there has been root avulsion. The following constellation indicates that root avulsion has occurred:

1. Denervation (fibrillation or positive sharp waves recorded from the paraspinal muscles)
2. A normal sensory nerve action potential
3. An unrecordable SEP
4. Absence of a histamine flare response

A recordable SEP is evidence of central-peripheral axonal continuity even in the face of active denervation or inability to record a sensory nerve action potential.[24,54,91,92] Root avulsion precludes reconstructive surgery.

The use of SEPs in nontraumatic plexopathies is less well delineated. The most common of these plexopathies are the nonneurogenic thoracic outlet syndromes. Their nosology is confused, but Swift and Nichols[90] have clearly defined at least one, probably the most common, variety. It predominantly affects young women and is typified by the following:

1. Droopy shoulders
2. Pain in the neck, shoulder, chest, arms, or hands aggravated by downward traction and relieved by propping up the arms
3. Tinel's sign over the brachial plexus
4. A radiologically visible T2 vertebra rostral to the shoulders on lateral cervical spine films

These patients have normal vascular, neurologic, and conventional electrodiagnostic findings. Results of SEP recording have been conflicting, partly because of the heterogeneity of nonneurogenic thoracic outlet syndromes.[65,96]

The "true," but rare, neurogenic thoracic outlet syndrome is characterized by the following electrophysiologic abnormalities:

1. A reduced compound motor action potential recorded from the thenar muscles but a normal amplitude motor action potential recorded from the hypothenar muscles
2. A small or absent ulnar sensory action potential but a normal median nerve sensory action potential
3. A small, absent, or delayed ulnar F-response despite a normal median F-wave
4. Motor unit abnormalities, characteristic of partial chronic denervation, on needle EMG of C8 and T1 muscles

Table 2-1. Peripheral nerves usefully stimulated to elicit SEPs in the evaluation of plexopathies

Plexus	Stimulation
Brachial	
Trunks	
Upper (C5/6)	Musculocutaneous
Middle (C7)	Median
Lower (C8/T1)	Ulnar
Cords	
Lateral (C5/6/7)	Musculocutaneous
Posterior (C5/6/7)	Radial
Medial (C8/T1)	Ulnar
Lumbar	
Upper (L2/3)	Lateral femoral cutaneous
Middle (L3/4)	Femoral
Lower (L4)	Femoral
Sacral	
Upper (L4/5)	Superior gluteal
Middle (S1/2)	Peroneal-tibial
Lower S3/4)	Pudendal

An abnormal SEP, evoked by ulnar nerve stimulation, may complement these characteristic electrodiagnostic abnormalities.

SEPs have also been helpful in radiation plexopathy and in the complex mixture of lower trunk plexopathy and ulnar neuropathy frequently complicating open-heart surgery. However, SEPs have not been of value in localizing paralytic brachial neuritis (neuralgic amyotrophy). This reflects the recently proposed anatomic basis of brachial neuritis, which is considered to lie in one or more peripheral nerves at their branching origin from the brachial plexus.[89]

Radiculopathies

Several reports have described use of SEPs in the assessment of disc disease.* The diagnostic yield has ranged from high to of little or no value. The major drawback to using SEPs in radiculopathies, especially those resulting from disc disease, is the short, few millimeter segment of diseased nerve (the root) relative to the long length of normally conducting nerve. Detection of slowing is precluded in most cases. This is true when using the F-wave or H-reflex to investigate radiculopathies. A variety of approaches have been developed in an attempt to render the SEP more sensitive in evaluating radiculopathies. They include cutaneous nerve stimulation, dermatomal stimulation, and motor point stimulation.

---

*References 3, 25, 27, 42, 44, 76, 87.

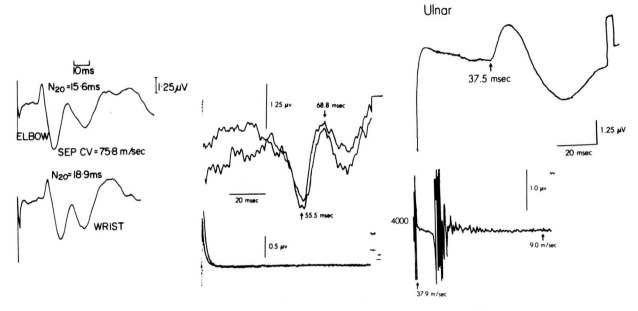

Figure 2-10. Segmental cutaneous stimulation to elicit SEPs. Examples indicate how cutaneous nerves can be selected for stimulation to match specific sensory roots. SEPs elicited are easily measurable. In each case, site of stimulation S is shown, as well as site R for simultaneous recording of sensory nerve action potential. SEPs were recorded using cephalic-bipolar montage (Cz-Fz). Values shown are mean ± SD for 50 normal subjects. Alternative techniques include dermatomal and motor point stimulation.

Table 2-2. Stimulation sites and normal latencies for SEPs elicited by segmental sensory stimulation

Cutaneous nerve	Stimulation site	Segment	Latency to N20 or P40 (mean ± SD [msec])
Musculocutaneous	Forearm	C5	17.4 ± 1.2
Median	Thumb	C6	22.5 ± 1.1
Median	Adjoining surfaces fingers 2 and 3	C7	21.2 ± 1.2
Ulnar	Finger 5	C8	22.5 ± 1.1
Lateral femoral cutaneous	Thigh	L2	31.8 ± 1.8
Saphenous	Knee	L3	37.6 ± 2.0
Saphenous	Ankle	L4	43.4 ± 2.2
Superficial peroneal	Above ankle	L5	39.9 ± 1.8
Sural	Ankle	S1	42.1 ± 1.4

Cutaneous nerve stimulation evokes a sizable and synchronous SEP, and nerves can be selected to reflect a reasonable degree of segmental specificity (Figure 2-10 and Table 2-2). However, for most cutaneous nerves the stimulation site is still too distal. Dermatomal stimulation, in which a patch of skin is innervated through a single dermatome, is even more segmentally specific.[55,78-80] However, the SEP evoked is small and desynchronized, making abnormalities difficult to interpret. Motor point stimulation is a new approach that is potentially the most relevant. In this technique the motor point is stimulated through a monopolar electrode. The stimulus should be sufficient to induce a visible muscle twitch. So doing excites the majority of muscle spindle Ia afferents. The procedure is painless because only motor terminals and Ia afferents are stimulated. Motor point stimulation is segmentally specific, allows very proximal stimulation, and permits stimulation of virtually any muscle.

Use of SEPs in disc disease complements but cannot replace needle EMG, which remains the single most useful electrophysiologic test. However, in patients whose needle EMG findings are normal and whose sensory complaints predominate or occur in isolation, an abnormal SEP can be helpful in confirming disease. A normal SEP study does not rule out root compression.

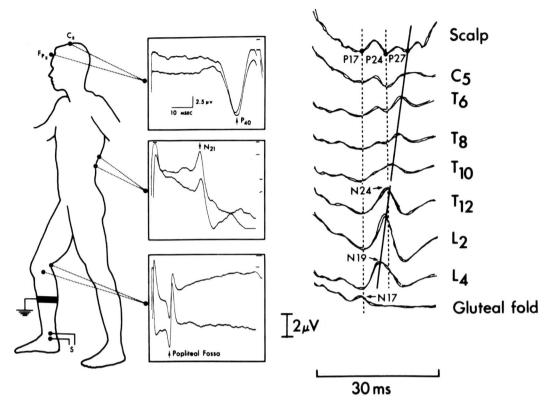

Figure 2-11. Spinal potentials (B) elicited by tibial nerve stimulation are shown. They are small and difficult to obtain above T10. This direct technique does, however, have localizing value and is useful in infants and children. The propagated volley ascends through the dorsal columns at about 60 m/sec. The short latency far-field potentials P17, P24, and P27 were recorded at the scalp (Cz-knee). They reflect changes in the volume conductor where the thigh joins the buttock (sacral plexus), spinal cord entry, and cervical-medullary junction respectively. The conduction time given by P40-N21 (A) is easily measured. Although incorporating the spinal cord, the technique has no localizing value.

SEPs are more useful in other types of radiculopathy. For example, in some radiculopathies there is severe loss of dorsal root ganglion cells. In these diseases, better termed ganglionopathies, the SEP and the peripheral sensory nerve action potential are usually unrecordable. Herpes zoster, diabetic radiculopathy, and an idiopathic variety are examples of true ganglionopathies.

Spinal cord disease

The ideal method of assessing spinal cord conduction has several prerequisites. The test must be noninvasive, free of discomfort, easy to perform, reproducible, and time and cost effective and must have localizing capability.

A variety of evoked potential methods have been used to evaluate afferent transmission through the spinal cord.[9,23] In essence, most methods either involve recording potentials over the spine that have been elicited by tibial nerve stimulation* or employ a combination of spinal and cortical

*References 6, 15, 16, 19, 21, 37, 53, 56, 62, 71, 81, 82, 94, 95.

evoked potentials elicited by tibial nerve stimulation (Figure 2-11).[28,74,88]

The theoretic advantage of recording spinal potentials, which allow the most direct measure of transmission through the cord, is severely limited by their small size. Without resorting to use of invasive techniques,[38-40,52,84-86] spinal potentials, especially those recorded over the upper adult spinal cord, require extensive averaging for recognition. Even then spinal potentials are frequently difficult or impossible to measure, which limits this technique in disease diagnosis. However, in infants and children spinal potentials are easily obtained and play a useful role.[7,10,11]

An easier but less direct approach is to measure the conduction time between the lumbar spinal potential (N21), which is sizable, and the much larger amplitude cortical evoked potential P40 (Figure 2-11). Doing so includes transmission through the spinal cord, brainstem, diencephalon, and cortex.[28,41,74,77,88] In common with other indirect methods, such as those that employ the F-wave or muscle movement potentials,[22,31,34] this method precludes localization of

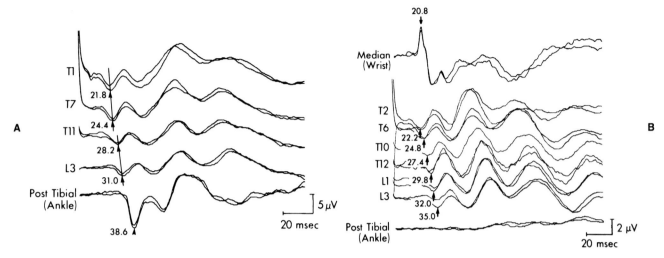

Figure 2-12. Paraspinal elicited SEPs. **A,** Normal subject. Paraspinal region was stimulated bilaterally at levels indicated, as well as tibial nerve at ankle. Note progressive shortening of latency allowing for localization of spinal lesion. **B,** Stimulation of tibial nerve failed to elicit SEP. Paraspinal SEPs below T12 are prolonged, but above this level they are of normal latency as is median elicited SEP. Patient had thoracolumbar arachnoid cyst surgically confirmed and removed.

disease. Thus it does not help to determine whether an abnormality is due to cord disease or brain disease or both.

Recently Goodrich, Eisen, and Hoirch[48] described a new method of eliciting SEPs by stimulation of the paraspinal region. The method meets many of the prerequisites of the ideal test listed previously. In essence simultaneous, percutaneous, bilateral paraspinal stimulation is applied about 2 cm lateral to the midline. Any spinal level can be stimulated. Routinely L3, T12, T7, and T1 are stimulated (Figure 2-12). The stimulus should be sufficient to induce a clearly visible muscle twitch. The intensity required is usually between 25 and 45 mA but is not uncomfortable. The evoked potential is recorded using a cephalic bipolar montage with electrodes placed at Cz (G1) and Fz (62). The volley initiated by paraspinal stimulation arises predominantly in the cutaneous branch of the dorsal primary ramus of the spinal nerve. Undoubtedly the muscle movement excites Ia afferents, which also contribute to the SEP.

The technique provides localizing information in both radiologically visible and nonvisible spinal lesions and is helpful in determining multisegmental disease (Figure 2-12). It is insufficiently sensitive to localize a lesion to a single spinal segment and therefore is unlikely to prove useful in the evaluation of radiculopathies. Also, because bilateral stimulation is employed to obtain the best results, unilateral cord disease is likely to be masked. Overall afferent cord conduction velocity with this method is about 60 m/sec. However, more important than documentation of slowed velocity is the ability to demonstrate a segment of focal slowing.

The ability to measure motor conduction through the spinal cord and more rostral central nervous system is also important. This has been achieved using electrical stimulation applied to either the brain or the spinal cord.[63,64,75] A modified stimulator capable of delivering a high-voltage shock (up to 2000 V) of brief duration (about 50 μsec) is required. Even then the method is uncomfortable and to some patients painful. Therefore it is unlikely to gain widespread acceptance. The recently developed nonpainful magnetic stimulator will probably be used in the future to stimulate the brain and spinal cord.[51] The main disadvantage of magnetic stimulation is its limited focus. For example, when the median nerve is stimulated at the elbow, the ulnar nerve is often stimulated too. Fortunately, the arm or leg cortical motor strips can be stimulated in isolation without difficulty.

Central nervous system diseases

Those who would use SEPs to assess central nervous system diseases must be cognizant of modern imaging techniques. Most structural diseases are identifiable by computerized tomography (CT) scanning. Brainstem and other deeply situated midline lesions are not always well recognized by CT scan, but magnetic resonance imaging (MRI) has proved singularly useful. Therefore SEPs seldom have a role in the anatomic localization of brain disease. Exceptions include small strokes involving the somatosensory pathways that are not visualized radiologically. This is particularly pertinent during the initial postictal days when the lesion is usually not visible on CT scan. The V potential

Table 2-3. Comparison of different abnormal test results in patients suspected to have multiple sclerosis

Test	Possible MS (N = 158)	Probable MS (N = 42)	Total (N = 200)
Magnetic resonance imaging	94 (59.5%)	32 (76.2%)	126 (63%)
Somatosensory evoked potential	73 (46.2%)	29 (69.0%)	102 (51%)
Visual evoked potential	68 (43.0%)	28 (66.6%)	96 (48%)
Cerebrospinal fluid oligoclonal bands	67 (42.4%)	29 (69.0%)	96 (48%)
Double-dose delayed contrast-enhanced computerized tomography	46 (29.1%)	9 (21.4%)	55 (27.5%)

may have a similar role in other deeply situated infarcts that do not involve the somatosensory pathways.

The real value of SEPs in central nervous system disease is in monitoring events in a comatose patient. Coma following trauma, infection, intoxication, and drug overdose can be monitored by serial SEPs. A progressive increase in central conduction times, usually measured as the difference between the median N20 and cervical spinal N14 peaks, frequently heralds a poor prognosis. On the other hand, unrecordable responses that improve usually indicate that recovery will be complete and rapid. The V potential, which has its origin in deep structures, appears to have equal validity and may be a more sensitive prognostic indicator in comatose patients.

Multiple sclerosis

MRI has had a significant impact on the diagnosis of multiple sclerosis (MS). Although the nature of the lesions visualized is unknown, they are sufficiently characteristic to be a reliable diagnostic mark of the disease.[5,46,50,66,69] If four or more typical lesions are seen, with one or more invading the periventricular region, the finding can be confidently equated with MS.[34] The diagnostic superiority of MRI over SEPs and other tests conventionally used in the diagnosis of MS is clearly established.[34] Eisen and co-workers[36] recently studied 200 patients with suspected MS and minimal or no neurologic deficit (mean Kurtzke scale below 2.5). Table 2-3 shows the diagnostic superiority of MRI compared with other tests in these patients. Double-dose delayed CT gave a poor diagnostic yield and should probably be dropped from the battery of diagnostic tests used for MS.

In patients with chronic progressive myelopathy the incidence of abnormal MRI and SEP results is higher (70%) than for other tests and is approximately equal. The larger number of abnormal SEPs is attributable to SEPs elicited by posterior tibial nerve stimulation, which were abnormal twice as frequently as median elicited SEPs. It is usually assumed that the higher yield of abnormal leg SEPs in MS reflects detection of additional lesions within the spinal cord.

However, if this explanation were entirely valid, one might anticipate a significantly higher incidence of abnormal SEP findings compared with MRI findings in progressive spinal MS, which was not the case in this study. An alternative or complementary explanation for abnormal tibial SEPs may reside in the preponderance of midperiventricular MRI-detected lesions involving the somatosensory pathways.

More than 60% of MS patients have autopsy-proven hydrocephalus ex vacuo attributable to loss of periventricular white matter. Appropriately placed lesions, as visualized by MRI, have been reported in all of 11 MS patients with CT-identified hydrocephalus.[30,72] Such lesions are more likely to involve the leg thalamocortical radiation because of its relatively larger surface proximity with the hydrocephalic ventricle.[49] Periventricular (thalamocortical) lesions are easily identifiable by MRI, but leg versus arm involvement can be difficult to determine. Accepting these limitations, the MRI findings raise the intriguing possibility that the "chronic myelopathy" in MS may in part be a misinterpretation, since the same clinical findings could be equally accounted for on the basis of periventricular lesions.

Careful analysis of SEP abnormalities in MS reveals altered morphology and reduced amplitude more commonly than prolonged latency. This is in keeping with the lesions seen on MRI, which viewed in both coronal and sagittal planes appear as thin slices in the periventricular regions and elsewhere. They are too thin to cause conduction slowing but would easily result in conduction block.

Tibial nerves P40 and N45 are often absent in MS, and the first measurable component is a positivity with a mean latency of 51.4 + 5.1 msec. This closely approximates the latency of the next normal positivity recorded with a bipolar-cephalic montage, namely P50. These early components, then, are subject to conduction block, which may be readily misinterpreted as conduction slowing.

SUMMARY

This chapter reviews current technology and clinical usage of SEPs. In day-to-day clinical practice, standardized reproducible and easily performed techniques are available to elicit SEPs from both the upper and lower limbs, stimulating both mixed and cutaneous nerves and also paraspinal musculature. In recent years the clinical role and usefulness of SEPs has become clarified, and its use should certainly be considered in the following situations: in the peripheral nervous system when one wants to measure a sensory conduction not available by standard techniques and to estimate conduction in proximal segments of sensory nerves, and in spinal cord and brain disease when there is no radiologically documented lesion. With the advent of magnetic resonance imaging, the role in multiple sclerosis has become less obvious. The role of SEPs and other evoked potentials in metabolic, postinfective, and posttraumatic encephalopathies, although not yet fully delineated, appears promising.

REFERENCES

1. Allison, T: Recovery functions of somatosensory evoked responses in man, Electroencephalogr Clin Neurophysiol 14:331, 1962.
2. Allison, T, et al: The scalp topography of human visual evoked potentials, Electroencephalogr Clin Neurophysiol 42:185, 1977.
3. Aminoff, MJ, et al: Dermatomal somatosensory evoked potentials in unilateral lumbosacral radiculopathy, Ann Neurol 17:171, 1985.
4. Angel, RW, et al: Decrement of somatosensory evoked potentials during repetitive stimulation, Electroencephalogr Clin Neurophysiol 60:335, 1985.
5. Buonanno, FS, et al: 'H nuclear magnetic resonance imaging in multiple sclerosis, Neurol Clin 1:757, 1983.
6. Cracco, RQ: Spinal evoked response: peripheral nerve stimulation in man, Electroencephalogr Clin Neurophysiol 35:379, 1973.
7. Cracco, J, Castells, S, and Mark, E: Spinal somatosensory evoked potentials in juvenile diabetes, Ann Neurol 15:55, 1984.
8. Cracco, RQ, and Cracco, JB: Somatosensory evoked potential in man: far field potentials, Electroencephalogr Clin Neurophysiol 41:460, 1976.
9. Cracco, RQ, and Cracco, JB: Spinal evoked potentials. In Buser, PA, Cobb, WA, and Okuma, T, editors: Kyoto symposium (EEG Suppl No 36), Amsterdam, 1982, Elsevier.
10. Cracco, JB, Cracco, RQ, and Graziani, LJ: The spinal evoked response in infants and children, Neurology 25:31, 1975.
11. Cracco, JB, Cracco, RQ, and Stolove, R: Spinal evoked potential in man: a maturational study, Electroencephalogr Clin Neurophysiol 46:58, 1979.
12. Davis, H, et al: Electrical reactions of the human brain to auditory stimulation during sleep, J Neurophysiol 2:500, 1939.
13. Davis, PA: Effects of acoustic stimuli on the waking human brain, J Neurophysiol 2:494, 1939.
14. Dawson, GD: A summation technique for the detection of small evoked potentials, Electroencephalogr Clin Neurophysiol 6:65, 1954.
15. Delbeke, J, McComas, AJ, and Kopec, SJ: Analysis of evoked lumbosacral potentials in man, J Neurol Neurosurg Psychiatry 41:293, 1978.
16. Delwaide, PJ, Schoenen, J, and DePasqua, V: Lumbosacral spinal evoked potentials in patients with multiple sclerosis, Neurology 35:174, 1985.
17. Desmedt, JE, and Cheron, G: Central somatosensory conduction in man: neural generators and interpeak latencies of the far-field components recorded from neck and right or left scalp and earlobes, Electroencephalogr Clin Neurophysiol 50:382, 1980.
18. Desmedt, JE, and Cheron, G: Prevertebral (oesophageal) recording of subcortical somatosensory evoked potentials in man: the spinal P13 component and the dual nature of the spinal generators, Electroencephalogr Clin Neurophysiol 52:257, 1981.

19. Desmedt, JE, and Cheron, G: Spinal and far field components of human somatosensory evoked potentials to posterior tibial nerve stimulation: analysis with oesophageal derivations and non-cephalic reference recording, Electroencephalogr Clin Neurophysiol 56:635, 1983.
20. Dimitrijevic, MR, et al: Evoked spinal cord and nerve root potentials in humans using a non-invasive recording technique, Electroencephalogr Clin Neurophysiol 45:331, 1978.
21. Dimitrijevic, M.R., et al: Characteristics of spinal cord evoked responses in man, Appl Neurophysiol 43:118, 1980.
22. Dorfman, LJ: Indirect estimation of spinal cord velocity in man, Electroencephalogr Clin Neurophysiol 43:26, 1977.
23. Eisen, A: Noninvasive measurement of spinal cord conduction: review of presently available methods, Muscle Nerve 9:95, 1986.
24. Eisen, A: SEPs in the evaluation of the peripheral nervous system. In Cracco, RQ, and Bodis-Wollner, I, editors: Frontiers of clinical neuroscience: evoked potentials, New York, 1986, Alan R Liss, Inc.
25. Eisen, A, and Aminoff, MJ: Somatosensory evoked potentials. In Aminoff, MJ, editor: Electrodiagnosis in clinical neurophysiology, ed 2, New York, 1986, Churchill Livingstone.
26. Eisen, A, and Cracco, RQ: Overuse of evoked potentials: caution, Neurology 33:618, 1983.
27. Eisen, A, Hoirch, M, and Moll, A: Evaluation of radiculopathies by segmental stimulation and somatosensory evoked potentials, Can J Neurol Sci 10:178, 1983.
28. Eisen, A, and Odusote, K: Central and peripheral conduction times in multiple sclerosis, Electroencephalogr Clin Neurophysiol 48:253, 1980.
29. Eisen, A, Purves, S, and Hoirch, M: Central nervous system amplification: its potential in the diagnosis of early multiple sclerosis, Neurology 32:359, 1982.
30. Eisen, A, Roberts, K, and Lawrence, P: Morphological measurement of the SEP using a dynamic time warping algorithm, Electroencephalogr Clin Neurophysiol 65:136, 1986.
31. Eisen, A, et al: A new indirect method for measuring spinal conduction velocity in man, Electroencephalogr Clin Neurophysiol 59:204, 1984.
32. Eisen, A, et al: Questions regarding the sequential neural generator theory of the somatosensory evoked potential raised by digital filtering, Electroencephalogr Clin Neurophysiol 59:388, 1984.
33. Eisen, A, et al: Sensory group Ia proximal conduction velocity, Muscle Nerve 7:636, 1984.
34. Eisen, A, et al: Non-invasive measurement of central sensory and motor conduction, Neurology 35:503, 1985.
35. Eisen, A, et al: Far-field potentials from peripheral nerve: generated at sites of muscle mass change, Neurology 36:815, 1986.
36. Eisen, A, et al: Comparison of magnetic resonance imaging with somatosensory testing in MS suspects, Muscle Nerve. In press.
37. El-Negamy, E, and Sedgwick, EM: Properties of a spinal somatosensory evoked potential recorded in man, J Neurol Neurosurg Psychiatry 41:762, 1978.
38. Ertekin, C: Human evoked electrospinogram. In Desmedt, JE, editor: New developments in electromyography and clinical neurophysiology, vol 2, Basel, 1973, Karger.
39. Ertekin, C: Studies on the human evoked electrospinogram. 1. The origin of the segmental evoked potentials, Acta Neurol Scand 53:3, 1976.
40. Ertekin, C: Evoked electrospinogram in spinal cord and peripheral nerve disorders, Acta Neurol Scand 57:329, 1978.
41. Ertekin, C, Sarica, Y, and Uckardesler, L: Somatosensory cerebral potentials evoked by stimulation of the lumbo-sacral spinal cord in normal subjects and in patients with conus medullaris and cauda equina lesions, Electroencephalogr Clin Neurophysiol 59:57, 1984.
42. Feinsod, M, et al: Somatosensory evoked potential to peroneal nerve stimulation in patients with herniated lumbar discs, Neurosurgery 11:506, 1982.

43. Frith, RW, Benstead, TJ, and Daube, JR: Stationary waves recorded at the shoulder after median nerve stimulation, Neurology 36:1458, 1986.

44. Ganes, T: Somatosensory conduction times and peripheral, cervical, and cortical evoked potentials in patients with cervical spondylosis, J Neurol Neurosurg Psychiatry 43:683, 1980.

45. Garudadri, H, et al: Application of smoothed Wigner distribution (WD) to speech signals, J Acoust Soc Am 79(suppl 1):94, 1986.

46. Gebarski, SS, et al: The initial diagnosis of multiple sclerosis: clinical impact of magnetic resonance imaging, Ann Neurol 17:469, 1985.

47. Goff, WR, et al: Neural origins of long latency evoked potentials recorded from the depth and from the cortical surface of the brain in man. In Desmedt, JE, editor: Clinical uses of cerebral, brainstem and spinal somatosensory evoked potentials, Prog Clin Neurophysiol, vol 7, Basel, 1980, Karger.

48. Goodridge, A, Eisen, A, and Hoirch, M: Paraspinal stimulation to elicit somatosensory evoked potentials: an approach to physiological localization of spinal lesions, Electroencephalogr Clin Neurophysiol 68:268, 1987.

49. Horne, MK, and Tracey, DJ: The afferents and projections of the ventroposterolateral thalamus in the monkey, Exp Brain Res 36:129, 1979.

50. Jacobs, L, et al: Correlations of nuclear magnetic imaging, computerized tomography, and clinical profiles in multiple sclerosis, Neurology 36:27, 1986.

51. Jarratt, JA: Magnetic stimulation for motor conduction. In International symposium on new concepts in electromyography, Boston, Rochester, Minn, 1986, Custom Printing, Inc.

52. Jones, SJ, Edgar, MA, and Ransford, AO: Sensory nerve conduction in the human spinal cord; epidural recordings made during scoliosis surgery, J Neurol Neurosurg Psychiatry 45:446, 1982.

53. Jones, SJ, and Small, DG: Spinal and sub-cortical evoked potentials following stimulation of the posterior tibial nerve in man, Electroencephalogr Clin Neurophysiol 44:299, 1978.

54. Jones, SJ, Wynn Parry, CB, and Landi, A: Diagnosis of brachial plexus traction lesions by sensory nerve action potentials and somatosensory evoked potentials, Injury 12:376, 1981.

55. Jorg, J, Dulberg, W, and Koeppen, S: Diagnostic value of segmental somatosensory evoked potentials in cases with chronic progressive para- or tetraspastic syndromes. In Courjon, J, Maugiere, F, and Revol, M, editors: Clinical applications of evoked potentials in neurology, New York, 1982, Raven Press.

56. Kakigi, R, et al: Short latency somatosensory evoked spinal and scalp recorded potentials following posterior tibial nerve stimulation in man, Electroencephalogr Clin Neurophysiol 53:602, 1982.

57. Kimura, J, et al: Far-field recording of the junctional potential generated by median nerve volleys at the wrist, Neurology 36:1451, 1986.

58. Kimura, J, et al: Model for far-field recordings of SEP. In Cracco, RQ, and Bodis-Wollner, I, editors: Evoked potentials, New York, 1986, Alan R Liss, Inc.

59. Kimura, J, et al: What determines the latency and amplitude of stationary peaks in far-field recordings? Ann Neurol 19:479, 1986.

60. Kimura, J, et al: Field distribution of antidromically activated digital nerve potentials: models for far-field recording, Neurology 33:1164, 1983.

61. King, D, and Ashby, P: Conduction velocity in the proximal segments of a motor nerve in the Guillain-Barré syndrome, J Neurol Neurosurg Psychiatry 39:538, 1976.

62. Lehmkuhl, D, Dimitrijevic, MR, and Renouf, F: Electrophysiological characteristics of lumbosacral evoked potentials in patients with established spinal cord injury, Electroencephalogr Clin Neurophysiol 59:142, 1984.

63. Levy, WJ: Spinal evoked potentials from the motor tracts, J Neurosurg 58:38, 1983.

64. Levy, WJ, and York, DH: Evoked potentials from the motor tracts in humans, Neurosurgery 12:422, 1983.

65. Livingstone, EF, aand DeLisa, JA: Electrodiagnostic values through the thoracic outlet using C8 root needle studies, F-wave, and cervical somatosensory evoked potentials, Arch Phys Med Rehabil 65:726, 1984.

66. Lukes, SA, et al: Nuclear magnetic imaging in multiple sclerosis, Ann Neurol 13:592, 1983.

67. Maccabee, P, Pinkhasov, EI, and Cracco, RQ: Short latency somatosensory evoked potentials to median nerve stimulation: effect of low frequency filter, Electroencephalogr Clin Neurophysiol 55:34, 1983.

68. Maccabee, PJ, et al: Short latency somatosensory and spinal evoked potentials: power spectra and comparison between high pass analog and digital filter, Electroencephalogr Clin Neurophysiol 65:177, 1986.

69. Noseworthy, JH, Paty, DW, and Ebers, GC: Neuroimaging in multiple sclerosis, Neurol. Clin. 2:759, 1984.

70. Pfurtscheller, G, Schwarz, G, and Gravenstein, N: Clinical relevance of long-latency SEPs and VEPs during coma and emergence from coma, Electroencephalogr Clin Neurophysiol 62:88, 1985.

71. Phillips, LH, II and Daube, JR: Lumbosacral spinal evoked potentials in humans, Neurology 30:1175, 1980.

72. Roberts, KB, Lawerence, PD, and Eisen, A: Dispersion of the somatosensory evoked potential (SEP) in multiple sclerosis, IEEE Trans Biomed Eng 30:360, 1983.

73. Rossini, P: Electrical stimulation for central motor tracts in man. In International symposium on new concepts in electromyography, Boston, Rochester, Minn, 1986, Custom Printing, Inc.

74. Rossini, PM, and Treviso, M: Central conduction velocity (lumbar-vertex) in man calculated by means of a new method, Eur Neurol 22:173, 1983.

75. Rossini, PM, et al: Transcutaneous stimulation of motor cerebral cortex and spine: noninvasive evaluation of central afferent transmission in normal subjects and patients with multiple sclerosis. In Cracco, RQ, and Bodis-Wollner, I, editors: Evoked potentials, New York, 1986, Alan R. Liss, Inc.

76. Scarff, TB, et al: Dermatomal somatosensory evoked potentials in the diagnosis of lumbar root entrapment, Surg Forum 32:489, 1981.

77. Schiff, JA, et al: Spine and scalp somatosensory evoked potentials in normal subjects and patients with spinal cord disease: evaluation of afferent transmission, Electroencephalogr Clin Electrophysiol 59:374, 1984.

78. Schramm, M: Clinical experience with objective localization of the lesion in myelopathy. In Grote, W, et al, editors: Advances in neurosurgery, vol 8, Berlin, 1980, Springer-Verlag.

79. Schramm, J, and Hashizame, K: Somatosensory evoked potentials (SEP) in patients with peripheral, spinal and supraspinal lesions of the sensory system. In Wullenburger, H, et al, editors: Advances in neurosurgery, vol 4, Berlin, 1977, Springer-Verlag.

80. Schramm, J, Oettle, GJ, and Pichert, T: Clinical application of segmental somatosensory evoked potentials (SEP)—experience in patients with non-space occupying lesions. In Barber, C, editor: Evoked potentials, Lancaster, Penn., 1980, MTP Press.

81. Seyal, M, Emerson, RG, and Pedley, TA: Spinal and early scalp-recorded components of the somatosensory evoked potential following stimulation of the posterior tibial nerve, Electroencephalogr Clin Neurophysiol 55:320, 1983.

82. Seyal, M, and Gabor, AJ: The human posterior tibial somatosensory evoked potential: synapse dependent and synapse independent spinal components, Electroencephalogr Clin Neurophysiol 62:323, 1985.

83. Sgro, JA, Emmerson, RG, and Pedley, TA: Real-time reconstruction of evoked potentials using a new two-dimensional filter method, Electroencephalogr Clin Neurophysiol 62:372, 1985.

84. Shimoji, K, Higashi, H, and Kano, T: Epidural recording of spinal electrogram in man, Electroencephalogr Clin Neurophysiol 30:236, 1971.

85. Shimoji, K, et al: Evoked spinal electrograms recorded from epidural space in man, J Appl Physiol 33:468, 1972.

86. Shimoji, K, et al: Evoked spinal electrogram in a quadriplegic patient, Electroencephalogr Clin Neurophysiol 35:659, 1973.

87. Siivola, J, Salg, I, and Heiskari, M: Somatosensory evoked potentials in diagnostics of cervical spondylosis and herniated disc, Electroencephalogr Clin Neurophysiol 52:276, 1981.

88. Small, M, and Matthews, WB: A method of calculating spinal cord transit time from potentials evoked by tibial nerve stimulation in normal subjects and in patients with spinal cord disease, Electroencephalogr Clin Neurophysiol 59:156, 1984.

89. Summner, A: Personal communication, 1987.

90. Swift, TR, and Nichols, T: The droopy shoulder syndrome, Neurology 34:212, 1984.

91. Synek, VM: Somatosensory evoked potentials from musculocutaneous nerve in the diagnosis of brachial plexus injuries, J Neurol Sci 61:443, 1983.

92. Synek, VM, and Cowan, JC: Somatosensory evoked potentials in patients with supraclavicular brachial plexus injuries, Neurology 32:1347, 1982.

93. Thomas, PK: Selective vulnerability of the centrifugal and centripetal axons of primary sensory neurons, Muscle Nerve 5:s117, 1982.

94. Tsuji, S, et al: Subcortical and cortical somatosensory potentials evoked by posterior tibial nerve stimulation: normative values, Electroencephalogr Clin Neurophysiol 59:214, 1984.

95. Yamada, T, Machida, M, and Kimura, J: Far field somatosensory evoked potentials after stimulation of the tibial nerve, Neurology 32:1151, 1982.

96. Yiannikis, C, and Walsh, JC: Somatosensory evoked responses in the diagnosis of thoracic outlet syndrome, J Neurol Neurosurg Psychiatry 46:234, 1983.

CHAPTER 3

Needle electromyography and nerve conduction study in clinical electrodiagnosis

DONG M. MA

Electrodiagnostic studies are an established multifaceted tool to study skeletal muscles, the nervous system, and neuromuscular transmission in normal and pathologic conditions. Knowledge of the physiologic characteristics of normal neuromuscular systems is a prerequisite for understanding the electrophysiologic abnormalities found in various disorders. In addition, the electromyographer must be thoroughly familiar with the electromyograph (EMG) and the electronics that may affect data and observations.

Before an electrodiagnostic examination the procedure should be carefully explained so the patient feels comfortable and cooperative. Nerve conduction studies using a magnetic beam for stimulation significantly reduce the patient's discomfort, but the method is still under development and investigation. A thorough medical history and physical examination are essential to the electromyographer in determining the best procedure for localizing the patient's problem. The performance of EMG examination requires adequate training and experience. There are considerable pitfalls for the novice.

Electromyographers may have difficulty differentiating between neuropathy and myopathy. For example, positive sharp waves, commonly encountered along with fibrillation potentials in denervated muscles, occur in a variety of acquired or hereditary myopathies, in motor neuron diseases, and at certain stages following upper motor neuron lesions such as stroke or spinal cord injury.[4,17,39] Positive sharp waves and fibrillation potentials can also be seen in disorders of neuromuscular transmission.[35]

Electromyographers must also be aware that certain single motor unit potentials resemble positive sharp waves and that, when end-plate spike potentials are picked up by an electrode outside the end-plate zone, they are indistinguishable from fibrillation potentials.[51]

Certain muscles such as facial, tongue, and anal sphincter normally have low-amplitude, short-duration motor unit potentials that may be erroneously interpreted as evidence of myopathic disease. In addition, motor unit potentials in an early stage of reinnervation are similar to the motor unit potentials seen in myopathy. In advanced myopathy, motor recruitment decreases.

Quantitative EMG may help in detection of mild axonal neuropathy or myopathy.

In this chapter electrophysiologic findings in various neuropathies, myopathies, and disorders of neuromuscular transmission are discussed. Information concerning instrumentation and technique of nerve conduction studies should be obtained from other sources, such as references 18, 25, and 28.

NEUROPATHY

Peripheral neuropathy can be divided into several categories depending on clinical pattern, histologic and electrophysiologic characteristics, or the anatomic involvement of the peripheral nervous system. It can also be divided simply into focal or generalized, and acquired or hereditary, neuropathy.

In this section several different neuropathies caused by axonal degeneration, segmental demyelination, and focal neuropathy including radiculopathy and a common compression neuropathy are discussed from the viewpoint of characteristic electrophysiologic observations.

Axonal degeneration

Axonal degeneration occurs not only from mechanical transection of the nerves, but also from death of perikarya as in motor neuron disease, from focal or systemic exposure to toxic substances, and from ischemic or cold injury.

Generally in this disorder motor and sensory conduction velocities are normal or close to normal in value because the myelin sheaths of the remaining nerves are not affected.

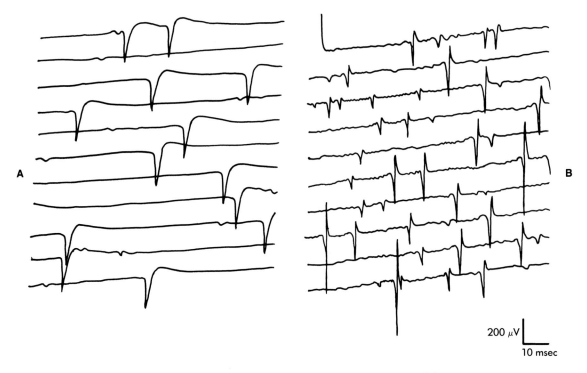

200 μV

10 msec

Figure 3-1. A, Positive sharp waves. **B,** Fibrillation potentials.

In severe cases, however, the velocities may be reduced to about 60% to 70% of average normal value owing to the loss of the fastest conducting fibers. Furthermore, because of loss of nerve fibers, compound muscle potentials and sensory nerve action potentials may be reduced in amplitude.

Motor neuron disease

Motor neuron disease is a group of disorders characterized by degeneration of lower motor neurons with or without upper motor neuron involvement. Included are such disorders as amyotrophic lateral sclerosis, spinal muscular atrophy, poliomyelitis, and syringomyelia.

EMG is an excellent tool to demonstrate involvement of the lower motor neuron, especially when this is subclinical or dominated by upper motor neuron disease. The EMG hallmark of these disorders is abnormal spontaneous activity: positive sharp waves and fibrillation potentials (Figure 3-1), decrease in number of motor units, and decrease in motor unit recruitment under voluntary control (Figure 3-2). However, in chronic stages motor unit potentials become polyphasic (Figure 3-3) and increase in amplitude and duration. Polyphasic motor unit potential changes in axonal neuropathy are due to the phenomenon of collateral sprouting. The increased duration of motor unit potentials reflects greater variability in length and conduction time along the sprouting terminal axons. The increased amplitude of the motor unit potential is due to the enlarged territory and increased fiber density.

The potentials of the individual motor units under voluntary control sometimes exhibit a variation in amplitude that indicates a failure of neuromuscular transmission in some of the synapses of the unit. This has been attributed to the presence of immature synapses associated with reinnervating axonal sprouts. It is also possible that variation of amplitudes is the expression of a dying motor neuron unable to maintain normal synaptic function. This defect of neuromuscular transmission can often be demonstrated by repetitive stimulation studies at rates of 2 or 3 per second. The abnormality is found more frequently in atrophied muscles.

In juvenile spinal muscular atrophy, EMG shows fibrillation potentials and positive sharp waves in one third of the patients, but most patients with infantile spinal muscular atrophy, amyotrophic lateral sclerosis, and poliomyelitis have abnormal spontaneous activity.[19] In syringomyelia, EMG abnormalities are commonly observed in only the atrophied muscles.

In poliomyelitis, positive sharp waves and fibrillation potentials subside as reinnervation by surviving motor neurons proceeds during recovery. However, in severely atrophied muscle the abnormal spontaneous activities can persist indefinitely and become extremely small (Figure 3-4).[12]

EMG in late progression of poliomyelitis may show large positive sharp waves and fibrillation potentials of recently denervated, hypertrophic muscle fibers in addition to the usual findings of old poliomyelitis. The pathophysiology of the later progression of old poliomyelitis is unclear but may be due to the failure of the sprouting axons that formed during initial recovery.[11]

In amyotrophic lateral sclerosis, fasciculations are more commonly observed than in other motor neuron diseases

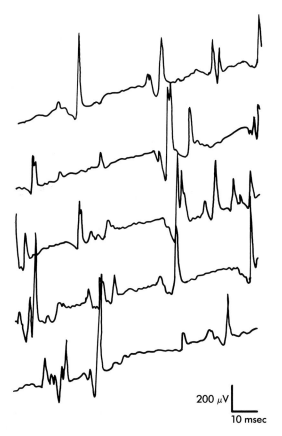

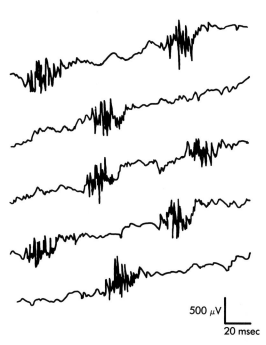

Figure 3-2. Discrete recruitment pattern. Reduced number of motor units firing under maximal volitional effort.

Figure 3-3. Long-duration polyphasic motor unit potentials in patient with chronic axonal neuropathy during reinnervation.

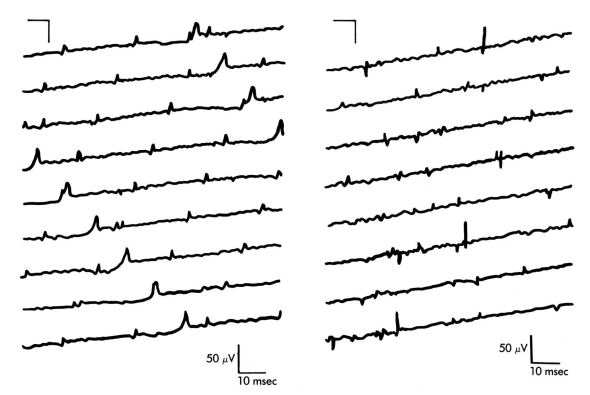

Figure 3-4. Small-amplitude positive sharp waves and fibrillation potentials in fibrotic muscles in "old" poliomyelitis.

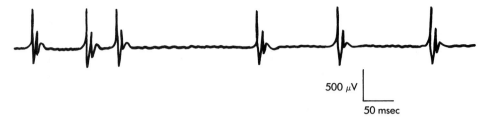

500 μV

50 msec

Figure 3-5. Fasciculation potentials recorded from patient with amyotrophic lateral sclerosis.

(Figure 3-5). Fasciculations are involuntary twitches of a bundle of muscle fibers[3] and can often be seen on the skin surface. The patients are often unaware of them. Fasciculation potentials are the electrical manifestation of this phenomenon. They are irregular in rate and rhythm, and their firing rate varies from 1 to 50 per minute. The shape of fasciculation potentials may be simple, diphasic, triphasic, or complex polyphasic waveforms. However, fasciculations by themselves are frequently seen in normal, healthy persons, particularly in calf muscles and small muscles of the hands and feet. These benign fasciculations are not identified with any neurologic abnormality. Some investigators have concluded that the fasciculations encountered in anterior horn cell diseases, nerve root lesions, and thyrotoxicosis are more polyphasic in shape and slower in rate, but this observation is not universally accepted. Fasciculation potentials originate in both the peripheral and the central portions of the motor neuron.[50]

Nerve conduction studies are important in motor neuron diseases to exclude other etiologies. In the former, motor and sensory nerve conduction velocities are generally within normal ranges. However, with compound muscle action potentials of low amplitude (usually less than 1 mV) motor conduction velocities may be moderately reduced.

Despite clinical sensory loss in syringomyelia, sensory nerve conductions and potentials are normal because the lesion is located proximal to the sensory ganglion.

Generalized peripheral axonal polyneuropathy

Neuropathy secondary to chronic alcoholism, uremia, overdosage of vincristine, carcinoma, thiamine deficiency, certain heavy metal poisoning, or intermittent porphyria belongs to the category of generalized axonal peripheral polyneuropathy.

In this neuropathy and motor neuron diseases, axonal degeneration initially occurs in the most distal segment of the longest peripheral nerve fibers and progresses centripetally. This is due to the "dying back" phenomenon.

Motor and sensory fibers are generally symmetrically attacked, and the distal muscles are initially involved. Nerve conduction is usually not affected in mild cases. In severe cases the amplitudes of compound muscle potentials are reduced because of loss of axons. EMG abnormalities are similar to those in motor neuron disease.

Segmental demyelination

Segmental demyelination is commonly seen in the Guillain-Barré syndrome, Charcot-Marie-Tooth disease, chronic relapsing polyneuropathy, certain cases of diabetic neuropathy, and heavy metal or diphtheric poisoning.

In demyelinating neuropathy, nerve conduction velocity is commonly reduced, although not always to more than 30% to 40% of average normal value. In addition, the responses are usually temporally dispersed and reduced in amplitude. EMG findings are normal unless axonal degeneration occurs secondarily.

Guillain-Barré syndrome

Guillain-Barré syndrome is a nonfamilial inflammatory demyelinating disease of peripheral nerves. Electrodiagnostic findings are variable depending on time after onset or severity and pattern of involvement of the peripheral nerves.

Segmental demyelination in Guillain-Barré syndrome can occur in the proximal or distal portion of the nerve, or there may be diffuse demyelination of the entire peripheral nerve. Since routine motor conduction studies cannot detect conduction defects in cases of proximal involvement, F-wave studies should be performed to unmask the proximate dysfunction (see Chapter 4).

In early stages of Guillain-Barré syndrome, only temporal dispersion of a compound muscle potential may be seen without slowing of motor conduction velocity or prolonged distal latencies.

Sensory nerve action potentials may be normal but have been reported as abnormal by some investigations.[16,31] Interestingly, sensory nerve action potentials may be abnormal or absent in median and ulnar nerves but normal in sural nerves. This may be due to particular susceptibilities at entrapment points. Nerve conduction abnormalities not initially present may appear subsequently, even during the clinical recovery phase.

In Guillain-Barré syndrome, two groups of patients are identified in view of electrophysiologic findings. One is characterized by gross abnormalities of conduction velocity without evidence of denervation on needle EMG. The other is characterized by evidence of extensive denervation with or without abnormalities of the nerve conduction velocities.[36] The patients in the latter group have limited recovery with pronounced residual deficits.

Charcot-Marie-Tooth disease

Charcot-Marie-Tooth disease is the common form of inherited neuropathy. The most prevalent type is the hypertrophic, which is usually inherited as an autosomal dominant trait with fairly marked penetrance but may also occur sporadically. It is characterized by enlargement of the peripheral nerve secondary to recurrent segmental demyelination and remyelination.

EMG and nerve biopsy are the most useful studies for the diagnosis of this illness. Motor conduction velocities are markedly reduced, and the distal latency is also prolonged, even in the early stages.

Sensory fibers are also affected, and sensory potentials, if recordable, are decreased in amplitude and prolonged in latency. Despite marked slowing, recorded potentials show minimal or no increase in temporal dispersion, indicating that nerve fibers of different calibers are equally affected. Needle EMG findings are normal except that motor unit recruitment may be decreased.

Other forms of Charcot-Marie-Tooth disease show a completely different EMG picture. The second form of Charcot-Marie-Tooth disease, the neuronal variety, is also inherited with an autosomal dominant pattern. It differs from the hypertrophic type in that nerve enlargement and segmental demyelination are not present but neuronal changes are prominent. Thus the nerve conductions are only slightly slowed whereas the amplitudes of the compound muscles and nerve action potentials are often reduced. EMG typically shows evidence of axonal degeneration.

The third type of Charcot-Marie-Tooth disease has been designated as a form of spinal muscle atrophy. Its clinical features resembles those of Charcot-Marie-Tooth disease, but nerve enlargement is not present and sensation is normal.

Compression neuropathy

Compression (entrapment) neuropathy represents a localized injury of a peripheral nerve caused by constant mechanical irritation from an impinging anatomic structure and less commonly by tumor, vascular aneurysm, hematoma, fracture, or another factor.

The peripheral nerves are generally buried deep within a muscle mass and protected from the trauma, but there are vulnerable sites, such as the radial nerve in the spiral groove of the humerus, ulnar nerve at the ulnar groove, and peroneal nerve at the head of the fibula.

Seddan[37] classified three grades of nerve injury—neuropraxia, axonotmesis, and neurotmesis—in terms of the different types of localized lesions.[37] In another classification, Sunderland[42] named five categories in which neurotmesis is divided into three, depending on the damage of the connective tissue sheath of the nerve.

Neuropraxia is a transient nerve conduction block without loss of continuity of the axon and without signs of denervation. Axonotmesis is characterized by a loss of continuity of axons but connective tissue and Schwann cell basement membrane that remain intact. Neurotmesis is damage to the axon and connective tissue or complete transection of the nerve.

In axonotmesis and neurotmesis, wallerian degeneration occurs distal to the injury. Recovery takes place by axonal regeneration and requires a few weeks to several months for complete return of function. When the nerve is transected, the best plan may be to suture it or to insert a graft to bridge the gap.

After transection of the nerve, no obvious morphologic changes in the distal segment are seen for 36 to 48 hours. Within this time axons continue to conduct and velocities remain near normal. As time passes, however, the evoked potentials decreased in amplitude until conduction fails finally. This usually occurs in about 7 to 9 days. Fibrillation potentials and positive sharp waves may not appear in denervated muscles for approximately the first 10 to 21 days. Thus certain EMG abnormalities do not appear for some time.

Within a few days after transection, sprouts of regenerative fibers appear at the proximal stump of the nerve. The sprouting fibers grow an average of 1 to 2 mm per day, but growth varies depending on the nerve involved and whether the site is proximal or distal. The regenerating fibers are unmyelinated and small in diameter. Maturation of the fibers subsequently takes place with a gradual return toward normal axon diameter and myelin thickness.

During the early phases of regeneration, electrical stimulation proximal to, at, or distal to the nerve damage produces no muscle response, although needle EMG may reveal a few voluntary motor unit potentials. These potentials are frequently of low amplitude and polyphasic, which can mislead the unwary into suggesting a myopathy (Figure 3-6).[2]

In partial denervation, nerve conduction velocities may be normal or near normal while the amplitude of the evoked potentials may be decreased.

Wallerian degeneration occurs in many neuromuscular diseases such as compression or radiation neuropathy, neuropathy resulting from burn, and ischemic neuropathy.

Neuropraxia commonly occurs in radial nerve palsy owing to injury in the spiral groove of the humerus. Saturday night palsy and tourniquet nerve palsy are examples of this. In classic neuropraxic neuropathy, EMG shows no abnormal spontaneous activity or decrease in motor unit recruitment. Nerve conduction studies show conduction defects of the motor or sensory nerve fibers across localized site of the lesion. Nerve conduction above and below the lesion is normal. The configuration of the compound muscle action potentials is commonly temporally dispersed and the amplitude of the evoked potentials is decreased when the nerve is stimulated above the lesion. If the compression is severe enough to cause degeneration of axons, EMG shows evidence of denervation of the muscles innervated by the nerve below the lesion. For example, in Saturday night palsy the distal muscles innervated by the radial nerves may be de-

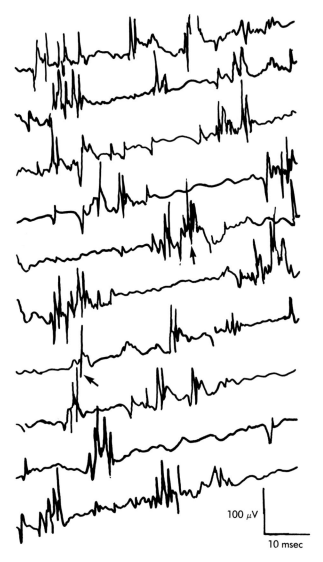

100 µV

10 msec

Figure 3-6. Low-amplitude, short-duration motor unit potentials and polyphasic motor unit potentials in patient in early stage of reinnervation.

nervated but the triceps brachii and anconeus muscles are usually normal, since their branches take origin proximally. Motor conduction velocity may be slightly decreased because of axonal degeneration.

Carpal tunnel syndrome

Carpal tunnel syndrome is the most common entrapment neuropathy and has been the subject of extensive electrophysiologic studies. Conduction abnormalities are often selectively localized in the carpal tunnel. The remaining distal nerve segment may show only mild or no abnormalities of sensory and motor conduction. To increase accuracy of diagnosis of carpal tunnel syndrome when clinical symptoms are minimal, palmar stimulation or inching technique should be used.[5,24]

In mild cases of carpal tunnel syndrome, only the sensory nerve conductions are abnormal. The distal sensory latency

is slightly prolonged, and the evoked potential amplitude is decreased with temporal dispersion. In most cases of carpal tunnel syndrome, distal motor and sensory latencies are prolonged without evidence of denervation of the median innervated muscles of the hand, but in more advanced cases EMG abnormalities are observed. In some instances, sensory nerve conduction is normal but the distal motor latency is prolonged. This may be due to separation of the carpal tunnel by a septum so that only the motor fibers are compressed.[23]

In our own study,[27] about 10% of patients with carpal tunnel syndrome showed conduction defects proximal to the wrist, especially when the distal motor latency was markedly prolonged.[44,45] This may be due to retrograde degeneration of median nerve motor fibers. About 40% of patients with carpal tunnel syndrome patients showed concurrent ipsilateral cervical radiculopathy (Table 3-1). The incidence of concurrent cervical radiculopathy was slightly higher in males (male/female 44.7%:36.6%) and was found to increase with age regardless of sex. Most (88%) of the carpal tunnel syndrome patients with radiculopathy showed EMG abnormalities in paravertebral muscles only. However, concurrent cervical radiculopathy was not observed in any patients with carpal tunnel syndrome below 30 years of age.

In 1973, Upton and McComas[47] postulated the hypothesis of the double crush syndrome in which axons, having been compressed in one region, become especially susceptible to damage at another distal site. In their study 70% of the patients with electrophysiologically proven entrapment neuropathy showed evidence of a cervical root lesion, which included x-ray findings of the cervical spine, clinical symptoms, results of sensory examination, and past history of neck injury.

The data derived from studies in our laboratory do not agree with the double crush hypothesis for the following reasons. First, EMG abnormalities were restricted to paravertebral muscles that are innervated by the posterior rami of the cervical roots. The median nerve fibers compressed in carpal tunnel syndrome arise from the anterior rami of the roots. Only 12% of the anterior rami were involved in concurrent carpal tunnel syndrome and radiculopathy cases. Second, in cases of motor and sensory fiber involvement of carpal tunnel syndrome, several cervical roots should be involved because the median nerve represents C6-T1 root distribution.

Therefore we conclude that cervical radiculopathy in carpal tunnel syndrome patients is a coincidental finding. Increased incidence of cervical radiculopathy may be due to degenerative change in the cervical spine, which is increased with age and more common in men. It follows that not all proximal pain in patients with carpal tunnel syndrome can be attributed to referral from the wrist; some may be due to cervical radiopathy. Thus performing EMG, especially on paravertebral muscles, is worthwhile to rule out concurrent cervical radiculopathy, since the treatment plan may be quite different.

Table 3-1. Incidence of ipsilateral cervical radiculopathy in patients with carpal tunnel syndrome according to age and sex

Age	Male		Female		Total	
	No. (CR/CTS)*	% (CR/CTS)	No. (CR/CTS)	% (CR/CTS)	No. (CR/CTS)	% (CR/CTS)
11-20	0/0	0	0/1	0	0/1	0
21-30	0/7	0	0/10	0	0/17	0
31-40	10/32	31.3	9/45	20.0	19/77	24.7
41-50	20/56	35.7	33/107	30.8	53/163	35.5
51-60	41/94	43.6	56/192	29.0	97/286	33.9
61-70	42/71	59.2	50/99	50.5	103/193	53.4
71-80	10/21	47.6	36/68	57.4	49/89	55.1
81-90	8/12	66.7	8/11	72.7	16/23	69.6
TOTAL	131/293	44.7	195/533	36.6	326/826	39.5

*CR, Cervical radiculopathy; CTS, carpal tunnel syndrome.

Pronator syndrome

The median nerve may be compressed as the nerve passes through the two heads of the pronator teres muscle or under the flexor digitorum sublimus bridge. This compression neuropathy is termed pronator syndrome.[32]

Nerve conduction velocities of the motor and sensory fibers across the lesion are usually slow, but the distal motor and sensory latencies are normal. In severe cases all median innervated muscles except the pronator teres may have signs of denervation. Occasionally the flexor carpi radialis is spared.

Anterior interosseous nerve syndrome

The median nerve gives rise to the anterior interosseous nerve just distal to its passage through the pronator teres muscle. The anterior interosseous nerve is a pure motor nerve and supplies the flexor pollicis longus, the radial portion of the flexor digitorum profundus, and the pronator quadratus. The most common symptoms are pain in the proximal forearm with distinct clinical sensory symptoms and inability to flex the distal phalanx of the thumb, index, and long fingers, such as an inability to hold a pencil or make a circle.[40]

EMG shows signs of denervation of the muscles innervated by the anterior interosseous nerve. Routine nerve conduction studies of the median motor and sensory fibers are normal, but motor latencies are prolonged when recorded from the involved muscles and stimulated above the lesion.[10]

Tardy ulnar neuropathy and cubital tunnel syndrome

The ulnar nerve is commonly injured at the elbow because of repeated trauma or fracture of the elbow. Segmental nerve conduction studies show decreased motor and sensory conduction velocities across the elbow. For accurate measurement of the velocities, the arm must be held in the same position during each study. The elbow should be flexed at 70 degrees, and the distance between stimulation sites above

and below the elbow should be more than 10 cm.[8,15,28] Sensory nerve action potentials of the main sensory branch and the dorsal cutaneous branch are decreased in amplitude.

In moderate or severe cases, EMG may show signs of denervation of all ulnar innervated muscles. In many cases, however, only the intrinsic hand muscles are denervated, since at the elbow the motor fibers innervating the intrinsic hand muscles are superficial to (and thus more vulnerable than) the motor fibers innervating the flexor carpi ulnaris and the flexor digitorum profundus.[43]

Ulnar neuropathy at Guyon's canal

Just before the ulnar nerve passes through Guyon's canal, the nerve divides into a deep muscular branch and a superficial cutaneous branch. Guyon's canal is bounded by the pisiform bone medially and the hook of the hamate laterally and is covered by the volar carpal ligament and the palmaris brevis muscle.

Entrapment of the ulnar nerve in Guyon's canal can be caused by pressure from a ganglion, repeated trauma in certain occupations, or rheumatoid arthritis.[38]

Electrophysiologic findings may be similar to those in carpal tunnel syndrome. The sensory nerve action potential of the dorsal cutaneous branch is normal because it arises about 5 cm above the wrist and does not pass through Guyon's canal.[21]

After the deep muscular branch supplies the hypothenar muscles, it may be damaged. In this situation EMG may show signs of denervation of the ulnar innervated intrinsic muscles of the hand except for the three hypothenar muscles. The motor conduction time of the deep branch to the first dorsal interosseous muscle may be prolonged.

Posterior interosseous syndrome

The radial nerve divides into a posterior interosseous branch and a superficial radial branch at the level of the lateral epicondyle. The posterior interosseous nerve usually innervates the extensor carpi radialis brevis and supinator muscles before it penetrates the latter. Radial nerve injury commonly results from trauma, fracture, tumor, or vascular anomaly at the arcade of Froshe between the two heads of the supinator.

When the posterior interosseous nerve is compressed before the nerve enters the supinator muscle. The condition is referred to as a posterior interosseous syndrome. When the nerve is compressed in the supinator muscle, supinator syndrome results.[7]

In the posterior interosseous syndrome all muscles supplied by the posterior interosseous nerve may be denervated, but in the supinator syndrome the extensor carpi radialis brevis and supinator muscles are spared. Motor conduction time of the posterior interosseous nerve to the affected muscles may be prolonged when the radial nerve is stimulated at the elbow. The compound muscle action potential is usually recorded from the extensor indicis proprius muscle because it is the last muscle innervated by the posterior interosseous nerve.

Sciatic neuropathy

The sciatic nerve may be injured in the pelvis and at the sciatic notch by a space-occupying tumor, abscess of the pelvic floor, fracture of the pelvis, iatrogenic complications of surgery, or compression by the piriformis muscle.

In traumatic sciatic neuropathy the peroneal portion of the sciatic nerve is generally much more damaged than the tibial portion. A common cause of damage is misplaced intramuscular injections in the buttocks.[22,43]

If the entire sciatic nerve is involved, regardless of etiology, EMG shows signs of denervation of the sciatic innervated muscles. In a partial lesion of the sciatic nerve the tibial and peroneal motor conduction velocities and sensory conduction velocity of the sural nerve may be normal or near normal with decreased amplitudes of the evoked potentials. F-wave latencies may be prolonged.

Peroneal neuropathy

The common peroneal nerve divides into the superficial, deep, and recurrent branches at the head of the fibula, where the nerve is most susceptible to compression. Compression is usually caused by direct trauma, leg-crossing, a tight cast, a ganglion, or a cyst. The deep branch is more frequently and severely affected by compression at this level.

EMG shows signs of denervation depending on which branch is affected. When only the deep branch is damaged, the peroneus longus and brevis are spared because they are innervated by the superficial branch. In some cases EMG examination of the tibialis posterior is useful to differentiate peroneal palsy from L5 radiculopathy because this muscle receives L5 root innervation through the tibial nerve.[20]

In compression (such as caused by crossed legs), motor conduction velocity of the nerve is slow across the head of the fibula and may be normal or near normal in the distal segment with decreased amplitude of the compound action potentials. If the extensor digitorum brevis muscle is severely atrophied, the response in the tibialis anterior can be studied to demonstrate the motor conduction defect across the head of the fibula. Although selective involvement of the superficial branch is rare, abnormal compound action potentials may be recorded from the peroneus longus muscle. Sensory nerve action potential of the superficial branch decreases in amplitude, but the distal latency is normal or near normal.

Tarsal tunnel syndrome

The tibial nerve may be compressed in the popliteal fossa by a cyst or arterial aneurysm, but more commonly the nerve is compressed within the tarsal tunnel by a fracture, a cyst, or tenosynovitis. The tarsal tunnel is posterior and inferior to the medial malleolus and is covered by the flexor retinaculum muscle. The tibial nerve divides into the medial and lateral plantar and calcaneal branches within the tunnel. The medial and lateral plantar nerves are mixed nerves.

In tarsal tunnel syndrome the medial or lateral plantar nerve or both may be damaged. EMG may show signs of denervation of the affected muscles. However, nerve conduction studies are more important in documenting the tarsal tunnel syndrome. Motor latencies of the medial or lateral plantar nerves increase with stimulation of the tibial nerve slightly above the medial malleolus.

In many cases it is difficult to demonstrate electrophysiologic evidence of nerve compression in the tunnel, especially when mainly the sensory fibers are compressed, because of technical difficulty in performing sensory nerve conduction studies of the medial and lateral plantar nerves.

Orthodromic sensory conduction studies show increased latencies of the medial or lateral plantar nerves with stimulation of the great toe or fifth toe, respectively, and recording from the tibial nerve at the ankle where it is usually stimulated in motor conduction studies.[33] For recording of the optimal sensory evoked potential, averaging is required in many cases.

Lateral femoral cutaneous neuropathy (meralgia paresthetica)

The lateral femoral cutaneous nerve is a pure sensory nerve that arises from the ventral rami of the second and third lumbar nerves. The nerve passes behind or through the inguinal ligament about 1 cm medial to the anterior superior iliac spine. It then passes in front of or through the sartorius muscle into the thigh, where it is commonly compressed.

Sensory nerve conduction study may show slow velocity across the compression site. However, this test is technically difficult. The evoked potential may be difficult to record because it is often obscured by the shock artifact and a motor response from the quadriceps muscles. In addition, determining the stimulation site is difficult, especially in a heavy person.[28] Because of the technical difficulties, no conclusions should be drawn if no evoked potential can be elicited. In this situation somatosensory evoked potential study may be helpful to demonstrate sensory conduction defect across the compression site.

EMG of the muscles innervated by L2-3 roots, including the lumbar paravertebral muscles, is useful to differentiate meralgia paresthetica from other neuropathy affecting mainly L2-3 roots.

Brachial plexus lesions

The brachial plexus is usually damaged by trauma, chronic compression, radiation therapy, or nontraumatic conditions.

Traumatic conditions affecting the brachial plexus most frequently are due to bullet wound and stretch injuries as occur in motorcycle accidents, birth injury, or fracture of the clavicle or during surgery in an unusual posture. Chronic compressive lesions of the brachial plexus include thoracic outlet syndrome and primary or metastatic nerve tumors. Nontraumatic brachial plexopathy is usually idiopathic.

In idiopathic brachial plexopathy the clinical picture is variable, but the disease commonly begins with severe pain in the shoulder and mild sensory impairment. Usually in a few days the pain subsides and the shoulder girdle muscles become weak and atrophied. The muscle weakness may be limited to the distribution of a single root, trunk, or cord of the brachial plexus or a peripheral nerve. The C5-C6 myotomes are most commonly involved, but occasionally the spinal accessory nerve is also affected.

In brachial plexus lesions, regardless of the cause, EMG is more informative than nerve conduction studies in delineating the degree and distribution. However, nerve conduction studies show decreased amplitude of motor and sensory nerve action potentials when the response to stimulation is recorded from the affected muscle and nerve. Frequently motor and sensory conductions are normal, even though stimulation of the nerves is carried out at the supraclavicular fossa. F-wave study may not be helpful except in some cases of thoracic outlet syndrome. In most thoracic outlet syndromes, vascular components but not nerves are generally compressed, so the F-wave latency and EMG findings are normal. However, if the lower trunk of the brachial plexus is compressed in the thoracic outlet syndrome, the F-wave latency is prolonged when the responses are recorded from the abductor digiti quinti or abductor pollicis brevis. The amplitude of the sensory nerve action potentials of the ulnar nerve may be reduced. Stimulation of the lower trunk of the brachial plexus may not be helpful for two reasons: Obtaining the response is painful and sometimes difficult, especially in a heavy or short-necked person. In addition, the site of the stimulation may be at or slightly distal to the compressed region. C8 root stimulation, however, may help to diagnosis thoracic outlet syndrome.[30]

In most brachial plexus lesions, EMG shows abnormal spontaneous activity and large, long-duration polyphasic motor unit potentials in the affected muscles. In brachial plexus lesions resulting from radiation therapy, myokymic discharges are commonly seen.[1] Myokymia is a special type of fasciculation, described as undulating, wormlike movements of muscles. It occurs spontaneously, recurs irregularly or regularly, is usually visible through the skin, and is thought to be caused by ephaptic activation of neighboring axons at a site of nerve injury.

Radiculopathy (nerve root lesion)

Nerve roots are commonly affected by mechanical compressions such as herniated disc, spondylosis, and trauma. However, they are also seen in diabetic polyradiculoneuropathy, metastatic carcinoma, infection such as abscess and herpes zoster, and other conditions.

Diagnosis of nerve root lesion is based on clinical examination and electrophysiologic studies that help delineate the distribution.

In nerve root lesions, distal motor and sensory conduction studies are generally normal, but in severe nerve root compression, significant axonal degeneration may occur and the amplitude of evoked potentials may be notably reduced. If F-wave studies are performed, the latency may be prolonged. However, practically all extremity muscles are innervated by two or more levels of root, so when only one root is involved, the F-wave latency may not be prolonged because the noninvolved roots conduct normally.

Sometimes sensory symptoms point to the presence of nerve root lesions but no weakness of muscles is noted and EMG findings are normal. In these cases, dermatomal somatosensory evoked potentials may be helpful to diagnose root compression. Because the sensory component encircles the motor component in the nerve root, only the sensory fibers may be compressed (Figure 3-7).[6]

Needle EMG is more important to correlate clinical localization of nerve root lesions. In classic cases, EMG of affected extremity muscles and paraspinal muscles shows abnormal spontaneous activity, reduced motor recruitment, and changes in motor unit potentials.

In radiculopathy, abnormal spontaneous activity includes not only fibrillation potentials and positive sharp waves, but also complex repetitive discharges. The last are commonly observed in paravertebral muscles and are also known as bizarre high-frequency discharges (Figure 3-8). They represent a phenomenon usually recorded in chronically denervated muscles, as well as in various myopathies, and are considered nonspecific evidence of dysfunction. They discharge repetitively at slow and fast rates, usually ranging from 5 to 150 impulses per second, and originate and terminate abruptly. The waveform is typically polyphasic and complex. They are triggered by movement of recording electrodes and are not abolished by nerve block or curare. Complex repetitive discharges are probably caused by

SUPERIOR

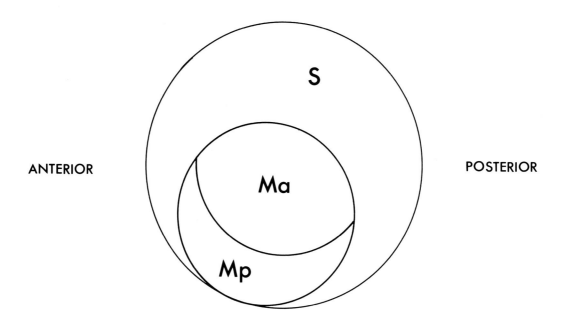

ANTERIOR   POSTERIOR

INFERIOR

Figure 3-7. Cross section of nerve root. *S*, Sensory fiber; *Ma*, anterior ramus of motor fiber; *Mp*, posterior ramus of motor fiber.

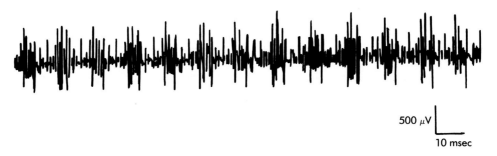

500 μV

10 msec

Figure 3-8. Complex repetitive discharges.

ephaptic transmission between muscle fibers, with one fiber acting as a pacemaker for neighboring muscle fibers.[6]

In many radiculopathies, especially in mild or early stages, EMG abnormalities may be found in only the paravertebral muscles. The relatively superficial layer of paravertebral muscles is innervated by nerve roots from multiple levels. Deeper paravertebral muscle innervation (for example, small rotators muscles) is more specifically related to a single nerve root. Therefore, with EMG abnormalities in paravertebral muscles, the level of nerve root compression cannot be easily judged, especially in the absence of peripheral muscle involvement.

An explanation for a radicular EMG abnormality found only in paravertebral muscles may be that posterior ramus fibers have a topographic location in the spinal root or intrinsic properties that make them more vulnerable to compression than anterior ramus fibers. It may be reasonable to hypothesize that the posterior ramus fibers are located peripheral to the anterior ramus fibers (Figure 3-7).

In traumatic root avulsions or cauda equina lesions resulting from mass lesions or other causes, distal sensory nerve conduction remains normal despite a complete loss of sensation because the lesions are proximal to the dorsal root ganglion.[46]

Dermatomal somatosensory evoked potentials help to localize the roots that are avulsed and to indicate whether the lesions are complete or incomplete. EMG also shows evidence of complete or partial denervation of the affected muscles depending on the severity of the root avulsion. In addition, myelography usually delineates the extent of root injury.

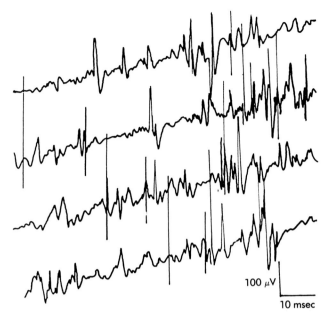

Figure 3-9. Low-amplitude, short-duration motor unit potentials and polyphasic motor unit potentials in patient with Duchenne muscular dystrophy.

MYOPATHY

Myopathies are primary muscle diseases that can be divided into hereditary and acquired categories. Hereditary myopathies include muscular dystrophy, myotonic disorders, congenital myopathy (nemaline and central core disease), and metabolic myopathy (for example, McArdle's disease and acid maltase deficiency). Among acquired myopathies are myositis, endocrine myopathy, myopathy resulting from collagen disease, and alcoholic myopathy.

EMG abnormalities in motor unit potentials are most valuable in differentiating myopathy from neuropathy. EMG shows changes in motor unit potential characteristics, especially in the proximal muscles. The motor unit potentials are generally reduced in amplitude and duration and become polyphasic (Figure 3-9). The total duration of polyphasic motor unit potentials usually does not exceed that of a normal motor unit potential, and the spikes of components of polyphasic motor unit potentials are all sharp. However, in Duchenne muscular dystrophy and polymyositis, large-amplitude motor unit potentials and long-duration polyphasic motor unit potentials may be seen.

The motor recruitment pattern may help distinguish myo-

pathic diseases from neuropathic diseases. Recruitment in myopathy is generally full at moderate muscle contraction, but in advanced myopathy the recruitment pattern may be decreased.

In addition, abnormal spontaneous activity including fibrillation potentials, positive sharp waves, and complex repetitive discharges may be observed, especially in polymyositis and Duchenne muscular dystrophy. The detailed findings are included in the discussion of individual entities.

Motor nerve conduction velocities are generally normal, but amplitude of compound muscle action potential may be decreased when recording from a proximal muscle. Sensory nerve conduction is normal.

Hereditary myopathy

Common types of muscular dystrophy including myotonia are discussed in this section. Duchenne muscular dystrophy is a sex-linked recessive disease that reveals not only characteristic features of myopathic motor unit potentials, but also neuropathic motor unit potentials of large amplitude. In addition, late components of motor unit potentials may be commonly observed in the distal muscles.[26,49] These late components are small potentials adjoining the main component of the motor unit potential by a constant interval (Figure 3-10). The late component may be due to various factors of desynchronization of motor unit potentials or collateral sprouting to segmental necrotized muscles.[9,13]

In Duchenne muscular dystrophy, fibrillation potentials and positive sharp waves are more commonly seen than in

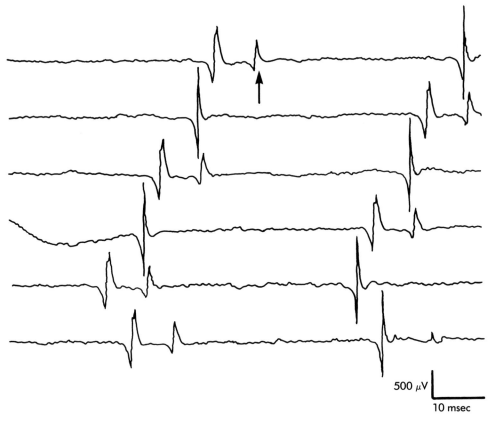

500 μV
10 msec

Figure 3-10. Late component of motor unit potential. Late portion of potential is marked by arrow. It follows main configuration.

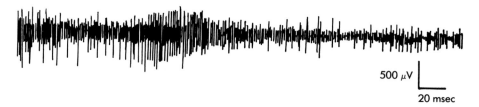

500 μV
20 msec

Figure 3-11. Myotonic discharge.

other muscular dystrophies but to a much lesser extent than in myositis. Repetitive complex discharges may also be observed. The abnormal spontaneous activity may occur in early stages but may be lost in the advanced stage when the muscles become fibrotic.

Other common muscular dystrophies are facioscapulo-humeral dystrophy and limb-girdle muscular dystrophy. Scapuloperoneal dystrophy is probably a variety of facio-scapulohumeral dystrophy. Patients with these muscular dystrophies show short-duration, low-amplitude, polyphasic motor unit potentials and full motor recruitment on moderate effort, but fibrillation potentials and positive sharp waves are rarely observed. The late components of motor unit potentials are not present.

Myotonic dystrophy, myotonia congenita, and paramyotonia congenita have somewhat different EMG characters from the previously mentioned muscular dystrophies. In these diseases EMG shows myotonic discharges in addition to myopathic characteristics of motor unit potentials and fibrillation potentials and positive sharp waves. Myotonic discharges are high-frequency repetitive discharges (20 to 80 per second) that characteristically wax and wane in amplitude and frequency (Figure 3-11).[18,25] They produce a dive-bomber-like sound. Myotonic discharges may be evoked by voluntary movement, mechanical irritation by needle electrode, or muscle percussion. The waveforms of myotonic discharges are positive waves resembling positive sharp waves and diphasic or triphasic spike potentials resembling fibrillation potentials.

Paramyotonia congenita resembles hyperkalemic periodic paralysis (adynamia episodica hereditaria) to such an extent that it has been postulated that the two really represent a single disease.[14] The episodic paralysis and myotonia may be precipitated by exposure to cold, as may occur when a swimmer afflicted with the disorder is submerged in cold water. The affected muscles do not respond to electrical stimulation of the appropriate nerve, and the EMG may show increased insertional activity, fibrillation potentials, and myotonic discharges. The individual motor unit potentials may show a small but distinct diminution of the mean duration.

In hereditary myopathy, motor and sensory conduction studies are normal, but myotonic dystrophy often shows mild motor conduction defects.[34]

Acquired myopathy
Myositis

Inflammation of muscles commonly occurs in polymyositis and dermatomyositis and may also occur in trichinosis, cysticercosis, annd sarcoidosis.

EMG shows fibrillation potentials, positive sharp waves, repetitive complex discharges, and short-duration, low-amplitude, polyphasic motor unit potentials with early recruitment. In some patients the short-duration, low-amplitude potentials are less prominent than the large-amplitude motor

units and long-duration polyphasic potentials that are more usually associated with neuropathic disease. This situation more commonly occurs in polymyositis. The abnormal spontaneous activity in polymyositis diminishes or disappears within a few weeks of successful steroid therapy. Frequently this is distinctively different from the activity observed in wallerian degeneration in peripheral neuropathy.

In some cases of polymyositis, repetitive stimulation of the nerve may elicit degrees of neuromuscular block similar to those seen in myasthenia gravis or myasthenic syndrome.[48]

Endocrine myopathy

Endocrine myopathy may develop in hyperthyroidism, hypothyroidism, parathyroid disease, Addison's disease, and Cushing's syndrome. EMG changes in motor unit potentials are similar to those in other myopathies. Abnormal spontaneous activity is unusual but is occasionally observed in hypothyroid myopathy. These EMG changes are also seen in the myopathy induced by systemic administration of steroids. Thus the treatment for myopathy (myosotic) induces myopathy and must be carefully evaluated.

DISORDERS OF NEUROMUSCULAR TRANSMISSION

The neuromuscular junction consists of the presynaptic nerve terminal, the synaptic cleft, and the postsynaptic region on the muscle fibers.

The most common disorder of neuromuscular transmission is myasthenia gravis, caused by a postsynaptic abnormality. Myasthenic syndrome (Lambert-Eaton syndrome), which sometimes occurs with bronchial carcinoma and botulinum poisoning, is associated with a presynaptic abnormality.

In myasthenia gravis, EMG of affected muscles shows variability in amplitude of motor unit potentials.[41] The amplitude of the first motor unit appears to be at a maximum followed by a series of three to 10 decreasing potentials. With somewhat stronger efforts the whole motor unit may fail. After a period of rest the motor unit potential may regain a normal range. In more pronounced myasthenia gravis, motor unit potentials are reduced in amplitude and duration, as in primary myopathy. This is due to dropout of muscle fibers from active motor units. This sign should not be misinterpreted as an indication of myopathic changes in myasthenia gravis.[41]

Fibrillation potentials and positive sharp waves may be present in severely affected muscles, probably reflecting loss of innervation. These low-amplitude, short-duration motor unit potentials and abnormal spontaneous activity also occur in disorders of presynaptic neuromuscular transmission.

Nerve conduction studies are normal in disorders of neuromuscular transmission. The study most commonly used

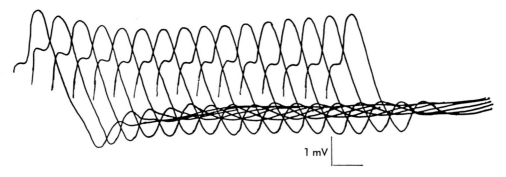

1 mV

Figure 3-12. Compound muscle action potential recorded from upper trapezius of patient with myasthenia gravis.

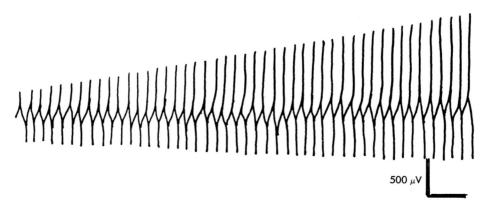

500 μV

Figure 3-13. Compound muscle action potentials recorded from abductor digiti quinti muscle of patient with myasthenia syndrome.

to diagnose neuromuscular transmission defects is repetitive stimulation of a motor nerve with recording of the compound muscle action potentials. In performing this test, particular precautions are necessary to avoid certain movements causing artifacts. The evoked potentials are significantly affected if the stimulating or recording electrodes are moved during stimulation. Therefore the electrodes and the extremity must be firmly immobilized. Stimulation intensity should remain supramaximal throughout the examination.

In myasthenia gravis, stimulation rates of 2 or 3 Hz are used. These low rates are less painful to patients and result in the least movement artifact. Higher rates (greater than 5 Hz) may produce an initial facilitation obscuring a defect. Between 4 and 8 stimuli are usually given, and the maximum defect of the response is usually seen between the first and fourth or fifth stimuli. The decrement should be reproducible.

After two or three trials of repetitive stimulation, voluntary activation of the rested muscles should be performed. An isometric contraction for 30 seconds or 1 minute is usually enough. Exercising initially enhances the compound muscle action potentials (postactivation facilitation) for 1

or 2 minutes. After 2 to 4 minutes there is a decrement owing to postactivation exhaustion.

In myasthenia gravis the incidence of electrophysiologic abnormalities is higher in clinically weak proximal or facial muscles than in distal muscles. In our laboratory the upper trapezius and facial muscles are usually tested with stimulation of the spinal accessory nerve or facial nerve.[28,29]

If the patient has been taking drugs that affect neuromuscular transmission, these drugs should be discontinued for at least 3 to 6 hours before examination. This time should be extended to more than 12 hours if the patient can tolerate it.

In myasthenia gravis the initial compound muscle action potential is usually in the normal range of amplitude. Successive action potentials decrease in amplitude until about the fourth or fifth response. Occasionally, in mild cases, decrement occurs when the test is repeated after the muscle is warmed or 1 or 2 minutes after a 30-second exercise period of the muscles being tested. When the amplitude of the fourth or fifth response is compared with the first one, reproducible decrement of 10% or more is generally considered significant (Figure 3-12). When conventional repetitive stimulation studies are equivocal, nerve stimulation under ischemic conditions or following regional administration of curare may be of diagnostic value.[29] Single-fiber EMG is among the most sensitive tests for myasthenia gravis, especially in ocular myasthenia.

A decrement of evoked potentials at low rates of stimulation may be observed in amyotrophic lateral sclerosis, poliomyelitis, and syringomyelia. In myotonia a decrement may occur during stimulation at low or high rates.

In disorders affecting presynaptic transmission, such as myasthenic syndrome and botulinum poisoning, the initial amplitude of the compound muscle action potential is usually very small; however, in mild cases the initial amplitude may be normal or in the low-normal range. In these disorders the distal muscles of the upper extremity are usually tested. At low rates of stimulation the decrement resembles that of myasthenia gravis, but at high rates (greater than 20 Hz) marked increase in amplitude (more than 50%) occurs (Figure 3-13).

REFERENCES

1. Albers, JB, et al: Limb myokymia, Muscle Nerve 4:494, 1981.
2. Borenstein, S, and Desmedt, DE: Range of variations in motor unit potentials during reinnervation after traumatic nerve lesions in humans, Ann Neurol 8:460, 1980.
3. Buchthal, F: Spontaneous electrical activity: an overview, Muscle Nerve 5:S52, 1982.
4. Buchthal, F, and Rosenfalk, P: Spontaneous electrical activity of human muscles, Electroencephalogr Clin Neurophysiol 20:321, 1966.
5. Buchthal, F, Rosenfalk, A, and Trojaberg, W: Electrophysiological findings in entrapment of the median nerve at wrist and elbow, J Neurol Neurosurg Psychiatry 37:340, 1974.
6. Calliet, K: Soft tissue pain and disability, Philadelphia, 1977, FA Davis Co.
7. Carfi, J, and Ma, DM: Posterior interosseous syndrome revisited, Muscle Nerve 8:499, 1985.
8. Checkles, NS, Russkar, AD, and Piero, DL: Ulnar nerve conduction velocity—effect of elbow position measurement, Arch Phys Med Rehabil 52:362, 1971.
9. Coers, C, and Telerman-Toppet, N: Morphological changes of motor units in Duchenne's muscular dystrophy, Arch Neurol 34:396, 1977.
10. Craft, S, Currier, DP, and Nelson, RM: Motor conduction of the anterior interosseous nerve, Phys Ther 57:1143, 1977.
11. Dalakas, MC, et al: A long-term follow-up study of patients with post-poliomyelitis neuromuscular symptoms, N Engl J Med 314:939, 1986.
12. Daube, JR: EMG in motor neuron disease, Minimonograph #18, Rochester, Minn. 1982, American Association of Electromyography and Electrodiagnosis.
13. Desmedt, JE, and Borenstein, S: Regeneration in Duchenne muscular dystrophy: electromyographic evidence, Arch Neurol 33:642, 1976.
14. Drager, GA, Hammill, JG, and Shy, GM: Paramyotonia congenita, Arch neurol Psychiatry 80:1, 1958.
15. Eisen, A: Early diagnosis of ulnar nerve palsy: an electrophysiologic study, Neurology 24:256, 1974.
16. Eisen, A, and Humphreys, P: The Guillain-Barré syndrome, Arch Neurol 30:438, 1974.
17. Goldkamp, O: Electromyography and nerve conduction studies in 116 patients with hemiplegia, Arth Phys Med Rehabil 48:59, 1967.
18. Goodgold, J, and Eberstein, A: Electrodiagnosis of neuromuscular diseases, ed 3, Baltimore, 1983, Williams & Wilkins.
19. Hausmaus-Petrosewieg, I, et al: Is Kugelberg-Welander spinal muscular atrophy a fetal defect? Muscle Nerve 3:389, 1980.
20. Hefferman, LPM: Electromyographic value of the tibialis posterior muscle, Arch Phys Med Rehabil 60:170, 1979.
21. Jabre, JF: Ulnar nerve lesions at the wrist: new technique for recording from the sensory dorsal branch of the ulnar nerve, Neurology 30:873, 1980.
22. Johnson, EW, and Raptou, AD: A study of intragluteal injection, Arch Phys Med 46:167, 1965.
23. Johnson, RK, and Shrewberry, MM: Anatomical course of the thenar branch of the median nerve—usually in a separate tunnel through the transverse carpal ligament, J Bone Joint Surg 52:269, 1970.
24. Kimura, J: The carpal tunnel syndrome: localization of conduction abnormalities within the distal segment of the median nerve, Brain 102:619, 1979.
25. Kimura, J: Electrodiagnosis in diseases of nerve and muscle: principles and practice, Philadelphia, 1983, FA Davis Co.
26. Lang, AH, and Pastanen, USJ: "Satellite potentials" and the duration of motor unit potentials in normal, neuropathic and myopathic muscles, J Neurol Sci 27:513, 1976.
27. Ma, DM, Kim, SH, and Spielholz, NI: Carpal tunnel syndrome and concurrent cervical radiculopathy. Unpublished.
28. Ma, DM, and Liveson, JA: Nerve conduction handbook, Philadelphia, 1983, FA Davis Co.
29. Ma, DM, Wasserman, EJL, and Giebfried, J: Repetitive stimulation of the trapezius muscle: its value in myasthenic testing (abstract), Electroencephalogr Clin Neurophysiol 50:243, 1980.
30. MacLean, IC: Nerve root stimulation to evaluate conduction across the brachial and lumbosacral plexuses, 3rd Annual Continuing Education Course, Philadelphia, Sept 25, 1980, American Association of Electromyography and Electrodiagnosis.
31. McLeod, JG: Electrophysiological studies in the Guillain-Barré syndrome, Ann Neurol 9(suppl):20, 1981.
32. Morris, HH, and Peters, BH: Pronator syndrome: clinical and electrophysiological features in seven cases, J Neurol Neurosurg Psychiatry 39:461, 1976.
33. Oh, SJ, et al: Tarsal tunnel syndrome: electrophysiological study, Ann Neurol 5:327, 1979.
34. Papagiotopoulos, LP, and Scarpalezos, S: Dystrophica myotonica: peripheral nerve involvement and pathogenic implications, J Neurol Sci 27:1, 1976.
35. Peterson, I, and Broman, AM: Electromyographic findings in a case of botulism, Nord Med 65:259, 1961.
36. Raman, PT, and Taori, GM: Prognostic significance of electrodiagnostic studies in the Guillain-Barré syndrome, J Neurol Neurosurg Psychiatry 25:321, 1968.
37. Seddan, HJ: Three types of nerve injury, Brain 66:237, 1943.
38. Shea, JD, and McClain, EJ: Ulnar nerve compression syndromes at and below wrist, J Bone Joint Surg 51A:1095, 1969.
39. Spielholz, NI, et al: Electrophysiological studies in patients with spinal cord lesions, Arch Phys Med Rehabil 53:558, 1972.
40. Spinner, M, and Spencer, PS: Nerve compression lesions of the upper extremity, Clin Orthop Rel Res 104:46, 1974.
41. Stalberg, E: Clinical electrophysiology in myasthenia gravis, J Neurol Neurosurg Psychiatry 43:622, 1980.
42. Sunderland, S: A classification of peripheral nerve injuries producing loss of function, Brain 74:491, 1951.
43. Sunderland, S: Nerve and nerve injuries, ed 2, Edinburgh, 1978, Churchill Livingstone.
44. Thomas, JE, Lambert, EH, and Csenz, KA: Electrodiagnostic aspects of the carpal tunnel syndrome, Arch Neurol 16:635, 1967.
45. Thomas, PK: Motor nerve conduction in the carpal tunnel syndrome, Neurology 10:1045, 1960.
46. Trontelj, J, and Stalberg, E: Bizarre repetitive discharges recorded with single fiber EMG, J Neurol Neurosurg Psychiatry 46:310, 1983.

47. Upton, ARM, and McComas, AJ: The double crush in nerve entrapment syndromes, Lancet 2:359, 1973.

48. Vasilescu, C, et al: Myasthenia in patients with dermatomyositis: clinical, electrophysiological and ultrastructural studies, J Neurol Sci 38:129, 1978.

49. Warren, J, et al: Electromyographic changes of brachial plexus root avulsion, J Neurosurg 31:137, 1969.

50. Wettstein, A: The origin of fasciculations in motor unit disease, Ann Neurol 5:295, 1979.

51. Wiederholt, WC: "End-place noise" in electromyography, Neurology 20:214, 1970.

CHAPTER 4

Reflex studies in humans

BHAGWAN T. SHAHANI

The work of Sir Charles Sherrington summarized in his Silliman lectures, "The Integrative Action of the Nervous System,"[52] marked a new era in the understanding of the fundamental principles of reflex physiology, which form a basis for modern concepts of nervous integration. Recent advances in electronic and computer technology have made it possible to study reflex activity quantitatively in intact human subjects. With electromyographic techniques it is possible to record most of the reflexes (both proprioceptive and exteroceptive) commonly studied in a clinical setting. These studies, in addition to providing better insights into the understanding of underlying physiologic mechanisms, give an objective and quantitative measure of function of the central and peripheral nervous systems in humans. Three useful physiologic parameters, the H-reflex, the F-response (which is not a reflex), and the "silent period," are briefly discussed in this chapter. H-reflex and F-response studies are widely used to evaluate the function of the peripheral nervous system. However, studies of these two late responses can also be useful in evaluating function of the central nervous system. Studies of the silent period can add a new dimension to electrodiagnostic testing because they can evaluate physiologic functions that cannot be assessed by conventional techniques.

H-REFLEX AND F-RESPONSES

In 1918, Hoffman[16] demonstrated that the compound muscle action potential (CMAP) associated with the ankle and knee jerk was comparable in latency and configuration to that evoked by submaximal electrical stimulation delivered percutaneously to the tibial or femoral nerve, respectively. He concluded that both tendon jerks and electrically induced late responses represent activity in the same kind of stretch reflex. On the basis of his findings, which included abolition of the late response with supramaximal stimulation

to the mixed nerve and relatively brief latency of the late response, he concluded that the afferent pathway of this reflex consists of very fast conducting nerve fibers and that the central delay is extremely short. The conclusions from Hoffman's remarkable experiments were confirmed in 1950 by Magladery and McDougal,[27] who designated the electrically induced late responses and the H-reflex after its discoverer. They called the shorter-latency CMAP evoked by direct electrical stimulation by motor axons the M-response. In contrast to the large-amplitude H-reflex, which could be easily recorded in calf muscles following submaximal stimulation, another type of late response was seen in intrinsic muscles of the hands and feet (Figure 4-1). This late response, which had a latency rather similar to that of the H-reflex but was not a reflex, was named the F-wave (or F-response). F-responses as recorded in the electromyography laboratory are due to centrifugal discharges from individual motor neurons, each of which is initiated by an antidromic volley.[9,29,31,56]

H-reflex and F-response studies in disorders of the central nervous system

H-reflex and F-response studies have been widely used to evaluate the function of the central nervous system,* as well as the peripheral nervous system.† The most commonly used tests for evaluation of the central nervous system are as follows:
1. Maximum amplitude of an H-reflex as compared with maximum amplitude of the compound action potential in the same muscle
2. Excitability curves of the H-reflex
3. Vibratory inhibition of the H-reflex

---

* References 6, 16, 17, 28, 34, 41, 43, 53, 54, 61, 63.
† References 1-5, 7-13, 15, 18-26, 30, 33, 35-42, 44-46, 50, 51, 57-60, 62.

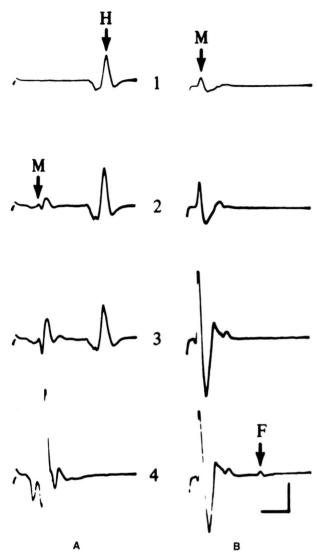

Figure 4-1. H-reflex (soleus). Increasing stimulus from traces 1 to 4. Note appearance of H-reflex in 1 before M-response is clearly seen in 2, 3, and 4. Calibration: traces 1 and 2 (vertical) 500 μV, traces 3 and 4 (vertical) 1 mV; horizontal, 10 msec (**B**) F-response (abductor pollicis brevis). Increasing stimulus and calibration as for **A.** (From Shahani, BT, and Sumner, AJ: Electrophysiological studies in peripheral neuropathy: early detection and monitoring. In Stalberg, E, and Young, RR, editors: Neurology, vol 1, Clinical neurophysiology, Boston, 1981, Butterworth.)

4. Mean F-response amplitude compared with the maximum amplitude of the compound muscle action potential
5. F-response persistence

Maximum amplitude H-reflex

Maximum amplitude H-reflex (H-max) is recorded by delivering a single electrical stimulus to the tibial nerve in

the popliteal fossa. The recording is made by placing surface electrodes over the soleus muscle. The stimulus intensity is adjusted to produce H-max. The maximum amplitude compound muscle action potential is produced in the usual manner by delivering a supramaximal stimulus to the tibial nerve in the popliteal fossa. H-max/M-max reflects the percentage of motor neurons in the motor neuron pool that can be activated by the H-reflex. When the excitability of the motor neuron pool is increased (as in upper motor neuron lesions), a greater percentage of motor neurons is activated and therefore amplitude of the H-reflex is increased. In conditions in which the excitability of the motor neuron pool is decreased (as in spinal shock) it may be impossible to record an H-reflex.

Excitability curves

H-reflex excitability curves following double stimulation of the tibial nerve in the popliteal fossa have been studied in various neurologic disorders. Such curves exhibit characteristic hypoexcitable and hyperexcitable phases in normal subjects,[34,53] which are often altered in patients with central nervous system lesions. It must be emphasized, however, that H-reflex excitability curves are markedly affected by such independent variables as the patient's position and the amount of background voluntary or reflex muscular activity. For reproducible results to be obtained, the subject must be still and relaxed in a comfortable position and the limb must be rigidly fixed at various joints at appropriate angles to avoid changes in proprioceptive input. In studies of H-reflex excitability curves, it is important to demonstrate a small preceding M-response of unchanging amplitude and shape from one stimulus to the next, as a proof of the stability of the relationship between the nerve and the stimulating electrode. Recent studies have shown that, when excitability curves are plotted by delivery of two stimuli (conditioning and test) at the same site in the nerve, they do not necessarily reflect changes in the central excitability.[37] Local changes of excitability in the peripheral nerve itself can give rise to excitability curves that resemble the H-reflex recovery curves described previously. Plotting of H-reflex excitability curves by giving double stimulation at the same site is therefore not recommended. If one wishes to study changes in excitability of the motor neuron pool by plotting H-reflex recovery curves, it is important that the conditioning stimulus be delivered at a different site in the same nerve or to a different nerve from that receiving the test stimulus for evoking the H-reflex.

Vibratory inhibition of the H-reflex

When a muscle of a normal subject is vibrated during elicitation of phasic proprioceptive reflexes, the reflexes are significantly inhibited. In contrast to normal subjects, patients with chronic spasticity have a diminished vibratory inhibition of the H-reflex. It has been suggested that the vibratory suppression of the H-reflex may be due to pre-

Table 4-1. Features distinguishing between H-reflex and F-response

H-reflex	F-response
Monosynaptic reflex in which afferent arc consists of group Ia afferent fibers from muscle spindles and efferent arc consists of alpha motor axons	Not a reflex; centrifugal discharge of small percentage of motor neurons initiated by antidromic volleys in their axons; both afferent and efferent arcs consist of alpha motor axons
Stimulus threshold lower than that required to evoke a direct M-response; supramaximal stimulation for M-response blocks H-reflex	Stimulus threshold usually higher than that required for H-reflex and M-response
Mean amplitude (5 to 10 responses) can be up to 50% to 100% of maximal M-response	Mean amplitude small, usually less than 5% of maximal M-response
Appearance and persistence rather constant at low rates of stimulation (1 every 10 to 30 seconds)	Appearance and persistence rather variable, even at low rates of stimulation
Easily recorded from soleus muscle and some proximal "postural" muscles in adults; present in intrinsic hand and foot muscles in newborn infants	Can be recorded easily from almost every skeletal muscle
Single motor units activated in H-reflex are different from those in preceding M-response	Single motor units activated in F-responses are same as those in M-response
Fluctuation of latency of single motor units activated in H-reflex is greater than for those in F- or M-response	Fluctuation of single motor unit latency in F-response is less than that in H-reflex but greater than that in M-response

From Shahani, BT: Late responses and the "silent period." In Aminoff, MJ, editor: Electrodiagnosis in clinical neurology, New York, 1986, Churchill Livingstone.

synaptic inhibition. However, effects of vibration as studied in human subjects are probably more complex.[48]

F-response amplitude and persistence

F-response studies can provide a measure of the central activity state of the spinal motor neurons.[14] In patients with an acute central nervous system lesion, F-responses occur with decreased persistence or amplitude, or both, on the clinically involved side. These abnormalities of F-responses correlate clinically with severity of the weakness, decreased tone, and decreased deep tendon reflexes. In patients with chronic spasticity, amplitude and persistence of F-responses may be increased.

H-reflex and F-response studies in disorders of the peripheral nervous system

Studies of the H-reflex and F-responses have proved useful in evaluating function of the peripheral nervous system. A clear distinction should be made between these two responses because they provide different types of information regarding the central and peripheral nervous system. Some of the features distinguishing these two responses are described in Table 4-1. H-reflexes in normal adult subjects can be easily recorded only in the soleus muscle and proximal postural muscles such as the quadriceps.[55] In contrast, F-responses can be recorded easily from almost every skeletal muscle, making the F-response more versatile for evaluating conduction in alpha motor axons. There is a direct relationship between the minimal latency of these two late responses and the height of the subject and length of the appropriate extremity. It is usually easier and more accurate to record heights rather than the distance between two anatomic landmarks. Nomograms with minimal latency plotted for different heights provide accurate information regarding conduction in entire segments of nerves from the motor neurons to the muscle. In addition to recording minimal latencies for the height of the subject, comparing minimal latencies of late responses on the two sides is often useful. In a given individual the minimal latency recorded on the two sides has a difference of less than 2 msec. It is also useful, sometimes, to compare the minimal latencies of F-responses in muscles innervated by two different nerves in the same limb. For example, there should be a difference of less than 2 msec in the minimal latencies recorded from the median-innervated abductor pollicis brevis muscle and from the ulnar-innervated abductor digiti minimi muscle in the same hand.

Other parameters of F-responses that have proved useful are minimum-maximum latency differences, F-response amplitude, and F-response persistence.[41,44] The minimum-maximum latency difference is useful because it provides information regarding conduction not only in the fastest conducting motor fibers (such as the maximum motor conduction velocity), but also in relatively slower conduction motor fibers. F-response studies therefore provide better information than the conventional motor conduction velocity studies. The amplitude of the F-response is increased in lesions of both the peripheral and the central nervous system. The reason for the increase in amplitude of F-response in lesions of the peripheral nervous system is that after denervation and reinnervation the individual motor units have an increased amplitude. This increase in amplitude is reflected in the increased F-response amplitude. In patients with lesions of the central nervous system, the increase in the amplitude of the F-response is due to synchronization of motor units seen in the F-response recorded with surface electrodes. The persistence of F-response is decreased in lesions of both the peripheral nervous system and the central nervous system. In acute lesions of the central nervous system such as a spinal shock after an injury to the spinal cord, decreased persistence is due to decreased excitability of the motoneuron pool. On the other hand, decreased persistence in the patients with peripheral neuropathies could be due to a conduction block in alpha motor axons.

Whenever late responses are recorded, changes in their latencies, amplitude, duration, and persistence must be interpreted in the light of the clinical context of the patient. Abnormalities of late responses are seen in patients with a variety of peripheral neuropathies. H-reflex and F-response studies have been useful in both the so-called axonal and the segmental demyelinating type of neuropathies. They have also proved useful in studying patients with entrapment neuropathies and root compression syndromes.[7,12,57] In neuropathies in which there is a specific disorder of sensory fibers (for example, Friedriech's ataxia) with preservation of alpha motor axons, the H-reflex is absent whereas F-responses can be recorded with normal latency. A combination of studies of the H-reflex and the F-response can document a lesion in the afferent or efferent arc of the reflex pathways. The minimal latency of the H-reflex is usually relatively prolonged when the ankle jerk is diminished.

Because F-responses can be recorded from a variety of skeletal muscles, they are valuable in providing information regarding motor conduction in the entire segment of peripheral nerves in different parts of the body. In many neuropathies of the metabolic nutritional type, such as alcoholic neuropathy, uremic neuropathy, and diabetic neuropathy, abnormalities of late responses can be demonstrated in the distribution of a nerve in which conventional methods of studying motor and sensory conduction do not show any abnormality. There are several possible reasons why late response studies are more sensitive than the conventional motor and sensory conduction studies. One explanation could be that the late response studies evaluate function along the entire course of the motor axon, so abnormality in any particular segment can be detected. Second, the range of normal values for late responses is relatively narrow compared with that for motor conduction velocities in different nerves, making it easier to detect abnormalities in individual patients. In patients with demyelinating neuropathies, such as Guillain-Barré syndrome, prolongation of late response latencies and decrease in their persistence may be the first objective recordable sign during early stages of the disease when the diagnosis is difficult and CSF protein and conventional motor and sensory conduction studies are normal. Significant prolongation of late response laten-

cies with minor changes in conventional motor conduction velocities helps to localize a lesion in proximal segments.

Recent studies have shown that measurement of late response latencies can be an important adjunct to routine motor and sensory motor conduction studies in establishing the diagnosis of entrapment neuropathies.[12] In patients with carpal tunnel syndrome the minimal latency of the F-response in the median innervated abductor pollicis brevis muscle may be prolonged (greater than 2 msec) when compared with the late response latency in the ulnar innervated abductor digiti minimi muscle in the same hand or median innervated abductor pollicis brevis muscle in the opposite hand. Similarly, in patients with an ulnar entrapment syndrome at the elbow, minimal latency of F-response in the abductor digiti minimi muscle becomes relatively prolonged (greater than 2 msec) when compared with the abductor pollicis brevis muscle in the same hand or the abductor digiti minimi muscle in the opposite hand.

H-reflex and F-response studies have also proved useful in documenting nerve root compression syndrome.[57] Minimal latency measurement for the H-reflex in the soleus muscle and F-response in other muscles of the lower extremity such as the extensor digitorum brevis (L5-S1) and abductor hallucis (S1-S2) provides useful information regarding lesions of appropriate roots. The minimal latency of the H-reflex in affected extremities is prolonged (and the amplitude decreased) when there is reduction in the clinically elicitable ankle jerk on the appropriate side. When the tendon jerk cannot be elicited, there is usually no H-reflex. If it is present, it is so small in amplitude that one cannot be certain, using surface electrodes, what percentage of late response is an H-reflex or an F-response. It must be recognized that a number of patients who have well-proven evidence of nerve root compression also have normal values for minimal latencies of late responses. As long as there are a few functional large-diameter axons with normal conduction velocity that can mediate the late response, the minimal latency for the particular response remains normal. However, when H-reflex and F-response studies are abnormal, they can be extremely useful in localizing a lesion in patients with cervical or lumbrosacral root disease. Patients who have a well-defined neurologic thoracic outlet syndrome also show abnormalities of late responses. The minimal latencies and the persistence of F-responses become abnormal in both median and ulnar innervated intrinsic hand muscles of patients with thoracic outlet syndrome.

SILENT PERIOD

The term "silent period" refers to a transitory, relative, or absolute decrease in electromyographic activity in the midst of an otherwise sustained contraction.[47] Although a silent period can be produced by a variety of different techniques, including stimulation of purely cutaneous nerves, shortening of muscles, and elicitation of phasic stretch ac-

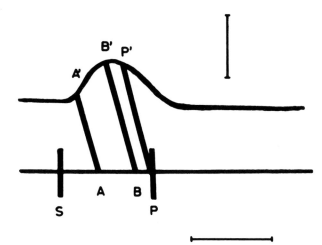

Figure 4-2. Schematic representation of factors presumably involved in silent period (S-P) where S is stimulus. Upper trace represents muscle twitch, and lower trace is time of EMG response. First 50 to 60 msec (S-A) is related to various antidromic factors including Renshaw recurrent inhibition. At A′ the muscle spindles begin to be unloaded and the Golgi tendon organs begin to be stimulated. At B′ the spindle pause ceases, and tendon organ firing may carry on until P′. Voluntary activity resumes at P. Calibrations are 100 msec and 1 kg. (From Shahani, BT, and Young, RR: Studies of the normal human silent period. In Desmedt, JE, editor: New developments in electromyography and clinical neurophysiology, vol 3, Basel, 1973, Karger.)

tivity (tendon jerks), the most commonly used method for its elicitation in a clinical setting is to deliver electrical stimulation to the mixed nerve as described by Merton.[32] When a supramaximal stimulus is delivered to a mixed nerve innervating a particular muscle, the silent period in different individuals ranges from 100 to 120 msec, when measured from the beginning of the stimulus artifact to the end of the silent period. The silent period is usually interrupted by the F-response at an appropriate latency after the stimulus. The initial part of the silent period, which is present even in completely deafferented human subjects, can be explained on the basis of collision of orthodromic and antidromic impulses in motor axons, Renshaw recurrent inhibition, and the refractory period of the motor neuron pool after its invasion by antidromic impulses (Figure 4-2). The second half of the silent period is produced by changes in the central nervous system related to modification of proprioceptive and cutaneous inputs resulting from direct stimulation of different types of nerve fibers and the muscle twitch. To avoid a cutaneously elicited silent period, it is important to reduce the stimulus amplitude and deliver a relatively low threshold stimulus to the mixed nerve. The silent period produced under these circumstances is termed proprioceptive silent period because it is due mostly to a pause in the primary muscle spindle afferent activity as a result of unloading of muscle spindles. In a recent study of a proprioceptive silent period (Figure 4-3) in different muscles of

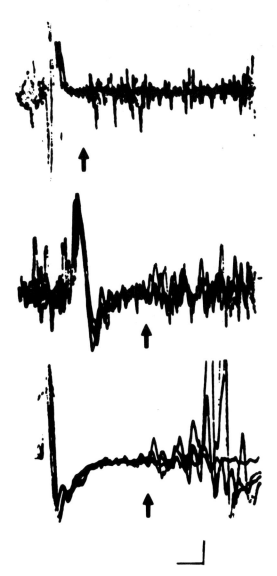

Figure 4-3. Silent periods recorded from abductor digiti minimi (*top*), wrist extensors (*center*), and biceps (*bottom*). In top, only early nonproprioceptive portion of silent period is seen. Center shows relative silent period, and bottom shows normal silent period. Arrows indicate end of silent period. (Stimulus is at beginning of sweep; calibration, 20 msec and 20 μV.) (From Ropper, AH, and Shahani, BT: Arch Neurol 40:537, 1983. Copyright 1983, American Medical Association.)

patients with Fisher's syndrome (Guillain-Barré polyneuritis with ophthalmoplegia, areflexia, and ataxia) there was mismatching of information from muscle spindle afferents and joint position receptors.[38,45] This mismatching of information resulted in ataxia that could not be differentiated from the true "cerebellar" type of ataxia. These studies have demonstrated that the "cerebellar" type of ataxia can be produced by a lesion of the peripheral nervous system and that it is not necessary to postulate a central nervous system disease in patients with Fisher's syndrome.

Other types of movement disorders, such as the "neuropathic tremor," can be produced by imbalance of sensory inputs.[49] Studies of the proprioceptive silent period therefore can be useful in documenting abnormalities in different afferent systems, leading to a better understanding of the pathophysiologic mechanisms responsible for certain disorders of the motor system.

SUMMARY

Electrophysiologic studies performed in the electromyography laboratory should no longer be limited to electromyography and conventional methods of measuring motor and sensory nerve conduction. H-reflex, F-response, and silent period studies have proved useful in early detection and documentation of various disorders of the peripheral and central nervous systems in individual patients. It must be emphasized that changes in different parameters of these responses can be seen under different physiologic conditions, as well as with disorders of the peripheral and central nervous systems. Proper interpretation of the results of these studies therefore requires a clear understanding of the underlying neural mechanisms that may alter these responses.

REFERENCES

1. Ackil, AA, Shahani, BT, and Young, RR: Late response and sural conduction studies: usefulness in patients with chronic renal failure, Arch Neurol 38:482, 1981.
2. Ackil, AA, Shahani, BT, and Young, RR: Sural conduction studies and late responses in children undergoing hemodialysis, Arch Phys Med Rehabil 62:487, 1981.
3. Adams, RD, Shahani, BT, and Young, RR: Tremor in association with polyneuropathy, Trans Am Neurol Assoc 95:44, 1972.
4. Adams, RD, Shahani, BT, and Young, RR: A severe pansensory familial neuropathy, Trans Am Neurol Assoc 98:67, 1973.
5. Albizzati, MG, et al: F-wave velocity in motor neurone disease, Acta Neurol Scand 54:269, 1976.
6. Angel, RW, and Hoffman, WW: The H reflex in normal, spastic rigid subjects, Arch Neurol 8:591, 1963.
7. Braddom, RI, and Johnson, EW: Standardization of H-reflex and diagnostic use in S-1 radiculopathy, Arch Phys Med Rehabil 55:161, 1974.
8. Conrad, B, Aschoff, JC, and Fischler, MD: Der diagnostische wert der F-Wellen-latenz, J Neurol 210:151, 1975.
9. Dawson, GD, and Merton, PA: Recurrent discharges from motoneurones, Proceedings of the Twentieth Congress on International Physiology, Brussels, 1956.
10. Dominque, JN, Shahani, BT, and Kolodney, E: Electrophysiological studies in Refsum's disease, Trans Am Neurol Assoc 106:173, 1982.
11. Drechsler, B, Lastouka, M, and Kalvodova, E: Electrophysiological study of patients with herniated intervertebral disc, Electromyography 6:187, 1966.
12. Egloff-Baer, S, Shahani, BT, and Young, RR: Usefulness of late response studies in diagnosis of entrapment neuropathies, Electroencephalogr Clin Neurophysiol 45:16P, 1978.
13. Eisen, A, Schomer, D, and Melmed, C: The application of F-wave measurements in the differentiation of proximal and distal upper limb entrapments, Neurology 27:662, 1977.
14. Fisher, MA, Shahani, BT, and Young, RR: Assessing segmental excitability after acute rostral lesions. I. The F response, Neurology 28:1265, 1978.
15. Fisher, MA, et al: Clinical and electrophysiological appraisal of the significance of radicular injury in back pain, J Neurol Neurosurg Psychiatry 41:303, 1978.
16. Hoffman, P: Uber die Beziehungen der Sehnenreflexe zur Willkurlichen Bewegung und zum Tonus, Z Biol 68:351, 1918.
17. Ioku, M, et al: Parkinsonism: electromyographic studies of monosynaptic reflex, Science 150:1472, 1965.
18. Kimura, J: F-wave velocity in the central segment of the median and ulnar nerves: a study in normal subjects and in patients with Charcot-Marie-Tooth disease, Neurology 24:539, 1974.
19. Kimura, J: Electrodiagnosis in diseases on nerve and muscle: principles and practice, Philadelphia, 1983, FA Davis Co.
20. Kimura, J, and Butzer, JF: F-wave conduction velocity in Guillain-Barré syndrome, Arch Neurol 32:524, 1975.
21. King, D, and Ashby, P: Conduction velocity in the proximal segments of a motor nerve in the Guillain-Barré syndrome, J Neurol Neurosurg Psychiatry 39:538, 1976.
22. Kneebone, CS, Shahani, BT, and Landis, D: Detecting small fibre axonal neuropathy in the presence of a severe demyelinating neuropathy, Arch Phys Med Rehabil 65:630, 1984.
23. Lachman, T, Shahani, BT, and Young, RR: Late responses as diagnostic aids in Landry-Guillain-Barré syndrome, Electroencephalogr Clin Neurophysiol 43:147, 1977.
24. Lachman, T, Shahani, BT, and Young, RR: Late responses as aids to diagnosis in peripheral neuropathy, J Neurol Neurosurg Psychiatry 43:156, 1980.
25. Lefebvre-D'Amour, M, et al: Importance of studying sural conduction and late responses in the evaluation of alcoholic subjects, Neurology 26:368, 1976.
26. Maccabee, PJ, Shahani, BT, and Young, RR: Usefulness of double simultaneous recording (DSR) and F response studies in the diagnosis of carpal tunnel syndrome (CTS), Electroencephalogr Clin Neurophysiol 49:17P, 1980.
27. Magladery, JW, and McDougal, DB: Electrophysiological studies of nerve and reflex activity in normal man. I. Identification of certain reflexes in electromyogram and the conduction velocity of peripheral nerves, Bull Johns Hopkins Hosp 86:265, 1950.
28. Magladery, JW, et al: Electrophysiological studies of spinal motoneurone excitability following afferent nerve volleys in normal persons and patients with upper motor neurone lesions, Bull Johns Hopkins Hosp 91:219, 1952.
29. Mayer, RF, and Feldman, RG: Observations on the nature of the F-wave in man, Neurology 17:147, 1967.
30. Mayer, RF, and Mawdsley, C: Studies in man and cat of the significance of the H-reflex, J Neurol Neurosurg Psychiatry 28:201, 1965.
31. McLeod, JG, and Wray, SH: An experimental study of the F-wave in the baboon, J Neurol Neurosurg Psychiatry 29:196, 1966.
32. Merton, PA: The silent period in a muscle of the human hand, J Physiol (Lond) 114:183, 1951.
33. Notermans, SLH, and Vingerhoets, HM: The importance of the Hoffmann reflex in the diagnosis of lumbar root lesions, Clin Neurol Neurosurg 1:54, 1974.
34. Paillard, J: Reflexes et regulations d'origine proprioceptive chex l'homme, Paris, 1955, Arnette.
35. Panayiotopoulos, CP, Scarpalezos, S, and Nastas, PE: F-wave studies in the deep peroneal nerve. 1. Control subjects, J Neurol Sci 31:319, 1977.
36. Panayiotopoulos, CP, Scarpalezos, S, and Nastas, PE: Sensory (Ia) and F-wave conduction velocity in the proximal segment of the tibial nerve, Muscle Nerve 1:181, 1978.
37. Potts, FA, and Young, RR: Can the early hyper and hypoexcitability phases of H reflex recovery curves be explained by changes in peripheral nerve excitability? Neurology 32:115, 1982.
38. Ropper, AH, and Shahani, BT: Proposed mechanisms of ataxia in Fisher's syndrome, Arch Neurol 40:537, 1983.

39. Ropper, AH, and Shahani, BT: Diagnosis and management of acute areflexia with emphasis in Guillain-Barré syndrome. In Asbury, A, and Gilliat, R, editors: Neurology 4: peripheral nerve disorders, Boston, 1984, Butterworth.

40. Shahani, BT: Flexor reflex afferent nerve fibres in man, J Neurol Neurosurg Psychiatry 33:786, 1970.

41. Shahani, BT: Application of newer F response parameters in the diagnosis of peripheral neuropathies, Muscle Nerve 5:1635, 1982.

42. Shahani, BT: Proximal and distal conduction velocities in neuropathies EEG Clin Neurophysiol 56:S29, 1983.

43. Shahani, BT, editor: Electromyography in CNS disorders, Boston, 1984, Butterworth.

44. Shahani, BT, Potts, F, and Dominque, J: F response studies in peripheral neuropathies, Neurology 30:409, 1980.

45. Shahani, BT, and Ropper, AH: Mechanism of ataxia in Fisher syndrome, Ann Neurol 12:77, 1982.

46. Shahani, BT, and Sumner, AJ: Electrophysiological studies in peripheral neuropathy: early detection and monitoring. In Stalbert, E, and Young, RR, editors: Neurology 1: clinical neurophysiology, London, 1981, Butterworth.

47. Shahani, BT, and Young, RR: Studies of the normal human silent period. In Desmedt, JE: New developments in EMG and clinical neurophysiology, vol 3, Basel, 1973, Karger.

48. Shahani, BT, and Young, RR: Effect of vibration on the F response. In Shahani, M, editor: The motor system: neurophysiology and muscle mechanisms, Amsterdam, 1976, Elsevier.

49. Shahani, BT, Young, RR, and Adams, RD: Neuropathic tremor, EEG Clin Neurophysiol 34:800, 1973.

50. Shahani, BT, Young, RR, and Lachman, T: Late responses as aids to diagnosis in peripheral neuropathy, J Postgrad Med 21:7, 1975.

51. Shahani, BT, et al: Terminal latency index (TLI) and late response studies in motor neuron disease (MND), peripheral neuropathies and entrapment syndromes, Acta Neurol Scand 60(suppl 73):118, 1979.

52. Sherrington, CS: The integrative action of the nervous system, New Haven, Conn, 1906, Yale University Press.

53. Taborikova, H, and Sax, DS: Conditioning of H-reflexes by a preceding subthreshold H-reflex stimulus, Brain 92:203, 1969.

54. Takamori, M: H reflex study in upper motoneuron diseases, Neurology 17:32, 1967.

55. Thomas, JE, and Lambert, EH: Ulnar nerve conduction velocity and H-reflex in infants and children, J Appl Physiol 15:1, 1960.

56. Thorne, J: Central responses to electrical activation of the peripheral nerves supplying the intrinsic hand muscles, J Neurol Neurosurg Psychiatry 28:482, 1965.

57. Tonzola, R, et al: Usefulness of electrophysiological studies in the diagnosis of lumbosacral root disease, Ann Neurol 9:305, 1981.

58. Wager, EE, Jr, and Buerger, AA: A linear relationship between the H-reflex latency and sensory conduction velocity in neuropathy, Neurology 24:711, 1974.

59. Wager, EE, Jr, and Buerger, AA: H-reflex latency and sensory conduction in normal and diabetic subjects, Arch Phys Med Rehabil 55:126, 1974.

60. Wechsler, LR, et al: Electrophysiological study of demyelinating neuropathy associated with systemic lupus erythematosus, Arch Phys Med Rehabil 65:634, 1984.

61. Yap, CB: Spinal segmental and long-loop reflexes on spinal motoneuron excitability in spasticity and rigidity, Brain 90:887, 1967.

62. Young, RR, and Shahani, BT: Clinical value and limitations of F-wave determination, Muscle Nerve I:248, 1978.

63. Zander Olsen, P, and Diamontopoulos, E: Excitability of spinal motor neurones in normal subjects and patients with spasticity, Parkinsonian rigidity and cerebellar hypotonia, J Neurol Neurosurg Psychiatry 30:325, 1967.

CHAPTER 5

Quantitative electromyography in clinical electrodiagnosis

SANJEEV D. NANDEDKAR

Sherrington[74] demonstrated that muscle fibers are organized into functional units that he called motor units (MUs). An MU consists of all muscle fibers innervated by a single motor neuron (Figure 5-1, *A*). The number of fibers in an MU, called the MU size, differs within a given muscle and from muscle to muscle.[26] We use the biceps muscle for most of the discussion to follow. MUs in the biceps muscle contain 50 to 163 muscle fibers.[20,30] They are scattered randomly within a circular territory of 3 to 10 mm diameter.[13,83] Thus a muscle fiber of one MU is surrounded by muscle fibers belonging to several other MUs. The individual muscle fiber diameter is in the range 25 to 85 μm, and the mean fiber diameter is 50 to 60 μm.[22] In the biceps muscle most endplates are distributed within a 10 mm wide zone near the center of the muscle.[6,15] The action potential (AP) propagation velocity of individual muscle fibers is in the range 2.2 to 6 M/sec, and the mean AP propagation velocity is 3.7 M/sec[79] to 4.7 M/sec.[15] The motor axon may form two or three major branches when it reaches the muscle (Figure 5-1, *A*). Each branch then innervates muscle fibers in different portions of the MU territory. These are called MU fractions.[83] The previously described features of the MU make up the MU architecture.

In diseased muscle the MU architecture is changed owing to one or more disease processes such as reinnervation, atrophy and hypertrophy of muscle fibers, and loss of muscle fibers. In clinical electromyography (EMG) the changes in the MU architecture are inferred from the electrical potentials recorded by using intramuscular or surface EMG electrodes. Recordings are made when the muscle is at rest (insertional activity, spontaneous activity, and so on), at minimal force levels (recordings of individual motor unit action potentials [MUAPs]), and at moderate to maximal force level (analysis of the EMG interference pattern, analysis of the compound muscle AP, and so on). These signals are usually assessed from their appearance on an oscilloscope screen and their sound on an audio monitor.

In quantitative EMG, certain features of the EMG signals are measured and compared with values obtained from normal muscles. Distinct patterns of the EMG features are seen in neurogenic and myopathic diseases, and these are used to establish the type of abnormality in the tested muscle. Quantitative EMG provides objective measures of the abnormality. By comparing the changes that occur in the EMG features with time, one can gain a better understanding of the disease progression. The use of abnormalities of the EMG features to infer changes in anatomy is a powerful tool to investigate the pathophysiology in different diseases of muscle and nerve.

The relationship between the EMG signals and their generators depends on the type of recording electrode and recording procedure used. By selecting an appropriate technique, one can focus the EMG examination on the MU abnormality of interest. In this chapter a variety of EMG recording and quantitation techniques are briefly reviewed. The emphasis is on the relationship between the EMG features and the MU and not on the technical aspects of the procedures. For details of recordings and quantitation, recent review articles and books are suggested. The techniques are divided into three groups of recordings: from individual MUs (analysis of MUAPs), from several MUs (analysis of the interference pattern), and from the whole muscle (surface EMG with nerve stimulation). Quantitative EMG studies in patients with different nerve and muscle diseases are described to show how the techniques can give better insight into the pathophysiology of the diseases.

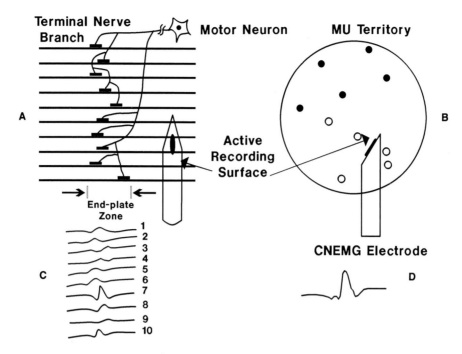

Figure 5-1. Schematic (**A**) longitudinal and (**B**) cross-sectional view of intramuscular needle electrode recording motor unit action potential (MUAP) from motor unit. Sum of action potentials of muscle fibers (**C**) is MUAP (**D**).

ANALYSIS OF MOTOR UNIT ACTION POTENTIALS

When a motor neuron is activated, each muscle fiber innervated by that motor neuron responds by producing an AP that propagates from the motor end-plate to the tendons (Figure 5-1, *C*). The waveform of the AP is triphasic when recorded by extracellular electrodes, and its amplitude decreases when the distance between the electrode and the muscle fiber increases.[4,60] The muscle fibers in a MU are at different distances from the recording electrode (Figure 5-1, *B*), and therefore their APs recorded by the electrode have different amplitudes. Furthermore, the APs from different muscle fibers in the MU are not synchronous (Figure 5-1, *C*). This is due to different lengths of the terminal nerve axons, differences in AP propagation velocity in terminal nerve axons, different distances from the electrode to the motor end-plates, and differences in the AP propagation velocity in the muscle fibers. The MUAP is the spatial and temporal summation of the APs of all muscle fibers in the MU (Figure 5-1, *D*). The MUAP waveform therefore depends on the MU architecture and changes when pathologic processes change the MU architecture.

Another important factor that affects the MUAP is the size and construction of the recording electrode, which differs among different recording techniques.[62] In general, when the size of the recording surface area is increased, both the amplitude of the AP and its rate of decline with distance from muscle fiber decrease.[55,89] If there is a rapid

decline of the AP amplitude with distance, the MUAP waveform is determined mainly by APs of the nearest few muscle fibers. Thus the recording procedure is selective. Recording techniques with the slowest rate of decline of AP amplitude with distance are the least selective, and the MUAP waveform is more likely to depend on APs of all muscle fibers in the MU.

We discuss four recording techniques that have different selectivity—single fiber EMG, concentric needle EMG, monopolar needle EMG, and macro EMG—and demonstrate their use in obtaining complementary information about the number, size, and distribution of muscle fibers in the MU territory. We then discuss some special techniques used to measure the AP propagation velocity in the muscle fibers and the diameter of the MU territory. Together these techniques provide information about the MU architecture.

Single fiber electromyography

The technique of single fiber EMG (SFEMG) was developed by Stalberg and Ekstedt in the mid-1960s. It has been used to study abnormalities of neuromuscular junction, reinnervation, reflexes, and so on. The details of the methods and interpretations are summarized in a monograph by Stalberg and Trontelj.[89]

Recording technique

In SFEMG the recording surface is a 25 μm diameter wire exposed at a side port on the cannula. The signals

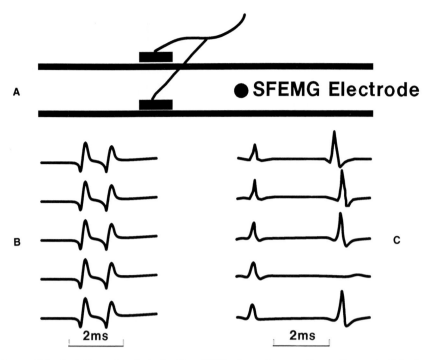

Figure 5-2. A, Schematic of single fiber EMG electrode recording action potentials from two muscle fibers of motor unit (MU). Five consecutive discharges of MU are shown, and jitter is normal in **B** and increased in **C.** Fourth discharge in **C** shows blocking.

measured are the difference between the electrical potential recorded by this surface and the electrode cannula, which acts as the reference electrode. The signals are filtered to exclude components below 500 Hz, which come predominantly from more distant fibers. Recordings are made from voluntarily activated MUs at minimal force levels. The position of the electrode is manipulated to record a sharply negative-going AP from one muscle fiber, which is used to trigger the oscilloscope sweep. The electronically delayed SFEMG signals are displayed on the oscilloscope. The trigger level on the oscilloscope is adjusted so the triggering AP appears stationary on the oscilloscope screen. The APs of muscle fibers belonging to the same MU as the triggering muscle fiber appear at a fixed position on the screen, whereas those from other active MUs appear randomly.

One may also stimulate the motor nerve fiber electrically to elicit APs from the muscle fibers it innervates.[94] The oscilloscope sweep is triggered by the stimulator, and SFEMG signals are displayed on the oscilloscope screen.

Quantitation

Three features of the SFEMG signals are measured: the neuromuscular jitter, the fiber density, and the mean interspike interval. To measure the jitter, the position of the electrode is manipulated to record APs from two or more muscle fibers from one MU (Figure 5-2, *A*). The interpotential interval (IPI), the time interval between a pair of selected APs, changes during successive discharges (Figure 5-2, *B* and *C*). This variability, the jitter, is quantitated as the mean value of consecutive differences of successive IPIs (MCD) and is calculated as

$$MCD = \frac{|IPI_2 - IPI_1| + |IPI_3 - IPI_2| + \ldots + |IPI_N - IPI_{N-1}|}{N - 1}$$

where IPIj is the IPI in the j-th of the N discharges recorded. While this is the formula most commonly used in automated systems,[5,85] simpler formulas based on the minimum and maximum IPIs in four to 10 successive discharges may be used when jitter is measured manually from photographed MUAP discharges.

In pathologic muscle some muscle fibers of the MU do not produce an AP with every discharge of the motor neuron (Figure 5-2, *C*). This is recognized when one AP of a pair is missing during some discharges and is called blocking. This phenomenon is quantitated by noting the percentage of end-plate pairs that showed blocking.

To measure the fiber density (FD), the electrode is positioned to maximize the amplitude of one AP, and the number of APs synchronous with this potential that have amplitude greater than 200 μV and rise time less than 300 μsec are counted. This number is determined for 20 different sites within a muscle, and the average of these 20 values is the FD. When more than one synchronous AP is seen at one site, the maximum IPI and the number of APs are

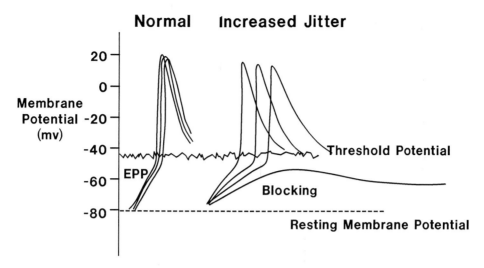

Figure 5-3. Schematic end-plate potentials and action potentials are shown to explain how low amplitude and slow rise of end-plate potentials is seen as increased jitter and blocking in single fiber EMG recordings.

measured. The interspike interval at that site is obtained by dividing the maximum IPI by the number of intervals, that is, the number of synchronous APs minus one. The mean of this value is called the mean interspike interval (MISI).

Relationship of features to motor unit

When the nerve AP reaches the nerve terminals, acetylcholine (ACh) is released into the synaptic cleft. It induces a depolarization of the muscle fiber membrane, called an end-plate potential. When the end-plate potential exceeds a threshold (which may vary slightly with time), an AP is produced and propagates from the end-plate toward the tendons (Figure 5-3). In a normal end-plate, sufficient ACh is released to produce a sharply rising end-plate potential that quickly reaches the threshold level, and an AP is elicited with every discharge of the motor neuron. When the quantity of ACh released from the nerve terminal is reduced, the end-plate potential is smaller and rises more slowly. Owing to the slow rise, the time to reach threshold is more variable, which is manifested as more variable IPIs. If the end-plate potential does not reach the threshold level, no AP is produced and this is noted as a block in the SFEMG recordings. Similar abnormalities are also seen when the number of ACh receptors in the end-plate is reduced. The jitter and blocking reflect the efficacy of neuromuscular transmission.

The SFEMG electrode records large amplitude APs (up to 20 mV) from muscle fibers close to the recording electrode. When the distance of the electrode from the muscle fiber is increased, the amplitude of the AP decreases rapidly. On average, when the muscle fiber is more than 300 μm from the electrode, the amplitude of its AP recorded by an SFEMG electrode is less than 200 μV.[87] Thus the number of synchronous APs counted in FD measurements is equal to the number of muscle fibers belonging to one MU that are within 300 μm of the recording surface. By virtue of the recording technique, the FD is always greater than or equal to 1. The neighboring fiber density (nFD) is obtained by subtracting 1 from the value of FD.[31] The nFD represents the average number of muscle fibers of one MU that are within 300 μm of one muscle fiber of that MU.

The MISI measures the time dispersion of APs of fibers belonging to one MU. It depends on a variety of MU features discussed earlier that affect the synchronicity of APs (Figure 5-1).

Normal values

Usually 20 or more sites are investigated in the tested muscle. The SFEMG features measured in normal subjects are summarized in Table 5-1.[32,89] Values within 2 standard deviations of the mean are considered normal. When the neuromuscular transmission is of interest, a study is called normal only if the mean MCD and at least 18 of 20 end-plates pairs have jitter within their corresponding normal limits. Note that a study may be normal even if one or two end-plate pairs have increased jitter. Blocking is usually not seen in a normal muscle. It should be emphasized that the normal values of jitter described in Table 5-1 reflect jitter measured between members of end-plate pairs. If electrical stimulation is used, one can measure jitter in individual end-plates and the normal values of jitter are smaller.[94] The FD increases with age and reflects the mild reinnervation known to occur in late decades.

Single fiber electromyography in pathologic muscle

SFEMG is the most sensitive technique for quantitating abnormalities of neuromuscular transmission, for example,

Table 5-1. Normal values of single fiber electromyography features

Muscle	Fiber density (mean ± standard deviation)			Mean MCD* (μsec) (mean ± standard deviation)	MCD in end-plate pair (μsec) (mean ± standard deviation)	MISI† (msec) (mean ± standard deviation)
	Age ≤ 60	60 < Age ≤ 70	Age > 70			
Extensor digitorum communis‡	1.46 ± 0.13	1.54 ± 0.16	2.01 ± 0.41	28.9 ± 4.7	27.4 ± 10.2	0.64 ± 0.3
Tongue§	1.48 ± 0.19			24.7 ± 4.4	25.5 ± 13.0	
Sternocleido-mastoid‡	1.64 ± 0.19			22.9 ± 5.4	22.8 ± 13.9	
Deltoid‡	1.32 ± 0.09			27.6 ± 4.7	27.4 ± 10.7	0.46 ± 0.17
Biceps‡	1.36 ± 0.13	1.45 ± 0.13	1.58 ± 0.19			0.42 ± 0.18
Adductor digiti quinti§	1.56 ± 0.17			30.8 ± 8.3	31.2 ± 12.9	
Tibialis anterior‡	1.62 ± 0.21	1.79 ± 0.35	1.83 ± 0.32	34.4 ± 4.9	34.8 ± 15.7	0.52 ± 0.13

Table compiled by J.M. Gilchrist.
*Mean value of consecutive differences of successive interpotential intervals.
†Mean interspike interval.
‡Data from E. Stalberg.
§Data from J.M. Gilchrist and D. Sanders.

in patients with myasthenia gravis or myasthenic syndrome. However, increased jitter does not always imply myasthenia.

In neurogenic diseases the jitter is increased and some blocking may also be seen.[88,89,93] This reflects the immaturity of the end-plates of muscle fibers undergoing reinnervation. In motor neuron disease, increased jitter may be seen before the FD increases.[47] In chronic reinnervated MUs the jitter is slightly increased and no blocking is seen. In patients with poliomyelitis, increased jitter and blocking are seen several years after the onset of the disease.[95] It is proposed that the reinnervated MUs are unable to maintain the enlarged pool of muscle fibers and some muscle fibers of the MU may lose their innervation. Increased jitter probably reflects this phenomenon.

In patients with myopathic diseases the jitter may be normal or sometimes increased.[38,89] In patients with muscular dystrophy the jitter is sometimes extremely low (less than 5 to 8 μsec). Low jitter is recorded when APs are recorded from two branches of a split muscle fiber that have a common motor end-plate.

In neurogenic diseases the FD increases because of reinnervation.[71,82,88,89,93] The FD also increases mildly in myopathic diseases (Figure 5-9) owing to regeneration of muscle fibers, split muscle fibers, and other factors.[80]

The changes in MISI in different diseases have not been investigated in detail. Other SFEMG abnormalities, such as concomitant jitter and blocking, recruitment, and interdischarge interval–dependent jitter, are seen in pathologic muscles,[89] but their details are beyond the scope of current discussion.

Concentric needle electromyography

The concentric needle EMG (CNEMG) electrode was developed by Adrian and Bronk[1] in 1929, the same year Sherrington[74] described the MU. More than 50 years later it is still the most widely used EMG electrode. Much of the earlier work on quantitation of CNEMG in normal and neuromuscular diseases and its relationship to the MU architecture was done by Buchthal and co-workers in the 1950s and later. The details of CNEMG recording techniques are described in most textbooks on EMG (see Chapter 3).[10,11,33,40]

Recording technique

The tip of the concentric needle (CN) electrode is ground to an angle of 15 degrees, exposing the elliptic recording surface (150 μm × 580 μm, 0.07 mm² surface area) of a 150 μm diameter central wire (Figure 5-4). The electrode cannula is used as the reference electrode. For distortion-free recordings the amplifier should have a high input impedance. Furthermore, the cutoff frequency of the low-pass and high-pass filters should be 10 kHz and 2 Hz, respectively.[11] Recordings are made at minimal force levels, and MUAPs from different MUs can be recognized visually.[11] With access to an electronic delay line, MUAP identification can be greatly simplified. The position of the electrode is slightly manipulated so MUAPs of only one MU trigger the oscilloscope sweep. When delayed signals are displayed on the oscilloscope screen, only the triggering MUAP appears stationary and other MUAPs occur randomly. The MUAP can be isolated by averaging these time-locked sweeps.

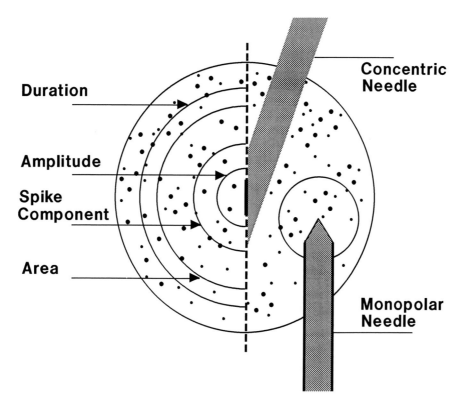

Figure 5-4. Schematic cross section of motor unit (MU) is shown. Active recording surface of concentric needle (CN) electrode, located in tip of needle, is at center of MU territory and records action potentials of muscle fibers that are in front of it (muscle fibers to left of dotted line). For different MUAP features, muscle fibers that mainly determine their numerical values are enclosed by semicircles. Radii of semicircles were estimated from computer simulation. Monopolar needle electrode is shown in right-hand side of MU territory. It has circular recording area, shown schematically by circle around electrode tip. Radius of circle has not been estimated, and therefore areas shown in figure should not be used to make comparisons between recording areas of CN and monopolar needle electrodes.

Recently a battery of techniques were developed that allow extraction of MUAPs from more than one MU recorded by the electrode.[3,51,85] The details of these techniques are beyond the scope of this discussion.

Quantitation

Usually 20 or more MUAPs are recorded from different sites in the tested muscle. The amplitude of the MUAP is defined from peak to peak. Phases of a MUAP (indicated by dots in Figure 5-5) are measured by adding 1 to the number of zero-crossings of the MUAP. A MUAP is called polyphasic when it has more than four phases. The beginning and end of the MUAP are assessed by visual inspection, and the time interval between these events is the duration of the MUAP. The subjective measurements of MUAP duration are sensitive to the display resolution, and therefore measurements are to be made under standard conditions of 100 μV/cm sensitivity.[11] In pathologic muscles the MUAP

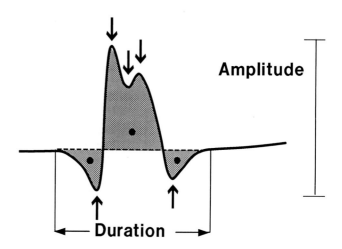

Figure 5-5. Schematic of motor unit action potential (MUAP) and its features. Arrows indicate turns, and filled circles indicate phases of MUAP.

waveform may change in successive discharges. The variability of the MUAP waveform is not quantitated, but the MUAPs are noted as being "unstable." New features of the MUAP have been proposed, such as number of turns (defined later and indicated by arrows in Figure 5-5), the area under the rectified MUAP waveform, area/amplitude ratio, and the duration of the spike component, which may increase the diagnostic sensitivity.[25,65,92]

Relationship to motor units

Computer simulations have been used to study the relationship between the features of the MUAP and the architecture of normal MUs.[3,54,64] The active recording surface of the CN electrode is surrounded by the metallic cannula on one side (Figure 5-4). The cannula acts as a shield; when it lies between the active recording surface and a muscle fiber, the AP of that muscle fiber is not recorded by the active surface. Thus the active recording surface records APs of all muscle fibers that lie in front of it, that is, to the left of the dotted line in Figure 5-4. The cannula, on the other hand, records APs from all muscle fibers in the MU. The portion of the MU territory that lies in front of the active surface is called the recording plane. If the electrode is rotated while its position is maintained, the fibers in the recording plane and the MUAP waveform change (unpublished observation). Therefore the CN electrode is directional and has a semicircular recording area.

Simulations indicate that the MUAP amplitude depends on the number and size of muscle fibers that are within 0.5 mm of the recording electrode and mainly on the size and distance of the closest muscle fiber (Figure 5-4).[64] When the dispersion of the APs of muscle fibers that are within 1 mm of the recording electrode increases, the MUAP waveform becomes polyphasic. The MUAP area and duration depend on the number of muscle fibers in the recording plane of the electrode and mainly on the fibers that are within 2 and 2.5 mm, respectively, of the electrode. The MUAP area also depends on the MUAP amplitude. Thus MUAP features provide complementary information about the MU architecture, and in a diseased muscle they do not always change in parallel. Furthermore, the above areas are smaller than the size of the MU territory. Therefore the MUAP waveform changes when recordings are made from different sites in the MU territory. This variability is best demonstrated by a technique called scanning EMG (discussed later). The instability of the MUAP reflects impaired neuromuscular transmission, which is quantitated by measuring jitter in SFEMG.

Normal values

Twenty or more MUAPs are recorded from the tested muscle. The mean amplitude, percentage of polyphasic MUAPs, and mean duration of MUAPs are calculated. The normal values of these features have been described by Rosenfalck and Rosenfalck,[69] and the mean duration values are reproduced in Table 5-2 for some muscles. The mean MUAP amplitude is in the range 100 to 400 μV. In most skeletal muscles less than 12% of MUAPs are polyphasic, and in deltoid and facial muscles up to 25% polyphasic MUAPs may be seen. The mean MUAP duration normally increases with age. MUAP durations are similar for different normal muscles, although the size of the muscles themselves, and perhaps the size of the MUs, is quite different. This is consistent with computer simulations showing that the MUAP duration depends mainly on the number of muscle fibers within a certain area around the electrode and not on all the muscle fibers in the MU.

When the MUAP duration is measured subjectively, the duration of the same MUAP measured by different operators is known to differ.[65,91] Even with automatic measurements the duration values vary owing to differences in the criteria for measurement.[91] Furthermore, the duration can be affected by technical factors such as the filter settings and the impedance of the amplifier.[14] Therefore it is of utmost importance for each laboratory to verify the values described in Table 5-2 or to define their own normal set of data.

Stewart and co-workers[92] have recorded MUAPs in the biceps muscle of 69 healthy subjects and have measured the features of the MUAPs using a computer-based automatic system. While the normal values of mean duration were similar to those in Table 5-2, the normal range of mean amplitude was from 200 μV to 800 μV. The data also showed a higher incidence of polyphasic MUAPs (15% to 20%) in some normal subjects.

The larger range of amplitude in normal subjects may be due to at least two factors. First, to facilitate MUAP extraction by a triggered delay line, the position of the electrode was manipulated to maximize the amplitude of each MUAP. Second, in this technique the larger MUAPs are selected for analysis in preference to smaller amplitude MUAPs. Rosenfalck and Rosenfalck[69] did not manipulate the electrode position and identified MUAPs by visual inspection. This allowed them to include the smaller amplitude MUAPs in analysis.

The sensitivity of MUAP amplitude to slight changes in the position of the recording electrode is demonstrated by two recordings of MUAPs from the same MU (Figure 5-6, *A*).

Findings in pathologic muscles

The typical changes in the EMG features in neurogenic and myopathic diseases are summarized by Buchthal and Kamieniecka (Table 5-3).[18] The abnormalities are also shown from waveforms of MUAPs recorded from the biceps muscle of a normal subject, a patient with myopathy and a patient with neuropathy (Figure 5-6).

In neurogenic diseases the time dispersion of APs may increase because of slow conducting terminal axon branches of the reinnervated MUs, slow propagation of APs in the reinnervated muscle fibers that had atrophied after dener-

Table 5-2. Mean duration of CNEMG MUAPs in normal subjects*

Muscle	Mean MUAP duration (msec)								
	Age: 5 yr	10	15	20	30	40	50	60	70
Extensor digitorum communis	7.8	8.4	8.8	9.2	9.8	10.2	10.5	11.0	11.4
Frontalis	4.5	4.8	5.1	5.3	5.4	5.5	5.6	5.7	5.8
Sternocleido-mastoid	7.1	7.6	8.1	8.4	8.9	9.3	9.6	10.0	10.4
Deltoid	8.6	9.3	9.8	10.2	10.7	11.3	11.6	12.1	12.6
Biceps	8.5	9.1	9.6	10.0	10.6	11.1	11.4	11.9	12.4
Triceps	9.9	10.6	11.2	11.6	12.0	12.2	12.4	12.6	12.8
Vastus lateralis	10.7	11.5	12.1	12.6	13.4	14.0	14.4	15.0	15.6
Tibialis anterior	10.5	11.2	11.7	12.3	13.1	13.6	14.0	14.7	15.3

From Rosenfalck, P, and Rosenfalck, A: Electromyography and sensory/motor conductions: findings in normal subjects, Copenhagen, 1975, Laboratory of Clinical Neurophysiology, Rigshospitalet.
*Deviations less than 20% are considered normal.

Table 5-3. Electromyographic criteria in neurogenic and myopathic diseases

EMG procedure	Myopathy	Neurogenic impairment owing to diseases of peripheral nerve or root	Anterior horn cell involvement
Motor unit potentials (weak effort)	Decrease in total duration*; increase in incidence of polyphasic MUAPs; decrease in amplitude	Increase in total duration*; increase in amplitude*; increased incidence of polyphasic MUAPs	Increase in total duration*; increase in amplitude (>200%)
Pattern of recruitment (full effort)	Full recruitment in a weak and wasted muscle*; decrease in amplitude*†	Discrete activity*; increase in amplitude*†	Increase in amplitude*†‡; discrete activity*
Pattern of recruitment (30% of maximum force)	Increase in number of turns (NT)*; decrease in amplitude between turns (MA); increase in NT/MA ratio*; increase in incidence of short intervals between turns	Decrease in NT/MA ratio*; increase in MA*; decrease in NT*; increase in incidence of long intervals between turns*	

From Buchthal, F, and Kamieniecka, Z: Muscle Nerve 5:265, 1982.
*Specific EMG criterion.
†Amplitude measured by envelope curves by negative and positive peaks, excluding high solitary peaks. Decreased when less than 2 mV.[69]
‡More than 6 mV.

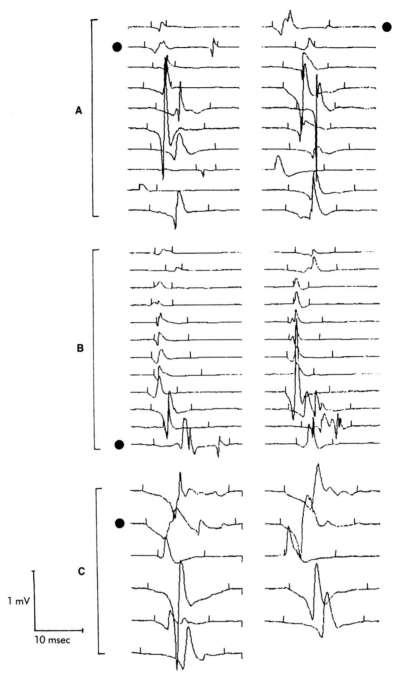

Figure 5-6. Concentric needle EMG motor unit action potentials (MUAPs) were recorded from biceps muscle of, **A,** normal subject, **B,** patient with polymyositis, and **C,** patient with motor neuron disease. All of them were 22 to 25 years old. Each muscle showed MUAPs with late components (indicated by filled circles next to their waveforms). In **A,** top MUAP in right column was recorded after manipulating electrode position to maximize amplitude of its negative peak. When position of electrode changed slightly, another MUAP was recorded from same MU (second MUAP from top in left column). In later position, MUAP amplitude fell and amplitude of late component increased, making it more prominent. This shows sensitivity of MUAP amplitude to slight changes in electrode position. MUAP amplitude shows great variability, and in this example it was from 120 μV to 2 mV. In **B,** mean duration of all MUAPs was normal. When polyphasic MUAPs (second and third last MUAPs in right column and also MUAP with late component in left column) were excluded, duration was reduced, indicating myopathy. MUAP amplitude and duration were increased in **C.**

vation, or increased width of the end-plate zone. In myopathic diseases the variability of fiber diameter and thus the variability of AP propagation velocity increase. Because of increased time dispersion the MUAPs are polyphasic in myopathy and neuropathy.

In myopathy the duration of MUAPs may increase owing to greatly increased time dispersion of APs (Figure 5-6, *B*).[66] Sometimes individual APs that occur several milliseconds after the main complex of the MUAP can be recognized. These are called satellite potentials or late components. Late components are also seen in neurogenic diseases and occasionally in normal muscle (Figure 5-6).[43] Since increased time dispersion of APs makes MUAP duration less dependent on the number of muscle fibers, perhaps the polyphasic MUAPs should not be included in duration measurements.[12,53a]

In neurogenic diseases the number of muscle fibers in the MU, and hence in the recording plane of the electrode, increases. Therefore the MUAP duration is greater. Conversely, in myopathic disease the individual muscle fibers in the MU are lost. Therefore the MUAP duration is reduced.

In neurogenic diseases, reinnervated MUs consist of groups of contiguous muscle fibers. Because of increased numbers of muscle fibers of the same MU near the electrode, the MUAP amplitude increases. Since a normal amplitude MUAP can be recorded even when only one muscle fiber is close to the recording electrode, this feature is not sensitive to loss of muscle fibers in myopathic diseases.[55] Occasionally, large amplitude MUAPs are recorded in a patient with myopathy, which probably reflects an increase in the size of the muscle fiber closest to the electrode.[92]

Normal values of features such as the number of turns, spike duration, area, and area/amplitude ratio have been described for the biceps muscle.[25,65,92] It would be premature to comment on their sensitivity for detecting disease processes.

Monopolar needle electromyography

The active recording surface of a monopolar needle electrode is the surface of a cone at the tip of a pointed wire (Figure 5-4). The wire is insulated except at the cone-shaped tip. The area of the recording surface can change because of deterioration of the insulation but is usually from 0.14 to 0.21 mm.[2] A remote surface or intramuscular needle electrode is used as reference. The MUAPs are recorded as in CNEMG. The amplitude, duration, and number of phases are used for quantitation and show the same patterns of abnormalities in pathologic MUs as the patterns seen in CNEMG MUAP analysis.[52]

The most important difference between the monopolar needle and CN electrode is in their recording areas. Because of the electrode cannula the CN electrode has directional properties and the MUAP waveform changes owing to rotation of the electrode. The monopolar needle electrode has a circular recording area (Figure 5-4), and the MUAP is not sensitive to the rotation of the electrode. Since the record-

ing surfaces are of similar sizes, the CN electrode and the monopolar needle electrode should record APs of similar amplitudes from muscle fibers that are at the same distance; that is, these electrodes have similar "selectivity." (Some differences would be expected because of geometry of the recording area, as described by Ekstedt and Stalberg.[23]) However, owing to its circular recording area, the monopolar needle records APs from more muscle fibers of the MU than does the CN electrode.

The cannula and the active CN electrode record APs of roughly the same amplitude from distant muscle fibers belonging to other active MUs. Their APs are cancelled when the cannula signals are subtracted to obtain the CNEMG MUAP. Thus CNEMG MUAPs have a better signal/noise ratio than do monopolar needle MUAPs. Since there is no corresponding cancellation of APs from the cannula in monopolar needle EMG, MUAPs also have longer duration.

Chu-Andrews, Bruyninckx, and Chan[21] have described the normal values of MUAP features recorded by a monopolar needle electrode. Compared with the CNEMG recordings, the MUAPs had higher amplitude, duration, and incidence of polyphasic MUAPs. We emphasize that the normal values of MUAP features described for CNEMG recordings should not be used to assess abnormalities of MUAPs recorded by a monopolar needle electrode.

With deterioration of insulation on the monopolar needle, the size of the recording surface increases and therefore the MUAP amplitude decreases.

Macro electromyography
Recording technique

In macro EMG the recording surface is the cannula of a modified SFEMG electrode that is insulated except for a length of 15 mm at the tip (Figure 5-7, *A*).[81] An SFEMG recording surface is located at the midpoint of the bared portion of the cannula and on the side opposite the beveled tip. The EMG is recorded as the potential difference between the cannula and a remote subcutaneous or surface electrode. The electrode is positioned to maximize the amplitude of the AP of a single muscle fiber recorded by the SFEMG recording surface. This signal (Figure 5-7, *B*) is used to trigger the oscilloscope, and the delayed cannula signals (Figure 5-7, *C*) are displayed on the oscilloscope screen. The macro EMG MUAP of the MU from which the triggering SFEMG signal is derived appears stationary on the screen during successive discharges. Several time-locked sweeps are averaged to extract the MUAP (Figure 5-7, *D*). MUs are selected based on the SFEMG potentials, and thus there is no bias in selecting MUAPs for averaging.

Quantitation

Usually 20 or more MUAPs are recorded from the tested muscle. The amplitude of an MUAP is defined from peak to peak. The complexity of the MUAP waveform is assessed by measuring the number of peaks. The area is measured from the rectified waveform.

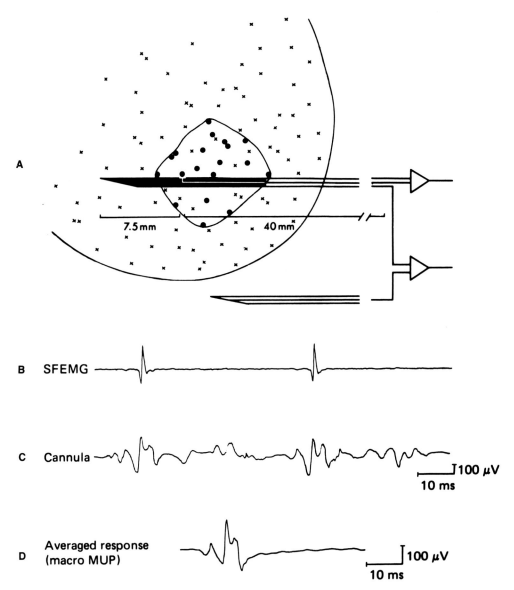

A

B   SFEMG

C   Cannula

100 μV
10 ms

D   Averaged response
(macro MUP)

100 μV
10 ms

Figure 5-7. A, Schematic of macro EMG electrode recording motor unit action potential (MUAP) from motor unit. Single fiber EMG signal **(B)** is used to trigger averager, and cannula signals **(C)** are averaged to obtain MUAP **(D).** (From Stalberg, E: J Neurol Neurosurg Psychiatry 43:475, 1980.)

Relationship to motor unit architecture

Computer simulations have been used to understand the relationship between the MU architecture and the macro EMG MUAP features.[61] The MUAP amplitude and area depend mainly on the number of muscle fibers in the MU and are less sensitive to the distribution of the muscle fibers in the MU territory. Therefore these features reflect the MU size. When recordings are made from different sites within one MU, the MUAP waveform is relatively constant (Figure 5-8). The MUAP area is less variable than the MUAP amplitude and therefore is a better choice for measuring the MU size. However, the area measurements are less accurate than the amplitude measurements when the signal/noise ratio is poor. When the end-plate zone or the variability of the muscle fiber diameters is increased, the MUAP waveform becomes complex. Complex MUAP waveforms were also produced when MU fractions were simulated.

The macro EMG MUAPs of the higher force threshold MUs have large amplitude.[83] This indicates the larger size of the higher force threshold MUs as indicated by the size principle.[37]

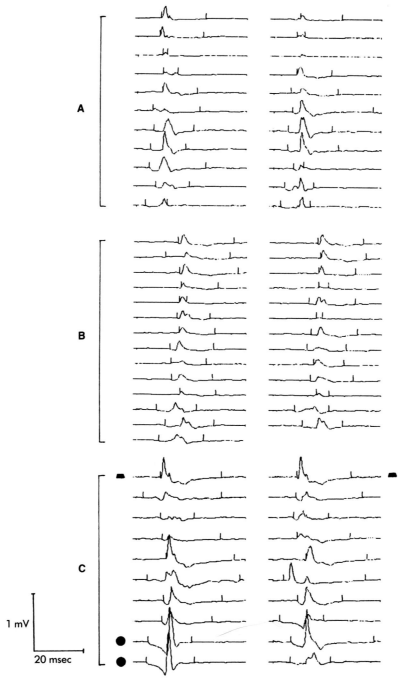

Figure 5-8. Macro EMG motor unit action potentials (MUAPs) were recorded from the biceps muscle of, **A,** normal subject, **B,** patient with polymyositis, and **C,** patient with motor neuron disease. When MUAP recordings are made repeatedly from same motor unit, MUAP waveforms are similar and can be identified by visual inspection. Two such pairs of MUAPs are seen in **C** and are identified by filled circles and filled rectangle. Median macro EMG MUAP amplitude was normal in **B** and increased in **C.** Fiber density was increased in both patients and was greater in **C.** Concentric needle EMG MUAPs recorded from same muscle are shown in Figure 5-6.

Normal values

The normal values of macro EMG MUAP features for different age groups and in different muscles (Table 5-4) have been described by Stalberg and Fawcett.[86] Most MUAPs had fewer than four peaks. Because of the skewed distribution of amplitude and area values in individual studies, median values were used rather than mean values. Normal limits were defined for the individual MUAP amplitudes and also for the median MUAP amplitude. A study is called abnormal if the median MUAP amplitude is outside the normal range or if two of 20 MUAPs have amplitude outside the normal range. The larger amplitude of macro EMG MUAPs in later decades reflects the mild reinnervation known to take place with age.

Pathologic findings

The changes in macro EMG MUAP amplitude reflect changes in the size of the MUs. In patients with neurogenic disease the amplitude increases because of increased MU size following reinnervation (Figure 5-8, *C*). In patients with chronic reinnervated MUs the individual MUAP amplitude has been found to be more than 10 times the mean amplitude of MUAPs in normal muscles.[82,88] When pattern recognition techniques were used to investigate waveform abnormalities, many MUAPs recorded from patients with amyotrophic lateral sclerosis had MUAPs with normal amplitude but increased area.[63] Furthermore, the MUAP waveforms were complex and less symmetric about the baseline.

In patients with myopathic disease the macro MUAP amplitude is usually normal or only slightly reduced (Figure 5-9, *C*).[39,81] When the data from patients with myopathy are pooled, the reduced MUAP amplitude is more obvious (Figure 5-9, *B* and *D*). The normal amplitude of macro EMG MUAPs, despite apparent loss of muscle fibers indicated by the smaller duration of CNEMG MUAPs, is rather surprising. This discrepancy is discussed in greater detail later in this chapter. In patients with disuse atrophy, as occurs with chronic immobilization of a limb, the MUAP amplitude is slightly reduced.[73]

MEASUREMENT OF MOTOR UNIT TERRITORY

The size of the MU territory is quantitated by measuring the longest distance over which muscle fibers belonging to one MU are found. If the MU territory is circular, this distance represents the diameter of the MU territory. The MU territory can be measured by two techniques: scanning EMG[84] and multielectrode EMG.[17]

Scanning electromyography
Recording technique

Scanning EMG requires two recording electrodes: an SFEMG electrode and usually a concentric needle electrode. The SFEMG electrode is used to record AP from one muscle fiber of an MU. This recording is used to identify the MU under investigation. The CNEMG electrode is then inserted into the muscle, and the EMG is recorded on a second channel. The SFEMG triggers an oscilloscope, and the delayed CNEMG signals are displayed. The CNEMG MUAPs of the MU from which the SFEMG is derived appear stationary on the screen. When such synchronized SFEMG and CNEMG signals are recorded, the CNEMG electrode is pushed deeper into the muscle so that its recording tip is beyond the MU territory. In this recording position an inverted MUAP with low amplitude is seen on the CNEMG channel (Figure 5-10, *A*).

When the MU discharges, the SFEMG signal triggers the oscilloscope and one CNEMG MUAP discharge is seen on the oscilloscope screen. Following each discharge the CN electrode is pulled a distance of 50 μm by a step motor, controlled by a computer that also acquires the MUAPs. Thus MUAPs are recorded from different positions in the MU territory with successive motor neuron firings (Figure 5-10, *B*). The procedure is continued until the tip of the electrode has been pulled through the entire MU territory.

Relationship to motor unit architecture

When the electrode has passed through the entire MU territory and the active recording tip is beyond the MU territory, no potential is recorded by the active electrode. The MUAP is then the inversion of the potential recorded by the cannula, that is, the macro EMG MUAP (Figure 5-10, *A*). When the tip of the electrode is within the MU territory, CN MUAPs are recorded (Figure 5-10, *B*). When the cannula and the active recording surface are both outside the MU territory, no MUAP is recorded. Thus the length of scan over which CN MUAPs are recorded is the diameter of the MU territory. (Usually, different positions of the CN electrode are tested to obtain the longest scan length. This ensures that the measured length is the diameter and not a chord of the MU territory.)

The scanning EMG is most impressive in demonstrating the variability of MUAP waveforms within one MU. Furthermore, the spike components of MUAPs have different latencies in different portions of the MU territory. It is inferred that the motor axon forms two or three main branches when it enters the muscle (Figure 5-10, *C*). Each branch innervates muscle fibers within a small portion of the MU territory. The muscle fibers innervated by one branch are called an MU fraction. As the electrode passes from one MU fraction to another, the latency of the spike component changes owing to differences in the length of the axon branches, differences in their AP propagation velocities, and perhaps differences in the end-plate zones for different fractions. It appears that the CN MUAP reflects the architecture of the MU fraction in which the recording tip is located.

As the tip of the CN electrode enters the MU territory,

Table 5-4. Normal limits of macro EMG MUAP amplitudes

	Biceps				Vastus lateralis				Tibialis anterior			
	Median		Individual		Median		Individual		Median		Individual	
Age (yr)	Min	Max	Min	Max	Min	Max	Min	Max	Min	Max	Min	Max
10-19	65	100	30	350	70	150	20	350	65	200	30	350
20-29	65	140	30	350	70	240	20	525	65	250	30	450
30-39	65	180	30	400	70	240	20	550	65	260	30	450
40-49	65	180	30	500	70	250	20	575	65	330	30	575
50-59	65	180	30	500	70	260	20	575	65	375	40	700
60-69	65	250	30	650	80	370	20	1250	120	375	45	700
70-79	65	250	30	650	90	600	20	1250	120	620	65	800

From Stalberg, E, and Fawcett, P: J Neurosurg Psychiatry 45:870, 1982.

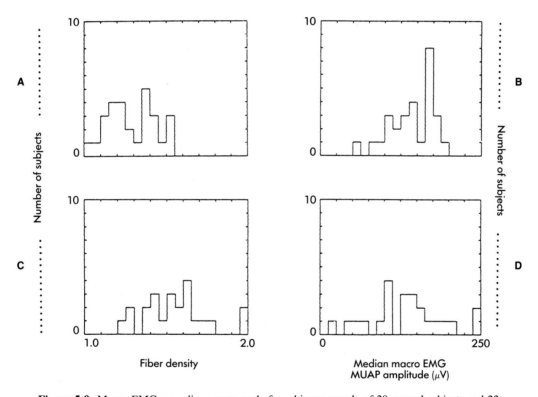

Figure 5-9. Macro EMG recordings were made from biceps muscle of 28 normal subjects and 23 patients with myopathy. Fiber density (FD) was also measured. Distribution of FD and median macro EMG motor unit action potential (MUAP) amplitude values in normal subjects are shown in **A** and **B**, respectively. In patients with myopathy, FD was increased **(C)**, but most patients had macro EMG MUAPs of normal amplitude **(D)**.

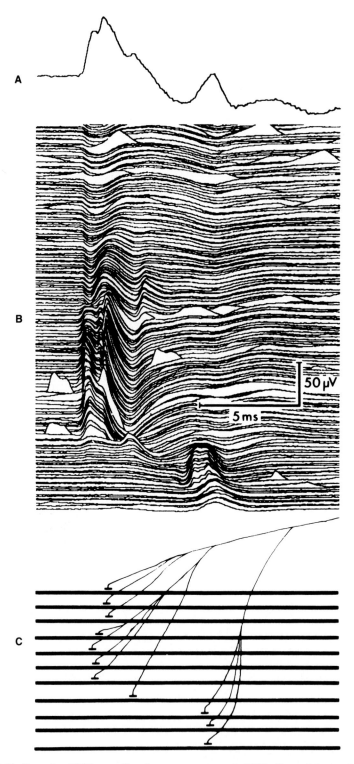

Figure 5-10. Scanning EMG recording from one motor unit (MU). Potential recorded by cannula before scan (**A**) represents macro EMG motor unit action potential (MUAP) from MU. Concentric needle EMG MUAPs recorded from MU when electrode was pulled through territory in steps of 50 μm (**B**) show variability of MUAP waveform. Model for innervation of muscle fibers in MU is proposed (**C**) to explain different latencies of spike component. (From Nandedkar, S, and Stalberg, E: EEG Clin Neurophysiol 56:52, 1983.)

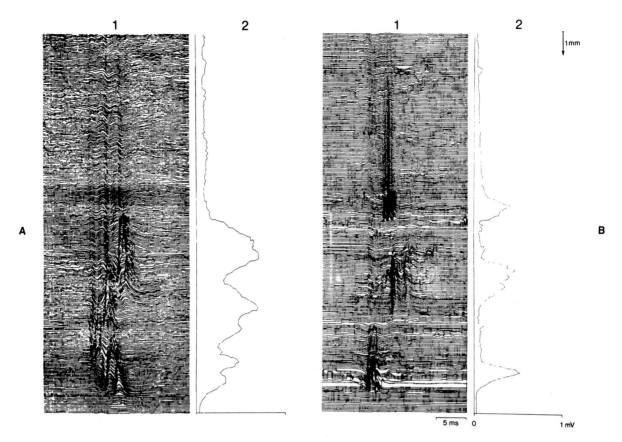

Figure 5-11. Motor unit action potentials (MUAPs) recorded in scanning EMG *(1)* from, **A,** normal motor unit (MU) and, **B,** MU from patient with muscular dystrophy. On right of potentials, variation in MUAP amplitude during scan *(2)* is indicated. Amplitude profile shows two silent areas in **B.** (From Hilton-Brown, P, and Stalberg, E: J Neurol Neurosurg Psychiatry 46:996, 1983.)

Table 5-5. Motor unit territory in normal subjects and patients with muscular dystrophy

Muscle	Total scan length (mm) (mean ± standard deviation)		Silent area/scan	
	Normal	**LG + FSH***	**Normal**	**LG + FSH***
Biceps	6.02 ± 3.91	7.87 ± 2.28	0.5	1.0
Tibialis anterior	7.87 ± 1.30	8.09 ± 3.10	0.2	1.2

From Hilton-Brown, P, and Stalberg, E: J Neurol Neurosurg Psychiatry 46:996, 1983.
*LG + FSH, Limb girdle and facioscapulohumeral dystrophy.

the amplitude of the MUAP increases. It varies as the scan is continued and then is reduced as the electrode leaves the MU territory. This variation of MUAP amplitude during a scan is shown in Figure 5-11, *A*. Occasionally, however, one may find an area in the MU territory where no MUAPs are seen. In such a case the amplitude profile shows areas of low amplitude (Figure 5-11, *B*). These so-called silent areas of the MU territory contain no muscle fiber of the MU in the immediate vicinity of the tip of the CN electrode.

Normal values

Each scan is quantitated by two features: the diameter of the MU territory and the number of silent areas. Their normal values are described in Table 5-5.[39]

Pathologic findings

In patients with neuropathy the scanning EMG reveals large-amplitude and long-duration MUAPs at different positions of the electrode. The MU territory is normal or mildly

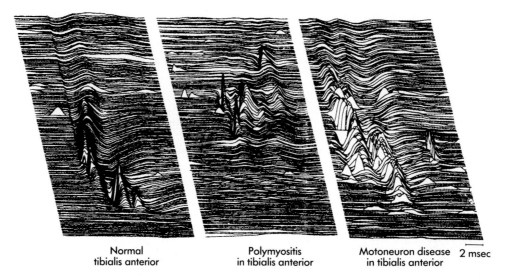

Normal
tibialis anterior

Polymyositis
in tibialis anterior

Motoneuron disease   2 msec
in tibialis anterior

Figure 5-12. Scanning EMG recordings from tibialis anterior muscle of normal subject *(left),* patient with polymyositis *(center),* and patient with motor neuron disease *(right).* Their interpretations are described in text. (From Stalberg, E, and Antoni, L: Computer-aided EMG analysis. In Desmedt, J, editor: Computer-aided electromyography, Basel, 1983, Karger.)

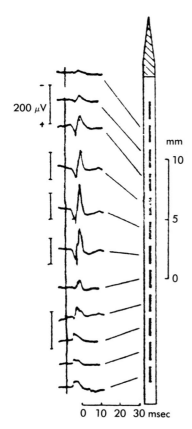

Figure 5-13. Schematic of multielectrode containing 12 recording surfaces that was used to measure motor unit (MU) territory. Motor unit action potentials from one MU recorded by each surface are shown on left. (From Buchthal, F, et al: Acta Physiol Scand 39:83, 1957.)

increased. The scanning EMG of an MU in a patient with motor neuron disease is shown in Figure 5-12. Note that the MUAPs appear normal in the beginning of the scan but become complex and long in duration in the second half of the scan. A late component is also seen. This shows ongoing reinnervation within a portion of the MU territory that overlaps with the territory of a lost MU.

In patients with myopathy, short-duration, polyphasic MUAPs are seen. The size of the MU territory is normal. In patients with muscular dystrophy, silent areas are more frequent than in normal MUs (Table 5-5).[39] A scan in a patient with polymyositis (Figure 5-12) shows simple MUAPs of short duration initially. This gives way to a silent area and then polyphasic MUAPs of long duration. These examples vividly demonstrate the variability of CNEMG MUAPs within one MU and also demonstrate that MUAPs may be normal and abnormal in different recording sites within the same MU.

Multielectrode electromyography

Instead of pulling a CNEMG electrode through the MU territory, Buchthal, Guld, and Rosenfalck[17] used an electrode containing 12 recording surfaces distributed over a length of 25 mm to examine the MUAP at different positions within the MU territory (Figure 5-13). The interelectrode distance was 0.5 mm. The MUAP of one MU was measured from each recording surface. The position of the electrode was adjusted so the central recording surfaces registered the largest amplitude MUAP. The occurrence of a positive-to-negative deflection in the potential of less than 0.2 msec duration, called a spike, was taken as evidence that an active

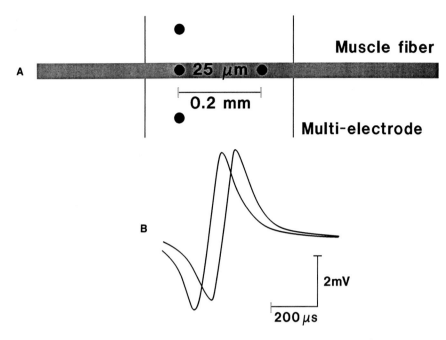

Figure 5-14. A, Schematic of multielectrode used to measure action potential (AP) propagation velocity of muscle fiber. For simplicity, three recording surfaces from one row and one recording surface from second row are shown. APs recorded by central recording surface in left row and by surface on right have similar shapes and amplitudes (**B**). Time interval between these APs is time for AP to travel distance between aforementioned two surfaces, that is, 200 μm.

muscle fiber was near the electrode. The distance between the extreme surfaces that recorded spikes was taken as the size of the MU territory.

The size of the MU territory thus measured in different muscles in normal subjects is summarized in Table 5-6.[13] In patients with neuropathy, Erminio, Buchthal, and Rosenfalck[24] found increased MU territory. The increase was greatest, up to 140%, in patients with anterior cell disease. In patients with limb-girdle and facioscapulohumeral dystrophies, Buchthal, Rosenfalck, and Erminio[19] found normal MU territory, as did Hilton-Brown and Stalberg (Table 5-6).[39] In progressive muscular dystrophies Buchthal and co-workers[19] found reduced MU territory.

MEASUREMENT OF ACTION POTENTIAL PROPAGATION VELOCITY

Two methods of measuring the AP propagation velocity are described. Buchthal, Guld, and Rosenfalck[15,16] recorded APs at different points along the muscle fibers. By dividing the distance between the recording sites by the time intervals between the APs, they calculated the AP propagation velocity. APs were elicited either by voluntary activation or by electrical stimulation. In the biceps muscle the mean AP propagation velocity was 4 M/sec during electrical stimulation[15] and 4.7 M/sec during voluntary activation.[16]

Table 5-6. Motor unit territory in normal muscles

Muscle	Mean MU territory (mm)
Biceps brachii	5.1
Tibialis anterior	7.0
Deltoid	6.7
Extensor digitorum communis	5.5

From Buchthal, F, Erminio, F, and Rosenfalck, P: Acta Physiol Scand 45:72, 1959.

No significant difference in AP propagation velocity was found between children and adults.

Stalberg[79] described another method of measuring AP propagation velocity. He used a multielectrode with two rows of SF recording surfaces along the electrode axis that were separated by about 200 μm (Figure 5-14, *A*). One row contained three (or one) recording surfaces and the other contained 11 (or 13). The position of the electrode was manipulated so a line connecting the neighboring electrodes from the two rows was parallel to the axis of the muscle fiber. In this position the two recording surfaces recorded

APs of similar amplitude and shape (Figure 5-14, *B*). The time difference between the APs recorded by the neighboring electrodes is the propagation time required for the AP to travel 200 μm. Thus the propagation velocity can be calculated. AP propagation velocity values for some muscles are described in Table 5-7. AP propagation velocity is lower in muscles that have smaller diameter muscle fibers. Stalberg[79] also found the AP propagation velocity to be lower in children and in an atrophied limb of an adult patient after immobilization in a cast.

ANALYSIS OF ELECTROMYOGRAPHIC INTERFERENCE PATTERN

The MUAPs can easily be recorded and analyzed when the subject exerts only minimal force. When the force of contraction is increased, more MUs are recruited and the firing rates of MUs also increase. The EMG signals become complex, and individual MUAPs cannot be recognized. The EMG recordings made at moderate and maximum contraction forces, called the interference pattern (IP), contain information about the number, size, and order of recruitment of the higher force threshold MUs. The IP signals are usually assessed by their appearance on the oscilloscope screen and their sound on an audio monitor. IP analysis includes assessment of the number of spikes and their size. The criteria for neurogenic and myopathic abnormalities of the IP have been described by Buchthal[18] and are summarized in Table 5-3.

Although a number of methods of quantitating the IP have been developed, we discuss only those based on the concept of so-called turns of the IP. Turns analysis is perhaps the most widely used quantitative technique of IP analysis in clinical EMG. It has been used to investigate different muscles, and thus normal values are available. It has a high diagnostic yield. Furthermore, the analysis is now being included in some commercially available electromyographs. The concept of a turn was first proposed by Willison.[96] The turns of an EMG signal are shown schematically in Figure 5-15 and have the following characteristics:

1. A turn occurs at a peak of the IP signal where the signal changes its direction.
2. If a turn occurs on a positive-going peak (for example, turn T2 in Figure 5-15), the preceding and the succeeding turns occur on negative-going peaks (for example, turns T1 and T3 in Figure 5-15), and vice versa.
3. Successive turns occur at peaks that differ by 100 μV or more in amplitude levels.

The EMG IP is usually recorded by a concentric needle or a monopolar needle electrode while the subject exerts a defined force of contraction. An epoch of defined duration is measured at a constant contraction level, and the number of turns (NT) is measured. The NT reflects the frequency of spikes in the IP. To quantitate the size of the spikes, the amplitude difference between successive turns is measured

Table 5-7. AP propagation velocity in normal muscles

Muscle	AP propagation velocity (M/sec) (mean ± standard deviation)
Biceps	3.69 ± 0.71
Frontalis	2.01 ± 0.39
Extensor digitorum communis	3.15 ± 0.75
Femoral quadriceps	3.39 ± 0.68

From Stalberg, E: Acta Physiol Scand 70(suppl 287):1, 1966.

and the mean value, called the mean amplitude (MA), is calculated. The MA increases with the force of contraction at all levels of activation. The NT reaches its maximum value when the force of contraction is roughly 50% of maximum. With further increase in the force of contraction, the NT increases very little or may even decrease slightly (Figure 5-16).[27,53]

Computer simulations have been used to study the relationship between the number, size, and firing rate of MUAPs and the IP features. Simulations indicated the following[56]:

1. The NT increases with the total number of MUAP discharges. Thus it depends on the number of active MUs and their firing rates. However, the rate of increase of NT decreases when the number of MUAP discharges is high. This explains the relatively constant values of NT at high levels of force of contraction when most MUs have been recruited and are firing at high rates. Furthermore, several MUs must be lost before the NT values recorded at maximum force of contraction are reduced.
2. The MA increases when the amplitude of the component MUAPs is increased. When the force of contraction is increased, more MUs are recruited, some of which also have large-amplitude MUAPs owing to their proximity to the recording electrode and larger size of muscle fibers belonging to the high force threshold MUs. Because of increased size of the component MUAPs, MA increases with force at all levels of contractions.

Clearly the patterns of abnormalities of IP features in pathologic muscles depend on the force of contraction at which IP recordings are made. This is demonstrated by the findings reported by different investigators and summarized in Table 5-8.

Stalberg and co-workers[90] have described a method of IP analysis, called turns and amplitude (TA), in which IP signals are recorded at different force levels ranging from minimal to maximal at each of six to 10 recording sites within a muscle. From each recording the NT and MA are calculated and a plot of MA versus NT is constructed (Figure 5-17). On this plot an area called a cloud is defined. The cloud contains more than 95% of the data points obtained

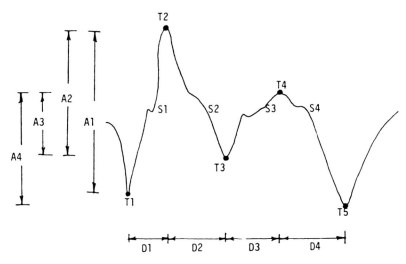

Figure 5-15. Schematic of EMG signal shows five turns *(T1 to T5)* that define four segments *(S1 to S4)* whose durations *(D1 to D4)* and amplitudes *(A1 to A4)* are indicated. (From Nandedkar, S, et al: Muscle Nerve 9:431, 1986.)

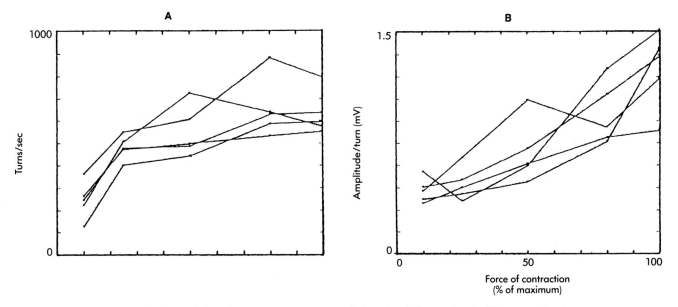

Figure 5-16. EMG interference pattern was recorded at five different sites in biceps muscle of normal subject when force of contraction was increased from 10% to 100% of maximum. Change in, **A,** number of turns (NT) and, **B,** mean amplitude (MA) with increasing force of contraction is shown. Data from each site are connected. NT increased until force was roughly 50% of maximum and thereafter increased slightly or decreased. MA increased with force at all levels of contraction.

Table 5-8. Comparison of interference pattern analysis when measured at different force levels in biceps brachii

Investigators	Force	Neuropathy	Myopathy
Rose and Willison[68]	2 kg	—	Increased number of turns
Hayward and Willison[36]	2 kg	Increased mean amplitude without significant change in number of turns	—
Fuglsang-Frederiksen, Scheel, and Buchthal[28,29]	30% of maximum	Increased mean amplitude and decreased number of turns	Increased and decreased number of turns
Sica, McComas, and Ferreira[76]	Maximum	Decreased number of turns in motor neuron disease only	Decreased mean amplitude; decreased number of turns

From Nandedkar, S, et al: Muscle Nerve 9:431, 1986.

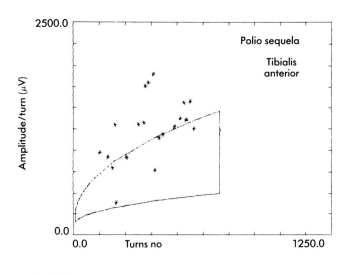

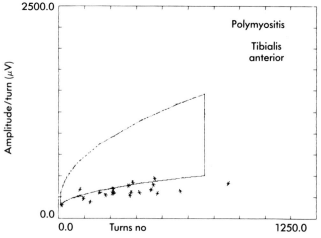

Figure 5-17. Results of interference pattern analysis in patients with old polio and polymyositis, using technique described by Stalberg and co-workers. For each recorded epoch, values of mean amplitude versus number of turns are plotted and superimposed on "cloud," which defines normal limits. (From Stalberg, E, et al: EEG Clin Neurophysiol 56:672, 1983.)

from a normal muscle. For each of the investigated muscle—biceps, tibialis anterior, extensor digitorum communis, and quadriceps—Stalberg and colleagues developed eight clouds representing combinations of three variables: sex, age, and the type of recording electrode (monopolar or concentric). A study is called normal only if more than 90% of the data points are inside the normal cloud. In patients with neuropathy, some data points lie outside and on the upper side of the cloud. In patients with myopathy, some data points lie below and outside the normal cloud. Because of contrasting patterns of distribution of data points (Figure 5-17), this technique is useful to differentiate between myopathy and neuropathy.

Fuglsang-Frederiksen, Scheel, and Buchthal[28,29] found the ratio NT/MA most useful to differentiate between myopathy and neuropathy. Smyth[78] used this feature to analyze IP recordings made in children in whom the force of contraction could not be controlled. The MA/NT ratio was calculated for each recording, and the mean of this value was found to be decreased in myopathy and increased in neuropathy. Haridasan[34] described the mean values of mean NT/MA ratio in the adductor digiti minimi, biceps brachii, and vastus medialis muscles of normal adults.

Kopec and co-workers[42] described an automatic method of analyzing the EMG signals using an analyzer of periodic noise discharges (ANOPS) computer. The reciprocal of the mean time interval between successive negative peaks, called density (measured in hertz), and the mean amplitude change between successive negative and positive peaks were measured.[35] The IP was analyzed when patients exerted maximal force of contraction.[41] Patients with myopathy had higher density and lower amplitudes compared with normal subjects. In patients with motor neuron disease the density was reduced while the amplitudes were higher.

The extraction of IP features described so far is very different from the way the IP signals are subjectively assessed. Nandedkar, Sanders, and Stalberg[58] described three

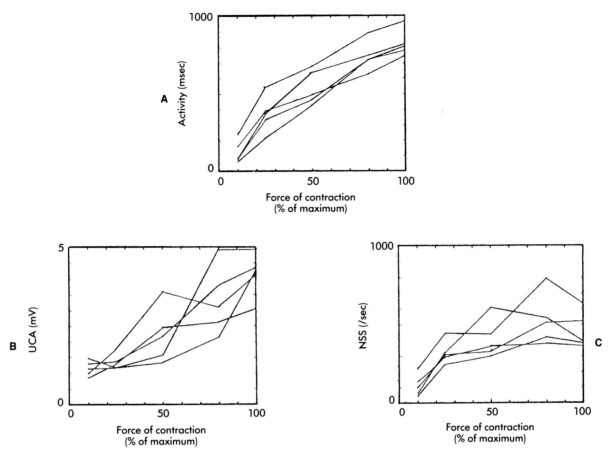

Figure 5-18. EMG interference pattern was recorded from five different sites in biceps muscle of normal subject when force of contraction was increased from 10% to 100% of maximum. **A,** Activity, **B,** upper centile amplitude (UCA), and, **C,** number of small segments (NSS) increased with force of contraction. Data from each site are connected. Change in number of turns and mean amplitude from same recordings are shown in Figure 5-16.

new features of IP signals, derived from the turns and amplitude measurements, which were developed to correspond to the IP features the electromyographer assesses subjectively. The *activity* feature measures the "fullness" of the IP. The activity has a value between 1 and 1000 msec and reflects the number of milliseconds within a 1-second epoch when spike components of MUAPs are found. At minimal force of contraction only a few MUs are active and activity value is low (Figure 5-18, *A*). When the force of contraction is increased, more MUs are activated and MUAP discharges occupy a greater portion of the IP signal. Therefore the activity value increases (Figure 5-18, *A*). When the activity values are more than 500 msec, the IP signals on the oscilloscope screen appear full to the electromyographer. Computer simulations indicate that this feature depends on the number of active MUs near the recording electrode and their discharge rates.[57]

A *segment* of the IP was defined as the portion of the IP signal between two successive turns (see Figure 5-15). The amplitude and duration of a segment are the difference in

amplitude levels and time of occurrence between the turns that define that segment. The *upper centile amplitude* (UCA) feature is the amplitude level that is exceeded by only 1% of segment amplitudes. It reflects the size of the largest spikes of the IP, excluding some occasional large spikes. In simpler terms it reflects the size of the EMG envelope. Computer simulations indicate that this feature represents the upper limit of the amplitude of the largest component MUAP in the IP.[57]

The *number of small segments* (NSS) feature measures the segments that have small amplitude and short duration. These segments represent the fast voltage changes in the IP signal that would correspond to the complexity of the IP signals on visual assessment and high-frequency components on an audio monitor.

When the force of contraction is increased from minimum to maximum, the IP becomes full, the size of the EMG signals increases, and the signals become complex. Therefore the values of the previously described features increased with the force of contraction (Figure 5-18).

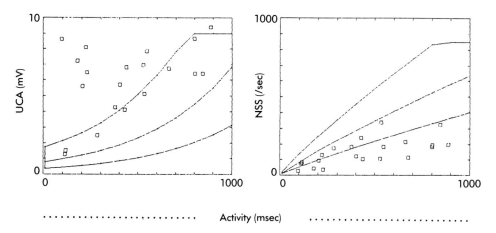

Figure 5-19. Analysis of interference pattern in male patient with spinal muscular atrophy shows neurogenic pattern of abnormality. Upper centile amplitude (UCA) is increased and number of small segments (NSS) is decreased relative to activity feature. Normal clouds for male subjects are superimposed. Lines through center of clouds represent mean UCA and NSS values at different activity.

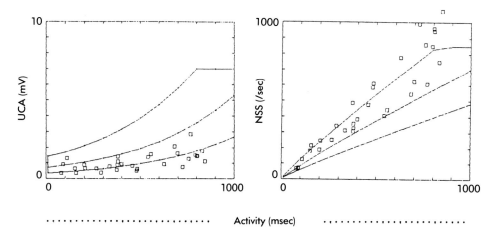

Figure 5-20. Analysis of interference pattern in female patient with polymyositis shows myopathic pattern of abnormality. Note smaller upper centile amplitude (UCA) values and higher number of small segments (NSS) values of normal clouds in females compared with males (Figure 5-19).

The concept of a "cloud" described by Stalberg and co-workers[90] was used to define the normal values of the IP features.[59] Two clouds were constructed defining the relationship between the UCA versus activity and NSS versus activity (Figures 5-19 and 5-20). The lower limit of the UCA value at maximum activity is almost 2 mV (Figures 5-19 and 5-20), which is similar to the lower normal limit of the size of the EMG envelope at maximum effort as described by Buchthal (Table 5-3).[18] A study is called normal if more than 90% of data points are inside both the clouds. Sometimes the data may lie within the cloud but are distributed toward the upper or lower boundary of the cloud. This tendency is quantitated by features DUCA and DNSS for the UCA activity and NSS activity clouds, re-

spectively (for details, see Nandedkar, Sanders, and Stalberg[59]). Values of tendency measure that are positive and large indicate that the data points lie toward the upper boundary of the cloud. For a study to be normal, the DUCA and DNSS features must also be within their normal range.

In patients with neuropathy the data points lie on the upper side of the UCA activity cloud and on the lower side of the NSS activity cloud (Figure 5-19). The DUCA values are increased, and the DNSS values are reduced. In patients with myopathy the patterns of the distribution of data points are exactly opposite to those in patients with neuropathy (Figure 5-20). The contrasting patterns of abnormalities make this technique a useful diagnostic tool.

The principal advantage of this approach is that the char-

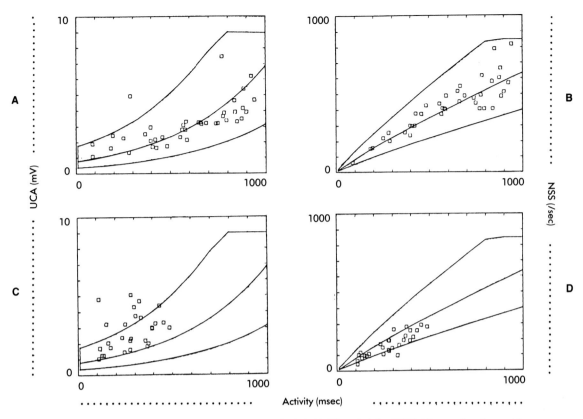

Figure 5-21. Analysis of interference pattern in left **(A,B)** and right **(C,D)** biceps of patient with amyotrophic lateral sclerosis. Neurogenic pattern was seen in right biceps, which was moderately weak. No abnormalities were seen on quantitative interference pattern analysis in left biceps, which had normal strength. Example demonstrates different degree of involvement of biceps muscles in same patient.

acteristics of the EMG signals assessed subjectively can be "read" from the distribution of data points. This is demonstrated by a few examples.

In a patient with amyotrophic lateral sclerosis (ALS), IP recordings were made in left and right biceps muscle. The right biceps was moderately weak (strength 3.5 on the Medical Research Council scale), and the left biceps had normal strength. Quantitative analysis of the IP in the left biceps was normal in that the IP was full (activity greater than 500 msec) and an orderly recruitment of MUAPs was indicated by larger UCA values at higher activity (Figure 5-21, *A* and *B*). More than 90% of data points lay inside the clouds. In the right biceps (Figure 5-21, *C* and *D*), the activity values were less than 500 msec even at maximum force of contraction. This indicated an incomplete IP. Furthermore, the UCA values were on the upper side of the cloud, and several were outside, indicating increased MUAP amplitude. This example demonstrates the different degree of involvement of the biceps muscles in a patient with ALS.

In a patient with spinal muscular atrophy the left biceps was moderately weak. Quantitative analysis showed that the UCA values were very high even at minimal activity and did not increase with further activation (Figure 5-19). The NSS values also remained relatively constant at all activity levels. It was inferred that the activity values increased with force of contraction because of increased firing rate of the MUs and not because of recruitment of additional MUs.

In a patient with myotonic dystrophy, quantitative analysis of the IP showed activity values greater than 500 msec, indicating a full IP (Figure 5-22). More than 10% of data points were outside and on the upper side of the UCA activity cloud, especially at maximal activity levels. When the activity values were less than 600 msec, most NSS data were distributed toward the upper boundary of the normal cloud, as would be seen in myopathy. Because of the contrasting distributions of data points at different levels of activation, the tendency features (DUCA and DNSS) were within the normal range. It was inferred that the IP showed myopathic and "neurogenic" features.

In a patient with postpoliomyelitis muscular atrophy, the UCA activity plot showed a pronounced neurogenic pattern (Figure 5-23). However, the NSS activity plot showed data points on the lower side of the cloud, as in neuropathy, and also on the upper side of the cloud, as in myopathy. It was inferred that the IP had mainly a neurogenic abnormality.

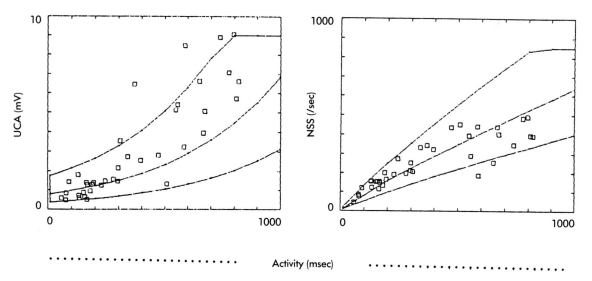

Figure 5-22. Interference pattern analysis in patient with myotonic dystrophy shows myopathic and "neurogenic" features.

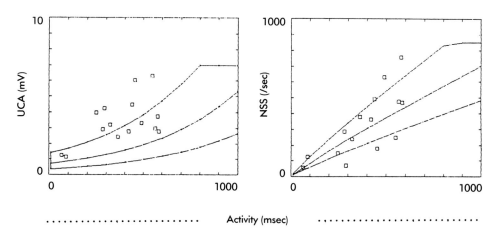

Figure 5-23. Analysis of interference pattern in patient with postpolio muscular atrophy shows neurogenic pattern on upper centile amplitude (UCA) activity plot and a mixed pattern on number of small segments (NSS) activity plot.

The increased NSS resulted from the complex shape of the MUAPs, which is seen in neuropathy but is seldom expressed so strongly on IP analysis. Indeed, when individual MUAPs were recorded, they had large amplitude and many had three to 10 small amplitude–linked potentials that contributed to the increased NSS.

The preceding analysis of the EMG signals made from plots in Figures 5-19 to 5-23 concurred with independent subjective analysis of the original signals made by an electromyographer. Thus the EMG findings can be communicated not only as a number, but also as a portrait of the raw EMG signal. This advantage makes the method attractive to compare and assess disease progression from serial studies.

Instead of quantitating the IP signals, McGill and Dorfman[51] have described a method to decompose the IP into discharges of component MUAPs. The MUAPs can then be analyzed by measuring their amplitude, duration, and other features. This technique allows one to extract and analyze as many as 15 MUAPs from a single recording. Furthermore, analysis is not restricted to the MUAPs recorded from the low force threshold MUs. By measuring the time interval between successive occurrences of the same MUAP in the IP signals, the firing rate of the MU can be calculated. Although of great interest, the analysis of firing pattern of MUs is beyond the scope of this discussion (for recent reviews see Andreassen[2] and Mambrito and De Luca[46]).

ANALYSIS OF SURFACE ELECTROMYOGRAPHIC RECORDINGS

The MUAPs can also be recorded by electrodes on the skin surface. However, because of the relatively large distance between the muscle fibers and the surface EMG recording electrode, the amplitude of individual MUAPs is much smaller than that recorded by intramuscular needle EMG electrodes. As the force of contraction is increased, an EMG IP can be recorded; the area under the rectified EMG signal is proportional to the force of contraction. The surface EMG can be quantitated by measuring the signal power in different frequency components of its power spectrum. The relationship between the power spectrum and the signal generators has recently been reviewed by Lindstrom and Petersen[45] and is briefly summarized as follows. In myopathic diseases the power in the higher frequencies of the spectrum increases, whereas in neurogenic diseases the power in the lower frequencies of the spectrum increases.[72] These changes can also be heard as a change in the pitch of the sound of the EMG signals on an audio monitor. The power in the lower frequency components also increases in a normal muscle when it fatigues.[44] Such a shift could be due to reduced AP propagation velocity during fatigue.[79] By identifying the so-called dip frequency of the power spectrum of EMG signals recorded by a bipolar suface electrode, the AP propagation velocity can be estimated.[44]

The EMG signals recorded in the aforementioned techniques were produced by voluntary activation of MUs. It is also possible to elicit muscle response by electrically stimulating the nerve that innervates the muscle. The oscilloscope sweep is triggered by the stimulator, and the evoked surface EMG signals are displayed on the oscilloscope screen. The active surface EMG electrode is placed at the motor point, and the reference electrode is placed at a distance. In this position the compound muscle action potential (CMAP) has a sharply negative-going initial phase (Figures 5-24 and 5-26). Nerve stimulation is the basis of two electrophysiologic techniques: motor unit counting and repetitive stimulation.

Motor unit counting

Motor unit counting was developed by McComas and coworkers in the 1970s to measure the number of MUs in the muscle. It was used initially to estimate the number of MUs in the extensor digitorum brevis (EDB) muscle of the foot[50] and later in the small muscles of hand.[77] To estimate the number of MUs in the EDB muscle, the stimulating electrode was placed over the deep peroneal nerve at a site just above the ankle. The recording surface electrode was placed over the end-plate zone of the muscle. The nerve was stimulated with increasing intensity until an evoked response was observed. This response represented one MUAP. When the stimulus intensity was increased further, another nerve fiber depolarized and the evoked response was the sum of two MUAPs. The increase in the evoked potential was

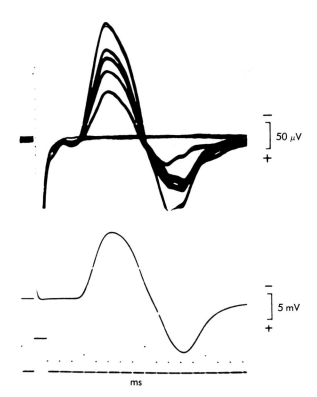

Figure 5-24. Surface EMG recordings made over thenar muscle show quantal increase in evoked potentials. Mean amplitude estimated from the five recordings was 72 μV. Amplitude of compound muscle action potential recorded by supramaximal stimulus *(lower trace)* was 22.5 mV. Hence estimated number of motor units was 313. Usually, mean amplitude is estimated from 10 to 11 motor unit action potentials. (From Sica, R, et al: J Neurol Neurosurg Psychiatry 37:55, 1974.)

"quantal" in that no response that was intermediate between one MUAP and the sum of two MUAPs was observed. When the stimulus intensity was increased further, the next quantal increase occurred when another nerve fiber depolarized and the evoked response was the sum of three MUAPs. Five such incremental responses are shown in Figure 5-24. Usually 10 reproducible increments could be observed. The amplitude of the last evoked response was then divided by the number of increments to estimate the mean MUAP amplitude. A supramaximal stimulus was then applied to the nerve to elicit the compound muscle action potential (CMAP). By dividing the amplitude of the CMAP by the average MUAP amplitude, researchers could estimate the total number of MUs in the muscle.

The number of MUs measured in a muscle on different occasions was reproducible.[50] The mean number of MUs in the EDB muscle of normal subjects was 199, which was similar to that estimated from counts of nerve fibers, and showed a great variation among subjects. Normal subjects who were more than 70 years old had fewer MUs and larger amplitude MUAPs than did younger subjects.[77]

This technique of estimating the number of MUs was used by McComas and co-workers in their electrophysiologic studies of various muscular dystrophies. Their observations were as follows.

In patients with Duchenne dystrophy,[49] the number of MUs in the EDB was reduced but was not related to patient age. The mean MUAP amplitude was also reduced, but some MUAPs had amplitude within normal range.

In patients with limb-girdle and facioscapulohumeral dystrophy,[75] the number of MUs in the EDB was reduced. The mean MUAP amplitude was increased, and some MUAPs with very large amplitude were seen. There was no correlation between the number of surviving MUs and the patient's age.

In patients with myotonic dystrophy,[48] the number of MUs was reduced and there was an inverse correlation between the number of MUs and the patient's age (that is, there were fewer MUs in older patients). The mean MUAP amplitude was decreased, but the potential amplitudes for the surviving units were within the normal range. When the data were separated into two groups based on twitch tension measurements in the extensor hallucis brevis muscle, there was no difference between the mean MUAP amplitudes in patients with "early dystrophy" (normal twitch tension) and those with "late dystrophy" (reduced tension).

Based on the reduced number of MUs, McComas and co-workers proposed that muscular dystrophy has a neurogenic basis.

The motor unit counting technique is based on four assumptions[50]:

1. The electrical activity is derived from a single muscle. This condition was satisfied by the EDB, thenar, and hypothenar muscles.
2. The incremental responses evoked by increasing stimulation intensity are produced by single MUs.
3. The MUAPs summate algebraically; that is, the sum of the amplitudes of the component MUAPs is equal to the amplitude of their summated waveform.
4. The MUAPs recorded to estimate mean MUAP amplitude are representative of the total population of MUs.

The validity of these assumptions and therefore that of the neuronal basis of muscular dystrophy has been questioned.

Panayiotopoulos, Scarpalezos, and Papapetropolos[67] argued that the 4 μV noise level[48] of the recording system was large enough to obscure small-amplitude MUAPs. They observed that the peak of the response occurred at different positions in the incremental responses and inferred that MUAP amplitude did not summate algebraically. Finally, they were not convinced that the sample of 10 or 11 MUAPs used to calculate the mean MUAP amplitude was a representative of the MU population in the muscle. Using a different instrumentation system (noise level 3 to 5 μV peak to peak), they estimated the mean number of MUs in normal EDB muscle to be 370, which is almost twice the number estimated by McComas and co-workers. In patients with Duchenne dystrophy they found the average number of MUs to be 295, which was not significantly different from normal. The mean MUAP amplitude, as well as the amplitude of the CMAP at supramaximal stimulation, was reduced compared with normal subjects.

Ballantyne and Hansen[7] developed a computer-based system to analyze the evoked potentials recorded during electrical stimulation and to estimate the number of MUs in the EDB muscle. The stimulus intensity was increased until an evoked potential was recorded that represented a single MUAP. This was stored in the computer as a template (Figure 5-25). The stimulus intensity was increased, and the evoked potential was compared with the first template. When it was different, it was stored in the computer as the second template. The second template contained the sum of MUAPs from the first two recruited MUs. The next response was compared with the first and second templates and, if different from both, was stored as the third template. The third template contained the sum of MUAPs from the first three recruited MUs. The procedure was continued until 10 to 15 templates were stored in the computer. The CMAP recorded by a supramaximal stimulus was stored as the last template. The number of MUs was calculated by the formula

$$n \times \frac{A(max)}{A(n)}$$

where A(max) was the area of the CMAP recorded by supramaximal stimulus, and A(n) was the area of the evoked potential in the penultimate template containing the sum of n MUAPs. The first template was also the MUAP of the first recruited MUAP, and by subtracting it from the second template, the MUAP of the second recruited MU was obtained. Similarly, by subtracting the second template from the third template, the MUAP of the third recruited MU was obtained. By continuing this procedure, the MUAPs of all recruited MUs could be obtained. A computer plot of templates and their component MUAPs thus obtained is shown in Figure 5-25.

Ballantyne and Hansen used this technique to estimate the number of MUs in the EDB muscle. Their measurements[7] in normal subjects concurred with those reported by McComas and co-workers: the normal EDB contained, on average, 197 MUs; the number of MUs was varied greatly among different subjects; and there was no loss of MUs until the age of 60 years. Also, in patients with myotonic dystrophy the number of MUs was reduced.[8] However, in patients with Duchenne, limb-girdle, and facioscapulohumeral dystrophy, the number of MUs was normal.[8]

In view of the conflicting measurements of the number of MUs, the neuronal basis for muscular dystrophy described by McComas and co-workers has not been universally accepted.

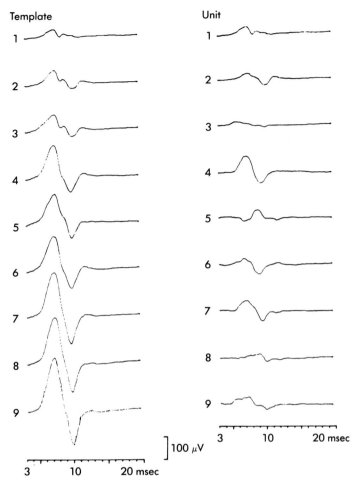

Figure 5-25. Surface EMG recordings made from extensor digitorum brevis muscle. Evoked responses containing up to nine motor unit action potentials (MUAPs), called templates, and individual MUAPs are shown. (From Ballantyne, J, and Hansen, S: J Neurol Neurosurg Psychiatry 37:1195, 1974.)

Repetitive nerve stimulation

When a supramaximal stimulus is applied to the nerve, all muscle fibers in the normal muscle produce an AP. The amplitude of the CMAP recorded by a surface EMG electrode reflects the number and size of the electrical generators, that is, the muscle fibers. In a normal muscle the CMAP remains constant when the stimulation is applied repeatedly at frequencies below 20 Hz. Should the number of AP generators change during a train of stimulation, the CMAP will change. This forms the basis of repetitive nerve stimulation studies, which have recently been reviewed by Sanders.[70]

The active recording electrode is placed at the motor point. The high- and low-pass frequencies on the amplifier are set at 2 and 5000 Hz, respectively. The nerve can be stimulated using surface electrodes or near-nerve needle electrodes. A stimulation rate of 2 to 5 Hz is most suitable. A train of 10 stimuli is given, and the CMAPs are recorded (Figure 5-26).

In a normal muscle the number of AP generators and the CMAP remain constant during the train of stimulation. With abnormalities of neuromuscular transmission, some muscle fibers do not produce an AP with each stimulus. Owing to reduced numbers of AP generators, the size of the CMAP, usually measured as the peak amplitude of the negative phase, decreases. The decrease in amplitude is most prominent in the fourth or fifth response (Figure 5-26). The amplitude difference between the fourth (or fifth) and the first CMAP is expressed as a percentage of the amplitude of the first CMAP and, if this is a negative value, is called the decrement. Some recovery of amplitude may be observed from the sixth to the tenth CMAP in diseases such

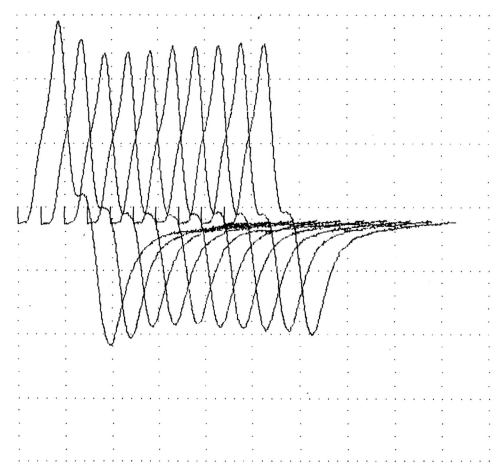

Figure 5-26. Compound muscle action potentials (CMAPs) recorded from patient with myasthenia gravis during train of 10 stimuli. Decrement is maximum in fourth response, followed by partial recovery of amplitude. Successive waveforms have been shifted to right to identify each CMAP.

as myasthenia gravis. A decrement of up to 10% is considered normal.

In patients with myasthenia gravis the decrement becomes less following muscle activation. The improved response is due to improved short-term neuromuscular transmission when acetylcholine (ACh) accumulates in the synaptic cleft. This response is called posttetanic facilitation. When the ACh has been removed from the synaptic cleft and the quantity of ACh in the nerve terminals has been reduced by the previous activation, the decrement worsens. This is the phase of postactivation exhaustion, which lasts for a few minutes after activation.

Abnormal decrement is seen in myasthenia gravis and the Lambert-Eaton syndrome but is also observed when neuromuscular transmission is impaired in conditions such as motor neuron disease and inflammatory myopathy. The decrement is less at low muscle temperature, and therefore a cold muscle must be warmed to at least 34° C to obtain the maximum diagnostic sensitivity with this technique.

DISCUSSION

Not all of the aforementioned quantitative techniques are performed in the clinical EMG laboratory. Routine EMG examination is usually restricted to recordings made by a concentric or monopolar needle electrode. Repetitive stimulation is used in virtually all laboratories. SFEMG is now performed in many laboratories. The remaining techniques are practiced mainly at the laboratories where they were developed.

Not every technique is diagnostically efficient in all diseases.[97] One must choose a technique that is most likely to reveal the abnormality of interest. Recordings of MUAPs and the EMG IP made by needle electrodes are most useful in differentiating between myopathy and neuropathy. A diagnostic yield in excess of 70% has been reported by Fuglsang-Frederiksen et al,[28,29] Hausmanowa-Petrusewicz and Kopec,[35] Buchthal and Kamieniecka,[18] Sica, McComas and Ferreira,[76] and Stewart and co-workers.[92] Considering that only the biceps muscle was tested and that it may not

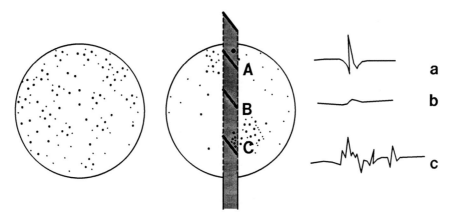

Figure 5-27. Schematic cross section of normal motor unit (MU) *(left)* and MU in muscular dystrophy *(center)*. Three positions of concentric needle electrode *(A, B, C)* in MU territory are shown, and motor unit action potentials at these positions are shown on right *(a, b, c)* to demonstrate their waveform differences.

have been involved by the disease process in all patients,[92] this diagnostic yield is quite impressive. SFEMG recordings and repetitive nerve stimulation studies are most useful in detecting abnormalities of neuromuscular junction. For example, SFEMG in the extensor digitorum communis and frontalis muscles showed the abnormality in 91% of patients with myasthenia gravis.[70]

As stated previously, the main objective of an EMG examination is to determine whether the patient has a disease. In most cases this can be determined by the conventional needle examination. The other techniques give us additional information about the MU that is not available from conventional needle examination. This can be extremely useful in understanding the pathophysiology of the disease and its progression. This is demonstrated by a few examples.

Motor unit architecture in muscular dystrophy

In patients with muscular dystrophy (MD) the CNEMG MUAP duration is reduced, which indicates loss of muscle fibers. Yet the size of macro EMG MUAPs is normal, indicating normal MU size. Furthermore, increased FD suggests increased numbers of muscle fibers. To explain these conflicting relationships, Stalberg and co-workers proposed a model for the MU architecture in muscular dystrophy (Figure 5-27) whereby the MU contains areas where muscle fibers are lost and other areas where the number of muscle fibers increases owing to regeneration or fiber splitting. By virtue of the recording technique, FD measurements cannot detect loss of muscle fibers. Increased FD reflects regeneration and grouping of muscle fibers. Low jitter is observed in some SFEMG recordings in MD, indicating that muscle fibers are split and share a common end-plate. The combination of muscle fiber loss and regeneration produces MU size that is relatively normal or reduced slightly. This would

explain the normal amplitude of macro EMG MUAPs. The shape of the CNEMG MUAPs depends on the muscle fibers in the immediate vicinity of the electrode. If the recording surface is located in a portion of MU territory where muscle fibers have been lost, the MUAP has a simple waveform and short duration (Figure 5-27, *A*). On the other hand, when the recording surface is in an area where the density of muscle fibers has increased, MUAPs may appear normal or have complex waveforms with linked potentials and long total duration (Figure 5-27, *C*). The scanning EMG (Figure 5-10) shows these waveform differences and will have silent areas when the electrode is in the portion of MU territory that does not contain muscle fibers (Figure 5-27, *B*).

Serial electromyographic studies in amyotrophic lateral sclerosis

In a patient with ALS the neighboring fiber density (nFD) and the amplitude of macro EMG MUAPs was increased when there was normal strength and remained so when mild weakness developed in the tested muscle (Figure 5-28). When the muscle became severely weak, the macro EMG MUAP amplitude was greatly increased while there continued to be only a mild increase in nFD. A few months later the nFD had increased while the macro EMG MUAP amplitude had fallen. The amplitude of CNEMG MUAPs changed in parallel with the nFD. Note that all EMG features had characteristics of neurogenic disease in individual studies. However, the features did not change in parallel as the disease progressed. Thus the degree of abnormality of individual EMG features at one point in time cannot be used to assess the stage or progression of motor neuron disease (MND).

The pattern of changes in the EMG features may be explained as follows. When the strength of the tested muscle was normal or slightly reduced, the increase in EMG fea-

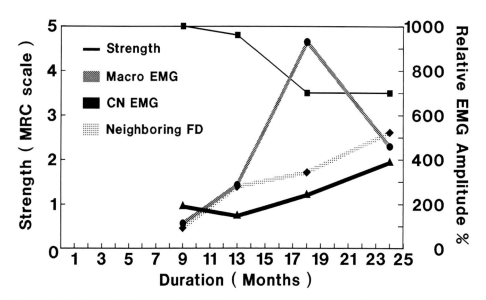

Figure 5-28. Macro EMG, single fiber EMG, and concentric needle EMG recordings were made in biceps muscle of patient with amyotrophic lateral sclerosis as disease progressed. Amplitude and neighboring fiber density values were expressed as percentages of mean values recorded from normal muscles. Strength was graded by Medical Research Council scale.

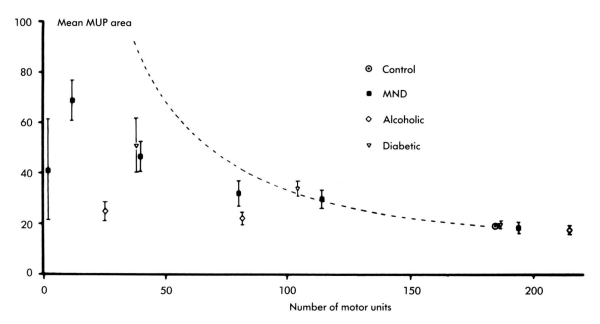

Figure 5-29. Number of motor units (MUs) and mean motor unit action potential (MUAP) area were measured in patients with neurogenic disease. Dotted line indicates mean MUAP area if all denervated muscle fibers, resulting from loss of MUs, were reinnervated. Data from patients were grouped, and mean values and 1 standard deviation range are shown. *MND*, Motor neuron disease. (From Ballantyne, J, and Hansen, S: Muscle Nerve 5:S127, 1982.)

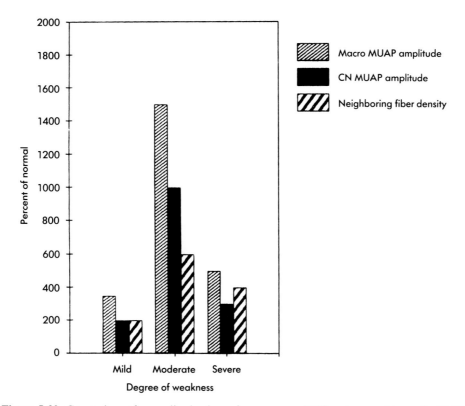

Figure 5-30. Comparison of normalized values of mean macro EMG and concentric needle EMG motor unit action potential amplitudes and neighboring fiber density in biceps muscle of patients with amyotrophic lateral sclerosis. All three measurements are increased and abnormal. However, maximum increase occurs in muscles with moderate weakness. (From Sanders, D, et al: Quantitive electromyography after poliomyelitis, Proceedings of Second Research Symposium on the Late Effects of Poliomyelitis, March of Dimes Birth Defect Foundation White Plains, NY, pp 182-200.)

tures reflected reinnervation changes. At the time of the third study there must have been a loss of MUs, so the later recordings were made from the larger MUs that are normally activated only at higher force levels. In normal muscle these MUs have large-amplitude macro EMG MUAPs.[83] Increased FD in the patient indicated that these MUs were reinnervated and therefore had even greater amplitude. Loss of MUs would also explain the marked progression of weakness seen at the time of the third study. The increase in nFD at the time of the fourth study indicated further reinnervation. Because of grouping of muscle fibers in the MU territory, the CNEMG MUAP amplitude also increased. At this time the overall MU size was decreased as indicated by smaller macro EMG MUAPs. Therefore reinnervation and loss of muscle fibers took place in the same MUs with the result that they contained fewer fibers that were packed densely in a smaller territory. This is called fractionation of MUs.[88]

Capacity for reinnervation

In neurogenic diseases, MUs are lost and their fibers are reinnervated by surviving MUs. Therefore the capacity for reinnervation of MUs is of great interest. Ballantyne and Hansen[9] measured the number of MUs and the mean area of MUAPs recorded from the EDB muscle of patients with MND and diabetic and alcoholic neuropathy. A plot of MUAP area against the number of MUs is shown in Figure 5-29. Superimposed on the data is a dotted line that indicates the theoretic size of the mean MUAP area if all fibers from lost MUs were reinnervated (that is, if the CMAP elicited by a supramaximal stimulus remained the same despite loss of MUs). The data points from patients with MND indicate that compensatory reinnervation occurred until 50% of MUs were lost. The MUAP area continued to increase with further loss of MUs but fell when there were fewer than 10 surviving MUs. The reinnervation capacity was poor in alcoholic neuropathy, which among the diseases was associated with least increase in MUAP area.

Macro EMG electrode records the activity from the entire MU and can also give information about reinnervation capacity. Sanders and co-workers[71] reported that in patients with MND the amplitude of macro EMG MUAPs was maximum in moderately weak muscles (Figure 5-30). In se-

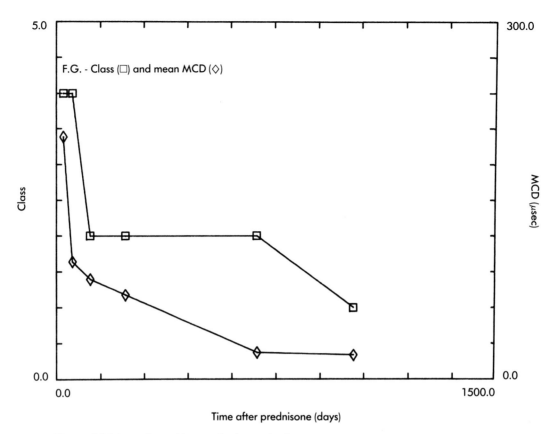

Figure 5-31. In patient with myasthenia gravis, jitter measured by single fiber EMG and severity of disease, called class, changed in parallel as patient improved.

verely weak muscles the amplitude was increased relative to normal but was smaller than that recorded in moderately weak muscle. Assuming that weakness is due to loss of functional MUs, the macro EMG abnormalities (Figure 5-30) concur with those from MU counting (Figure 5-29).

Stalberg[82] observed maximum reinnervation capacity in patients with spinal muscular atrophy and in patients with sequelae after poliomyelitis. Individual macro EMG MUAP amplitude exceeded the normal value by more than 25 times.

Serial single fiber electromyography in myasthenia gravis

Quantitative EMG measurements can also be useful in assessing the effect of treatment of some neuromuscular diseases. Jitter was measured from SFEMG recordings in the extensor digitorum communis muscle of a patient with myasthenia gravis who was being treated with prednisone. At each examination the severity of disease was assessed subjectively and assigned a "class" from 1 (normal) to 5 (severely abnormal). As the patient improved and became clinically normal, the jitter values returned to normal (Figure 5-31). The jitter and subjective assessment changed in parallel during recovery, demonstrating the usefulness of jitter as an objective measure to assess the response to treatment in myasthenia gravis.

CONCLUSION

In this chapter different techniques of recording and quantitating EMG signals have been described to indicate the complementary information they provide. Their use in diagnosis and in understanding of pathophysiology of nerve and muscle disease is discussed. Most of those techniques have been developed in the last two decades, and there is great interest in developing even more sensitive techniques. Recent advances in computer technology will certainly stimulate progress in quantitative EMG. Advanced signal processing techniques will allow us to derive more information from the EMG signals than ever before. Not only will EMG signals be quantitated more efficiently, but the analysis techniques will also be different. Already the feasibility of so-called expert systems is being investigated. Such a system would not only make statistical decisions about abnormalities, but could also indicate additional tests that would improve the reliability of diagnosis. Such a system could retain each study in its "memory" and learn from it to become a better "expert."

This does not imply that computers are necessary for quantitative EMG. In fact, most of the work by the pioneers, Buchthal and Stalberg, was accomplished without the sophistication of modern computers. The triggered delay line, averager, and a hard copy device (a plotter or camera) are standard features on most current electromyographs, and by using them one can record and analyze MUAPs recorded by concentric needle, monopolar needle, macro EMG, and single fiber EMG electrodes. Many new models of electromyographs also have the hardware (and software) necessary to analyze the IP.

Finally, quantitative EMG is not a substitute for good EMG recordings. If the signals are not acquired properly, it is more likely that quantitative measurements will be misleading. Many clinicians have mistakenly diagnosed themselves as having abnormal neuromuscular transmission while learning SFEMG.

ACKNOWLEDGMENT

Many of the ideas regarding the MU architecture that are presented in this chapter are a result of numerous discussions with Drs. D.B. Sanders and E.V. Stalberg. Along with them, I would like to thank Drs. P. Barkhaus, J. Gilchrist, J. Massey, and C. Stewart for their help in making EMG recordings and reviewing the manuscript. This work was supported in part by a grant from the Muscular Dystrophy Association of America.

REFERENCES

1. Adrian, E, and Bronk D: Discharge of impulse in motor nerve fiber, J Physiol 67:119, 1929.
2. Andreassen, S: Computerized analysis of motor unit firing. In Desmedt, J, editor: Computer-aided electromyography, Basel, 1983, Karger.
3. Andreassen, S: Method for computer-aided measurement of motor unit parameters. In Ellingson, RJ, Murray, N, and Halliday, AM, editors: The London Symposia, EEG Suppl 39, pp 13-20, 1987.
4. Andreassen, S, and Rosenfalck, A: Relationship between intracellular and extracellular action potential of skeletal muscle fiber, CRC Crit Rev Bioeng 6:267, 1981.
5. Antoni, L, Stalberg, E, and Sanders, D: Automated analysis of neuromuscular "jitter," Computer Programs Biomed. 16:175, 1983.
6. Aquilonius, S, et al: Topographical localization of motor endplates in cryosections of whole human muscles, Muscle Nerve 7:287, 1984.
7. Ballantyne, J, and Hansen, S: Computer method for the analysis of evoked motor unit potentials. I. Control subjects and patients with myasthenia gravis, J Neurol Neurosurg Psychiatry 37:1187, 1974.
8. Ballantyne, J, and Hansen, S: New method for the estimation of the number of motor units in a muscle. II. Duchenne, limb-girdle and facioscapulohumeral, and myotonic muscular dystrophies, J Neurol Neurosurg Psychiatry 37:1195, 1974.
9. Ballantyne, J, and Hansen, S: A quantitative assessment of reinnervation in polyneuropathies, Muscle Nerve 5:S127, 1982.
10. Brown, W: The physiological and technical basis of electromyography, Stoneham, Mass, 1984, Butterworth Publishers.
11. Buchthal, F: An introduction to electromyography, Copenhagen, 1957, Scandinavian University Books.
12. Buchthal, F: Electrophysiological signs of myopathy as related with muscle biopsy, Acta Neurol 32:1, 1977.
13. Buchthal, F, Erminio, F, and Rosenfalck, P: Motor unit territory in different human muscles, Acta Physiol Scand 45:72, 1959.
14. Buchthal, F, Guld, C, and Rosenfalck, P: Action potential parameters in normal human muscle and their dependence on physical variables, Acta Physiol Scand 32:200, 1954.
15. Buchthal, F, Guld, C, and Rosenfalck, P: Innervation zone and propagation velocity in human muscles, Acta Physiol Scand 35:174, 1955.
16. Buchthal, F, Guld, C, and Rosenfalck, P: Propagation velocity in electrically activated muscle fibers in man, Acta Physiol Scand 34:75, 1955.
17. Buchthal, F, Guld, C, and Rosenfalck, P: Multielectrode study of the territory of a motor unit, Acta Physiol Scand 39:83, 1957.
18. Buchthal, F, and Kamieniecka, Z: The diagnostic yield of quantified electromyography and quantified muscle biopsy in neuromuscular disorders, Muscle Nerve 5:265, 1982.
19. Buchthal, F, Rosenfalck, P, and Erminio, F: Motor unit territory and fiber density in myopathies, Neurology 10:398, 1960.
20. Christensen, E: Topography of terminal motor innervation in striated muscle from still born infants, Am J Phys Med 38:65, 1959.
21. Chu-Andrews, J, Bruyninckx, F, and Chan, R: Personal experience on quantitative analysis of the MUAP on minimal contraction. In Chu-Andrews, J, and Johnson, R, editors: Electrodiagnosis: an anatomical and clinical approach, Philadelphia, 1986, J.B. Lippincott Co.
22. Dubowitz, V, and Brooke, M: Muscle biopsy: a modern approach, Philadelphia, 1973, WB Saunders Co.
23. Ekstedt, J, and Stalberg, E: How the size of the needle electrode leading-off surface influences the shape of the single muscle fiber potentials in electromyography, Computer Programs Biomed 3:204, 1973.
24. Erminio, F, Buchthal, F, and Rosenfalck, P: Motor unit territory and muscle fiber concentration in paresis due to peripheral nerve injury and anterior cell involvement, Neurology 9:657, 1959.
25. Falck, B: Automatic analysis of individual motor unit potentials recorded with a special two channel electrode, Academic dissertation, Turku, Finland, 1983, University of Turku.
26. Feinstein, B, et al: Morphologic studies of motor units in normal human muscles, Acta Anat. 23:127, 1955.
27. Fuglsang-Frederiksen, A, and Mansson, A: Analysis of electrical activity of normal muscle in man at different degrees of voluntary effort, J Neurol Neurosurg Psychiatry 38:683, 1975.
28. Fuglsang-Frederiksen, A, Scheel, U, and Buchthal, F: Diagnostic yield of analysis of the pattern of electrical activity and of individual motor unit potentials in myopathy, J Neurol Neurosurg Psychiatry 39:742, 1976.
29. Fuglsang-Frederiksen, A, Scheel, U, and Buchthal, F: Diagnostic yield of the analysis of the pattern of electrical activity of muscle and of individual motor unit potentials in neurogenic involvement, J Neurol Neurosurg Psychiatry 40:544, 1977.
30. Gath, I, and Stalberg, E: In situ measurement of the innervation ratio of motor units in human muscle, Exp Brain Res 43:377, 1981.
31. Gath, I, and Stalberg, E: On the measurement of fiber density in human muscles, EEG Clin Neurophysiol 54:699, 1982.
32. Gilchrist, J M: Personal communication, 1987.
33. Goodgold, J, and Eberstein, A: Electrodiagnosis of neuromuscular diseases, Baltimore, 1977, Williams & Wilkins Co.
34. Haridasan, G: Quantitative electromyography using automatic analysis, Proceedings of the Eighth Annual Conference of the IEEE Engineering in Medicine and Biology Society, Fort Worth, Tex, Nov 7-10, 1986, vol 1, New York, 1986, IEEE Publishing Services.
35. Hausmanowa-Petrusewicz, I, and Kopec, J: The value of automatic analysis for quantitative electromyography, Acta Physiol Pol 30:231, 1979.
36. Hayward, M, and Willison, R: Automatic analysis of the electromyogram in patients with chronic partial denervation, J Neurol Sci 33:415, 1977.
37. Henneman, E: Recruitment of motoneurons: the size principle. In Desmedt, J, editor: Motor unit types, recruitment and plasticity in health and disease, Basel, 1981, Karger.
38. Hilton-Brown, P, and Stalberg, E: Motor unit in muscular dystrophy, a single fiber EMG and scanning EMG study, J Neurol Neurosurg Psychiatry 46:981, 1983.
39. Hilton-Brown, P, and Stalberg, E: Motor unit size in muscular dystrophy, a macro EMG and scanning EMG study, J Neurol Neurosurg Psychiatry 46:996, 1983.
40. Kimura, J: Electrodiagnosis in diseases of nerve and muscle: principles and practice, Philadelphia, 1983, FA Davis Co.
41. Kopec, J, and Hausmanowa-Petrusewicz, I: Diagnostic yield of an automated method of quantitative electromyography, EMG Clin Neurophysiol 25:567, 1985.

42. Kopec, J, et al: Automatic analysis in electromyography. In Desmedt, J, editor: New developments in electromyography and clinical neurophysiology, vol 2, Basel, 1973, Karger.

43. Lang, A, and Partanen, V: "Satellite potentials" and the duration of motor unit potentials in normal, neuropathic and myopathic muscles, J Neurol Sci 27:513, 1976.

44. Lindstrom, L, Magnusson, R, and Petersen, I: Muscular fatigue and action potential conduction velocity studied with frequency analysis of EMG signals, Electromyography 10:341, 1970.

45. Lindstrom, L, and Petersen, I: Power spectrum analysis of EMG signals and its applications. In Desmedt, J, editor: Computer-aided electromyography, Basel, 1983, Karger.

46. Mambrito, B, and De Luca, C: Acquisition and decomposition of the EMG signal. In Desmedt, J, editor: Computer-aided electromyography, Basel, 1983, Karger.

47. Massey, J, Sanders, D, and Nandedkar, S: Sensitivity of various EMG techniques in motor neuron disease, EEG Clin Neurophysiol 61:S74, 1985.

48. McComas, A, Campbell, M, and Sica, R: Electrophysiological study of dystrophia myotonica, J Neurol Neurosurg Psychiatry 34:132, 1971.

49. McComas, A, Sica, R, and Currie, S: An electrophysiological study of Duchenne dystrophy, J Neurol Neurosurg Psychiatry 34:461, 1971.

50. McComas, A, et al: Electrophysiological estimation of the number of motor units within a human muscle, J Neurol Neurosurg Psychiatry 34:121, 1971.

51. McGill, K, and Dorfman, L: Automatic decomposition electromyography (ADEMG): validation and normative data in brachial biceps, EEG Clin Neurophysiol 61:453, 1985.

52. Middleton, L, and Lovelace, R: Use of monopolar electrodes in automatic EMG analysis with ANOPS computer, EMG Clin Neurophysiol 25:539, 1985.

53. Nandedkar, S, and Sanders, D: Number of turns in the EMG interference pattern measured at different force levels in biceps, Muscle Nerve 7:561, 1984.

53a. Nandedkar, S, and Sanders, D: Simulation of myopathic motor unit action potentials. Submitted for publication.

54. Nandedkar, S, Sanders, D, and Stalberg, E: Simulation of concentric needle EMG motor unit action potentials, Muscle Nerve 7:562, 1984.

55. Nandedkar, S, Sanders, D, and Stalberg, E: Selectivity of the electromyographic recording techniques: a simulation study, Med Biol Engineering Computing 23:536, 1985.

56. Nandedkar, S, Sanders, D, and Stalberg, E: Simulation and analysis of the electromyographic interference pattern in normal muscle. I. Turns and amplitude measurements, Muscle Nerve 9:423, 1986.

57. Nandedkar, S, Sanders, D, and Stalberg, E: Simulation and analysis of the electromyographic interference pattern in normal muscle. II. Activity, upper centile amplitude and number of small segments, Muscle Nerve 9:486, 1986.

58. Nandedkar, S, Sanders, D, and Stalberg, E: Automatic analysis of the electromyographic interference pattern. I. Development of quantitative features, Muscle Nerve 9:431, 1986.

59. Nandedkar, S, Sanders, D, and Stalberg, E: Automatic analysis of the electromyographic interference pattern. II. Findings in control subjects and in some neuromuscular diseases, Muscle Nerve 9:491, 1986.

60. Nandedkar, S, and Stalberg, E: Simulation of single muscle fiber action potentials, Med Biol Engineering Computing 21:158, 1983.

61. Nandedkar, S, and Stalberg, E: Simulation of macro EMG motor unit potentials, EEG Clin Neurophysiol 56:52, 1983.

62. Nandedkar, S, Stalberg, E, and Sanders, D: Simulation techniques in electromyography, IEEE Trans Biomed Eng 32:775, 1985.

63. Nandedkar, S, et al: Use of signal representation to identify abnormal motor unit potentials in macro EMG, IEEE Trans Biomed Eng 31:220, 1984.

64. Nandedkar, S, et al: Simulation of concentric needle EMG motor action potentials, Muscle Nerve. In press.

65. Nandedkar, S, et al: Analysis of amplitude and area of concentric needle EMG motor unit action potentials, EEG Clin Neurophysiol. In press.

66. Reference deleted in proofs.

67. Panayiotopoulos, C, Scarpalezos, S, and Papapetropolos, T: Electrophysiological estimation of motor units in Duchenne muscular dystrophy, J Neurol Sci 23:89 1974.

68. Rose, A, and Willison, R: Quantitative electromyography using automatic analysis: studies in healthy subjects and patients with primary muscle disease, J Neurol Neurosurg Psychiatry 30:403, 1967.

69. Rosenfalck, P, and Rosenfalck, A: Electromyography and sensory/motor conductions: findings in normal subjects, Copenhagen, 1975, Laboratory of Clinical Neurophysiology, Rigshospitalet.

70. Sanders, D: Electrophysiologic study of disorders of neuromuscular transmission. In Aminoff, M, editor: Electrodiagnosis in clinical neurology, New York, 1986, Churchill Livingstone.

71. Sanders, D, Massey, J, and Nandedkar, S: Quantitative electromyography after poliomyelitis, Proceedings of the Second Research Symposium on the Late Effects of Poliomyelitis, March of Dimes Birth Defect Foundation, White Plains, NY, pp 189-200.

72. Sanstedt, P: Quantitative examination in neuromuscular disorders studied by muscle biopsy and electromyography, Medical dissertation, No 121, Linkoping, Sweden, 1981, Linkoping University.

73. Sellman, M, et al: Macro electromyography (macro EMG) after limb immobilization, Muscle Nerve 4:440, 1981.

74. Sherrington, C: Some functional problems attaching to convergence, Proc R Soc (B) 105:332, 1929.

75. Sica, R, and McComas, A: An electrophysiological investigation of limb-girdle and facioscapulohumeral dystrophy, J Neurol Neurosurg Psychiatry 34:469, 1971.

76. Sica, R, McComas, A, and Ferreira, J: Evaluation of an automated method for analyzing the electromyogram, Can J Neurol Sci 5:275, 1978.

77. Sica, R, et al: Motor unit estimation in small muscle of the hand, J Neurol Neurosurg Psychiatry 37:55, 1974.

78. Smyth, D: Quantitative electromyography in babies and young children with primary muscle disease and neurogenic lesions, J Neurol Sci 56:199, 1982.

79. Stalberg, E: Propagation velocity in human muscle fibers in situ, Acta Physiol Scand 70(suppl 287):1, 1966.

80. Stalberg, E: Electrodiagnosis in dystrophic muscle. In Rowland, L, editor: Pathogenesis of human muscular dystrophies, Amsterdam, 1977, Excerpta Medica.

81. Stalberg, E: Macro EMG, a new recording technique, J Neurol Neurosurg Psychiatry 43:475, 1980.

82. Stalberg, E: Macro electromyography in reinnervation, Muscle Nerve 5:S135, 1982.

83. Stalberg, E: Personal communication, 1982.

84. Stalberg, E, and Antoni, L: Electrophysiologic cross section of the motor unit, J Neurol Neurosurg Psychiatry 43:469, 1980.

85. Stalberg, E, and Antoni, L: Computer-aided EMG analysis. In Desmedt, J, editor: Computer-aided electromyography, Basel, 1983, Karger.

86. Stalberg, E, and Fawcett, P: Macro EMG in healthy subjects of different ages, J Neurol Neurosurg Psychiatry 45:870, 1982.

87. Stalberg, E, and Gath, I: Measurement of the uptake area of small size electromyographic electrodes, IEEE Trans Biomed Engineering 26:374, 1979.

88. Stalberg, E, and Sanders, D: The motor unit in ALS studied with different neurophysiological techniques. In Rose, C, editor: Progress in motor neuron disease, London, 1983, Pitman Books.

89. Stalberg, E, and Trontelj, J: Single fibre electromyography, Old Woking, Surrey, Eng, 1979, Mirvalle Press Ltd.

90. Stalberg, E, et al: Automatic analysis of the EMG interference pattern, EEG Clin Neurophysiol 56:672, 1983.

91. Stalberg, E, et al: Quantitative analysis of individual motor unit potentials: a proposition for standardized terminology and criteria for measurement J. Clin Neurophysiol 3:313, 1986.

92. Stewart, C, et al: Evaluation of an automatic method off measuring features of motor unit action potentials, Muscle Nerve. In press.

93. Swash, M, and Schwartz, M: A longitudinal study of changes in motor units in motor neuron disease, J Neurol Sci 56:185, 1982.

94. Trontelj, J, et al: Axonal stimulation for end-plate jitter studies, J Neurol Neurosurg Psychiatry 49:677, 1986.

95. Wiechers, D, and Hubbell, S: Late changes in motor unit after acute poliomyelitis, Muscle Nerve 4:524, 1981.

96. Willison, R: Analysis of the electrical activity in healthy and dystrophic muscle in man, J Neurol Neurosurg Psychiatry 27:386, 1964.

97. Yu, Y, and Murray, N: A comparison of concentric needle electromyography, quantitative EMG and single fiber EMG in the diagnosis of neuromuscular diseases, J Neurol Neurosurg Psychiatry 58:220, 1984.

PART II | BRAIN DAMAGE AND STROKE

CHAPTER 6

Specific medical management of stroke and the rehabilitation physician

SARAN JONAS

The rehabilitation physician taking care of a patient who has had a stroke can think about *specific* medical management in two ways: (1) What should be done to prevent further strokes in patients stable or improving after a stroke? (2) If another stroke occurs, what *acute* treatment is relevant (before the patient is transferred to the care of a neurologist)?

The following sections review and interpret the results of *controlled studies in which completed or progressing stroke patients were randomized for a specific treatment or for management without that treatment.* Data other than those from such randomized controlled studies are ignored, as are unsubstantiated opinions and recommendations. Results from studies of patients with transient ischemia are not reviewed here.

In the recording of outcomes the term "stroke" means a new stroke occurring during treatment or observation.

INHIBITORS OF PLATELET AGGREGATION

Aspirin. Bousser and co-workers[6] administered aspirin (ASA), 990 mg daily, or a placebo to 342 patients who had had a stroke within the previous year. Of this group, 11% had no sequelae and 89% had mild to moderate sequelae. At 3 years 11% of 168 ASA-treated patients and 18% of 173 placebo-treated controls had had a new ischemic stroke. (Rates for cerebral hemorrhage are not presented; there were no more than two such events in either group, according to the authors.)

Britton and co-workers[7] studied 505 patients who had had a stroke (44% minor, 56% major) in the previous 3 weeks. The patients received ASA, 1500 mg daily, or a placebo. At 2 years, total death rates (13%) and nonlethal recurrent stroke rates (9%) were identical among the 253 treated and the 252 control patients.

Dipyridamole. Acheson, Danta, and Hutchinson[1] reported on 106 stroke patients who had been given dipyridamole (DP), 400 to 800 mg a day, or placebo. During follow-up averaging 25 months, 35% of 52 patients receiving DP had a stroke or died; the rate was 32% among the 54 controls.

Aspirin plus dipyridamole. Bousser and co-workers[6] also included in their study a cohort of 169 stroke patients who received ASA, 100 mg daily, plus DP, 225 mg daily. The 3-year ischemic stroke recurrence rate was 11%, identical with the rate for ASA alone.

Suloctidil. Suloctidil is an inhibitor of platelet aggregation and an antagonist of arterial spasm. Gent and co-workers[15] studied 438 patients who had had a thromboembolic stroke of more than mild degree in the period 2 weeks to 4 months before entry to the study. The patients were administered either suloctidil, 600 mg daily, or placebo. Follow-up averaged 20 months. The stroke recurrence rate was 15% among the 218 treated patients and 15% among the 220 controls.

Summary of results. The results of Bousser and co-workers[6] indicate that ASA has value; the results of Britton and co-workers[8] show no value but no evidence of harm. Further ASA-versus-no-ASA trials are needed; until then, ASA treatment after stroke is justifiable. There is no evidence to favor the use of DP or suloctidil.

ANTICOAGULATION THERAPY

Marshall and Shaw[18] described 51 patients who had had nonembolic cerebral infarction no more than 72 hours before entry into the study. The patients underwent 21 days of anticoagulation therapy (ACT) or control management. By 6 weeks there had been six deaths in the ACT group and three deaths plus two further ischemic episodes among the controls.

The Veterans Administration Cooperative Study[28] randomized 155 cerebral ischemia patients to ACT (follow-up average 9.3 months) or to control management (follow-up average 12.8 months). Most patients entered the study within 1 month of their (most recent) episode; more than 50% entered within 2 weeks. Of the 155 patients, 118 had entered because of cerebral ischemia (defined by the authors as a deficit lasting more than 12 hours). The annualized rates of stroke or death (based on the above follow-up averages) were 35% among 56 cerebral infarction patients treated with ACT and approximately 15% among 62 controls.

Carter[9] studied 76 patients with progressing stroke who received either 4 weeks of ACT (intravenously administered heparin followed by phenindione) or control treatment. At 6 months 32% of the 38 ACT patients were not improved or were dead; for the 38 controls the figure was 50%.

Hill and co-workers[16] studied nonhypertensive patients considered to have had a stroke because of cervical or intracranial arterial disease 14 or more days earlier. Sixty-six were given phenindione, 50 mg daily; 65 were given what the authors apparently considered an ineffectual dose of phenindione (1 mg daily) and were considered to be the controls. Follow-up averaged 28 months for the anticoagulated patients and 31 months for the controls. The annualized stroke or death rate was 11.8% for the anticoagulated patients and 13.1% among the controls.

In the National Cooperative Study of Baker and co-workers[3] ACT or control management was provided to 271 patients considered to have had thrombotic or embolic stroke (manifestations lasting more than 1 hour; see Fisher[13]). Sixty-six percent entered the study within 7 days of their (most recent) episode. Annualized stroke or death rates were 49% among 137 ACT patients (based on 8.89 months of average follow-up) and 33% among 132 controls (average follow-up of 15.19 months).

The National Cooperative Study also included the administration of ACT (apparently intravenously administered heparin followed by dicumarol) to 128 patients considered to be having a stroke in evolution. The subsequent annualized stroke or death rate was 33% for 61 ACT patients (average follow-up 12.05 months) and 47% for 67 controls (average of 14.64 months' follow-up).

McDowell and co-workers[21] reported on the treatment of 190 ischemic stroke patients with warfarin or control management. Follow-up averaged 30 months; the treated patients received warfarin during 41% of the observation time. The stroke or death rate was 54% among the 90 treated patients and 58% among the 100 controls.

Wallace[29] studied 52 patients who had had a nonembolic ischemic stroke 14 or more days earlier. During an average follow-up of 21 months, 37% of 27 patients treated with phenindione and 72% of 25 controls had another stroke or died (p between .05 and .02 by Yates-corrected chi-square analysis).

Enger and Boyesen[12] provided ACT to 50 patients with cerebral infarction not of cardiac origin (and also one patient with transient ischemic attacks [TIAs]); they gave control management to 47 cerebral infarction (plus two TIA) patients. ACT was given for an average of 22.8 months, at which time the new stroke or death rate was 18% to 20% (allowing for the removal of the TIA patient, whose actual outcome is not specified) for ACT, and 26% to 30% (TIA patients here handled similarly) for control management. Final follow-up averaged 38.4 months; the new stroke or death rates were 46% to 48% for ACT and 47% to 51% among the controls.

The Cerebral Embolism Study Group[10] conducted a randomized trial of intravenously administered heparin versus no ACT in patients thought to have had brain infarction secondary to embolization from the heart during the previous 48 hours. The 24 ACT patients began to receive heparin at an average of 32 hours after onset; five of the 24 had had large infarcts when CT scanned an average of 20 hours after onset. Among these 24, no deaths, new strokes, or hemorrhages occurred during 14 days of treatment. Among 21 controls, two had new ischemic infarcts (on days 2 and 7) and two others died, yielding a stroke or death rate of 17% for 14 days. Two other control patients had hemorrhagic transformations in their infarcts (without clinical deterioration; the transformations were detected on CT scanning on days 6 and 8). The two new strokes and the two hemorrhagic transformations occurred among the eight control patients who had had large infarcts on prerandomization scanning.

Duke and co-workers[11] randomized 220 patients stable after a partial (motor deficit less than complete) thrombotic stroke of less than 48 hours' duration. Atrial fibrillation, cardiac source for emboli, and progression of deficit in the hour before assignment of treatment were grounds for exclusion. Heparin was given intravenously to 109 patients for 7 days; 111 patients received placebo. At 7 days mean neurologic scores showed a 27% improvement with heparin (two patients died) and a 24% improvement with placebo (one patient died).

Summary of results. The results of the National Cooperative Study, of Carter, and of the Cerebral Embolism Study Group indicate that ACT is of value for patients with stroke in evolution or with emboli of cardiac origin.

Among patients not deteriorating after a stroke, ACT patients did worse than controls in the Veterans Administration and the National Cooperative studies and slightly worse in the study of Marshall and Shaw.[18] The ACT patients of Hill[16] and McDowell[21] and their co-workers did marginally better than the controls. Enger and Boyesen[12] found benefit during treatment, as did Wallace.[29] An overview of these seven results (three worse, four better) indicates that ACT has not been shown to be advantageous for patients stable after a stroke.

ENDARTERECTOMY

Bauer and co-workers[4] gave results of endarterectomy (mostly carotid) versus nonsurgical management in random samples of patients after completed stroke. Follow-up ranged up to 42 months. Any patient with a poor outcome was listed either as worse or as dead. Among 37 patients stable after an "old" stroke, 57% were worse or dead at final follow-up; the comparable proportion was 35% for 34 controls. Among 31 patients operated after a "recent" stroke (but with surgery usually deferred at least 2 weeks) the worse or dead rate was 39% at final follow-up; among 39 recent stroke patients who were not treated surgically, the worse or dead rate was 33%.

These authors subsequently[5] published more extensive survival (but not "worsening") data, which included the cases previously described. Among patients who had had completed stroke (the majority had severe neurologic deficits), the death rate at average follow-up of 42 months was 52% for the 186 treated surgically and 29% for the 203 controls.

Summary of results. The available randomized data show that endarterectomy has been dangerous for patients with completed stroke and give no justification for its use in such circumstances.

DEXAMETHASONE

Patten and co-workers[24] described the administration of dexamethasone or placebo to 31 patients who had had a stroke within the previous 24 hours. The treated patients received 10 mg of dexamethasone intravenously initially and 4 mg intramuscularly every 6 hours for 10 days; the doses were tapered to zero over the next 7 days. Final evaluation was on day 17. Among the treated patients (12 cerebral infarcts, two brainstem infarcts) 64% improved; the average neurologic assessment score for all 14 patients was 12% better. Among the controls (14 cerebral infarcts, three cerebral hemorrhages) 41% improved; the average score for all 17 was 12% worse.

Mulley, Wilcox, and Mitchell[22] reported on 118 patients who had had a first stroke within the previous 48 hours. The treated patients received dexamethasone, 4.2 mg intramuscularly every 6 hours for 10 days, tapering to discontinuation at 14 days. By the tenth day of treatment, 41% of 61 dexamethasone patients and 47% of 57 controls, who had received placebo, were dead. At 1 year 16% of the treated patients and 14% of the controls were independent in their activities; all others had disabling residua or were dead.

Norris and Hachinski[23] studied the administration of dexamethasone, 40 mg daily for 12 days, or placebo to 113 patients who had had a cerebral infarction within the preceding 48 hours. At the end of 21 days of observation the 54 treated patients did not differ significantly from the 59 placebo patients in deaths (13 in each group), or in stroke recurrence among survivors.

Summary of results. The small study of Patten and co-workers[24] suggested that dexamethasone produced short-term benefit; however, this was not found in the larger studies of Mulley, Wilcox, and Mitchell[22] or of Norris and Hachinski.[23] In addition, no long-term benefit could be demonstrated by Mulley and co-workers. Dexamethasone treatment is therefore not considered useful for acute stroke management.

GLYCEROL

Mathew and co-workers[20] studied 54 ischemic and eight hemorrhagic stroke patients (all strokes of less than 96 hours' duration). The patients were given antiedema treatment with glycerol, 50 g intravenously daily for 4 to 6 days, or placebo. At 14 days 18% of 34 treated patients and 21% of 28 controls were worse or dead. For cerebral infarcts only, neurologic assessment at 14 days implied that treatment was beneficial: 76% of 29 treated, versus 56% of 25 control patients, were improved (p less than .01).

Treatment similar to that just described was also given for 6 days by Gelmers[13c] (50 patients seen in the first 12 hours); Larsson, Marinovich, and Barber[17a] (27 patients seen in the first 6 hours; none had subsequently cleared by 24 hours); Friedli and co-workers[13b] (56 patients seen in the first 24 hours); and Bayer, Pathy, and Newcombe[5a] (173 patients seen in the first 24 hours). Gelmers noted neither survival nor neurologic score benefit at 4 weeks, nor did Larsson and associates at 10 days or at 3 months. Overall, Friedli and co-workers saw less neurologic deficit at 2 weeks (p less than .02) but not at 6 months; mortality was not reduced. Bayer and associates noted increased survival at 1 week and at 12 months but no neurologic or functional recovery benefit.

Frei and co-workers[13a] reported a randomized study of 61 patients who, beginning 24 hours to 1 week after a stroke, received intravenous glycerol, glycerol plus dextran, or placebo. Neither treatment produced survival or neurologic score benefit at 1, 6, 12, or 24 weeks.

Summary of results. Glycerol treatment has not been shown to produce consistent benefit.

DEXTRAN

Intravenous dextran 40 or placebo was given for 3 days by Gilroy, Barnhart, and Meyer[15a] to 50 patients first seen 24 to 72 hours after a stroke, and by Spudis, de la Torre, and Pikula[26a] to 58 patients seen within 24 hours of a stroke. The former authors noted survival and neurologic status benefit from treatment at 10 days; the latter found no survival benefit at 3 weeks.

Dextran combined with glycerol was of no benefit in the study of Frei and associates[13a] (see previous discussion).

Summary of results. Dextran has not been demonstrated to be beneficial.

AMINOPHYLLINE

Britton and co-workers[8] reported on 46 acute (under 48 hours) ischemic stroke patients who were given aminophylline intravenously for 3 days or placebo. At discharge, 27% of 22 treated patients and 29% of 24 controls were worse or dead.

Summary of results. On the basis of this one small study there is no reason to consider aminophylline useful in stroke treatment.

HEMODILUTION THERAPY

Strand and co-workers[27] conducted a study of patients who had had ischemic stroke in the preceding 48 hours. Some of the patients received hemodilution therapy (HDT) consisting of removal of 250 to 650 ml of venous blood in the first 24 hours, with 10% dextran (Rheomacrodex) infusions on days 0, 1, 2, 4, and 6. The following outcomes were noted among 52 HDT patients and 50 controls: 85% of HDT patients improved in neurologic scoring at 10 days, versus 64% of controls; 46% of HDT patients were alive and able to walk without technical aid at 3 months, versus 38% of controls.

Asplund[2] performed another randomized study of similar nature and reported the results for 334 patients. At 3 months the mortality was 16% for HDT, versus 13% among the controls, and there were no benefits in terms of neurologic scoring, activities of daily living, or need for long-term hospital care.

Summary of results. The extended study makes it clear that HDT has not been shown to be valuable in stroke treatment.

PROSTACYCLIN

Martin and co-workers[19] described the use of prostacyclin or placebo for 31 patients with ischemic stroke. Treatment began within 24 to 36 hours of onset and was carried out over 2.5 days. At 2 weeks deaths and disability scores were similar in the two groups.

Huczynski and co-workers[17] reported on prostacyclin or placebo in 26 patients with cerebral infarction. Treatment began within 2 to 5 days of onset and was carried out over 2.5 days. There were no deaths; neurologic status in the two groups was similar at 2 weeks.

Summary of results. Prostacyclin has not been shown of value for patients with recent stroke.

NIMODIPINE

Gelmers and co-workers[14] studied 186 acute ischemic stroke patients who were treated with the calcium channel blocker nimodipine or with placebo. (All patients also received Rheomacrodex and low-dose heparin.) At 4 weeks 90% of 79 nimodipine-treated patients, versus 79% of 85 controls, were still alive (p less than .02); by neurologic scoring the nimodipine group had a better outcome than the controls (p less than .003).

Summary of results. Acute treatment with nimodipine seems to be of value for ischemic stroke patients.

TRAZADONE

Ramirez-Lassepas and co-workers[26] gave trazadone (an antidepressant that blocks serotonin reuptake in the central nervous system), 10 mg intravenously every 12 hours for 7 days, or placebo to 49 patients who had had cerebral infarction within the 24 hours preceding entry into the randomized trial. All patients also received 5000 units of heparin subcutaneously every 12 hours. Among the 25 treated patients there occurred one death and one extension of cerebral infarction during an average of 22.9 days of hospitalization; among 24 controls the comparable occurrences were one and none during an average of 25.6 days of hospitalization.

Summary of results. Trazadone was of no value as an early treatment of cerebral infarction.

PENTOXIFYLLINE

Pentoxifylline, which increases red cell deformability and decreases fibrinogen levels and platelet aggregation, was given to ischemic stroke patients by the Pentoxifylline Study Group[25] under a randomized double-blind placebo-controlled protocol. The patients (mean age 69 years; 58% men) began treatment within 15 hours of stroke onset. Pentoxifylline, 16 mg/kg/day, was given intravenously for 3 to 7 days; the agent was then continued at 400 mg orally three times a day for the remainder of 28 days. Neurologic deficit scores among the 139 treated patients were better than among the 131 controls during the first few days, but the two groups did not differ in either neurologic status or survival at 28 days.

Summary of results. Pentoxifylline showed no sustained benefit in patients with acute ischemic infarct.

GENERAL SUMMARY

Aspirin was of value for poststroke treatment in one large study but not in another. Since the latter study showed no evidence of harm, long-term therapy with ASA, 990 mg per day, is recommended pending further evidence on the issue.

Immediate anticoagulation therapy, beginning with intravenously administered heparin, is of value for stroke in evolution (two studies) and may be of value (one small study) in the acute treatment of ischemic stroke secondary to emboli of cardiac origin. ACT has not been demonstrated to be of value, early or late, for the general patient with a nondeteriorating ischemic stroke.

Nimodipine (one study) may improve outcome in acute ischemic stroke.

Glycerol, dextran, aminophylline, dexamethasone, dipyridamole, hemodilution therapy, pentoxifylline, prostacyclin, suloctidil, and trazadone have all failed to show benefit in stroke treatment.

Endarterectomy after completed stroke is dangerous, according to the evidence available from randomized observation, and should not be performed.

REFERENCES

1. Acheson, J, Danta, G, and Hutchinson, EC: Controlled trial of dipyridamole in cerebral vascular disease, Br Med J 1:614, 1969.
2. Asplund, K: Hemodilution in acute ischemic stroke—a randomized multicenter trial, Stroke 17:143, 1986.
3. Baker, RN, et al: Anticoagulant therapy in cerebral infarction: report on cooperative study, Neurology 12:823, 1962.
4. Bauer, RB, et al: A controlled study of surgical treatment of cerebrovascular disease—42 months experience with 183 cases. In Millikan, CH, Siekert, RG, and Whisnant, JP, editors: Cerebral vascular diseases, New York 1966, Grune & Stratton, Inc.
5. Bauer, RB, et al: Joint study of extracranial arterial occlusion. III. Progress report of controlled study of long-term survival in patients with and without operation, JAMA 208:509, 1969.
5a. Bayer, AJ, Pathy, MSJ, and Newcombe, R: Double-blind randomised trial of intravenous glycerol in acute stroke, Lancet 1:405, 1987.
6. Bousser, MG, et al: "AICLA" controlled trial of aspirin and dipyridamole in the secondary prevention of athero-thrombotic cerebral ischemia, Stroke 14:5, 1983.
7. Britton, M, Helmers, C, and Samuelsson, K: High dose acetylsalicylic acid after cerebral infarction: a Swedish cooperative study, Stroke 17:132, 1986.
8. Britton, M, et al: Lack of effect of theophylline on the outcome of acute cerebral infarction, Acta Neurol Scand 62:116, 1980.
9. Carter, AB: Anticoagulant treatment in progressing stroke, Br Med J 2:70, 1961.
10. Cerebral Embolism Study Group: Immediate anticoagulation of embolic stroke: a randomized trial, Stroke 14:127, 1983.
11. Duke, RJ, et al: Intravenous heparin for the prevention of stroke progression in acute partial stable stroke: a randomized controlled trial, Ann Intern Med 105:825, 1986.
12. Enger, E, and Boyesen, S: Long-term anticoagulant therapy in patients with cerebral infarction, Acta Med Scand 178(suppl 438):7, 1965.

13. Fisher, CM: Anticoagulant therapy in cerebral thrombosis and cerebral embolism: a national cooperative study, interim report, Neurology 11(Part II):119, 1961.
13a. Frei, A, et al: Glycerol and dextran combined in the therapy of acute stroke: a placebo-controlled double-blind trial with a planned interim analysis, Stroke 18:373, 1987.
13b. Friedli, W, et al: Infusionsbehandlung des akuten ischaemischen hirninfarktes mit glycerin 10%: doppelblindstudie, Schweiz Med Wschr 109:737, 1979.
13c. Gelmers, HJ: Effect of glycerol treatment on the natural history of acute cerebral infarction, Clin Neurol Neurosurg 4:277, 1975.
14. Gelmers, HJ, et al: Effect of nimodipine on clinical outcome in patients with acute ischemic stroke, Stroke 17:145, 1986.
15. Gent, M, et al: A secondary prevention, randomized trial of suloctidil in patients with a recent history of thromboembolic stroke, Stroke 16:416, 1985.
15a. Gilroy, J, Barnhart, MI, and Meyer, JS: Treatment of acute stroke with dextran 40, JAMA 210:293, 1969.
16. Hill, AB, Marshall, J, and Shaw, DA: Cerebrovascular disease: trial of long-term anticoagulant therapy, Br Med J 2:1003, 1962.
17. Huczynski, J, et al: Double-blind trial controlled trial of the therapeutic effects of prostacyclin in patients with completed ischaemic stroke, Stroke 16:810, 1985.
17a. Larsson, O, Marinovich, N, and Barber, K: Double-blind trial of glycerol therapy in early stroke, Lancet 1:832, 1976.
18. Marshall, J, and Shaw, DA: Anticoagulant therapy in acute cerebrovascular accidents: a controlled trial, Lancet 1:995, 1960.
19. Martin, JF, et al: Double-blind controlled trial of prostacyclin in cerebral infarction, Stroke 16:386, 1985.
20. Mathew, NT, et al: Double-blind evaluation of glycerol therapy in acute cerebral infarction, Lancet 2:1327, 1972.
21. McDowell, F, McDevitt, E, and Wright, IS: Anticoagulant therapy: five years experience with the patient with an established cerebrovascular accident, Arch Neurol 8:209, 1963.
22. Mulley, G, Wilcox, RG, and Mitchell, JRA: Dexamethasone in acute stroke, Br Med J 2:994, 1978.
23. Norris, JW, and Hachinski, VC: High dose steroid treatment in cerebral infarction, Br Med J 292:21, 1986.
24. Patten, BM, et al: Double-blind study of the effects of dexamethasone on acute stroke, Neurology 22:377, 1972.
25. Pentoxifylline Study Group: Pentoxifylline (PTX) in acute ischemic stroke, Stroke 18:298, 1987. (Additional details given at 12th International Joint Conference on Stroke and Cerebral Circulation, Tampa, Fla, Feb 28, 1987.)
26. Ramirez-Lassepas, M, et al: Failure of central nervous system serotonin blockage to influence outcome in acute cerebral infarction, Stroke 17:953, 1986.
26a. Spudis, EV, de la Torre, E, and Pikula, L: Management of completed strokes with dextran 40: a community hospital failure, Stroke 4:895, 1973.
27. Strand, T, et al: A randomized controlled trial of hemodilution therapy in acute ischemic stroke, Stroke 15:980, 1984.
28. Veterans Administration Cooperative Study of Atherosclerosis, Neurology Section: An evaluation of anticoagulant therapy in the treatment of cerebrovascular disease, Neurology 11(Part II):132, 1961.
29. Wallace, DC: Cerebral vascular disease in relation to long-term anticoagulant therapy, J Chron Dis 17:527, 1964.

CHAPTER 7 | Brain plasticity

PAUL BACH-Y-RITA

Following nonfatal brain damage, some recovery of function usually occurs, and progress can continue for years. The degree of recovery depends on many factors, including age, the brain area and amount of tissue damaged, rapidity of the damage, the rehabilitation program, and environmental and psychosocial factors. These and other aspects have been examined extensively elsewhere.[2,3,6,23]

In recent years the brain's ability to modify functions and compensate for damage has been shown to play a role in recovery. However, the importance of this ability has only recently been appreciated. In the middle of the last century Broca[17] identified a specific area in the left temporal lobe that is related to speech. This discovery was the focal point for the coalescence of neuroscience around a concept of strict localization. A plethora of studies describing the identification of specific areas in the brain related to specific functions followed; the subject is still being studied.

It was an appropriate time for Broca's discovery. Exciting developments in physics, chemistry, and biology revealed much of nature's design, and descriptive science flourished. As morphologic, physiologic, and neurochemical techniques improved, more and more details of the brain's structure and functional connectivity were revealed. The enormous complexity of the brain may have contributed to the conceptual rigidity that developed. To organize all that was known into a cohesive and understandable whole, anatomists had to compartmentalize (as is evident in Brodmann's division of the cortex into 52 regions),[18] and the descriptions and illustrations of those components (each clearly separated from the others) resulted in a concept of a rigid, sharply divided brain. This, coupled with the connectivity studies and the absence of any sign of significant regeneration in the brain (in contrast to organs such as the liver that have

the capability of mitotic duplication), combined to create an impression of a divided, nonmalleable organ with little ability to recover from damage. Few anatomists, physiologists, or clinicians projected a concept of dynamic adaptability. Thus significant recovery was rarely expected or sought through well-founded, ambitious rehabilitation programs. The fact that so few persons showed significant recovery reinforced the fashionable concept of a rigid brain. In this there is an element of what Merton[33] has called the "self-fulfilling prophecy."

Home programs developed by nonprofessional family members who had no knowledge of prevailing beliefs (or "conceptual substance"; see Frank[25]), which at the time were that little or no recovery could be expected, may have been successful *because* of this ignorance: they did not *know* that recovery was impossible after a certain period of time (for example, 6 months) and thus proceeded to work toward, and to obtain, recovery.[2,26]

How can the nihilism of neurologic specialists (and many rehabilitation specialists) be counteracted? Solid, well-founded studies of brain rehabilitation are needed, despite the methodologic difficulties in developing such studies.[3] This field is in a stage comparable to that of nerve physiology when the usefulness of the giant axon of the squid was discovered. The accessibility of this axon enabled axonal physiology to make major advances with techniques then available, and as newer techniques emerged, the basic properties of the squid axon generalized to smaller and less accessible axons. In rehabilitation we are still in a stage when the intensive study of single, unusual cases (such as that discussed in Bach-y-Rita[2]) may produce results that can lead to the design of broader-scale studies. However, the premature reliance on broad-scale studies when the methodologies and statistical comparisons are questionable may result in not only misleading conclusions, but also the masking of the unusual cases of recovery.

The rationale for reliance on brain plasticity to obtain significant recovery following brain damage is still insufficiently developed. The evidence has been evaluated elsewhere.[1,2,3,8,23] Some of this evidence is discussed in the context of cultural, methodologic, and philosophic factors relating to the current status of the concept of brain plasticity.

CONCEPT OF BRAIN PLASTICITY

A *synapse* can be considered a morphologic and physiologic entity, but it is also a concept in evolution.[28] Similarly, brain plasticity is a concept, although one that is less well supported by a body of specific scientific literature than is the synapse. Concepts we develop are significantly influenced by social, technologic, and scientific·factors. Fleck[24] showed that even a well-studied "fact" such as the cause of syphilis is a concept that is a product of these factors.* He stated:

> Evidence conforms to conceptions just as often as conceptions conform to evidence. After all, conceptions are not logical systems. . . . They are stylized units which either develop or atrophy just as they are or merge with their proofs into others. Analogously to social structures, every age has its own dominant conceptions as well as remnants of past ages and rudiments of those of the future.†

A fact can be manufactured by prevailing conceptions. For example, a *prion* has never been shown to exist. It is, as far as has been demonstrated to date, a concept advanced by a scientist who has predicted its existence and has been interpreting his and other data in that context. The broad use of the term *prion* (a short version of "proteinaceous infectious particles," a postulated subviral structure that is purported to be the cause of certain "slow virus" diseases) in popular and scientific literature has led many to consider it a fact.[37] Frank, in a discussion of the development of techniques, noted that "the popular image of science formed largely by the elegant conceptual intricacies of theoretical physics portrays *ideas* as pre-eminently important. . . . On the contrary. . . techniques are intimately bound up with both the conceptual substance and the social process of the experimental biological sciences."[25] Similarly, the concept

of brain plasticity is bound in social context, technology, and scientific fashion.

Brain plasticity can be defined broadly or narrowly. In the first case, all learning can be included in the concept. In the second case, evidence of morphologic changes such as sprouting is required. I consider a middle position to be appropriate and have defined brain plasticity as "the adaptive capacities of the central nervous system—its ability to modify its own structural organization and functioning."[2] It permits an adaptive (or a maladaptive) response to functional demand. Konorski[30] considered plasticity to be one of the two fundamental properties of the nervous system: it permits enduring functional changes to take place. He considered the other fundamental property to be excitability, which relates to rapid changes that leave no trace in the nervous system. Mechanisms of brain plasticity can include neurochemical, end-plate, receptor, and neuronal structural changes.

The "conceptual substance" of neuroscience has, since Broca's time, been inhospitable to plasticity concepts. However, during this time a few significant results have been obtained.* These studies and the conclusions that are commonly drawn from them were not in fashion at that time. Since plasticity was not an important part of the conceptual substance, evidence supporting it was generally ignored. Similarly, the ability to influence neural function through mental activity was not a significant part of the conceptual substance, except in the case of the placebo effect, when the effect was of interest (and thus widely studied) because the placebo is a major "contaminant" of drug studies. It would thus appear that mental activity has been of interest more for its negative than its positive effects (for example, its role in recovery from brain damage). However, interesting results were obtained in this area also. Walter Cannon,[20] whose studies of homeostasis have been widely quoted, published an article in 1941 titled "Voodoo Death," apparently because of his interest in the ability of mental activity to influence homeostatic mechanisms—even to the point of producing death in otherwise healthy persons. More recently Rosenzweig[36] reviewed the literature on animal studies related to the role of the environment on developmental measures and on recovery from brain damage. This is pertinent to a study of brain rehabilitation, since it must be related to the mechanisms of action of environmental and psychosocial factors in influencing recovery.

It is important to determine the limitations of brain plasticity in obtaining recovery. Different systems in the brain may require different amounts of viable tissue, and some structures may be more important than others.[1,2,15] Also, techniques applicable to one system may not work in another.[11] Thus this discussion of brain plasticity mechanisms should be interpreted in the context of a concept in devel-

---

*In the fifteenth century syphilis was considered a scourge brought on by sin and was associated with the blood. The idea of bad blood took on mystical-ethical overtones. With the discovery of the agent of the disease and the development of the blood tests, the association with the blood became scientifically sound. In a chapter titled "How the Modern Concept of Syphilis Originated," Fleck[24] notes how the current scientific thought at each stage influenced the concept. For example, astrologic interpretations were conditioned by the high status astrology held at the time.

†Fleck, L: Genesis and development of a scientific fact, Chicago, 1979, University of Chicago Press.

*References 14, 19, 31, 32, 34, 38.

opment. By no means does this diminish its usefulness or its relevance to the rehabilitation of brain-damaged patients.

SOME MECHANISMS UNDERLYING BRAIN PLASTICITY

Bach-y-Rita and co-workers[8] recently reviewed the literature on mechanisms of recovery, and it has been discussed extensively elsewhere.[2-4,23] Therefore only a brief summary is provided here.

Sprouting

Sprouting is the growth from a cell body to another cell as a result of normal growth, a vacancy at a particular site, or a return to a particular site. Collateral sprouts are new axonal processes that have budded off an uninjured axon and have grown to a vacated synaptic site. Sprouting has been shown to occur in the central nervous system (CNS). However, it can be adaptive or maladaptive, and its role in recovery from brain damage is still uncertain.

Denervation supersensitivity

Denervation supersensitivity results in a permanent increase in neuronal responsivity to diminished input. The receptor site may become more sensitive to a neurotransmitter, or the receptors may increase in number. This may be a factor in CNS reorganization.

Behavior compensation

Following brain damage, new combinations of behaviors can develop. For example, a patient may use different groups of muscles or cognitive strategies.

Unmasking

Quiescent neuronal connections that are inhibited in the normal state may be unmasked following brain damage. This may be an important mechanism of recovery of function. Negative effects of unmasking may also occur. For example, the appearance of "pathologic" reflexes (such as a Babinski reflex) following brain injury may be due to the unmasking of reflexes that were normal in infancy but became inhibited during development.

MODELS OF BRAIN PLASTICITY

A few selected human and animal models of brain plasticity are discussed. The further development of these and other models is necessary for the concept to be more generally understood and accepted.

Animal models

The application of animal models to brain rehabilitation is discussed extensively in other texts[2,23] and is noted briefly here.

Rehabilitation of amblyopic cats

Hubel and Wiesel[27] demonstrated that, if the eyelids of one eye of a kitten are sutured closed for the duration of the critical period of normal visual development, that eye is permanently amblyopic following the removal of the sutures—even if the cat lives for 5 years or more with the eyelids functioning normally. However, Chow and Steward[19] asked the critical question: can recovery of vision be obtained with an appropriate training (rehabilitation) program? They were able to demonstrate that it is possible to obtain some function (vision), but they also recorded concomitant physiologic changes (increased numbers of binocular cells in the visual cortex) and morphologic changes (in the lateral geniculate body). This study is one of the most important animal studies to date in the field of rehabilitation. In addition to the brain plasticity findings, the description of procedures is pertinent to human rehabilitation. For example, it was noted that commonly used rewards were insufficient; the cats required periods of "gentling" and petting (to establish an affectionate bond with the experimenters), and the experimenters' approach to developing a demanding and intensive rehabilitation program while avoiding frustration is of interest.

Chow and Steward's findings may also be relevant to human amblyopia.[19] Although amblyopia is usually not successfully treated when a good eye is present, Romero-Apis and others[35] cited eight cases in which patients between 16 and 69 years of age with amblyopia lost their good eye or had it severely damaged. In all cases vision in the amblyopic eye improved markedly, thus revealing plasticity of the adult brain.

Environmental enrichment in a rat model

Rosenzweig[36] analyzed pertinent animal studies from the perspective of possible applications to human rehabilitation. Rats were placed in enriched environments consisting of cages with a number of toys and other stimuli, which resulted in morphologic, physiologic, neurochemical, and behavioral changes. A number of intriguing possibilities for human studies emerge from these findings. For example, 2 hours per day of enriched environment was found to be as effective as 24 hours per day, which suggests the need for a human study of quality versus quantity in a rehabilitation program.

Role of neurotransmitters in recovery from brain damage

Feeney and co-workers[22] showed in rats that stimulation of catecholamines in the brain following a sensorimotor cortex lesion, combined with a "rehabilitation" program, significantly hastens motor recovery. Further studies have shown the roles of the locus cereuleus and the cerebellum in this phenomenon.[8,15,16] This is of considerable interest to those in the field of brain rehabilitation, and human studies are under way. A pilot study has already shown that neurotransmitter manipulation can produce increased recovery in stroke patients when combined with rehabilitation.[21]

Human models
Late rehabilitation

Most brain-damaged rehabilitation patients receive rehabilitation during a stage (which may last 2 years or more) when they would have demonstrated some spontaneous recovery even in the absence of specific rehabilitation, especially if some of the complications had been prevented (for example, by passive movements to prevent contractures). Therefore it is difficult to quantify accurately the effect of the rehabilitation program, since its results proceed simultaneously with the spontaneous recovery. Thus we have designed rehabilitation programs that can be provided after spontaneous recovery ceases to be a factor. After three complete baseline studies over a period of a year, the specifically designed late rehabilitation program is initiated. Objective measures include positron emission tomography (PET) scans and the analysis of cerebral electrical activity, as well as functional measures. The goals are to obtain objective correlates of functional improvement and evidence for brain plasticity and to develop scientifically validated rehabilitation procedures.[8]

Facial paralysis rehabilitation is one area where late rehabilitation has been successful. Persons who lose motor control of the facial musculature on one side because of the destruction of the facial nerve (often caused by a tumor such as an acoustic neuroma) are excellent models for the evaluation of brain plasticity concepts. This is especially true of those who undergo anastomosis of cranial nerves VII and XII, since in these cases there is direct surgical evidence of a complete section of the facial nerve and the attachment of its peripheral portion to the central portion of nerve XII. In these cases the reinnervation of facial muscles by nerves genetically programmed to control tongue muscles leads to excellent muscle tone (and thus a relatively symmetric face at rest) but dysfunction that is apparent on movement and often results in inhibition of the uninvolved side and diminished affect. For example, during a smile, one side of the face does not rise, and during eating, facial movements occur on one side of the face. The selection of a group of persons whose dysfunction has been evident for several years has enabled us to evaluate rehabilitation programs specifically designed to obtain reorganization of function by reprogramming the motor neurons of nerve XII on the operated side to become included in facial motor programs.[10,13]

Improvement of vision in a longstanding amblyopic eye following loss of the good eye (discussed previously) could be considered late rehabilitation. In this case the need to see leads to self-rehabilitation. In all eight cases reported by Romero-Apis and co-workers,[35] improvement occurred over a period of up to 2 years and was maintained.

Voluntary ocular torsion

The ability of normal research subjects to develop voluntary control over movements that do not exist genetically was studied by means of training voluntary ocular torsion around an anterior-posterior axis.[12] Subjects were trained to produce voluntary saccades and slow movements up to 20 degrees. (Larger torsion movements were considered unsafe.) The development of new motor programs by means of training not only supports the concept of "brain plasticity" but also raises the possibility that in the rehabilitation of patients with paralysis, one mechanism of recovery might be the development of entirely new motor programs. Of course, other possible interpretations are not ruled out. For example, the motor rehabilitation may be related to changes in neurotransmitter release or in the balance of excitation and inhibition.

Sensory substitution

Adults born blind have used their remaining senses and brain mechanisms to develop motor, conceptual, and social behavior. However, the congenitally blind person has not had the experience of receiving and interpreting visual information and developing visual percepts. Such a person offers an ideal model for studying the development of visuospatial perception and behavior. The experimenter can control all facets of the development, and it can occur only with the use of the sensory substitution equipment. In contrast, a hemiparetic patient can practice at home or in the hospital room following therapy sessions, and so in those cases it is less possible to evaluate all the factors that enter into motor rehabilitation.

Tactile vision substitution systems deliver visual information to the brain via the skin. The output of a small television camera (controlled by the blind subject) is displayed on an area of skin, after transduction to a form of energy (delivered by vibrotactors or electrotactors) that can activate the skin sensory receptors. Blind persons not only develop the ability to perceive visual information but also learn to use visual means of analysis (parallax, looming and zooming, monocular clues of depth and perspective, and subjective spatial localization). This model has provided considerable information on brain plasticity, perceptual mechanisms, and the coordination of sensory and motor factors in the development of a "perceptual organ," as well as on other subjects.[1,5,7] It is also being used as a means to develop visuospatial concepts in congenitally blind children. Tactile sensory substitution systems are under development for persons with other sensory losses and for sensory augmentation (for example, for space suit gloves for extravehicular space activities of astronauts[9]).

Intensive study of unusual cases of recovery following brain damage

This model is briefly discussed above. Its broad-scale application in brain rehabilitation will provide the basis for the future design of larger studies. Single case statistical techniques (for example, those described by Kazdin[29]) can be applied to prospective studies such as the testing of a specific rehabilitation methodology. Retrospective individual case studies require interpretation and analysis of objective findings. For example, in the case discussed by Bach-y-Rita,[2] premorbid and postmorbid functional information, as well as medical and autopsy findings, were available. Reliable data on the extent of the neural damage in cases of excellent recovery are particularly important in developing an understanding of compensatory mechanisms and of the capacity for reorganization of the CNS. Noninvasive techniques such as nuclear magnetic resonance and computerized tomography (CT) scan data are valuable. Dynamic measures such as PET scanning to evaluate metabolic activity in specific brain regions and sophisticated electrical activity evaluation techniques (evoked potentials, analysis of ongoing electrical activity) provide objective evidence of change associated with brain rehabilitation.

CONCLUSIONS

The concept of brain plasticity and evidence of its importance in brain rehabilitation are presented. Extensive studies are needed to strengthen the concept and to develop appropriate "conceptual substance" and methodologies leading to maximum recovery. It is apparent that, although spontaneous improvement occurs, specific rehabilitation programs are necessary. (As a comparison, although some adults learn new languages merely by being in the appropriate environment, specific language training is often required.)

The appropriate conditions for rehabilitation are only briefly mentioned here, since they have been discussed in other publications.[2,3,8] Beyond appropriate therapy, environmental, psychosocial, and other factors are important, as is the development of functional rehabilitation programs. The clinical mandate for the field of brain rehabilitation—recovery of function following brain damage—is broad and important. The efforts required to bring it to maturity through the development of a strong theoretic foundation and scientifically based and validated rehabilitation procedures are fully justified.

REFERENCES

1. Bach-y-Rita, P: Brain mechanisms in sensory substitution, New York, 1972, Academic Press, Inc.
2. Bach-y-Rita, P, editor: Recovery of function: theoretical considerations for brain injury rehabilitation, Baltimore, 1980, University Park Press.
3. Bach-y-Rita, P: Brain plasticity as a basis for the development of rehabilitation procedures for hemiplegia, Scand J Rehabil Med 13:73, 1981.
4. Bach-y-Rita, P: Central nervous system lesions: sprouting and unmasking in rehabilitation, Arch Phys Med Rehabil 62:413, 1981.
5. Bach-y-Rita, P: Sensory substitution and recovery from "brain damage." In Finger, S, et al: Theoretical and controversial issues in recovery after brain damage, New York, Plenum Press. In press.
6. Bach-y-Rita, P, and Balliet, R: Recovery from stroke. In Duncan, PW, and Badke, MB, editors: Motor deficits following stroke, Chicago, 1987, Year Book Medical Publishers.
7. Bach-y-Rita, P, and Hughes, B: Tactile vision substitution: some instrumentation and perceptual considerations. In Warren, C, and Strelow, E, editors: Electronic spatial sensing for the blind, Dordrecht, The Netherlands, 1985, Martinus-Nijhoff Publishers.
8. Bach-y-Rita, P, et al: Neural aspects of motor function as a basis of early and post-acute rehabilitation. In DeLisa, JA, et al: Principles and practice of rehabilitation medicine, JB Lippincott. In press.
9. Bach-y-Rita, P, et al: Sensory substitution for space gloves and for space robotics. In Rodriquez, G, editor: Proceedings of the 1986 Space Telerobotics Workshop, Pub No 87-13, vol II, Pasadena, Calif, 1987, Jet Propulsion Laboratories.
10. Balliet, R: Facial paralysis and other neuromuscular dysfunctions of the peripheral nervous system. In Payton, OD, editor: Manual of physical therapy techniques, New York, 1987, Churchill Livingston Inc, Publishers. In press.
11. Balliet, R, Blood, K, and Bach-y-Rita, P: Visual field rehabilitation in the cortically blind? J Neurol Neurosurg Psychiatry 48:1113, 1985.
12. Balliet, R, and Nakayama, K: Training of voluntary torsion, Invest Ophthalmol Vis Sci 17:303, 1978.
13. Balliet, R, Shinn, JB, and Bach-y-Rita, P: Facial paralysis rehabilitation: retraining selective muscle control, Int Rehabil Med 4:67, 1982.
14. Bethe, A: Plastizitat und Zentrenlehre, Handb Norm Pathol Physiol 15(11):1175, 1930.
15. Boyeson, MG, Krobert, KA, and Hughes, JM: Norepinephrine infusions into the cerebellum facilitate recovery from sensorimotor cortex injury, Neuroscience (abstract) 12:1120, 1986.
16. Boyeson, MG, and Feeney, DM: The role of norepinephrine in recovery from brain injury, Neuroscience (abstract) 10:68, 1984.
17. Broca, P: Nouvelle observation dáphémie produite par une lésion de la zème circonvolution frontale. Bull Soc Anat 6(Zème Série), 1861.
18. Brodman, K: Vergleichende Lokalisationslehre der Groshirninde, Leipzig, 1909, Barth.
19. Chow, KL, and Steward, DL: Reversal of structural and functional effects of long-term visual deprivation in cats, Exp Neurol 34:409, 1972.
20. Cannon, W: Voodoo death, Am Anthropol 44:1076, 1942.
21. Davis JN, et al: Amphetamine and physical therapy facilitate recovery from stroke: correlative animal and human studies. In the 15th Princeton Conference on Cerebrovascular Disease, New York, Raven Press. In press.
22. Feeney, DM, Gonzalez, A, and Law, WA: Amphetamine, haloperidol, and experience interact to affect rate of recovery after a motor cortex injury, Science 217:855, 1982.
23. Finger, S, and Stein, DG: Brain damage and recovery: research and clinical perspectives, Orlando, Fla, 1982, Academic Press, Inc.
24. Fleck, L: Genesis and development of a scientific fact, Chicago, 1979, University of Chicago Press.
25. Frank, RG: The Columbian Exchange: American physiologists and neuroscience techniques, Fed Proc 45:2665, 1986.
26. Griffith, VE: A stroke in the family, New York, 1970, Delacorte Press.
27. Hubel, DH, and Wiesel, TN: The period of susceptibility to the physiological effects of unilateral eye closure in kittens, J Physiol (Lond) 206:419, 1970.
28. Johnson, JE: Editorial, Synapse 1:1, 1987.
29. Kazdin, AE: Single case research designs: methods for clinical and applied settings, New York, 1982, Oxford University Press.
30. Konorski, J: The physiological approach to the problem of recent memory. In Fessard, A, editor: Brain mechanisms and learning, Oxford, 1961, Blackwell Press.
31. Lashley, KS: Functional determinants of cerebral localization, Arch Neurol Psychiatry 38:371, 1937.
32. Lashley, KS: Cerebral organization and behavior. In Jeffress, LA, editor: Cerebral mechanisms in behavior, New York, 1951, John Wiley & Sons.

33. Merton, RK: The self-fulfilling prophecy. In Merton, RK, editor: Social theory and social structure, New York, 1968, Free Press.

34. Ogden, R, and Franz, SI: On cerebral motor control: the recovery from experimentally produced hemiplegia, Psychobiology 1:33, 1917.

35. Romero-Apis, D, et al: Perdida del ojo fijador en ambliopia adulta, Ann Soc Mexicana Oftalmol 56:445, 1982.

36. Rosenzweig, M: Animal models for effects of brain lesions and for rehabilitation. In Bach-y-Rita, P, editor: Recovery of function: theoretical considerations for brain injury rehabilitation, Baltimore, 1980, University Park Press.

37. Taubes, G: the name of the game is fame: but is it science? The Discover 7:28, 1986.

38. Zulch, KJ: Otfrid Foerster—physician and naturalist, Berlin, 1969, Springer Verlag.

CHAPTER 8

Rehabilitation of patients with stroke and traumatic brain damage

PAUL KAPLAN AND SANTOSH LAL

HISTORICAL OVERVIEW

Lehmann and co-workers' series on stroke rehabilitation highlights the early, modern history of this area of rehabilitation.[62,63] These authors collected functional outcomes and analyzed cost benefits. Certain medical factors (such as heart failure and atherosclerosis) and other factors (such as age) had predictive values regarding functional outcome after rehabilitation. Indeed, these items had a significant impact on cost-benefit measurements.

Soon thereafter, Bach-y-Rita published his book on recovery of function.[7] Although his text, which presented work published during the 1970s, was about patients with brain injury, his conclusions emphasizing that the brain was a multipotential "malleable organ" provided the theoretic and neurophysiologic explanations for both stroke and brain damage rehabilitation. Bach-y-Rita's studies of "sensory substitution" and "vestibular limb control" techniques complemented Lehmann's proposed theories about improvements in functional abilities that were observed. Bach-y-Rita discussed two hypotheses: "sprouting" from undamaged neurons and "unmasking" previously dormant synapses.[8,9] The effects of sensory and motor reeducation could thus be measured by applying reproducible methods that studied functional advances. In fact, theories had been proposed to explain the observed improvements with specific hypotheses that could be proved or disproved.[7-9,62,63] Bach-y-Rita's and Lehmann's studies were presented at virtually the same time and complemented each other. Technologic advances have permitted a more immediate and exacting observation of both areas.

To measure evolution of the brain damage and later the outcome of management techniques, several scales were devised.* The first was the Glasgow Coma Scale, which rated coma by examining eye opening, motor response, and verbal response. This scale was meant to be general and global, not fine or very specific. The second type of scale was comprehensive and measured the amount of disability. The Rancho Scale and the Glasgow Outcome Scale come to mind.[45] In them the patient is categorized into stages. The lower the stage, the worse the functional ability profile and the higher the disability. Patients with too low a score were not supposed to be candidates for rehabilitation because their disability was too great. Patients with a high score were not supposed to need rehabilitation. The process yielded cost-benefit implications that frequently became an excuse for denying therapy.

CLINICAL PATHOPHYSIOLOGY
Motor and sensory reverberating circuits

Throughout the 1970s and 1980s, detailed studies of central nervous system structures were published. Cayaffa[16] has reviewed much of this literature. Certain specific observations have become relevant to functional gains after central nervous system lesions. The precentral motor cortex of the cerebral hemispheres receives fibers from the thalamus—especially from the ventrolateral nucleus and the posterior portion of the ventroanterior nucleus. These nuclei in turn receive fibers from the lenticular nuclei. Efferent fibers not only go to the corticospinal tracts but also pass through the frontal lobes and terminate in the lenticular nuclei. Therefore a motor reverberating circuit is naturally present. Reverberating loops are prominent in hypotheses concerning cen-

---

*References 51, 52, 68, 86, 97-99.

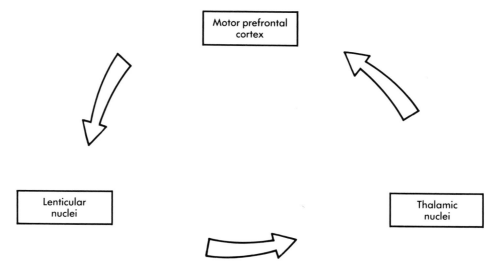

Figure 8-1. Motor reverberating circuit.

tral nervous system structural or functional deficits.[15,49,50,87] The motor reverberating circuit described above probably has connections—direct or indirect—with the internal capsule, the red nucleus, the cerebellum, the reticular formation, and other brainstem areas. Its basic interactions, however, remain cyclic (Figure 8-1).

The somatosensory system has the same cyclic structure. The postcentral cortex receives fibers from the medial and lateral ventral posterior nuclei of the thalamus.[16] Efferent fibers are widely scattered throughout the central nervous system but include tracts directed through the frontal lobes to the lenticular nuclei. Efferent fibers also terminate directly in thalamic nuclei to give an added element of reciprocal control or feedback. Fibers from the lenticular nuclei terminate in thalamic nuclei. Since two sensory and two motor loops are present, if one set is damaged, the remaining intact circuits can take over the function of the lost loops.[101] However, many brain-damaged patients have extensive involvement over both cerebral hemispheres, precluding this (Figure 8-2).

The loops have specific types of chemical receptors. Endogenous opioids are active after both stroke and brain damage.[30] Indeed, thyrotropin-releasing hormone—an opioid antagonist—has been effectively applied to the treatment of patients with brain damage.[30,40,105]

The integrity of the motor loop and therefore of praxic function depends on intact subcortical tracts.[2,22] When stroke or brain damage interrupts these circuits, deficits in the motor reverberating circuit generate clumsiness far outweighing any residual muscular power. The affected extremity is functionally disabled.

When the somatosensory cyclic system is interrupted, deficits are noted in dynamic sensation even if static sensation is intact.[54] Even when light touch and pinprick sensations remain, deficits are still noted in two-point discrimination, stereognosis, and relative velocity determination. Consequently the extremity is effectively blinded. The patient does not know through what space that arm or leg moves. That extremity cannot be used as efficiently, even though its muscular power is preserved. This deficit exhaustively complements that noted after the interruption of the motor circuit, and in fact they are nearly always noted together.[61] The motor deficit is especially prominent in patients with lesions in the left cerebral hemisphere. The left hemisphere initiates or activates both reverberating circuits when deliberate actions are required. Neglect is itself an understatement; affected patients avoid touching the involved extremity and a few actually abuse it because it is no longer responsive. When action is begun, it is delayed and sequences are slowed. Slow motion represents augmented inertial resistance to any change. The following outline presents deficits after interruption of cyclic systems:

I. Isolated deficit
   A. Motor circuit—kinetic apraxia
   B. Somatosensory circuit—deficit of dynamic sensation
II. Combined deficit
   A. Motor neglect
     1. High inertial resistance to quick movements
      a. All movements performed in slow motion
      b. Difficulty in changing or stopping motion
     2. Involved extremity avoided or neglected

It probably does not matter whether the interruption is traumatic or vascular in origin. Other factors are more important. Thrombotic vascular events linger longer than hemorrhagic incidents. An arterial spasm, similar to that noted in coronary arteries, can be as devastating as thrombosis.[91] The completeness and extent of the lesion are also important.

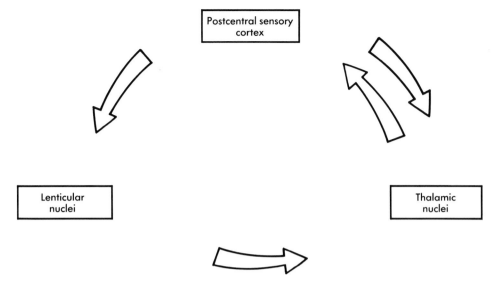

Figure 8-2. Somatosensory reverberating circuit.

Necrotic lesions create more permanent sequelae than those that cause ischemia of the neurons. Lesions therefore differ in their ability to abolish the cyclic systems.

Leipmann[65] noted that frontal lobe lesions generate "limb kinetic apraxia." When an extremity is commanded to perform a specific motor act or sequence of acts, it is unable to respond. Consequently, lesions in the cortical gray matter or subcortical white matter can produce apraxia.[39]

Spasticity

Classical concepts of the origin of spasticity stressed release of cortical inhibition and the action of muscle spindles.[107,108] It was thought that the spindle was the primary site of the disorder that resulted in spasticity. However, more recent studies of spindle activity by neuroelectrode impalement of selected nerve trunks have shown that spindle activity does not correlate well with hyperactive tendon reflexes.[14,43,44] Instead, the hyperactivity of long tracts—corticospinal, vestibulospinal, reticulospinal—does seem to correlate with reflex excitability.[14,107]

Inhibition has always been difficult to prove. Like the emperor's new clothes, it is demonstrated only by its absence. The long spinal tracts mentioned previously are organized by areas and have many connections with the pool of internuncial neurons.[87] The activity of these neurons can also be manipulated. Decerebrate rigidity in cats is increased during, and markedly reduced after, vibration stimuli—the tonic vibration reflex. Motor output and force only slowly reach previbration levels.[50] The complex effects of sensory stimuli and motor response involve interneuronal activity[88] and direct spinal motor neuron contributions,[49] and serotonin augments this reflex by modifying spinal neuronal depolarization.[15]

When the long spinal tracts become hyperactive, the func-

tion of the spinal internuncial neurons increases in the affected spinal cord segments.[58,59] Possibly this is a negative control mechanism through a posterior horn gating system similar to that postulated for pain control.[74] A spasticity gate control would help explain why spasticity often decreases in an involved joint after isolated, volitional motor control has been restored across that joint. This method naturally reduces spasticity, but it is not invariable. Many patients recover isolated motion across a joint but experience only a minimal reduction in spasticity.

The frequency of motor unit discharges is reduced in spastic muscles.[5,85] A study of electromyographic surface activity and isometric force relationships has also produced results consistent with reductions in motor unit discharge frequency in spastic paretic arms.[96] The origin of this abnormal muscle control lies, at least in part, in long tract dysfunction. Figure 8-3 is a diagram of the polyvariant causes of spasticity.

When patients have had extensive and bilateral cortical lesions, they spontaneously place themselves in symmetric or asymmetric tonic neck reflex positions in bed. Usually these postures are accompanied by increases in flexor muscular tone. The patients are decorticate. Electromyographic and vestibular studies performed on decerebrate cats have demonstrated vestibulocolic reflexes and described the role of the semicircular canal, inner ear macular receptors, vestibular nuclei, and the reticular formation on the brainstem.[104] The reflex response stabilizes head position involuntarily and permits quantitative studies of the resulting head motion.[12] The reflex is potentiated by normal head rotation and controls head placement in space in a normal cat.[25] Since body positions are determined by reactions to vestibular reflexive head placement by lumbar interneurons, head positioning also determines the placement of the rest of the

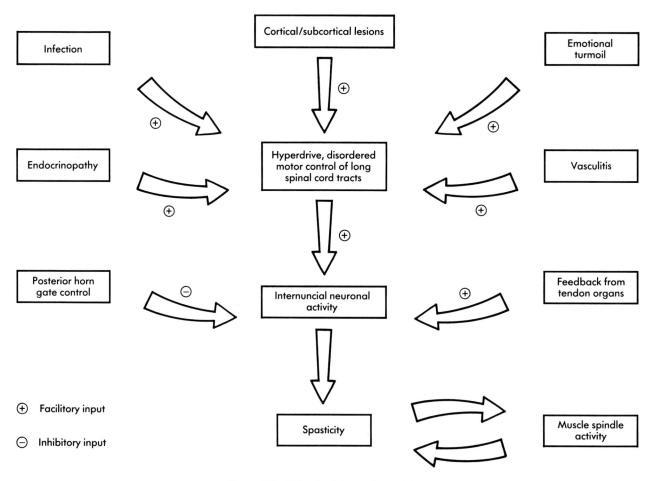

Figure 8-3. Pathophysiology of spasticity.

animal.[95] These studies provide a basis for therapeutic application in rehabilitation, where reflex responses are used repetitively to stimulate the patient to form a new engram or motor pattern even if the patient is essentially decorticate.[58,59] Indeed, the process is normal in motor learning—for example, learning to bat, pitch, type, or sew. We are merely juxtaposing a functional action with an approximate sequence of reflexive positionings.

NONINVASIVE EVALUATION OF BRAIN DYSFUNCTION

Computerized tomographic (CT) scans and positron emission tomographic (PET) scans have made it possible to correlate clinicopathologic observations with exact anatomic areas of dysfunction. Three particular types of study using these methods[81] have been reported:

1. The natural history of stroke syndromes
2. Patients with more widespread areas of metabolic abnormalities than those areas with infarcted tissue; these patients include individuals with spontaneous posturing, aphasic patients, and brain-damaged patients with significant problems of memory or emotion

3. Prognostic implications—for example, which patients require greater perfusion

CT scans in patients with widespread cerebral lesions can demonstrate development of hydrocephalus.[98] PET scanning and F-18-2 fluorodeoxyglucose have been used to map loci of human cerebral metabolism.[71] PET scanning with ^{15}O can differentiate ischemically injured brain tissue from metabolically impaired tissue in stroke patients.[1]

The conventional repertoire of neurologic examination and scans is augmented by cerebral evoked potential studies (auditory, visual, somatosensory), magnetic resonance imaging or nuclear magnetic resonance, and digital subtraction angiography. We are now in a much better position to determine noninvasively what the structure looks like, how its metabolism is functioning, and what electrical activity is being generated.[75] The use of these new procedures in patients referred for rehabilitation permits a more precise localization of cerebral lesions and a definition of their extensiveness. Some patients referred with incomplete study have been found to have tumors, hematomas, multiple sclerosis, or Wilson's disease.[55] The procedures are particularly useful for patients with deficits in speech and cognition. Patient populations can be selected in a much more homogeneous manner, and outcomes can be correlated with laboratory results clinicopathologically.

Magnetic resonance imaging (MRI) is very sensitive to a wide range of vascular abnormalities.[22] MRI cannot be performed when the patient has metal implants. Digital subtraction angiography is a good screening test for abnormalities in cerebral or cervical blood vessels.[18] It has a very low complication rate, but it is also relatively nonspecific.

In one study on aphasia, CT scanning, cerebral angiography, and ^{133}Xe intracarotid regional blood flow measurements were applied.[81] The tests suggested that "subcortical" aphasia was secondary to decreased blood flow in the cortical speech areas. Establishment of collateral circulation accompanied recovery of language function. The extension and correlation of these studies may help in distinguishing whether specific tests of aphasia could differentiate lesions in the parietal area from those in the frontal cerebral area. One specific test is fluency. Fluency seemed relevant, but auditory repetition proved less useful.[83] Nonetheless, cortical location of the lesion is important. An extensive rolandic lesion is usually associated with persistent nonfluency.[57] PET scanning has revealed decreased glucose metabolism in these cortical areas in patients with aphasia.[72] These noninvasive scanning examinations could also provide a morphologic correlation for memory,[64] neuropsychologic,[38] and semantic[109] testing and should provide some morphologic correlates to the study of the role emotional turmoil plays in stroke and brain injury.[13,36,77,78,82]

MANAGEMENT

Survivors of stroke and traumatic brain damage are left with a variable degree of physical, cognitive, and psychosocial impairment. These two diagnostic groups have some similarities and some differences in disabilities and the therapeutic approaches used in their management. Both groups suffer from fragmented care, lack of validated therapeutic programs, and outcome of treatment approaches. Their progress, residual disability, and adjustment to disability vary depending on the severity of the impairment and on available resources for acute care, rehabilitation program, and long-term care.[34] Not all the patients affected by these disabilities participate in specialized treatment programs. Lack of uniform and appropriate care adversely affects the neurophysical and psychosocial recovery of these patients and inhibits the development of a reliable database for use in planning improvements in care.

Traumatic brain damage
Acute care

The patient in coma after brain damage must have an intact airway and must be monitored to establish the level of coma. Although these needs can be met by the ambulance team, brain damage is frequently accompanied by multiple trauma, which makes care at the scene of injury complex.

Initial hospital management is also difficult. The clinician must quickly determine the origin of the coma, the extent of the brain damage, the stability of the patient's neurologic and general clinical condition, whether there are open or closed injuries to be treated, and whether there is seizure activity. Diagnostic procedures include electroencephalography (EEG), CT scanning, and MRI scanning.

For an unconscious patient an airway must be cleared and maintained. At first endotracheal intubation can be applied, but often a tracheostomy must be performed. The opening created is then often attached to a ventilator. Suctioning of the tracheostomy is required regularly and should be preceded by 5 minutes of 100% oxygen administration. Inspired air needs humidification to prevent desiccation of mucosal secretions. If airway obstruction is present, bronchoscopy is required. Levels of arterial blood gases should be obtained at regular intervals and used to monitor the oxygen level. The volume- and pressure-regulated ventilator can be triggered by the patient as uninterrupted ventilation is discontinued.

Whether mechanical ventilation in and of itself aids recovery from severe brain damage is uncertain. Certainly with time and continued ventilation, alveolar dead space is augmented and lung compliance is reduced. Hyperventilation has been used with mixed results in severely brain-injured adults. EEG slow wave activity can be observed after hyperventilation.

Since hypotension can actually extend the area of damage centrally, monitoring central venous pressure readings to assess right ventricular and atrial function during neurosurgical procedures has become more common. Regular blood pressure and pulse readings are routine. Many patients with severe blood loss require transfusions.

Regulation of fluid and electrolyte balance becomes important once the patient has survived the initial stages. Sodium imbalance and osmolar dysfunction are common after brain damage. A Foley indwelling catheter is used so urinary output can be monitored. It should be taped to the patient's abdomen and changed every 2 weeks. A feeding tube is required. Percutaneous gastrostomy techniques have minor side effects and offer a durable feeding portal. Several commercial feeding solutions, supplying protein, electrolytes, and calories, are available.

The risk of coagulation thrombotic disorders can be alleviated with regular subcutaneous heparin injections. These should be used cautiously in hemorrhagic central disorders but are otherwise effective as a preventive measure. Disseminated intravascular coagulopathies and deep venous thrombophlebitis or pulmonary embolism require more vigorous anticoagulant therapy.

Differential diagnosis of fever is commonly needed. Elevated temperatures can accompany infection and hypothalamic brain damage. These infections can be fatal if not vigorously treated. Urinary tract infections are the most common source of infective pyrexia, but atelectasis and bronchopneumonia are also common in patients attached to respirators.

Because brain damage is stressful, ulcerations frequently cause gastrointestinal bleeding. Cimetidine either alone or with antacids is usually effective, but it should not be given for more than 12 weeks at a time. Fiberoptic endoscopy is extremely valuable in establishing a diagnosis.

Seizure disorders and raised intracranial pressure are two significant neurologic complications of brain damage. Early monitoring and detection are important, since seizures can be managed medically and intracranial pressure surgically. Seizures can be partial, petit mal, grand mal, temporal, or in combinations. If they occur when the patient is unsupervised, they can lead to death by suffocation. Low-pressure hydrocephalus is a nonspecific response to diverse trauma and can cause a subtle dementia. Newer scanning techniques have facilitated diagnosis by physicians alert to these potential problems.

Multiple fractures including spinal injuries can complicate traumatic brain damage. Patients who have unconscious periods after spinal cord injury should be evaluated for brain damage.

Rehabilitation

The rehabilitation of brain-damaged patients is a complex process involving a multidisciplinary approach to reduce disability and improve the function and the quality of life for the patient and family.[4,60,63,100] The rehabilitation process and its outcome depend on the severity of disability, the medical stability of the patient, and the skills of all members of the rehabilitation team. Some reports in the literature describe accurate assessment and benefit of rehabilitation[93] for stroke[75,87] and traumatic brain damage. Early involvement of the rehabilitation team in the care of these patients to improve function and reduce disability and complications is essential and needs to be accepted by all persons in the decision-making process: the physician, family, and representatives of financial agencies.[20,48,53]

During the acute stage, even in intensive care, range-of-motion and strengthening exercises, and cognitive-communication therapy can be started. This approach reduces complications and side effects. It introduces the patient and the family gradually to the long-term implications of the problem and facilitates the transition from acute to chronic rehabilitative care. It is at this early stage that a decision must be made, for example, whether the patient has recovered from the coma enough to profit from acute rehabilitation care or whether another type of facility is required at this time.

Stroke

Rehabilitative intervention within the first 72 hours after admission to the hospital following stroke has resulted in increased ambulatory ability, independence in function, and a shortened hospital stay.[32,48,53] Early rehabilitation team involvement prevents complications and deconditioning.[4,17,33,101] It also improves the patient's functioning and determines the level of safety in long-term care.

A state of coma may occur in both stroke and traumatic brain damage, but the presence of various tubes (tracheostomy tube, nasogastric tube, arterial line, and indwelling catheters) and the use of a respirator is not a contraindication to initiation of therapy. Patients with problems of persistent vegetative stage (PVS), akinetic mutism, and locked-in syndrome might need gastrostomies for a prolonged period to prevent complications, provide safety, and make care management easier for the family or attendant at home. Sometimes premorbid undiagnosed congenital anomalies make it necessary to continue use of a tube. For example, we have experience in managing a brain trauma patient with redundant epiglottis that necessitated a tracheostomy tube to protect the airway, although the patient had achieved partial independence in ambulation and daily care and was living at home. A long-term tracheostomy tube is also needed if the patient is unable to cough and manage oropharyngeal and respiratory secretions appropriately; there is a high risk of complicating aspiration pneumonia. Any medical complication prolongs rehabilitation and adversely affects the process and outcome.[86]

Complications of prolonged ostomies have also been reported. The possibility of repeated infections, stricture stenosis, and fistulas dictates removal of all the tubes as soon as possible. The care of a patient in a coma or PVS mainly requires maintenance of hydration, nutrition, and prevention of complications[106] such as contractures and pressure sores. Lack of prevention of the latter complications necessitates further surgical procedures to correct the deformities for positioning and proper nursing care (Figures 8-4 to 8-7). Periodic monitoring is required for complications and their management; these include hydrocephalus,[56] heterotopic ossification (Figures 8-8 and 8-9),[35] and metabolic disturbances such as hyponatremia and hypoproteinemia.

The continued life support of patients with prolonged coma, PVS, or akinetic mutism has raised moral, ethical, social, and legal controversy during the last few years and has resulted in decisions such as the "living will" and "do not resuscitate" policies.[11,37] These same issues exist for the patients with locked-in syndrome who have the potential to recover.[37,46,94]

Acute intensive rehabilitative care

Cerebrovascular disease and traumatic brain damage are the two leading causes for morbidity and mortality in middle-aged and young adults. The annual U.S. incidence of stroke and head trauma is 500,000 and 450,000, respectively. The estimated cost of stroke is 6 to 8 billion dollars per year, and the cost of brain trauma is even higher. Early and appropriate rehabilitation application can greatly reduce this cost and therefore is cost effective in the long run.[26,34]

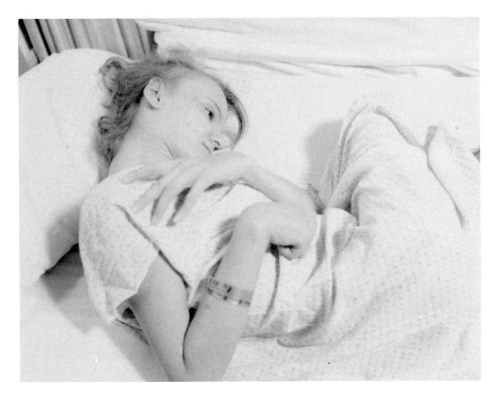

Figure 8-4. Contractures in head trauma.

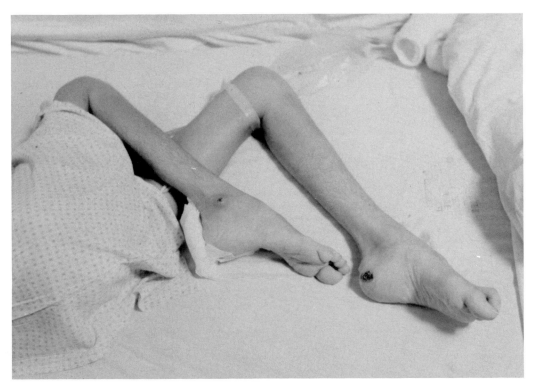

Figure 8-5. Contractures and pressure sores in head trauma.

Figure 8-6. Neck contractures in head trauma.

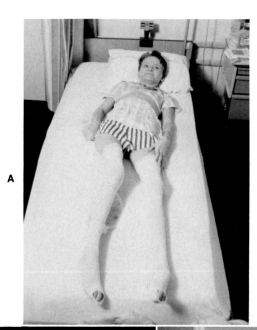

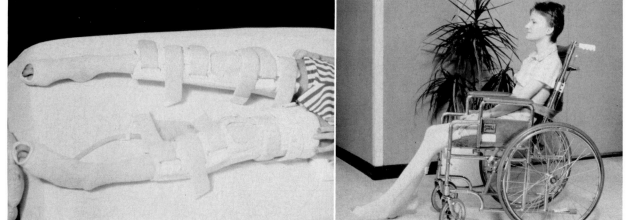

Figure 8-7. A, Postsurgical correction of contractures. **B,** Maintenance of correction with splints.
C, Position in wheelchair after contracture correction.

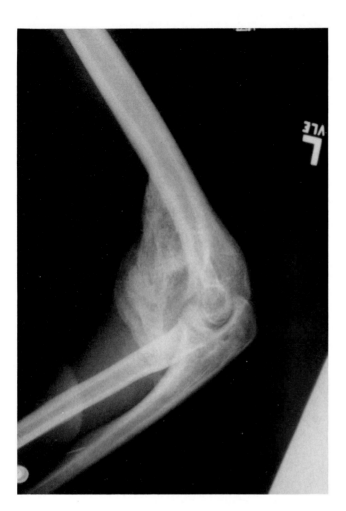

Figure 8-8. Heterotopic ossification in elbow in head trauma.

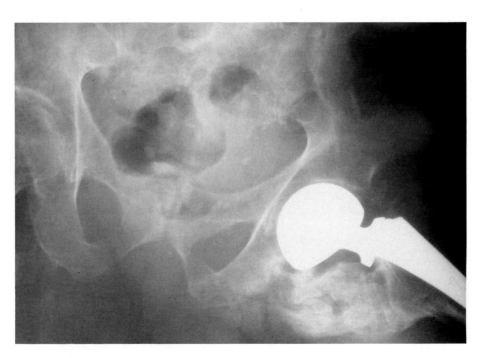

Figure 8-9. Heterotopic ossification with total hip prosthesis in stroke patient.

The major goals of rehabilitation remain the same with any disability: to improve function and independence to the patient's best possible potential, to reduce complications, and to provide an accessible environment. Education and assistance enable the family to pursue the same goals at home. With changes in technology, the possibility of severely disabled individuals gaining independence is increasing. Consequently, community placement education and development are essential in inpatient rehabilitation programs to improve the patient's emotional, physical, and psychosocial coping mechanisms. The major limiting factor in this process is lack of appropriate alternative residential and vocational education arrangements.

According to the National Head Injury Foundation, 14 different categories of care are required for patients with head injury, depending on the stage and severity of injury.[20,21] Different programmatic approaches are needed depending on the stage of recovery. These approaches include subacute care, coma stimulation, physical rehabilitation, and cognitive retraining program. Therefore chronic care for long-term living and transitional living arrangements with pursuit of vocational and educational goals, is important as an available resource. Physical and cognitive rehabilitation, family education, and social integration must be continued at all levels. Traditional extended care facilities cannot fulfill the needs of these patients, who often have severe behavior problems. An increasing need for appropriate long-term living institutions, transitional living centers, day-care programs, special schools, workshops, and job opportunities are encouraging health professionals to develop new programs. Some of the programs are well developed, others are changing, and some are in the process of development. These programs have to be flexible to fulfill the patients' needs. The brain is an ever-adapting dynamic organ that responds to internal and environmental influences.[7-9]

Recovery of control

Stroke and brainstem shock can resolve spontaneously, but the extent and completeness of the resolution are variable. Effectiveness of subsequent therapy depends in part on the extent to which the motor and sensory reverberating circuits are intact. Therapy in this special context has specific characteristics. At an early stage patients must be taught to manage their own therapeutic effort. The rehabilitative effort must be efficient, safe, and in effect throughout the entire 24-hour day.

Tasks must be broken down to units small enough that the patient can master them. In this way the patient is programmed for success and also learns to deal with sequential cause-and-effect functions. Wheelchair transfers, for example, can be divided into a number of smaller, sequential tasks that can be individually practiced and then combined.

Trunk and head control and mobility exercises are crucial at an early stage, especially when trunk- and head-righting responses are impaired. Only after mastering the full developmental mat exercise sequence will the patient be able to tackle midline and vertical spatial orientation programs and finally balance and weight-shifting exercises. Although control of the patient's legs may return relatively fast, use of postural reflex mechanisms is vital to the patient's mastering of motion of the body through his nearby environment. Millions of repetitions could well be needed for any progress. As developmental progress usually proceeds from head to tail, trunk control will help lower extremity control. Full control of the body evolves only after some basic stability of the body position in space has been achieved. Selective fine motor control supplants gross patterned control only after isolated repetition leads to isolated, willed volitional control. Random bilateral motion precedes evolution toward unilateral skilled movement.

In the developmental process the patient must first understand the correlation between his residual skill and the new developmental action to be achieved. He must then experience the performance required from him. Then the patient must learn to extend these recognitions and proprioceptions into an automatic motor response—an active, functional, motor plan or program. Throughout this therapeutic sequence the patient must receive biofeedback on a regular basis. In addition, increased muscular tone, abnormal positional reflexes and defective reciprocal coordination are discouraged so they do not effectively block evolving motor control. Modalities—especially vibration, hydrotherapy, and therapeutic massage—can help discourage these adversive processes and therefore aid the total developmental effort.

Gait therapy

For the usual stroke or brain injury patient, gait therapy is reasonably successful. At the most a plastic ankle-foot orthosis of relatively moderate rigidity is needed. The exceptions are patients with dense central ataxia or anterior cerebral artery distribution lesions. These patients have involvement of the feet that is similar to the parietal hand. Indeed, these strokes are commonly associated with fractured hips in the elderly. Gait therapy will be unsuccessful and inadvisable.

Therapy for dysfunctional sensation

Deficits of dynamic sensation noted after interruption of the sensory reverberating circuit (see Table 8-1) impair motion of that extremity through space. Visually substituted activities are a therapeutic alternative. These usually involve working with the patient to compensate for visual field defect by increased concentration and neck motion. Activities such as weaving are particularly valuable, since large looms demand reciprocal activities as well as horizontal activities crossing the midline.

Sensory retraining activities are the other alternative. Brief, intensive sessions should be held throughout the day so the patient experiences repetitively a wide variety of textures, temperatures, hardness, softness, vibrations, and positions. These should lead to kinetic coordinative exercises, such as guiding a ball through a maze on a tilt board with holes. Some biofeedback should be provided with a light or a buzzer. Repetitive kinetic exercise uses perception, thus aiding the functional recovery of sensation.

Positioning exercises are also valuable for patients with widespread central nervous system lesions. An extension of tactile function, positioning exercises must be coordinated with the developmental sequences described previously.

Natural history

The pattern and course for each lesion of the central nervous system are unique and affect rehabilitation. For example, a stroke patient with a hemorrhagic cerebral lesion generally has a better neurologic recovery than one with a thrombotic lesion. Generally, the farther caudally one travels in the central nervous system, the better the chances are for neurologic recovery but the greater the chances for recurrence. Hypertensive brainstem strokes are far more likely to return than are cerebral thromboses. On the other hand, if the patient's blood pressure is kept stable, neurologic recovery can be dramatic. Aneurysms with subarachnoid hemorrhage generally have a pattern similar to hemorrhagic strokes.

Traumatic brain injury has a pattern of its own. Almost 300 of each 100,000 hospital admissions in the United States are for traumatic brain injury.[51,52,97-99] An estimated 18 deaths from traumatic brain injury occur per 10,000 population. Worldwide, the combination of fast transportation, alcohol, drugs, and youthful operators is both frequent and fatal.[41] Programs to prevent head and spinal cord injuries are important and can take several forms:

1. Intensive and multidisciplinary programs aimed at junior and senior high school students. These audiences respond well to films and television programs and also to meeting patients who have had these injuries and have experienced rehabilitation. Follow-up of these audiences is essential to the efficacy of this type of program. For example, high school students could visit or volunteer at rehabilitation centers.
2. Well-being clinics to promote athletic activities and moderate exercise and diet activities in young adults. This is the time to call attention to health, sports, and sports medicine concerns. Since physiatrists are experts in care of the muscles, they are the natural leaders for these interdisciplinary activities.
3. Day-care centers for elderly patients so inpatient regimens can be continued on an outpatient basis. Again, since multidisciplinary team efforts must be coordinated, physiatrists should be active in these projects.[76]

Cognitive and communicative therapy

Most important in the rehabilitation of the patient with brain damage resulting from trauma or stroke is the location of and extent of the insult. Damage in a cerebrovascular accident is usually focal, whereas in a traumatic insult it is often widespread. Trauma results in a more extensive psychologic disability and a greater impairment in concentration in addition to localized physical disabilities. Patients with minor head injuries with no or transitory impaired consciousness might not receive an appropriate evaluation and follow-up observation. Most of the evaluation scales — Glasgow Coma Scale, Glasgow Outcome Scale,[86,98,99] and Glasgow Assessment Schedule[68] — are biased toward more severely injured patients.

Candidacy for rehabilitation treatment continues to be controversial. Usually, all the patients or patients with a specific level of impairment, for example, Glasgow Coma Scale rating of 7 to 9 or higher, receive comprehensive rehabilitation treatment. The brain is a dynamic organ and does respond to external stimuli; this underlines the need for individualization of intensity of therapy and continued evaluation to redefine the goals and length of stay in a rehabilitation setting. Early and late goals for individual patients can be developed using the cognitive level model established at Ranchos Los Amigos Head Trauma service in California.[45]

Neurophysical sequelae owing to a hemispheric and subcortical involvement resulting in cranial nerve deficits, paralysis, spasticity, speech impairments, swallowing problems, ataxia, and movement disorders can be assessed in stroke and head trauma victims. The maximum physical and mental recovery takes place in 3 to 6 months. Recovery does continue after 6 months but at a slower rate. At this stage the final level of disability is established and the patient and family are assisted to develop permanent adaptation skills called coping behavior.

There are major differences in coping behavior between stroke patients and their families and brain-injured patients and their families. The survivors of stroke are usually mature, taxpaying, middle-aged individuals with a family consisting of a spouse and adult children. They have some type of financial security that they have earned during their life. The chances of a stroke survivor going back to work in some capacity are 10% to 15%.[24] The behavior reaction of a stroke-disabled person often is depression. Some families require short-term psychologic counseling.

The reactions of patients with brain injury and their families have been described as "locked in grief." These individuals are between 15 and 35 years of age, socially maladapted before the injury, with aging parents, a young spouse, and small children. Financial support is a major problem. An individual who could have been a taxpayer becomes a tax burden. The family lives in guilt, grief, and frustration. The survivors face a life of disorientation, disorganization, poor memory, frustration, and despair.[67,105] Continuous monitoring, counseling, and support by well-trained psychologists or behavior therapists is essential to the patient and family.[23]

Patients with brain damage resulting from trauma or stroke usually respond well to a warm, familiar, relatively structured environment. The team needs to be sensitive and well organized and to present a consistent yet relaxed appearance. Signs and notations should be used to improve the patient's orientation to time, place, and person, and these must be coordinated with oral and visual cues. The floor staff must be helpful, friendly, and optimistic so they can encourage these attitudes in their patients. Frequent consultation among the clinicians and dialogue between patient and clinician will produce a consistent group performance. The staff should encourage the patient to recognize himself, his family, and his background. Photographs, posters, and cards help as long as they are not so numerous or poorly positioned as to distract. Television and radio programs not only divert patients but also remind them of past programs. Patient diaries, communication books, and activity cards are likewise adaptive environmental devices. Organization of time—for therapy, meals, recreation, and sleep—is fundamental. Laissez-faire ambience can be destructive, since the patient usually cannot provide inner discipline. The rehabilitation team must meet frequently to keep the program running smoothly, but the results are well worth the effort.

The speech pathologist should be heavily involved in therapy. Many patients with brain damage require swallowing examination, fluoroscopy, swallowing exercises, swallowing diets, and therapy. Gastrostomy buys time for these efforts. Aspiration is always a problem with the nasogastric tube, and the tubes are often forcibly ejected by agitated patients in the middle of the night. A simple abdominal binder protects the gastrostomy.

Aphasia is frequently a problem with both dominant and nondominant strokes. Even lesions confined to the thalamus have produced aphasia. Therapy proceeds after a thorough, cautious evaluation that includes graded repetitive exercises alone and with the therapist. Auditory evaluation should also be performed, since hearing deficits contribute to the total language dysfunction found in aphasia. During therapy for aphasia, melodic techniques accompany gestures and auditory and visual cues. Adjusting to the patient's new language abilities is a task for both patient and family. The therapist acts as an advisor—a function extending beyond the initial inpatient stay. Occasionally, digital computers, speech prostheses, or other adaptive devices are prescribed to help with communication functions.

Articulation problems should be treated separately. Lungs and vocal facilities might be poorly coordinated. With paralysis or paresis and abnormal muscular tone, words could be poorly pronounced. Exercises of the oral musculature can be specifically prescribed for special deficits. Obviously, flaccid deficits—which usually recover at least partially—have a better prognosis than spastic dysfunction.

At the very least, some type of communication aid can be introduced that the patient can use appropriately and consistently. The system can be as simple as pointing to a picture or as complex as using a computer to scan and present patterns of signals. Many communication deficits departments have specialized language laboratories for this very aspect.

Cognitive rehabilitation

Cognitive rehabilitation changes the patient's behavior as he tries to go from acute hospital care to inpatient rehabilitation to the outpatient environmental setting. In the process, cognitive training becomes personal counseling, and later small psychotherapy group therapy becomes community activity groups. Within each group the patient progresses from therapy directed toward concentration and orientation to improving cause-effect perceptive relationships and later from personalized and supported individual explorations to restoration to the patient's home and vocational environment.

At each level of cognitive therapy a job is chosen for the patient that has its own demands. To meet these demands, the patient has to exercise some higher judgmental discrimination. As the jobs become harder, the judgmental activities required become more complex. One way of structuring this complexity is through the methods and materials the patient has to use to solve the problem. Another is whether the chore involves an action or first requires a set of mental or emotional activities so the job can be solved appropriately.

Any exercise or routine the patient is given should follow a basic general pattern. The patient first has to give some evidence of examining the problem and stating what that problem is. The patient has to devise and then perform a specific plan. Then the patient should evaluate the results and be able to learn some lessons for the next time. During this time the therapist works on capturing the patient's concentration, prompting the patient, and generating a satisfactory closure.

Progress depends on several factors. How rapidly is the patient recovering neurologically? How well can he remember information? How easily can he apply it to different sequences? Psychosis can interfere with this process at any stage. Progress is followed through sequential neuropsychiatric evaluations. The team targets specific behaviors and plans for a specific set of contingencies. One contingency involves positive reinforcement for the desired behavior. Eventually, as behavior became self-reinforcing and external, group reinforcement fades.

During this process a patient's behavior "rises" to successive levels and behavior is shaped presumably as water flows into canal locks. There comes a point, however, when the patient is saturated and a timeout period is entered to give both patient and therapist time to decompress. This therapy, as noted above, begins as limited therapy on the rehabilitation floor. Sooner or later, it extends to the family and community. Outpatient therapy consisting of follow-up and group psychotherapeutic techniques is required, since cognitive development usually lags far behind physical accomplishments.

The behavior modification and cognitive remediation in management of brain-injured patients is the most challenging goal for the rehabilitation team.[10,103,105] The primary goal is to complete the neuropsychologic assessment. This goal may be elusive because of poor patient tolerance. Extensive test batteries (Halstead Reitan Battery, Luria Neuropsychological Investigation, Luria Nebraska Neuropsychological Battery, and Boston Veterans Administration Approach) are commonly needed. There could be a localization of specific behavior problems in specific brain areas, which can be mapped by magnetic resonance imaging or PET scanning.

In management of neurobehavioral disturbances, behavioral techniques, token economy,[3] positive and negative reinforcement, repetition, and overlearning are implemented initially. Pharmacologic agents that have shown some effects are psychostimulants[66,103] for lethargy, apathy, and abulia and antidepressants for depression, disruptive behavior, and vegetative signs. Propranolol has also been used for belligerent behavior, psychomotor agitation, and tremors in these patients.[28] Use of neuroleptics, benzodiazepines, and lithium continues to be controversial[29-31,80] because of their effects on the level of alertness, cognition, and seizure activity.

Use of other drugs such as baclofen and diazepam for spasticity affects behavior and cognition.[107,108] Local treatment for spasticity control in this situation can be useful with motor point phenol block (Figure 8-10). Recent animal and human research with the use of amines and neurotransmitters in functional and cognitive recovery of brain injury is encouraging.*

Drug therapy

The neurobehavioral sequelae of traumatic brain damage are the most challenging of long-term disabilities. Use of pharmacologic agents,[28,31,38] especially amines and neurotransmitters,[30,42,47,68,102] has not been fully explored in the process of awakening, cognitive retraining, and behavior modification.[69,80] The drug therapy used is mainly for seizure control,[40,79] spasticity management,[30,31,107,108] behavior modification, and prevention of some complications such as heterotopic ossification.[35] There are no universal guidelines for use of all these drugs.

Stroke survivors do suffer from some of these problems, but they are usually treated with combination therapy for associated medical conditions such as hypertension or diabetes. They are treated for spasticity, but seizure prophylaxis is uncommon even though the incidence of poststroke seizures is not low[19,90] and these seizures could be responsible for falls and complicating fractures.

Ongoing seizure prophylaxis should be evaluated on an individual basis for long-term management with consideration of choice of drugs and their side effects. Commonly used drugs such as phenytoin and phenobarbital might not be ideal for these patients because of their cognitive and behavioral side effects.[40,70,84] Sometimes they can contribute to seizure frequency. Phenobarbital can cause hyperactivity. However, it is of great value in status epilepticus. Carbamazepine, an anticonvulsant that is increasingly used for long-term, nonemergency situations, might improve mental processes but causes blood and gastrointestinal side effects,

*References 27, 42, 47, 60, 68, 84, 93.

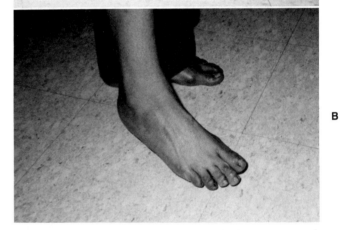

Figure 8-10. Patient with stroke and hemiplegia. **A,** Before phenol block. **B,** After phenol block.

headaches, diplopia, heart failure, and equilibrium disturbances. Valproic acid has also been shown to cause cognitive disturbances. The incidence of posttraumatic seizures varies from less than 3% to more than 60%,[86] depending on the type and site of injury. Since the risk factors for seizures are well known, a systematic approach in monitoring documented seizure prophylaxis needs to be developed as a priority.

Sexual function

Sexual problems in stroke and brain injury are not addressed as part of the regular protocol as they are for spinal cord–injured individuals. Hypersexuality or hyposexuality and inappropriate social sexual behavior are major problems in both stroke survivors and brain-injured patients. Disturbance in sexual behavior is sometimes due to involvement of the temporal lobe and hypothalamus.[73] The problems of eating disorder, temperature and blood pressure control,[89] and sexual and mood disorder could all be related to an injury to the hypothalamus. Use of stereotaxis surgery to control some of the brainstem syndromes has been recommended,[6] especially for movement disorder seizure and tone management. Surgical procedures are essential to correct contractures, hydrocephalus, and related problems. Impaired bladder and bowel function (frequency, lack of inhibition, and so on) often remains a lifelong problem.

SUMMARY

Ninety-seven percent of brain-injured patients have some form of mental or physical deficit.[52] The physical disability predominates in less than one third. By contrast, two thirds of brain-injured patients exhibit changes in personality and cognitive ability. These disabilities often improve slowly.[77,78] Prospects of normal life, that is, unsupervised living, complete independence in mobility (driving),[92] and employment, seem dim to the patient and his family. The clinician develops individual treatment strategies after acquiring an understanding of the patient's weaknesses, idiosyncrasies, and strengths. Rehabilitation teams must improve management of these patients with innovative approaches to improve function, cognitive skills, and socioeconomic adjustments.

REFERENCES

1. Ackerman, RH, et al: Positron imaging in ischemic stroke disease using compounds labeled with oxygen 15: initial results of clinico-pathologic correlations, Arch Neurol 38:537, 1981.
2. Agostini, E, et al: Apraxia in deep cerebral lesions, J Neurol Neurosurg Psychiatry 46:804, 1983.
3. Allyn, T, and Azrin, NH: The token economy: a motivational system for therapy and rehabilitation, New York, 1968, Appleton-Century-Crofts.
4. Anderson, TP, and Kottke, FJ: Stroke rehabilitation: reconsideration of some common attitudes, Arch Phys Med Rehabil 59:175, 1978.
5. Andreassen, S: Interval patterns of single motor units (thesis), Copenhagen, 1977, Institute of Neurophysiology, University of Copenhagen.
6. Andrew, J. Fowler, C, and Harrison, MJ: Tremor after head injury and its treatment by stereotaxic surgery, J Neurol Neurosurg Psychiatry 48:815, 1982.
7. Bach-y-Rita, P: Recovery of function: theoretical considerations for brain injury rehabilitation, Baltimore, 1980, University Park Press.
8. Bach-y-Rita, P: Brain plasticity as a basis of the development of rehabilitation procedures for hemiplegia, Scand J Rehabil Med 13:73, 1981.
9. Bach-y-Rita, P: Central nervous system lesions: sprouting and unmasking in rehabilitation, Arch Phys Med Rehabil 62:413, 1981.
10. Ben-Yishay, Y, editor: Working approaches to remediation of cognitive deficits in brain damaged persons, IRM Rehab Monograph No. 62, New York, 1981, New York University Medical Center.
11. Berrol, S: Consideration for management of the persistent vegetative state, Arch Phys Med Rehabil 67:283, 1986.
12. Bilotto, G, et al: Dynamic prospectus of vestibular reflexes in the decerebrate cat, Exp Brain Res 47:343, 1982.
13. Binder, LM: Emotional problems after stroke, Stroke 15:174, 1984.
14. Burke, D: A reassessment of the muscle spindle contribution to muscle tone in normal and spastic man. In Feldman, RG, Young, RR, and Koella, WP, editors: Spasticity: disordered motor control, Chicago, 1980, Year Book Medical Publishers, Inc.

15. Casp, JS, and Rymer, WZ: Enhancement by serotonin of tonic vibration reflex and stretch reflexes in the decerebrate cat, Exp Brain Res 62:111, 1986.
16. Cayaffa, JJ: Cortical and subcortical cerebral structures related to motility and somatic sensation. In Kaplan, P, and Cerullo, L, editors: Stroke rehabilitation, Boston, 1986, Butterworths.
17. Chaudhuri, G: Rehabilitation of stroke patient, Geriatrics 35:45, 1980.
18. Chilcote, WA, et al: Digital subtraction and angiography of the carotid arteries: a comparative study in 100 patients, Radiology 139:287, 1981.
19. Cocito, L, Favele, E, and Reni, L: Epileptic seizures in cerebral arterial occlusive disease, Stroke 13:189, 1982.
20. Cope, DN: Head injury rehabilitation: benefit of early intervention, Arch Phys Med Rehabil 63:433, 1982.
21. Cope, N: Brain injury rehabilitation, Rehabil Rep 2:18, 1984.
22. Crooks, LE, et al: Nuclear magnetic resonance, visualization of cerebral and vascular abnormalities by NMR imagery: the effect of imaging parameters on contrast, Radiology 144:842, 1982.
23. Diller, L, and Gordon, WA: Intervention for cognitive deficit in brain injured adults, J Consult Clin Psychol 49:822, 1981.
24. Dombovy, ML, Sandok, BA, and Basford, JR: Rehabilitation for stroke: a review, Stroke 17:363, 1986.
25. Duria, MB, and Hunter, MJ: The sagittal vestibulocolic reflex and its interaction with neck proprioceptive afferents in the decerebrate cat, J Physiol 359:17, 1985.
26. Eazell, DE, and Johnston, MV: Cost benefits of stroke rehabilitation, NARF Monograph Series 4, McLean, Va, 1981, NARF.
27. Elliott, D, and Street, RM: Akinetic mutism from hypothalamic damage: successful treatment with dopamin agonist, Neurology 31:1435, 1981.
28. Elliott, FA: Propranolol for the control of belligerent behavior following acute brain damage, Ann Neurol 1:489, 1977.
29. Erwin, CW, et al: Lithium carbonate and convulsive disorders, Arch Gen Psychiatry 28:646, 1973.
30. Faden, AI: Neuropeptides and central nervous system injury: clinical implications, Arch Neurol 42:501, 1986.
31. Feeney, DM, Gonsolez, A, and Law, WA: Amphetamine, haloperide, and experience interact to affect rate of recovery after motor cortex injury, Science 217:855, 1982.
32. Feigenson, JS: Stroke rehabilitation: effectiveness, benefits and cost: some practical considerations, Stroke 10:1, 1979.
33. Feigenson, JS: Stroke rehabilitation: outcome studies and guidelines for alternative level of care, Stroke 12:372, 1981.
34. Feigenson, JS, et al: Factors influencing outcome and length of stay in stroke rehabilitation unit, Parts I and II, Stroke 8:651, 657, 1977.
35. Finerman, GAM, and Stover, S: Heterotopic ossification following hip replacement or spinal cord injury, Metab Bone Dis Relat Res 3:337, 1981.
36. Finkelstein, S, et al: Mood, vegetative disturbance, and dexamethasone suppression test after stroke, Ann Neurol 12:463, 1982.
37. Franklin, C: Commentary, Hastings Center Report, December 1985, pp 14-15.
38. Gentilini, M, et al: Neuropsychological evaluation of mild head injury, J Neurol Neurosurg Psychiatry 48:137, 1985.
39. Geschwind, N: The apraxias: neural mechanisms of disorders of learned movements, Am Sci 63:188, 1975.
40. Glenn, MB: Update on pharmacology, Head Trauma Rehabil 1:73, 1986.
41. Glenn, MB, and Rosenthal, M: Rehabilitation following severe traumatic brain injury, Semin Neurol 5:233, 1985.
42. Guidice, MA, et al: Improvement in motor functioning with levodopa and bromocriptine following closed head injury, Neurology 36: 1986.
43. Hagbarth, K-E, Wallin, G, and Lofstedt, L: Muscle spindle responses to stretch in normal and spastic subjects, Scand J Rehabil Med 5:156, 1973.

44. Hagbarth, K-E, et al: Muscle spindle activity in alternating tremor of parkinsonism and in clonus, J Neurol Neurosurg Psychiatry 38:636, 1975.

45. Hagen, B, et al: Levels of cognitive functioning. In Rehabilitation of the head-injured adult, Comprehensive Physical Management, Professional Staff Association of Rancho Los Amigos Hospital, Downey, Calif, 1979.

46. Haig, A, Katz, R, and Sahgal, V: "Locked-in syndrome": a review, Curr Concepts Rehabil Med 3:12, 1986.

47. Hayes, RL, Stonnington, HH, and Lyeth, BG: Pharmacological treatment of head injury—a new challenge, Brain Injury 1:1, 1987.

48. Hayes, SH, and Carroll, SR: Early intervention care in the acute stroke patient, Arch Phys Med Rehabil 67:319, 1986.

49. Hounsgaard, J, et al: Intrinsic membrane properties causing a bistable behavior of alpha-motorneurons, Exp Brain Res 55:391, 1984.

50. Hultborn, H, Wigstrom, H, and Wangberg, B: Prolonged activation of soleus motorneurons blowing a conditioning train in soleus IA afferents: a case for a reverberating loop? Neurosci Lett 1:147, 1975.

51. Jennett, B: Post traumatic epilepsy. In Rosenthal, M, et al, editors: Rehabilitation of head injured adult, Philadelphia, 1984, FA Davis Co.

52. Jennett, B, and Bond, M: Assessment of outcome after severe brain damage, Lancet 1:480, 1975.

53. Jongbloed, L: Prediction of function after stroke: a critical review, Stroke 17:765, 1986.

54. Kaplan, PE: Rehabilitation of the lower extremity. In Kaplan, P, and Cerullo, L, editors: Stroke rehabilitation, Boston, 1986, Butterworths.

55. Kaplan, PE, et al: Glioblastoma multiforme presenting as stroke: electrophysiological and clinicopathological case report, Arch Phys Med Rehabil 60:74, 1979.

56. Kishore, PR, et al: Delayed development of hydrocephalus in patients with severe head injury, Neuroradiology 16:261, 1978.

57. Knopman, DS, et al: A longitudinal study of speech fluency in aphasia: CT correlates of recovery and persistent nonfluency, Neurology (Cleveland) 33:1110, 1983.

58. Kottke, F: Historia obscura hemiplegiae, Arch Phys Med Rehabil 55:623, 1974.

59. Kottke, F: Neurophysiologic therapy for stroke. In Licht, S, editor: Stroke and its rehabilitation, New Haven, Conn, 1974, E Licht, Publisher.

60. Lal, Moerbitz, and Grip: Modification of function in head injury patients with Sinemet, Poster presentation ACRM & AAPM & R, 1986.

61. LaPlane, D, and Degan, JD: Motor neglect, J Neurol Neurosurg Psychiatry 46:152, 1983.

62. Lehmann, JF, et al: Stroke: does rehabilitation affect outcome? Arch Phys Med Rehabil 56:375, 1975.

63. Lehmann, JF, et al: Stroke rehabilitation: outcome and prediction, Arch Phys Med Rehabil 56:383, 1975.

64. Levin, HS, High, WM, and Meyers, CA: Impairment of remote memory after closed head injury, J Neurol Neurosurg Psychiatry 48:556, 1985.

65. Liepmann, H: Apraxia, Ergeb Ges Med 1:516, 1920.

66. Lipper, S, and Tuchman, MM: Treatment of chronic post-traumatic organic brain syndrome with dextroamphetamine: first reported case. J Nerv Ment Dis 162:366, 1976.

67. Lishman, WA: The psychiatric sequelae of head injury: a review, Psychiatr Med 3:304, 1973.

68. Lyeth, BG, et al: Neurological deficits following experimental cerebral concussions in the rat attenuated by scopolaurine pre-treatment, Soc Neurosci 11:432, 1985.

69. Mansheim, P: Treatment with propranolol of the behavioral sequelae of brain damage, J Clin Psychiatry 42:132, 1981.

70. Mattson, RH, et al: Comparison of carbamazepine, phenobarbital, phenytoin, and primidone in partial and secondarily generalized tonic, clonic seizures, N Engl J Med 313:145, 1985.

71. Mazziotta, JC, et al: Tomographic mapping of human cerebral metabolism: normal unstimulated state, Neurology (New York) 31:503, 1981.

72. Metter, EJ, et al: 18 F/D G positron emission computed tomography of aphasia, Ann Neurol 10:173, 1981.

73. Monga, TN, et al: Hypersexuality in stroke, Arch Phys Med Rehabil 67:415, 1986.

74. Nathan, PW: The gate-control theory of pain: a critical review, Brain 99:123, 1976.

75. Newlon, PG, Greenberg, RP: Assessment of brain function with multimodal evoked potentials. In Rosenthal, M, et al, editors: Rehabilitation of the head-injured adult, Philadelphia, 1983, FA Davis Co.

76. Norris, JW, and Hachinski, VC: Units or stroke centres, Stroke 17: 360, 1986.

77. Oddy, M, and Humphrey, M: Social recovery during the year following severe head injury, J Neurol Neurosurg Psychiatry 43:798, 1980.

78. Oddy, M, et al: Social adjustment after closed head injury: a further follow-up seven years after injury, J Neurosurg Psychiatry 48:564, 1985.

79. Oles, KS, and Penry, JK: Pharmacological prophylaxis of post-traumatic seizures. In Johnson, RT, editor: Convulsive-therapy in neurologic disease, 1985-86, Toronto, 1985, BC Decker.

80. Oyewumi, LK, and Lapierre, YD: Efficacy of lithium in treating mood disorder occurring after brain stem injury, Am J Psychiatry 138:110, 1981.

81. Phelps, MW, Schelbert, HR, and Mazziotta, JC: Positron computed tomography for studies of myocardial and cerebral function, Ann Intern Med 98:339, 1983.

82. Reading, M, et al: The dexamethasone suppression test: an indicator of depression in stroke but not a predictor of rehabilitation outcome, Arch Neurol 42:209, 1985.

83. Reinvang, I, and Dugstad, G: Aphasia typology and lesion localization with computed axial tomography, Scand J Rehabil Med 13:85, 1981.

84. Reynolds, EH, and Trimble, MR: Adverse neuropsychiatric effects of anticonvulsant drugs, Drugs 29:570, 1985.

85. Rosenfalck, A, and Andreassen, S: Impaired regulation of force and firing pattern of single motor units in patients with spasticity, J Neurol Neurosurg Psychiatry 43:907, 1980.

86. Rosenthal, M, et al, editors: Rehabilitation of the head-injured adult, Philadelphia, 1984, FA Davis Co.

87. Ruch, TC, and Patton, HD: Physiology and biophysics, ed 19, Philadelphia, 1960, WB Saunders Co.

88. Rymer, WZ, and Hansan, Z: Prolonged time course for vibratory suppression of stretch reflex in decerebrate cat, Exp Brain Res 44:101, 1981.

89. Sandel, ME, Abrahms, PL, and Horn, LJ: Hypertension after brain injury, Arch Phys Med Rehabil 67:469, 1986.

90. Schold, C, Yarnell, PR, and Earnest, MP: Origin of seizures in elderly patients, JAMA 238:1177, 1977.

91. Shimokawa, H, et al: Coronary artery spasm induced in atherosclerotic miniature swine, Science 221:560, 1983.

92. Simms, B: The assessment of the disabled for driving: a preliminary report, Int Rehabil Med 7:187, 1985.

93. Sivenius, J, et al: The significance of rehabilitation of stroke—a controlled trial, Stroke 16:928, 1985.

94. Steffen, GE: Who speaks for the patient with the locked-in syndrome? Hastings Center Report December 1985, pp 13-14.

95. Suzuki, I, Timerick, SJB, and Wilson, VJ: Body position with respect to the head or body position in space is coded by lumbar interneurons, J Neurophysiol 54:123, 1985.

96. Tang, A, and Rymer, WZ: Abnormal force—EMG relations in paretic limbs of hemiparetic human subjects, J Neurol Neurosurg Psychiatry 44:690, 1981.

97. Teasdale, E, et al: CT scan in severe diffuse head injury: physiological and clinical correlations, J Neurol Neurosurg Psychiatry 47:600, 1984.

98. Teasdale, G, and Jennett, B: Assessment of coma and impaired consciousness: a practical scale, Lancet 2:81, 1974.

99. Teasdale, G, and Jennett, B: Assessment of severity of head injury, J Neurol Neurosurg Psychiatry 39:574, 1976.

100. Truscott, BL, et al: Early rehabilitative care in community hospitals: effect on quality of survivorship following stroke, Stroke 5:623, 1974.

101. Valenstein, E, and Heilman, KM: Unilateral hypokinesia and motor extinction, Neurology (New York) 31:445, 1981.

102. Van Woerkom, TCAM, et al: Neurotransmitters in the treatment of patients with severe head injuries, Eur Neurol 21:227, 1982.

103. Weinstein, GS, and Wells, CE: Case studies in neuropsychiatry: posttraumatic psychiatric dysfunction—diagnosis and treatment, J Clin Psychiatry 42:120, 1981.

104. Wilson, VJ, and Melville Jones, G: Mammalian vestibular physiology, New York, 1979, Plenum Press.

105. Wood, RL: Behaviour disorders following severe brain injury: their presentation and psychological management. In Brooks, N, editor: Closed head injury: psychological, social and family consequences, Oxford, Eng., 1984, Oxford University Press.

106. Yarkony, GM, Betts, HB, and Sahgal, V: Rehabilitation of craniocerebral trauma, Ann Acad Med 12:417, 1983.

107. Young, RR, and Delwaide, PJ: Drug therapy: spasticity (first of two parts), N Engl J Med 304:28, 1981.

108. Young, RR, and Delwaide, PJ: Drug therapy: spasticity (second of two parts), N Engl J Med 304:96, 1981.

109. Zaudel, DW: Memory for scenes in stroke patients: hemisphere processing of semantic organization in pictures, Brain 109:547, 1986.

ADDITIONAL READINGS

Bond, M: Head Injury Symposium: the stages of recovery from severe head injury with special reference to late outcome, Int Rehabil Med 1:155, 1978.

Garland, HO: Incidence, location, and management in rehabilitation of the head injured adult, J Bone Joint Surg 52:1143, 1980.

Henderson, VW, Alexander, MP, and Naeser, MA: Right thalamic injury, impaired visuospatial perception, and alexia, Neurology 32:235, 1982.

Livingston, MG, and Livingston, HM: The Glasgow assessment schedule: clinical and research assessment of head injury outcome, Int Rehabil Med 7:145, 1985.

Newcombe, F, Brooks, N, and Baddeley, A: Rehabilitation after brain damage: an overview, Int Rehabil Med 2:133, 1980.

Olsen, TS, Bruhn, P, and Oberg, RGE: Cortical hypoperfusion as a possible cause of subcortical aphasia, Brain 109:393, 1986.

Reimberr, FW, Wood, DR, and Wender, PH: An open clinical trial of L-dopa and carbidopa in adults with minimal brain dysfunction, Am J Psychiatry 137:73, 1980.

Weddell, R, Oddy, M, and Jenkins, D: Social adjustment after rehabilitation: a two year follow-up of patients with severe head injury, Psychol Med 10:257, 1980.

CHAPTER 9

Stroke and traumatic brain injury

BEHAVIORAL AND PSYCHOSOCIAL CONSIDERATIONS

LEONARD DILLER AND YEHUDA BEN-YISHAY

The incidence and nature of cognitive-behavioral problems in stroke and traumatic brain injury (TBI) rehabilitation are difficult to pin down because of the wide variation of sequelae following brain damage. The sequelae may be considered as a vector of three interacting sets of considerations: premorbid individual differences in biologic, psychologic, and sociologic factors in patients; different syndromal patterns of brain damage; and the nature of rehabilitation with its emphasis on enhancing recovery and optimizing adaptation to the demands of daily living for all patients whenever possible. While individual differences are usually subsumed under considerations of demographic information and characteristics of brain syndromes are readily grasped in clinical diagnosis, the perspective cast by rehabilitation is more subtle. To a neurobiologist or neuropsychologist, the term "function" refers to a property emanating from nervous system activity, as in vision, audition, or motion. In rehabilitation, "function" refers to a dimension of behavior that is manifested in naturalistic settings, in contrast to test or laboratory settings. Thus functional recovery takes on different meanings depending on the context.

In addition, cognitive-behavioral problems may influence rehabilitation both indirectly as correlands of rehabilitation, (for example, perceptual competence is related to ambulation in hemiplegics) and directly as targets of rehabilitation treatment (for example, in attempts to treat visual perceptual problems as disorders unto themselves).[8]

In this chapter we consider first some of the relationships of basic factors such as age, sex, education, time since onset, and parameters of brain damage to stroke and TBI. Then we consider the cognitive-behavioral sequelae in stroke and TBI. We conclude with a brief, state of the art review of interventions for the management of stroke and TBI. Our focus is cognitive-behavioral problems.

AGE AT ONSET

The incidence of stroke peaks at 60 to 65 years of age, whereas the incidence of TBI peaks in the early twenties. Age at onset is important in the following ways.

Brain damage has a different effect on skills that existed before brain damage than on skills acquired after brain damage. For example, traumatically brain-damaged adults perform better when tasks involve the application of old learning than when they demand new learning. Thus, performance on intelligence subtests that reflect previously acquired knowledge (such as tests of cultural information) may be intact, while performance on tasks requiring processing and organizing new information or the integration of different kinds of information may be impaired. On psychologic tests, as well as in life, skilled behaviors often involve combinations of old and new learning. Clinically this may be manifested in two ways: people with a stroke may be able to function competently at seemingly high-level tasks when the tasks have been overlearned and are familiar to the point of being automatic. Yet they may act unintelligently when confronted with seemingly simpler tasks that are unfamiliar. When confronted with an arithmetic problem, a child who had acquired arithmetic skills before TBI responds differently from one who had not.

Lateralization of hemispheric functions and age have received great emphasis in recent years. For example, for right-handed people and half of left-handers, the left hemisphere is associated with language, analytic, and serial thinking while the right hemisphere is associated with visual perception, metaphor, and parallel and simultaneous thinking.[23] Some have argued that lateralization is programmed at birth, whereas others believe that it evolves with age. The ability of one hemisphere to take over the functions of the other hemisphere indicates the existence of cerebral plasticity. Some theorists have argued that right hemispheric abilities (for example, visual spatial skills) mature and decline more rapidly than do left hemispheric abilities.[25] Furthermore, damage to the same area of the brain impairs cognitive operations differently at different ages. Thus damage to the same area of the brain results in different kinds of language disturbances at different ages. Types of aphasia tend to peak at different ages. Thus Wernicke's aphasia peaks at older ages than Broca's aphasia in men.[31]

Studies conducted with stroke and TBI populations suggest that age at onset has little differential effect on mental functioning from adolescence to age 50. Past this age, patients with brain damage show differential decline.[4,9,57] The decline with age in both right- and left-sided stroke patients is seen in tests of motor speed (such as finger tapping) and cognitive flexibility but not in visual information processing and measures of arousal and depression.[13] Thus an individual with acquired brain damage may be able to continue working on a job that requires a high level of skill because the skills are overlearned and because cognitive flexibility or a high degree of alertness is no longer required.

EDUCATION

Years of schooling are highly correlated with performance on neuropsychologic tests.[45] The power of this relationship may be seen by the fact that language tests administered to a sample of aphasic patients showed a correlation with years of schooling.[68] Clinically, two points may be noted. First, norms for tests used for clinical populations should be comparable in educational attainment.[45] Second, premorbid educational attainment may be used as a predictor of expected performance on neuropsychologic tests. Significant deviations from expected, that is, normative, levels of performance may therefore be used as a sign of mental impairment resulting from brain damage. Levin and co-workers[44] found that intellectual outcome after TBI is predictable from premorbid estimate of IQ and from the Glasgow Coma Scale.

A person's preinjury education is important from another vantage point in rehabilitation. Individuals with more education have more skills and more diverse occupational choices than those with fewer educational attainments. However, for highly educated TBI individuals who held down jobs that require high degrees of mental flexibility or executive skills, in addition to factual knowledge, the chances of return to work may be better than for lesser educated ones, but the return to work at the same level is uncommon. Educational factors enter in yet another way, particularly with regard to traumatic brain damage. Epidemiologic data suggest a higher incidence of premorbid sociopathy and learning disability in this population.[60] Therefore a preinjury history of poor adjustment coupled with poor education prognosticates poor vocational rehabilitation.

GENDER

Concerning the relationship between gender and cognitive functions in brain damage the following must be noted: (1) The generalizations concerning laterality of hemispheric functions have been based on studies conducted with populations of men, such as patients in Veterans Administration hospitals. They do not necessarily apply to women.[25] (2) Although stroke occurs with approximately equal frequency in men and women, traumatic brain injury occurs more often (2.5:1) among men than women.[41]

PREMORBID PERSONALITY

Personality usually refers to the enduring and persistent style of attitudes and behaviors that serve as distinguishing characteristics of the individual.

The relationship between premorbid personality and behaviors manifested after brain damage is difficult to delineate because the study of premorbid personality can be carried out only retrospectively. Psychologic tests of personality administered after brain damage are influenced by the presence of brain damage. Nevertheless, methods and logic difficulties notwithstanding, there is evidence that a premorbid tendency to deny unpleasant events such as the presence of illness is related to the presence of anasognosia (denial of paralysis) in stroke patients.[67] This relationship between premorbid personality and behavioral manifestations following a brain injury has been reaffirmed in clinical psychiatric interviews and studies.[62] Such notions also fit with the idea that after brain damage an individual under stress falls back on established neurotic or maladaptive patterns of behavior. However, great caution must be exercised lest such notions are carried too far, since there is ample clinical evidence that direct disruption of brain functions resulting from different brain syndromes can produce organically based alterations in an individual's personality, as in frontal lobe damage.

TIME SINCE ONSET

In the case of stroke and TBI the greatest recovery in cognitive function occurs during the first 6 months from onset or emergence from coma.[9] Performance on tests plateaus more quickly than does performance on measures of functional skills or in naturalistic settings. Van Buskirk and Webster,[63] working with sensory motor tests in hemiplegic patients, and Sarno and Levita,[58] working with aphasic patients, found improvement in functional measures even after scores on formal tests plateaued.

Whether there is a natural priority in the order of return of cognitive deficits is still an open question. There is some evidence that return of function on a battery of visual-perceptual measures follows a logical hierarchy of recovery in the case of TBI.[50] The point at which recovery stops is uncertain. Earlier studies suggested that little recovery occurs on neuropsychologic tests after 6 months.[48] However, Dikman, Reitan, and Temkin[12] found continued improvement on a battery of neuropsychologic tests in their population of patients with TBIs 18 months after injury. Plateaus in recovery curves are based on group averages. However, when individual patients with TBIs were followed over time, observers noted that some patients continued to improve but others became even worse over the years.[40] Levin and co-workers[43] suggested that magnetic resonance imaging (MRI) administered soon after TBI can predict deterioration.

SIZE AND LOCATION OF LESION AS PARAMETERS OF BRAIN DAMAGE

The extent and locus of brain damage and their effects on cognitive function are beyond the scope of this chapter. The interested reader will find summaries pertinent to stroke[33] and traumatic brain damage[9,41] in other texts. While size and locus of lesion are important, other dimensions might be relevant. For example, Birch and Diller[7] tested Hebb's theory that distinguished between subtractive and additive lesions.[32] Subtractive lesions occur when parts of the brain are destroyed, causing a loss of specific abilities associated with specific areas. Additive lesions interfere with abilities usually thought to pertain to the intact areas of the brain as well and therefore may be more disruptive. An example of an additive lesion is scar tissue formation, which causes epilepsy and confused mental state. Subtractive lesions, such as those in hemispherectomy wherein an entire hemisphere is removed, may cause specific and circumscribed losses in function and yet not disrupt cognitive function despite the removal of an entire hemisphere.

With regard to TBI, various measures have been used as indicators of severity of brain damage. These include the Glasgow Coma Scale,[38] length of posttraumatic amnesia, and specific neurologic indicators of focal damage.[41] In addition, measures of certain patterns of behavioral disturbance and cognitive deficit associated with particular neurologic syndromes (such as frontal lobe damage) have been used as gauges of the severity of injury. Imaging techniques such as computerized tomography (CT) and nuclear magnetic resonance scans have been used to predict rehabilitation outcomes in medical rehabilitation programs for patients with moderately severe and severe TBIs, but these have not proved as successful in the case of individuals with only mild head injury. A recent report suggests that MRI has some usefulness in distinguishing patients who will probably improve from those who are likely to become worse.[44]

With regard to stroke, location and severity of brain dam-

age are salient. Although the cause of damage (for example, thrombosis, hemorrhage, or embolism) is of course important for considerations of medical management, it is less pertinent for gauging behavioral progress and predicting outcome. In one group of stroke patients with damage to the right side of the brain, CT scans were of limited value in detecting cognitive-perceptual problems.[21]

BEHAVIORAL RESPONSES AFTER STROKE

Right-handed individuals with damage to the left side of the brain tend to have aphasia. Since diagnosis and management of language disorders are discussed elsewhere in this text, they are not discussed further here. However, several points concerning behavioral responses may be noted.

Left-sided brain damage

There appears to be a high incidence of emotional disturbance associated with aphasia. Goldstein[24] pointed to the "catastrophic reaction" in aphasia accompanied by anxiety and depression. Although it is readily apparent that this reaction may be a response to loss of language, more recent students of the problem have argued that the emotional disturbance has a neurologic basis; that is, the hemispheres mediate emotions differently, so emotional responses may be related to locus of lesion.[34] Methods for the management of emotional problems use supportive counseling, environmental management (including groups for patients and significant others), and pharmacologic treatment. However, as yet no definitive studies have demonstrated the superiority of a particular approach. The general therapeutic strategy in dealing with loss is to have the patient identify the object of the loss (speech, paralysis, job), attempt to have the patient contain the spread of feelings of loss (that is, separate the patient as a person from the loss of a given function—the language problem, the paralyzed arm, the inability to resume work), and attempt to have the patient focus on other areas capable of providing satisfaction or meaning to the patient's life. This approach is intended as a paradigm for therapeutic strategies. The feelings of loss are said to resemble the grief over the loss of a person.

Cognitive problems may also occur with damage to the left hemisphere. For example, there may be difficulty in learning to adapt to changing stimuli or situations.[15,17] This difficulty may be related to specific disturbances in the ability to process information. Thus for left brain–damaged people, auditory information is retained less well than visual information and sequential information is retained less well than information that makes no demands on sequencing.[18] One possible reason for this is a slowing in the rate at which information can be absorbed. This pattern of deficits suggests that, for left brain–damaged people, material presented visually can be absorbed more readily than material presented auditorily and that material can be absorbed better if presented slowly.

Right-sided brain damage

Over the past century, cognitive and behavioral problems associated with right-sided brain damage have received attention from neurologists and neuropsychologists, most of whom have described deficits and syndromes and developed theories and techniques to assist in diagnosis. The rehabilitation of patients with right-sided damage was ignored for many years. Even the textbooks failed to view the neurologic examination from a rehabilitation perspective.[61] However, in the past two decades these problems have received increasing attention in medical rehabilitation, since it has become apparent that they could become critical determinants of rehabilitation outcome. Among the difficulties associated with cognitive deficits in right brain–damaged people are mental confusion, perceptual problems, problems in arousal and awareness, problems with comprehension and expression, problems in abstract thinking, and emotional problems.

Mental confusion

Patients with right-sided brain damage may be so mentally confused that they cannot respond to questions about gross aspects of their environment. Such patients have difficulty learning and retaining functional skills. Brief mental screening devices are useful in detecting these severe disturbances, which occur more often in bilaterally brain-damaged people.[47] These patients make slower progress in rehabilitation. Patients who fail the short mental status examination may be unable to utilize the full 3 hours daily of required physical and occupational therapy. Such patients are slow to master a fundamental skill such as learning to transfer to and from a wheelchair and tend to regress when there is a change in physical therapists or program schedules.[15] Recent attempts to develop valid mental status screening techniques promise to provide a powerful screening tool for physiatrists.

Perceptual problems

Visual-perceptual problems have been commonly associated with right-sided brain damage. Although descriptions of these disturbances and their status as syndromes have been discussed by neurologists for the past century, in rehabilitation work began soon after World War II with gross descriptions of disturbances and correlands of ambulation and activities of daily living.[46] The methodologies, including descriptions of populations, tests used, statistical analyses, and criterion measures, have varied from study to study. More recently visual-perceptual disorders have been broken down in terms of sensory loss and visual field cuts, hemi-inattention and hemispatial neglect, hemiperceptual deficits,

and gaze and visual pursuit disorders. Perhaps the most extensive work has been directed at analyzing and treating disorders in hemi-inattention and visual-spatial neglect.[28] Researchers have demonstrated that individuals with severe forms of these problems constitute 30% to 40% of an inpatient population with right-sided brain damage.[20] Their disturbances are manifested not only on psychologic tests that involve the detection and organization of stimuli, but also in daily experiences such as frequency of accidents while in a rehabilitation program,[19] failure to eat food on the left side of a tray, failure to check off items on the left side of a menu, failure to correctly count money spread out on a table, difficulty in reading newspapers, problems in grooming (uneven shaving in men, poor application of makeup in women), and problems in academic skills of spelling and arithmetic. These problems are associated with patients' denial of their errors of omission in response to stimuli on the left side of space.[20] Although some of the problems may resolve spontaneously, many persist for a long time.

Many of the visual-perceptual problems associated with right-sided brain damage can be successfully treated by systematic scanning exercises designed to alter faulty gazing habits. These exercises have been built on the following principles:

1. Anchoring—defining and orienting a starting point for visual search
2. Pacing—preventing errors of omission by having the subject recite the stimuli aloud to slow down performance
3. Feedback—pointing out the errors of omission to patients who are unaware of them
4. Stimulus load—increasing or decreasing the complexity of the task by varying the stimulus load

A series of studies showed that such exercises offered for a minimum of 20 hours can improve performance on tests that are sensitive to visual neglect, improve reading, writing, and arithmetic, improve solving of complex problems in space, and increase spatial-sensory awareness.[64-66] Follow-up monitoring revealed that gains were maintained. Although a control group who received conventional treatment tended to catch up with the experimental patients on criterion test scores, patients who received the special training continued to read more on follow-up.[26] In replications by other investigative teams, improvements were noted when the exercises were supplemented by other training experiences in the actual functional situations; for example, scanning training, plus mobile scanning and space estimation, improved wheelchair navigation.[28] One common problem is that the patient must be reminded to apply the newly learned skill to new situations. Varying the training procedures to encourage generalization might be helpful.

Training procedures may also be organized in a hierarchic fashion so that one set of procedures, such as training in visual scanning, is used to build skills for retraining sensory awareness and body image, as well as skills for spatial analysis and synthesis.[66] The fact that results can be demonstrated across training programs suggests that the above principles (anchoring, pacing, feedback, and stimulus load) in retraining are useful.[16] Furthermore, the tasks of the remediator and the learner can be organized around three major areas: identification of the problem (explaining the task, having the patient understand its relevance to the clinical problem); organization of activities (calibrating task difficulty, plateaus, feedback, number and frequency of training sessions), and generalization (self-monitoring, developing exposure of skills to new situations).

Alertness and arousal

Difficulties in alertness and arousal are nearly as common as difficulties in visual perception, occurring in over 75% of a population of patients with right-sided brain damage and 60% of those with left-sided damage.[13] Such problems are manifested clinically when patients fall asleep while waiting for the therapist or, more subtly, in slowness in finger tapping and reaction time and failure to explore space in search tasks. Although some researchers have attributed alertness problems to hypokinesia for the side of space contralateral to the damaged hemisphere, particularly for visual-perceptual problems associated with the parietal lobes,[33] others have noted a skill reduction in movement in other type of tasks, for example, in performing block design tasks.[4] The issue of whether it is possible to improve arousal through training, much as one improves visual-perceptual functioning, is being explored. On a clinical level a patient with limited alertness and arousal should be presented with tasks that do not require much energy. In the verbal area a patient who falls asleep during a therapeutic session may be kept stimulated by having him discuss familiar subjects such as sports or hobbies. Such a patient may be aroused motorically by simple automatic tapping procedures.

Comprehension and expression

Ross[55] noted that patients with right-sided brain damage have difficulty understanding and expressing affect. Such a patient with frontal damage is more likely to have difficulty expressing affect. A patient with damage to the posterior right side of the brain has difficulty comprehending affect. This phenomenon, aprosodia, is alleged to be the right hemisphere analog of aphasia wherein the frontal part of the left hemisphere is concerned with language expression and the posterior part with language reception. However, clinical data suggest that difficulties in comprehension of affect occur in more than half of hemiplegic patients with either right or left brain damage. Problems in aprosodia may have important clinical consequences in that patients may respond in an affectively inappropriate manner. A patient's family and staff members may therefore mistakenly believe that the patient is not depressed. Treatment strategies for problems associated with aprosodia have not been tested.

Impairment in logical and abstract reasoning

For many years it was thought that patients with right-sided brain damage had intact verbal-ideational skills. However, more recent analyses suggest that these patients do in fact experience impairments in abstract thinking, reasoning in novel situations, and solving verbal problems involving metaphor. Impairment in cognitive flexibility may cause a patient to dwell on the losses associated with the disability, to have a narrow perspective with regard to future prospects, and to be concerned with only the immediate and the present. These types of verbal-ideational responses are typically obscured by verbal intelligence tests when test items draw on a mixture of old, overlearned facts and skills and do not call for dealing with novel situations. Special analyses are therefore needed to tease apart old and new learning. The problem becomes particularly salient when one is trying to judge whether a patient is capable of managing a business, signing a check, or making a financial decision. It may also appear when a patient misinterprets the significance and intent of the behavior of other people because of the inability to shift perspective to see things from another person's vantage point.

Mood and emotional state

The classical literature indicates that patients with right-sided brain damage show denial and tend to be cheerful and optimistic. However, more recent evidence indicates that depression is present in approximately 75% of those with right or left brain damage. This depression is unrelated to other dimensions of cognitive disturbance and tends to be reported in follow-up studies.

TRAUMATIC BRAIN INJURY
Assessment of functional disability

While the cognitive-behavioral sequelae of TBI are diverse with regard to both quantity and quality, so generalizations are difficult, a major problem has been to develop instruments that can measure the results of recovery and rehabilitation efforts. Forer[22] lists 18 methods for assessing functional disability that have been developed with other populations in rehabilitation settings but can be applied to TBI patients. Among the specific approaches and methods developed for TBI exclusively are the following:

1. Glasgow Coma Scale (GCS).[38] This tool has been widely adopted as a way of quantifying the severity of and recovery from coma. The predictive validity of the GCS is useful for groups of patients.
2. Galveston Orientation and Amnesia Test (GOAT).[42] This test is useful for tracking recovery from post-traumatic amnesia. Like the GCS, it is most useful

for patients before they enter rehabilitation programs.

3. Level of Cognitive Functioning Scale, also known as the Rancho Los Amigos Scale.[30] This is the most widely publicized of the scales developed for tracking recovery in inpatient settings. It describes severity of disability in terms of cognitive-behavioral organization and intactness, which are judged by the staff's scaling of spontaneous responses, as well as standardized tests. It has recently been compared with other scales such as the Glasgow Outcome Scale, the Disability Rating Scale, and the Stover-Zieger Scales.[27] All of them demonstrate reliability of ratings and validity in terms of being sensitive to individual differences before and after inpatient treatment. These approaches designed specifically for TBI inpatients may be compared with more traditional approaches. The most thorough approach, using conventional ratings by therapists in different areas, has been presented by Sehgal and Heineman.[56]

4. Glasgow Outcome Scale (GOS)[37] and its modified version, the Disability Rating Scale (DRS).[52] These scales have been adapted as an instrument to track improvement. The DRS is more sensitive than the GOS to individual differences in outcome. The GOS, although useful for tracking groups of patients during recovery from TBI, is too crude a measure to be useful for rehabilitation purposes. These instruments have been useful mainly to provide data for evaluating programs, rather than measures useful in case management.

From a clinical standpoint it is necessary to integrate information from several different domains. In addition to gathering data for various assessment methods used in clinical neurology, the rehabilitation team must be alert for medical complications and sequelae, which appear with a high degree of frequency in inpatient medical rehabilitation programs.[39] Finally, rehabilitation itself requires the integration of information concerning impairments (deficits in motor, cognitive, sensory, and language functions) that need to be assessed by testing procedures, disabilities (deficits in functional skills), and handicaps (deficits in roles that prevent the person from conducting conventional activities).

Impairment measures in different domains may be found in a recent volume edited by Rosenthal and others.[54] In the neuropsychologic area the following critical domains should be assessed:

1. Basic arousal functions (by psychomotor tests of vigilance, focused attention, and concentration)
2. Eye-hand coordination with finger dexterity
3. Visuoconstructive ability
4. Visual information–processing ability
5. Language
6. Memory functions and ability to assimilate and recall new information
7. High-level abstract thinking and ''executive'' skills
8. Academic skills
9. Interpersonal skills and appropriateness of judgment
10. Emotional responsiveness and self-control
11. Acceptance or denial of disability
12. Degree of inability, that is, response to remedial interventions

Detailed discussion of these impairments and their measurements may be found in texts by Ben-Yishay and Diller,[1,2] Lezak,[45] and Levin, Benton, and Grossman.[41]

Many conventional tests such as the Wechsler Adult Intelligence Scale are less sensitive than specialized targeted tests to impairments in TBI. For example, the processes in passing or failing items on intelligence tests may be multiply determined. A test of vocabulary differs from a test of block design performance not only because the former is verbal and the latter is visual-spatial in content, but also because answering questions on a vocabulary test depends on old learning, whereas solving a block design problem requires the analysis, synthesis, and handling of essentially novel stimuli. Furthermore, whereas a vocabulary test is untimed, a block design test is timed; hence, in addition to being a novel visuoconstructional task, it is also a time-efficiency test.

Many patients emerging from coma cannot respond to standard stimuli because of confusion, apathy, or disturbed emotional state. Ingalls[35] found that 21% of inpatient TBIs cannot respond to conventional neuropsychologic tests because of motor-sensory or language disturbances that impair response modalities. Special test batteries for such patients are under study.[35]

Disability assessment should include assessment not only of conventional activities of daily living (ADLs) that are motorically based, but also of daily life activities in which failure may not be due to a motoric disturbance. The Behavior Competence Index, for example, rates 16 areas of naturalistic (home) life activities, including the ability to handle utensils, do chores, orient oneself in familiar and unfamiliar environments, manage routines of daily life, plan and organize activities, behave with social appropriateness, regulate emotions, and others.[5] Mayer and his colleagues[49] pointed out that even the assessment of conventional ADL tasks such as toothbrushing may have to be different for a TBI patient. The individual may need assistance not because of muscle weakness but because of the organizational and sequential qualities required for the vast number of subactivities from removing the cover of the toothpaste and picking up the toothbrush to replacing the toothbrush at the end.

Patients with TBI have handicaps in two major areas of life, the capacity to live intimately in a family and vocational adjustment. Rosenbaum and Najenson[53] reported that wives of TBI patients had greater adjustment problems than did wives of spinal cord–injured patients. A detailed review of family adjustment problems may be found in Rosenthal[54] and Brooks.[9] Recent research in this area has focused on the concept of family burden, which includes both objective and subjective problems posed by TBI. Vocational problems occur in a high percentage of TBI patients, with estimates varying depending in part on the severity of the brain damage. In a prospective study of individuals discharged from a hospital after severe head trauma, only 25% were employed at the end of 1 year and 50% at the end of a second year.[14] Dikman, McLean, and Temkin[11] found similar results for a group of patients with minor head injury. Ben-Yishay and co-workers[6] reviewed vocational outcome studies in TBI and found that high unemployment was a major problem. Brooks[9] noted that unemployment is more likely when severe head injury is accompanied by physical disability.

Treatment

The treatment strategy for TBI is chosen on the basis of the severity of the brain damage and the specific constellation of posttrauma sequelae. An individual with severe TBI may go through various stages of recovery from coma through unresponsive vigil, responsive mutism, confusion, independence in self-care, and independence in social and vocational functioning, to complete social reintegration. These stages usually span several years after the injury occurs. The treatment goals and strategies differ at these different stages. Cognitive and behavioral disturbances, which are typical of TBI, may make conventional rehabilitation services less effective for the patient. Modifying programmatic aspects and developing a team approach may therefore be necessary. In this approach a dedicated team of professionals works together on the same patients, according to a holistic philosophy of treatment, to respond to specific functional problems beyond the traditional approaches.[49] The team develops specific interventional techniques to deal systematically with problems that appear more frequently among TBI patients than in other groups of disabled people, such as problems of program compliance, awareness of problems, and understanding of the disability and its consequences. The team also applies specially designed techniques for the acquisition of skills; these programs often follow different patterns from those used for other disability groups. These features of treatment require agreement among team members not only on goals but also on strategies of management. Team members must communicate frequently to recalibrate therapeutic activities in order to meet the fluctuations in performance and cope with difficulties that arise on a daily basis. Principles of team management for outpatients may be found in Ben-Yishay and Piasetsky,[3] Prigatano,[51] and Grimm and Bleiberg.[29]

Because a number of studies have shown that increases in family burden are a major problem in TBI,[36] special attention must be paid to the development of effective methods of dealing with the family as part of the management of the patient's problems. Family support groups, often run by local chapters of state head injury associations, may be helpful. The National Head Injury Foundation has developed informational resources and reading materials that are helpful to families.

Various approaches to the management of cognitive and behavioral problems have been offered. Ben-Yishay and co-workers[5] presented methods for retraining in diverse cognitive domains ranging from basic attention, psychomotor dexterity, visuomotor integration, and abstract and logical reasoning to interpersonal skills and prevocational preparation. These methods have been developed to interconnect and have been systematically incorporated in a holistic framework. All of the various routines have been translated into specific activities that others can observe and measure.

Grimm and Bleiberg[29] presented clinical strategies for the management of behavioral problems as they appear in inpatient rehabilitation.

Conventional behavioral modification techniques have been applied with some success in the management of severe behavioral disturbances,[69] but such approaches by themselves have only a limited (that is, symptom-specific) utility and have been of less use in the overall management of TBI, particularly in dealing with the multitude of cognitive or behavioral problems. Similarly, conventional psychotherapy approaches with this population must be modified to take into account the particular nature of the underlying cognitive problems. Ben-Yishay[5] developed a special technique suitable for TBI. The approach takes into account the fact that patients with impaired ego functioning associated with TBI profit from directive, structured therapeutic activities but respond poorly to the task demands of conventional psychotherapy, which depend on inferential reasoning, free association, and insight.

Pharmacologic approaches have been reported in different case studies as aids to management; however, these approaches await further controlled study.

In recent years various computer-assisted remedial approaches have been proposed and in some instances successfully applied with TBI in different settings. Their use will probably remain limited to an adjunct rather than primary role in the overall rehabilitation of TBI patients. This is because in the majority of TBI patients with moderate and severe impairments, the most severe impairments for the functional reintegration of the patient are problems in self-activation or self-modulation, in persistence, and in executive skills (the ability to plan, set priorities, implement, self-monitor and self-correct behavior) rather than the absence of skills per se. The amelioration of such problems requires the guidance of a clinician, plus a variety of carefully orchestrated remedial activities, none of which can be computerized.

A major question is whether there is any evidence for the efficacy of interventions with TBI patients. While the task in trying to prove the efficacy of intervention programs in human service programs may really be a fool's errand,[10] studies supporting some of the approaches are beginning to appear. For example, Prigatano[51] and Scherzer[59] demonstrated the benefits of a holistic intervention program when compared with no treatment in a control group. In their study Ben-Yishay and co-workers[5] used statistical methods of control instead of pure control groups. They accepted for treatment patients with chronic TBI, averaging 2.7 years postinjury, and administered a battery of tests on two occasions separated by a 3-month interval to serve as a double-baseline before treatment commenced. They varied types of treatment in three different groups of equated patients so that some patients received more cognitive remedial interventions, some received more social group–oriented interventions, and others received equal amounts of both. All groups improved to about the same extent in regard to return to work, but the cognitive remediation group improved more on psychometric tests and the social skills training group improved more on measures of self-esteem and interpersonal effectiveness. In short, there were some carryover effects of this holistic intensive remedial approach under all three conditions, with regard to the major dimension of productivity and implied improvement in morale, compliance, and executive functions related to successful return to productive work, and there were certain improvements that were treatment specific. Whether such results would be achieved by direct application of the principles in the workplace without prior remedial intervention remains to be tested.

REFERENCES

1. Ben-Yishay, Y, and Diller, L: Cognitive deficits. In Rosenthal, M, editor: Rehabilitation of the head injured adult, Philadelphia, 1983, FA Davis Co.
2. Ben-Yishay, Y, and Diller, L: Cognitive remediation. In Rosenthal, M, editor: Rehabilitation of the head injured adult, Philadelphia, 1983, FA Davis Co.
3. Ben-Yishay, Y, and Piasetsky, E: Neurologic rehabilitation: quest for a holistic approach, Semin Neurol 5:252, 1985.
4. Ben-Yishay, Y, et al: Similarities and differences in block design performance between older normal and brain injured persons: a task analysis, J Abnorm Psychol 15:17, 1970.
5. Ben-Yishay, Y, et al: Working approaches to remediation of cognitive deficits in brain damage, Rehabilitation monographs, published annually, 1977-1983, Rusk Institute of Rehabilitation Medicine, New York University Medical Center, New York.
6. Ben-Yishay, Y, et al: Relationship between employability and vocational outcome after intensive holistic cognitive rehabilitation, J Head Trauma Rehabil 2:35, 1987.
7. Birch, HG, and Diller, L: Rorschach signs of organicity: a psychological basis for perceptual disturbance, J Project Technol 23:184, 1959
8. Birch, HG, et al: Visual verticality in hemiplegia, Arch Neurol 5:441, 1961.
9. Brooks, N, editor: Closed head injury: psychological, social and family consequences, New York, 1984, Oxford University Press.
10. Cronbach, LJ: Beyond the two disciplines of scientific psychology, Am Psychol 30:116, 1975.
11. Dikman, S, McLean, A, and Tremkin, NR: A one month follow-up in recovery from head trauma, Arch Phys Med Rehabil 68:53, 1986.
12. Dikman, S, Reitan, R, and Temkin, NR: Neuropsychological recovery in head injury, Arch Neurol 40:333, 1983.
13. Diller, L: Progress report—NYU Research and Training Center: improving rehabilitation potential in brain trauma and stroke, Washington, DC, 1986, Dept of Education, National Institute for Disability and Rehabilitation Research.
14. Diller, L, and Ben-Yishay, Y: Severe head trauma: a comprehensive approach and medical approach to rehabilitation, Final Report GT #13P59082, National Institutes of Handicapped Research, New York, 1983, New York University.
15. Diller, L, Buxbaum, J, and Chiotelis, S: Relearning motor skills in hemiplegia: error analysis, Genet Psychol Monogr 85:249, 1972.
16. Diller, L, and Gordon, WA: Interventions for cognitive deficits in brain injured adults, J Consult Clin Psychol 49:822, 1981.
17. Diller, L, and Weinberg, J: Learning in hemiplegia, Proceedings of the Annual Meeting, New York, Sept 1962, American Psychological Association, 1962.
18. Diller, L, and Weinberg, J: Attention patterns in hemiplegia, J Education, 1968, p 68.
19. Diller, L, and Weinberg, J: Evidence for accident prone behavior in hemiplegic patients, Arch Phys Med Rehabil 51:358, 1970.
20. Diller, L, et al: Studies in cognition and rehabilitation in hemiplegia, Rehabilitation Monograph #50, New York, 1974, Institute of Rehabilitation Medicine, New York University Medical Center, New York, 1974.
21. Egelko, S, et al: The relationship between CT scan and visual perceptual performance in right brain damage. In press.
22. Forer, S: Rehabilitation outcomes and evaluation systems for traumatic brain injury, J Organization Rehab Eval 5:52, 1985.
23. Gazzaniga, N: The bisected brain, Neuroscience Series #2, New York, 1970, Appleton-Century-Crofts.
24. Goldstein, K: Brain damage. In Arieti, S, editor: American handbook of psychiatry, New York, 1959, Basic Books.
25. Goldstein, G, and Shelly, C: Does the right hemisphere age more rapidly than the left? J Clin Neuropsychol 3:65, 1981.
26. Gordon, WA, et al: Perceptual remediation in patients with right brain damage: a comprehensive program, Arch Phys Med Rehabil 66:353, 1985.
27. Gouvier, WD, Blanton, PD, and LaPorte, KK: Rehabilitation and validity of cognitive functioning scales in monitoring recovery from severe head injury, Arch Phys Med Rehabil 68:90, 1987.
28. Gouvier, WD, Webster, JS, and Warner, MS: Treatment of acquired visuoperceptual and hemiattentional disorders, Ann Behav Med 8:15, 1986.
29. Grimm, PB, and Bleiberg, J: Psychological rehabilitation on traumatic brain injury. In Filskov, S, and Boll, T, editors: Handbook of clinical neuropsychology, vol 2, New York, 1986, John Wiley & Sons, Inc.
30. Hagen, C: Language and cognitive disorganization following severe closed head. In Trexler, L, editor: Cognitive rehabilitation, New York, 1982, Plenum Press.
31. Harasymou, S, and Halper, A: Sex age, age and aphasia type, Brain Language 12:190, 1981.
32. Hebb, DO: Organization of behavior—a neuropsychological theory, New York, 1949, John Wiley & Sons, Inc.
33. Heilman, K, and Valenstein, E, editors: Clinical neuropsychology, ed 2, New York, 1984, Oxford University Press.
34. Hibbard, MR, Gordon, WA, and Diller, L: Affective disturbance associated with right brain damage. In Filskov, S, and Boll, T, editors: Handbook of clinical neuropsychology, vol 2, New York, 1986, John Wiley & Sons, Inc.
35. Ingalls, C: Neuropsychological assessment of the severely handicapped brain injured person, Forum 2:5, 1987.
36. Jacobs, H: The family as therapeutic agent: long term rehabilitation for traumatic brain injury patient, final report, Washington, DC, 1984, National Institute for Handicapped Research.
37. Jennett, B, and Bond, M: Assessment of outcome after severe brain damage, Lancet 6:480, 1975.
38. Jennett, B, and Teasdale, G: Management of head injuries, Philadelphia, 1981, FA Davis Co.
39. Kalisky, Z, et al: Medical problems encountered with patients with closed head injury, Arch Phys Med Rehab 60:25, 1985.

40. Kay, T: Consistency of individual recovery after closed head injury. In Proceedings of the National Head Injury Conference, Chicago, Nov 16, 1986.

41. Levin, HS, Benton, A, and Grossman, RG: Neurobehavioral consequences of closed head injury, New York, 1982, Oxford University Press.

42. Levin, HS, O'Donnell, VM, and Grossman, RG: The Galveston Orientation and Amnesia Test: A practical scale to assess cognition after head injury, J New Ment Disord 167:675, 1979.

43. Levin, HS, et al: Magnetic reasonance imaging and correlated neuropsychological findings in long term survivors of severe closed head injury, J Clin Exp Neuropsychol 8:118, 1987.

44. Levin, HS, et al: Predictors of intellectual outcome after closed head injury, J Clin Exp Neuropsychol 8:123, 1987.

45. Lezak, MD: Neuropsychological assessment, New York, 1983, Oxford University Press.

46. Lorenz, E, and Cancro, R: Dysfunction in visual perception with hemiplegia: its relation to activities of daily living, Arch Phys Med Rehabil 43:512, 1962.

47. Luxenberg, JS, and Feigenbaum, LZ: Cognitive impairment in a rehabilitation setting, Arch Phys Med Rehabil 67:797, 1986.

48. Mandleberg, I: Cognitive recovery after severe head trauma—Wechsler Adult Intelligence Scale during post traumatic amnesia, J Neurol Neurosurg Psychiatry 38:1127, 1975.

49. Mayer, N, Keating, DJ, and Rapp, D: Skills routines, and activity patterns of daily living: a nested approach. In Uzzell, BP, and Gross, Y, editors: Clinical neuropsychology of intervention, Boston, 1986, Nijhoff Publishers.

50. Meeder, DL: Cognitive perceptual motor evaluation research findings for adult head injured. In Trexler, LE, editor: Cognitive rehabilitation, New York, 1982, Plenum Press.

51. Prigitano, G: Neuropsychological rehabilitation after brain injury, Baltimore, 1986, Johns Hopkins University Press.

52. Rappaport, M, et al: Disability rating scale for severe head trauma: coma to community, Arch Phys Med Rehabil 63:118, 1982.

53. Rosenbaum, M, and Najeson, T: Changes in life patterns and symptoms as reported by wives of severely brain injured soldiers, J Consult Clin Psychol 44:881, 1976.

54. Rosenthal, M, et al, editors: Rehabilitation in brain damage, Philadelphia, 1983, FA Davis Co.

55. Ross, E: The aprosodias: functional anatomic organization of affective componants of language in the right hemisphere, Arch Neurol 38:581, 1981.

56. Sehgal, V, and Heinemann, A: Outcome of rehabilitation in traumatic brain damage. Paper presented at a meeting of the National Association of Rehabilitation Research and Training Centers, Kansas City, May 14, 1986.

57. Sands, E, Sarno, MT, and Shankweiler, D: Long term assessment of language function due to stroke, Arch Phys Med Rehabil 50:203, 1973.

58. Sarno, MT, and Levita, E: Natural course of recovery in severe aphasia, Arch Phys Med Rehabil 52:175, 1971.

59. Scherzer, BP: Rehabilitation following severe head trauma: results of a three year program, Arch Phys Med Rehabil 67:366, 1986.

60. Tobis, JS, Puri, KB, and Sheridan, J: Rehabilitation of the severely brain injured patients, Scand J Rehabil Med 14:83, 1982.

61. Turney, TM, Garraway, WM, and Sinak, M: Neurologic examination in stroke rehabilitation: adequacy of its description in clinical textbooks, Arch Phys Med Rehabil 66:92, 1987.

62. Ullman, M: Behavioral changes in patients after stroke, Springfield, Ill, 1962, Charles C Thomas, Publisher.

63. Van Buskirk, D, and Webster, D: Prognostic value of sensory defect in rehabilitation of hemiplegia, Neurology 5:407, 1955.

64. Weinberg, J, et al: Visual scanning training on reading related tasks in acquired right brain damage, Arch Phys Med Rehabil 58:480, 1977.

65. Weinberg, J, et al: Training sensory awareness and spatial organization in people with right brain damage, Arch Phys Med Rehabil 60:491, 1979.

66. Weinberg, J, et al: Treating perceptual organization deficits in non neglecting RBD stroke patients, J Clin Neuropsychol 4:59, 1982.

67. Weinstein, E, and Kahn, R: The denial of illness, Springfield, Ill, 1955, Charles C Thomas, Publisher.

68. Weinstein, S, and Teuber, HL: The role of preinjury education and intelligence level in intellectual loss after brain injury, J Comp Physiol Psychol 50:535, 1957.

69. Wood, RL: Behavior disorder following severe head injury: their presentations and psychological management. In Brooks, N, editor: Closed head injury: psychological, social and family consequences, New York, 1984, Oxford University Press.

PART III | # SPINAL CORD TRAUMA

CHAPTER 10

Medical and rehabilitation management in spinal cord trauma

JUNG H. AHN AND RICHARD SULLIVAN

Physicians involved in the care of patients with spinal cord injury (SCI) deal not only with the physical disability but also with socioeconomic and vocational aspects of the problem. Secondary medical complications such as diminished pulmonary function, interrupted pathways of the autonomic nervous system, sensory loss, immobility, diminished sexuality, osteoporosis, and urinary-bowel dysfunction are common.

The past 10 years have seen significant changes in the epidemiology of spinal cord injury, great progress in medical management of injury-related complications, and enormous progress in research in rehabilitation engineering aimed at alleviating secondary functional deficits resulting from the permanent injury. Studies during the past decade have shown a decline in the incidence of complete spinal cord injuries resulting from accidental injury; partial recovery of function below the level of injury is now more commonly seen. Instances of chronic renal failure have declined, and it is no longer the main cause of death in these patients.

Recently developed computerized electrical stimulating apparatus is permitting aerobic exercise of the lower extremities for the first time. The development of computer-assisted reciprocating orthoses (which offer hope for greater ambulation ability on a functional level) is under experimentation. Newly designed wheelchairs are more acceptable cosmetically than older model wheelchairs and offer greater comfort and mobility. We are in an era when much can be offered the SCI patient to provide comfort and an acceptable life-style. However, there are many gray areas in the pathophysiology of injury to the spinal cord that must be explored in order to reduce morbidity resulting from trauma to the central nervous system. Even more important is the need for public education programs (especially for young adults, who are most vulnerable) to prevent accidents that lead to spinal cord injuries.

Guttmann, the English physician who has been a pioneer in the care and treatment of SCI patients, put it succinctly when he said, "Of the many forms of disability which can beset mankind, a severe injury or disease of the spinal cord undoubtedly constitutes one of the most devastating calamities in human life."[6] The best treatment therefore continues to be prevention.

DEMOGRAPHICS

The most current—and perhaps the most accurate—demographics on spinal cord injury come from the National Spinal Injury Database, which consists of data collected from the Model Spinal Cord Injury Systems Program between 1973 and 1985. The following statistics resulted from an analysis of data from 19 centers across the United States, all of which have or have had designation as Spinal Cord Injury Model Systems.[13]

Age of injury: 61.1% of spinal cord injuries occur between the ages of 16 and 30.

Analysis by age groups:

0 to 15 years	4.9%
16 to 30 years	61.1%
31 to 45 years	19.4%
46 to 60 years	9.2%
61 to 75 years	4.4%
76 to 90 years	1.0%

Distribution by sex:

Male	82%
Female	18%

Distribution by race:

White	73.9%
Black	16.0%
Other	10.1%

Distribution by etiology:

Motor vehicle accidents	47.7%
Falls	20.8%
Sports	14.2%
Acts of violence	14.6%
Other	2.7%

Relative to the month of injury, the study shows a gradual rise in incidence from January to a peak (11.5%) in July, followed by a gradual decline in incidence throughout the rest of the year. A total of 53.1% of injuries occurred from Friday to Sunday.

The most frequently recorded level of neurologic injury is cervical vertebra V (15.8%), followed by cervical IV (12.5%), cervical VI (12.5%), and thoracic XII (7.5%). Cervical injuries accounted for 53.2% of injuries, thoracic 35.6%, and lumbosacral 10.1%.

ANATOMY

The central nervous system is composed of the brain and the spinal cord. Injury to either results in such specific physical changes that it is often easy to determine the site of the injury.

The spinal cord originates at the foramen magnum just below the medulla oblongata. It extends to the base of L1 in the adult. The cord terminates near L3 at birth and with growth attains the L1 level. The area below, called the filum terminale, extends and anchors to the first coccygeal segment (Figure 10-1). Surrounding the filum terminale are peripheral nerve roots emanating from the axons of the anterior horn cells below the T12 level, as well as the returning sensory nerve roots. These combine to form the cauda equina. Because of this dichotomy, elements of the central and peripheral nervous systems are susceptible to injury depending on the site of the trauma. Therefore injuries to the spinal column above the T12 and L1 level result in an upper motor neuron type of injury, whereas trauma below this level results in lower motor symptoms.

The term "upper motor neuron injury" suggests trauma to the central nervous system, in this case the spinal cord. Such an injury results in motor and sensory paralysis below the level of the injury if the lesion is complete. In addition, physical examination reveals hyperreflexia, spasticity, and pathologic reflexes, as well as bowel, bladder, and sexual abnormalities. These findings imply that there has been an interruption of the ascending and descending pathways in the white matter of the cord, as well as local destruction of the gray matter, with a loss of cortical control of function below the level of the lesion.

"Lower motor neuron lesion" suggests injury to the peripheral nerve roots of the cauda equina. Symptoms include flaccidity, muscular atrophy, areflexia, and absence of pathologic reflexes, as well as bowel, bladder, and sexual abnormalities different from those of upper motor neuron injuries.

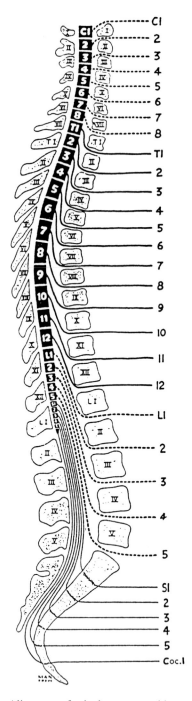

Figure 10-1. Alignment of spinal segments with vertebrae. Bodies and spinous processes of vertebrae are indicated by Roman numerals. (From Haymaker, W, and Woodhall, B: Peripheral nerve injuries: principles and diagnosis, Philadelphia, 1953, WB Saunders.)

Incomplete injuries to the spinal cord result in specific syndromes: Brown-Séquard syndrome, central cord syndrome, and anterior and posterior spinal cord syndromes.

The Brown-Séquard syndrome occurs most often in knife or gunshot wounds that result in a hemisection of the spinal cord. The result is ipsilateral motor paralysis, loss of proprioception, and contralateral loss of pain and temperature sensation. When the cervical or lumbar cord is hemisected, damage of the anterior horn cells leads to lower motor neuron signs in the affected muscles that correspond to the neurologic level of the lesion on the same side.

The central cord syndrome, as the name implies, involves injury to the internal regions of the cord (gray matter) at the site, with sparing of the surrounding elements (white matter). The degree of involvement can vary. Examination shows fewer neurologic defects in the lower extremities than in the upper extremities. In addition, sacral sensory sparing is evident, and there is often functional return of bowel and bladder control.

Anterior and posterior spinal cord syndromes have also been described, with the former meaning the preservation of posterior column sensory function in association with the paralysis and the latter meaning that there is retention of motor function and temperature and pain sensation, with partial loss of posterior column function.

Lesions above C4 result in total paralysis and respirator dependency.

The conus medullaris syndrome suggests injury to the tapered end of the spinal cord in the upper lumbar spine. The result is a lower motor neuron syndrome that includes areflexia of both bowel and bladder because of the destruction of the second, third, and fourth sacral cord segments. A spinal injury damaging the conus medullaris frequently involves the surrounding lumbar and sacral nerve rootlets. According to the severity of the lesion, muscle weakness or paralysis in the lower extremities occurs.

The cauda equina syndrome is similar to the conus medullaris syndrome but involves the destruction of the lumber and sacral roots. The physiologic results are the same although different anatomic areas are involved.

MODEL SYSTEMS

Awareness of the importance of early and long-term management of spinal cord injuries has resulted in the development of Model System of Care, a program funded by the U.S. Department of Education through the National Institute on Disability and Rehabilitation Research. Thirteen systems across the country are striving to develop and encourage superior medical and fiscal management in the care and treatment of SCI patients. Each system has four components:

1. An emergency medical service in radio contact with a level 1 trauma center emergency room. The ambulance personnel must be trained medics who are fully knowledgeable in the care that must be taken when moving and transporting injured patients. This includes proper stabilization of the fracture site for transfer, as well as emergency medical management of the patient via radio contact with the trauma center.

In some centers, air transport of patients is also available.

2. An affiliated acute care hospital with level 1 trauma center emergency room capability, as well as the equipment and personnel necessary to provide acute medical and surgical care to injured patients

3. An affiliated rehabilitation hospital with a designated service area that can provide ongoing physical rehabilitation to SCI patients. Comprehensive services available for the care and treatment of these patients must consist of full medical, therapeutic, vocational, and social services, with the added support of orthotic and rehabilitation nursing expertise. The rehabilitation hospital must provide patients and their families with a comprehensive discharge plan that sets attainable goals and provides outpatient services after discharge to complete the program of rehabilitation and attain the highest level of functional return.

4. Lifetime follow-up services of care and treatment

In this chapter we discuss the acute care and rehabilitation of patients with spinal cord trauma.

ACUTE CARE
Quadriplegic patients (C2 to T1 injury)

After an SCI patient's arrival at the acute care hospital, medical stabilization is first achieved. This includes treatment for shock (should it exist), stabilization of cardiopulmonary problems, catheterization of the urinary bladder, and evaluation for evidence of paralysis, as well as treatment of head and other bony or internal injuries. Radiographic evaluation of the spinal fracture and a decision of whether surgical stabilization is necessary must be made. Initial realignment of cervical fractures is usually achieved with the use of skeletal tongs with weights.

If fracture instability is found, a decision must be made for either invasive or noninvasive stabilization techniques. The invasive techniques are these:

1. Anterior cervical fusion with or without decompression

2. Posterior cervical fusion with or without wiring of the posterior elements

The noninvasive techniques consist of the following:

1. Continued cervical tong traction until healing is achieved

2. Halo traction

In the use of invasive techniques, decompressive laminectomy is no longer the treatment of choice. The more common treatment is fusion, followed by placement in halo immobilization. Every effort is made to achieve (as closely as possible) normal alignment of the vertebral segments with traction.

In the noninvasive stabilization techniques, halo traction is the treatment of choice if feasible. Its use avoids the long period of bed confinement necessitated by the use of cervical tong traction, thus allowing the transfer of the patient to the active phase of rehabilitation at a much earlier time. Halo traction allows the patient to be up in a wheelchair and active in the program of physical restoration.

The halo vest has been widely used to stabilize the fractured cervical spine in the last decade, although its complications (discussed in the section on physiatric evaluation) occur more frequently during rehabilitation. The pin locks should be checked daily. If they appear to be loose, this should be verified by a radiographic examination to check the pin's depth in the skull before tightening. Pin sites should be dressed with povidone-iodine solution at least once daily. If a reddened area, blister, or open wound is noted in the skin under the vest, extra padding should be placed under the plastic, or a small area of the plastic should be partly removed. In case of an emergency requiring cardiopulmonary resuscitation, the anterior portion of the vest should be removed to provide access to the chest while the patient is placed in a supine position.

Paraplegic patients (injury to T2 and below)

As is the case with SCI quadriplegics when first brought to the acute care hospital, medical stabilization and the evaluation and treatment of associated injuries of SCI paraplegics after arrival at the hospital should be accomplished. After that, a decision regarding stabilization of the spinal fracture must be made. Treatment depends on the severity of the fracture of the vertebrae and the presence or absence of any dislocation of the elements.

The invasive treatment techniques consist of bony fusion of the site of fracture with posterior spinal instrumentation for two levels above and below the injury or decompression laminectomy, followed by both of the other measures.

The noninvasive techniques consist of the use of orthotic stabilization devices: Knight braces for fracture below L2, Knight-Taylor braces for midthoracic fractures, hyperextension braces for lower thoracic–upper lumbar level fractures, and plaster or plastic laminated body jackets for thoracolumbar fractures.

Decompression laminectomy is no longer the treatment of choice. Some physicians employ laminectomy to relieve bony fragments or pressure against the cord by bony parts, although many disagree with this surgical solution and doubt its value. In most cases of high-thoracic and midthoracic fracture, surgical stabilization is usually unnecessary because of the inherent stability of the area involved. Harrington rod instrumentation with bone grafts seems to be the most common surgical procedure for thoracolumbar fractures. In both paraplegic and quadriplegic patients the stabilizing force, if external, is kept in place for varying lengths of time, depending on the extent of the injury and the progress of healing. The decision for removal of the orthosis is made jointly by the orthopedic and rehabilitation medicine physicians.

General comments

Intensive nursing care by personnel trained in the problems of SCI patients is essential. Skin ulcerations must be prevented by means of position changes at least every 2 hours. Areas of redness suggesting pressure must receive prompt attention. Early intervention by physical and occupational therapists to avoid flexion contractions (through the use of range of motion exercises and positional orthoses) must be understood and carried out.

Proper bowel and bladder care must be instituted from the onset of treatment. The use of a Foley catheter during the period when intravenous fluids are required must be followed as promptly as possible by institution of a program of intermittent catheterization to protect the bladder from overdistention and reduce the possibility of infection. Bowel management includes the judicious use of enemas and proper hydration to prevent constipation, followed by a program of scheduled bowel evacuations at least every other night through the use of stool softeners, stimulating suppositories, and proper diet. Early care in a general hospital is best provided in a surgical or neurosurgical intensive care unit. Once the patient is stabilized and ready for transfer, it is better to make the transfer directly to a spinal cord unit at a rehabilitation hospital rather than to the general hospital floor.

Radiographic evaluation including plain radiographs and computerized tomograms (CT scans) of the spine is done. Myelo-CT and magnetic resonance imaging (MRI) may be used to assess the severity of external pressure on the cord or the amount of cord swelling. The patient should be meticulously examined for injuries such as head trauma, intrathoracic, intra-abdominal, intrapelvic, and retroperitoneal organ damage, and bony fractures.

Cardiopulmonary monitoring is essential in quadriplegic and high-paraplegic patients. If there is no medical contraindication, heparin in low dosage is recommended to prevent deep venous thrombosis. Either elastic stockings or external pneumatic compression should be applied. Even with no signs of respiratory distress, intermittent positive pressure breathing or incentive spirometry should be used. The patient should be log-rolled every 2 hours and should wear ankle pads to prevent pressure sores. Routine blood and urine tests are performed as needed. Stress ulcers are relatively common, and preventive measures must be instituted promptly. When steroid therapy is instituted, prophylactic measures for steroid-induced ulcers, drug-induced diabetes mellitus, and serum electrolyte changes should be considered. Intravenous hydration and antimicrobial therapy may be needed.

Functional classification

Because of the diversity of injury resulting from spinal cord trauma, many attempts have been made to develop a functional scheme to classify patients on admission according to the severity of their injury and to evaluate neurologic

Table 10-1. Levels of paralysis compatible with functional capabilities

Neurologic level	Functional capabilities
C2-3	Totally dependent in activities of daily living (ADLs); respirator dependent (or needs phrenic nerve pacemakers)
C4	Totally dependent in ADLs except for driving powered wheelchair by using chin control unit or sip-puff control unit
C5	Self-feeds and brushes teeth with assistive devices; drives powered wheelchair with hand control unit
C6	Pushes manual wheelchair with vertical tips on hand rim; potential independence in self-care activities by using natural wrist tenodesis mechanism; able to do pushups while sitting in wheelchair without elbow flexion contractures; independent in sliding board transfers; drives van with hand control device and powered door lift
C7	Self-care activities easier than for patient with C6 paralysis; true pushups; manual wheelchair sufficient for locomotion
C8-T1	Fully independent from wheelchair level excluding high-level wheelchair activities; self–urinary catheterization and self-insertion of rectal suppositories
T2-10	Not candidate for functional ambulation training with bilateral knee-ankle orthoses and crutches, which may be used for exercise and strengthening
T11-L1	Borderline candidate for ambulation with orthoses in community
L2-3	Able to walk with bilateral ankle-knee orthoses requiring four-point crutch gait—wheelchair is still necessary
L4-5	Able to walk with ankle-foot orthoses and crutches
S1	May have some mild residual lower extremity weakness (innervation); requires walking aids (braces, crutches); because of neurogenic bladder and bowel requires intermittent catheterization (or spontaneous voiding or Credé maneuver) and regular bowel program

progress periodically. One of the most commonly used is the Frankel classification, which also defines injuries anatomically.[5] This classification is summarized as follows:

1. Complete (A). The lesion was found to be complete, with motor and sensory loss below the segment marked. If there was an alteration of level but the lesion remained complete below the new level, then an arrow would point up or down the "complete" column.
2. Sensory only (B). Some sensation was present below the level of the lesion but the motor paralysis was complete below that level. The column does not apply when there is a slight discrepancy between the motor and sensory level but does apply to sacral sparing.
3. Motor useless (C). Some motor power was present below the lesion but it was of no practical use to the patient.
4. Motor useful (D). There was useful motor power below the level of lesion. Patients in this group could move the lower limbs, and many could walk, with or without aids.
5. Recovery (E). The patient was free of neurologic symptoms; that is, there was no weakness, sensory loss, or sphincter disturbance. Abnormal reflexes may have been present.

In another way, based on the neurologic level, functional levels of independence can be expected following spinal cord injury (Table 10-1).

REHABILITATION PHASE
Physiatric evaluation

In the next phase, rehabilitation, a thorough physical examination should be performed. It should include vital signs, general appearance, mental status, skin, lungs, heart, abdomen, gross appearance of the extremities, range of motion, muscle strength, sensation, tendon reflexes, anal reflex, bulbocavernosus reflex, and evidence of sacral sparing.

The halo apparatus should be checked daily. Because of the increasing application of the halo vest for cervical spinal fracture subluxation, side effects of the halo must be addressed. These include loosening the halo pins, soft tissue infection or even osteomyelitis at the pin site, crooking of a plastic vest, and decubitus ulceration under the vest. Pain at the pin site is usually due to pin loosening but can result from the mislocation of a pin, particularly in the supraorbital region, which causes pinching of a small nerve. Although the common cause of pin loosening is suboptimal insertion into the outer table of the skull, one should be aware of the possibility of unrecognized osteomyelitis at the pin site, in which case tightening of the pin may result in a dural puncture or intracranial damage.

Spinal radiographs should be reviewed on admission to the hospital. The spinal level of the injury, spinal alignment at the fracture site, fracture healing, status of a bone graft or surgically placed metallic materials, evidence of a laminectomy, and distance between spinous processes at the injured site should be carefully assessed. Radiographic evidence of ligamentous injury without a surgical fusion, regardless of neurologic completeness, is indication of an unstable spine. Spinal instability may cause pain at the fractured level secondary to root irritation. Even during the period of halo immobilization, follow-up radiographs should be obtained. Polytomography is often needed to evaluate the upper and midthoracic spine, which is overshadowed by intrathoracic organs and adjacent bony structures on a plain film. Spinal CT scan is indicated when neurologic status deteriorates.

A comprehensive urologic evaluation, including urodynamic studies, kidney, ureter, and bladder (KUB), cystourethrography, intravenous pyelography, and cystoscopy, should be completed. Laboratory tests to be performed include serum electrolyte and protein levels, complete blood count, prothrombin time/partial thromboplastin time, liver enzyme levels, urinalysis, and urine culture and sensitivity. Optional tests of use include pulmonary function tests, venous Doppler ultrasonography and venous occlusive plethysmography, and somatosensory evoked potentials.

Functional evaluations, including determination of neurologic level (Frankel classification[5]), functional rehabilitative potential, equipment needs and attendant help, home planning, vocational potential, social status, and financial coverage are likewise in order.

Rehabilitation

The concentrated team effort begins when the patient is admitted to the rehabilitation hospital. Fracture healing is monitored, and the external stabilization system—be it halo traction or body jacket—is removed at the appropriate time. During the healing phase the patient is able to carry out an intensive program of exercise aimed at increasing strength and endurance in the spared musculature while maintaining range of motion in the paralyzed limbs. The tilt table is also used for hemodynamic purposes to prevent orthostatic hypotension. Mat exercise routines are gradually intensified as the patient's strength and endurance increase to allow, where feasible, independence in bed and transfer activities (Figure 10-2). Such exercises include mobilization with side-to-prone-to-supine turning, seated pushups, exercises to improve sitting balance, and resistive exercises with weights.

In occupational therapy the quadriplegic patient is given exercises aimed at increasing functional use of the upper extremities. The patient is provided with static or dynamic hand splints and is trained in their use. For a higher level quadriplegic patient, environmental control systems designed to meet the specific demands and needs of the patient in the home are available. These can be breath operated if the patient has insufficient functional ability in the arms and hands. The patient is shown how to use these devices and receives training in homemaking techniques and in other activities of daily living. Devices for the home such as

wheelchairs, tub and shower benches, commodes, Hoyer lifts, and self-help devices for the kitchen are provided as needed.

Psychologic services are likewise available. There is a recognized need for peer support and group therapy sessions. Family counseling for injury-related sexual adjustments is also provided for the paralyzed patient and spouse. The social needs of the patient and family are assessed, and referrals are made to appropriate social agencies. Special needs for home services are handled by the social services department.

Vocational services in the form of an assessment of the past work and educational experiences of the patient are instituted early. As the rehabilitation process proceeds, a more intense effort is made to determine the patient's employability and the need for further education. The ultimate goal is a work activity compatible with the disability.

Ambulation training with or without orthoses is provided when indicated, as is hand control driver training. Two-door sedans are recommended for the paraplegic patients (Figure 10-3). They can be set up easily for hand controls. The seat next to the driver can be moved forward to allow the patient to pull the wheelchair into the automobile. For quadriplegic patients, specially equipped vans allow independence of access and various accommodations for the wheelchair and the steering wheel to allow safe independent driving.

Special clinics

Specialized clinics exist within the rehabilitation hospital setting: upper extremity orthotics (Figures 10-4 to 10-8), lower extremity orthotics (see box on p. 156), hand, wheelchair seating (Figure 10-9), urology, and spinal cord follow-up. Each of these clinics combines the expertise of several health care professionals (Table 10-3).

AREAS OF SPECIAL CONSIDERATION
Autonomic dysreflexia

Autonomic dysreflexia occurs in quadriplegic and high-paraplegic patients with lesions above T5. These lesions are located above the splanchnic outflow of the sympathetic nervous system. Also called sympathetic dysreflexia, the condition is caused by any unusual irritation or noxious stimuli that cause reflex stimulation of the sympathetic nervous system. The most common cause in SCI patients is urinary retention and overdistention of the urinary bladder. Other causes are bowel distention secondary to constipation, digital stimulation of the rectum, decubitus ulceration, ingrown toenail, menstrual cramps, labor and delivery, and genital stimulation during sexual activity in both sexes. When it occurs, it is an acute crisis requiring vigorous treatment, the focus of which is removal of the irritant. Relief of the stimulus causes an immediate reversal of symptoms.

The symptom complex consists of a sudden elevation of

Text continued on p. 157.

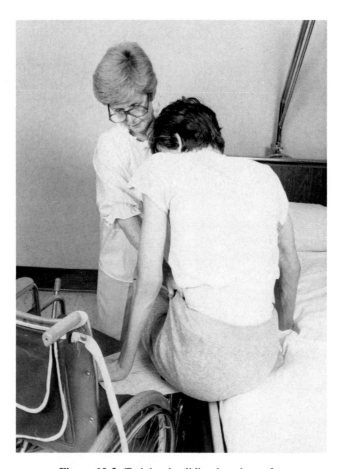

Figure 10-2. Training in sliding board transfer.

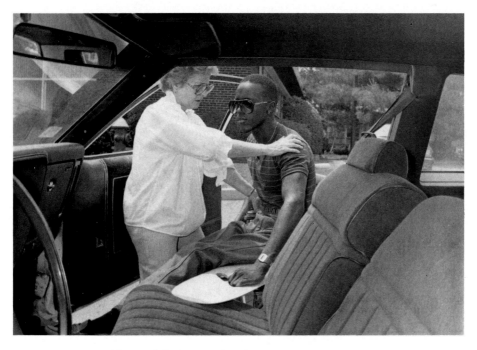

Figure 10-3. Car transfer with sliding board in place.

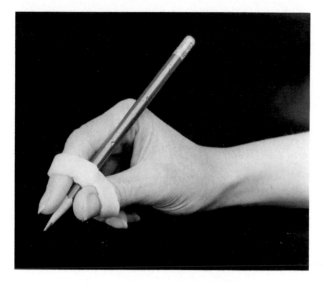

Figure 10-4. Plastic writing device.

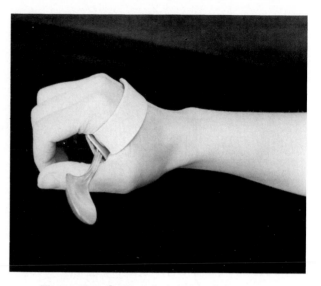

Figure 10-5. C-clip swivel ADL cuff (Universal).

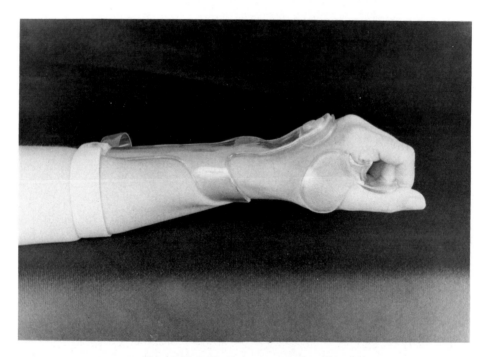

Figure 10-6. Plastic long opponens splint.

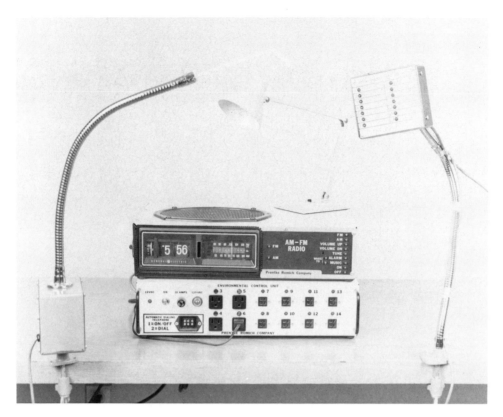

Figure 10-7. Environmental control unit.

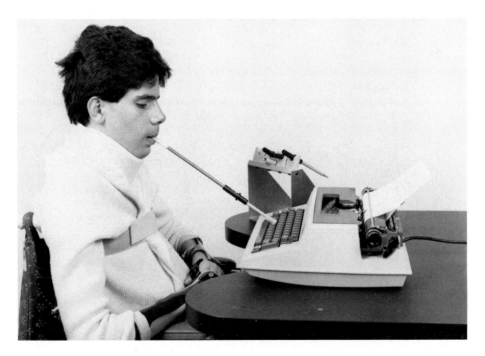

Figure 10-8. Mouth stick for typing in high quadriplegia.

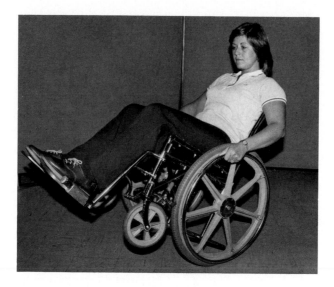

Figure 10-9. Wheelies.

ORTHOSES USED IN SPINAL CORD INJURY

I. Upper extremity orthoses for self-care
   A. Balanced forearm orthosis
   B. Long opponens orthosis
   C. Wrist-driven prehension orthosis
   D. Short opponens orthosis
   E. Metacarpophalangeal flexion (or extension) orthosis
II. Lower extremity orthoses for ambulation
   A. Conventional double-bar, long leg brace with dropping locks at knee and 90-dgree posterior stop at ankle
   B. Scott-Craig orthosis
   C. Reciprocating lower extremity orthosis
   D. Ankle-foot orthosis—plastic laminated
   E. Posterior leaf spring orthosis
   F. Solid ankle orthosis
   G. Spiral orthosis
   H. Conventional ankle-foot orthosis with variable ankle strap
III. Spinal orthoses for stabilization
   A. Collars
      1. Soft cervical collar
      2. 4-Poster cervical collar
      3. Philadelphia collar
   B. Minerva jacket
   C. Sterno-occipitomandibular immobilizer (SOMI)
   D. Knight-Taylor orthosis with shoulder straps
   E. Total contact thoracolumbar plastic molded orthosis
   F. Hyperextension brace
   G. Knight lumbar brace
IV. Other equipment available for quadriplegic patients
   A. Environmental control unit
   B. Cock-up splint
   C. Occupational therapy utensils for eating and writing
      1. Peg handle
      2. Finger loop device
      3. C-clip
      4. Vertical activities of daily living (ADL) holder
      5. ADL universal staff
      6. Swivel spoon

Table 10-3. Special clinics

Clinic	Staff	Purpose
Upper extremity orthotics (Figures 10-4 to 10-8)	Physiatrist, orthotist, therapists	Provision of passive and active upper extremity orthoses to prevent deformity and increase functional potential of patient
Lower extremity orthotics	Physiatrist, orthotist, therapists	Stabilization of ankle, knee, and hip to allow standing and in some instances ambulation, be it functional or exercise related
Hand	Physiatrist, hand surgeon, occupational therapist	Evaluation of quadriparetic hand and wrist to estimate level of residual functional muscle power, assessment of feasibility of tendon transfers combined with joint fusions for more functional hand (voluntary pinch mechanism)
Wheelchair seating (Figure 10-9)	Physiatrist, physical and occupational therapists, wheelchair vendor	Evaluation of patient for wheelchair that provides greatest functional ability, and in the case of higher level quadriplegic patients, safe sitting balance and stability to permit use of upper extremities
Urology	Physiatrist, urologist, urology nurse technician	Assessment of entire urinary tract at scheduled intervals
Spinal cord follow-up	Physiatrist, spinal cord injury nurse, psychologist, social worker	Physical examination of patient, laboratory and radiograph evaluations as required, patient equipment checked and repaired or replaced as necessary

blood pressure in the range of over 200 mm Hg systolic to 140 to 160 mm Hg diastolic. The hypertension is accompanied by a severe pounding headache, bradycardia, flushing of the skin, gooseflesh, nasal congestion, and visual blurring. If allowed to continue, it can result in a seizure or cerebrovascular accident.

Treatment of autonomic dysreflexia consists primarily of finding the cause (if possible) and relieving it, for example, emptying the bladder or removing the constipated stool. Treatment with anticholinergic medications such as propantheline (Pro-Banthine) or oxybutinin (Ditropan) or in more severe cases ganglionic blocking agents such as mecamylamine (Inversine) is possible, although such medications are rarely necessary. To date, alpha-blocking agents have not proved of value in the syndrome. If the irritation is secondary to skin ulcerations or rectal sphincter irritation, the use of topical anesthetics can help control the symptoms.

Cardiovascular complications

During the acute stage of cervical spinal cord injury, sinus bradycardia and sinus arrest are often noted on cardiac monitoring. The conceivable mechanism is sudden loss of supraspinal sympathetic control to the heart, while the parasympathetic vagal system remains intact. Bradycardia may be managed by administering atropine, but frequent sinus arrest requires a temporary or permanent cardiac pacemaker.

Because of muscular paralysis with flaccidity and immobility following SCI, venous flow in the paralyzed lower limbs is sluggish. Slow venous return is exacerbated by

hypercoagulability associated with SCI. Therefore SCI patients are at high risk for the development of deep venous thrombosis (DVT), particularly for 6 weeks following the injury. The incidence of DVT in SCI patients ranges from 25% to 100%, depending on which diagnostic methods are used.[2,8,14] Fatal pulmonary embolism, which is the most serious complication of DVT, has been reported in over 1% of these patients. This catastrophic event may occur even without clinical evidence of DVT. Swelling of a paralyzed lower limb requires a thorough clinical evaluation to rule out DVT, intramuscular hemorrhage, cellulitis, heterotopic ossification, and long-bone fracture.

When DVT is suspected, further diagnostic procedures should be performed. Both the venous Doppler study and plethysmography are reasonably reliable and can be done quickly.[2] If results of these studies are equivocal for DVT, venography should be performed (Figure 10-10). ^{125}I-labeled fibrinogen scanning is infrequently used because it requires time and does not reveal formed clots. DVT is treated intravenously with heparin, followed by oral doses of warfarin and conservative measures including bed rest, warm soaks, elevation of the affected leg, and gradient elastic stockings. Prophylactic miniheparin is believed to be effective in reducing DVT. External pneumatic compression or gradient elastic stockings should be applied to increase venous return from the paralyzed lower extremities.

The mechanical support of elastic stockings is also beneficial in preventing dependent edema of the feet and ankles and orthostatic hypotension, which is caused by poor venous

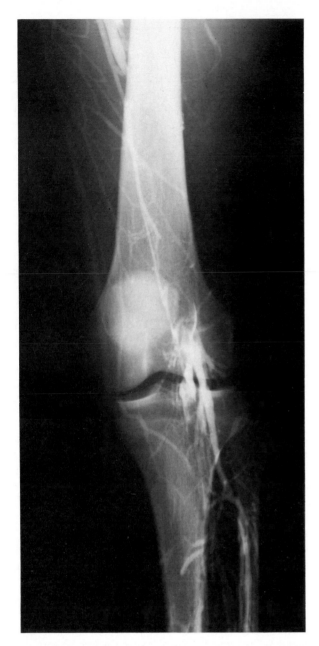

Figure 10-10. Venogram revealing multiple intraluminal filling defects in the deep tibial and popliteal veins, consistent with deep venous thrombosis.

blood return to the heart and subsequently to the brain. Quadriplegic and high-paraplegic patients should begin their rehabilitation with tilt table training. Before they get up, they should wear elastic stockings and an abdominal binder. If orthostatic hypotension develops, the head should be tilted down immediately. In the long run, spasticity is considered to be helpful in the management of orthostatic hypotension. Infrequently, sympathomimetic agents such as pseudo-ephedrine and ephedrine become necessary to prevent hypotensive episodes in quadriplegic patients.

Neurogenic bladder

Immediately after spinal cord injury, urinary retention in the bladder is inevitable because of interruption of the autonomic nervous pathway and lack of sensory feedback. Shortly after suprasacral cord injury, a patient's urinary bladder appears enlarged and smoothly outlined (flaccid), and the bladder neck is flat on the cystogram. A cystometric curve is flat, while external sphincter activities are sporadic or invisible on the urodynamics. These findings are also seen with a neurogenic bladder secondary to conus medullaris or cauda equina injury (lower motor neuron injury).

A patient with spinal cord injury above the level of the conus medullaris eventually develops a small, contracted, diverticulated bladder because of spasticity. There is often dyssynergia between the external sphincter and bladder activities in micturition. This is called detrusor–external sphincter dyssynergia. For SCI patients, intermittent catheterization is widely applied to lessen urinary complications during bladder training[7] and to achieve a reflex-emptying bladder. The intermittent catheterization program starts on a 4-hour schedule between 6 AM and midnight.[7] If the catheterized urine volume decreases in conjunction with the gradual increase in spontaneous reflex voiding through an external collection device, the time interval is increased as follows:

Residuals (ml)	Frequency of catheterization
400 (350-450)	Four times a day
300 (250-350)	Three times a day
200 (150-250)	Twice a day
100 (75-150)	Daily

If residual amounts are consistently less than 75 ml with good spontaneous voiding, catheterization is gradually discontinued.

In females, reflex voiding is problematic. Urine leakage between catheterizations sometimes can be successfully prevented with use of uropharmacologic agents.[1] Administration of oxybutynin, 5 mg two or three times a day, helps reduce bladder spasms that can result in wetting. Pseudoephedrine (a sympathomimetic), 30 mg three times a day, may be added to flatten the bladder neck. If a female patient is physically incapable of performing self-catheterization, indwelling catheterization may be necessary. Patients using long-term indwelling catheterization should take anticholinergic agents to prevent bladder contracture. Individuals for whom self-catheterization is impractical during the daytime are advised to insert a Foley catheter in the morning, remove it in the evening, and then void any residual urine before going to bed. Women who must use Foley catheters on a long-term basis commonly complain of urine leakage and catheter slippage. If uropharmacologic therapy fails, uroplasty may be considered.

Urinary tract infection

During indwelling or intermittent catheterization, bacteriuria is frequently noted on urinalysis. A single catheterization carries a risk of bacteriuria estimated to be between 2% and 10%. However, the presence of bacteriuria alone is not an indicator of the severity of urinary tract infection (UTI). Pyuria with more than 20 white blood cells per high-power field associated with proteinuria and bacteriuria is usually indicative of significant UTI, depending on whether fever is present. There is now a trend toward treating asymptomatic (afebrile) UTI with short-term use of broad-spectrum antibiotics in SCI patients to prevent fever during bladder training with intermittent catheterization. The urine culture and sensitivity test may be ordered to identify microbes and to choose the most effective and appropriate antibiotics. During indwelling catheterization, however, prophylactic therapy does not seem to be beneficial for asymptomatic UTI.

UTI with high fever (higher than 102° F) should be treated with intravenous administration of antibiotics, hydration, and short-term indwelling catheterization. A blood culture may be done, but findings are negative in most cases. As soon as the temperature drops to normal, intermittent catheterization and easy rehabilitative therapy may be resumed. Once the urine becomes sterile, antibiotics can be discontinued. At this point, orally administered acidifying agents or small doses of broad-spectrum antibiotics may be used as a prophylactic measure. UTI with mild fever can be treated successfully with orally administered antibiotics, which may be selected by the best-guess principle or on the basis of the results of the urine culture and sensitivity tests. Periodic follow-up urinalysis and urine cultures and sensitivities are useful, especially when intermittent catheterization continues, to diagnose early UTI and help select antibiotics. When UTI recurs frequently, bladder stones and vesicoureteral reflux should be ruled out. Of course, other causes of fever should also be ruled out, that is, penile-scrotal fistula, kidney stones, and urethral diverticulum (Figures 10-11 to 10-13).

Neurogenic bowel

Loss of anal sphincteric function and lack of sensory feedback from the colon and rectosigmoid are believed to be the primary pathogenesis of a neurogenic bowel following spinal cord injury. In the suprasacral lesion, the sacral spinal–neural arc for colonic peristalsis is still intact, but the conus medullaris is uncontrolled by the hypothalamus. Peristalsis of the proximal digestive system down to the ascending colon is carried out by the intact vagus nerve which is not affected by the cord lesion. During the stage of spinal shock, temporal abolition of the sacral parasympathetic tone seems to be responsible for absence of contractility of the intrinsic muscle fibers in the wall of the transverse and descending colon until return of local reflexes begins.

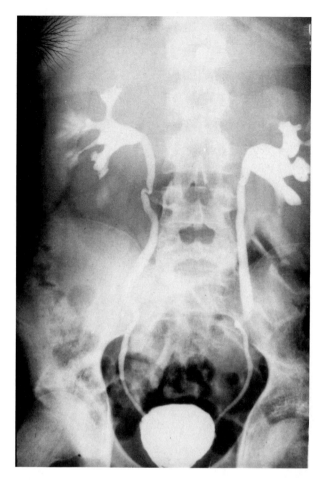

Figure 10-11. Cystogram showing bilateral vesicoureteral reflux.

In the lower motor neuron type of neurogenic bowel, absence of distal colonic contractility is permanent. During the spinal shock or in the lower motor neuron type of neurogenic bowel, fecal impaction at the high colonic level is common and often troublesome. Parasympathetic denervation of the colon after an injury to the conus medullaris or cauda equina can paradoxically cause frequent fecal oozing through the atonic anal sphincter because of poor fluid absorption in the denervated colon. In this case a bulky agent in conjunction with a high colonic enema is helpful to prevent fecal incontinence. Patients with low paraplegia should use abdominal straining to increase intra-abdominal pressure and subsequently to facilitate passage of the colonic contents.

When return of anal sphincteric tone (which indicates isolated function of the pudendal nerves) is noticeable, the pelvic nerves have presumably begun firing the myenteric plexus in the colon, resulting in the increase of colonic peristalsis and water absorption. At this stage satisfied settlement of bowel routine is usually achieved by using pharmacologic agents such as emulsifying stool softeners, colon stimulants, and rectal suppositories. Digital stimulation or

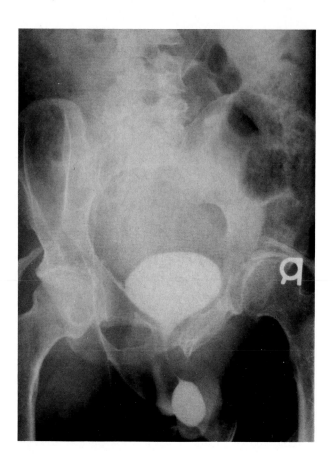

Figure 10-12. Huge diverticulum at penoscrotal junction on voiding cystourethrogram. Extra-articular heterotopic ossification of hip is incidentally noted on both sides.

Figure 10-13. KUB demonstrating staghorn stone in left kidney.

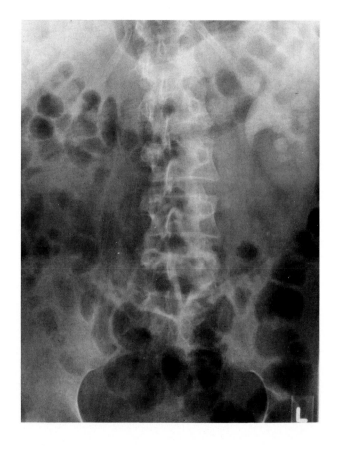

enema may be added. It is important to remember that a colon stimulant should be used 6 to 8 hours before the designated time for bowel movements and that the actual routine is executed by insertion of a rectal suppository, use of an enema, or digital stimulation of the hypertonic anal sphincter.

Heterotopic ossification

Heterotopic ossification (HO) is not life threatening but can be disabling. It is relatively common following spinal cord injury. In most cases the hip joint is involved, although any joints below the level of cord lesion can be affected. The ossification occurs in the connective tissue of skeletal muscle close to a joint. Thus in Europe this condition is called para-articular ossification.

The pathogenesis of HO is not fully understood. There is a correlation between the activity of osteoblasts and the level of serum alkaline phosphatase (SAP). Abnormal mineral metabolism and hormone changes secondary to spinal cord injury play important roles.

Individual, age, and geographic differences may be factors in terms of morbidity of HO. Early clinical detection frequently is not possible owing to sensory loss. It is usually asymptomatic and incidentally noted on a radiograph such as KUB or a cystogram (Figure 10-14). When symptomatic, its classic inflammatory signs include local heat, redness and swelling, mimic thrombophlebitis, and cellulitis. During the acute stage, a three-phase bone scan demonstrates increased vascularity in the involved soft tissue area secondary to arteriovenous shunts. Sometimes early HO is suspected because of the significant elevation of SAP shown on routine blood tests, with absence of hepatic diseases or long bone fractures. It should also be noted that spinal bony fusion may increase the SAP level slightly and that the severity of HO may not be related to the SAP level.

Once acute HO is confirmed, aggressive passive range of motion exercises to the affected joint[11] and etidronate disodium therapy should begin. Recommended dosage of this medication for HO in SCI patients is 20 mg/kg/day for 2 weeks, followed by 10 mg/kg/day for an additional 10 weeks. As ossification is completed, the SAP level gradually decreases.

HO can result in the immobilization of an affected joint because of severe extra-articular calcification and lead to difficulty with lower extremity positioning. Prophylactic use of etidronate disodium following spinal cord injury has been advocated as a countermeasure to this calcification because it can inhibit crystal growth of calcium hydroxyapatite through chemisorption. If HO is extensive and has caused ankylosis of the affected joint, surgery can be considered after completion of bone maturity. Preoperative and postoperative administration of etidronate disodium may be necessary to prevent new bone formation.[12]

Pathologic fractures

Osteoporosis of bones below the level of cord lesion following spinal cord injury is inevitable in time. Increased urinary excretion of calcium and hydroxyproline is found during the 18 months after injury, which reflects demineralization of bones and loss of collagen matrix.[3] Muscle paralysis, autonomic changes, and decreased physical activity seem to be responsible for these metabolic changes

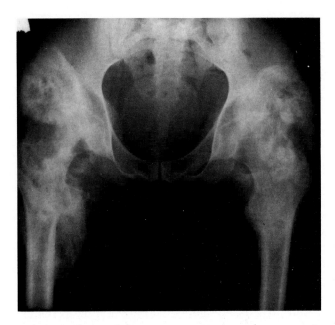

Figure 10-14. Severe heterotopic ossification in quadriplegic patient.

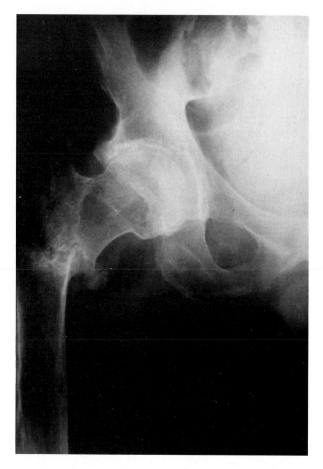

Figure 10-15. Intertrochanteric (pathologic) fracture and severe osteoporosis in quadriplegia.

in quadriplegia and paraplegia. Minor trauma during transfer and wheelchair activities can cause fracture of osteoporotic bone (frequently a femur, either proximal or distal) in patients with chronic SCI. Healing of pathologic fracture is good with conservative treatment.[9] Prolonged cast immobilization may result in decubitus ulcers and ankylosis of an adjacent joint secondary to exuberant callus formation. Surgical internal fixation is seldom necessary (Figure 10-15).

Sexuality and fertility

Sexual functioning of a normal man is dependent on a highly complex interaction of neurologic, hormonal, and psychologic factors. Penile erections following SCI are frequently noted and are usually reflexogenic.[4] Patients with cord lesions above the conus medullaris have intact sacral spinal–peripheral reflex arcs. Spontaneous activation of the sacral parasympathetic nerves results in opening of the arteriovenous shunts and dilatation of the arterioles within the corpora and subsequently erection of the penis. In lower motor neuron lesions the ability to have reflexogenic erections is lost. These patients may experience psychogenic

erections, which are rare and unpredictable. Successful ejaculations resulting from the use of an electric vibrator on the glans penis or an intrarectal electroejaculator have been reported in SCI individuals. Even if ejaculation is possible in some male SCI patients, the possibility of fertilization remains unlikely because of the reduced number and reduced motility, and the changed morphology of spermatozoa. Infertility in male SCI patients is possibly secondary to germinal cell degeneration, failure of ductal conduction, changes in production of sex hormones (luteinizing and follicle stimulating), and retrograde ejaculation. Paretic impotence can be evaluated by monitoring of nocturnal penile tumescence and may be helped by surgical implantation of an inflatable or semirigid penile prosthesis.

In female SCI patients, menstruation returns after a transient period of amenorrhea, and therefore pregnancy is possible. During labor and delivery, particularly in quadriplegia and high paraplegia, signs of autonomic hyperreflexia should be carefully monitored. The incidence of postpartum thrombophlebitis may be higher in SCI individuals. Possible teratogenic effects of certain medications being taken daily for SCI-related problems should be discussed with the patient and her spouse. During pregnancy, autonomic hyperreflexia may mimic toxemia.

Regardless of sex, no patient with a complete SCI can have an orgasm.

Spasticity

Spasticity can best be defined as an abnormal increase in the resistance of an extremity to passive stretch. In spinal cord injury it is associated with hyperactive deep tendon reflexes and pathologic reflexes. Spasticity is present in all upper motor neuron spinal cord injuries, that is, injuries that involve direct trauma to the spinal cord. Its intensity can vary in patients with similar injuries. Emotional factors are certainly involved.

When the degree of spasticity suddenly increases, a search must be made for a secondary cause, which must be attended to when found. Simply increasing antispasmodic medication is not the solution. Secondary causes can include fecal impactions, acute ingrown toenails, decubitus ulcers, acute fractures, urinary tract infections, or the passage of kidney stones. Specific activities can also result in increased spasticity, and the reason for this must be evaluated and then corrected. If a single muscle group or a group of muscles around a single joint are found to be the cause, selective nerve blocks may be the solution.

In many cases mild to moderate spasticity is of value to the patient and can be of assistance in carrying out specific functional tasks, such as in turning from side to side in bed, for independence in position changing, or in transfer activities. Intensive treatment is indicated only when the spasticity is of such a degree that it interferes with function or causes pain and discomfort requiring analgesic medications. Other positive considerations are a delay in the development

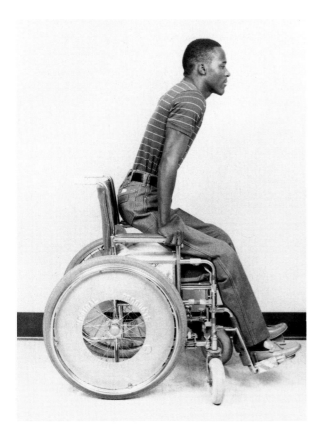

Figure 10-16. Push-up for pressure relief while sitting in wheelchair.

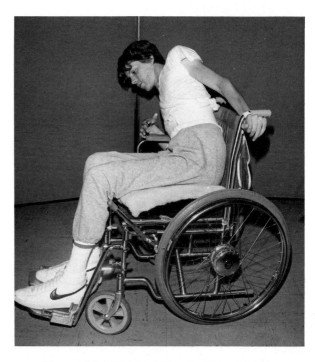

Figure 10-17. Weight shifting in C6 quadriplegia.

of muscular atrophy in the extremities, a delay in the tendency to develop severe osteoporosis, and assistance in standing and in the performance of pivot transfers. Even controlled spasticity requires some medication to maintain it at a reasonable level. The medications available today are these:

1. Diazepam, a benzodiazepine derivative that enhances release of gamma-aminobutyric acid (GABA) presynaptically and potentiates GABA postsynaptically
2. Dantrolene sodium, which acts directly on the skeletal muscles and does not affect neuromuscular transmission. It suppresses the release of the calcium ion needed to activate the contractile apparatus of the muscle.
3. Baclofen, a derivative of GABA, which acts on the neurons in the spinal cord presynaptically. It decreases excitatory synaptic transmission and therefore decreases reflexes. In addition, it acts as an antagonist to substance P, an excitatory peptide.

Experience with usage suggests only limited results with most of the medications used today. Side effects (such as the potential danger to the liver from dantrolene sodium in certain individuals) make it important that the medications be monitored closely to prevent problems. Drowsiness and diminished mental alertness are also factors when diazepam

is used. The ideal drug, which is yet to be found, would reduce spasticity without causing dependence, drowsiness, muscle weakness, and liver toxicity.

Decubitus ulcers

Decubitus ulceration of the skin resulting from improper skin care is among the most common of morbidities of the SCI patient, and it is totally preventable. Proper nursing care and proper training of the patient and the patient's family in the care and treatment of the skin are essential if such ulcers are to be avoided. The need for continual repositioning by the patient while in the wheelchair must be stressed, as must the need for turning the patient in bed every 2 hours. Meticulous care of the skin and avoidance of pressure from clothing, catheters, and drainage tubes, excessive skin traction while performing sliding board transfers, and burns from cigarettes or coffee held between the legs, is essential. There must be an intensive education program to develop the patient's awareness of these dangers. The best treatment continues to be avoidance (Figures 10-16 and 10-17).

Metabolic factors such as negative nitrogen balance, anemia, and dependent edema, in addition to the problem of sensory loss and the ischemia secondary to pressure over bony prominences, are the major causes of decubitus ul-

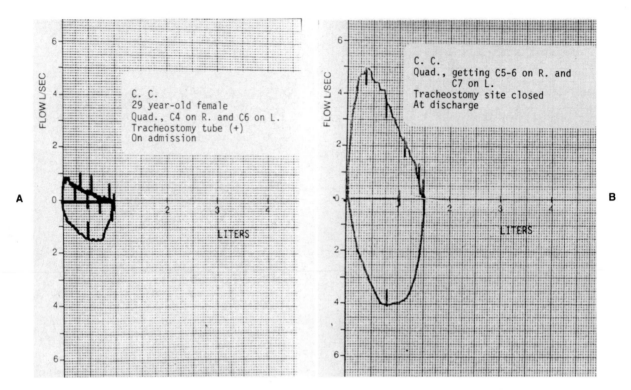

Figure 10-18. A, Severely contracted airflow volume loop obtained during acute stage of cervical spinal cord injury with resultant C4 quadriplegia. **B,** Follow-up study (3 months later) showing improved inspiratory and expiratory flow volumes in same patient.

ceration. The cost in time and money if the problem is not avoided is enormous. This issue is covered completely in Chapter 11 of this text.

Respiratory care

Injuries above the level of T10 can result in diminished pulmonary function. The muscles of inspiration are the accessory muscles of respiration, that is, the sternocleidomastoid and the scalenus (anterior, middle, and posterior). They improve pulmonary function through the elevation of the sternum and the elevation and fixation of the upper ribs. In addition, the intercostal muscles, the parasternal intercartilaginous muscles, and the diaphragm combine to allow full inspiration to occur.

Expiration can occur passively, with more forceful expiration taking advantage of the effort of the intercostal and abdominal muscles. The higher the lesion, the greater the embarrassment of both inspiration and expiration. Exercise to increase the strength of the pectoralis major muscle is recommended as a means of improving cough in quadriplegia below the level of C5. Evaluations of vital capacity and expiratory reserve volume should be carried out routinely, especially in quadriplegic patients. Breathing exercises stressing deep inspiration and expiration should be carried out at intervals throughout the day. The use of the simple but readily manageable incentive spirometer should

also be encouraged. Most of these exercise activities, when combined with the basic physical exercise routines, can substantially increase the vital capacity of a patient. This results in greater mental alertness, as well as in increased strength and ability to function (Figure 10-18).

Fluid intake must be maintained at between 2 and 3 L a day, with greater amounts allowable in the heat of the summer or when there is an acute upper respiratory infection. High fluid intake helps loosen secretions and allows easier expectoration but may leave higher residual urinary volume in the bladder. Frequent position changes aid in secretion elimination and management. Acute upper respiratory infections that result in fever, chest congestion, and cough require immediate medical attention to reduce potential morbidity. Chest radiographs, blood counts, sputum cultures, and sensitivity evaluations are required, and prompt treatment with appropriate antibiotics is necessary to prevent pneumonia and severe respiratory embarrassment. Oxygen supplementation may also be required with motor and sensory loss above the C4 level, and portable respirators or tracheostomies may be required. Vaccinations for influenza are of benefit to this patient population.

Phrenic pacemakers are being used in many instances in patients with high cervical lesions that have resulted in paralysis of the diaphragm. Placement of the pacemakers is not possible if the phrenic nerve is transected or if C3 to

C5 anterior horn cell damage is present. Pacemakers are placed bilaterally. Problems with mechanism failure and the fatiguing of the phrenic nerve have limited use of the diaphragm. In most rehabilitation centers the portable respirator is the treatment of choice.

Functional electrical stimulation

In recent years there has been a rekindling of interest in the control of the motor system by application of electrical stimulation. The basic definition of functional electrical stimulation (FES) concerns the application of an electric stimulus to muscle to allow it to be used in a purposeful manner—to perform work. The renewed interest in and application of this modality is undoubtedly due to the revolutionary changes in design and efficiency of electronic devices, especially the microminiaturization made possible by the fabrication of integrated circuits.

The spectrum of application is rapidly expanding, but some examples of current interest are as follows:

1. Physical conditioning of paralyzed muscles in patients who have sustained spinal cord trauma
2. Stimulation of muscles to effect a functional state of the limb, for example, stimulation of the quadriceps muscles to extend and maintain the thighs in a fixed position to support standing erect
3. Control of bracing devices by FES, for example, peroneal footdrop braces and the provision of wrist tenodesis and prehension in quadriplegic patients
4. The stimulation of ambulation in paraplegia and low quadriplegia with radio-controlled and computer-assisted sequencing of stimulation of the appropriate muscles

The reports that have appeared on FES are of great interest and offer hope that the application of electrical stimulation holds promise for the treatment of neuromusculoskeletal disorders. However, there still exist many neurophysiologic impediments that have to be overcome, including control of the force and speed of contraction and feedback of spatial information. There are favorable reports on the cardiovascular effects of FES, but the superiority of electrical stimulation in this regard has to be measured against the accomplishment of the same results in the traditional manner of exercising. In a paraplegic patient, for example, one must ask whether anything more can be gained from FES than what a normal exercise routine for the upper extremities provides. The need for further research and careful evaluation is obvious.

C1 or C2 quadriplegia

Individuals with C1 or C2 quadriplegia suffer respiratory paralysis but usually have intact phrenic nerves. In the acute stage these patients are managed by being attached to a mechanical ventilator connected to a tracheostomy tube. As described in the section of this chapter on respiratory care, diaphragm pacing may be considered in selected cases. Continued simultaneous pacing of both hemidiaphragms with low-frequency stimulation at a slow respiratory rate reportedly provides adequate ventilation to high quadriplegics at rest and decreases susceptibility to diaphragm fatigue.[14] Patients with the diaphragm pacer may have a tracheostomy tube plugged or replaced by a button when suctioning is not required.

In terms of functional rehabilitation, C1 and C2 quadriplegics should be given the opportunity to be trained in the use of various adaptive equipment. They may become able to use a mouth stick for page turning or typing or to drive a powered wheelchair by using a suction cup chin control fastened to a chest harness. A full lap-board support of the upper extremities and the phrenic nerve stimulator are essential to their wheelchair mobility. Lateral side supports may be added to provide some stabilization while sitting. Barrier-free housing is certainly required, in which case the patient should have full-time nursing at home by private duty nurses who are familiar with the pacemaker (or ventilator), skin care, neurogenic bowel, neurogenic bladder, and if needed, airway suctioning and tracheostomy care.

REFERENCES

1. Bissada, NK, and Finkbeiner, AE: Pharmacology of continence and micturition, Am Fam Physician 20(5):128, 1979.
2. Chu, DA, et al: Deep venous thrombosis: diagnosis in spinal cord injured patients, Arch Phys Med Rehabil 66:365, 1985.
3. Claus-Walker, J, et al: Bone metabolism in quadriplegia: dissociation between calciuria and hydroxyprolinuria, Arch Phys Med Rehabil 56:327, 1975.
4. Cressy, JM, and Comarr, AE: Sexuality and spinal cord injury, Sci Dig 23, Spring, 1981.
5. Frankel, HL, et al: The value of postural reduction in the initial management of closed injuries of the spine with paraplegia and tetraplegia. Part 1, Paraplegia 7:179, 1969.
6. Guttmann, L: Spinal cord injury, Oxford, Eng, 1976, Blackwell Scientific Publications.
7. Guttmann, L, and Frankel, H: The value of intermittent catheterization in the early management of traumatic paraplegia and tetraplegia, Paraplegia 4:63, 1966.
8. Perkash, A, Perkash, V, and Perkash, I: Experience with management of thromboembolism in patients with spinal cord injury. I. Incidence, diagnosis and role of some risk factors, Paraplegia 16:322, 1978.
9. Ragnarsson, KT, and Sell, H: Lower extremity fractures after spinal cord injury: a retrospective study, Arch Phys Med Rehabil 62:418, 1981.
10. Silver, J: The prophylactic use of anticoagulant therapy in the prevention of pulmonary emboli in one hundred consecutive spinal injury patients, Paraplegia 12:188, 1974.
11. Stover, S: Heterotopic ossification in spinal cord injured patients, Arch Phys Med Rehabil 56:199, 1975.
12. Stover, SL, Niemann, KM, and Miller, JM III: Disodium etidronate in the prevention of postoperative recurrence of heterotopic ossification in spinal cord injured patients, J Bone Joint Surg [Am] 58:683, 1976.
13. Stover, SL, et al: Spinal cord injury: the facts and figures, Birmingham, 1986, The University of Alabama at Birmingham.
14. Todd, JW, et al: Deep venous thrombosis in acute spinal cord injury: a comparison of 125I fibrinogen leg scanning, impedance plethysmography and venography, Paraplegia 14:50, 1976.

ADDITIONAL READINGS

Abramson, AS: Advances in the management of the neurogenic bladder, Arch Phys Med Rehabil 52:143, 1971.

Ahn, JH: Current trends in stabilizing high thoracic and thoracolumbar spinal fractures, Arch Phys Med Rehabil 65:366, 1984.

Amelar, RD, and Dubin, L: Sexual function and fertility in paraplegic males, Urology 20:62, 1982.

Bellamy, R: Respiratory complications in traumatic quadriplegia: analysis of 20 years experience, J Neurosurg 39:596, 1973.

Brindley, GS: The fertility of men with spinal injuries, Paraplegia 22:337, 1984.

Cheshire, D: The complete and centralized treatment of paraplegia, Paraplegia 6:59, 1967.

Comarr, AE: Bowel regulation for patients with spinal cord injury, JAMA 167:18, 1958.

Glenn, WWL, et al: Ventilatory support by pacing of the conditioned diaphragm in quadriplegia, New Engl J Med 310:1150, 1984.

Green, BA, et al: Acute spinal cord injury: current concepts, Clin Orthop 154:125, 1981.

Griffith, ER, and Trieschmann, RB: Sexual functioning in women with spinal cord injury, Arch Phys Med Rehabil 56:18, 1975.

Hachen, HJ: Anticoagulant therapy in patients with spinal cord injury, Paraplegia 12:176, 1974.

Keys, TF, and Edson, RS: Antimicrobial agents in urinary tract infections, Mayo Clin Proc 58:165, 1983.

Kosiak, M: Etiology and pathology of ischemic ulcers, Arch Phys Med Rehabil 40:62, 1959.

Lance, JW, and Burke, D: Mechanics of spasticity, Arch Phys Med Rehabil 55:344, 1974.

Long, C, and Lawton, E: Functional significance of spinal cord lesion levels, Arch Phys Med Rehabil 36:249, 1955.

Maryniak, O, and Nicholson, CG: Doppler ultrasonography for detection of deep vein thrombosis in lower extremities, Arch Phys Med Rehabil 60:277, 1979.

Merritt, JL: Urinary tract infections, causes and management with particular reference to the patient with spinal cord injury: a review, Arch Phys Med Rehabil 57:365, 1976.

Nicholas, JJ: Ectopic bone formation in patients with spinal cord injury, Arch Phys Med Rehabil 54:354, 1973.

Pederson, E: Clinical assessment and pharmacologic treatment of spasticity, Arch Phys Med Rehabil 55:344, 1974.

Perkash, I: Intermittent catheterization failure and an approach to bladder rehabilitation in spinal cord injured patients, Arch Phys Med Rehabil 59:9, 1978.

Prolo, D, and Hanberg, J: Cervical stabilization-traction board, JAMA 224(5):615, 1973.

Scott, FB, et al: Erectile impotence treated with an implantable, inflatable prosthesis, JAMA 241:2609, 1979.

Silver, JR: Immediate management of spinal cord injury, Br J Hosp Med 29:412, 1983.

Sullivan, RA: Role of the psychiatrist in the care and treatment of the spinal cord injured patient, J Med Soc NJ 72:189, 1975.

Viera, A, Merritt, J, and Erickson, R: Renal function in spinal cord injury: a preliminary report, Arch Phys Med Rehabil 67:257, 1980.

Welch, RD, et al: Functional independence in quadriplegia: critical levels, Arch Phys Med Rehabil 67:235, 1968.

Wharton, G, and Morgan, TH: Ankylosis in paralyzed patients, J Bone Joint Surg [Am] 52:105, 1970.

CHAPTER 11 | Pressure sores

STEPHEN R. COLEN

The terms "pressure sore," "bedsore," and "decubitus ulcer" are frequently used interchangeably to describe ischemic tissue loss resulting from pressure, usually over a bony prominence. "Bedsore" and "decubitus," which comes from the Latin *decumbre,* "to lie down," do not account for the commonly seen pressure ulceration in the ischial region from prolonged sitting. "Pressure sore" is the more accurate term, since it reflects the current belief that the cause is excessive pressure on the skin, which eventuates in tissue necrosis and ulceration. Paget in 1873 was among the first to ascribe bedsores to pressure, saying that such sores were "the sloughing and mortification" or death of a part produced by pressure. The spectrum of clinical presentations is broad, ranging from superficial skin loss to the progressive destruction of underlying fat, muscle, bone, and joints. If bedsores are allowed to progress untreated, infection and sepsis may develop and death may ensue.

ETIOLOGY

Although neuropathology, shear, and pressure have all been implicated as etiologic factors in the development of pressure sores, the single most important factor is excessive pressure. Unrelieved pressure for periods variously estimated at 1 to 12 hours is the major etiologic agent. Landis[38] in 1930, using a microinjection method to study capillary blood pressure, reported an average pressure of 32 mm Hg in the arteriolar limb, 22 mm Hg in the midcapillary bed, and 12 mm Hg in the venous side. Distribution of pressure points in the lying and sitting positions has been documented by Lindan, Greenway, and Piazza[8] in their study using a "bed of springs and nails" (Figure 11-1). In the supine position the sacrum, buttocks, heels, and occiput are subject to greatest pressures, in the range of 40 to 60 mm Hg. In the prone position the knees and chest sustain approximately 50 mm Hg. In the sitting position the ischial tuberosities receive pressures up to 75 mm Hg. Pressures are transmitted from the surface to the underlying bone, compressing all of the underlying tissues. Pressures are greatest over the bone, gradually decreasing toward the periphery. The greatest extent of tissue ischemia and necrosis would therefore be deep at the bony interface and not at the skin surface. Husain[33] demonstrated that when pressures are altered, even for periods lasting only 5 minutes, tissues are able to withstand greater pressures.

The lowering of the nutritional status of the patient, whether by infection, starvation, or inanition, plays a role in the formation of pressure sores. Hubay, Kiehn, and Drucker[32] felt that a disturbed metabolic state is necessary for both their formation and chronicity. Although one might agree with chronicity, it is not essential that the metabolic state be altered for their formation. Pressure sores have been known to develop in healthy young men suddenly immobilized because of accident or disease.

That neurotrophic factors are important in causing pressure ulceration has not been substantiated. Charcot in 1879 and Munro as recently as 1940 placed great emphasis on the neurotrophic explanation for tissue ischemia and necrosis leading to ulceration.

Dinsdale[17] in 1974 concluded from pressure and friction studies on paraplegic pigs that friction was additive to pressure in producing skin ulceration. The shear theory postulates that stretching and compression of muscle-perforating vessels to the skin result in subsequent ischemic necrosis.

Reproduced in part from Colen, SR: Pressure sores. In McCarthy, J, editor: Reconstructive plastic surgery: principles and procedures in correction, reconstruction, and transplantation, ed 3, Philadelphia, 1988, WB Saunders Co.

167

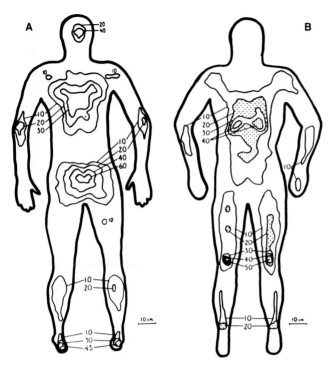

Figure 11-1. Comparison of pressure distribution in healthy adult maly lying, **A,** supine and, **B,** prone with feet hanging over edge of bed. Isobar values are in mm Hg. (From Lindan, O, Greenway, RM, and Piazza, JM: Arch Phys Med Rehabil 46:378; 1965.)

Dinsdale demonstrated that shear effect did not effect tissue injury by this mechanism but instead contributed to skin ulceration by direct application of mechanical forces to the epidermis.

From examination of all available data it appears that pressure plays the key role in formation of pressure sores. The critical questions clinically are how much pressure over what period of time is required to predictably produce ulceration and which tissues are at greatest risk.

Research into the effects of pressure has been reported by Groth,[23] Kosiak,[35] and Dinsdale.[17] In a series of experiments in rabbits, Groth applied direct pressure to the posterior ischii. Pressure was transmitted by a single lever device for varying periods of time. The effect on the treated areas was examined both macroscopically and microscopically. Animals weighing 2 to 3 kg were exposed to a surface pressure of 143 mm Hg for 3 to 4 hours. Macroscopic changes were seen after a few days. The changes consisted of slight swelling, redness, and small hemorrhages and progressed to well-circumscribed foci of necrosis, surrounded by a narrow reddish zone. At times the well-circumscribed foci were missing and the changes appeared as distinct stripes running in the direction of the muscle fibers. No changes were apparent in the nerves and larger blood vessels of the area. On microscopic examination there were capillary hemorrhages, waxy degeneration of Zenker, vacuola-

tion, or loss of striation, followed, on the second or third day after pressure application, by calcification in some of the necrotic muscle fibers. Phagocytosis with beginning interstitial proliferation producing granulation tissue that formed a wall of demarcation around the necrotic musculature was also observed. Seven days after the application of pressure a collagenous ground substance developed, leading to scar formation. Even in the animals that showed no macroscopic changes, there were microscopic alterations such as described previously. The longer the duration of pressure, the greater the extent of changes. Additional investigations on the role of sepsis and spinal transection were reported. Among the conclusions drawn by Groth were the following:

1. Pressure sores simulating those in humans can be produced experimentally in animals.
2. Decubiti occur more frequently in flaccid paralytic patients than in spastic patients.
3. The larger the muscle mass, the greater the ability to withstand pressure.
4. The effective pressure force increases toward the smaller surface. This accounts for the greater destruction of tissue at the base of the inverted cone, typified by the small area of skin redness or destruction overlying a bony prominence. This condition is frequently observed in both ischial and trochanteric ulcers and even to a lesser degree over the sacrum.
5. Generalized sepsis in an animal leads to local infection at the site of pressure, with abscess formation, extension of inflammation, thrombosis of the larger vessels, and consequently broader distribution of tissue necrosis. However, large vessel thrombosis per se is not a cause of ulceration because of the extensive collateral circulation usually present.

Kosiak[35] conducted a well-controlled experiment using healthy dogs subjected to accurately controlled pressure ranging from 100 to 550 mm Hg for periods of 1 to 12 hours. He also came to the conclusion that prolonged pressure was the direct and main cause of pressure sores.[35] Microscopic examination of tissue obtained 24 hours after the application of 60 mm Hg pressure for only 1 hour showed cellular infiltration, extravasation, and hyaline degeneration. Tissues subjected to higher pressures for longer periods of time showed, in addition, muscular degeneration and venous thrombosis. Kosiak concluded that intense pressure of short duration was as injurious to tissues as lower pressure of longer duration. In both cases the tissue ischemia led to irreversible cellular changes and ultimately to necrosis and ulceration.

Kosiak disagreed with Groth in regard to the location and severity of the changes, stating that they extended equally throughout the area under pressure instead of being most severe at the deepest part overlying the bony prominence. He concluded that skin and subcutaneous tissue provide a sling or suspension effect, with the result that only a fraction of the applied pressure is transmitted to the deep tissues.

Husain[33] reported microscopic changes in rat muscle subjected to a pressure of 100 mm Hg for as little as 1 hour. His microscopic findings were essentially similar to those reported by Groth and Kosiak.

Keane[34] noted that muscle is more susceptible to pressure injury than skin and pointed out that body weight is borne on superficial, weight-bearing bony prominences, which are covered only with skin and superficial fascia. He believed that in this way muscle was protected from the effects of pressure. Nola and Vistnes[44] supported Keane's ideas by documenting significant areas of muscle necrosis histologically in rats when pressure was applied to a transposed muscle flap over a bone. Daniel,[13] in cadaver dissections, found that in normal human weight-bearing positions over bony prominences, muscle is seldom interposed between bone and skin.

In 1974 Dinsdale[17] analyzed the role of pressure and friction in the production of pressure sores in normal and paralyzed pigs. Pressure of 160 to 1120 mm Hg was mechanically applied with and without friction for 3 hours. Ulcerations produced extended into the dermis and were present after 24 hours. Dinsdale concluded that "friction is a factor in the pathogenesis of decubitus ulcers since it applied mechanical force in the epidermis." He cautioned against blindly accepting the pressure-ischemia relationship as the only cause for ulceration. In 1974 Dinsdale concluded that a constant pressure of 70 mm Hg applied for greater than 2 hours produced irreversible tissue damage. If the pressure was intermittently relieved, minimal changes occurred even at pressures of 240 mm Hg.[17]

The preceding studies suggest that pressure equaling approximately two times the end-capillary arterial pressures (that is, 70 mm Hg), unrelieved for between 1 and 2 hours, can produce ischemia.

Paraplegia in relation to pressure sores

Paraplegia may be caused by trauma or disease. Holdsworth[30] made important observations on traumatic paraplegia that might have some bearing on knowledge of the problem of ulcer development at certain sites and might influence the management of patients from the inception of the paraplegia. His study of 71 patients showed that correct nursing care, careful attention to simple bladder drainage, and proper rehabilitation measures resulted in an avoidance of all serious complications, maintenance of the patients' general health, and a reduction in hospitalization to an average of 9 to 10 months. In these patients not one serious bedsore developed, and in reviewing his paper, one is impressed with the care exercised in the diagnostic asessment of the injury, a factor that must have been reflected in the notable results achieved.

During the initial period of spinal shock the paralysis is flaccid. As a result many of these patients are left in the supine position in which undue pressure against the bony prominences of the occiput, thorax, sacrum, and heels may be allowed to develop. Pressure sores may appear rapidly at these points unless care is taken to prevent prolonged pressure. In a patient with injury but without transection, some function may return after several weeks. Isolated cord segments may regain some function, and reflexes may reappear. The paralysis that was flaccid during the shock period becomes spastic or of the upper motor neuron type and may lead to the development of ulcers in quite different sites. If still restricted to bed, the patient may be placed in a side-lying position, incurring the risk of ulcers over the greater trochanters, or there may be spastic pressure of knee rubbing against knee or medial malleolus against medial malleolus, which combined with friction and maceration may result in ulcers in these areas. If the patient has been allowed to assume a sitting position and is not carefully instructed concerning the avoidance of pressure, ischial ulcers may develop, as well as ulcers along the margins of the plantar surface of the heel and foot.

PATHOLOGY OF PRESSURE SORES
Gross pathology

Although these lesions are often discussed only in terms of their chronicity, there is an acute phase (Figure 11-2). This may take the form of erythema or redness, caused by pressure, then pass through the stages of swelling, blistering, cyanosis, and beginning tissue necrosis. Frequently the acute phase can be reversed by relief of pressure and other measures. Although Campbell and Delgado[6a] recommended moderate heat to accompany the relief of pressure, Kosiak and associates[36] believe that it should not be used because it increases the metabolic requirements in an area whose blood supply is already impoverished and thus may lead to additional tissue ischemia.

An incipient pressure sore may be mistaken for an ischiorectal or other form of acute abscess and may be incised for drainage of pus that is not present. Instead of pus, grayish yellow necrotic fat may be exposed. This may become infected after incision, resulting in further destruction of tissue and the development of a craterlike defect. If an infection is present elsewhere in the body, organisms may settle in the traumatized area, even though the skin covering may be intact. In such cases pus and necrotic fat may be apparent after incision of the area.

In chronic ulcers, deep destruction generally extends from skin and fat through fascia, muscle, and synovial membrane, if adjacent to a joint, and even into the joint. Osteitis or osteomyelitis with bone destruction may be present. In the most advanced cases dislocations and pathologic fractures may occur.

A long-standing ulcer that has passed through periods of repeated healing and breakdown may show considerable growth of a thin, shiny, marginal scar epithelium with wide surrounding zones of dense scar tissue. The granulation

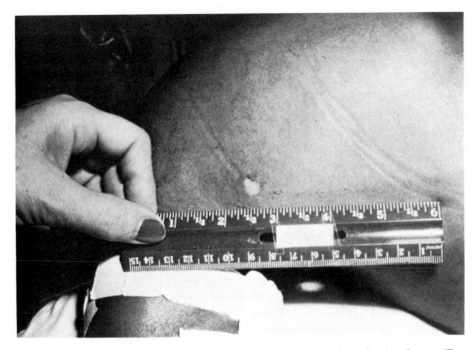

Figure 11-2. Early pressure sore of axillary fold region resulting from Stryker frame. (From Converse, JM, editor: Reconstructive plastic surgery: principles and procedures in correction, reconstruction, and transplantation, ed 2, Philadelphia, 1977, WB Saunders Co.)

tissue may be pale and purulent with little or no sign of activity because of the gradual impairment of the blood supply by the progressive vascular constriction caused by the dense scarring at the base. Some chronic ulcers show evidence of arrested epithelial ingrowth from the margin, resulting in turned-in, curled margins. This is especially true of a deep ulcer in which it is impossible for the epithelium to line the edges of the ulcer, owing to the failure of granulation tissue to grow upward and thus eliminate deep pockets.

The products of bacterial invasion and tissue breakdown form a foul-smelling, purulent discharge that in itself destroys new epithelium. The continuous discharge of proteolyzed material leads to protein deficiency, anemia, temperature fluctuation, malaise, and a general lowering of the constitutional status.

The infecting organisms include staphylococci, streptococci, *Pseudomonas aeruginosa*, *Escherichia coli*, *Bacillus proteus*, and others, often in combination. The consistency and color of the purulent exudate depend on the major infecting organism. Systemic administration of antibiotics, selectively matched to the infecting organism, is useful at times. However, their value is questionable in older chronic ulcers with heavy scarring and thrombosed vessels, which prevent an antibiotic's access to the ulcer.

The suppurative process may track great distances along fascial planes, establishing ramifying sinus tracts,[40] penetrating bursae, entering joint cavities through the destruction of the joint capsule, and causing septic arthritis or joint destruction and dislocation (Figure 11-3). Genitourinary complications, septicemia, and death may occur.[6]

In a retrospective autopsy study of paraplegic patients, secondary amyloidosis was found in 40% of those surviving the initial injury by at least 1 year.[12] Of this subgroup, 70% died of renal failure secondary to renal amyloidosis. Chronic bedsores were a major factor in the development of amyloidosis in the paraplegic.

In summary, pressure sore ulcers may take two major forms or may represent a combination of the two. They may start as superficial lesions involving skin alone or skin and fat. In the early stages they may be treated conservatively because the condition is reversible if the ischemic tissue receives pressure relief and an enhanced oxygen supply. For the latter, serial transfusions increase the oxygen-carrying component.[35,41] The use of hyperbaric oxygen has been described by Fischer[19] in diabetic ulcers, stasis ulcers, and pressure sores of varying sizes with reported encouraging results. The second form may appear as an area of reddening of the skin with a small opening or no opening at all. Beneath the surface, however, is a cone-shaped area of widespread destruction extending through all layers of tissue down to and even including bone.

Histopathology

Pressure sores are indistinguishable from other (nonspecific chronic) ulcers except in their extent. In the early stages

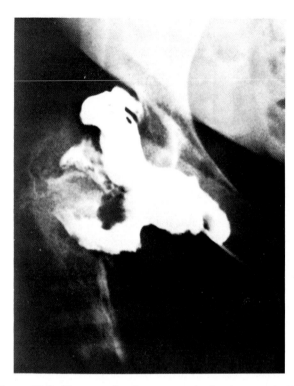

Figure 11-3. Sinogram showing communication between ischial pressure sore and hip joint. (Courtesy Dr JM McCarthy, Institute of Reconstructive Plastic Surgery. From McCarthy, J, editor: Reconstructive plastic surgery: principles and procedures in correction, reconstruction, and transplantation, ed 3, Philadelphia, 1988, WB Saunders Co.)

Table 11-1. Sites of pressure sores in paraplegic patients

Site	Number	Percentage
Ischium	68	28
Sacrum	64	27
Heel	44	18
Trochanter	27	12
External malleoli	20	8
Tibial crest	10	4
Anterosuperior spine	5	2
Costal margin	2	1
TOTAL	240	100

In a review of 1604 pressure sores in paraplegics, Dansereau and Conway[14] reported the following anatomic distribution:

Site	Percentage
Ischial tuberosity	28.0
Trochanter	19.0
Sacrum	17.0
Heel	9.0
Malleolus	5.0
Pretibial	5.0
Patella	4.0
Foot	3.0
Anterosuperior spine	2.5
Elbow	1.5
Miscellaneous	6.0

Petersen and Bittman,[47] in a study of pressure sores in patients in and around the County of Aarhus, Denmark, found that in 63% they developed while the patient was hospitalized. Sacral, ischial, and trochanteric sores were the most common; 10% of the sores were found in ambulatory patients, 37% were in wheelchair patients, and 53% were in bedridden patients.

The factors determining the site of involvement are many, including the state of paralysis (whether flaccid or spastic), whether the patient is bedridden, and if so, whether the patient is supine or prone. If the patient is in a wheelchair or wears braces, certain sites are more subject to pressure than others. The location of a patient's bed in relation to roommates[20] or to a television set or window may determine the site of involvement, since the patient may spend long hours watching the television screen or view or facing away from a wall and conversing with roommates.

The early weeks after an accident or the onset of disease are generally a period of flaccid paralysis and loss of vasomotor control, factors that contribute to tissue breakdown. The patient generally lies supine, with changes of position to the side. Thus the development of sacral ulcers can be expected, followed closely in frequency by trochanteric ulcers. Calcaneal, thoracic, and even occipital sores may also occur. Pressure sores involving the anterosuperior spine of

of redness and swelling the patient has vascular dilatation and interstitial edema, followed by epidermal separation, capillary clotting and hemorrhage, Zenker's waxy degeneration of muscle fibers, vacuolation, and death of tissue cells. Neutrophils and lymphocytes infiltrate the affected tissues. Phagocytosis is increased, and a wall of demarcation formed by interstitial proliferation develops around the necrotic area.

Deposition of collagen in the granulation tissue at the base and margins of the ulcer may become so heavy that wound healing is seriously impaired. Thrombosis of larger vessels progresses, with the development of successively greater areas of tissue necrosis. Sometimes calcific deposits may be identified in necrotic muscle fibers.

CLINICAL ASPECTS
Site of occurrence

Knowledge of the sites of predilection is useful from the standpoint of prophylaxis. Yeoman and Hardy[60] in a detailed analysis of 240 pressure sores in paraplegic patients reported eight sites of involvement (Table 11-1).

the ilium, knees, tibial crests, elbows, and dorsum of the foot have a much smaller incidence because the patient generally is not placed in the prone position, or if placed in this position, does not remain there long because it is tolerated so poorly by most patients.

If spasticity develops in a bedridden patient, medial condylar and medial malleolar sores may appear with great rapidity owing to repeated rubbing of these parts against each other through spasm. There may also be associated trochanteric and sacral ulcers.

When the patient is finally allowed to sit up in bed, pressure occurs in new sites, notably the ischial tuberosities, where a rapid breakdown of skin and subjacent tissues may follow the assumption of this position. Guttman[24] and Reichel[49] have both referred to shearing stress exerted on sacral and buttock skin by the elevation of the bed to a sitting position as a possible major cause of sacral pressure sores.

Sitting in a wheelchair may expose the thoracic or sacral regions to some pressure, but more generally the pressure is exerted against the buttocks; thus the ischial tuberosities, where a major portion of the weight is borne, may break down. The dependent feet, which frequently become edematous and less able to withstand the pressure of resting on a footpiece, may show tissue necrosis on the plantar and posterior aspects of the heels and the lateral margins of the toes unless adequate protection is provided.

No surface of the body is immune to the development of ulcers. They have been observed in soft tissue areas such as the midthigh, calf, upper arms, and forearms, and the incidence is of course much greater in the quadriplegic population.

Pressure sores generally develop more quickly in patients whose nutritional status is lowered. In long-standing ulcers the copious discharge of the products of proteolysis results in a nitrogen imbalance with a lowering of the serum protein levels, anemia, and vitamin deficiency. When any or all of these situations are present, fat and lean body mass and the ability to heal traumatized areas are reduced. These changes encourage the breakdown processes, and a vicious cycle may be instituted unless steps are taken to interrupt it.

TREATMENT

Treatment can be divided into two major categories: systemic and local. Local intervention may be conservative or surgical.

Systemic treatment
Nutritional measures

The prime concern after relief of pressure and wound toilet is restoration of the patient's nutritional status. The measures undertaken vary according to the chronicity of the lesion and the patient's general physical state. Of prime importance is the administration of a high-protein, high-

caloric, high-vitamin diet. In the presence of hypoproteinemia, development of ulcers is rapid and healing is slow. Restoring a positive nitrogen balance facilitates the healing of damaged tissue.

Measures to correct the nutritional imbalance must be instituted early and must show results before any but life-saving surgery is attempted. A daily intake of 135 g of protein in the form of lean meats, cheese, skim milk, protein hydrolysate, and amino acids is effective. Vegetable protein is important, but animal protein is preferable. It may be necessary to supplement oral feedings by the use of a nasogastric tube or by hyperalimentation.

If fat occupies too great a proportion of a patient's diet, the patient may be unable to ingest adequate protein. Reducing the fat and increasing the carbohydrate content of the diet may be wise.

If blenderized diets are impractical, high-protein liquid diets are commercially available. However, they are relatively more expensive and are hyperosmolar.

Intravenous hyperalimentation with a long-term, indwelling, centrally placed venous catheter is possible. Amino acid glucose and fat emulsion are available for this purpose. The procedure for alimentation by this route has been standardized.

It is generally less expensive, less complicated, and more effective to feed the patient by the oral route.

In the case of vitamin deficiency, some restoration occurs as a result of the dietary measures, but these should be supplemented by the administration of multivitamins. A geriatric formula type of vitamin compound is useful for patients with pressure sores.

Unless the serum protein level is above 6 mg/dl, surgery should not be undertaken except as a life-conserving measure.

Treatment of anemia

The correction of anemia accompanies the correction of the protein deficiency. A combination of diet, drugs, and blood transfusion may be required. Liver should be a regular item on the menu. Iron preparations, which may have the additional beneficial effect of reducing the frequency of loose stools and thus helping maintain cleanliness in certain affected regions, are given by mouth or injection.

Transfusions of whole blood two or three times a week may be necessary, not only before but also during and after surgery. By the judicious use of these measures, an effort is made to raise the hemoglobin level to a minimum of 12 g, although some physicians prefer a level of 15 g.[41] At any rate the red cell mass should be increased as much as possible preoperatively and should be maintained at this level in the postoperative period.

Relief of spasm

The presence of spasm in close to 50% of paraplegic patients must be of serious concern to all who treat them.

Cannon and co-workers[7] reported that spasm was serious enough to interfere with surgery in one third of their patients with spastic paraplegia.

When no ulcers are present, measures to correct spasm must be considered from the standpoint of prophylaxis. When there are sores, the continued spasmodic movement of the parts usually prevents healing. If surgical treatment is contemplated, the spasm must first be eliminated or the surgery will fail almost certainly.

Any consideration of the correction of spasm must take into account the fact that such measures as anterior rhizotomy and alcohol injection may destroy reflex sexual activity and bladder control, greatly reducing the patient's sense of adequacy and social acceptance. As emphasized by Chase and White,[25] paraplegic patients have been robbed of so many functions that preservation of sexual function is an important aspect of rehabilitation. In connection with sexual ability, Talbot,[54,55] Munro,[43] and Zietlin, Cottrel, and Lloyd[61] have reported complete erection in 66% to 74% of paraplegic men. Talbot reported that anterior rhizotomy destroyed reflex sexual activity in six out of 10 of his patients, and alcohol injection abolished erection in 28 out of 30 patients studied by Bors.[3] This disadvantage led Chase and White[8] to support the use of bilateral high-thigh amputation in patients with spastic paraplegia rather than subjecting them to neurosurgical intervention. Harding[25] was of the opinion that intrathecal alcohol blocks and dorsal rhizotomy, which in his series yielded only temporary improvement in about half the cases, should be abandoned. He believed that procaine block, which Munro[43] showed controlled mass reflex spasm permanently in selected patients, should be more widely used. When this fails, selective anterior rootlet rhizotomy and bilateral anterior dorsolumbosacral rhizotomy should be considered. Bors[4] relieved spinal reflexes by peripheral obturator neurectomy combined with adductor myotomy.

Pharmacologic agents that relieve spasm include diazepam, baclofen, dantrolene sodium, mephenesin carbonate, dimethothiazine, and orciprenaline. Specific medical contraindications must be carefully evaluated before administering these drugs.

Clearly, many factors must be considered in spasm relief. The merits and demerits of each method must be weighed carefully in light of the overall situation. Only after such deliberation and after discussion with the patient should a course of treatment that is permanently damaging to his physical status be performed. However, a hard choice must often be made; retaining bladder and erectile function would be of little advantage if the procedure failed to control a gross ulcer that might cause the patient to be incapacitated and bedridden and might possibly lead to his death.

Relief of pressure

The field of pressure relief is still being explored and developed. The expense involved in this form of therapy is a major drawback and has prevented widespread adoption.

Formerly the main method of pressure relief was the extensive use of bulky nonabsorbent dressings applied to the affected parts. Springy, synthetic, nonabsorbent fibers, such as Acrilan and Dacron, encased in an absorbent cover of cotton were employed in preference to the flat absorbent dressings frequently seen in hospital wards. However, the work involved in changing the bulky dressings in a time of high labor costs, plus their overall inefficiency, led to a search for more efficient methods. These newer methods have not yet come into general use because of their high cost; the older methods of pressure relief are still widely used and are reviewed here.

A dressing of sterile Acrilan or Dacron fiber, built up to a thickness of 5 to 7.5 cm over a regular absorbent gauze dressing and held in place by Elastoplast or Montgomery straps, produces a light, airy, resilient dressing that diffuses heat, allows air to circulate, and does not become sodden. It may be necessary to protect the skin under the Elastoplast or the straps by painting it with tincture of benzoin, collodion, or one of the aerosol sprays.

Another method of pressure relief that has been used is sheepskin[18,46] placed beneath the patient or applied to specific areas such as the feet in the form of easily removed bootees.[5] This was a step forward, but laundering caused the sheepskin to either disintegrate or become too hard to serve its purpose. Easily washed, synthetic, deep-piled pads were substituted successfully.

Another substitute material is silicone gel used in a cushion or pad.[52] These pads provide fairly good weight distribution but are expensive, and some patients find them hard to use. The Jobst Hydro-float flotation pad is somewhat cheaper and fits wheelchairs of all sizes. The cost may be further reduced by using air cushions filled with water.

The water bed was first described by Arnott in 1838 and mentioned by Paget in 1873 but was more or less ignored until Weinstein and Davidson[58] published a report of an updated modern version for the prevention and treatment of decubitus ulcers. They described both a bed and a seat. Harris[27,28] and Dewis, Caplan, and Pache[16] reported favorably on the use of a bed with a plastic bladder to hold the water, which was contained in a Styrofoam form contoured to the body.

Pfandler[48] reviewed the entire subject of flotation for pressure relief, describing the principle (Archimedes'), variations, and experience with its use at the University of Rochester Rehabilitation Center. A lifting device to make nursing care easier is incorporated into the contoured fiberglass bed, and the patient lies on a free-floating vinyl sheet called Staph-check, which is impregnated with a chemical formula designed to inhibit the growth of *Staphylococcus* organisms. The depth of the water varies from 1 foot at the shoulders to 2½ feet at the buttocks. This allows the patient to assume a sitting position while still floating freely.

Thornhill and Williams[56] reported their experiences with the water mattress in a large city hospital. They described

10 patients who had satisfactory results: all ulcers showed signs of healing, no new ulcers or lesions were observed in any patient while on the water mattress, and the healing time was accelerated. Dewis, Caplan, and Pache[16] reported that routine nursing care was continued, and only dry sterile dressings were applied to the ulcers. The patients were turned to increase their comfort and aid pulmonary drainage. Frequent turning proved to be unnecessary, since the fluid support eliminated many of the pressure points.

Some of the commercial preparations developed during the 1960s were the DePuy Flote-bed (DePuy, Inc.), the Hydro-float (Jobst), and variations of these making use of such equipment as sports air cushions and camping mattresses filled with water to reduce the expense. One difficulty with the latter is that leaks occur frequently. They can be patched, but considerable water escapes before the leak is discovered.

One difficulty encountered with water beds was patients' inability to adjust to a jiggling, constantly moving surface. Other problems occurred in changing position and with difficulty in breathing because of limited movement or limited activity. An unexpected effect was that patients became accustomed to water beds and resisted being moved to regular beds.

Kosiak and co-workers[36] compared the pressures exerted at 12 points on the thigh, ischium, and coccyx when the patient was positioned on various materials. Kosiak found that pressure on a flat board varied from 50 to 500 mm Hg, pressure on a wooden office seat varied from 97 to 200 mm Hg, and pressure on a board with a 2-inch foam rubber pad varied from 53 to 160 mm Hg. These findings were recorded in 11 spinal injury patients, and the highest pressures were exerted over the ischia and coccyx.

When patients sat on an alternating pressure pad at $\frac{1}{2}$-inch excursion, pressures in the inflated position ranged from 100 to 275 mm Hg. In the deflated position, pressures at critical sites were about equal to or below the level of the arterial diastolic pressure in all but four sites around the ischia and coccyx. Pressure greater than capillary pressure was exerted at least half the time at all sites and constantly in four critical areas.

Weinstein and Davidson[59] found water bed pressures of 18 mm Hg (average) against the heels, 19 mm Hg against the sacrum, and about 25 mm Hg against the trochanters when the patient was in a side-lying position. These pressures are below capillary pressures at heart level, which range from 20 to 30 mm Hg, so the vicious circle of pressure producing vascular occlusion, anemia, and tissue necrosis is broken.

Baran and associates,[2] using a new mattress of a specially engineered polyurethane foam and a regular hospital mattress, compared various site pressures in five patients and noted that they differed significantly. Another study of 16 patients by the same investigators, using a different method of recording pressures and adding an additional element of

recommended support (the water mattress), yielded even stronger evidence in favor of the polyurethane mattress.

Although pressure was considerably relieved by these methods, the ultimate goal of weightlessness or total pressure relief remains elusive. The British Hover bed, following the principle of the British Hovercraft in which jets of air are used to support a mass above ground or sea level, supports the body in reverse on jets of air directed upward. A disadvantage of this method is the intensely disagreeable noise produced by the powerful fans that provide the supporting jets. The desiccating effect of blowing warm air over wounds is undesirable, and there is the hazard that electrical or mechanical failure might allow the patient to slide to the hard, flat surface below.

The noise factor was also encountered at first with the latest development in flotation therapy, the air-fluidized bed developed by Artz and Hargest[1] and others at the Medical College of South Carolina. The use of this bed is described in *The Air Fluidized Bed, Clinical and Research Symposium,* edited by Artz and Hargest.[1]

The basic principle of the air-fluidized bed involves supporting the body on a bed whose fluid consists of air and ceramic spheres. (The fluid is not to be confused with liquid, which is wet.) An object of any size or shape can be supported in an airstream if the volume and pressure of the stream are sufficient. Through the use of hundreds of millions of ceramic spheres, 74 to 125 μm in size and made of crown optical glass with no free silica present, the density of the supporting medium is increased and the volume of air necessary to support the body is markedly decreased. The volume of air is approximately 6% of that required for the British Hover bed. Thus the motor is less powerful and much quieter than that of the Hover bed. The patient is separated from direct contact with the spheres by a sheet of square-weave monofilament polyester woven to a controlled 37 μm porosity.[26] This keeps the spheres in the bed, with the exception of an insignificant number of undersized spheres. The latter may cause a slight dust problem for a few days, but they permit free passage of warmed, humidified air that can be closely controlled to obtain the optimum temperature and humidity for the patient, creating an environment that inhibits bacterial growth.[51] The bed of spheres is approximately 12 inches deep at rest. When the blower is activated, the depth of the spheres is increased only $\frac{1}{2}$ inch, and yet it provides the flotation equivalent to 17 inches of water for a 250-pound body. The body mass resting on the ceramic sphere and air bed penetrates to a distance of only 4 inches. Because of the penetration effect of the mass, the surface pressures are less than those obtained when the body rests on a foam mattress or water-filled bladder. Since the polyester sheet provides no support but moves freely to contour itself to the depression, no shearing forces are developed to damage the tissues.

Body wastes and secretions, which ordinarily would be considered sources of autocontamination cross-contamination, have not been a problem. Sharbaugh and Hargest[51] have shown that sequestration and desiccation of microorganisms within the air-fluidized bed system constitute the main contributing factor in the bactericidal and fungicidal ability of the system, a factor making it of incalculable value in the hospital environment. Because of the very low pressures exerted on the body, the bed can be used for paraplegic and other decubitus-prone patients immediately after surgery. Lying on skin grafts and flaps has not been harmful, and dressing changes are simple.[29]

The air-fluidized bed has some disadvantages: active suction is sometimes necessary to maintain urinary drainage, the noise may annoy the patient and other patients in the same room, the bed is heavy, necessitating reinforcement at the corners, and it is costly.

Favorable aspects of air-fluidized beds, as reported by Hofstra,[29] are that patient comfort is increased, the need for medication to control restlessness and aid sleep is greatly reduced, the patient shows physiologic improvement and has an improved appetite, the skin remains dry and does not become macerated, and skin lesions are cleaner and heal faster.

The use of foam rubber rings is unsatisfactory. They may lead to a false sense of security on the part of the nursing staff, with a possible reduction in the frequency of position changes ordered by the physician. In addition, while relieving pressure at one point, they may produce an annular area of pressure around that point, which can lead to vascular constriction and disastrous results.

Blocks of foam rubber used as seats on wheelchairs may be either solid or cored. They afford some protection, but they inhibit air circulation and tend to sag if laid on a canvas wheelchair seat. The sagging can be eliminated by placing a piece of plywood across the canvas seat. It might be preferable to substitute as a seat pad one of the light, porous, foamed plastics in a block 7.5 to 10 cm thick. These plastics have great resilience and shock absorption power and form an effective protective pad beneath the ischial tuberosities for a patient who is in a wheelchair. Patients in wheelchairs should be urged by all who see them to shift position frequently until it becomes an ingrained habit. Houle[31] evaluated a number of seat devices designed to prevent ischemia, which leads to ulceration. The many types of seat cushions are all aimed at the same objective: the greatest possible reduction of pressure on the ischial tuberosities.

For bedridden patients the foam rubber or plastic sectional mattress has properly replaced the usual types of innerspring mattress. A more refined development is the alternating pressure mattress, although it is rather costly. The principle is sound and these mattresses have proved helpful, but I consider the previously described support systems to be superior.

The Stryker frame has the disadvantage that the canvas surfaces of the mattress are relatively unyielding. If the patient is left too long in the prone position, ulcers may develop through pressure in the anterior axillary folds (Figure 11-2). In addition, the patient must be turned regularly by an attendant, who may unconsciously resent or fail to adhere to a rigid timetable.

The revolving bed (Circo-Lectric) may be helpful not only in reducing direct pressure to sensitive sites but also in maintaining vascular and muscular tone. The bed is particularly useful in the postoperative period to turn a patient after flap coverage of a sacral, ischial, or trochanteric defect.

However, too much reliance must not be placed on any automatic instrument, which cannot be a substitute for human care and attention. While pressure is being relieved in the area of an ulcer, other areas must not be subjected to undue pressure, especially during the postoperative period. Therefore special care in the positioning and padding of the unaffected parts must be taken.

Radiographic studies

If there are sinus tracts and infected bursae, it is advisable to take radiographs using a contrast medium instilled into the tracts (Figure 11-3). The devious paths of the sinus tracts can thus be identified before surgery, and their presence may be an indication for more extensive surgery. The degree of involvement revealed by the radiograph is often astounding. An ischial ulcer may show osteomyelitis of the tuberosity, but in addition the suppurative process may track medially and anteriorly toward the pubis, especially in a patient who has been placed in the prone position. A trochanteric ulcer may show peripheral extensions around the thigh in the fascial and muscle planes. There may be extensions upward from the trochanter to the femoral neck and into the hip joint, producing septic arthritis or pyarthrosis. A sacral decubitus may communicate with the hip joint.[40] Heterotopic bone can be demonstrated in many ulcers of long standing, with some deposits reaching a large size. Although simple superficial periostitis is no contraindication to surgery when joints are involved, the problem of treatment may be complex and orthopedic consultation should be obtained. Resection of the femoral head may be indicated if a sinus tract is communicating with the hip joint.

Local treatment
Conservative treatment

Local treatment is aimed at securing a surgically clean wound. If the ulcer is not too large, it fills in from below and epidermal growth from the sides produces a closed wound. However, coverage by scar epithelium is unsatisfactory because the new skin is vulnerable to the minimal trauma of daily activities.

Most pressure sores initially require surgical debridement of all of the necrotic material, including skin, fat, and muscle. Fragments of dead bone may be found lying free at the wound base, and if not removed they continue to cause drainage. Fibrous septa are broken down, and unilocular or multilocular infected bursae are opened for free drainage.

Devitalized fascia or tendons should be excised. Such simple surgical measures can generally be performed at the patient's bedside with only an occasional complication such as mild bleeding. Extensive debridement should be performed in the operating room, and the procedure may have to be repeated several times. The surgeon must have cross-matched blood available in the operating room to replace excessive blood loss.

Modest success with enzymatic debridement was reported by Morrison and Casal,[42] although surgical debridement is more reliable. Some patients have had skin irritation with the prolonged use of this preparation, but the irritation disappeared when the medication was stopped and saline dressings were substituted. In addition to helping clean up the wound, enzyme preparations helped to supress the associated foul odor. Other enzyme preparations have been described, among them a proteolytic enzyme-antibiotic mixture that was reported to be effective in chronic leg ulcers.[53]

Frequent dressing changes are preferable, and wet-to-dry fluff gauze dressings are particularly suited to the rapid removal of necrotic material from the wound.

Irrigations of the depths of the ulcer, particularly those in the trochanteric and ischial areas, should be done daily or with each dressing change. I prefer a mixture of hydrogen peroxide and saline in equal parts. It is relatively bland, and the foaming action of the hydrogen peroxide provides a satisfactory mechanical flushing effect. Plain saline wet dressings and dilute acetic acid dressings have their advantages, and the use of 1.5% Dakin's solution applied in the form of continuous moist dressings has shown good results.[22] The surrounding skin may be protected by preparations such as a thick film of zinc oxide ointment or silicone cream to prevent maceration.

Clark and Rusk[9] have reported positive results with the use of dried blood plasma applied locally; others have recommended the local application of antiseptic or antibiotic substances. My preference is for the use of simple measures known to be effective, economical, and relatively certain. If an exceedingly large ulcer surface is moderately clean, a simple split-thickness skin graft is often applied to obtain a closed wound before performing a definitive flap procedure. This helps immeasurably in preventing inordinate protein loss and in restoring the hematocrit and the nutritional balance to levels that enhance the chances for success.

Immersion in tepid water with soapsuds may be instituted 3 to 7 days before operation with beneficial effects on the wound. Padding the bottom of the tub is generally unnecessary, especially if one recalls that the weight of the totally immersed adult is reduced to about 10 to 15 pounds on the average. Nyquist[45] recommended brine baths. Moist saline dressings alone or combined with an antibiotic, applied for 24 to 48 hours before operation, have been effective in providing a clean granulating surface with a relatively low bacteria count.

At the commencement of local therapy, cultures of the ulcer drainage should be taken, the organisms identified, and their sensitivity to various antibiotics determined. The local use or application of antibiotics is usually ineffective, but the systemic use of an effective drug matched to the organism may be of value initially. It is used as a therapeutic measure when the organism has invaded other parts of the body. However, antibiotics are of little use in the older chronic ulcers with heavy scarring and thrombosed vessels in the area of inflammation, for the simple reason that these conditions prevent access of the therapeutic agent to the ulcerated sites.

The foregoing methods of conservative therapy may result in the healing of small or medium-sized ulcers after a period of time. It is unusual for a large ulcer to resurface itself, but on occasion this has been seen. In many instances, particularly when the level of the healed surface is below that of the surrounding skin and is not subject to pressure, healing may be adequate. As a general rule, however, the new skin covering is of low quality without sebaceous or sweat glands or well-developed dermal and subdermal layers. Such scar epithelium is generally dry and thin with a poor blood supply and must be lubricated by the application of petrolatum, cocoa butter, cold cream, lanolin, or similar preparations. Areas thus healed are more subject to breakdown on slight trauma than is normal skin because of poor vascularity and quality; healing is generally slower when the continuity of such a skin surface has been disrupted.

With the conservative method of treatment, not only is the initial healing time lengthy, but also repeated periods of morbidity may occur owing to minor trauma and tissue breakdown. Because of these factors, physicians treating pressure sores believe that relatively early surgical therapy offers the best hope in the form of earlier closure and improved ability to withstand subsequent trauma. In addition, the successful overall rehabilitation of the patient is a factor of the greatest importance economically, socially, and psychologically. Only a very small percentage of pressure sores can be treated adequately by conservative therapy.

Surgical treatment

The history of the surgical closure of bedsores began with the report of four cases by Davis[15] in 1938. The importance of the excision of the underlying bony prominence was also appreciated toward the end of World War II. This surgical concept was significant for two reasons: first, it eliminated an important element of infection, since microscopic studies demonstrated that changes ranging from fibrosis to osteomyelitis were present in the affected bone; second, it also provided for the elimination of the projecting bony eminence, a significant factor in the recurrence of ulcers.[37] In the same year the Plastic Surgery Service at the Bronx Veterans Administration Hospital suggested the use of split-thickness skin grafts to resurface the donor defects created by the rotation of large flaps.[11] In 1948 Bors and Comarr,[4] in a report on the treatment of ischial ulcers, advocated covering the open bony surface with flaps of nonfunctioning muscle. In 1956 Georgiade, Pickrell, and Maguire[21] reported bilateral high-thigh amputation for "end stages" of decubiti. Current understanding of flap anatomy and physiology allows the surgeon several alternatives when faced with the task of reconstruction in a patient with pressure sores. The surgical strategy must be carefully planned. Future flap requirements must be considered when treating the initial pressure sore. Flap design must not violate other vascular territories or pedicles, since that would make future flaps impossible.

The patient's rehabilitative potential must be considered from the outset. The patient's potential for sitting, lying, and ambulating must be understood when planning the initial procedure for a pressure sore. The treatment of a sacral pressure sore in a quadriplegic patient with minimal use of the upper extremities is quite different from that in a paraplegic patient with strong, well-functioning upper extremities. In the former patient, recurrent sacral, trochanteric, and ischial breakdown is far more common than in the second individual, and multiple flaps are therefore more likely to be required.

Current knowledge about myocutaneous, fasciocutaneous, and skin axial territories gives the treating surgeon many alternatives for flap design. The more complete this understanding is, the more creative and precise the surgeon can be when planning a flap to close a specific area of pressure ulceration.

The surgical principles in the treatment of pressure sores described in 1956 by Conway and Griffith[10] have been modified and include the following:

1. Total excision of the ulcer, surrounding scar tissue bursae, and any soft tissue calcification that may be present
2. Complete removal of all infected bone with recontouring of bony prominences to alleviate discrete pressure points. Removal of bone during treatment of an ischial pressure sore should redistribute pressure evenly over both ischii when the patient is sitting
3. Careful hemostasis and appropriate suction drainage. Delaying closure for 24 hours following an extensive debridement frequently ensures hemostasis
4. Obliteration of all potential "dead space" by use of muscle flaps, myocutaneous flaps, or deepithelialized skin flaps
5. Closure of the wound using well-vascularized flaps designed so the suture line is not over areas of pressure and does not disturb the vascular supply to other flaps that may be required in the future
6. Achievement of a primary, tension-free closure of the donor site, or the use of split-thickness skin grafts

Timing of surgery. Elective reconstructive surgery should not be contemplated unless the patient's general condition has stabilized and the ulcer shows the following signs of improvement: clearance of all necrotic tissue, appearance of healthy granulation tissue, and a tendency for the ulcer to shrink by diminution of the extent of the undermining or evidence of advancing epithelial margins.

General principles of surgical treatment

PREOPERATIVE PREPARATION OF THE PATIENT. Assumption of the prone position for increasing lengths of time in the preoperative period prepares the patient for the prolonged positioning required following surgery for sacral, ischial, and in some instances trochanteric ulcers. The majority of patients initially find the position disagreeable or even intolerable, but they can be persuaded into assuming it. They should do this preoperatively so they know what to expect after the operation and become accustomed to feeding themselves in this position. It is also a training period for bowel evacuation, which may pose a problem following surgery.

ANESTHESIA. General endotracheal anesthesia is preferred to local infiltration or sedation alone, since it prevents spasmodic reflex muscle movements. However, some surgeons find sedation alone acceptable provided an anesthesiologist is in attendance to monitor the patient's physiologic status.

A competent anesthesiologist, who can supervise fluid and whole blood replacement and is capable of warning the surgeon in ample time of the beginning of shock or the development of cardiac complications, is essential to the proper functioning of the surgical team. Paraplegic patients have wide fluctuations in blood pressure and pulse rate and lack the usual compensatory physiologic (sympathetic) responses to hypovolemia. There is often considerable blood loss despite the most exacting techniques. From a psychologic standpoint a conscious patient may be unduly worried or concerned about chance remarks made by the surgical team or may become extremely restless through fear that he or she is lying too long in one position and may incur an additional pressure sore. Under general anesthesia these worries are eliminated, and the surgeon can concentrate totally on the problem of coverage.

OPERATING ROOM CONDUCT AND PREPARATION. On the morning of surgery the ulcer is cleaned and a dry dressing applied. A new indwelling Foley catheter should be introduced to prevent changes in position while the patient's mobility is restricted during the postoperative period. The catheter is allowed to drain freely into a recipient closed system container.

Once the patient is in the operating room, anesthesia is induced and the endotracheal tube is placed while the patient is on the stretcher. The patient is positioned on the operating table, and the surgeon is particularly careful to provide abundant cushioned support to the exterior bony prominences, anterior superior iliac spines, knees, tibial crests, and dorsum of the feet. The patient's position must provide adequate exposure not only of the defect but also of the adjacent donor area.

The skin is prepared with the antiseptic solution of choice. Care is exercised to prevent the solution from running down

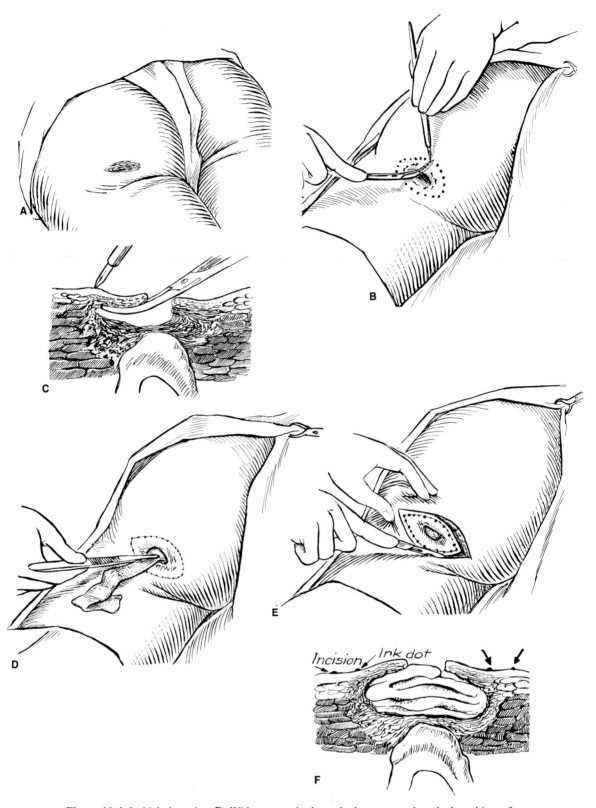

Figure 11-4. Ischial ulcer. **A** to **D,** Widest extent is shown by hemostat and marked on skin surface with ink. Defect is filled with Betadine-soaked packing. **E** and **F,** Extent of soft tissue resection. (From Converse, JM, editor: Reconstructive plastic surgery: principles and procedures in correction, reconstruction, and transplantation, ed 2, Philadelphia, 1977, WB Saunders Co.)

and forming a pool on the dependent surface, possibly the groin, where signs of irrigation develop in susceptible patients.

The entire area is draped to provide ample exposure, and no towel clips are used on the skin. If necessary a few sutures may be placed for fixation of the surgical drapes.

The next step is to outline the extent of the ulceration, which is clearly evident on external examination. However, in many patients a variable degree of undermining is present around the periphery of the ulcer. The surgeon must determine the extent of the undermining by exploring with the finger or probing with a curved clamp in all directions. When slight upward pressure is applied to the clamp, its tip may be felt or seen projecting through the skin; at that point a mark is made with ink (Figure 11-4). In this manner a series of dots outline the extent of the undermining. This is a necessary maneuver because the surface above is covered by a pale, shiny granulation tissue, which is the source

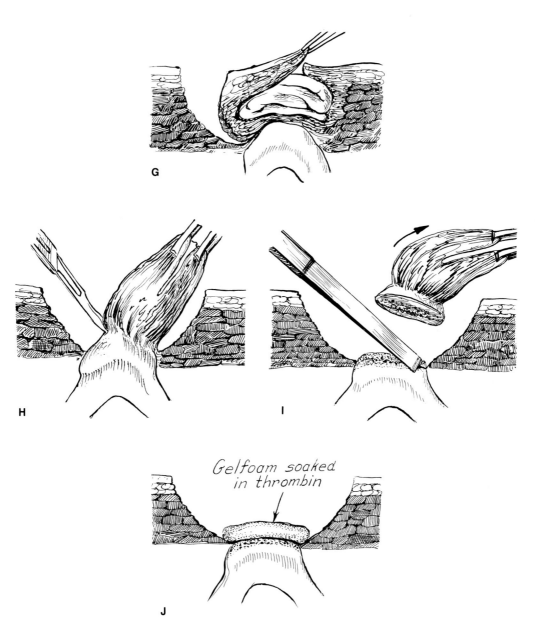

Figure 11-4, cont'd. G to **I,** Partial removal of ischial tuberosity. **J,** Hemostasis is facilitated by application of Gelfoam (soaked in thrombin) on bony surface.

of serous drainage. The surface has the appearance of an endothelial lining. This tissue should be carefully removed either by including it with the ulcer, if it is of limited extent, or by means of surface excision down to the normal-appearing tissue if the undermining is extensive. If any of the tissue of the undermined area is left behind, the risk of seroma formation under the flap and its sequelae of delayed adherence or nonadherence of the flap to the undersurface is considerably increased.

Postoperative care. The postoperative care in the treatment of a pressure sore is of the utmost importance. From the time the patient is transferred from the operating table, care must be exercised to prevent motion or shearing forces in the region of the flap. When an air-fluidized bed is used, the patient is allowed to lie supine for 2 weeks before being wedged into a semisitting position. The patient may be transferred to a regular bed by the end of the third week and then requires the usual frequent repositioning and turning. When the air-fluidized bed is unavailable, the patient is placed on a regular bed in the prone position. Adequate padding with cushions, pillows, and foam rubber pads is used to make this position as comfortable as possible. The position can be changed from the prone slightly to the side position by the careful use of props inserted under the hips and chest. Control of any residual spasms that may be present is mandatory during the immediate postoperative period.

A check of the hematocrit to determine the need for additional blood replacement is made in the recovery room and again within the first 12 hours.

Closed suction drainage is maintained for 7 to 10 days, at which time it is removed providing there is no significant drainage.

If loose bowel movements are soiling and contaminating the surgical area, an effort is made to constipate the patient. Low-residue diets and codeine are helpful in this regard. However, if the stool is formed, inducing constipation is unnecessary.

The skin sutures are left in place for approximately 2 weeks unless there is evidence of skin reaction.

During the fourth postoperative week the patient can gradually be exposed to pressure on the repaired area, beginning with 10-minute periods and progressively increasing the time by daily increments of 5 to 10 minutes or more. The patient in particular, as well as the personnel involved in care, must be told that all areas subjected to pressure must be inspected carefully each morning and after each pressure period. If there is any evidence of skin discoloration, pressure should be immediately relieved and discontinued until all redness disappears.

In addition to the daily inspection, the patient should be instructed to make frequent changes in position while in a wheelchair or in bed. This point is absolutely essential, and it should be constantly stressed to the patient that this is a lifelong concern whenever any area of the body is subjected to pressure, especially if it has been surgically repaired.

Ulcer excision. It is not the purpose of this chapter to present the details of surgical intervention for ulcer excision. This subject is adequately discussed in the additional readings at the end of this chapter. However, complications are addressed in the following section.

COMPLICATIONS
Malignant degeneration

Malignant degeneration does occur in chronic, long-standing pressure ulcers. Generally 10 to 15 years is required for this degeneration to occur. In most cases the prognosis is poor. Malignant degeneration should be suspected whenever the ulceration shows a cauliflower-type appearance. The treatment has generally been radical excision and regional lymphadenectomy when possible.[57]

Postsurgical complications
Flap necrosis

With increased understanding of regional blood supply and the almost routine use of muscle and musculocutaneous flaps, the incidence of flap loss and partial necrosis has markedly decreased. These flaps are more vigorous than traditional skin flaps, and flap necrosis is rare when a major vascular pedicle is included in the flap design.

Hematoma

Hematoma is the most common complication of surgery for pressure sores, and frequently its presence predisposes the patient to other complications. Flap necrosis, wound infection, bursa formation, and subsequent pressure sore recurrence can all be influenced by postoperative hematoma formation. When discovered in the postoperative period, a hematoma should be immediately evacuated. When there has been extensive debridement and bony resection, definitive flap closures should be delayed for 24 hours to ensure adequate hemostasis.

Seroma

Seroma formation is common after flap closure of pressure sores. Inadequate immobilization with resultant shearing forces is usually responsible. Inadequate resection of the bursa can also predispose the patient to seroma formation. Suction drainage should remain postoperatively for 7 to 10 days. If a seroma develops, repeated needle aspiration usually controls it, but the space established by the seroma may create a bursa unless remobilization of the patient is delayed until adequate wound healing can be achieved.

Wound infection

Despite appropriate preoperative wound cultures and adequate soft tissue and bony debridement, wound infection remains a significant postoperative complication. It should be aggressively treated with wide drainage and appropriate antibiotics. Frequently an unrecognized hematoma predisposes a patient to wound infection.

Wound separation

Wound separation occurs occasionally, particularly in a debilitated patient or when the flap is sutured under tension. When debilitation is a factor, extra efforts should be made to improve the patient's nutritional status. Wound tension generally indicates improper planning of the flap or an effort to close the donor wound without using a skin graft.

Recurrence

The recurrence rate following the surgical repair of pressure sores is high despite continual improvements in technique. In a follow-up study of 100 paraplegic patients, the recurrence rate was 44% with 4 years of surgery.[25] In the series reported by Griffith and Schultz,[22] 49 of the 73 ulcers surgically treated were recurrent; the three troublesome sites of recurrent ulceration were the sacrum,[12] the trochanter,[18] and the ischium.[19]

Despite the introduction of muscle and myocutaneous flaps, recurrences still take place. The main reasons for recurrence are the same as for the initial ulceration. They frequently reflect the fact that these patients are unable to assume responsibility for their own care, including meticulous skin care and avoidance of all of the etiologic factors of skin ulcers. The behavioral problems of the severely disabled often involve an underlying anger and self-destructive force that must be dealt with and controlled if these patients are to be truly rehabilitated. Under these circumstances the pressure sores often seem to be a symptom of underlying psychosocial problems rather than a disease. The physician must always remember these complex issues when treating patients with pressure sores.

REFERENCES

1. Artz, CP, and Hargest, TS: Air-fluidized bed. In Artz, CP, and Hargest, TS, editors: Clinical and research symposium, Medical University of South Carolina, 1971, Milton Roy Co.
2. Baran, E, et al: Deforming pressure measurements and a new type of mattress, Paper presented at American Congress of Rehabilitation Medicine, Denver, Colo, Aug 20-25, 1972.
3. Bors, E: Veterans Administration Technical Bulletin, TB 10-503, Washington, DC, Dec 15, 1948.
4. Bors, E, and Comarr, AE: Ischial decubitus ulcer, Surgery 24:680, 1948.
5. Butterworth, RF, and Golding, C: A device for treating pressure sores around the ankles, Geriatrics 20:413, 1965.
6. Campbell, RM: The surgical management of pressure sores, Surg Clin North Am 39:509, 1959.
6a. Campbell, RM, and Delgado, JP: Pressure sores. In Converse, JM, editor: Reconstructive plastic surgery, Philadelphia, 1977, WB Saunders Co.
7. Cannon, B, et al: An approach to the treatment of pressure sores, Ann Surg 132:760, 1950.
8. Chase, RA, and White, WJ: Bilateral amputation in rehabilitation of paraplegics, Plast Reconstr Surg 24:445, 1959.
9. Clark, AB, and Rusk, HA: Decubitus ulcers treated with dried blood plasma: preliminary report, JAMA 153:787, 1953.
10. Conway, H, and Griffith, BH: Plastic surgery for closure of decubitus ulcers in patients with paraplegia: based on experience with 1000 cases, Am J Surg 91:946, 1956.
11. Conway, H, et al: Complications of decubitus ulcers in patients with paraplegia, Plast Reconstr Surg 7:117, 1951.
12. Dalton, JJ, Jr, Hackler, RH, and Bunts, RC: Amyloidosis in the paraplegic: incidence and significance, J Urol 93:553, 1965.
13. Daniel, RK: Muscle coverage of pressure points: the role of myocutaneous flaps, Ann Plast Surg 8:446, 1982.
14. Dansereau, JG, and Conway, H: Closure of decubiti in paraplegics: report on 2000 cases, Plast Reconstr Surg 33:474, 1964.
15. Davis, JS: Operative treatment of scars following bed sores, Surgery 3:1, 1938.
16. Dewis, LS, Caplan, HI, and Pache, HL: Treatment of decubitus ulcers by use of a water mattress, Arch Phys Med 49:290, 1968.
17. Dinsdale, SM: Decubitus ulcers: role of pressure and friction in causation, Arch Phys Med Rehabil 55:147, 1974.
18. Ewing, MR, et al: Further experiences in the rise of sheepskins as an aid in nursing, Med J Aust 2:139, 1964.
19. Fischer, BH: Topical hyperbaric oxygen treatment of pressure sores and skin ulcers, Lancet 2:405, 1969.
20. Gelb, J: Plastic surgical closure of decubitus ulcers in paraplegics as result of civilian injuries, Plast Reconstr Surg 9:525, 1952.
21. Georgiade, N, Pickrell, K, and Maguire, C: Total thigh flaps for extensive decubitus ulcer, Plast Reconstr Surg 17:220, 1956.
22. Griffith, BH, and Schultz, RC: The prevention and surgical treatment of recurrent decubitus ulcers in patients with paraplegia, Plast Reconstr Surg 27:248, 1961.
23. Groth, KE: Clinical observations and experimental studies of the pathogenesis of decubitus ulcers, Acta Clin Scand 87(suppl 76):207, 1942.
24. Guttmann, L: The problem of treatment of pressure sores in spinal paraplegics, Br J Plast Surg 7:196, 1955.
25. Harding, RL: An analysis of 100 rehabilitated paraplegics, Plast Reconstr Surg 27:235, 1961.
26. Hargest, TS: A ceramic application in patient care, Presented at a symposium on Use of Ceramics in Surgical Implants, Jan 31-Feb 1, 1969, Clemson University and South Carolina State Development Board.
27. Harris, C: Decubitus ulcers in the sick aged, J Am Geriatr Soc 13:538, 1965.
28. Harris, C: Flotation as an aid in the treatment of decubitus ulcers, J Am Geriatr Soc 15:605, 1967.
29. Hofstra, PC: The air-fluidized bed for spinal injuries. In Artz, CP, and Hargest, TS, editors: Clinical and Research Symposium, Medical University of South Carolina, 1971.
30. Holdsworth, FW: Traumatic paraplegia, Ann R Coll Surgeons 15:281, 1954.
31. Houle, RJ: Evaluation of seat devices designed to prevent ischemic ulcers in paraplegic patients, Arch Phys Med 90:587, 1969.
32. Hubay, CA, Kiehn, CL, and Drucker, WR: Surgical management of decubitus ulcers in the post-traumatic patient, Am J Surg 93:705, 1957.
33. Husain, T: Experimental study of some pressure effects on tissues, with reference to bed-sore problem, J Pathol Bacteriol 66:347, 1953.
34. Keane, FX: The function of the rump in relation to sitting and the Keane reciprocating wheelchair seat, Paraplegia 16:390, 1978.
35. Kosiak, M: Etiology and pathology of ischemic ulcers, Arch Phys Med 40:62, 1959.
36. Kosiak, M, et al: Evaluation of pressure as a factor in the production of ischial ulcers, Arch Phys Med 39:623, 1958.

37. Kostrubala, JC, and Greeley, PW: The problem of decubitus ulcers in paraplegics, Plast Reconstr Surg 2:403, 1947.

38. Landis, EM: Micro-injection studies of capillary blood pressure in human skin, Heart 15:209, 1930.

39. Lindan, O, Greenway, RM, and Piazza, JM: Pressure distribution on the surface of the human body. I. Evaluation in lying and sitting positions using a "bed of springs and nails," Arch Phys Med Rehabil 46:378, 1965.

40. Lopez, EM, and Aranha, GV: The value of sinography in the management of decubitus ulcers, Plast Reconstr Surg 53:208, 1974.

41. Matheson, AT, and Lipschitz, R: Nature and treatment of trophic pressure sores, S Afr Med J 30:1129, 1956.

42. Morrison, JE, and Casali, JL: Continuous proteolytic therapy for decubitus ulcers, Am J Surg 93:446, 1957.

43. Munro, D: The rehabilitation of patients totally paralyzed below the waist, with special reference to making them ambulatory and capable of earning their own living: end result study of 445 cases, N Engl J Med 250:4, 1954.

44. Nola, GT, and Vistnes, LM: Differential response of skin and muscle in the experimental production of pressure sores, Plast Reconstr Surg 66:728, 1980.

45. Nyquist, RH: Brine bath treatments for decubitus ulcers, JAMA 169:927, 1959.

46. Nyquist, RH, and Bors, E: Useful appliances in spastic patients following spinal cord injury, Paraplegia 2:120, 1964.

47. Peterson, NC, and Bittmann, S: The epidemiology of pressure sores, Scand J Plast Surg 5:62, 1971.

48. Pflandler, M: Flotation, displacement and decubitus ulcers, Am J Nurs 68:2351, 1968.

49. Reichel, SM: Shearing force as a factor in decubitus ulcers in paraplegics, JAMA 166:762, 1958.

50. Rusk, HA: New horizons in rehabilitative medicine. In Proceedings of the Seventeenth V.A. Spinal Cord Injury Conference, Bronx, NY, Sept 29, 30, Oct 1, 1969.

51. Sharbaugh, RJ, and Hargest, TS: The effects of air-fluidized systems on microbial growth, Clinical and Research Symposium, Medical University of South Carolina, 1971.

52. Spence, WR, Burke, RO, and Rae, JW, Jr: Gel support for prevention of decubitus ulcers, Arch Phys Med 48:283, 1967.

53. Spencer, MC: Treatment of chronic skin ulcers by a proteolytic enzyme-antibiotic preparation, J Am Geriatr Soc 15:219, 1967.

54. Talbot, HS: Report on sexual function in paraplegics, J Urol 61:265, 1949.

55. Talbot, HS: Sexual function in paraplegics, J Urol 73:91, 1955.

56. Thornhill, HL, and Williams, ML: Experience with the water mattress in a large city hospital, Am J Nurs 68:2356, 1968.

57. Vasconez, LO, Bostwick, J, and Pendergrast, J: Marjolin's ulcer: an immunologically privileged tumor, Plast Reconstr Surg 57:66, 1976.

58. Weinstein, JD, and Davidson, BA: A fluid support mattress and seat for the prevention and treatment of decubitus ulcers, Lancet 2:625, 1965.

59. Weinstein, JD, and Davidson, BA: Fluid support in the prevention and treatment of decubitus ulcers, Am J Phys Med 45:283, 1966.

60. Yeoman, MP, and Hardy, AG: The pathology and treatment of pressure sores in paraplegics, Br J Plast Surg 7:179, 1954.

61. Zeitlin, AB, Cottrell, TL, and Lloyd, FA: Sexology of the paraplegic male, Fertil Steril 8:337, 1957.

ADDITIONAL READINGS

Auregui, J, et al: Long-term evaluation of ischiectomy in the treatment of pressure ulcers, Plast Reconstr Surg 36:583, 1965.

Becker, H: The distally-based gluteus maximus muscle flap, Plast Reconstr Surg 63:653, 1979.

Bovet, JL, et al: The vastus lateralis musculocutaneous flap in the repair of trochanteric pressure sores: technique and indications, Plast Reconstr Surg 69:830, 1982.

Cochran, JH, Jr, Edstrom, LE, and Dibbell, DG: Usefulness of the innervated tensor fascia flap in paraplegic patients, Ann Plast Surg 7:286, 1981.

Conway, H, et al: Complications of decubitus ulcers in patients with paraplegia, Plast Reconstr Surg 7:117, 1951.

Comarr, AE, and Bors, E: Perineal urethral diverticulum: complications of removal of ischium, JAMA 168:2000, 1958.

Daniel, RK, Terzis, JK, and Cunningham, DM: Sensory skin flaps for coverage of pressure sores in paraplegic patients: a preliminary report, Plast Reconstr Surg 58:317, 1976.

Dibbell, DG: Use of a long island flap to bring sensation to the sacral area of young paraplegics, Plast Reconstr Surg 54:220, 1974.

Dibbell, DG, McCraw, JB, and Edstrom, LE: Providing useful and protective sensibility to the sitting area in patients with meningomyelocele, Plast Reconstr Surg 64:796, 1979.

Dowden, RV, and McCraw, JB: The vastus lateralis muscle flap: technique and applications, Ann Plast Surg 4:396, 1980.

Ger, R: The surgical management of decubitus ulcers, Surgery 69:106, 1971.

Ger, R, and Levine, SA: The management of decubitus ulcers by muscle transposition: an eight year review, Plast Reconstr Surg 58:419, 1976.

Guthrie, RH, and Conway, H: Surgical management of decubiti in paraplegics. In Proceedings of the Seventeenth V.A. Spinal Cord Injury Conference, Bronx, NY, Sept 29, 30, Oct 1, 1969.

Hauben, DJ, et al: The use of the vastus lateralis musculocutaneous flap for the repair of trochanteric pressure sores, Ann Plast Surg 10:359, 1983.

Hill, HL, Brown, RG, and Turkiewicz, MJ: The transverse lumbosacral back flap, Plast Reconstr Surg 62:177, 1978.

Hurteau, JE, et al: V-Y advancement of hamstring musculocutaneous flap for coverage of ischial pressure sores, Plast Reconstr Surg 68:539, 1981.

Hurwitz, DJ, Swartz, WM, and Mathes, SJ: The gluteal thigh flap: a reliable sensate flap for the closure of buttock and perineal wounds, Plast Reconstr Surg 68:521, 1981.

Krupp, S, Kuhn, W, and Zaech, GA: The use of innervated flaps for the closure of ischial pressure sores, Paraplegia 21:119, 1983.

Lewis, VL, Jr, Cunningham, BL, and Hugo, NE: The tensor fascia lata V-Y retroposition flap, Ann Plast Surg 6:34, 1981.

Maruyama, Y, et al: A gluteus maximus myocutaneous island flap for repair of sacral decubitus ulcer, Br J Plast Surg 33:150, 1980.

Minami, RT, Hentz, VR, and Vistnes, LM: Use of vastus lateralis muscle flap for repair of trochanteric pressure sores, Plast Reconstr Surg 60:364, 1977.

Minami, RT, Mills, R, and Pardoe, R: Gluteus maximus myocutaneous flaps for repair of pressure sores, Plast Reconstr Surg 60:242, 1977.

Nahai, F, Hill, HL, and Hester, TR: Experiences with the tensor fascia lata flap, Plast Reconstr Surg 63:788, 1979.

Nahai, F, et al: The tensor fascia lata musculocutaneous flap, Ann Plast Surg 1:372, 1978.

Parry, SW, and Mathes, SJ: Bilateral gluteus maximus myocutaneous advancement flaps: sacral coverage for ambulatory patients, Ann Plast Surg 8:443, 1982.

Royer, J, et al: Total thigh flaps for extensive decubitus ulcers: a 16 year review of 41 total thigh flaps, Plast Reconstr Surg 44:109, 1969.

Schulman, NH: Primary closure of trochanteric decubitus ulcers: the bipedicle tensor fascia lata musculocutaneous flap, Plast Reconstr Surg 66:740, 1980.

Snyder, GB, and Edgerton, MT: The principle of the island neurovascular flap in the management of ulcerated anesthetic weight bearing areas of the lower extremity, Plast Reconstr Surg 36:518, 1965.

Stallings, JO, Delgado, JP, and Converse, JM: Turnover island flap of gluteus maximus muscle for the repair of sacral decubitus ulcer, Plast Reconstr Surg 54:52, 1974.

Tobin, GR, et al: The biceps femoris myocutaneous advancement flap: a useful modification for ischial pressure ulcer reconstruction, Ann Plast Surg 6:396, 1981.

Vasconez, LO, Schneider, WJ, and Trukiewicz, MJ: Pressure sores, Curr Probl Surg 24:23, 1977.

Weeks, PM, and Brower, TD: Island flap coverage of extensive decubitus ulcers, Plast Reconstr Surg 42:433, 1968.

Wesser, DR, and Kahn, S: The reversed dermis graft in the repair of decubitus ulcers, Plast Reconstr Surg 40:252, 1967.

White, JC, and Hamm, WG: Primary closure of bedsores by plastic surgery, Ann Surg 124:1136, 1946.

Wingate, GB, and Friedland, JA: Repair of ischial pressure ulcers with gracilis myocutaneous island flaps, Plast Reconstr Surg 62:245, 1978.

Withers, EH, et al: Further experience with the tensor fascia lata musculocutaneous flap, Ann Plast Surg 4:31, 1980.

CHAPTER 12

Urologic management of the spinal cord injury patient

PABLO MORALES

The long-term survival of a patient with complete spinal cord transection depends greatly on the prevention of urologic complications that arise from physiologic alterations in the bladder. Until recently, renal failure was the main cause of death among spinal cord–injured patients.[5]

The sacral segments of the spinal cord (S2-4) containing the parasympathetic neurons to the bladder lie opposite the body of the first lumbar vertebra. Transection of the spinal cord above these sacral segments leaving them undamaged and free of higher cerebral control eventually leads to the development of reflex micturition. With complete destruction of the spinal cord segments or their outflow tracts, the bladder becomes a sac that can be emptied only by a rise in intra-abdominal pressure.

CLASSIFICATION OF NEUROGENIC VESICAL DYSFUNCTION

Classifications of neurogenic bladder disturbance following spinal cord injury have been based either on the anatomic location of the neurologic lesion or on a description of the detrusor dysfunction. A bladder disturbance may be called a suprasacral or sacral lesion depending on whether the sacral micturition center in the sacral cord is preserved or damaged. A bladder may be a reflex bladder because it contracts involuntarily by virtue of preservation of the sacral micturition reflex arc, or it may be an autonomous bladder because it is incapable of reflex detrusor contraction following interruption of the sacral micturition reflex arc. The terms "upper motor neuron lesion bladder" and "lower motor neuron lesion bladder" are synonymous with reflex and autonomous bladder, respectively. Thus one can predict that a suprasacral lesion would be associated with a reflex bladder, and a sacral lesion with an autonomous bladder. However, clinical experience and urodynamic findings have shown that this is not invariably true because even with high

cord lesions there may be an autonomous or lower motor neuron lesion bladder. Since the purpose of classification is to serve as a guide to treatment, a classification based on the type of bladder disturbance itself rather than the site of the neurologic lesion is more meaningful.

Urodynamic classification

With the advent of urodynamic techniques, bladder disturbances in spinal cord–injured patients are now categorized as detrusor hyperreflexia and detrusor areflexia. The bladder and its urethral sphincters are now also recognized as a conjoint unit and the dynamic and pathologic interactions between them have been more clearly defined.

Detrusor hyperreflexia

Cystometric findings are characterized by reflex detrusor contractions during bladder filling that cannot be consciously suppressed. The contractions may be intermittent, in close succession, or sustained. The cystometric volume before the detrusor contraction is usually below the volume a normal individual has when the sensation of impending micturition develops (Figure 12-1).

Detrusor hyperreflexia is generally found in patients with suprasacral neurologic lesions. It is believed that the micturitional center is located in the pons and that the normal micturitional reflex involves synapsing of long spinal cord tracts afferent and efferent to the micturitional center.[4] Following transection of the spinal cord above the sacral segments the micturitional reflex converts from a long tract reflex to a segmental reflex organized in the sacral spinal cord with no supraspinal afferent or efferent connections. Whether the appearance of this reflex voiding results from the formation of new neural pathways by collateral sprouting or the removal of inhibitory influence on an existing pathway is unknown. The end result is a new micturitional reflex center located in the sacral cord, whose threshold for firing is reduced, thus accounting for reflex detrusor contractions at low bladder volumes.

Likewise, the center responsible for coordination between the detrusor and external sphincter is located in the pons. Bladder contractions are normally associated with reflex inhibition of external urethral sphincter activity, but in a spinal cord–injured patient with a lesion between the sacral cord and the pons, there is a lack of appropriate coordination between the detrusor and external striated muscle sphincter, or detrusor sphincter dyssynergia. There may also be a dyssynergic closure of the internal smooth muscle sphincter at the time of a detrusor contraction in some patients when the internal sphincter responds to increased sympathetic reflex from the thoracolumbar spinal cord.[7]

Detrusor areflexia

Cystometric findings are characterized by absence of reflex detrusor activity during vesical filling. There is a slow upward progression in intravesical pressure with filling (Figure 12-2).

Detrusor areflexia is found in patients with sacral cord or cauda equina lesions. The disturbance also occurs in patients

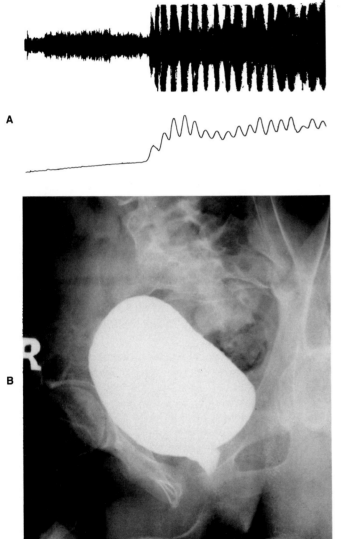

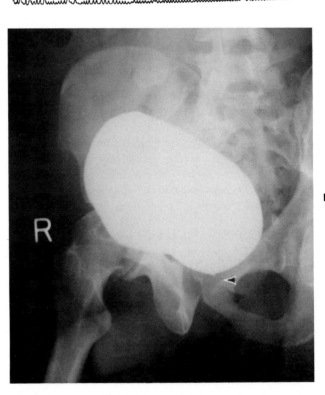

Figure 12-1. Man, 18 years of age, with complete paraplegia (lesion at T8) 12 months after injury. **A,** Cystometrogram shows detrusor hyperreflexia with vesicosphincteric dyssynergia. **B,** Voiding cystogram demonstrates spasm at external sphincter area.

Figure 12-2. Man, 26 years of age, with complete quadriplegia (lesion at C4-5) 4 months after injury. **A,** Cystometrogram shows detrusor areflexia with no external sphincter activity during vesical filling. **B,** Voiding cystogram demonstrates failure to void. Arrow points to vesical neck.

with high cord lesions because there may be complete infarction of the cord below the lesion. Patients with high spinal cord lesions and initial hyperreflexia may also have a second subclinical lesion involving the lumbosacral cord as a result of a "shock wave" effect by the cerebrospinal fluid occurring at the initial injury.[9]

When the innervation of the external sphincter has been compromised as a result of a lesion of the pudendal nucleus in the sacral cord or of the pudendal nerves, there is no external sphincteric activity during vesical filling. In other patients the external sphincter retains its innervation and may not relax appropriately during attempts at voiding. As with detrusor hyperreflexia, detrusor areflexia may be associated with an uncoordinated interaction between the detrusor and the internal smooth muscle sphincter that can result in functional obstruction.[7]

STAGES OF RECOVERY
Spinal shock

Immediately after severe spinal cord injury the patient enters a stage of spinal shock. All neuronal activity is depressed below the level of the lesion. The patient is unaware of vesical distention and is incapable of voiding spontaneously. If the retention is not relieved, the bladder distends until the pressure overcomes the resistance of the urethral sphincters and overflow incontinence occurs. Spinal shock lasts several days to several weeks.

Cystometrograms demonstrate an areflexic bladder. Vesical filling continues without any sense of distention being perceived. Generally the detrusor has an intrinsic resistance to vesical filling and is not atonic. No reflex activity of the detrusor is seen despite overfilling of the bladder. Concomitant electromyography of the external sphincter demonstrates little or no activity with the bladder empty or during filling. Despite the generalized areflexia, however, there is evidence that the internal smooth muscle sphincter mechanism still functions and may be a contributing factor to the retention.[1]

Recovery phase

After a period ranging from a few days to 3 months or more, reflex activity may return to the bladder if the cord lesion does not involve the sacral segments. If these segments or the cauda equina is damaged, reflex activity does not return to the bladder unless the lesion is incomplete. In general, patients with cervical lesions regain detrusor activity more slowly than those with thoracolumbar lesions.

With full return of reflex activity in the intact sacral cord segments, detrusor and external sphincter contractions can be demonstrated urodynamically. Micturition is reflex or involuntary; that is, the patient cannot start or stop micturition in a normal way. Most patients cannot recognize vesical distention, but some learn to detect a full bladder by a vague sensation of fullness in the abdomen. Other patients learn to initiate reflex micturition by tapping on the bladder or by abdominal straining.

Micturition does not necessarily occur with return of reflex detrusor contractions; this is because of inappropriate simultaneous contractions of the external sphincter. In some patients the spasticity of the external sphincter may be insufficient to cause urinary retention, but voiding in this circumstance may occur with abnormally high intravesical pressures. Quadriplegic patients with lesions above T6 develop autonomic dysreflexia manifested by bradycardia, paroxysmal hypertension, severe headache, and "gooseflesh" during distention of the bladder.

The vesicosphincteric dyssynergia is an almost constant feature of the hyperreflexic bladder. The extent of the imbalance generally parallels the completeness of the cord transection. Patients with incomplete cord lesions are more likely to overcome the functional obstruction. Although usually associated with high residual urine volumes, dyssynergia also occurs in patients with low residual urine. The degree of dyssynergia not only varies between individual patients but also changes over the months following injury in individual patients.

When the spinal cord regains function in the patient with injury to sacral cord segments or cauda equina, the bladder function depends on the absence or presence of a permanent lesion. Detrusor areflexia persists if the lesion is complete. The patient cannot recognize bladder fullness and voids by straining with his abdominal muscles or applying manual pressure directly to the bladder in the suprapubic region. During straining or manual pressure, urine is expelled from the urethra but stops as the patient relaxes or the application of manual pressure ceases.

External sphincteric activity may or may not be present during vesical filling. Patients with sphincteric activity cannot appropriately relax the external sphincter during attempts at voiding and consequently develop high intravesical pressure when voiding and retain considerable residual volumes. Patients with sphincteric denervation as occurs with more extensive lesions can void at low intravesical pressure with abdominal straining or manual pressure.

Irrespective of the level of the neurologic lesion, the bladder retains its tone, which is reflected by the slow rise in intravesical pressure during filling in the early stage of recovery. However, bladder function varies with time. Hypertonicity develops, and the increase in intravesical pressure during filling becomes greater compared with that in a normal bladder. Hypertonicity has been ascribed to hypersensitivity of the detrusor muscle itself or of the preganglionic neural fibers. Later, detrusor compliance to filling is further aggravated with the development of bladder wall hypertrophy secondary to hyperreflexia or vesical fibrosis from infection.

The ultimate fate of the upper urinary tract in spinal cord–injured patients depends on the severity of the detrusor sphincter dyssynergia and the resultant high intravesical pressure state of the bladder. The higher the outlet resistance is, the higher the detrusor pressure must be to push urine across it. This high-pressure response interferes with the free flow of urine from the ureters,[12] and induces vesicoureteral reflux and dilation of the upper urinary tract. The sequence of events is inevitable but can be slowed significantly by appropriate treatment at the proper time. Spinal cord–injured patients now survive longer and reach an age at which other diseases pose a greater threat to their lives.

EARLY BLADDER MANAGEMENT

Immediately after spinal cord injury the aims of urologic management are prevention of damage to the detrusor musculature from overdistention and prevention of urinary tract infection. Since urinary retention usually occurs, a Foley catheter, Fr. 14-16, is initially inserted into the bladder and left indwelling. As soon as the injured patient becomes stable, a decision is made whether to continue indwelling catheter drainage or institute intermittent catheterization.

Intermittent catheterization

Intermittent catheterization is currently the method of choice in the early bladder management of spinal cord–injured patients. Its value was demonstrated in 1966 by Guttman and Frankel,[6] who showed that it reduced early complications associated with prolonged indwelling catheters, such as penoscrotal abscess, fistula, epididymitis, and urinary infection. It may also stimulate earlier return of bladder activity.

Intermittent catheterization programs should be performed by nurses or technicians proficient in catheterization. Sterile, gloved, nontouch technique is followed, using disposable catheterization packs and Fr. 14 catheters. Depending on the urinary output, the patient is catheterized three times and more if needed. The fluid intake should be restricted to adjust the catheterized volume to between 500 to 600 ml. Repeated overdistention impairs recovery of reflex vesical function and appears to be associated with an increased risk of bacteriuria and symptomatic urinary infection.

As reflex detrusor activity returns, the patient starts to void involuntarily and has to wear a condom catheter between catheterizations. Measurement of the catheterized urine volumes shows a reduction in amount, and if the volume is below 300 ml, the frequency of catheterization can be reduced to twice a day and then to once daily as long as the catheterized residual volumes remain below 300 ml. Finally intermittent catheterization is discontinued, but periodic residual urine measurements are still advisable.

Indwelling catheter

When there is lack of trained personnel to implement an intermittent catheterization program, indwelling catheter drainage may be continued. The Fr. 14 Foley catheter is changed every 7 to 10 days, and fluid intake is maximized. The catheter is connected to a closed drainage system, and the drainage bag should always be below the level of the bladder to prevent retrograde flow of urine. In males the catheter is taped over the anterior abdomen to prevent penoscrotal complications such as abscess and fistula. Bladder irrigation may be necessary to help clear clots or debris and prevent catheter blockage, but irrigation should be avoided if possible because it can be a source of infection by breaking the closed drainage system and permitting entry of bacteria into the bladder.

Although instituting intermittent catheterization soon after spinal cord injury is preferable, indwelling catheter drainage is an acceptable method for the short-term acute care of spinal cord–injured patients in community hospitals before transfer to a rehabilitation center. Some data suggest that early intermittent catheterization has no long-term advantage over continuous catheterization in terms of urinary infection rates, upper tract pathologic conditions, or ultimate bladder function.[10] Intermittent catheterization can therefore be initiated when the patient is admitted to rehabilitation centers where programs are well established.

Control of infection

In normal bladders the incidence of bacteriuria is 6.6% and 50% after 24 hours and 72 hours of catheterization, respectively.[3] Spinal cord–injured patients managed with indwelling catheters invariably develop urinary infection. Despite earlier reports that intermittent catheterization reduces the incidence of infection, bacteriuria is still common among patients undergoing intermittent catheterization and is not infrequent even among those who have achieved urethral voiding.

Prophylactic antibacterial therapy has been advocated by many, especially when an indwelling catheter is present. Ascorbic acid (1 to 4 g daily) has been recommended to keep the urine pH in the acidic range. The following medications have been used prophylactically:
1. Methenamine mandelate, 1 g four times daily
2. Methenamine hippurate, 1 g twice daily
3. Trimethroprim-sulfamethoxasole, 40/800 mg twice daily
4. Nitrofurantoin, 50 mg three times daily
5. Nalidixic acid, 500 mg four times daily

In a study of urinary infection in spinal cord–injured patients, we reported in 1962 that prophylactic doses of antibacterials were ineffective in preventing bacteriuria in patients with and without indwelling catheters, and we demonstrated that in the majority of patients bacteriuria was confined to the bladder and not identified in the renal pelvis.[11] Others have arrived at the same conclusion that bacteriuria per se in a spinal cord–injured patient does not require prophylactic antibacterial therapy.[8] However, symptomatic episodes of urinary tract infection should be treated with the ever-broadening armamentarium of antibiotics.

LATER TREATMENT

Further treatment is based on the magnitude of the detrusor response (intravesical pressure) during the filling and voiding phases and on the effects of the altered bladder physiology on the upper urinary tract. Measurement of residual urine volume should be another consideration because retention not only is conducive to infection but also sustains a high pressure state in the bladder. However, some patients have low residual urine with high intravesical pressure and deterioration of the upper urinary tract.

Reducing urethral sphincteric resistance

Since high intravesical pressure is potentially dangerous to the upper urinary tract and high residual urine volume is associated with symptomatic infection, a logical approach to treatment is to reduce the urethral sphincteric resistance to the outflow of urine from the bladder. This can be accomplished by pharmacologic agents or transurethral sphincterotomy.

Clinical experience with the use of pharmacologic agents in reducing urethral sphincteric resistance has been disappointing. Phenoxybenzamine, an alpha-adrenergic blocker,

has been used in dosages of 20 mg/day to relax the internal smooth muscle sphincter,[7] but it seems ineffective. Similarly, dantrolene (25 mg in divided doses up to 100 mg/day) and baclofen (10 mg in divided doses up to 80 to 100 mg/day) have been shown to decrease external striated muscle sphincteric activity in selected cases, but the effects are unreliable and transient. Bethanechol, a parasympathomimetic agent, can enhance detrusor tone but is ineffective in producing micturition because the sphincters remain closed.

A reliable way of reducing sphincteric resistance is transurethral sphincterotomy. However, there is disagreement on the timing of sphincterotomy: whether it should be performed on identification of high intravesical pressure (more than 40 cm H_2O) before complications occur, or whether beginning deterioration of the upper tract should be identified first (Fig. 12-3). There are no conclusive data to prove that high intravesical pressure, when documented by the nonphysiologic technique of rapid filling cystometry currently in use, inevitably is followed by upper tract deterioration, but there is clinical evidence that early upper tract deterioration secondary to the bladder alterations can be reversed by sphincterotomy.

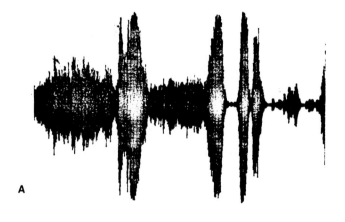

A

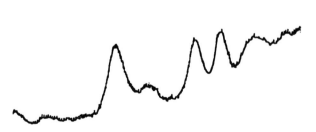

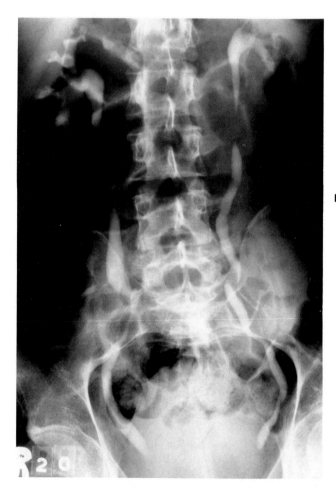

B

Figure 12-3. Man, 20 years of age, with complete quadriplegia (lesion at C5) 6 months after injury. Patient has autonomic dysreflexia. **A,** Cystometrogram shows detrusor hyperreflexia with severe vesicosphincteric dyssynergia and high intravesical pressure. **B,** Intravenous pyelogram reveals early ureteral and calyceal dilation. Transurethral sphincterotomy was performed.

Our policy at the Rusk Institute of Rehabilitation Medicine is to perform sphincterotomy on a spinal cord–injured patient who cannot void or has large residual urine volumes (more than 300 ml) at least 3 months after the injury. Rehabilitation treatments proceed better when uninterrupted by intermittent catheterization, and bladder management in the home setting, especially in quadriplegic patients, is less of a problem with a condom catheter than with intermittent or continuous catheterization.

For a patient who can void, intravesical pressures should be monitored with cystometrograms, and upper tract changes with intravenous pyelograms and cystograms. The demonstration of a high intravesical pressure should be a warning and calls for increased vigilance. Sphincterotomy should not be delayed when upper tract deterioration is demonstrated. However, if the patient refuses sphincterotomy, intermittent catheterization together with an anticholinergic drug can be an option. Sphincterotomy can also diminish significantly the frequency and magnitude of autonomic dysreflexia.

In performing the transurethral sphincterotomy we are not overly concerned about which elements of the urethral sphincteric mechanism still function because we weaken both the internal smooth muscle sphincter and the external striated muscle sphincter by incisions with a knife electrode at 12, 3, and 9 o'clock positions from the vesical neck through the prostatic and membranous urethra, down to the beginning of the bulb. We believe that total sphincterotomy more effectively reduces sphincteric resistance than does selective sphincterotomy. Moreover, there is usually uncertainty as to where the main area of resistance lies.

Increasing vesical compliance

Since there is no efficient urinary collecting device for women, an alternative to sphincterotomy is to increase vesical compliance without diminishing urethral sphincteric resistance and to continue with intermittent catheterization. Diminished intravesical response to increasing volumes may be obtained with anticholinergic agents such as oxybutynin (5 mg two or three times daily), dicyclomine (20 mg three times daily), and imipramine (50 mg twice daily). However, although anticholinergic drugs are usually effective in suppressing detrusor activity during early recovery, they become less effective when detrusor activity or bladder wall hypertonicity is increased. Incontinence then recurs, and the female patient may have to resort to continuous catheterization with no assurance that she will keep dry permanently.

Augmentation cystoplasty to increase the reservoir capacity of the bladder should be considered when urinary incontinence becomes intolerable despite intermittent catheterization, indwelling catheter drainage, and anticholinergic drugs. The fibrotic or hypertonic bladder is partially excised, and a substitute reservoir is constructed with ileum, cecum, or sigmoid colon (Figure 12-4). Intermittent catheterization is often required after augmentation cystoplasty

because the procedure may diminish the ability to void spontaneously.

Increasing outlet resistance

A method for the treatment of incontinence in spinal cord–injured patients is to increase outlet resistance by implanting an artificial urinary sphincter. Before an artificial sphincter implantation, however, it is important to determine whether the bladder has adequate storage capacity and can empty urine effectively. If the bladder cannot store a reasonable amount of urine and intravesical pressure rises precipitously with increasing volumes, vesical compliance must be increased by either pharmacologic agents or augmentation cystoplasty. If residual urine volume is large, a preliminary sphincterotomy is required.

The AMS Sphincter 800 is the newest generation of artificial urinary sphincters (Figure 12-5).[2] It is made of silicone rubber and consists of three parts: a cuff, a pump, and a balloon. The parts are filled with fluid and connected by silicone tubing. In a man the cuff is wrapped around the bulbous urethra and the pump lies in the scrotum. In a woman the cuff wraps around the vesical neck and the pump is in one of the labia. The balloon lies inside the body near the bladder. At rest the cuff, which is filled with fluid, gently compresses the bulbous urethra or vesical neck and retains the urine in the bladder. To urinate, the patient squeezes the pump, which causes the fluid in the cuff to move to the balloon. Thus the cuff opens, and the patient can empty the bladder. When the pump is no longer being squeezed, the fluid from the balloon slowly flows back into the cuff and continence is once again maintained.

In selected cases of intolerable urinary incontinence the patient's satisfaction following successful implantation of an artificial urinary sphincter is immeasurable. However, the long-term successes with artificial sphincters are variable. Malfunctions have followed cuff erosion, fluid loss, tube kink, and interruption of tubing connection. The quality of the product is constantly being improved, and with wider surgical experience and better comprehension of the bladder disturbance, artificial sphincters may play a more effective role in management.

Vesicoureteral reflux and dilation of the upper urinary tract

Beginning vesicoureteral reflux diagnosed by cystography is a warning signal of upper urinary tract deterioration and may precede recognition of upper tract dilation by intravenous pyelography. Reflux is a manifestation of poor vesical compliance aggravated by increased sphincteric resistance. Treatment should be either intermittent catheterization combined with anticholinergic agents or transurethral sphincterotomy. If reflux persists, surgical correction with ureteroneocystostomy should be considered. However, the results of ureteral reimplantation have not been as good as in the normal population. The operation is more difficult in

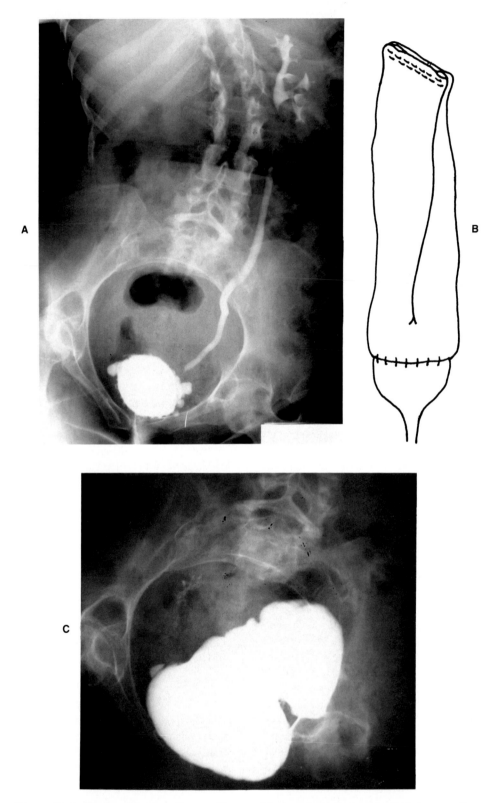

Figure 12-4. Woman, 39 years of age, with complete paraplegia (lesion at T8-9) 6 years after injury. Patient is incontinent during intermittent catheterization owing to poor vesical compliance. **A,** Cystogram shows small bladder capacity with diverticula and left reflux. **B,** Bladder augmented with ileal segment folded to form a U compartment. **C,** Cystogram 11 months after surgery demonstrates increased reservoir capacity. Continence is maintained with intermittent catheterization.

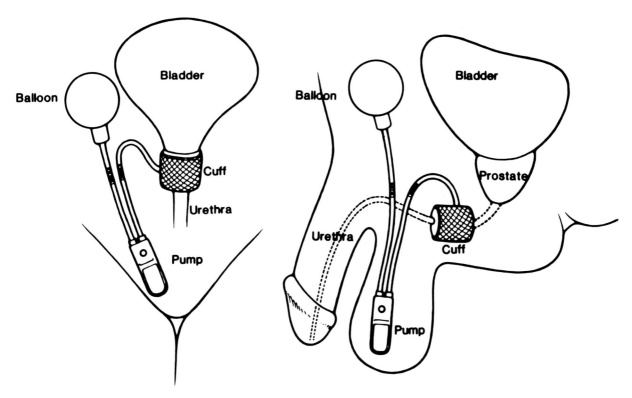

Figure 12-5. AMS Artificial Urinary Sphincter 800. (Courtesy American Medical Systems.)

the presence of bladder wall fibrosis and trabeculation. Failure is also more likely if the high pressure in the bladder is not successfully relieved. In such circumstance, ureteroneocystostomy should be combined with augmentation cystoplasty.

Progressive dilation of the ureter, pelvis, and calyces also calls for more aggressive treatment. Again, either intermittent catheterization combined with anticholinergic agents or transurethral sphincterotomy is indicated. If the dilation is severe, our policy is to institute continuous catheterization for 3 months to ascertain that the dilation is the result of outlet resistance rather than blockage in the bladder wall. Moreover, restoration of the upper tract dilation to a normal state gives the patient a margin of safety should the sphincterotomy fail.

Intestinal conduit urinary diversion

In the past, intestinal urinary diversion was performed mostly to achieve urinary continence and in some cases to forestall further deterioration of the upper urinary tract. The procedure is now performed less often because the long-term results with ileal loop diversion indicated an alarming incidence of renal deterioration attributable to stomal stenosis, reflux from the ileal loop, and ureteroileal stricture. In some situations, however, such as repeated episodes of febrile urinary infection, high-grade vesicoureteral reflux or hydronephrosis, and markedly hypertonic or fibrotic blad-

der, urinary diversion is still performed as a last resort with the hope that the remaining renal function can be preserved. If we decide to perform a diversion, we prefer a nonrefluxing ileocecal conduit because complications from stomal stenosis and reflux are less.

Creation of a continent ileostomy that is emptied by intermittent catheterization and requires no urinary bag has been advocated in recent years, but the frequency of surgical revisions with this operation has been discouraging. Furthermore, it does not offer substantial advantages over intermittent catheterization of a bladder with adequate storage capacity or even over augmentation cystoplasty of a small bladder to relieve a high pressure state.

Urologic surveillance

One goal in the rehabilitation of a spinal cord injury patient is to send the patient home catheter free with sterile urine and little residual urine volume. However, this goal is often not completely achieved. Even when it is, there is a constant risk of recurrent urinary infection and other urologic complications that may threaten renal function. Continual urologic assessment is therefore of paramount importance in the long-term management of a spinal injury patient.

Follow-up monitoring should ideally be scheduled in the rehabilitation center where the patient received the initial treatments, but if this is logistically difficult, the responsibility for the follow-up should be with the urologist in the patient's local hospital.

Our policy at the Rusk Institute of Rehabilitation Medicine is to schedule annual urologic checkups that include intravenous pyelography, cystography, cystoscopy, urodynamic testing, residual urine volume measurement, and urine culture. Intravenous pyelograms detect stone formation and early dilation of the upper urinary tract; cystography demonstrates evidence of bladder decompensation (trabeculation and diverticula) and reflux; cystoscopy reveals urinary calculi sometimes missed radiographically and easily removed; urodynamic testing alerts the urologist to potentially dangerous high intravesical pressure states and increased severity of vesicosphincteric dyssynergia that may develop in time; and high volumes of infected residual urine may necessitate surgical reduction of outlet resistance.

Objections have been raised to the routine use of intravenous pyelograms because of allergic reactions, nephrotoxicity, radiation exposure, and unreliability as a renal function test. Consequently, scintigraphic measurement of effective renal plasma flow has been advocated as a sensitive test capable of detecting renal function changes resulting not only from anatomic obstruction in the urinary tract but also from chronic pyelonephritis. However, measurement of effective renal plasma flow does not determine whether the cause of renal deterioration is correctable and intravenous pyelography must still be performed; this procedure is not only more expensive but also not easily available. If there is significant fear of radiation exposure, intravenous pyelograms can be limited or tailored to minimize radiation. Renal sonography has also been advocated, but the test is inferior in the detection of early or mild obstruction in the upper urinary tract.

REFERENCES

1. Awad, SA, et al: Urethral pressure profile during spinal shock stage in man: a preliminary report, J Urol 117:91, 1977.
2. Brown, J, and Morales, P: Artificial urinary sphincter 800, Urology 23:479, 1984.
3. Cox, CE, and Winman, F: Incidence of bacteriuria with indwelling catheters in normal bladders, JAMA 178:919, 1961.
4. DeGroat, WC: Nervous control of the urinary bladder of the cat, Brain Res 87:201, 1975.
5. DeVivo, JJ, Fine, PR, and Stover, SL: Cause of death following spinal cord injury, Arch Phys Med Rehabil 65:622, 1984.
6. Guttman, L, and Frakel, H: The value of intermittent catheterization in the early management of traumatic paraplegia and tetraplegia, Paraplegia 4:63, 1966.
7. Krane, RJ, and Olsson, CA: Phenoxybenzamine in neurogenic bladder dysfunction. II. Clinical considerations, J Urol 110:653, 1973.
8. Kuhlemeier, KV, Stover, SL, and Lloyd, LK: Prophylactic antibacterial therapy for preventing urinary tract infections in spinal cord injury patients, J Urol 134:514, 1985.
9. Light, JK, Faganel, J, and Berk: Detrusor areflexia in supravesical spinal cord injuries, J Urol 134:295, 1985.
10. Lloyd, LK, et al: Initial bladder management in spinal cord injury: does it make a difference? J Urol 135:523, 1986.
11. Morales, P, and Tsou, AY: Quantitative bacteriologic study of urinary infection among paraplegics, J Urol 87:191, 1962.
12. Shalit, S, and Morales, P: Ureteral activity in paraplegia, J Urol 96:815, 1966.

PART IV

SYSTEMIC DISORDERS AND SPECIAL SERVICES

CHAPTER 13

Arthritis and related disorders

MEDICAL MANAGEMENT

THOMAS KANTOR

The arthritides may be distinguished as being inflammatory and noninflammatory conditions, although this may not be entirely relevant. The inflammatory group may be divided into those with primarily joint involvement and those with a more systemic involvement. A further subdivision of this group would include the crystal-induced and metabolic conditions.

INFLAMMATORY ARTHRITIDES
Rheumatoid arthritis

Rheumatoid arthritis affects the joints symmetrically but is a systemic disease in which anemia, fatigability, weight loss, and fever are prominent features. All of the inflammatory diseases may lead to joint destruction and deformity, and rheumatoid disease is almost certain to do so.

Rheumatoid arthritis often begins in the proximal interphalangeal and metacarpophalangeal joints and is usually more severe on the dominant side of the body. The usual onset of the disease is in the spring or fall. The onset may be explosive, with many if not all of the peripheral joints involved, and with high fever and severe inanition. However, the onset may be insidious, with the disease taking a year or more to become fully present in the joints involved. Frequently a polycyclic course is noted, with progressive attacks involving more and more joints. In the classic situation both wrists are inflamed. The symmetry may not become apparent for many months.

While rheumatoid disease is essentially not life threatening, several severe and morbid complications may occur. These include involvement of the joint between the cervical atlas and the odontoid process of C2, which can lead to platybasia or endangerment of the spinal cord. Death or paraplegia may result. Occasionally rheumatoid disease is complicated by vasculitis, which can occur in almost any organ system, although the skin is most often affected. Vasculitic ulcerations around the ankle joints and elsewhere are not rare and may be an entrance for systemic infection. Likewise, subcutaneous nodules over bony prominences are not uncommon and are vasculitic in origin. They have been found in visceral organs, may be seen in the lung, and have even been reported to destroy the conduction system of the heart.

As a result of a compilation of data from several thousand cases,[6] it has been found that active rheumatoid disease lasts for a mean period of 21 years. Because no rational curative treatment is available, management of the disease is empiric.

Etiology

The cause of rheumatoid disease is unknown. Various viral etiologies have been suggested, but none have withstood application of Koch's principles. Adjuvant-induced arthritis and injection of collagen fragments into joints of experimental animals mimic the disease but are not acceptable as true models. There has been considerable difficulty in finding evidence of the disease in ancient human skeletal remains, although recent discoveries in Mexico and Central America suggest that the disease was known within a few centuries after the birth of Christ.

Histocompatibility cell markers show a predominance of HLA-DRW4 in severe cases of the disease.[1] However, there is no clear evidence of genetic inheritability.

Laboratory diagnosis and pathogenesis

There are known immunopathic phenomena in rheumatoid arthritis, at least one of which has provided diagnostic precision. The inflammation that affects the synovial lining of joints and tendon sheaths is made up primarily of round cells and lymphocytes, plasma cells, and macrophages. The lymphocytes may be T-helper (OKT4) or T-suppressor

(OKT8), with the former predominating. The macrophages and T cells are in an activated form, which means that lymphokines (interleukins 1 and 2, various interferons, and other, less well characterized substances) are produced by these activated cells and interact with other cells that make up both the humoral and cellular immune systems. An aggregate form of gamma globulin (IgM) is produced and is unrecognized by the immune system, which makes an IgG antibody to it. This complex of ingestion by macrophages results in the production of enzymes destructive to connective tissue and of further mediators of inflammation. Proteases including collagenase destroy the cartilage of joints and cause bony erosions. Prostaglandins and bradykinin amplify the inflammation and cause the pain of arthritis. Substance P, an 11 amino acid neuropeptide, is secreted by the dorsal ganglion cells of the nerves carrying the pain signal. It acts as a neurotransmitter, and by antidromal flow down microtubules in the pain nerves, it activates mast cells to produce histamine, which further amplifies the inflammation.

The IgM immunoglobulin noted previously is the basis for the latex rheumatoid factor test. Immunoglobulin G (IgG) specific for this IgM is produced in rabbits, stuck to latex particles, and exposed to the patient's serum. If IgM of the specific type is present in the serum, the latex particles stick to it and to each other, and the resulting larger mass precipitates from the test solution in which it is suspended. Dilutions of the test serum give a titer determination. This latex test is not a good diagnostic test, since the results are often negative in the early stages when most needed. It is better as a prognostic indicator—the earlier it becomes positive and the higher the titer, the worse the prognosis for joint destruction and deformity.

An iron-deficiency anemia (the anemia of chronic disease) is frequently present in rheumatoid arthritis, and the white blood cell count may be elevated. Both the erythrocyte sedimentation rate (ESR) and the platelet count are commonly elevated and act as excellent markers for either the progress of disease or its modulation by treatment.

Joint fluid is easily obtained, especially from the knee joint, by needle aspiration. White blood cell (WBC) counts and differential counts may be performed using saline rather than Hayem's solution as a diluent. Hayem's solution, which contains acetic acid, precipitates the mucin in the fluid, traps the white cells, and produces a falsely low count. However, the WBC count and differential count vary widely in rheumatoid arthritis and are not helpful diagnostically. The mucin clot test may be of greater use. Normal joint fluid, when subjected to weak acetic acid solution, forms a single firm clot of the hyaluronic acid–protein complex found in joint fluid. Rheumatoid fluid, on the other hand, forms a fragmented precipitate in this test because of the inflammatory enzymes that partially digest the complex.

About 15% to 25% of patients with rheumatoid arthritis have positive results on a antinuclear antibody test, which is usually diffuse or speckled. This may cause considerable diagnostic confusion. Raynaud's phenomenon may occur.

In the early stages of rheumatoid arthritis radiographs are rarely useful, since the impact of the disease is on soft tissues. As the disease progresses, juxta-articular osteoporosis becomes evident, and as the inflammatory pannus takes hold, cartilage loss occurs. Eventually osteoarthropathy with bone loss at the joint margins is noted. If extensive use of corticosteroids has been necessary, more severe, generalized osteoporosis occurs, and a vasculitic form of bone destruction, osteonecrosis, may also be noted especially at weight-bearing joints such as the hip and knee.

Another clinical feature of systemic rheumatoid disease is a rarely noted pleural effusion. The glucose content of this fluid is considerably lower than that of a simultaneously drawn blood sample, which is a diagnostic indicator of rheumatoid disease if infection can be ruled out.

Treatment

Treatment of rheumatoid arthritis is empiric in that, as noted previously, there are no rational treatments for a disease whose cause is unknown. Therefore the physician must take those measures that will maintain the patient in his or her normal socioeconomic milieu as much as possible. The physician must be understanding and compassionate to carry the patient through the ups and downs of a chronic disease. The pain must be relieved and an attempt made to arrest or repair the ravages resulting from deterioration. This therapeutic process is often shown as a pyramid, with lesser, first-line therapies at the bottom and more aggressive and potentially dangerous therapies at the top.

Nonsteroidal anti-inflammatory drugs. The nonsteroidal anti-inflammatory drugs (NSAIDs), including salicylates, form the base of the therapeutic pyramid. There are 16 of these available in the United States and at least that many more awaiting approval from the Food and Drug Administration. The market for these drugs is a lucrative one, and there seem to be idiosyncratic responses to them so that patients are frequently switched from one to another because of side effects or lack of activity. They are listed in Table 13-1 according to their chemical class and elimination half-life. In general, the residence time in the body for any one dose of a drug is six to seven times the half-life. This allows a wide range of dose schedules for these drugs, as Table 13-1 shows.

The major pharmacologic feature of NSAIDs is the inhibition of the enzyme cyclo-oxygenase; this ordinarily acts on arachidonic acid, which is in turn liberated from the fatty acids of perturbed membranes by the enzyme phospholipase A. The end products of cyclo-oxygenase action on arachidonic acid include endoperoxides, thromboxane, prostacyclin, and prostaglandin E 1 and 2. These latter sensitize neurologic pain receptors in and around joints to the further action of histamine and bradykinin, which causes pain. Therefore all the NSAIDs have potential as analgesic agents.

Table 13-1. Half-lives of available NSAIDs

	Half-life (hr)	Suggested top daily dose	
		Manufacturers' recommendation (mg)	Author's recommendation (mg)
Pyrazoles			
Oxyphenbutazone (Oxalid, Tandearil)	72-96	400	200
Phenylbutazone	84-96	400	200
Indole acetic acids			
Indomethacin (Indocin)	3-4½	200	200
Sulindac (Clinoril)	13 (active metabolite)	400	400
Tolmetin (Tolectin)	1	2000	2000
Phenylalkanoic acids			
Fenoprofen (Nalfon)	3	3200	3600
Ibuprofen (Motrin, Rufen)	2-3	2400	4800
Ketoprofen (Orudis)	2-3	300	300
Naproxen (Naprosyn)	13	1000	1000
Naproxen sodium (Anaprox)			
Fenamic acids			
Meclofenamate (Meclomen)	2-5	400	300
Mefenamic acid (Ponstel)	2-5	1250	1000
Oxicams			
Piroxicam (Feldene)	44-50	20	20
Salicylates			
Aspirin	3-16	3600	5200
Choline magnesium trisalicylate (Trilisate)	7-18	3000	3000
Diflunisal (Dolobid)	8	1500	1500
Magnesium salicylate	2-2½	3000	5000
Salsalate (Arcylate, Disalcid)	8	3000	3000

Aspirin is a special case in that its acetyl group is donated to the cyclo-oxygenase that destroys the enzyme.

Since there seems to be no particular advantage of one NSAID over another regarding efficacy in the therapy for any rheumatologic disease, the drug to be used must be chosen on other grounds. A patient's compliance with an effective dose schedule is most often governed by whether there are adverse effects. Gastric irritation is unacceptable in 10% to 30% of patients for any one drug tried because of the mechanism outlined previously. They may consciously or unconsciously reduce dosage to alleviate symptoms of gastric irritation, which would undermine efficacy. A patient may not report this to the physician, who would then prescribe another drug, convinced that the first had been inactive.

The first choice for NSAID is probably governed by the elimination half-life of the drug. All of the NSAIDs are metabolized by the liver, and conjugates are excreted by the kidney. Older people may have half or less the renal capacity of young patients but may have normal blood urea nitrogen and serum creatinine values. This could greatly prolong the elimination half-life beyond those stated in Table 13-1, and hepatic disease would make matters even worse. Therefore the very old (80 years and beyond) should not be given drugs with half-lives much beyond 12 hours.

Unfortunately, the very old are frequently taking a basketful of drugs—digoxin, a diuretic, a stool softener, an oral hypoglycemic agent, and so on—for other conditions. Requesting them to take an NSAID with a low half-life (such as tolmetin) three times a day may be asking too much. This dilemma is not an easy one to solve and may require considerable interaction between the physician, the patient, and a third party living with the patient.

Detailed discussion of each drug is beyond the scope of this chapter, but standard texts in rheumatology and package inserts for the drugs are helpful.

Table 13-2. Disease-modifying drugs

Drug	Dose
Gold (aurothioglucose in oil suspension) (Solganal)	1 g in 50 mg weekly doses intramuscularly
Gold (Auranofin)	6 to 9 mg/day orally
Oxychloroquine (Plaquenil)	200 mg/day orally
Penicillamine	250-750 mg/day orally

Table 13-3. Antineoplastic drugs

Drug	Dose
Methotrexate	7.5-15 mg weekly orally or intramuscularly
Azathiaprine (Imuran)	Up to 200 mg/day orally
Cyclophosphamide (Cytoxan)	Up to 200 mg/day orally
	Up to 1 g monthly by pulse infusion

Second-line drugs. The so-called disease-modifying drugs or DMARDS are listed in Table 13-2. Among them, injected gold is believed to be the most reliable for rheumatoid arthritis, with penicillamine a close second. The reliability of orally administered gold (auranofin) is undetermined but may be less than either injected gold or penicillamine. Oral gold may be useful as maintenance therapy for those who have gained considerable benefit from a course of injected gold. Antimalarial treatment is perceived to be the weakest of these therapies.

It is important that the physician understand that all drugs in this group take up to 3 months to achieve a recognizable clinical effect, thus requiring perseverance on the part of both patient and physician, as well as interim therapy (NSAIDs or low-dose steroids) to keep the patient functioning.

These drugs have greater danger for side effects than the NSAIDs and should be used with great caution and a full understanding of the tests and examinations necessary for monitoring patients (Table 13-2). Combinations of drugs in this group are not recommended but have been prescribed by rheumatologists.

Third-line drugs. Third-line drugs are all antineoplastic drugs and are considered by some to modulate the aberrant immune events that make up the pathophysiology of rheumatoid disease. A simpler explanation is that without white cells in a joint there can be no inflammation, and the third-line drugs (Table 13-3) are all toxic to granulocytes, lymphocytes, and monocytes, limiting their ability to respond to chemotactic factors that would draw them into a joint.

An important feature of second- and third-line drugs is that their adverse effects are potentially fatal, whereas the disease being treated is not. Using these drugs should be a last resort. Constant attention to their potential for bone marrow depression is important.

In order of effectiveness, cyclophosphamide is the most reliable, but it is also the most toxic and has been associated with an increased incidence of tumors, especially lymphomas some years after onset of treatment. Loss of hair is a less hazardous but particularly devastating problem for women, who make up the majority of rheumatoid arthritis patients. American rheumatologists consider chlorambucil

and levamisole to be too toxic for use. Azathioprine is the weakest of the group but the least toxic.

The use of methotrexate is becoming favored by rheumatologists as fear of its hepatotoxicity recedes in the face of reduced dosage schedules used at present. It is not yet known, however, whether the reduced dosage schedules may be prolonging the time it takes to produce significant and possibly fatal toxicity. Cyclosporine is too new to make any statement about.

Other therapies. Such heroic treatments as lymphopheresis or plasmopheresis and total body irradiation have not withstood the test of time and are not cost effective but may be used in selected situations.

OTHER POTENTIALLY CRIPPLING DISEASES
Ankylosing spondylitis (Marie-Strümpell disease)

Although ankylosing spondylitis is primarily a spondyloarthropathy, often there is enough peripheral disease to make it resemble rheumatoid arthritis. Characteristically it affects patients in their late twenties or early thirties, and in contrast to rheumatoid arthritis it involves men up to 15 times more often than women. Its cause is unknown, but there is a strong association between ankylosing spondylitis and the histocompatibility marker HLA-B27[3]; over 90% of patients with the disease test positive for HLA-B27.

The disease commonly begins at the sacroiliac joints and then ascends the spine, causing inflammation of the anterior and posterior spinal ligaments. These eventually calcify and become visible on radiographs as characteristic "bambooing" of the spine. By then the sacroiliac joints are often obliterated. The calcific ligaments limit joint motion so that loss of the normal lumbar lordosis occurs, and eventually the disease may work its way up the spine to the neck. The end result for some unfortunate patients is total rigidity of the spine, including the cervical portion.

The costovertebral joints are often involved in ankylosing spondylitis, and one of the hallmarks of the disease is reduced chest expansion. Aortic insufficiency is a rare but significant feature of the disease. Peripheral joint involvement is common in the hips and shoulders, although other medium-sized joints may become affected. The hip involvement is compounded by lumbar lordosis, flexion deformities of the hips, and gluteus medius weaknesses, which lead to a Trendelenburg gait.

Laboratory findings

Since the disease is inflammatory, an iron-deficiency-type anemia is often present, and the ESR rises. Latex and antinuclear antibody (ANA) tests are negative. The joint fluid is like that in rheumatoid disease. As noted previously, HLA-B27 positivity is common.

Treatment

The treatment is primarily use of the NSAIDs. As in a few other rheumatic conditions, there may be some advantage for certain drugs. Indomethacin and phenylbutazone seem to have some specificity for the spondyloarthropathies, although others may work as well. Long-term use of phenylbutazone should be avoided if possible because of its unique adverse effects, but doses up to 200 mg a day may be effective and tolerated for years by many patients.

The second- and third-line drugs used to treat rheumatoid arthritis are not as useful in ankylosing spondylitis, although they may be of some benefit. Physical therapy is extremely important to prevent deformity.

Reiter's syndrome

Reiter's syndrome, named after a World War I German Army physician who described it in a German officer, is considered to be one of the reactive arthritides, since it seems to follow certain infections. It is almost certain that the original case followed a *Salmonella* bowel infection. *Yersinia, Chlamydia,* and *Campylobacter* bowel infections have also been implicated.[11] The syndrome may also follow urethritis, either specific (gonococcal) or nonspecific.

Reiter's syndrome is so classified because conjunctivitis (sometimes iritis), urethritis, balanitis, and a rare productive skin disease, keratoderma blennorrhagica, often coexist with the joints. Occasionally, psoriatic skin patches are seen. The link between the infections and the various elements of the syndrome is obscure. The disease may be a destructive one to joints—most often those of the lower extremities. Asymmetry is common, as is spondyloarthropathy with sacroiliac joint involvement. The normal course of the disease includes recurrent attacks with periods of almost complete remission.

Laboratory findings

Laboratory tests are nonspecific, as in ankylosing spondylitis.

Treatment

Surprisingly, given the relationship to bacteria noted previously, antibiotic treatment of Reiter's syndrome is unrewarding. NSAIDs are most effective, with local therapy for iritis or iridocyclitis (as necessary) an important adjunct. In resistant cases injected gold and steroids may be helpful. There was a recent report of success with azathioprine. Any long-term therapeutic claim must be weighed against the cyclic nature of the disease.

Psoriatic arthritis

About 15% of patients with psoriasis develop an arthritis that, at its worst, is extremely destructive to bone. Involvement with a destructive lesion of the terminal phalanges of fingers and toes is common and is usually found on digits with psoriatic nail involvement. However, onset of psoriatic arthritis with knee joint arthritis is the most common presentation. In some cases the joint disease seems to wax and wane with the skin lesions, but there have been many recorded instances of the joint disease preceding the onset of the skin disorder, as well as arthritis appearing years after the skin lesions appear. Spondyloarthropathy is fairly common, but as with Reiter's syndrome, it rarely causes the endpoint rigidity of spinal motion common to ankylosing spondylitis.

Laboratory findings

Laboratory values are not specific in blood or joint fluid, which show only the characteristic anemia and ESR elevation of chronic disease.

Treatment

NSAIDs again are the first-line therapy, with resistant cases treated with gold, antimalarial agents, and various third-line drugs, the most common of which has been methotrexate. However, higher doses of methotrexate than those successful with rheumatoid arthritis are necessary to control psoriasis and psoriatic arthritis, and therefore toxicity is more common and more severe in psoriasis. Aggressive attention to the skin (occlusive dressing, light box therapy, PUVA*) is also of benefit to the arthritic component.

Juvenile arthritis

Once called juvenile rheumatoid arthritis, this disease frequently deviates from rheumatoid disease so that the new terminology seems more precise. It has been divided into several components (Table 13-4), with the last one so similar to rheumatoid arthritis as to be indistinguishable except for the age at onset. Most of the other components separate themselves into well-defined syndromes as noted in the table.

As a further complication of classification for this disease, rather characteristic cases of adult onset juvenile arthritis have been reported with generalized lymphadenopathy and fever accompanying the arthritis. The major subdivisions are Still's disease (with high fever and an evanescent rash in the very young), a pauciarticular form more prevalent in girls that is associated with iritis, a polyarticular form with

---

*Oral administration of psoralen and exposure to ultraviolet light.

Table 13-4. Classes of juvenile arthritis

Characteristic	Oligoarthritis or pauciarthritis	Systemic disease (Still's disease)	Polyarthritis
Number of joints	Four or fewer	Usually more than two	Usually more than five
Uveitis	20% (especially girls)	Unusual	5%
Involvement other than joints	Unusual	Frequent	Some
RA factor	Unusual	Very unusual	At least 10%
Antinuclear antibody	75% or more	10% or less	50%
Prognosis for joints	Fairly good	Good	Fair

Modified from Kelley, WN, et al, editors: Textbook of rheumatology, ed 2, Philadelphia, 1985, WB Saunders Co.

equal sex incidence that has more frequent involvement of the knees, and finally a polyarticular form in adolescence with frequent extension into adult life that is the only one that tests positive in latex tests.

Laboratory findings

Except for the adolescent symmetrically involved group, the latex test result is negative, but other tests of chronic disease show positive findings.

Treatment

High-dose salicylate therapy and rare periods of corticosteroids are the accepted therapies. Tolmetin is approved among the NSAIDs. Third-line drugs are almost never prescribed for these patients with evolving cell development, but the second-line drugs have been used.

Behçet's syndrome

Behçet's syndrome is a polyarthritic condition found primarily among patients from the eastern Mediterranean basin and Japan. It is characterized by painful mucosal ulcerations of the mouth, vaginal, and rectal areas and rarely by meningoencephalitis and polyneuropathy. NSAIDs are the treatment of choice, but colchicine has also been used.

Lyme disease

Our knowledge about Lyme disease is a tribute to American rheumatologic research in that the disease was described, its etiology was determined, and a successful treatment plan for it was devised all within 5 years.[9] It is caused by a spirochete borne by a biting deer tick. In most cases a characteristic pale, centered, red blotch appears at the bite site. Cardiac conduction problems, meningoencephalitis, and peripheral neuritis can occur. Courses of tetracycline and penicillin treatment are successful.[10] An arthritis may not appear until months after an untreated infection.

Infection arthritides

Infection arthritides caused by bacteria or higher organisms are treated parenterally with an appropriate antibiotic that invariably reaches a satisfactory drug level in the joint. In weight-bearing joints, sterile effusions may continue for weeks after the infection is arrested. Staphylococcal infection must be considered in elderly, diabetic, or immunosuppressed patients. Gonococcal infections may begin as polyarthritis, but they later settle into one or two joints. Dermal-infected lesions, especially between the digits, are also characteristic. Since all of the infections are treatable, failure to tap and culture an available joint is inexcusable.

Metabolic and crystal arthritides
Gout

Although we still do not know the cause of gout, we know enough about its pathophysiologic characteristics to treat the condition. Clearly, a large increase of uric acid in the body is the fundamental problem. It would be a reasonable deduction that this is caused by an overproduction of urate or an underexcretion by the kidney and bowel. Although the details of the purine synthesis and metabolic pathways are known, no enzyme defect has been found, nor have any consistent defects in the urinary excretion of urate been noted, despite vigorous investigation.[7]

The disease is considered to be predominantly a genetic problem with incomplete penetrance, since it is noted to occur in families. Women rarely have onset until menopause, whereas men begin to get the disease at puberty, with the peak incidence during middle life. In general men have higher serum urate levels than women, but it is possible to have one's first attack of gout with a normal serum uric acid level. As the disease progresses, the serum urate level rises.

Primary gout is a recognizable entity, but secondary gout may come from a variety of conditions. Prolonged renal failure can result in a buildup of urate leading to attacks of gout. So can rapid replacement of tissue, which presents an untenable load of nuclear material to the purine metabolic pathway. This situation occurs in proliferative disorders of bone marrow elements such as leukemia, lymphomas, and polycythemia. Tumors under treatment with cytotoxic agents can also dump more nuclear material than can be handled. Drugs such as diuretics can interfere with urate excretion by the kidney. Lead poisoning causes a renal lesion that holds back urate and can cause gout.

The tissue pathogenesis of the gouty attack depends on a supersaturated solution of urate in the connective tissue interstitium. Urate solubility is greatly reduced when the pH is lower than 7. In areas of minor trauma, white cells that are cut off from oxygen supply depend on nonoxygen metabolism, which produces lactic acid. This lowers the pH level, bringing uric acid out of solution in the form of monosodium urate, a needlelike crystal. When this crystal is engulfed by a polymorphonuclear leukocyte, the ensuing phagosome bursts and allows digestive enzymes to roam free in the cytosol, thus destroying the cell. This further reduces the pH level, and the crystal is left intact to be swallowed by another leukocyte. It is difficult to understand why gouty attacks terminate spontaneously—usually in 5 to 7 days. Characteristically the joint affected is the base of the big toe, in which case the condition is called podagra, although the knee or foot is often affected. Any joint can be subject to a gouty attack.

If the defect that increases the body's urate burden is a large one, the supersaturated connective tissue solution of urate (called the miscible pool because it is in equilibrium with the serum) may deposit solid concretions of urate crystals in and around joints. This may activate prostaglandins to erode bone around joints, which may be very destructive. This condition is called tophaceous gout, and the first manifestation of it may be in the pinna of the ear.

Treatment. Treatment can be divided into control of the acute attack and long-term management. Colchicine can be used specifically to terminate acute attacks and can also be used as a diagnostic test; if the joint responds quickly, the diagnosis is practically established. However, this drug's major toxic effect on the gastrointestinal tract, diarrhea, comes around the time of beneficial effect, and once the diagnosis is established, NSAIDs (which are equally effective, if less specific) are kinder to the patient. If more than two attacks a year occur, prophylaxis with 1 or 2 colchicine tablets daily is helpful. If tophi occur or if the serum urate level rises over 10 mg/dl, further measures are necessary. First, there are the uricosuric agents, probenecid, sulfinpyrazone, and benbromarone, which interfere with urate reabsorption by the renal tubule after complete glomerular filtration. These drugs present large amounts of urate to the urine, and there is danger of renal urate stone formation in the acid pH of urine. A high intake of fluid is necessary to dilute the urine.

THERAPY FOR GOUT

Acute attack

  I. Colchicine
    A. Oral—0.6 mg ql-2h until diarrhea or pain relief
    B. IV—3 mg slow bolus, another 3 mg in 8 hours if necessary
  II. NSAIDs—all oral, doses in package inserts
  III. Corticosteroids
    A. Prednisone—oral, 15 mg TID for 2 days
    B. Solu-Medrol—IV, 40 mg ql2h × 2

Chronic tophaceous gout

  I. Allopurinol—300 mg orally every day for 1 year
  II. Colchicine—0.6 mg BID, then allopurinol 300 mg orally every day for life
  III. Uricosuric agent
    A. Probenecid—0.25 g BID for 7 days, then orally 0.5 g BID or
    B. Sulfinpyrazone—200-400 mg BID orally

It is also possible to curtail much of the production of urate by the use of allopurinol, which blocks the conversion of xanthine and hypoxanthine to uric acid.

Uricosuric agents and allopurinol are useful together in reducing joint-destructive tophi, but each group may cause an increase in gouty attacks for 3 months to a year after introduction. The mechanism for this is unknown. The problem can be solved by giving 1 or 2 tablets of colchicine daily, which is withdrawn after 6 to 12 months. Uricosuric and allopurinol therapy is lifelong—the disease is controllable, not curable. See the box above for a therapeutic summary.

Pseudogout

Various crystals can come out of solution in joint fluid to create symptoms much like those of gout, although less severe. Calcium pyrophosphate and apatite can be ingested by polymorphonuclear leukocytes, leading to inflammation. This problem is often associated with other arthritides. Colchicine is useful for the acute attacks and NSAIDs for the more common, low-level, chronic episodes. When calcium pyrophosphate is the causative agent, a characteristic line of calcium density may be seen in the cartilage on radiographs. Examination of joint fluid revealing positively birefringent crystals is the basis for the diagnosis.

Ochronosis

Ochronosis associated with alkaptonuria can cause a form of osteoarthritis, usually limited to the spine, that is amenable to NSAID therapy.

Inflammatory bowel disorders

Inflammatory bowel disorders such as regional ileitis (Crohn's disease), granulomatous colitis, and ulcerative colitis may be accompanied by an inflammatory destructive arthritis affecting medium-sized joints. Spondyloarthropathy may also be present.

Sjögren's syndrome

Sjögren's syndrome or sicca syndrome is often associated with various rheumatologic inflammatory diseases but can stand alone. Characteristically, it is marked by dry eyes, dry mouth, or dry vagina, which requires artificial lubrication. Parotid and lachrymal gland swelling is common, and the disease can progress to one of a variety of lymphomas. Oral mucosal biopsy shows atrophied salivary glands and a lymphatic cell reaction. Antinuclear antigens Ro and La are elevated in the serum.

ARTHRITIC CONDITIONS THAT DO NOT DESTROY JOINTS

Rheumatic fever is believed to be an immunologic disease caused by antibodies produced to combat hemolytic streptococcus, a bacterium that has components similar to cardiac and synovial tissue. The total sensitivity of beta-streptococci to penicillin and other antibiotics has almost wiped out the disease in the United States, but endemic areas still exist, particularly in Haiti.

The disease is characterized by a sore throat, following which a migratory polyarthritis occurs, occasionally with cardiac conduction or valvular defects and a central nervous system feature called chorea.

The diagnosis is based on the discovery of beta-streptococci in the throat and a rising titer of streptozyme antibodies in the serum, as well as on the clinical picture.

Low doses of aspirin (under 3 g/day) wipe out the arthritic component, but it is also necessary to destroy the beta-streptococci using long-acting penicillin or other antibiotics. In the case of carditis, corticosteroids are used for 1 to 3 months along with aspirin, which is continued for 6 months or more. The ESR and C-reactive protein values in the serum are useful to follow, since they are elevated during activity. Antibiotic prophylaxis is then used for an indefinite period to preclude further streptococcal infection.

SARCOID

A form of sarcoidosis can also cause migratory polyarthritis and enlarged hilar lymph nodes. Sometimes sarcoid can cause a mildly destructive osteoarthropathy around joints. Corticosteroid therapy plus antituberculosis therapy is the preferred treatment, with NSAIDs used as an adjunct therapy.

CONNECTIVE TISSUE DISORDERS

Connective tissue conditions are considered rheumatologic disorders because arthritis is often a prominent feature. However, only very rarely do they cause actual joint destruction and crippling, and arthritis, although inflammatory, is usually the least of the patient's problems.

Systemic lupus erythematosus[5]

Systemic lupus erythematosus is a systemic disease affecting young women, although increasingly women have an onset of the disease in their fifties and sixties. Women with lupus predominate at least 10:1 over men, which suggests hormonal influences. The disease is considered to be a model of autoimmune disease but on a very broad scale. Something triggers a breakdown of the immune regulating apparatus so that antibody is formed to normal body constituents. This can be caused by a failure of the T-suppressor cells, an augmented effect of the T-helper cells, or an abnormal hyperresponse on the part of the antibody producing B cells. In any case the hallmark of the disease is antibodies to various nuclear components forming immune complexes that, because of their size, lodge in various organs that require a large vascular bed. These are the kidney, brain, and skin, but other organs may be affected. When these complexes are caught in a small vessel, they cause endothelial cell damage and the beginning of an inflammation in which inflammatory mediators of the platelets, macrophages, lymphocytes, and polymorphonuclear leukocytes are produced. The ensuing inflammatory action destroys the vessel, and if enough vessels are destroyed, the organ fails.

Considering the preceding, it is not surprising that antibodies against thyroid tissue, various cells of the bone marrow, and components of both the nuclei and cytosol of many other body tissues are seen. The antibody most commonly sought in clinical diagnosis is ANA, which is reported in titer and in qualitative terms. The test is performed by raising an antibody to human gamma-globulin that is then tagged with a fluorescent dye. The patient's serum is layered onto frozen sections of mouse liver tissue, where circulating antibody to nuclei bind to the nuclear components of the liver cells. The fluorescent antiglobulin is then layered over that and combines with the patient's serum and globulin on the nucleus. The fluorescein is activated by ultraviolet light and appears yellow. A positive result may be diffuse staining of the whole nucleus, a stippled pattern, or a staining only of the periphery or rim of the nucleus. The last is considered to be almost specific for lupus, although the other patterns may be seen in proven cases. Antibody to certain cytosol components such as the Sm antigen are considered even more specific.

Clinical syndromes in lupus may be a skin rash that is most often malar in position, alopecia, Raynaud's phenomenon, vasculitis, hemolytic anemia, polyserositis affecting the pleura, peritoneal lining, and pericardium, encephalitis, nephritis, arthritis, and a severe, febrile acute illness called crisis. Other hematologic problems such as thrombocytopenia and leukopenia may also be present. About 15% of lupus patients are extremely sun sensitive and may have severe systemic flares after minimal sun exposure. The disease is characterized by periods of remission and flares of greater or lesser severity.

The nephritis is divided into three general syndromes. First is the focal glomenulonephritis, which sometimes reverses itself spontaneously or after small doses of prednisone. Second is a membranous nephropathy characterized by nephrotic syndrome, and third is diffuse, proliferative glomerulonephritis. The focal form may change into the others. The membranous form may also be successfully treated with prednisone in high doses. The diffuse proliferative disease is the least amenable to treatment and frequently has an inexorable course leading to uremia and the necessity for dialysis.

There is no unanimously accepted therapy for diffuse, proliferative nephritis. High-dose corticosteroid therapy, sometimes by intravenous (IV) pulses of 1 g of methylprednisolone (Solu-Medrol), supplemented by cyclophosphamide either orally or by IV pulse, are favored at present. However, hair loss and severe bone marrow depression may be consequences of the cyclophosphamide. Milder cases can be treated successfully with orally administered prednisone and azathioprine. Prednisone is the corticosteroid of choice for long-term treatment because it has a lesser myopathic effect than other corticosteroids. The clinician must remember that a characteristic of this disease is immunoincompetence and that corticosteroids only aggravate this feature. There may be long periods in the course of lupus when no treatment is necessary.

There is a variety of lupus called discoid lupus that is primarily a destructive skin disease without systemic involvement. However, about 15% of patients with discoid lupus eventually develop systemic disease.

A recently discovered syndrome of lupus patients is found in women who have a history of spontaneous abortions and of multiple deep vein thromboses. An antibody to cardiolipin is frequently found in such patients. No special therapy is known.

Other connective tissue disorders

Other connective tissue syndromes include scleroderma, polymyositis, dermatomyositis, polyarteritis nodosa, and thrombotic thrombocytopenia. Each may be associated with arthritis or arthralgia, which is rarely destructive or crippling.

Scleroderma

Scleroderma is primarily a skin disease that often begins as Raynaud's phenomenon and progresses from dermal edema to a bound-down, heavily collagenized subdermis that does not allow movement of the epidermis over the deeper tissues. This process most often occurs first in the skin of the hands and forearms, then the upper chest and face, and finally the lower extremities. While arthritis is a feature of the disease, the binding of the skin is most often the lesion that restricts joint motion. Visceral involvement of the lungs, heart, gastrointestinal tract, and the kidney (in rare cases) is also seen. ANA test results of the speckled or diffuse pattern are common.

The CRST syndrome is a variant of scleroderma that is considered to be more benign. Its clinical features of calcinosis, Raynaud's phenomenon, sclerodactyly, and telangiectasia of the skin are reflected in the abbreviation that makes up its name.

There are few satisfactory treatments for CRST syndrome. Prednisone reduces the edematous phase and may seem to improve lung function without change in pulmonary function tests. Recently, penicillamine therapy has been said to at least arrest visceral involvement.

Eosinophilic fasciitis may be a variant of scleroderma. It is characterized by an "orange peel edema" of the epidermis. However, the pathologic factor is an eosinophil-rich inflammation in the deep fascia overlying muscle. The condition often appears after extreme exertion and may be associated with various bone marrow syndromes. It is successfully treated with prednisone.

Polymyositis (dermatomyositis)

Polymyositis or dermatomyositis may be accompanied by a nonspecific rash affecting the eyelids with a violaceous color, thinning of the skin over extensor areas of joints, and paronycheal vasculitis. The main thrust of the disease is an inflammation of the muscle sarcolemma, with an infiltration of T lymphocytes. This causes weakness of skeletal muscle and sometimes atrophy. Axial muscles are most often involved, but weakness of respiratory and cardiac muscles may lead to dire results. ANA positivity is fairly common, but the main laboratory features are high serum levels of muscle enzymes such as creatine phosphokinase, serum glutamic-oxaloacetic transaminase, and aldolase released from damaged muscle cells. Biopsy of muscle is helpful for diagnosis, and there is a characteristic electromyographic pattern.

Pharmacologic treatment of polymyositis is prednisone in doses sufficient to reduce the abnormal serum enzyme levels. Cytotoxic therapy with azathioprine, cyclophosphamide, and chlorambucil is necessary on occasion. Children with the disease frequently have accompanying calcinosis. For reasons that are unclear, 40% to 60% of adults with polymyositis have concurrent carcinoma of any organ. Accompanying carcinoma is almost unheard of in children.

Polyarteritis

Polyarteritis is a rare condition that is the most severe of a group of vasculitides of unknown cause. In some cases an allergic reaction to drugs is suspected to be the cause, and 5% to 15% of patients have eosinophilia. An inflammation attacks medium-sized and small arteries in any organ, although kidney, bowel, and peripheral nerves are most often affected.

Treatment consists of high-dose corticosteroid therapy, although cytotoxic drugs are occasionally necessary.

Thrombotic thrombocytopenia

Thrombotic thrombocytopenia affects the brain with a peculiar dementia and can cause thrombotic lesions anywhere in the body. It is characterized by low thrombocyte counts, which are not due to autoimmunity. The cause is unknown, and no rational treatment has been developed, although infusions of fresh plasma occasionally have been helpful.

Mixed connective tissue disease

Some patients have a mixture of scleroderma, lupus, and polymyositis. This condition is called mixed connective tissue disease and is somewhat more benign than the individual disease conditions.

Fibrositis

Fibrositis is an increasingly diagnosed disease that occurs primarily in females and has been reported in children. Its clinical picture consists of vague musculoskeletal pain, morning stiffness, trigger points of painful nodules (paraspinally in the back and at the costochondral junctions anteriorly), nonrestorative sleep disturbances, and in some cases, benign colitis.[12] It is successfully treated with low doses of tricyclic antidepressants such as amitriptyline given at bedtime, along with NSAIDs and local injection of cortisone or procaine at trigger points. Injection at costochondral junctions must be done carefully to avoid causing cartilage necrosis.

Polymyalgia rheumatica

Polymyalgia rheumatica affects men and women equally and usually occurs after 60 years of age. Patients have profound morning stiffness, greater or lesser muscular pain, anemia, and a greatly elevated ESR. The muscles are not weak, and there is no elevation of serum muscle enzymes, which distinguishes polymyalgia rheumatica from polymyositis. Arteritis, particularly in the head and neck, is a rare complication and may lead to sudden blindness in one or both eyes.[4] The disease disappears spontaneously in 1 to 3 years.

The myopathic component of polymyalgia rheumatica is readily treatable with low doses of corticosteroids; 2.5 to 5 mg of prednisone daily is often all that is necessary to correct the symptoms, the anemia, and the elevated ESR. The arteritic complication requires much higher doses of steroids, and its diagnosis should be reinforced with temporal artery biopsy.

NONINFLAMMATORY ARTHRITIS—OSTEOARTHRITIS

Osteoarthritis, often called osteoarthrosis in Europe, is best considered two separate conditions, since the treatment and the prognosis are quite different. The division is between non-weight-bearing and weight-bearing joints, including the lower spine. In general the condition is often considered to be part of the normal aging process in that it is triggered by a wearing away of the joint cartilage. The process may be initiated by a previous injury, congenital malalignment of joints, poor muscular or ligamentous stabilization of the joint, or prior infection or inflammation injuring the cartilage. There seems to be some genetic propensity for early osteoarthritis,[8] but almost everyone over 60 years of age has some amount of the disease in one or more joints. American rheumatologists prefer to call it osteoarthritis because in many cases there are accelerated attacks that involve redness, tenderness, and swelling of the joint.

Disease in non-weight-bearing joints

The disease most often begins in the distal phalangeal joints and is accompanied by soft synovial swelling on either side of the joint. This eventually generates outcroppings of bone called osteophytes, which are characteristic of the disease and in this case are called Heberden's nodes. A similar, somewhat less common, process in the proximal interphalangeal joints is called Bouchard's nodes. On radiographs, the cartilaginous region between the bones is clearly worn away. It is as if the bones were trying to spread the load of joint motion over a larger surface area when the resiliency of the cartilage is lost. When the cartilage begins to wear down, frequently it frays, and small pieces of it may enter the joint space, causing further abnormal wear and occasional but brief locking of the joint. This description holds for both weight-bearing and non-weight-bearing joints.

A frequently involved joint in the hand is the first metacarpophalangeal joint, where a shelf of extra bone can be palpated.

The elbow can be involved, and only rarely are the joints of the shoulder complex involved, unless the patient has used them for bearing weight (by using crutches, for example). Under those conditions the acromioclavicular joint is usually affected. The apophyseal joints of the cervical spine can be part of the osteoarthritic process, particularly if disc degeneration has changed the anatomy sufficiently to place stress on the apophyseal joints. Flexion-extension injuries (whiplash) may cause osteoarthritic changes and symptoms many years after the incident.

In general, the disease in the non-weight-bearing joints has a self-limited course if the joints are rested and treated for pain. The joints appear gnarled because of productive, osteophytic changes, and there is some deformation, but the process of cartilage wear, possible osteophyte formation, and inflammation usually takes place over months and years, with frequent pain and stiffness. At the end of that time the situation stabilizes and the disease becomes asymptomatic, and often there is little or no loss of effective function.

The pharmacologic treatment is the use of NSAIDs and occasional injections into the joint of corticosteroid preparations.

Disease in weight-bearing joints

Weight-bearing joints in the osteoarthritic process demand different treatment than non-weight-bearing joints. In weight-bearing joints the process is continuous and often unrelenting, possibly because the wear and tear is greater.

In the feet and ankles, prior injury or genetically poor weight-bearing structures are often associated with osteoarthritis. Jogging also results in early disease on imperfect weight-bearing joints. In the knee, prior loss or loosening of the menisci, rupture of the cruciate ligaments, or strain on the collateral ligaments sets up conditions for later osteoarthritis. Most cases of hip osteoarthritis are also probably due to congenital malalignment. Occasionally osteonecrosis of the femoral head associated with previous hip fracture or steroid therapy causes a form of osteoarthritis. Rickets and Paget's disease can cause enough bowing of the tibia to produce malalignment of the knees, ankles, and hips, leading to early osteoarthritis.

Osteoarthritis has no positive laboratory tests, and the joint fluid examination is usually unrevealing. Radiographs showing cartilage loss and osteophyte formation are helpful.

In the early stages, NSAIDs and judicious use of injected steroids are the drug treatments of choice, but physical medicine adjuncts are extremely important.[2] At end-stage conditions, surgical replacement of hip and knees is now a successful treatment modality. Ankle replacement is still in its infancy and is not recommended generally. Various midfoot and forefoot procedures are available and have been quite successful.

REFERENCES

1. Bennett, JC: The etiology of rheumatoid arthritis. In Kelley, WN, et al, editors: Textbook of rheumatology, ed 2, Philadelphia, 1985, WB Saunders Co.
2. Brandt, KD: Management of osteoarthritis. In Kelley, WN, et al, editors: Textbook of rheumatology, ed 2, Philadelphia, 1985, WB Saunders Co.
3. Brewerton, DA, and James, DCO: The histocompatibility antigen (HLA-B27) and disease, Semin Arthritis Rheum 4:191, 1975.
4. Dixon, AS, et al: Polymyalgia rheumatica and temporal arteritis, Ann Rheum Dis 25:203, 1966.
5. Dubois, EL, editor: Lupus erythematosus, ed 2, Los Angeles, 1974, University of Southern California Press.
6. Fries, J: Personal communication, 1986.
7. Kelley, WN, and Fox, IM: Gout and related disorders of purine metabolism. In Kelley, WN, et al, editors: Textbook of rheumatology, ed 2, Philadelphia, 1985, WB Saunders Co.
8. Stecher, RM: Heberden's nodes: heredity in hypertrophic arthritis of the finger joints, Am J Med Sci 201:801, 1941.
9. Steere, AC, et al: Curing Lyme arthritis: successful antibiotic therapy of established joint involvement, Arthritis Rheum 27:26, 1984.
10. Steere, AC, Pachner, A, and Malawista, SE: Neurologic abnormalities of Lyme disease: successful treatment with high-dose intravenous penicillin, Ann Intern Med 99:767, 1983.
11. Willkens, RF, et al: Reiter's syndrome: evaluation of preliminary criteria of definite disease, Arthritis Rheum 24:844, 1981.
12. Yunus, M, et al: Primary fibromyalgia (fibrositis): clinical study of 50 patients with matched normal controls, Semin Arthritis Rheum 11:151, 1981.

CHAPTER 14

Rehabilitation management in arthritis and related disorders

VALERY F. LANYI

The often unpredictable, remitting, and exacerbating nature of rheumatic diseases poses a special challenge to the physiatrist. Although a single plan of therapeutic approach might suffice for some disabling conditions, arthritis and related disorders require a series of assessments that may result in a variety of treatment methods during the natural course of the disease. Rehabilitation must provide a broad range of procedures to help patients who have arthritis achieve the maximum potential for normal living.[39] Whereas Chapter 13 discussed classification and pharmacologic treatment of rheumatic diseases, this chapter focuses on the necessity of and the timing for rehabilitation intervention, as well as its applications to and effect on inflammatory and noninflammatory arthritic manifestations.

Increased diagnostic acuity and sophisticated laboratory testing have led to earlier recognition and more precise diagnosis of rheumatic diseases. This permits the introduction of rehabilitation interventions at an earlier stage and their more effective use at various stages of rheumatic disease. In addition, functional scales provide a more accurate way to measure the effects of the disease at the time of initial evaluation.[7,28] Such scales enable physicians to assess the patient's functional ability at any given point during the course of the illness; they also measure the efficiency of various treatments.[43,44]

Rehabilitation treatment methods include physical modalities, pain modification techniques, physical therapy, and therapeutic exercises. They also involve functional occupational therapy, splinting, energy conservation, joint protection, and work simplification methods that require an understanding of the effects of joint loading during activities of daily living. In addition, they include aids ranging from readily available and often inexpensive self-help devices to complex electronic instruments, environmental modifications, and robotics.

The chronic pain, disfigurement, and diminished physical capabilities that result from most forms of arthritis are likely to have a profound psychologic effect on patients. An understanding of this effect is necessary to educate patients and their families about the nature and stages of the illness, to plan vocational and avocational activities, and most important, to help patients feel and function better in the environment.

The treatment plan for any stage of the disease begins with a physical examination, which may also reveal complications stemming from unrelated disorders. The recording of the static and kinetic state of the musculoskeletal system serves as a baseline for rehabilitation assessment. A standard range-of-motion evaluation should be augmented by a description of the signs of inflammation if present, for instance, heat, swelling, redness, and fluid accumulation. Muscle testing must also reflect the state of the joints. It should be noted whether contracture or joint instability has affected the arc of motion. Gait analysis measures body motion in three dimensions. Computerized gait analysis records gait events and ground reactive forces, making it possible to pinpoint both the locus and effect of the disorder.[34]*

Careful evaluation of the activities of daily living provides the widest range of information regarding the patient's level of self-care and locomotion. The ability to perform a task with precision and the strength and stamina involved in performing these tasks is evaluated and documented. In addition, homemaking skills are reviewed, and leisure activities and social interactions are appraised.

The most difficult evaluation is the objective measurement of pain in patients with arthritis; however, research studies indicate a close correlation between the disease activity and how patients experience the effect of pain on their lives

---

*Currently, computerized gait analysis is used primarily as a research tool.

("pain behavior").[4,63] Psychosocial evaluation identifies the patient's emotional reaction and adaptability to pain, stiffness, disfigurement, and deformity and permits an estimate of the impact of arthritis on social and sexual roles. Vocational and educational evaluation complete the assessment.

RHEUMATOID ARTHRITIS

The rehabilitative management of rheumatoid arthritis depends on the stage of inflammation in the disease (that is, acute, subacute, and chronic), the number of joints involved, the severity of joint involvement, and the interrelationship of contiguous joints. When inflammation is acute, patients tend to assume positions for comfort that may lead to contractures unless appropriate interventions are used. These contractures may interfere with function.

Acute stage

When the disease is acute, it is most beneficial for patients to rest the joint or joints as close to the position of function as tolerated.[16,54] Support of the neck in physiologic lordosis provides the best maintenance of usual posture. Shoulders should be abducted at about 45 degrees with wedge pillows. Elbows should not be flexed beyond 75 degrees. The dominant wrist should be extended at 20 degrees, and the nondominant wrist should be kept in neutral or slight flexion. Finger flexion (to retain the position of function for chuck, pinch, grip, and grasp) is 35 to 45 degrees of flexion at the metacarpophalangeal (MCP) joints, 25 to 30 degrees of flexion of the proximal interphalangeal (PIP) joints, and 15 degrees at the distal interphalangeal (DIP) joints. The thumb should be abducted with the interphalangeal (IP) joint flexed at 25 degrees and opposed to the forefinger. Hips should be abducted at 45 degrees and flexed no more than 5 degrees. The knees should be supported in the fully extended position, the ankle at the 90 degree angle, and the feet in neutral.

In my experience, resting splints in the active rheumatoid patient have been well tolerated and comfortable when they are made to conform to the patient's contours. Serial splints made of lightweight plastics with memory are used to stretch soft tissue contractures and to change joint positions gradually. Splints can be worn 24 hours a day for a week to 10 days without danger of contracture. Since the splint is custom made for the patient, it is a great improvement over the early bivalved casts.[26,36] Partridge and Duthie[62] in 1963 demonstrated that immobilization in splints, even at the end of 4 weeks, caused no loss of significant range of motion when compared with patients whose splints were removed twice daily.

The acute stage usually subsides in a week to 10 days with the use of proper pharmacologic agents and by resting the acutely involved joint in as close to the position of function as possible with splints, slings, or wedge pillows. Resting the joint was shown to be beneficial in animals with

crystal-induced arthritis.[13] Reports on studies of patients who have had strokes or poliomyelitis show that arthritis does not occur in neurologically impaired limbs.[19,20,68,71]

Short-term rest by immobilization has not shown the adverse reactions brought about by prolonged immobilization, such as decreases in lean body mass, total body water, total intracellular fluid volume, and metabolic rate.[23,38,65] For instance, in one study, immobilizing joints in animals led to stiffening of the joints and decreased water concentration after 3 months.[1] However, weight bearing on joints immobilized for 4 weeks did not prevent the development of edema and adhesions in animal experiments.[57]

The ideal exercise for the patient whose joints are immobilized during the acute phase is static isometric exercise, which produces minimum muscle shortening and maximum muscle tension without moving the joint.[16,46] Motion through the joint is undesirable because it leads to an increase in disease activity as demonstrated by the increase in joint temperature and in the white blood cell (WBC) count of the joint fluids.[53] In recent animal experiments the use of transcutaneous electrical nerve stimulation (TENS) decreased the intracellular fluid volume and WBC count.[42] These findings may explain the analgesic effect of TENS.

Subacute stage

When inflammation becomes subacute, it is essential to begin assisted active range-of-motion exercises to initiate a smooth gliding movement of the joint. An assistant helps the patient move the joint through a tolerated range of motion. This motion acts as a pump to reduce edema. The motion should create neither pain nor stress to the joint. Night splinting also prevents pain by supporting the target joint against the pull of gravity and involuntary motion. For example, functional splints support the wrist in subacute synovitis and provide reinforcement for the ligaments against relaxation. The splint is designed to protect the carpal bones from subluxation and radial deviation. Reinforcement on the ulnar side of the MCP and PIP joints can provide resistance to ulnar deviation.[17]

Balancing rest and exercise in the subacute period is the greatest challenge in rehabilitative management. The reduction of inflammation by means of rest must be carefully weighed against the adverse local and systemic responses to the effect of prolonged rest.[2] This can be avoided by the timely introduction of exercise, which not only helps prevent localized weakness but also combats the systemic effect of immobilization.[54] (Pools are useful when beginning exercises during the subacute stage because the bouyancy of the water combats gravitational pull and reduces body weight by as much as it displaces.) Assisted active range-of-motion exercises can be effectively initiated and enhanced with the use of superficial heat modalities (for instance, hot packs, hydrotherapy, and paraffin baths). Superficial heat[48] helps by increasing surface blood flow and reflex cooling of the joint surface,[28,31,41] whereas cold packs elevate joint temperature.[30] However, prolonged superficial heating in animal experiments results in an elevated WBC count in the synovial fluid, indicating increased inflammatory activity.[13] Deep heating modalities (for example, ultrasonography and diathermy) are also contraindicated in acute rheumatoid arthritis because they have the potential to raise intercellular temperature, increase collagenase activity, and induce inflammation.[25] By contrast, studies show that superficial heat does not cause the disease to progress.[6]

Passive isotonic (stretching) exercise should be discouraged in the subacute stage to avoid overstretching the joint. Resistive exercises must also be avoided because they increase intra-articular pressure and joint temperature.[66]

In this stage the introduction of energy conservation, joint protection, and work simplification methods in both the home and the workplace is timely. Patients with rheumatoid arthritis may have difficulty accepting these methods, which necessitate rearranging priorities and altering life-styles. They fear these stopgap measures in their treatment because they see them as the stigma of end-stage disability. Physicians need to understand the fear and problems of patients who have morning stiffness, significant pain, and fatigue, and patient education must be sensitive to these fears to encourage compliance. Altering homemaking habits, adapting work surfaces and storage areas, and step-by-step analysis of body mechanics is most helpful. The elimination of bending, lifting, and carrying (by using carts or trays with casters) at chest level is both helpful and cost effective. Budgeting time, eliminating unnecessary walking, and using lightweight equipment, tools with large gripping surfaces, and lightweight utensils with built-up handles help prevent stresses on the joints.[70]

Adaptive devices and self-care aids during this period of reduced but still active joint involvement include lightweight clothing that can easily be donned and doffed and shoes of the slip-on variety or with Velcro straps. The poor heel-toe walking pattern of a rheumatoid patient with subacute metatarsal involvement can be successfully managed with metatarsal rocker bars. Although custom-molded shoes to accommodate cock-up toes are expensive, soft Spenco and Plastazote inserts in extra-depth shoes can reduce weight-bearing pain and improve walking cadence and speed. Patients have to decide whether to use awkward stocking-pulling aids or to not wear stockings and whether to use complicated long-handled combs and brushes or to cut their hair short. Long-handled reachers and grippers can be put to multiple uses. Independence in personal hygiene may be aided with nonskid strips in the bathtub and nonskid (Vikem) gripping aids for handling toileting articles, as well as other items.

Patients tend to look on the introduction of ambulatory aids in the subacute stage as a stigma of end-stage disability as well; to ensure that patients do not reject these aids, an explanation of their joint-sparing properties is necessary. The aids also provide greater flexibility in day-to-day ac-

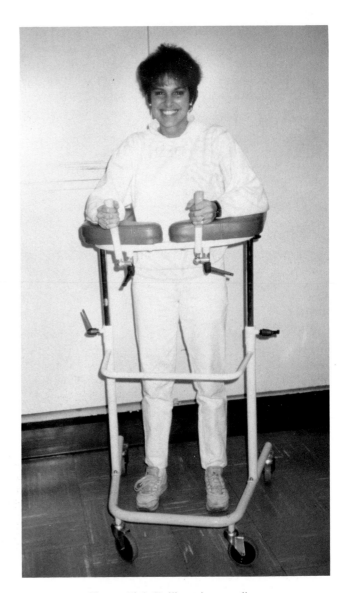

Figure 14-1. Rolling triceps walker.

tivities. For a patient with symmetric arthritis, however, standard ambulatory aids (for example, canes, crutches, and standard wheelchair) may be insufficient. When the upper and lower extremities are equally involved, the use of an electrically operated wheelchair as a temporary measure, however expensive (and at times threatening to the patient), may still be the best device for joint protection. When the arthritic manifestations are asymmetric, the effect of loading must be carefully considered in choosing ambulatory aids. Weight bearing on involved hands may hasten deformities. With the exception of an electric wheelchair, a rolling walker with triceps attachment is the most efficient aid for reducing weight bearing on all four extremities (Figure 14-1). The addition of easy grip or custom-designed handles extends the width of the hand's gripping surface and divides the load more evenly among the joints of the hand and wrist.

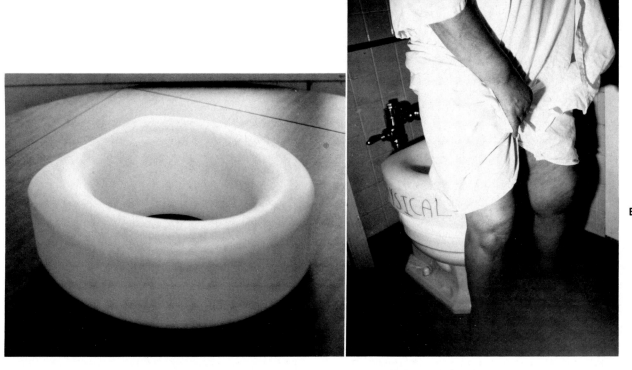

Figure 14-2. A, Elevated toilet seat. **B,** Getting up off elevated toilet seat.

These ambulatory aids minimize fatigability and lack of endurance, the most common complaints of arthritic patients.

Architectural barriers may disable a patient with multiarticular inflammatory arthritis in the subacute stage. When joints are distended, arising from a low chair requires the assistance of the upper extremities because the hip and knee extensor muscles are weak. However, this increases the stress placed on the wrist, elbow, and shoulder. Elevated toilet seats (Figure 14-2), chair leg extenders on ordinary household chairs, and tall shower stools with suction attachments make getting up easier (Figure 14-3).

Chronic stage

Chronic rheumatoid arthritis is disabling, even when it is "burnt out." Occasional flare-ups may result from inappropriate loading[10] and impaired alignment. On the other hand, the disease can persist unremittingly, with increases in joint destruction, deformities, and severe disability. These results are invariably associated with atrophy and weakness adjacent to the involved joints.

The classic deformity of the rheumatoid neck is forward flexion and foreshortening. The characteristic rheumatoid posture of the shoulder is in adduction, internal rotation, and forward flexion. Semiflexed elbow, pronated forearm,

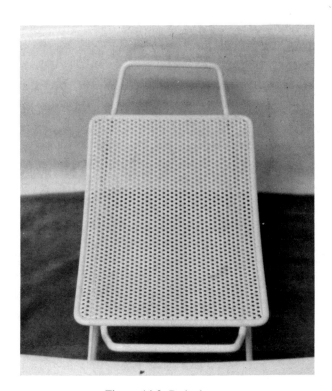

Figure 14-3. Bathtub seat.

flexed wrist, semiflexed MCP, PIPs, and DIP joints, and adducted thumb are also hallmarks of rheumatoid arthritis. Radial deviation of the wrist, ulnar deviation of the MCP joints, swan-neck deformities, boutonnière deformities of the fingers, and boutonnière deformity of the thumb occur most frequently in the hand. The hip becomes contracted in flexion and external rotation, and the knee in flexion. Feet become pronated, and frequently hallux valgus, subluxation of the metatarsals, and cock-up toes occur. These positions are assumed for greater comfort because they reduce intra-articular pressure.[32]

Chronic pain further interferes with functional activity. The selection of pain modification in this chronic stage includes the use of a transcutaneous nerve stimulator,[52,73] in addition to the traditional modes of delivering pain relief through pharmacologic and physical agents. In my experience, ice is not well tolerated by arthritic patients.

The treatment of choice is gentle stretching to increase joint motion and stretch soft tissue contractures. This is guided by the establishment of joint damage in the physical examination and radiologic findings. When inflammation and pain are controlled and sufficient isometric static strength has been achieved, the exercise of choice is dynamic, repetitive, low-resistance isotonic exercise.[10,11] The best forms of this exercise are lifting light weights through short arcs of motion or such activities as swimming, bicycling, gardening, and weaving.[15,58-59,60] Patients with chronic inactive rheumatoid arthritis are troubled by the appearance of their deformed joints and atrophic muscles, and some may appeal to the physician for a more vigorous

exercise prescription. Vigorous, highly resistive exercises and the use of devices providing active resistive forces (for example, Nautilus or Cybex) should be discouraged.[9,49] Resistance, sustained through the range of motion, increases strain on periarticular structures, intra-articular pressure, and joint temperature and is likely to induce arthritic flares.[29]

Swimming pools are excellent for increasing endurance and are a pleasurable adjuvant for recreational exercises. To help prevent osteoporosis—a common complication of chronic (especially steroid-treated) rheumatoid arthritis—walking with the arms swinging at the sides is recommended. However, speed walking increases stress on hips, knees, feet, and ankles and is potentially harmful. It is important to remember that only repetitive performance of task leads to increased endurance in that task.[27]

Ambulatory aids are selected not only for their joint-sparing role in chronic rheumatoid arthritis but also to compensate for gait abnormalities. These abnormalities are a result of established joint contractures, subsequent instabilities, compensatory mechanisms, and disturbances in cadence and speed of locomotion. In addition, upper extremity contractures frequently necessitate adaptations to walkers and crutches. Triceps attachments to axillary crutches or walkers can compensate for elbow flexion contractures or biceps weakness. The addition of ambulatory aids increases energy expenditure and decreases the speed of walking. A reduction in the weight of crutches and canes or walkers made of lightweight alloys or rosewood can minimize the extreme fatigue and decreased stamina that are so disabling for arthritis patients. Motorized wheelchairs

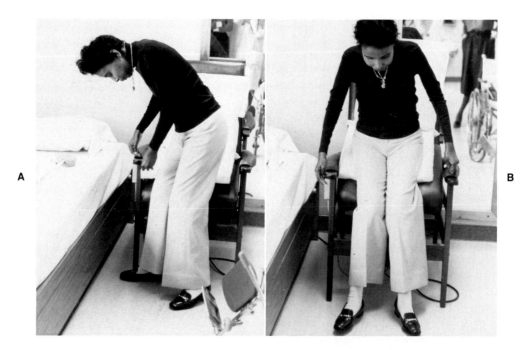

Figure 14-4. A, Self-rising armchair. **B,** Getting up out of self-rising chair.

and "Amigos" allow severely disabled patients with chronically active rheumatoid arthritis to participate in activities away from the isolation of their rooms, elevating their sense of worth by permitting them to play an active role in society. Electronically operated self-rising chairs eliminate the need to employ a home attendant and not only enhance the patient's feeling of well-being and sense of independence but also are cost effective (Figure 14-4). These interventions may make gainful employment possible, which would improve the socioeconomic status of disabled arthritic patients and their families.

Splints are the most frequently used orthotic devices. Resting splints may be employed for a few hours at a time by patients in the active chronic stage. Splints that address specific problems include ring splints for swan-neck and boutonnière deformities, ulnar deviation splints, postoperative dynamic splints, and thumb spicas for reduction of stress on the carpometacarpal (CMC) joint. The best resting splints for the knee are custom constructed and extend up to the midthigh to support the large thigh muscles with the knee in full extension and the foot and ankle at a right angle. Commercially available knee immobilizers also are useful in a flare-up in the chronic phase of arthritis.

Bracing has rarely been acceptable to patients with inflammatory arthritis because the swelling that changes from day to day creates pain. Knee cages may reduce the patient's sense of instability at that joint. In addition, because chronic cervical subluxation can cause death or spinal cord transection if the patient falls or stumbles, cervical orthoses (for example, soft collars or modified Philadelphia collars) are used. They minimize the risk of falls and subsequent spinal cord injury. Peripheral neuropathy, an uncommon and self-limited event in rheumatoid arthritis, can be managed with the use of posterior leaf splints. (Electrodiagnostic studies also are particularly helpful in the differentiation of carpal and tarsal tunnel syndromes from peripheral neuropathy.) The weight of orthoses increases caloric demands and further impairs the agility of patients with rheumatoid arthritis. Attempts at correcting deformities through force (that is, by turnbuckles) may result in subluxation.

Aids to transfer an arthritic patient from a wheelchair to a car, elevated and swiveled car seats, and car door openers improve the patient's ability to function independently. The use of wide-angle rearview mirrors compensates for neck disabilities. Special adaptations to the steering wheel reduce stresses on the rheumatoid hand. Citizen band (CB) radios help patients to arrange barrier-free travel accommodations.

Surgical interventions, such as joint reconstruction, joint replacement, and salvage procedures, are an integral part of rehabilitation (see Chapter 33).

Rheumatoid arthritis is often pauciarticular and mild and does not require complex and extensive intervention. Early recognition of the need for rehabilitation management of soft tissue contractures, and its timely introduction, may be all that is required. However, even the best intentions and informed, timely, and skilled interventions cannot always save patients from profound disability.

SYSTEMIC LUPUS ERYTHEMATOSUS

The characteristic musculoskeletal manifestations of systemic lupus erythematosus (SLE) are arthralgia and tenosynovitis. Spontaneous rupture of tendons can be managed with temporary immobilization.[72] When arthritis occurs in this multisystem disease, it resembles rheumatoid arthritis and is managed similarly. The deformities are frequently reducible; functional splints are well tolerated. Weakness and ligamentous laxity are hallmarks of this disease; genu recurvatum is manageable with posterior leaf splints, gait retraining, and quadriceps-setting exercises.

The physical management of SLE requires an understanding of the overwhelming systemic involvement. Neurologic manifestations vary depending on the locus of vasculitis in the nervous system[8]; with the aid of electromyography, myopathy can be differentiated from neuropathy.[21] Transverse myelitis frequently leads to paraplegia[37]; major strokes result in hemiplegia. These impairments require modification of the management of the disabilities of SLE. Psychosis may greatly complicate active rehabilitation intervention. Cognitive rehabilitation measures may be helpful in the management of lupus patients with organic brain damage and progressive dementia.

Avascular necrosis, a complication of long-standing SLE, occurs most commonly in the femoral head, tibia, humerus, and mandible but may occur in any joint. Rest, proper positioning of the involved limb to reduce pain and motion, and the maintenance of muscle power with isometric exercises is the management of choice and resembles the physical regimen of acute inflammatory arthritis. On occasion, elimination of weight bearing may salvage weight-bearing joints. When muscle wasting occurs and the disease has come to a standstill, resistive exercises may restore muscle bulk. Joint regeneration rarely occurs, and surgical rehabilitation is often successful.

PROGRESSIVE SYSTEMIC SCLEROSIS

Progressive systemic sclerosis, or scleroderma, is a gradually developing form of restrictive skin disease. The restrictions caused by the tightening of the skin and underlying connective tissue interfere with the patient's functioning. Limitation of motion in the upper limbs can interfere with dressing, grooming, grip, grasp, and fine hand motions. Depending on the extent of the lower extremity involvement, ambulation and elevation activities may be impeded. Opening the mouth and chewing can be affected. Function also becomes impaired by Raynaud's phenomenon. Frequent paraffin applications and home use of whirlpools help reduce stiffness and provide excellent preliminary modalities for stretching and range-of-motion exercises of the limbs. The innovative use of commercially available clothing (for example, silk underwear, down mittens, electrically heated socks, and face masks) keeps skin warm and joints movable, enabling the patient to be socially active and employable. Stretching of the mouth and mandible manually improves bite. When lower extremities are restricted, hydraulically operated elevating chairs and Stairolators increase independence. The use of relaxation tapes and temperature biofeedback has been reported beneficial in the treatment of Raynaud's phenomenon.[18]

Dermatomyositis and mixed connective tissue disease pose essentially the same problems as progressive systemic sclerosis. The rehabilitation goal is maintenance of range of motion and physical comfort to allow active exercises.

Polymyositis causes symmetric weakness and atrophy of the limb girdles, neck, and pharynx. Electromyographic evidence supported by muscle biopsy is decisive in establishing the diagnosis. In the active stage of the disease, proximal muscle weakness necessitates the introduction of self-help devices to substitute for the lack of overhead motion and difficulty in rising from low surfaces and climbing stairs. Muscle-strengthening exercises are prescribed when the disease is in remission and the serum enzyme levels are low. In chronic polymyositis, contractures may occur but can be reduced by the range-of-motion exercises.

SERONEGATIVE SPONDYLOARTHROPATHIES
Ankylosing spondylitis

The clinical course of ankylosing spondylitis—the gradual loss of motion in the entire spine—should be managed with rehabilitation intervention as early as possible. Dixon's statement, "It's the doctor's job to control the pain and the patient's job to keep moving," is particularly appropriate here.[12] Because motion in the spine decreases with the progression of enthesopathy, the upright position is harder to maintain as the disease progresses. However, the upright position can be maintained for a longer time if the patient rests in the fully extended position and receives postural training and therapeutic exercises. Pharmacologic pain relief can be supplemented with superficial and deep heating. Underwater ultrasound treatment in Hubbard tanks is also useful. Isometric and resistive exercises to the hip girdle and the neck and trunk extensors help the patient regain height and some mobility. Breathing exercises maintain chest expansion. It is also useful to change positions from upright to prone several times a day.

Evaluation of body mechanics includes the position of the head at work to prevent both flexion and hyperextension deformities. The patient's sitting position, as well as the chairs used at work and for relaxation, should be modified to provide positive postural reinforcement. If the patient sits during the working day, periodic assumption of the upright and the prone positions helps minimize flexion contractures of the hip and knees. Work efficiency and lifting techniques

to maximize mobility and minimize disability can be individually designed for patients. Environmental modifications include specially designed seating to support the neck and back and tilted work surfaces, such as drawing boards, which assist in performing tasks at home and in the workplace. Reading with the aid of prism glasses relieves the boredom of gravity stretching (when lying completely flat) and encourages patient compliance. Because of this disease's particular disabling quality, clarification of sexual positions assists in adjustment to sexual problems.

Recreational exercises, especially swimming, help maintain joint mobility and assist in stretching soft tissue contractures. Contact sports should be avoided to prevent osteoporotic fractures. Low-impact aerobic exercises in well-cushioned shoes on resilient surfaces promote general well-being and improve cardiac capacity and pulmonary capacity in patients with restricted chest expansion.

Psoriatic arthritis

Psoriasis may be accompanied by symmetric or asymmetric peripheral arthritis, which frequently involves the joints of the spine. Management is more difficult than in ankylosing spondylitis because of incomplete fusion and pain at the site of the motion. The aims of intervention are maintenance of trunk mobility and avoidance of contractures.

The peripheral arthritis, characterized by DIP joint involvement and "sausage fingers," is often complicated by extension contractures. Short-term splinting or immobilization must be followed by frequent and vigorous range of motion exercises. Severe destructive changes may occur in the hand, causing loss of bone, severe joint instability, and poor grip. Specially designed adaptive equipment serves to maintain the patient's independence in personal hygiene and self-care and assists in most activities of daily living.

Destructive changes in the feet and ankles may be especially disabling. In patients with chronic synovitis, subluxation of the ankles can be made less painful and more functional with a brief application of Unna boots. The destructive changes and the resulting subluxation of the metatarsophalangeal (MTP) joints, as well as the swollen and deformed toes, can be managed with high toe-boxed shoes, soft resilient soles, and soft Spenco or Plastazote inserts. Pain on weight bearing caused by heel spurs and plantar fasciitis can be reduced by heel cups and soft foam rubber inserts with cutouts.

Spinal orthoses have limited use in inflammatory arthritis; the psoriatic arthritic patient with cervical spondylitis, however, requires support by means of a soft collar and cervical pillows to reduce the pull of gravity. Semirigid back supports offer comfort and prevent painful motion.

Reiter's disease

The arthritis of Reiter's disease is similar to other inflammatory arthritides. The axial skeletal involvement is often indistinguishable from ankylosing spondylitis or psoriatic spondylitis; however, there may be only sacroiliitis. The disease is often self-limited. The severe and painful Achilles tendonitis specific to this disease responds to management with an Ace bandage wrapping, high-laced soft-soled athletic shoes, or the temporary use of air splints. When keratoderma blennorrhagica occurs on the sole of the foot, padding a postoperative boot with a soft foam rubber insert may keep the patient functioning.

• • •

Arthritides accompanying inflammatory bowel disease (for example, ulcerative colitis and Crohn's disease) come to the physician's attention because of associated sacroiliitis or spondylitis and are managed accordingly.

JUVENILE RHEUMATOID POLYARTHRITIS (JUVENILE RHEUMATOID ARTHRITIS)

Children with pauciarticular arthritis have an excellent chance for complete recovery. Palmar flexion of the wrist, one of the most common sites of involvement, and compensatory extension contracture of the MCP joints respond well to early management with a resting cock-up splint at the wrist combined with functional splints to increase MCP joint flexion and thumb motion.[6] The knee is often affected by relatively pain-free effusion. The resulting valgus or varus deformity can be treated with hinge splints, allowing full extension and free flexion to 90 degrees.[69]

Children with polyarticular arthritis, chronic synovitis, and generalized malaise present a greater challenge in maintaining joint position and function. Joint contractures occur early unless range-of-motion exercises, interrupted by short periods of splinting, are carefully monitored by a responsible person (for example, a teacher or family member). Serial casting to reduce soft tissue contractures is well tolerated by children. Swimming in pools for therapeutic exercises and active play for maintenance of functional motion (for instance, ball playing for overhead motion and bicycling for hip, knee, and ankle function) serve best as an exercise program.

Orthotic devices are introduced into the child's daily activity to prevent flexion deformity of the neck and torticollis.[6] Soft collars serve this purpose and are used, for instance, when doing homework. There is insidious onset of flexion contractures of the hip in children with multiarticular disease. These contractures are often associated with knee flexion contractures. If gravity stretching with prolonged maintenance of the prone position and serial splinting does not succeed in reducing the contractures, soft tissue surgical release may be successful. If the hip joint shows radiologic evidence of destruction, total joint replacement, despite skeletal immaturity, should be contemplated (see Chapter 33).

The volatile emotional states of teenagers often make it difficult for them to comply with the prescribed management. In addition, children in whom the disease occurs early may be particularly sensitive about and preoccupied with their appearance, especially when growth has been retarded. This is seen most clearly in the "china doll" syndrome in young girls with multiarticular arthritis. They may deny the deformity to the point that they refuse help. In some cases they may develop a disability of such severity that it requires management in a wheelchair.

The education of the child, parent, and teacher regarding the disease is more complex than in the adult. Realistic vocational goals need to be approached with particular sensitivity. Pain or dysfunction may interfere with sexual pleasure or performance, and line drawings and discussions of pain-free positions can be extremely helpful.

OSTEOARTHRITIS (DEGENERATIVE ARTHRITIS)

The chief complaints of patients with osteoarthritis are restriction of movement, pain on movement, pain on changes of position, and interference with daily activities. Degenerative arthritis is usually limited to one or a few joints. Understanding the effects provides the rationale for management. Loss of elasticity, biomechanical alterations of the cartilage resulting from biochemical changes, and osteophyte formation lead to abnormal biomechanics.[56] The articular cartilage becomes too thin to be an effective shock absorber during impact loading.[31,64] At times of snyovial effusion, pain and limitation of motion can mimic rheumatoid arthritis.[61] It is helpful to explain to patients that osteoarthritis is not a systemic illness and that limitations can be dealt with by specific procedures. The patient can cope better with stiffness and pain if given an explanation of body mechanics, for example, how the stiffness and pain are brought about by changes of position. Single joint involvement requires changes only in a few specific activities of daily living.

Carpometacarpal joint involvement interferes with many functions that require accurate pinch. For instance, a patient so altered could not hold a pen. The use of thumb spicas reduces joint pain and maintains web space. Writing may become painful, in which case help may be provided by a universal cuff that holds the writing article or by a tape recorder. The gelling phenomenon and morning stiffness in the hands may be reduced by wearing stretch gloves at night.

The use of paraffin or other superficial heat modalities may also reduce disabling pain and stiffness in the hand. Paresthesia in the hand may represent entrapment syndromes at the cervical root or along the course of the brachial plexus. Differential diagnosis is greatly aided by electrodiagnostic studies because osteoarthritis frequently causes double crush syndrome. When carpal tunnel syndrome is caused by degenerative joint disease of the wrist, cock-up splints with or without local injection of steroids can relieve the patient from disturbing, often bizarre night pain in the hand.

Osteoarthritis of the hips can lead to pain during motion, loss of motion, and shortening of the extremities. Pain relief is often achieved with rest, local heat, and reduction of weight bearing using ambulatory aids. Isometric exercises of the hip girdle help combat atrophy. Excess body weight, by increasing repetitive loading forces in walking, can increase pain and interfere with function. Weight reduction, when no destructive changes complicate the hip involvement, may preserve unimpeded locomotion. However, if the joint is destroyed, only total joint replacement eliminates pain and restores function.

Degenerative joint disease of the knee may affect part or all of the knee joint. Unicompartmental disease or mild patellofemoral arthritis responds well to temporary reduction of weight bearing, local heat, and quadriceps-setting exercises. Sometimes elimination of stair climbing is all that is needed. Hinged knee cages, sometimes with attached patella-stabilizing pads, cut down on the painful effect of walking. Ligamentous laxities and lateral and medial instability can be lessened with the use of derotation braces (for example, a Lenox Hill brace). Local heat modalities moderate pain and stiffness and allow strengthening of the quadriceps muscle to ensure greater stability. Elevated seats at home and in the workplace, elevated toilet seats, and reduced walking time often permit a return to otherwise unimpeded function. When valgus or varus deformities cause severe instability, surgical interventions are indicated.

Metatarsophalangeal subluxation, rigid toes, or hallux valgus can hinder walking. Thick resilient soles on comfortable walking shoes (for example, Vibram soles or soft crepe soles) can lessen this pain. Pain caused by heel spurs may be alleviated by wearing soft heel cups. Swelling produced by osteoarthritic changes can be reduced by high-laced athletic shoes and intermittent elevation of the lower limbs.

The management of neck pain and cervical radiculopathy, back pain, and lumbosacral radiculopathies is discussed in Chapters 38 and 39.

Systemic elimination of the motion causing the greatest pain is often all that is needed to curtail disability in patients with single joint osteoarthritis. Understanding body mechanics and evaluating postural work and recreational habits assist in isolating the untoward motion, which leads to pain relief and significantly reduces morbidity. The physician's role is to identify the causes of the disability, specific techniques to reduce morbidity, and alternative avenues of management.

Recreational exercises should always be preceded by warm-up and proceeded by cool-down. If mild degenerative changes are not accompanied by signs of inflammation, if the joint spaces are well maintained (despite some spur formation), and if the joints are stable, repetitive joint-loading sports (for example, jogging, tennis, and fencing) can be resumed. Should signs of inflammation return or

weakness occur, the exercise was too vigorous. Pain that occurs for over 2 hours after exercise is a warning signal.

INFECTIOUS AND METABOLIC ARTHRITIS

According to Ehrlich, "Arthritis is a multiplicity of disorders masquerading under a single expression . . . insults of joints, from whatever cause, express themselves similarly."[14] Infectious arthritis is curable, and metabolic arthritis (such as gout) is self-limited; both are usually monarticular. Rehabilitative intervention consists of immediate immobilization of the "red hot" target joint. Once the inflammation has subsided, vigorous range-of-motion exercise is needed to restore complete function.

FIBROMYOSITIS

In fibromyositis the painful trigger points—palpable nodules frequently occurring in the trapezius muscles, costoscapular junction, paraspinal regions, and backs of the knees—respond well to the combined effects of pharmacologic agents and injection of a local anesthetic and/or corticosteroids into the trigger points, as well as use of relaxation tapes and transcutaneous nerve stimulation. Acupuncture and acupressure have been reported to be useful.[51] The use of hydrotherapy and deep-heating methods (such as ultrasound) may relieve pain.

BURSITIS

Bursitis is a syndrome frequently appearing in conjunction with osteoarthritis. Most bursae are congenital and reduce friction between interlaced muscles and tendons. Some bursae are created, possibly by repeated microtrauma to aging muscles, tendons, or fibrous tissues.[40] The physician's role is to review body mechanics, pinpoint abnormal kinesiologic events (for example, recognize "self-bracing" in low back pain that leads to trochanteric bursitis), and suggest changes that will prevent recurrences. Local injection of steroids with or without a local anesthetic often results in immediate cure. In addition, application of ultrasound was reported to be successful in cases of persistent discomfort.[22] Untreated subacromial bursitis, which is frequently associated with adhesive capsulitis of the shoulder, severely interferes with self-care and motion. Spray-stretch methods and vigorous physical therapy, including joint mobilization, require persistence on the part of the patient and the therapist.

SUMMARY

This chapter focuses on the rehabilitation management of patients with arthritis or allied conditions, which is accomplished by targeting rehabilitation interventions at various stages of inflammatory arthritides. The management of rheumatoid arthritis is described at length, and the management of other conditions is discussed only insofar as it differs from this model.

The aim of rehabilitation interventions is to prevent disability, enhance performance, supplement functions with adaptive aids, and substitute lost abilities with others. The factors influencing function are multifaceted,[3,5] and an assessment of function should identify the patient's state and the treatment modalities that are most beneficial for the patient's disabilities. Functional assessments are increasingly more sophisticated; their purposes, comprehensiveness, credibility, accuracy, sensitivity to change, and feasibility are examined in this chapter. Physiatrists have been the innovators of functional assessments.[45,47,55,67] Currently, functional assessment variables are studied to document specific performance improvements, which can have an impact on program costs. Standardization of the assessment methods is quantified and related to outcome measures.[24,33,50]

REFERENCES

1. Akeson, WH, et al: The connective tissue response to immobility: an accelerated aging response? Exp Gerontol 3:289, 1968.
2. Alexander, GJM, Hortas, C, and Bacon, PA: Bed rest activity and the inflammation of rheumatoid arthritis, Br J Rheumatol 22:134, 1983.
3. American Medical Association: Guide to the evaluation of permanent impairment, ed 2, Chicago, 1984, The Association.
4. Anderson, KO, et al: The assessment of pain in rheumatoid arthritis: validity of behavioral observation method in arthritis and rheumatism, Arthritis Rheum 30:36, 1987.
5. Anderson, TP: Trochanteric bursitis: diagnostic criteria and clinical significance, Arch Phys Med Rehabil 39:617, 1958.
6. Ansell, BA: Handbook on rehabilitation rheumatology, New York, 1985, Council on Rehabilitative Neurology. In press.
7. Bombardier, C, and Tugwell, P: A methodologic framework to develop and select indices for clinical trial: statistical and judgemental approaches, J Rheumatol 9:753, 1982.
8. Bresnehan, B, et al: The neuropsychiatric disorder in SLE: evidence for both vascular and immune mechanism, Ann Rheum Dis 38:301, 1979.
9. Castello, BA, El Sallab, RA, and Scott, JT: Physical activity, cystic erosion, and osteoporosis in rheumatoid arthritis, Ann Rheum Dis 24:522, 1965.
10. DeLateur, BJ: Exercise for strength and endurance. In Basmajain, JV, editor: Therapeutic exercise, ed 4, Baltimore, 1984, Williams & Wilkins Co.
11. DeLateur, BJ, et al: Isotonic versus isometric exercise: double shift transfer of training study, Arch Phys Med Rehabil 53:212, 1971.
12. Dixon, A: Ankylosing spondylitis and spinal osteotomy, Proc Soc Lond 70:53, 1977.
13. Dorwart, BB, Hansell, A, Jr, and Schumacher, HR, Jr: Effects of cold and heat on urate crystal-induced synovitis in the dog, Arthritis Rheum 17:563, 1974.
14. Ehrlich, G: Rehabilitation management in rheumatic diseases, Baltimore, 1986, Williams & Wilkins Co.
15. Ekblom, B, et al: Effect of short-term physical training on patients with rheumatoid arthritis, Scand J Rheumatol 5:70, 1976.
16. Gault, SJ, and Spyker, JM: Beneficial effect of immobilization of joints in rheumatoid and related arthritides: a splint study using sequential analysis, Arthritis Rheum 12:34, 1969.
17. Gerber, LH: Rehabilitation of patients with rheumatic diseases, In Kelley, WV, et al, editors: Textbook of rheumatology, ed 2, Philadelphia, 1985, WB Saunders Co.
18. Gerber, LH, et al: Autogenic training in the treatment of *Raynaud's* phenomenon, Arch Phys Med Rehabil 59:522, 1978.
19. Glick, LN: Asymmetrical rheumatoid arthritis after poliomyelitis, Br Med J 3:26, 1967.
20. Glynn, JJ, and Clayton, ML: Sparing effect of hemiplegia on tophaceous gout, Ann Rheum Dis 35:534, 1977.
21. Goodgold, J, and Eberstein, A: Electrodiagnosis of neuromuscular diseases, ed 3, Baltimore, 1983, Williams & Wilkins Co.
22. Gorkiewicz, R: Ultra-sound for subacromial bursitis, Phys Ther 64:24, 1984.
23. Greenleaf, JE, et al: Effects of exercise on fluid exchange and body composition in man during 14-day bed rest, J Appl Physiol 43:126, 1977.
24. Gresham, GE, and Labi, MLC: Functional assessment instruments currently available for documenting outcomes in rehabilitation medicine. In Granger, CV, and Gresham, GE, eds: Functional assessment in rehabilitation medicine, Baltimore, 1984, Williams & Wilkins Co.
25. Harris, ED, Jr, and McCroskery, PA: The influence of temperature and fibril stability on degradation of cartilage collagen by rheumatoid synovial collagenase, N Engl J Med 290:1, 1974.
26. Harris, R, and Copp, EP: Immobilization of the knee joint in rheumatoid arthritis, Ann Rheum Dis 21:353, 1962.
27. Hicks, J, and Nicholas, FF: Handbook on rehabilitation rheumatology, New York, 1985, Council on Rehabilitation Rheumatism. In press.
28. Himmel, PB: In Granger, C, and Gresham, G, editors: Functional assessment in rehabilitation medicine, Baltimore, 1984, Williams & Wilkins Co.
29. Hollander, JL, and Horvath, SM: Changes in joint temperature produced by diseases and by physical therapy, Arch Phys Med Rehabil 30:437, 1949.
30. Horvath, SM, and Hollander, SL: Intra-articular temperature as a measure of joint reaction, J Clin Invest 28:469, 1949.
31. Howell, DS, and Talbott, JH, editors: Osteoarthritis symposium, Florida, Palme Aire, Oct 20-22, 1980, Semin Arth Rheum II (suppl 1) 1981.
32. Jayson, MIV, and Dixon, ASJ: Intra-articular pressure in rheumatoid arthritis of the knee III: pressure changes during joint use, Ann Rheum Dis 29:401, 1970.
33. Jette, AM: Functional status index: reliability of the chronic disease evaluation influence, Arch Phys Med Rehabil 61:395, 1980.
34. Karanya, et al: Ergomatic evaluation of pathological gait, J Appl Physiol 55:607, 1983.
35. Kelly, M: The prevention of deformity in rheumatic disease, Med J Aust 2:1, 1950.
36. Kelly, M: Rheumatoid arthritis: the active immobilization of acutely inflamed joints, NZ Med J 60:311, 1961.
37. Klippel, JH, and Zvaifler, NJ: Neuropsychiatric abnormalities in systemic lupus erythematosus, Clin Rheum Dis 1:621, 1975.
38. Kohke, F: The effects of limitation of activity upon the human body, JAMA 196:825, 1966.
39. Krusen, FH: The scope of physical medicine and rehabilitation. In Krusen, FH, Kottke, FJ, and Ellwood, PM, editors: Handbook of physical medicine and rehabilitation, Philadelphia, 1971, WB Saunders Co.
40. Larsson, LG, and Baum, J: Bull Rheum Dis, vol 36, no 1, 1986.
41. Lehmann, JF, et al: Temperature distributions in the human thigh, produced by infrared, hot pack and microwave application, Arch Phys Med Rehabil 47:291, 1966.
42. Levy, A, et al: Transcutaneous electrical nerve stimulation in experimental acute arthritis, Arch Phys Med Rehabil 68:75, 1987.
43. Liang, MH, and Jette, AJ: Measuring functional ability in chronic arthritis: a critical review, Arthritis Rheum 24:80, 1981.

44. Liang, MH, et al: Comparative measurement efficiency and sensitivity of five health status instruments for arthritis research, Arthritis Rheum 28:542, 1985.

45. Lowman, EW: Rehabilitation of the rheumatoid cripple: a five-year study, Arthritis Rheum, vol 1, no 1, 1958.

46. Machover, S, and Sapecky, AJ: Effect of isometric exercise on the quadriceps muscle in patients with rheumatoid arthritis, Arch Phys Med Rehabil 47:737, 1966.

47. Mahoney, FI, and Barthel, DW: Functional evaluation—the Barthel index. In Rehabilitation notes, Baltimore, 1965, Baltimore City Medical Society.

48. Mainardi, CM, et al: Rheumatoid arthritis: failure of daily heat therapy to affect its progression, Arch Phys Med Rehabil 60:390, 1979.

49. McMorris, RO, and Elkins, EC: A study of production and evaluation of muscular hypertrophy, 35:420, 1954.

50. Meenan, RF, Gertman, PM, and Mason, FH: Measuring health status in arthritis: the arthritis impact measurement scales, Arthritis Rheum 23:146, 1980.

51. Melzack, R: Myotacial trigger points: relation to acupuncture and mechanism of pain, Arch Phys Med Rehabil 62:114, 1981.

52. Melzack, R, and Wahl, PD: Pain mechanism: a new theory, Science 150:971, 1965.

53. Merritt, JL, and Hunder, GG: Passive range of motion, not isometric exercise, amplifies acute urate synovitis, Arch Phys Med Rehabil 64:130, 1983.

54. Mills, JA, et al: Value of bed rest in patients with rheumatoid arthritis, N Engl J Med 284:453, 1971.

55. Moskowitz, E, and McCann, CB: Classification of disability in the chronically ill and aging, J Chronic Dis 5:342, 1957.

56. Moskowitz, RW: Treatment of osteoarthritis. In McCarty, DJ, editor: Textbook of rheumatology, ed 9, Philadelphia, 1979, Lea & Febiger.

57. Muray, DG: Modification of experimental arthritis in rabbits by tenotomy, J Surg Res 6:488, 1966.

58. Nordemar, R: Physical training in rheumatoid arthritis: a controlled long term study. II. Functional capacity and general attitudes, Scand J Rheumatol 10:25, 1981.

59. Nordemar, R, Edstrom, L, and Ekblom, B: Changes in muscle fibre size and physical performance in patients with rheumatoid arthritis after short term physical training, Scand J Rheumatol 5:70, 1976.

60. Nordemar, R, et al: Changes in muscle fibre size and physical performance in patients with rheumatoid arthritis after 7 month's physical training, Scand J Rheumatol 5:233, 1976.

61. Palmoski, MJ, and Brandt, KD: Immobilization of the knee prevents osteoarthritis after anterior cruciate ligament transection, Arthritis Rheum 25:1201, 1982.

62. Partridge, REH, and Duthie, IJR: Controlled trial of the effect of complete immobilization of the joints in rheumatoid arthritis, Ann Rheum Dis 22:91, 1963.

63. Pincus, T, et al: Elevated MMPI scores for hypochondriasis, depression, and hysteria in patients with rheumatoid arthritis reflect disease rather than psychological status, Arthritis Rheum 29:1456, 1986.

64. Radin, EL: Mechanical aspects of osteoarthrosis, Bull Rheum Dis 26:862, 1976.

65. Saltin, B, et al: Response to exercise after bed rest and after training, American Heart Association Monograph, No 23, 1968.

66. Smith, RD, and Palley, HF: Rest therapy for rheumatoid arthritis, Mayo Clin Proc 53:141, 1978.

67. Sokolow, J, et al: A method for the functional evaluation of disability, Arch Phys Med Rehabil 40:421, 1959.

68. Stecher, RM, and Karnach, LJ: Herberden's nodes IV: the effect of nerve injury upon formulation of degenerative joint disease of the fingers, Am J Med Sci 213:181, 1947.

69. Stein, H, and Kickson, RA: Reversed dynamic slings for knee flexion contractures in the hemophiliac, J Bone Joint Surg 51A:282, 1975.

70. Swezey, DL: Arthritis: rational therapy and rehabilitation, Philadelphia, 1978, WB Saunders Co.

71. Thompson, M, and Bywaters, EGL: Unilateral rheumatoid arthritis following hemiplegia, Ann Rheum Dis 21:370, 1962.

72. Twining, RH, Marcus, WY, and Garey, JL: Tendon rupture in SLE, JAMA 189:377, 1964.

73. Wahl, PD, and Cronly-Dillon, JR: Pain, itch and vibration, Arch Neurol 2:365, 1960.

CHAPTER 15

Cardiac rehabilitation

COMPONENTS OF A REHABILITATION PROGRAM FOR CORONARY PATIENTS

NANETTE KASS WENGER

GOALS FOR REHABILITATION OF CORONARY PATIENTS

The rehabilitative approach to the care of the coronary patient is designed to help that individual, by his or her own efforts, rapidly resume a normal or preillness life-style and return to a productive, active, and satisfying role in society.[115] The components of rehabilitative care include assessment of functional and psychologic status, efforts to limit the progression of the disease, the restoration, maintenance, and enhancement of physical capability, and social, educational, and vocational abilities.[103]

CATEGORIES OF CORONARY PATIENTS ELIGIBLE FOR REHABILITATIVE SERVICES

In the early years of coronary rehabilitative programs most patients enrolled for exercise training were recovered from a relatively uncomplicated myocardial infarction. In subsequent years patients with a more complicated clinical course were considered for more gradual or limited exercise rehabilitation. Currently a considerable number of patients receiving rehabilitative services have had coronary bypass surgery and coronary angioplasty.[31,46,54,64,67]

There is a growing trend toward providing rehabilitative services to a greater proportion of elderly patients and those with significant complications of their coronary disease — patients with compensated congestive heart failure, controlled but serious arrhythmias, permanent pacemakers, and so on. Patients with angina pectoris, who may or may not have had myocardial infarction or myocardial revascularization, are likely to comprise an increased proportion of those receiving rehabilitative care; this subgroup of coronary patients, who typically have significant functional impairments, has been underrepresented in most rehabilitation programs. Increasingly, categories of patients once excluded

from rehabilitation services (particularly exercise rehabilitation services) may be considered to require the most protracted and supervised rehabilitative care. Providing rehabilitative services to elderly coronary patients may prove the most economical approach to limiting or delaying the need for costly custodial care.

Exercise training has been progressively included in the management of patients with diabetes, hypertension, and end-stage renal disease, most of whom are likely to have concomitant coronary disease. Finally, coronary patients who have undergone cardiac transplantation (and possibly artificial heart implantation) will constitute a greater proportion of those who receive rehabilitation services.[32]

NEW CONCEPTS IN THE DELIVERY OF REHABILITATIVE SERVICES[79,107]

In the early years of rehabilitative care for coronary patients, the program itself was the preeminent feature. Highly structured, gradually progressive, prescriptive exercise training was the major component, and stringent guidelines were imposed for this fledgling form of care.

At that time exercise testing had relatively limited application in clinical practice and was a major service offered by cardiac rehabilitation programs. It was used to determine the eligibility for exercise, to formulate an exercise prescription, as a component of work evaluation, and to serially evaluate the patient's functional capacity.

Exercise testing is far more widely used in contemporary clinical practice, with exercise testing for risk stratification characteristic for patients after myocardial infarction in the 1980s.[21,62,106] A low-level exercise test before discharge from the hospital is used to identify patients who are at increased risk for an early recurrent coronary event and thus need invasive diagnostic and therapeutic procedures. The results of this exercise test are typically available when the patient is referred for cardiac rehabilitation services, and they can guide recommendations for physical activity and return to work. In addition, serial exercise tests have become part of the long-term clinical assessment of the coronary patient, with test data used to determine the adequacy of medical and surgical therapies in limiting myocardial ischemia, arrhythmias, and so on. Thus the results of serial exercise tests are also often available outside the context of a rehabilitation program, but this information can be used to guide rehabilitative physical activity as well.

Standards for rehabilitation programs have been promulgated by the American Heart Association, the American College of Sports Medicine, and scientific committees of the American Medical Association and other organizations.[3,4,17,81] These have delineated the appropriate components and expectations of rehabilitative care and have offered guidelines for facilities and personnel. However, the emphasis was on guidelines for the exercise testing and training components. More recently, the American College of Sports Medicine[58,113] has categorized coronary patients who are likely to be able to exercise safely without supervision.

The trend is toward delivery of specific rehabilitative services required by a patient, rather than requiring that the patient conform to a highly structured, relatively inflexible, multi-interventional program. An individualized approach is more acceptable to patients, referring physicians, and insurance carriers. Recent emphasis on the value of coronary risk reduction, on the importance of psychosocial assessment and interventions, and on the role of work assessment and vocational counseling mandates that these components, which can be offered in conjunction with supervised exercise rehabilitation programs, also be available for appropriate patients.

Quality assurance, as well as evaluations of effectiveness and cost effectiveness, must be task specific; that is, standards must be set for each service to be delivered and outcome measures must be specifically identified and related to the goals of intervention for the individual patient. For example, in the rehabilitation of elderly nonemployed patients, some would undergo a progressive physical activity regimen with the goal of an appropriately active life-style—they would be able to live and function independently and to enjoy leisure and recreational activities for a longer time. Other elderly patients would undergo a low-intensity activity regimen and would learn work simplification techniques with the goal of helping them maintain their independence. Both goals differ from the major rationale of exercise training in younger patients, where a decrease in symptoms and improvement in functional status is anticipated to enable a return to remunerative employment.

An increasing number of patients perform rehabilitative prescribed exercise regimens with limited or intermittent supervision or independently at home. Programs must address the nonexercise educational needs of these patients. In addition to exercise-related education and counseling, the other informational and learning needs of these patients must be met. Technologic advances such as computer-assisted education and interactive video systems may enable teaching, reinforcement of education, and tracking of accomplishments at sites distant from the rehabilitation program—perhaps at work, in the home, in a senior citizen facility, or in a community clinic.[105]

SPECIFIC SERVICES IN CORONARY REHABILITATION SETTINGS[108]
Exercise testing

As previously noted, exercise testing may be performed as a service of a coronary rehabilitation program, but exercise test data obtained for other components of clinical care—at predischarge testing during a hospitalization[17,36,106] or for serial assessment in a physician's office—may also guide rehabilitative physical activity in a supervised or an unsupervised setting. Similarly, exercise test data obtained in the rehabilitation setting for exercise prescription and for evaluation of the effect of training should be promptly transmitted to the primary care physician, who can use it to make decisions about alteration of therapy and the need for evaluative procedures. Exercise test data are often used to determine the efficacy of medical and surgical strategies designed to limit myocardial ischemia; exercise rehabilitation is included among the medical modalities that may do so.

Exercise training[3,4,17]
Appropriate goals—survival versus functional improvement

The previously published goals of exercise training require reexamination and revision. In the past, the focus of most controlled clinical trials of exercise was on reduction of mortality and morbidity; the specific component of morbidity most often assessed was nonfatal reinfarction. Most physicians currently recommend exercise, and most patients currently engage in exercise rehabilitation with the goal of decreasing symptoms and improving function and sense of well-being—a goal that is common to other medical and surgical interventions for symptomatic coronary disease. A recent position report of the American College of Cardiology defines cardiovascular rehabilitation as "those exercise and counseling services which will reduce symptoms or improve cardiac function."[73]

Many other therapies are variably applied in the care of coronary patients: myocardial revascularization procedures, anti-ischemic drug therapies, drugs designed to limit platelet aggregation or clotting, and modifications of a variety of conventional coronary risk factors. It is unrealistic to assess exercise training as a sole feature for its effect on future cardiac events, mortality, or reinfarction. Exercise training may engender other favorable risk modifications[9] or may reveal evidence of activity-induced myocardial ischemia or its complications, thus enabling earlier treatment. Despite these problems of multiple concomitant interventions, most randomized clinical trials of exercise training have demonstrated a 24% to 32% trend favoring survival,* with a statistically significant survival advantage for exercising subjects evident only when all trial data were pooled.[56,65] This improved survival is comparable to that described with beta-blockade following myocardial infarction. A statistically significant decrease in recurrent coronary events was also evident from the pooled trial data.[56] Morbidity and mortality data from individual studies were limited by methodologic weaknesses that included small sample sizes, the preponderance of low-risk patients in many studies, late time of enrollment after acute events, lack of consideration of multiple and confounding endpoints, and problems of compliance, dropouts, contamination, and the like. Clinical trial requirements for strictly standardized interventions may have encouraged dropouts and lack of compliance in excess of that occurring with clinical care, and systematic neglect of the control group's activity program in an exercise-aware society may have encouraged these individuals to undertake physical activity outside the randomized trial. In fact, the sole randomized clinical trial that individually showed a favorable effect on mortality, done by Kallio and associates,[45] not only was an exercise trial, but also entailed multifactorial interventions that were begun shortly after discharge from the hospital following myocardial infarction. The predominant favorable effect was a reduction in sudden death, particularly in the first 6 months after infarction. Furthermore, mortality and morbidity endpoints (with the morbidity feature assessed being nonfatal infarction), although amenable to evaluation in a clinical trial, are less appropriate than consideration of a decrease in symptoms, an increase in the exercise threshold required to precipitate angina, an augmentation of function, an improvement in the sense of well-being, and their consequences—the major goals of exercise rehabilitation regimens. The efficacy of exercise training should be assessed against these goals.

There is no evidence that the short-term, modest-intensity aerobic exercise characteristic of most rehabilitation programs for coronary patients increases the coronary collateral circulation, improves myocardial oxygen supply or myocardial perfusion, or alters the angiographic appearance of coronary artery lesions.[28,47,85,98] The primary beneficial effect is on the peripheral (skeletal) musculature. However, an improvement in exercise tolerance has been maintained among exercising patients for 4 years or more after infarction.[66]

Changes in initiation, design, and duration of exercise training

Exercise training regimens for coronary patients have changed greatly since the earlier years, in part because of the general acceptance of early ambulation during the hospital stay for myocardial infarction and myocardial revascularization procedures.[108] Patients are less likely to have protracted deconditioning resulting from immobilization during their hospital stay. The decrease in the interval between discharge from the hospital after an acute event and enrollment in exercise rehabilitation has further limited the deconditioning related to inactivity. Rehabilitation programs usually commence as soon as possible following discharge from the hospital.[73] For patients with angina pectoris that significantly limits activity[80] or those who have had major complications of myocardial infarction or myocardial revascularization surgery necessitating a prolonged hospital stay, an exercise regimen that begins with very low-level, supervised activity may be warranted.

The "compression of morbidity"[34] characteristic of the accelerated contemporary acute interventions often no longer warrants differentiation between phases II and III of exercise rehabilitation; many patients, particularly those after coronary angioplasty or coronary bypass surgery without prior protracted angina or prior infarction, may enter immediately into what is traditionally considered a phase III program, without an intermediate phase II component. Progression in the intensity and duration of exercise training is usually more rapid for these patients as well.[74] In contrast, patients with severe angina pectoris or complications of myocardial infarction or of coronary bypass surgery, those who are elderly and may have significant co-morbidity, and those who remain high-risk coronary patients by virtue of continuing myocardial ischemia or serious arrhythmias may require what is now characterized as a phase II program for a protracted period. Therefore it would seem more appropriate that exercise rehabilitation be divided into hospital and posthospital components and that the out-of-hospital characteristics of the exercise training, surveillance, and electrocardiographic (ECG) monitoring be individualized for the patient's clinical and risk status, rather than be divided into traditional phases of relatively fixed composition and duration. The total duration of exercise rehabilitation also varies considerably depending on the goal of exercise training and the characteristics of the patient. This underlines the importance of responding to the individual patient's exercise rehabilitation needs, rather than having the patient conform to program phases or requirements.

Need for routine electrocardiographic monitoring: new data

Although in the early years of exercise rehabilitation most patients did not have continuous ECG monitoring because ECG telemetry was not generally available, continuous ECG monitoring has become increasingly prevalent for the early weeks to months of many coronary exercise rehabilitation programs. This was encouraged by the increased availability of the technology for ECG telemetry, the requirements and reimbursement practices of insurance carriers, and concerns for patient safety. The duration of ECG monitoring during recent years has decrementally paralleled the reimbursement patterns of most insurance carriers (decreasing serially from 2 years to 1 year to 6 months and most recently to 3 months),

---

*References 7, 72, 78, 87, 88, 110.

which suggests that it was not determined primarily by medical criteria or by the level of exercise attained. Indeed, another subset of patients at high risk for an adverse event during exercise typically had this complication 1 to 2 years after infarction. This group was characterized by an above-average exercise performance, marked and asymptomatic ST depression during exercise testing, and habitual exceeding of their recommended exercise prescription during training[42]; the mean duration of exercise training before an adverse event was 224 ± 235 hours.

A number of surveys have been undertaken to assess the safety of medically supervised exercise rehabilitation for coronary patients. From 1960 to 1977, one death occurred on average in 116,402 patient exercise hours and one myocardial infarction per 232,805 patients hours; one cardiac arrest was described per 32,593 hours, typically associated with successful resuscitation without resulting infarction.[38] Early data suggested that the risks of medically supervised exercise training were greater in patients who were not ECG monitored; however, characteristics of the program other than ECG monitoring, including exercise intensity and characteristics of the participants, were not analyzed. Thus, even though data from ECG monitoring resulted in changes in exercise prescription or medication,[60] the benefits of routine ECG monitoring have not been substantiated. Furthermore, none of these data encompassed current concepts of risk stratification; most programs at that time included few patients after myocardial revascularization and none who were receiving the current medical therapies. The combination of high cost, increased requirements for equipment and professional services, and suboptimal availability and accessibility of ECG-monitored exercise programs has resulted in challenges to the need for costly, routine, and protracted ECG monitoring during exercise training.[42,60,73,95,97]

A more recent study of cardiovascular complications of supervised outpatient exercise rehabilitation (encompassing the years 1980 to 1984) showed a considerably lower exercise risk; the number of cardiac arrests was one fourth and the fatality rate one seventh of those previously reported.[97] Neither the extent of ECG monitoring nor the size or experience of the exercise rehabilitation program appeared to influence the complication rate. These data suggest that routine ECG monitoring does not offer a significant safety advantage and does not warrant the considerable increase in cost and associated requirement for equipment and trained personnel. However, the sizeable percentage of successful resuscitations from cardiac arrest that occurred in the supervised exercise settings contributing to the survey warrants delineation of the patient subgroups who might benefit from supervised exercise; this has yet to be done. Similar data emphasizing safety are also reported from Australia.[27] The occurrence of cardiac events ranged in time from 1 to 4 months, and most coincided with the warm-up or cool-down period of exercise. It is not known whether better patient selection, improved medical or surgical therapies, better patient education and adherence to the exercise

prescription, or yet other features have contributed to the recent improved safety of exercise for coronary patients.

Supervised versus unsupervised exercise training

There has been a trend toward initially independent exercise or rapid transfer of patients from a supervised to an unsupervised exercise setting. This may decrease the cost and increase the availability of rehabilitative physical activity for these low-risk patients. Because economic or logistic constraints often limit the availability of supervised exercise programs, preliminary criteria have been developed to identify patients who require at least initial medical supervision (and probably ECG monitoring) of exercise because of their increased risk status[58,113]; patients lacking these high-risk characteristics often exercise independently. Several studies have documented the efficacy of home exercise in improving functional capacity for appropriately selected patients after myocardial infarction,[20,59] although greater improvements in functional capacity were associated with more intense exercise supervision.[19] Transtelephonic ECG monitoring appears to be a promising alternative for patients who live in areas remote from exercise centers.[19,29] Some patients intermittently exercise in supervised and unsupervised settings. Even in supervised exercise settings, economic constraints may mandate that a larger number of patients exercise together to reduce the personnel-to-patient ratio.

The challenge presented to exercise programs is considerable but may favorably affect the economics of exercise rehabilitation. About half of all survivors of myocardial infarction are at low risk. These low-risk patients can rapidly and safely resume an active life-style and exercise independently but often have had no exercise experience as an adult; the prescribing physician or rehabilitation program must be prepared to teach them how to exercise; signs and symptoms of exercise intolerance; how to self-monitor their exercise, including techniques of pulse counting and the use of the rating of perceived exertion to gauge training intensity[10]; safety features to limit orthopedic complications; how to select appropriate shoes, clothing, and equipment; and environmental considerations in exercising. The program must also offer opportunities to practice exercise skills and provide the support needed for maintenance of an exercise regimen. Since exercise rehabilitation should be designed to motivate patients to maintain a lifelong pattern of physical activity, patients leaving supervised exercise programs require counseling to help them select and initiate unsupervised exercise in the community.

In the supervised, ECG-monitored programs of exercise rehabilitation, the patients are likely to be sicker, to be at higher risk, and to require more protracted periods of ECG monitoring than those described previously. Current recommendations concerning the patients requiring medical supervision of exercise, probably with ECG monitoring, include those with a markedly reduced exercise capacity, severely depressed left ventricular function, or complex ventricular rhythm disturbances; those who develop angina pectoris, marked ST segment depression, QT prolongation, or exercise-induced hypotension (as evidence of ischemia-induced ventricular dysfunction) at low levels of exercise; and those unable to self-monitor their exercise heart rates.[58,113] At least until comparative safety data are available, patients with congestive heart failure,[15,112] controlled serious arrhythmias, and persistent evidence of ischemia at low levels of activity should probably receive protracted exercise surveillance; patients in the ECG-monitored programs may be in categories that previously were excluded from exercise rehabilitation.

The recent data cited above should encourage the restructuring of models for delivery of exercise rehabilitation services. Additional new information may also modify the characteristics of the exercise recommended. Postoperative patients especially need range-of-motion exercises for the upper extremities to restore flexibility and maintain muscle tone.[74] Isometric activities, particularly for low-risk patients who have progressed beyond low-intensity levels of dynamic exercise, do not appear to impose additional risk and may improve the patient's ability to return to active occupational and recreational life-styles.[48] As dynamic exercise intensity progressively increases, addition of isometric activities, including weight training, will become more common.

High-intensity exercise training

In a selected subgroup of patients, high-intensity, long-term exercise training may be appropriate, with the goal of improving cardiac function.[23,35,44] Individuals in this category are likely to resemble the small subset of coronary patients currently engaged in marathon running and those studied by Ehsani and associates.[23] High-intensity, prolonged exercise is not recommended for most middle-aged patients with symptomatic coronary atherosclerotic heart disease but may fit the desired life-styles of some patients.

Benefits of exercise rehabilitation

Benefits of exercise rehabilitation, in addition to augmentation of functional capacity, include favorable metabolic changes: decrease in triglyceride levels,[69] increased sensitivity to insulin, and improved HDL/LDL cholesterol ratios.[39,114] Exercise also improves joint mobility and stability, enhances neuromuscular coordination, and makes weight control easier. Improved psychosocial status is manifest as a lessening of fear, depression, and dependency and an increase in self-confidence and self-esteem.[92] Improved work attendance and increase in leisure activities are also described.[14,87] As myocardial oxygen demand lessens for the workload of specific activities, the number and dosage of medications needed may decrease.

Coronary risk reduction—education and counseling[41,84,94]

Modification of coronary risk factors is designed to retard the progression of atherosclerosis or potentially cause regression of atherosclerotic obstructive lesions.[6,11] Hyperlipidemia, hypertension, and cigarette smoking all adversely affect outcome in patients recovered from myocardial infarction.[86] Despite the lack of definitive evidence that risk modifications can retard or reverse coronary atherosclerosis, reduce recurrent coronary events, or prolong survival in an *individual* patient, the minimal expense and risk relative to the potential benefit have generated enthusiasm for its clinical implementation. This component of rehabilitative care does not involve simply the transmission of cognitive information, but rather the teaching of the skills needed for life-style modifications, the ability to practice these techniques, and the provision of the reinforcement and motivation needed for the maintenance of desired changes.[8] Many facets of care after myocardial infarction entail modifications of life-style; education and counseling can provide insight into behaviors that may reduce the risk of reinfarction. Risk reduction education and counseling in a structured setting may be appropriate for patients who are not eligible for exercise rehabilitation because of concurrent medical illnesses or for those with low-risk status for exercise who may exercise independently and participate only in formal or structured cardiac educational services. A number of reports describe better risk modification among participants in organized rehabilitation programs than with usual care, as well as a favorable effect on psychosocial adjustment,[24,63,99] possibly because of the repetitive educational counseling offered. However, there has not been adequate comparison of the efficacy in changing risk-related behaviors between structured group instruction and the informal counseling given by an individual physician. A group or class educational setting has been described as less threatening, allowing the patient to maintain self-esteem while learning, to participate in the group and help others, and to assume control and responsibility. The ideal way to provide information and support to coronary patients and their families in the early months after infarction or coronary surgery is unknown. Although the response to the teaching of cardiopulmonary resuscitation (CPR) techniques to patients and their families has been generally favorable, one study described CPR training for family members as having an adverse psychologic effect on high-risk cardiac patients.[22]

The major goal of secondary prevention is to limit or delay recurrent events in patients with clinical manifestations of coronary atherosclerosis. Traditional coronary risk modification has been addressed most extensively in survivors of myocardial infarction. Cigarette smoking, uncontrolled hypertension, and hypercholesterolemia contribute to the increased risk of patients who have recovered from myocardial infarction; all these risk components are modifiable.* Because patients who have required coronary bypass surgery or coronary angioplasty are those with accelerated atherosclerosis, risk reduction is also appropriate for

---

*References 5, 40, 55, 76, 83, 86, 102.

these populations. The postoperative recurrence of symptoms and deterioration of function in patients after coronary saphenous vein graft bypass surgery appears to be due predominantly to progression of atherosclerosis both in the graft vessels and in the native circulation.[12,13,16,52,71] In a number of studies, coronary surgery did not appear to encourage favorable modification of the coronary risk profile of patients after the operation.[16,49]

Cessation of cigarette smoking

Cessation of cigarette smoking may be the most effective single risk intervention for patients following myocardial infarction.[1,18,61,111] Several studies have unequivocally documented a substantially improved prognosis of both younger and older patients with angina and following myocardial infarction associated with discontinuation of cigarette smoking. A 20% to 50% lowering of total mortality was described, with a concomitant decrease in sudden death and fatal reinfarction. The favorable effect is most prominent in the early years following infarction. Dietary counseling can limit the adverse effect of weight gain that often occurs with smoking cessation.

Nutritional counseling

Dietary assessment and modification is appropriate for patients with hyperlipidemia, obesity, and hypertension.

Hypercholesterolemia is an adverse prognostic factor for patients after myocardial infarction and unfavorably affects the patency of vein grafts following coronary bypass surgery. The initial management of hyperlipidemia is dietary[50] and involves not only information about food consumption, but also learning about food preparation and eating outside the home.

Although obesity is not a powerful independent coronary risk factor, weight reduction favorably affects the level of blood pressure, blood glucose and lipids, and uric acid, as well as lessening cardiac work, limiting angina, and improving exercise tolerance. Education should include information about caloric restriction and exercise.

Sodium restriction for patients with hypertension has beneficial effects in limiting the hypokalemia associated with diuretic therapy and potentially lessening the needed dosage of antihypertensive drugs.

Control of hypertension

Control of elevated blood pressure, in addition to decreasing the occurrence of cerebrovascular accident and congestive heart failure, decreases cardiac work; it thus may lessen angina and improve functional capacity.[30] Control of hypertension involves dietary sodium restriction, weight control, limitation of excessive alcohol intake, and physical activity recommendations, in addition to pharmacotherapy.

Psychosocial services

Many patients who have angina pectoris, have had myocardial infarction, or have undergone myocardial revascularization surgery are more disabled by psychologic problems than by the physiologic consequences of their coronary illness.[77,108] However, only during the past two decades have there been systemic efforts to define the type and severity of psychologic problems in coronary patients, their frequency, and their influence on outcome. Rehabilitation requires limiting and reversing these psychologic complications. Because many adverse psychosocial outcomes appear to be related to the patient's perception of personal health status, this potential barrier to recovery may be favorably affected by education and counseling. Many patients consider that they have received inadequate or ambiguous information from their physicians and other health professionals about their prognosis and long-term care plans.[37,57] Educational programs that provide information and correct misinformation or misunderstanding about the illness help alleviate the fear and anxiety that often cause unwarranted invalidism after a coronary event.

Physical activity is also an important intervention strategy to limit the incidence and severity of psychosocial complications.[53,87,92] Patients who exercise generally have an improved self-image, are better able to cope with life stresses, and are more likely to renounce the sick role. An improvement in family, occupational, and community relationships has been described among exercising patients, with the influence on peer reinforcement in a group exercise setting and an educational-counseling group or club seen as contributory. Exercising patients in randomized exercise trials returned more rapidly to sexual activity,[87] to a near-normal life-style, and to work[93] and had improvement in work capacity, income, and job responsibility. Indeed, in this study considerable physical and psychosocial benefit occurred with very low-level exercise, previously believed to be of "placebo" level; these data have important implications for the low-level exercise appropriate for elderly and sicker populations.[92]

A major component of psychosocial distress is the fear that physical exertion may cause a recurrence of anginal symptoms, precipitate myocardial infarction, or result in sudden death; this fear can cause prolonged abstinence from activity, including sexual activity and work activity. Interpreting the results of exercise testing to patients, with extrapolation of test results to apparently dissimilar activities, often improved their view of their physical capabilities.[25,26] Helping postsurgical patients differentiate normal postoperative chest discomfort or the symptoms of postoperative pericarditis from myocardial ischemic pain encourages resumption of activity.

The role of the family has been neglected in rehabilitation; the characteristics of the family and the resultant social support system may influence the success or failure of rehabilitative activities. Although in a recent study husbands underestimated their ability to perform treadmill exercise following myocardial infarction, wives rated their husbands' abilities at even lower levels. Watching her husband perform treadmill exercise tests did not significantly alter the wife's perception of her husband's cardiac capabilities following infarction; walking on the treadmill at the highest level accomplished by her husband increased the wife's perception of his ability to be physically active after infarction.[96]

Involving patients in planning for recovery, both during the hospital stay and afterward, teaching self-monitoring of the heart rate response to activity, and identifying areas of patient decision and responsibility are components of education and counseling that return control to the patient, improve self-image, and help patients renounce the sick role.

Although few adequate controlled studies are available,[70,75] combinations of structured exercise training, education, and counseling appear to provide modest but consistent psychosocial benefit. The specific contribution of the peer support available in a group setting has not been defined.

Friedman and associates[33] described a significant decrease in nonfatal reinfarction attributable to alteration of type A behavior by patients after myocardial infarction. Although less attention is currently directed to the classical type A personality, the components of persistent hostility and suppressed anger appear to increase the risk of coronary events. Most therapeutic interventions have been neither well characterized nor adequately evaluated. The role of stress management also requires elucidation, although preliminary reports seem encouraging.[68] However, because the pattern of coping with an acute illness is comparable to that seen with other prior major illnesses or life crises, patients with habitual unsuccessful adaptation to stress should be anticipated to require added support and counseling following myocardial infarction or myocardial revascularization procedures.

Vocational assessment and guidance

A major goal of rehabilitation for patients recovered from myocardial infarction or coronary bypass surgery is to help them resume prior gainful employment, change jobs if needed, and participate in desired avocational or retirement activities. Coronary heart disease remains the leading cause for which persons receive premature disability benefits under the U.S. Social Security system[90]; during the past decade almost one fourth of the men and women receiving Social Security disability allowances were considered permanently disabled by coronary disease. Both after myocardial infarction and following myocardial revascularization, symptomatic and functional improvements correlate poorly with return to work and with general resumption of preillness life-style; psychosocial status appears to be an important determinant of these latter features.[101] Because of the major economic implications of failure to resume work, there is considerable interest in the psychosocial benefits of rehabilitative care.

Exercise testing to assess a patient's functional capacity for work, exercise training to enhance functional capacity, and on-the-job ECG monitoring if needed may help the patient return to work. Because an overwhelming determinant of return to work following coronary bypass surgery is the patient's preoperative perception of the ability to do so,[91] preoperative and postoperative counseling may be helpful. However, since improved functional status and absence of angina favorably influence employment,[89,100] medical and surgical therapies (including exercise training as a component of medical therapy) may also prove helpful.

Gauging the efficacy of rehabilitative physical activity by a return to work outcome may not be appropriate. The beneficial effect on resumption of employment associated with an improved physical work capacity as a result of exercise training may be overshadowed by more compelling nonmedical determinants of failure to return to work, including the financial, social, disability, and compensation benefits of remaining unemployed. In general, the greater the social benefits available, the less the incentive to return to work after a coronary event.[2,109]

Results of exercise testing, by documenting the functional impact of coronary disease on the patient, can guide recommendations for occupational activity levels. Currently most low-risk patients whose occupations do not include heavy labor return to work within 2 months after infarction. Exercise test data relate moderately well to work demands of jobs when differences in temperature, environment, intellectual demands, relationship to food intake and other activities, and emotional stress are considered. The adequate performance of an exercise test may encourage patients to return to work, since they no longer fear that their heart cannot tolerate the physical and emotional demands of the job.[25,26] Patients free of symptoms or evidence of myocardial ischemia and arrhythmia at exercise testing typically are free of these adverse consequences even when static and dynamic effort are combined, as at work.[44] Indeed, even the concern about heavy labor has been challenged, since more than 95% of patients who experienced a recurrent coronary event after infarction did not engage in strenuous activity in proximity to the event; however, more data are needed to document the safety of early resumption of high-intensity work.

The patient's perception of personal physical capabilities and the expectations of return to work following myocardial infarction are powerful predictors of the ability to do so. Counseling as to how the intensity of occupational or recreational activities compares to that of the exercise test may extend the patient's perceived ability to engage in these activities.[25] This can readily be done in a rehabilitation program or following exercise testing and has been associated with improved work resumption.

For elderly or more impaired patients, where return to remunerative work is not the desired rehabilitation outcome, resumption of self-care and of avocational or leisure activities should be the goal of exercise testing, exercise training, and counseling. Teaching of work simplification and energy-conserving techniques may be beneficial for selected patients.[104]

EVALUATION OF EFFECTIVENESS AND COST EFFECTIVENESS—REHABILITATION OF THE CORONARY PATIENT

A rehabilitation program should not be evaluated as a unit, nor should it be evaluated against the traditional biomedical outcome measures of improved survival or freedom from reinfarction. With a chronic symptomatic illness such as coronary atherosclerotic heart disease, limitation of symptoms and improvement of function, as well as limitation of progression of the disease, may be more desired outcomes and thus more appropriate outcome measures.[51] For example, 20% of survivors of myocardial infarction have varying degrees of residual physiologic, psychosocial, and vocational disabilities,[82] and many patients following coronary bypass surgery and coronary angioplasty have a suboptimal recovery because of psychologic or social complications. The rehabilitative approach should be designed to limit the physical, psychosocial, and vocational invalidism. As each patient undertakes rehabilitative services, the goal of each service should be defined for that patient and the outcome measured in relation to that specific goal.

In an assessment of the cost effectiveness of individual rehabilitation services, outcome measures for different patients may include improvement in functional capacity, return to work, changes in life-style, improved quality of life, risk reduction, and others. Cost effectiveness may differ for individual or combinations of these outcome measures, and the importance of each may differ in different settings.

Unfortunately, there are no widely accepted psychosocial outcome criteria for the evaluation of rehabilitative services, and most current nonmedical assessments have been based on return to remunerative employment. Arbitrary levels of improvement in functional capacity are often used as exit criteria from structured exercise rehabilitation programs, rather than adjusting the exit criteria to the activity level appropriate for an individual patient, including the high-risk characteristics of one subset of coronary patients with above-average physical capabilities.[42]

Other criteria of successful rehabilitation amenable to assessment include life quality aspects such as the patient's perception of physical improvement, rather than solely objective data about functional capacity, favorable modifications of preillness life-style (coronary risk reduction) and degree of satisfaction with these new behaviors, psychosocial adjustments in family, sexual, and interpersonal roles, and potential for promotion and advancement at work, the level of pay, the job prestige, and the extent to which the work resumed is commensurate with the patient's knowledge, skill, and abilities, and the facilitation of functional independence, prevention of premature disability, and delay or lessening of the need for custodial care for elderly patients.

REFERENCES

1. Aberg, A, et al: Cessation of smoking after myocardial infarction: effects of mortality after 10 years, Br Heart J 49:416, 1983.
2. Almeida, D, et al: Return to work after coronary bypass surgery. Circulation 68(suppl II):II-205, 1983.
3. American College of Sports Medicine: Guidelines for exercise testing and prescription, ed 3, Philadelphia, 1986, Lea & Febiger.
4. American Heart Association: The exercise standards book, Dallas, 1979 (revised 1981), The Association.
5. Berg, KG, Canner, PL, and Hainline, A, Jr: Coronary Drug Project Research Group: high-density lipoprotein cholesterol and prognosis after myocardial infarction, Circulation 66:1176, 1982.
6. Blankenhorn, DH: The prevention, deceleration and possible regression of coronary atherosclerosis. In Hurst, JW, editor: The heart, update III, New York, 1980, McGraw-Hill Book Co.
7. Blomqvist, CG: Role of exercise training in secondary prevention of ischemic heart disease, Prevent Med 12:228, 1983.
8. Blumenthal, JA, et al: Cardiac rehabilitation: a new frontier for behavioral medicine, J Cardiac Rehabil 3:637, 1983.
9. Bonanno, JA, and Lies, JA: Effects of physical training on coronary risk factors, Am J Cardiol 33:760, 1974.
10. Borg, G, Psychophysical bases of perceived exertion, Med Sci Sports Exerc 14:377, 1982.
11. Borhani, NO: Prevention of coronary heart disease in practice: implications of the results of recent trials, JAMA 254:257, 1985.
12. Bourassa, MG, et al: Progression of atherosclerosis in coronary arteries and bypass grafts: ten years later, Am J Cardiol 53:102C, 1984.
13. Campeau, L, et al: Loss of improvement and recurrence of angina 1 to 12 years after CABG: role of preoperative variables, degree of correction and changes in grafts or in coronary arteries, Circulation 70(suppl 2):II-20, 1984.
14. Carson, P: Activity after myocardial infarction, Br Med J 288:1, 1984.
15. Conn, EH, Williams, RS, and Wallace, AG: Exercise responses before and after physical conditioning in patients with severely depressed left ventricular function, Am J Cardiol 49:296, 1982.
16. CASS principal investigators and their associates: Coronary Artery Surgery Study (CASS): a randomized trial of coronary artery bypass surgery: quality of life in patients randomly assigned to treatment groups, Circulation 68:951, 1983.
17. Council on Scientific Affairs: Physician-supervised exercise programs in rehabilitation of patients with coronary heart disease, JAMA 245:1463, 1981.
18. Daly, E, et al: Long-term effect on mortality of stopping smoking after unstable angina or myocardial infarction, Br Med J 287:324, 1983.
19. DeBusk, RF, et al: Exercise training soon after myocardial infarction, Am J Cardiol 44:1223, 1979.
20. DeBusk, RF, et al: Medically directed at-home rehabilitation soon after clinically uncomplicated acute myocardial infarction: a new model for patient care, Am J Cardiol 55:251, 1985.
21. DeBusk, RF, et al: Identification and treatment of low-risk patients after acute myocardial infarction and coronary-artery bypass graft surgery, N Engl J Med 314:161, 1986.
22. Dracup, K, et al: Cardiopulmonary resuscitation (CPR) training: consequences for family members of high-risk cardiac patients, Arch Intern Med 146:1757, 1986.
23. Ehsani, AA, et al: Cardiac effects of prolonged and intense exercise training in patients with coronary artery disease, Am J Cardiol 50:246, 1982.
24. Erdman, RA, and Duivenvoorden, HJ: Psychological evaluation of a cardiac rehab program: a randomized clinical trial in patients with myocardial infarction, J Cardiac Rehabil 3:696, 1983.

25. Ewart, CK, and Taylor, CB: The effects of early post-myocardial infarction exercise testing on subsequent quality of life, Quality Life Cardiovasc Care 1:162, 1985.

26. Ewart, CK, et al: Effects of early postmyocardial infarction exercise testing on self-perception and subsequent physical activity, Am J Cardiol 51:1076, 1983.

27. Fagan, ET, et al: Serious ventricular arrhythmias in a cardiac rehabilitation programme, Med J Aust 141:421, 1984.

28. Ferguson, RJ, et al: Effect of physical training on treadmill exercise capacity, collateral circulation, and progression of coronary disease, Am J Cardiol 34:764, 1974.

29. Fletcher, GF, et al: Telephonically-monitored home exercise early after coronary artery bypass surgery, Chest 86:198, 1984.

30. Forman, S, et al: Blood pressure in survivors of myocardial infarction, J Am Coll Cardiol 4:1135, 1984.

31. Foster, C, et al: Work capacity and left ventricular function during rehabilitation after myocardial revascularization surgery, Circulation 69:748, 1984.

32. Franklin, BA, and Hellerstein, HK: Exercise testing and training of coronary patients with selected additional problems. In Wenger, NK, and Hellerstein, HK, editors: Rehabilitation of the coronary patient, ed 2, New York, 1984, John Wiley & Sons.

33. Friedman, M, et al: Feasibility of altering type A behavior pattern after myocardial infarction, Circulation 66:83, 1982.

34. Fries, JJ: Aging, natural death, and the compression of morbidity, N Engl J Med 303:130, 1980.

35. Hagberg, JM, Ehsani, AA, and Hollosky, JO: Effect of 12 months of intense exercise training on stroke volume in patients with coronary artery disease, Circulation 67:1194, 1983.

36. Hamm, LF, Stull, GA, and Crow, RS: Exercise testing early after myocardial infarction: historic perspective and current uses, Prog Cardiovasc Dis 28:463, 1986.

37. Harris, L, et al: Americans and their doctors, 1985.

38. Haskell, WL: Cardiovascular complications during exercise training of cardiac patients, Circulation 57:920, 1978.

39. Heath, GW, et al: Exercise training improves lipoprotein lipid profiles in patients with coronary artery disease, Am Heart J 105:889, 1983.

40. Heliovaara, M, et al: Importance of coronary risk factors in the presence or absence of myocardial ischemia, Am J Cardiol 50:1248, 1983.

41. Hogan, CA, and Neill, WA: Effects of a teaching program on knowledge, physical activity, and socialization in patients disabled by stable angina pectoris, J Cardiac Rehabil 2:379, 1982.

42. Hossack, KF, and Hartwig, R: Cardiac arrest associated with supervised cardiac rehabilitation, J Cardiac Rehabil 2:402, 1982.

43. Hung, J, et al: Comparison of cardiovascular response to combined static-dynamic effort, postprandial dynamic effort and dynamic effort alone in patients with chronic ischemic heart disease, Circulation 65:1411, 1982.

44. Hung, J, et al: Changes in rest and exercise myocardial perfusion and left ventricular function 3 to 26 weeks after clinically uncomplicated acute myocardial infarction: effects of exercise training, Am J Cardiol 54:943, 1984.

45. Kallio, V, et al: Reduction in sudden deaths by a multifactorial intervention programme afer acute myocardial infarction, Lancet 2:1091, 1979.

46. Kappagoda, CT, and Greenwood, PV: Physical training with minimal hospital supervision of patients after coronary artery bypass surgery, Arch Phys Med Rehabil 65:57, 1984.

47. Kennedy, CC, et al: One-year graduated exercise program for men with angina pectoris: evaluation by physiologic studies and coronary arteriography, Mayo Clin Proc 51:231, 1976.

48. Kilbom, A, and Persson, J: Cardiovascular response to combined dynamic and static exercise, Circ Res 48(suppl I):I-93, 1981.

49. Leaman, DM, Brower, RW, and Meester, GT: Coronary artery bypass surgery: a stimulus to modify existing risk factors? Chest 81:16, 1982.

50. Levy, RI, Hyperlipoproteinemia and its management, J Cardiovasc Med 5:435, 1980.

51. Luginbuhl, WH, et al: Prevention and rehabilitation as a means of cost containment: the example of myocardial infarction, J Public Health Policy 2:103, 1981.

52. McIntosh, HD: Aortocoronary bypass grafting: an internist's perspective, Circulation 65(suppl 2):II-77, 1982.

53. McPherson, BD, et al: Psychological effects of an exercise program for post-infarct and normal adult men, J Sports Med Phys Fitness 7:95, 1967.

54. Maresh, CM, et al: Comparison of rehabilitation benefits after percutaneous transluminal coronary angioplasty and coronary artery bypass graft surgery, J Cardiac Rehabil 5:124, 1985.

55. Marmor, A, et al: Recurrent myocardial infarction: clinical predictors and prognostic implications, Circulation 66:415, 1982.

56. May, GS, et al: Secondary prevention after myocardial infarction: a review of long-term trials, Prog Cardiovasc Dis 24:331, 1982.

57. Mayou, R, Foster, A, and Williamson, B: Medical care after myocardial infarction, J Psychosom Res 23:23, 1979.

58. Miller, HS, Jr: Supervised versus nonsupervised exercise rehabilitation of coronary patients. In Wenger, NK, editor: Exercise and the heart, ed 2, (Cardiovascular Clinics vol 15, pt 2), Philadelphia, 1984, FA Davis Co.

59. Miller, NH, et al: Home versus group exercise training for increasing functional capacity after myocardial infarction, Circulation 70:645, 1984.

60. Mitchell, M, et al: Cardiac exercise programs: role of continuous electrocardiographic monitoring, Arch Phys Med Rehabil 65:463, 1984.

61. Mulcahy, R: Influence of cigarette smoking on morbidity and mortality after myocardial infarction, Br Heart J 49:410, 1983.

62. Multicenter Postinfarction Research Group: Risk stratification and survival after myocardial infarction, N Engl J Med 309:331, 1983.

63. Mumford, E, Schlesinger, HJ, and Glass, GV: The effect of psychological intervention on recovery from surgery and heart attacks: an analysis of the literature, Am J Public Health 72:141, 1982.

64. Murray, GC, and Beller, GA: Cardiac rehabilitation following coronary artery bypass surgery, Am Heart J 105:1009, 1983.

65. O'Connor, GT, et al: An overview of randomized trials of exercise after myocardial infarction, Clin Res 34:379A, 1986.

66. Oldridge, NB, Cunningham, DL, and Jones, NL: Central cardiovascular function before and after four years of exercise following myocardial infarction, Circulation 72(suppl III):III-268, 1985.

67. Oldridge, NB, et al: Aortocoronary bypass surgery: effects of surgery and 32 months of physical conditioning on treadmill performance, Arch Phys Med Rehabil 59:268, 1978.

68. Ornish, D, et al: Effects of stress management training and dietary changes in treating ischemic heart disease, JAMA 249:54, 1983.

69. Oscai, LB, et al: Normalization of serum triglycerides and lipoprotein electrophoretic patterns by exercise, Am J Cardiol 30:775, 1972.

70. Ott, CR, et al: A controlled randomized study of early cardiac rehabilitation: The Sickness Impact Profile as an assessment tool, Heart Lung 12:162, 1983.

71. Palac, RT, et al: Risk factors related to progressive narrowing in aortocoronary vein grafts studied 1 and 5 years after surgery, Circulation 66(suppl I):I-40, 1982.

72. Palatsi, I: Feasibility of physical training after myocardial infarction and its effect on return to work, morbidity, and mortality, Acta Med Scand (suppl)599-602:1-84, 1976.

73. Parmley, WW: Position report on cardiac rehabilitation: recommendations of the American College of Cardiology on cardiovascular rehabilitation, JACC 7:451, 1986.

74. Pollock, ML: Exercise regimens after myocardial revascularization surgery: rationale and results. In Wenger, NK, editor: Exercise and the heart, ed 2, Philadelphia, 1984, FA Davis Co.

75. Pozen, MV, et al: A nurse rehabilitator's impact on patients with myocardial infarction, Med Care 15:830, 1977.

76. Pyorala, K, et al, editors: Secondary prevention of coronary heart disease: workshop of the International Society and Federation of Cardiology, Titisee, Oct 21-24, 1983, New York, Stuttgart, 1983, Thieme-Stratton.

77. Razin, Am: Psychosocial intervention in coronary artery disease: a review, Psychosom Med 44:363, 1982.

78. Rechnitzer, PA, et al: Relation of exercise to recurrence rate of myocardial infarction in men: Ontario Exercise-Heart Collaborative Study, Am J Cardiol 51:65, 1983.

79. Recommendation of the American College of Cardiology on cardiovascular rehabilitation, JACC 7:451, 1986.

80. Redwood, D, et al: Circulatory and sympathetic effects of physical training in patients with coronary-artery disease and angina pectoris, N Engl J Med 286:959, 1972.

81. Report of the Inter-Society Commission for Heart Disease Resources: Optimal resources for the care of patients with acute myocardial infarction and chronic coronary heart disease, Circulation 65:654B, 1982.

82. Report of the Working Group on Arteriosclerosis of the National Heart, Lung, and Blood Institute: Summary, conclusions, and recommendations. In Arteriosclerosis 1981 (NIH Pub. no 81-2034), vol 1, Washington, DC, 1981, US Department of Health and Human Services, Public Health Service.

83. Rose, G, et al: Myocardial ischaemia, risk factors and death from coronary heart disease, Lancet 1:105, 1977.

84. Roviaro, S, Holmes, DS, and Holmsten, RD: Influence of a cardiac rehabilitation program on the cardiovascular, physiologic, and social functioning of cardiac patients, J Behav Med 7:61, 1984.

85. Scheuer, J: Effects of physical training on myocardial vascularity and perfusion, Circulation 66:491, 1982.

86. Schlant, RC, et al: The Coronary Drug Project Research Group: The natural history of coronary heart disease: prognostic factors after recovery from myocardial infarction in 2789 men: the 5-year findings of the Coronary Drug Project, Circulation 66:401, 1982.

87. Shaw, LW: Effects of a prescribed supervised exercise program on mortality and cardiovascular morbidity in patients after myocardial infarction: the National Exercise and Heart Disease Project, Am J Cardiol 48:39, 1981.

88. Shephard, RJ: The value of exercise in ischemic heart disease: a cumulative analysis, J Cardiac Rehabil 3:294, 1983.

89. Smith, HC, et al: Employment status after coronary artery bypass surgery, Circulation 65(suppl 2):120, 1982.

90. Social Security Administration: Social Security disability applicant statistics 1970, Washington, DC, 1974, US Department of Health, Education, and Welfare Pub No (SSA) 75-11911.

91. Stanton, BA, et al: Predictors of employment status after cardiac surgery, JAMA 249:907, 1983.

92. Stern, MJ, and Cleary, P: The National Exercise and Heart Disease Project: psychosocial changes observed during a low-level exercise program, Arch Intern Med 141:1463, 1981.

93. Stern, MJ, and Cleary, P: The National Exercise and Heart Disease Project: long-term psychological outcome, Arch Inter Med 142:1093, 1982.

94. Stern, MJ, Plionis, E, and Kaslow, L: Group process expectations and outcome with post-myocardial infarction patients, Gen Hosp Psychiatry 6:101, 1984.

95. Stevens, R, and Hanson, P: Comparison of supervised and unsupervised training after coronary bypass surgery, Am J Cardiol 53:1524, 1984.

96. Taylor, CB, et al: Exercise testing to enhance wives' confidence of their husband's capability soon after clinically uncomplicated myocardial infarction, Am J Cardiol 55:635, 1985.

97. VanCamp, SP, and Peterson, RA: Cardiovascular complications of outpatient cardiac rehabilitation programs, JAMA 256:1160, 1986.

98. Verani, MS, et al: Effects of exercise training on left ventricular performance and myocardial perfusion in patients with coronary artery disease, Am J Cardiol 47:797, 1981.

99. Vermeulen, A, Lie, KI, and Durrer, D: Effects of cardiac rehabilitation after MI: changes in coronary risk factors and long-term prognosis, Am Heart J 105:798, 1983.

100. Wallwork, J, Potter, B, and Caves, PK: Return to work after coronary artery surgery for angina, Br Med J 2:1680, 1978.

101. Walter, PJ, editor: Return to work after coronary bypass surgery: psychosocial and economic aspects, Berlin, 1985, Springer-Verlag.

102. Weinblatt, E, et al: Prognosis of men after first myocardial infarction: mortality and first recurrence in relation to selected parameters, Am J Public Health 58:1329, 1968.

103. Wenger, NK: Coronary care: rehabilitation of the patient with symptomatic coronary atherosclerotic heart disease, prepared for the Coronary Care Committee Council on Clinical Cardiology, and the Committee on Medical Education–American Heart Association, 70-002-F, Dallas, 1981.

104. Wenger, NK: The elderly coronary patient, In Wenger, NK, and Hellerstein, HK, editors: Rehabilitation of the coronary patient, ed 2, New York, 1984, John Wiley & Sons.

105. Wenger, NK, editor: The education of the patient with cardiac disease in the twenty-first century, New York, 1986, LeJacq Publishing, Inc.

106. Wenger, NK: Risk stratification after myocardial infarction: learning center highlights, American College of Cardiology 1:14, 1986.

107. Wenger, NK: Future directions in cardiovascular rehabilitation, J Cardiac Rehabil 7:168, 1987.

108. Wenger, NK, et al: Physician practice in the management of patients with uncomplicated myocardial infarction: changes in the past decade, Circulation 65:421, 1982.

109. Wiklund, I, et al: Sick-role and attitude towards disease and working life two months after a myocardial infarction, Scand J Rehabil Med 16:57, 1984.

110. Wilhelmsen, L, et al: A controlled trial of physical training after myocardial infarction: effects on risk factors, nonfatal reinfarction, and death, Prev Med 4:491, 1975.

111. Wilhelmsen, L, et al: Effects of infarct size, smoking, physical activity, and some psychological factors on prognosis after myocardial infarction, Adv Cardiol 29:119, 1982.

112. Williams, RS: Exercise training of patients with ventricular dysfunction and heart failure. In Wenger, NK, editor: Exercise and the heart, ed 2, Philadelphia, 1985, F.A. Davis Co.

113. Williams, RS, et al: Guidelines for unsupervised exercise in patients with ischemic heart disease, J Cardiac Rehabil 1:213, 1981.

114. Wood, PD, and Haskell, WL: The effect of exercise on plasma high-density lipoprotein, Lipids 14:417, 1979.

115. World Health Organization, Regional Office for Europe, Copenhagen: The rehabilitation of patients with cardiovascular diseases (EURO 0381), 1969.

CHAPTER 16

Nutrition and cardiovascular disease

SANFORD J. FRIEDMAN

Although the clinical manifestations of atheromatosis may not appear for decades, they are devastating when they do appear. In the United States, atheromatosis results in 550,000 deaths per year, 1,000,000 heart attacks per year, and 400,000 strokes per year. The estimated cost of cardiovascular disease to our economy is $80,000,000,000 per year; the estimated suffering is incalculable. According to some accounts fully one quarter of the first manifestations of coronary artery disease is sudden death.

Still, the United States seems to be doing something right. In the decade ending in 1978, there were 25% fewer cardiovascular deaths in the 35- to 65-year-old age group than in the previous decade. Since 1968 there has been a 50% reduction in the number of strokes and a 30% reduction in the number of cases of coronary artery disease.[11,31,32] It is surmised that this trend results from a rising health consciousness among Americans. Americans exercise more, eat less animal fat,[7] smoke less, and have lower blood pressures. We also benefit from the more highly advanced technology in cardiology.

If atheromatosis, like some cancers, is considered a disease state long before its manifestations appear, one could convincingly make the case that Americans have been rehabilitating themselves with better relative results than any other country, with the possible exceptions of Canada and Israel. The role of nutrition in retarding progression of the atheromatous plaque is the focus of this review. The following paragraphs consider the roles of animal fat, vitamins, and fish oils.

ANIMAL FATS

Fats move around the body by attaching themselves to proteins. The resultant complexes, lipoproteins, are char-acterized by their relative densities: high-density lipoprotein (HDL), intermediate-density lipoprotein (IDL), low-density lipoprotein (LDL), and very low-density lipoprotein (VLDL). Each has a different protein component, or apolipoprotein, and varying concentrations of cholesterol, cholesterol esters, triglycerides, fatty acids, and phospholipids. An excellent review by Grundy[14] of fat metabolism provides a useful overview.

Prior to their incorporation into lipoproteins, triglycerides and cholesterol are absorbed through the gut. Triglycerides are broken down in the intestinal lumen to glycerol and monoglycerides and transported and reconstituted in the lymph, where large triglyceride-rich particles called chylomicrons pass into the bloodstream via the thoracic duct. The chylomicrons can certainly contribute to lipemia but are believed to be too large to enter the endothelium and hence do not appear to increase the risk for atheromatosis.

VLDLs are large, triglyceride-laden particles. These are heterogeneous in size and are manufactured in the liver. In prospective epidemiologic studies triglycerides and VLDLs do not seem to be risk factors for coronary disease. They are probably too large to penetrate vascular endothelium. Some investigators, however, have found evidence incriminating VLDLs and triglyceride in the angiographic severity of coronary artery disease in smaller population samples.[41] It may be that in select patients there are VLDLs small enough to contribute to the plaque. Moreover, VLDLs carry cholesterol esters and are the eventual precursors of LDL, the principal lipid component of the atherosclerotic plaque. The companion protein in the VLDLs is apolipoprotein B-100. This molecule, also found in the LDLs, increases the stability of these fatty particles and contributes to atherosclerosis.[48] The clinical utility of measuring apolipoproteins in individual patients has yet to be determined.

The chylomicrons and VLDLs are metabolized in the blood by lipoprotein lipase. Apolipoprotein C (apo C) is necessary for the function of this enzyme.[18] When apo C is deficient, large molecules of VLDL, which are not believed to be atherogenic, build up in the serum. This can result in gross lipemia and pancreatitis.

The normal by-products of lipoprotein lipase action are chylomicron remnants, fatty acids, glycerol, and VLDL remnants, otherwise known as IDL. IDL either can attach to the liver receptors for metabolism by means of its apo E or can be converted to LDL. LDL and IDL are catabolized by the same liver receptors.

Therefore, on a metabolic scheme hypercholesterolemia can occur by the depressed catabolism of LDL by the liver (the most common malady), by overproduction of LDL as a by-product of decreased catabolism of IDL,[19] or by consumption of too much animal fat. Patients with familial hypercholesterolemia have a marked deficiency of hepatic LDL and IDL receptors. IDL catabolism is impaired, increasing LDL precursors, and of course LDL catabolism is impaired. In these patients, traditional drug and dietary therapy has not been optimal. They often have cholesterol levels higher than 350 mg/dl when seen initially.

In patients with too much LDL, the major determinant of risk might be the HDLs.[17] These small particles are the garbage trucks for body fat. Enough HDLs can compensate for too much LDL—up to a point. They consist of cholesterol ester, cholesterol, triglycerides, a coating of apolipoproteins and phospholipids, which permit partial water solubility.

Apo A1 and A2, the main protein components of HDL, are secreted in the gut and liver.[18] They are the principal components of "nascent HDL," which enlarges into HDL by picking up cholesterol from peripheral tissues. The operative enzyme is lecithin-cholesterol acyltransferase (LCAT), which requires apo A1 to function. The HDL can accrue additional cholesterol from the action of lipoprotein lipase on VLDL.

Therapy is aimed at reducing total cholesterol generally and LDL cholesterol specifically. Diet changes usually decrease the total cholesterol by no more than 20% to 25%. Bile sequestrants (cholestyramine and colestipol) accentuate intrahepatic transformation of cholesterol to bile.[38] Neomycin inhibits intestinal cholesterol absorbtion.[27] A new class of drugs diminishes hepatic cholesterol formation by inhibiting the key enzyme, 3-hydroxymethyl-3-glutamyl coenzyme A (HMG-CoA).[30,35] All of these, by decreasing total hepatic cholesterol, increase hepatic LDL receptor sites and therefore LDL catabolism.[6] A decrease in LDL cholesterol can also be achieved by decreasing VLDL formation. Gemfibrozil[25] and nicotinic acid[20] are effective agents for this purpose.

A more challenging task is to increase the HDL levels of patients who are at risk from hypercholesterolemia. Aerobic exercise in amounts as little as half an hour three times a week increases HDL and lowers cholesterol.[20] Patients who smoke do not enjoy this benefit of exercise,[10] and they have markedly reduced HDLs.[40] Small quantities of alcohol inhibit hepatic lipase and therefore decrease HDL catabolism.[21] Ironically, diets high in animal fat increase HDL, and vegetarian diets high in polyunsaturates decrease HDL.[43] In the former case the attendant increase in LDL easily negates whatever benefit a rising HDL confers, and in the latter case the very low LDL achieved probably negates the lower HDL. Weight loss increases HDL.

Epidemiologists have observed that in countries such as Greece and Italy, where large quantities of olive oil are consumed, there is a low incidence of coronary artery disease. These diets are high in monounsaturated fatty acids, particularly oleic acid. When a diet high in oleic acid and low in carbohydrates is compared with a diet low in saturated fat but high in carbohydrate, there are comparable reductions in total cholesterol. The former diet, however, does not cause a drop in HDL, whereas the latter, as mentioned in the previous paragraph, does cause a drop in HDL. The implication of course is that calories on a low saturated fat diet might be better replaced with monounsaturated fatty acids than with carbohydrates.[15]

Bile sequestrants result in modest increases in HDL.[28] Nicotinic acid reduces catabolism of HDL.[4] Gemfibrozil facilitates addition of cholesterol from HDL2 to HDL3, resulting in a net increase in HDL. Dilantin stimulates HDL synthesis.[32] Finally estrogens, like ethanol, inhibit catabolism of HDL by inhibiting hepatic lipase.[37] Conversely, anabolic steroids and most drugs employed in the treatment of hypertension (for example, thiazide and loop diuretics, reserpine, aldomet, and selective and nonselective beta-blockers) decrease HDLs.[11] So far, captopril, enalopril, labetalol, and prazocin do not seem to decrease HDL formation. The nonselective beta-blockers adversely affect HDL more than the selective beta-blockers. Pindolol, a beta-blocker with intrinsic sympathomimetic activity, may even increase HDLs.

Much can be learned from the few large prospective trials concerning primary and secondary prevention of atherosclerosis from manipulation of fats. The Framingham study strongly supported the observations of the danger of high cholesterol and the protective effect of high HDLs.[20] A total cholesterol level of above 200 mg/dl (an LDL level greater than 125 mg/dl) in the absence of other risk factors is associated with longevity. The risk of atherosclerosis increases twofold for cholesterol levels of 225 to 275 mg/dl; the risk increases from twofold to fourfold for cholesterol levels of 275 to 325 mg/dl and from fourfold to eightfold for cholesterol levels greater than 325 mg/dl.

The Framingham study also demonstrated that the total cholesterol level alone is not completely predictive. The mean cholesterol levels of patients with coronary disease was only 245 mg/dl, the level of large numbers of healthy people. Low HDLs in the population with high average

LDLs was two times more predictive of coronary artery disease than total cholesterol level.[9]

Recently Brunner and co-workers[8] published their prospective findings of the effect of the HDL/cholesterol ratio in a cohort of 3000 men and women over a 20-year period. A ratio of HDL/total cholesterol less than 14% was associated with a 28% incidence of total coronary events. With an HDL/total cholesterol ratio greater than 21% the incidence was 7%. These researchers were able to define a subset of patients with two to four times the coronary risk even within the subset of patients with total cholesterol levels less than 200 mg/dl. In men with cholesterol levels greater than 265 mg/dl, coronary risk varied from one and one-third to four times that of men with cholesterol levels of 210 mg/dl, depending on the HDL level.

Many other studies have made important contributions to knowledge of the role of nutrition in cardiovascular disease. Four large primary prevention trials and three secondary prevention trials are reviewed here.

In the Oslo Study Group patients were encouraged to quit smoking and decrease their consumption of saturated fat.[23] The intervention group lowered total cholesterol of 1200 hypercholesterolemic men by only 14% over 5 years. Yet in this group there was a 47% lower incidence of sudden death and myocardial infarction. It was estimated that 60% of the benefit came from improved diet and 40% from discontinuing cigarettes.

The U.S. MR FIT[2] study looked at the effect of reducing hypertension, hypercholesterolemia, and cigarette abuse in 12,000 men. There was a 50% reduction in the mortality of normotensive cigarette smokers with initial high cholesterol levels. The overall results of the study were inconclusive because of an unexpectedly low incidence of coronary morbidity and mortality in the control group.[46]

The Helsinki Heart Study included over 4000 men with average baseline cholesterol levels of 288 mg/dl and HDL levels of 49 mg/dl, randomly assigned to placebo and gemfibrozil (Lopid) groups.[13] The rate of total cardiac events was 27.3/1000 in the treatment group and 41.4/1000 in the placebo group. There was a 26% reduction in cardiovascular events. The drug was well tolerated, and there was no increase in cancer incidence. The treatment group had a 10% increase in HDL levels, a 43% reduction in triglyceride levels, and a 10% reduction in LDL cholesterol levels.

The Lipid Research Clinic Coronary Primary Prevention Trial (LRC-CPPT) studied the bile sequestrant cholestyramine in 3806 men between the ages of 35 and 59 years without evidence of coronary artery disease but with serum cholesterol levels over 265 mg/dl.[32] The treated group, despite only an 8.5% decrease in cholesterol levels and an 18% drop in LDL levels, had 19% fewer myocardial infarctions and coronary deaths. Benefit was seen after only 2 years of treatment. There were 20% less angina, 25% less positive results of exercise tolerance tests, and 21% less coronary artery bypass grafts. With full adherence to the regimen, a 25% reduction in cholesterol could be achieved, resulting in a 50% reduction in risk. For each 1% reduction in cholesterol level, there was a 2% reduction in risk.

The Leiden Intervention Trial is a secondary prevention study of 39 patients with stable angina and at least single-vessel disease of greater than 50% occlusion.[1] Patients were given a vegetarian diet with a polyunsaturate/saturate ratio of 2:1. The total cholesterol allowed per day was 100 mg. There were significant decreases in weight, systolic blood pressure, and total cholesterol levels and an increase in the HDL/total cholesterol ratio. Angiography was repeated in 6 months. No patients who initially had an HDL/total cholesterol ratio less than 6.9 and after the trial had a ratio above 6.9 had angiographic progression of disease.

The NHLBI Type II Coronary Intervention Study looked at 143 individuals with type II hyperlipidemia, clinically significant coronary artery disease, and at least one occlusion of at least 20% in at least one coronary artery.[5] Patients were treated with cholestyramine (24 g/day) plus diet changes or diet changes alone. In the treatment group there was a 17% drop in total cholesterol, a 26% drop in LDL, and an 8% increase in HDL. If those with probable and definite angiographic progression of disease are considered in one group, the placebo group had a 49% incidence of progression versus a 32% incidence in the treated group, a statistically significant difference.

Blankenhorn and co-workers[3] in the Cholesterol-Lowering Atherosclerotic Study (CLAS) studied 162 nonsmoking men who had received coronary bypass grafts. The trial was a prospective placebo-controlled effort to study the effects of combined niacin-colestipol therapy using endpoints of changes in coronary angiography. Compliant patients had a 26% reduction in total cholesterol and a 37% elevation in HDL. There was a statistically significant decrease in the progression of disease in the treatment group. In 16% of the patients there was evidence of regression of plaque. Unfortunately, there was no difference in progression to total occlusion. Mineral oil was used prophylactically to mitigate the constipating effects of the colestid.

There are no data yet concerning the clinical effectiveness of lovastatin. The drug is well tolerated and gives a remarkable, dose-related reduction in LDL from 24% at 5 mg/day to 39% at 20 mg twice a day.[30] In addition, the HDL level increases. Complications so far are rare and include a myositis syndrome. Reports of corneal opacities associated with this drug are controversial, and liver enzyme elevations are benign and reversible.

The skeptic at this point might argue that by the time a person experienced a myocardial infarction or an incapacitating atherosclerotic stroke, the natural history of the organ damage, the advanced nature of the vascular angiopathy that produced the damage, or simply the advanced age of those patients most likely to have these conditions makes therapeutic efforts to alter serum lipoprotein levels not cost effective. This is probably so, but one cannot be sure. In any case a young, productive patient should certainly receive every potential advantage.

FISH OIL

Epidemiologists have long observed that coronary artery disease is almost nonexistent among the Eskimos who consume huge quantities of oily fish. A recent study revealed the protective effect of eating only 30 g of fish per day, or one tenth the amount of fish consumed by Eskimos. The protective effect is greater than would be expected from the reduction of lipids alone.[44]

Investigators focused on the omega-3 fatty acid called eicosapentanoic acid. This compound can compete with arachidonic acid in the cyclo-oxygenase pathway. Normally arachidonic acid is converted either to prostacyclin, a potent vasodilator and platelet deaggregant, or thromboxane A_2. The latter is a potent vasoconstrictor and platelet aggregator. Increased levels of thromboxane A_2 have been found in peripheral blood of patients with coronary insufficiency.

Large doses of eicosapentanoic acid were given to volunteers to simulate the Eskimo diet.[28] The fatty acid was incorporated into the phospholipid of the red blood cells; some antiplatelet effect, as well as significant diminution in thromboxane A_2, was observed. At lower, more usual doses the antiplatelet effect was lost. Aspirin was believed to be more potent in this regard. However, some significant effects of eicosapentanoic acid that might not be reflected in peripheral platelet function should not be ignored.

Investigators working in Japan, a country with an obviously high per capita ingestion of fish, found that free arachidonic acid/eicosapentanoic acid ratios formed a separate risk factor for coronary artery disease without relation to HDLs.[29]

Fish oil can be obtained commercially in the form of flavored cod liver oil or fish oil tablets such as Promega, Omega-500, or Maxepa. Whether these oils are free of the carcinogenic potential known to exist in oily sea fish is an open question. In patients with markedly increased risk of atherosclerosis or with known coronary artery disease, these tablets might prove a useful supplement.

VITAMINS

The evidence that vitamin supplementation impedes atherosclerotic progression is problematic at best. For example, vitamin B_6 facilitates the catabolism of homocysteine. In homocysteinuria, an inherited disease of metabolism, children die before their late teens from diffuse and malignant atherosclerosis. The large quantities of this amino acid presumably damage endothelium and allow fats to enter the vessel walls, thus initiating the vicious cycle of plaque formation. Researchers have posited that, in young adults with coronary artery disease and few risk factors, there might be a forme fruste of homocysteinuria. To test this hypothesis,

patients received intravenous administration of methionine, a precursor of homocysteine.[36] Urine samples revealed an unexpectedly high amount of homocysteine in 25% of the patients with coronary artery disease compared to the control groups. However, there have not yet been reliable trials employing vitamin B_6 in this population.

Scurvy is the well-known and rarely occurring vitamin C deficiency state. Laboratory animals made deficient in vitamin C develop early lesions of atherosclerosis.[49] Animals on a vitamin C–deficient diet have hypercholesterolemia before demonstrating evidence of scurvy.[14] Humans with normal levels of vitamin C do not seem to have improvement in their cholesterol profiles with supplementation.[39] Finally, investigators have discovered that vitamin C decreases platelet adhesiveness and platelet aggregation in patients with coronary artery disease, particularly after a fatty meal.[4] No clinical trials with vitamin C as an antiplaque agent have been reported.

Lecithin has long been touted as a useful prophylactic agent. It is a phospholipid that confers solubility to lipoproteins. It is present in high concentrations in HDL and has been shown to elevate HDL levels and lower LDL levels by one investigator. Moreover, by acting as an emulsifier, lecithin helps dissolve the cholesterol esters formed by lecithin-cholesterol acyltransferase. Thus lecithin may help move cholesterol from peripheral tissue into HDL particles. Unfortunately, it is not clear how much of this substance can be absorbed through the gut. Moreover, as with the vitamins discussed previously, no convincing trials employing lecithin as an antiatherosclerotic agent exist.

CONCLUSION

There is some controversy over the ideal regimen to retard the atherosclerotic process. In my opinion, physicians should make every effort to lower LDL levels and elevate HDL levels in susceptible patients. Gemfibrozil (Lopid) can be given to patients with low LDL levels and low HDL levels to elevate the HDL levels. However, pending further data, this is a question of judgment and hunch. I favor more liberal use of antihyperlipidemic agents, am inclined to prescribe fish oils, and would not dissuade patients from using nontoxic vitamin supplements, despite fragile evidence for their effectiveness.

REFERENCES

1. Arntzenius, AC, et al: Diet: ioproteins and the progression of coronary atherosclerosis—the Leiden Intervention Trial, N Engl J Med 312:805, 1985.
2. Benfari, RC, and Sherwin, R: The multiple risk intervention trial (MR FIT): the methods and impact of intervention over four years, Prev Med 10:387, 1981.
3. Blankenhorn, DH, et al: Beneficial effect of combined colestipol-niacin therapy on coronary atherosclerosis and coronary venous bypass grafts, JAMA 257:3233, 1987.
4. Bordia, A, and Verma, SK: Effect of vitamin C on platelet adhesiveness and platelet aggregating in coronary artery disease patients, Clin Cardiol 8:552, 1985.

5. Brensike, JF, et al: Effects of therapy with cholestyramine on progression of coronary atherosclerosis: results of the NHLBI type II coronary intervention study, Circulation 69:313, 1984.

6. Brown, MS, and Godstein, JL: Lipoprotein receptors in the liver: control signals for plasma cholesterol traffic, J Clin Invest 72:743, 1983.

7. Brown, WV, Ginsberg, H, and Karmally, W: Diet and the decrease of coronary heart disease, Am J Cardiol 54:27c, 1984.

8. Brunner, D, et al: Relation of serum total cholesterol and high density lipoprotein cholesterol percentage to the incidence of definite coronary events: twenty-year follow-up of the Donolo–Tel Aviv Prospective Coronary Artery Disease Study, Am J Cardiol 59:1271, 1987.

9. Castelli, WP, et al: The incidence of coronary heart disease and lipoprotein cholesterol levels: the Framingham Study, JAMA, 256:2835, 1986.

10. Cowan, GO: Influence of exercise on high-density lipoproteins, Am J Cardiol 52:13B, 1983.

11. Feinleib, M: The magnitude and nature of the decrease in coronary heart disease mortality rate, Am J Cardiol 54:2c, 1984.

12. Frick, HM, et al: The Helsinki Heart Study: primary prevention trial with gemfibrozil in middle-aged men with dyslipidemia; safety of treatment, changes in risk factors, and incidence of coronary heart disease, N Engl J Med 317:1237, 1987.

13. Ginsberg, H, and Karmally, W: Diet and the decrease of coronary heart disease, Am J Cardiol 54:27c, 1984.

14. Ginter, E, et al: Lowered cholesterol catabolism in guinea pigs with chronic ascorbic acid deficiency, Am J Clin Nutr 24:1238, 1971.

15. Glueck, CJ: Nonpharmacologic and pharmacologic alteration of high-density lipoprotein cholesterol: therapeutic approaches to prevention of atherosclerosis, Am Heart J 110(5):1107, 1985.

16. Goldstein, JL, and Brown, MS: Familial hypercholesterolemia. In The metabolic basis of inherited disease, ed 8, Philadelphia, 1980, WB Saunders Co.

17. Gordon, T, et al: High-density lipoprotein as a protective factor against coronary heart disease: the Framingham study, Am J Med 62:707, 1977.

18. Gotto, AM: High-density lipoproteins: biochemical and metabolic factors, Am J Cardiol 52:2b, 1983.

19. Grundy, SM: Hyperlipoproteinemia: metabolic basis and rationale for therapy, Am J Cardiol 54:20c, 1984.

20. Grundy, SM: Comparison of monounsaturated fatty acids and carbohydrates for lowering plasma cholesterol, N Engl J Med 314:745, 1986.

21. Grundy, SM, Mok, HY, and Zech, L: Influence of nicotinic acid on metabolism of cholesterol and triglycerides in man, J Lipid Res 22:24, 1981.

22. Haskel, WL, et al: The effect of cessation and resumption of moderate alcohol intake on serum high density lipoprotein subfractions, N Engl J Med 310:805, 1984.

23. Hjermann, I, Byre, KV, and Holme, I: Effect of diet and smoking intervention on the incidence of coronary heart disease: report from the Oslo Study Group of a randomized trial in healthy men, Lancet 2:1303, 1981.

24. Huttunen, JK, et al: The effect of moderate physical exercise on serum lipoproteins: a controlled trial with special reference to serum high density lipoproteins, Circulation 60:1220, 1979.

25. Kannel, WB, et al: Cholesterol in the prediction of atherosclerotic disease: new perspectives based on the Framingham Study, Ann Intern Med 90:85, 1979.

26. Kesaniemi, YA, and Grundy, SM: Influence of gemfibrozil on metabolism of cholesterol and plasma triglycerides in man, JAMA 251:2241, 1984.

27. Kesaniemi, YA, and Grundy, SM: Turnover of low density lipoproteins during inhibition of cholesterol absorption by neomycin, Arteriosclerosis 4:41, 1984.

28. Knapp, HR, Reilly, IA, and Alessandrini, P: In vivo indexes of platelet and vascular function during fish oil administration in patients with atherosclerosis, N Engl J Med 314:937, 1986.

29. Kondo, T, et al: Plasma free eicosapentaenoic acid/arachidonic acid ratio: a possible new coronary risk factor, Clin Cardiol 9:413, 1986.

30. The Lovastatin Study Group II: Therapeutic response to lovastatin (Mevinolin) in nonfamilial hypercholesterolemia: a multicenter study, JAMA 256:2829, 1986.

31. Levy, RI, Cardiovascular reserarch: decades of progress, a decade of promise, Science 217:121, 1982.

32. Levy, RI: Causes of the decrease in cardiovascular mortality, Am J Cardiol 54:7c, 1984.

33. Lipid Research Clinics Program: The lipid research clinics coronary primary prevention trial results. I. Reduction in incidence of coronary heart disease to cholesterol lowering, JAMA 251:351, 1984.

34. Lipid Research Clinics Program: The lipid research clinics coronary primary prevention trial results. II. The relationship of reduction in incidence of coronary heart disease to cholesterol lowering, JAMA 251:365, 1984.

35. Mabuchi, H, et al: Effect of an inhibitor of 3-hydroxy-3-methylglutaryl coenzyme: a reductase on serum lipoproteins and ubiquinone-10-levels in patients with familial hypercholesterolemia, N Engl J Med 305(9):478, 1981.

36. Murphy-Chutorian, DR, Wexman, MD, and Grieco, AJ: Methionine intolerance: a possible risk factor for coronary artery disease, J Am Coll Cardiol 16:725, 1985.

37. Nikkila, EA, Kaste, M, and Ehnholm, C: Increase in serum high-density lipoproteins in phenytoin users, Br Med J 2:99, 1978.

38. Packard, CJ, and Shepherd, J: The hepatobiliary axis and lipoprotein metabolism: effects of bile acid sequestrants and ileal bypass surgery, J Lipid Res 23:1081, 1982.

39. Peterson, VE, et al: Quantification of plasma cholesterol and triglyceride levels in hypercholesterolemic subjects receiving ascorbic acid supplements, Am J Clin Nutr 28:584, 1975.

40. Rablin, SW, Boyko, E, and Streja, DA: Relationship of weight loss and cigarette smoking to changes in high-density lipoprotein cholesterol, Am J Clin Nutr 34:975, 1981.

41. Reardon, MR, et al: Lipoprotein predictors of the severity of coronary artery disease in men and women, Circulation 71:881, 1985.

42. Ross, RK, et al: Menopausal oestrogen therapy and protection from death from ischemic heart disease, Lancet 1:858, 1981.

43. Sacks, S, et al: Plasma-lipids and lipoproteins in vegetarians and controls, N Engl J Med 292:1148, 1975.

44. Shekelle, RB, et al: Fish consumption and mortality from coronary disease, N Engl J Med 31:820, 1985.

45. Shepherd, J, et al: Effects of nicotinic acid therapy on plasma high-density lipoprotein subfraction distribution and composition on apolipoprotein metabolism, J Clin Invest 63:858, 1979.

46. Stamler, J, Wentworth, D, and Newton, JD: Is the relationship between serum cholesterol and the risk of premature death from coronary heart disease continuous or graded? JAMA 256:2823, 1986.

47. Weidmann, P, Uehlinger, DE, and Gerber, AJ: Antihypertensive treatment and serum lipoproteins, Hypertension 3:297, 1985.

48. Whayne, TF, et al.: Plasma apolipoprotein B and VLDL, LDL, and HDL cholesterol as risk factors in the development of coronary artery disease in male patients examined by angiography, Atherosclerosis 39:411, 1981.

49. Willis, GC: The reversibility of atherosclerosis, Can Med Assoc J 77:106, 1957.

CHAPTER 17

Physiologic principles of an effective cardiac rehabilitation program

ROY J. SHEPHARD

Both empiric evidence from cardiac rehabilitation centers[8,18] and cumulative analysis of controlled trials[19] support the use of a regimen of progressive and vigorous physical activity in the treatment of patients who have had a myocardial infarction. However, physiologic arguments in favor of such therapy are equally strong. This chapter looks briefly at the benefits of a practical rehabilitation program, particularly considering the physiologic mechanisms of benefit.

BENEFITS FROM PROGRESSIVE ENDURANCE EXERCISE

Uncontrolled trials have long suggested a substantial reduction in both morbidity and mortality among patients who have had a myocardial infarction and who participated in programs of progressive endurance exercise.[18] The benefit of exercise persists after adjustment for differences of risk factors between exercised and nonexercised series; moreover, the advantage seems closely linked to exercise adherence.[20]

Controlled trials have now confirmed these conclusions. Whereas individual trials have included too few subjects to attain statistical significance, a majority of investigators have reported a 20% to 30% improvement in the prognosis of patients engaging in a progressive exercise program. A cumulative analysis of the various published results shows a significant patient response to these programs.[19] The one major randomized trial that failed to confirm this was our own multicenter trial in Southern Ontario.[17,17a] However, critics have rightly pointed out that the mortality among our "light activity" group was surprisingly low, suggesting that this group also received some benefit from physical activity.[2] The explanation of our aberrant data seems to be that many in our control group decided to exercise, whereas many in the exercise group failed to adhere to the prescribed activity program. Although statisticians wince at the idea, the only fair approach to evaluating the effects of exercise using this set of data is to reclassify subjects post hoc on the basis of their actual activity behavior. When this is done, those patients who have exercised have a 26% better prognosis, an increase similar to other series from around the world.[3]

POSSIBLE MECHANISMS OF BENEFIT FROM EXERCISE THERAPY

Some 20 years ago, Fox and Haskell[4] presented a comprehensive listing of the possible mechanisms whereby physical activity might improve the prognoses of patients prone to myocardial infarction. These are listed in the following outline.[4] Benefits are listed under the intensity of activity at which they first occur.

I. Light activity
   A. Life-style advice
   B. Psychosocial effects
      1. Camaraderie
      2. Joie de vivre
      3. Relaxation
      4. Eu-stress
II. Moderate activity
   A. Reduced cardiac work rate
      1. Lower heart rate
      2. Lower blood pressure
      3. Increased myocardial efficiency and muscle force
   B. Improved O_2 transport
      1. Increased blood volume
      2. Better flow distribution
      3. Increased capillarity
      4. Increased tissue enzymes

5. ? Increased hemoglobin
6. ? Increased arterial O_2 content
C. Hormonal changes
  1. Decreased catecholamines
  2. Increased growth hormone and thyroid hormone
D. Blood coagulability
  1. Increased fibrinolysis
  2. Decreased platelet stickiness
III. Intense activity
  A. Habituation
  B. Enlargement of coronary arteries and ? collaterals
IV. Increased energy usage
  A. Decreased body mass
    1. Lower work rate
    2. Easier heat loss
  B. Muscles strengthened—less afterload
  C. Blood profile
    1. Increased HDL cholesterol
    2. Decreased triglycerides
    3. Improved glucose tolerance

There is little need to expand this list, although it is useful to distinguish between responses that might be anticipated from the general support of membership in an exercise rehabilitation class, relatively low intensities of exercise that nevertheless augment daily energy expenditures, moderate endurance exercise of the type usually found in a cardiac conditioning class, and very intensive or prolonged exercise bouts (such as preparation for marathon events).

Hopes that regular exercise would induce an enlargement of the coronary arteries or an increase of collateral blood flow have now largely faded—at least with respect to the intensities of activity possible for patients who have had a myocardial infarction. Instead, the improved prognoses of these patients come from a general improvement in lifestyle, a checking of the disease process, a reduction in myocardial irritability, a reduction in cardiac work rate for a given level of physical activity, and an improvement of coronary oxygen delivery despite unchanged coronary vascular dimensions.

General improvement of life-style

The patient's attendance at an exercise class provides an opportunity for the physician to reinforce medical advice on diet, smoking withdrawal, and a more relaxed attitude to life. Studies of class participants have shown them to have relatively low average levels of blood lipids, with about 35% of the participants continuing to smoke.[11] Little further change of cardiac risk factors is seen when follow-up examinations of such patients are made during their membership in the exercise class. Although at first the number of smokers seems discouraging, the initial percentage of smokers in a cardiac rehabilitation class is much lower than the percentage before infarction. The exercise class thus may play an important role in checking recidivism. There have been suggestions that exercise has more specific value in helping the process of smoking withdrawal (Table 17-1); this is probably true only when subjects are running quite long distances.[14]

Checking the disease process

Exercise cannot reverse the destruction of infarcted segments of the ventricular wall. However, it may prevent further myocardial damage by countering risk factors and checking the spread of the disease. Risk factors after infarction are summarized in Table 17-2.

The recent Lipid Research Trial demonstrated fairly clearly that the prognosis of an average, middle-aged person can be helped by a chemically induced reduction in serum cholesterol.[13] Less is known of the situation after infarction. In the Southern Ontario Multicentre Exercise–Heart Trial, very few patients had persistent high serum cholesterol levels. Nevertheless, the average serum cholesterol level was 5% higher in those patients who experienced another infarction.[17] Some evidence seems to indicate that a persistently elevated serum cholesterol level worsens the patient's prognosis, particularly in those who are exercising (Table 17-2). Thus if physical activity corrects the adverse lipid profile, it is anticipated that there will be a proportionate reduction in the chances of the patient having another infarction. Unfortunately, the mileage that a patient must run to improve the lipid profile is relatively high (around 20 kilometers/week[1] in the Toronto Rehabilitation Centre data and other recent trials).[7,12,26] Given the fairly slow rate of exercise progression possible for average patients who have had an infarction, it is unlikely that an improved lipid profile contributes to benefit, at least in the first year of rehabilitation. There are possible acute responses to vigorous exercise that could check the disease process—an increase of fibrinolysis and a decrease in platelet stickiness—but again it is unlikely that these are primarily responsible for the benefit observed with exercise rehabilitation.

Table 17-1. Smoking status of participants in Masters' distance running events

Smoking status	Percentage of runners in each class, by age	
	<21 yr	>21 yr
Never	56	36
Former	36	60
Current	8	4

Modified from data from Morgan, P, Gildiner, M, and Wright, GR: CAHPER J 42:39, 1976.

Table 17-2. Influence of selected risk factors on response to exercise program (incidence of fatal or nonfatal recurrence relative to incidence in those free of risk factor)

Risk factor	Sedentary	TRC program (3 years)	Southern Ontario Multicentre	
			High intensity	Low intensity
Continued smoking	2.00	1.30	1.52	2.02
Angina (final test)	1.93	1.93	1.95	2.79
Aneurysm	1.80	2.05	—	—
Enlarged heart	2.32	2.40	—	—
Serum cholesterol 270 mg/dl^{-1}	1.05	1.98	1.56*	0*
Hypertension 150/100 mm Hg	2.55	0.98	0.14*	0.62*
Resting ECG abnormalities	2.47	1.02	0.68*	1.05*
Exercise ST depression 0.2 mV	1.23	1.82	1.11*	0.7*
Polyfocal PVCs (three in 10 seconds)	1.61	1.53	0.37*	0.53*

Modified from Shephard, RJ, et al: Br J Sports Med 15:6, 1981.
*For these variables, the incidence is known only in those sustaining a recurrence; the overall incidence has been assumed to correspond with that for the Toronto Rehabilitation Center (TRC) "post-coronary" exercise program.

Reduced myocardial irritability

Fatal recurrence of myocardial infarction is often associated with sudden arrhythmia. The prognoses of these patients can be improved by reducing the irritability of the myocardium. Irritability reflects, among other factors, the relative oxygen supply to the myocardium, the secretion of catecholamines, and the adverse effects of smoking. Mechanisms whereby exercise might improve the relative oxygen supply of the myocardium (a decrease in cardiac work rate or an increase in coronary oxygen delivery) are discussed in the next two sections of this chapter.

Catecholamine output depends on both the relative intensity of the exercise and any associated emotional stress. Blood catecholamine levels are much higher if the subject is facing business or domestic anxieties or is engaged in competitive forms of exercise. The patient who has had an infarction must be advised to avoid competitive exercise and to find relaxation from business and social problems. A well-run exercise class can offer many helpful suggestions in this regard. A sharp increase in catecholamine output occurs as maximum oxygen intake is approached.[25] However, if the patient's maximum oxygen intake has been increased by 22% (the average response observed over 3 years of conditioning in the Toronto Rehabilitation Centre series),[11] the intensity of activities of everyday living may well be brought below the level at which dangerous amounts of catecholamine are secreted.

Smoking increases myocardial irritability in several ways. Nicotine has a direct stimulating effect on the cardiac pacemaker. By increasing heart rate and causing cutaneous vasoconstriction, it also increases cardiac work rate; at the same time, it reduces oxygen delivery to the myocardium by provoking coronary vascular spasm, forming carboxyhemoglobin, and modifying the shape of the oxygen dissociation curve of the blood. Because regular exercise may help in smoking withdrawal, it can reduce these problems.

Reduced cardiac work rate

At any given end-diastolic volume, the cardiac work rate is approximated by the double product (heart rate times systolic blood pressure). A decrease in heart rate at any intensity of exercise is one of the more obvious responses to cardiac rehabilitation. For a 22% increase in maximum oxygen intake, one anticipates at least a 15% to 20% reduction of heart rate during heavy effort (or a larger effect if emotional tachycardia is reduced). This leads in turn to a proportional reduction of cardiac work rate.

The impact of conditioning on blood pressure is complex. Most authors agree that regular exercise produces a therapeutically useful 5 to 10 mm Hg reduction in resting blood pressure levels.[24] However, patients who have had an infarction and who are active may actually achieve a higher systolic blood pressure during maximum exercise. This is because the patient is now capable of more vigorous activity. If the intensity of effort is matched before and after conditioning, a reduction of the blood pressure during exercise can be demonstrated in response to rehabilitation. This reflects both a lower secretion of catecholamines and a reduction of afterloading secondary to a strengthening of the active muscles. The importance of blood pressure levels is illustrated by a dramatic improvement in the prognoses of hypertensive patients when they become involved in an exercise program (Table 17-2).

The cardiac demand also is reduced when body mass is decreased or when heat elimination is facilitated by a decrease in subcutaneous fat. However, the patients attending the Toronto Rehabilitation Centre initially had no more fat than the average Torontonian of comparable age, and we found no evidence that the percentage of body fat changed materially over 3 years of progressive exercise rehabilitation.[21]

Endurance training generally increases myocardial contractility. The direct effect of this change is to increase cardiac oxygen consumption per unit of time. At the same time, the relative duration of systole is shortened. This facilitates coronary perfusion, which is largely a diastolic phenomenon. Moreover, for any given afterload, the heart is emptied more completely after training, so that by Laplace's law, the tension developed by the myocardial fibers is diminished. The time course of changes in myocardial contractility remains the subject of debate. Paterson and associates[16] found that, over the first 6 months of rehabilitation, the main response was an increase in peripheral oxygen extraction (reflecting such changes as an increase in muscle enzyme activity, a greater capillarization, and a more ready perfusion of the working muscles as they became stronger). Over the second 6 months of rehabilitation, there was also an increase in cardiac stroke volume. It is less clear whether this reflected an increased contractility of undamaged tissue, a recovery of function in partially damaged areas of the myocardium, or a reduction of afterloading as the leg muscles became stronger.

Improved coronary oxygen supply

The overall coronary oxygen supply depends on the rate of blood flow through the coronary system and the oxygen content per unit volume of blood. Training may induce some increases in blood hemoglobin levels, but this is usually a second-order effect. Likewise, coronary vasodilatation is unlikely to create any major increase in blood flow if the vessels are already rigidly sclerosed. On the other hand, coronary flow can be substantially augmented by a reduction in heart rate, and it can also be influenced less directly by a change in myocardial contractility.

Left ventricular perfusion occurs almost exclusively during the diastolic phase of the cardiac cycle.[6] If the heart rate decreases at any intensity of exercise, most of the increased cycle length is added to the diastolic phase. A 20% decrease in heart rate could, in itself, improve left ventricular perfusion by 30% to 40%.

An increase in myocardial contractility also shortens the systolic phase of the cardiac cycle at any given heart rate. Moreover, it decreases ventricular volume and thus the wall tension opposing coronary flow. This last change is particularly important for subendocardial tissue, since perfusion of this part of the heart is dependent on perforating branches of the coronary arteries that traverse the entire thickness of the ventricular wall. The prognostic importance of improvements in the coronary oxygen supply is suggested by a high incidence of recurrent infarction and sudden death in patients initially showing an exercise-induced myocardial ischemia (angina or ST depression) (Table 17-3).[18] The concept that regular conditioning can improve myocardial oxygen supply is further supported by reports showing a reduction in ST depression at any given heart rate–blood pressure product and scintigraphic evidence of improved myocardial perfusion after exercise rehabilitation.[5]

DIFFERENCES IN CLINICAL STATUS

Much of the early work on cardiac rehabilitation was oversimplified because it failed to distinguish between types and degrees of ischemic heart disease. Exercise trials often included a poorly defined heterogeneous mixture of patients, both those with symptomatic and electrocardiographic ischemia and those with minor infarcts. Patients with severe myocardial damage, pump failure, and conduction abnormalities were often underrepresented, and the average patient age was sometimes as low as 45 years.

Such a bias in the selection of patients inevitably contributed to the favorable results of exercise series over conservative treatment series. Moreover, since controlled trials suffer from a similar patient-selection bias, it raises the question of whether the benefits that have been demonstrated in controlled trials with random allocation of the exercise treatment apply only to young patients with small infarcts and not older persons with more extensive damage of the myocardium and the conduction system. Some recent research has suggested that patients with continuing myocardial ischemia (possibly because of pump failure) respond poorly to exercise programs.[5] Both the Southern Ontario Multi-Centre Trial and the Toronto Rehabilitation Centre data show greater risk of fatal and nonfatal recurrences in patients with exercise-induced ST segmental depression (high-intensity exercise), angina (recreational exercise), aneurysm, cardiac enlargement, or a history of repeated infarction (Table 17-2).[11,18] Furthermore, older patients seem less likely to progress to an adequate training mileage and are less likely to demonstrate substantial gains of oxygen transport with reversal of ST segmental depression as rehabilitation progresses.[10]

On the other hand, we have found that patients with angina can increase their maximum oxygen intake as much as patients without angina if they become involved in an appropriate type of interval training regimen.[9] Some of the gains may be peripheral (for instance, a strengthening of the skeletal muscles and a reduction of systemic blood pressure). However, if subjects are matched carefully for cardiovascular status before they begin training, date of entry into a rehabilitation program, and duration of training, the gains of cardiac stroke volume shown by patients with angina may be as great as in patients without angina.[15,16]

PRACTICAL IMPLICATIONS FOR EXERCISE PROGRAMMING
Group versus individual programming

Significant advantages are gained from a group program: camaraderie, mutual support, and advice on improvements in life-style. The patient develops confidence because exercising is conducted initially under close medical supervision; the physician can observe the patient in the gymnasium and thus regulate the speed of training. Exercise adherence is also strongly influenced by spousal support, and a group setting allows spouses to be trained for this supportive role.[1]

The disadvantages of group exercise for patients are the time occupied in traveling to and from the rehabilitation center and the substantial costs of exercise classes, which are unlikely to be met by insurance carriers on a continuing basis. Shift work and business commitments can also have an adverse effect on class adherence if the hours of attendance are rigidly defined.

The optimum arrangement varies somewhat with the intelligence and personality of the patient. Typically, there should be an initial 3-month period when the patient attends the rehabilitation center at least twice per week to build confidence, while learning techniques of exercise, pulse counting, and symptom recognition. For the next year attendance can be reduced to one supervised session per week, with four additional home sessions monitored by weekly diary sheets. In this way regular exercise habits are formed and the patient's rate of progression can be closely watched by the rehabilitation center. Finally, the patient can graduate to one session of supervised exercise every 8 weeks; this is sufficient to provide continuing motivation, while allowing periodic discussion of any problems and necessary adjustments of the exercise prescription.

Energy balance

The gains from a substantial expenditure of energy (lower body mass, more ready elimination of heat, improved glucose tolerance, reduced serum cholesterol level, and increased HDL cholesterol level) can probably be realized by walking or jogging 3 miles five times per week. It is the policy of the Toronto Rehabilitation Centre to encourage patients to reach at least this level of activity.

Moderate endurance activity

Most of the postulated mechanisms of benefit from exercise can be realized through moderate endurance activity. In a young patient with a small infarction, the intensity of the prescribed exercise can progress rapidly to the normal cardiorespiratory training zone (60% to 70% of maximum oxygen intake), but in an older person with complicated or advanced disease, it may be necessary to begin training at no more than 50% of maximum oxygen intake. Since many patients have been extremely inactive immediately before beginning rehabilitation, even these low intensities of effort usually have a training effect. If there are symptoms such as anginal pain, training is begun at the corresponding percentage of the symptom-limited maximum effort.

A typical home exercise prescription specifies a daily distance to be covered by walking or jogging with a specific

time, a heart rate ceiling corresponding to the desired percentage of maximum oxygen intake at the patient's age, any warning symptoms that call for a slowing of activity (for example, anginal pain or extrasystoles), instructions regarding any medications, and the duration of the exercise prescription (for example, "to be reevaluated after 4 weeks").

The patient must learn techniques of fine tuning an exercise prescription, using such indications as heart rate, breathlessness, and sweating. The patient must also be aware of appreciable day-to-day variations in maximum oxygen intake resulting from factors such as weather conditions (for example, an increase in central blood volume but a progressive decrease in total blood volume can occur during a cold spell). The energy cost of even a simple task such as a brisk walk can depart widely from that stated in metabolic tables, resulting from differences in techniques of movement, weather conditions (for example, a strong head wind), and ground conditions (a smooth road versus a rough field or dry versus wet snowy roads).

Intense or prolonged activity

Much controversy has been generated by the participation in marathon races of selected patients who have had a myocardial infarction. Some of these individuals have completed the 42 km course in a little over 3¼ hours.[23] At least a third of the patients attending the Toronto Rehabilitation Centre have the minimum physiologic and psychologic characteristics needed to participate in a marathon event, although a much smaller number (about 1%) choose to do so. To date, the prognosis of the marathon participants has been favorable, relative to the group as a whole. While the prospect of such an accomplishment provides motivation for a number of patients, other patients who are more seriously disabled are also encouraged by the success of their fellow class members. However, it is clear from the outline on pp. 232 and 233 that, once a substantial daily energy expenditure has been established and the individual intensity of activity is passing the training threshold on a regular basis, there is no strong physiologic argument in favor of progressing to the very prolonged and intensive preparation required for safe participation in a marathon.

Typical class

An exercise class should begin with a 5- to 10-minute discussion session, when problems of interest to the group can be discussed, unusual symptoms requiring a review of the exercise prescription can be reported, and special instructions can be given.

A warm-up period of at least 10 minutes follows. This is important to avoid provoking both arrhythmias and musculoskeletal injuries. This phase of the class can include not only slow walking but also some light calisthenics, for instance, gentle stretching of the joints to be exercised and some brief (5- to 10-second) isometric or loaded contractions of the arm muscles. Prolonged isometric contractions cause an undesirable rise of blood pressure; the extent of the hypertensive response is almost directly proportional to the period for which a contraction is held. Brief isometric efforts avoid the loss of arm muscle liable to occur during a rehabilitation program that focuses exclusively on walking and jogging.

The main part of the exercise session (at least 30 minutes) alternates slow and fast walking or jogging. The speed is individually prescribed and is designed to develop the patient's target heart rate. A brief ball game (10 to 15 minutes) may follow to provide fun and create a group spirit. However, the game must not become competitive. If the instructor perceives that the contest is developing too rapid a pace, he or she can delay proceedings, for instance, by seizing the ball and demonstrating some point of technique.

Finally, the class must include a cool-down of at least 5 minutes of slow walking. There is a strong tendency for peripheral pooling of blood after vigorous exercise, and if venous return is not maintained at this stage by a gentle contraction of the leg muscles, hypotension can cut coronary flow and provoke a cardiac crisis. Several authors have described cardiac emergencies arising in the showers and changing areas immediately after exercise classes.

SUMMARY

The patient who has had a myocardial infarction is helped by a rehabilitation program that stresses progressive endurance exercise. The main physiologic mechanisms of benefit include a reduction in myocardial irritability, secondary to smoking withdrawal and a lesser secretion of catecholamines at any given intensity of exercise; a reduction in cardiac work rate resulting from a training bradycardia and a lesser rise of blood pressure during exercise; and an improved coronary perfusion, largely attributable to the training bradycardia. General advice on life-style and (after due progression of the exercise prescription) an improvement in lipid profile are other ways in which exercise may modify the disease process. The chapter describes a practical program that maximizes these benefits.

REFERENCES

1. Andrew, GM, et al: Reasons for drop-out from exercise programs in post-coronary patients, Med Sci Sports Exerc 13:164, 1981.
2. Cunningham, DA, et al: Effect of a 2-year program of exercise training on cardiovascular fitness and recurrence rates in past myocardial infarction patients: an interim report, Cardiology 62:136, 1977.
3. Cunningham, DA, et al: Stratification by compliance following an exercise trial is fallacious. Unpublished.
4. Fox, SM, and Haskell, WL: Physical activity and the prevention of coronary heart disease, Bull NY Acad Med 44:950, 1968.
5. Froelicher, V, et al: A randomized trial of exercise training in patients with coronary heart disease, JAMA 252:1291, 1984.
6. Gregg, DE, and Fisher, LC: Blood supply to the heart. In Hamilton, WF, editor: Handbook of physiology—circulation II, Washington, DC, 1963, American Physiological Society.
7. Haskel, WL: The influence of exercise on the concentrations of triglyceride and cholesterol in human plasma, Exerc Sport Sci Rev 12:205, 1984.
8. Kavanagh, T: The healthy heart programme, Toronto, 1980, Van Nostrand Reinhold.
9. Kavanagh, T, and Shephard, RJ: Conditioning of post-coronary patients: comparison of continuous and interval training, Arch Phys Med Rehabil 56:72, 1975.
10. Kavanagh, T, et al: Intensive exercise in coronary rehabilitation, Med Sci Sports Exerc 5:34, 1973.
11. Kavanagh, T, et al: Prognostic indexes for patients with ischaemic heart disease enrolled in an exercise-centered rehabilitation program, Am J Cardiol 44:1230, 1979.
12. Kavanagh, T, et al: Influence of exercise and lifestyle variables upon high density lipoprotein cholesterol after myocardial infarction, Arteriosclerosis 3:249, 1983.
13. Lipid Research Clinics Program: The Lipid Research Clinic's coronary primary prevention trial results. JAMA 251:351, 1984.
14. Morgan, P, Gildiner, M, and Wright, GR: Smoking reduction in adults who take up exercise: a survey of running clubs for adults, CAHPER J 42:39, 1976.
15. Paterson, DH, et al: Effects of physical training upon cardiovascular function following myocardial infarction, J Appl Physiol 47:482, 1977.
16. Paterson, DH, et al: Influence of age, angina, and time since infarction upon the cardiovascular response to physical training. Med Sci Sports Exerc 12:100, 1980.
17. Rechnitzer, PA, et al: Characteristics that predict recurrence of infarction within 3 years in the Ontario Exercise–Heart Collaborative Study, Can Med Assoc J 128:1287, 1983.
17a. Rechnitzer, PA, et al: Relation of exercise to the recurrence rate of myocardial infarction in men: Ontario Exercise–Heart Collaborative Study, Am J Cardiol 51:65, 1983.
18. Shephard, RJ: Ischemic heart disease and exercise, Chicago, 1982, Year Book Medical Publishers, Inc.
19. Shephard, RJ: The value of exercise in ischaemic heart disease—a cumulative analysis, J Cardiac Rehabil 3:294, 1983.
20. Shephard, RJ, Corey, R, and Kavanagh, T: Exercise compliance and the prevention of myocardial infarction, Med Sci Sports Exerc 13:1, 1981.
21. Shephard, RJ, Cox, M, and Kavanagh, T: Post-coronary rehabilitation and risk factors, with special reference to diet. Can J Appl Sport Sci 5:250, 1980.
22. Shephard, RJ, et al: Prognosis in myocardial infarction: the benefits of exercise as seen in non-randomized trials, Br J Sports Med 15:6, 1981.
23. Shephard, RJ, et al: Marathon jogging in post-myocardial infarction patients, J Cardiac Rehabil 3:321, 1983.
24. Tipton, C: Exercise, training and hypertension, Exerc Sport Sci Rev 12:254, 1984.
25. Vendsalu, A: Studies on adrenaline and noradrenaline in human plasma, Acta Physiol Scand 49(suppl 173):1, 1960.
26. Wood, PD, et al: The distribution of plasma lipoprotein in middle-aged male runners, Metabolism 11:1249, 1976.

CHAPTER 18

Cardiac rehabilitation exercise programs after coronary artery bypass surgery

OBSERVATIONS AS PATIENT AND PHYSICIAN

GAVRIL URSU

On the evening of September 4, 1981, during a brisk walk, I felt a strange chest discomfort that increased as I walked faster and disappeared when I stopped. After a few minutes of such "exercising," I realized the unthinkable: I was experiencing effort-related chest pain. My lifelong record of "never feeling fatigued" on exertion was at an end. On that night my pleasant memories of skiing from 9 AM to 5 PM with no break, of swimming and walking indefinitely, and of driving days and nights on end while vacationing became history. In fact, I had just spent 2 days and 2 nights on a driving trip to see my father and to bring him some medication (Nitro-Bid) for the chest discomfort he had recently experienced after climbing two flights of stairs. He was 83 years old.

I entered the hospital for a complete workup 2 weeks later. The finding was a severely stenotic left anterior descending artery (proximally and distally). Suddenly, I had to accept and adapt to a new life-style, to walk "as if your leg is casted," as a physician put it. I decided to undergo surgery, and on the night of November 2, 1981, I went peacefully to sleep, knowing that within a few hours I would be under very good surgical hands. I underwent a double coronary artery bypass graft, using internal mammary and saphenous vein, the next day. In about 2 weeks I was home, and except for some episodes of supraventricular tachycardia the immediate postsurgical course was quiet.

My integration to a new life-style began. Although I had heard about cardiac rehabilitation, nothing concrete was offered to me at that time. Therefore I started a program on my own. For exercise modalities I chose gradually increased walking outdoors and a cycle ergometer indoors. At the same time I started reviewing and slowly altering my diet and my habits in a painful adjustment (as is any undesirable change) to a new life-style. Later I enrolled in a periodically monitored cardiac rehabilitation program at home.

This chapter reflects opinions from literature and my own impressions of a suitable cardiac rehabilitation program after coronary artery bypass graft surgery, based on personal experience as a patient and participant and later as a profesional involved in this discipline. Interposed in this presentation are personal comments that emphasize my own experience and conclusions about a postsurgical cardiac rehabilitation program aimed toward preventing a secondary event.

I believe that the future trends in this field will emphasize cardiac prevention (primary prevention) and rehabilitation, involving apparently healthy people, as well as those who have had coronary artery bypass surgery (secondary prevention). In many respects the best therapeutic medicine is preventive medicine. It is also my belief that prevention and rehabilitation of coronary artery disease will evolve mainly based upon genetics, diet, control of stress, exercise, and leisure-time activity (in this order).

NATURAL HISTORY OF SURGICAL INTERVENTION

The benefits of coronary artery bypass surgery (CABS) range from complete pain relief (in 50% to 70% of patients for at least 3 to 5 years)[96] to significantly improved conditions (for 90% of patients).[74] The greatest improvements are gained by patients in whom all grafts remain patent[57] and who experience complete revascularization.[85] A significant number of postsurgical patients (perhaps 20%) experience no improvement or deteriorate despite being free of angina or having only mild residual symptoms.[61,77] Neural deafferentation, postoperative infarction of a previously ischemic segment,[7] has been implicated in this salutary effect of anginal symptoms.[7,8,40] Relief of chest pain in general has been shown to correlate with graft patency[45,49] and stabilization of the process that inhibits occlusion in both grafted and

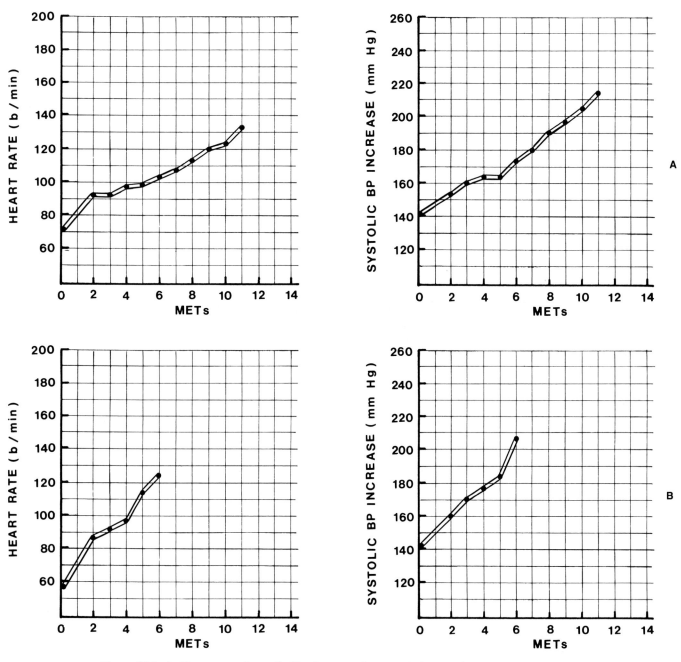

Figure 18-1. A, Heart rate and systolic blood pressure increase during exercise testing 15 months after coronary bypass surgery (CABS). At 11 METs workload, double product (pick systolic blood pressure times heart rate) was 278 and the ST segment depression was 1.3 mm. No symptoms occurred during test, which was conducted on patient receiving beta-blockade medication. **B,** Heart rate and systolic blood pressure increase during exercise testing 3 years after CABS. At 6 METs workload, double product was 258 and ST segment depression was 1.8 mm. No symptoms appeared during test; patient was not taking medication.

Continued.

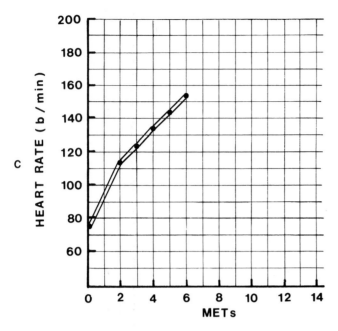

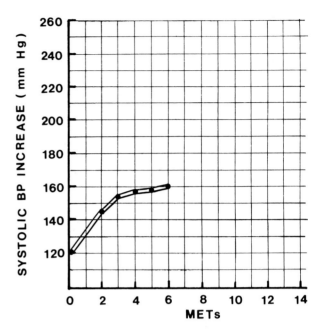

Figure 18-1, cont'd. C, Heart rate and systolic blood pressure during the exercise test 4 years after CABS. At 6 METs workload, double product was 258 and ST segment depression was 2.4 mm. No symptoms occurred during test. Patient was receiving beta-blockers and long-acting nitrate medication.

ungrafted vessels.[46] With the passage of time, the proportion of asymptomatic patients gradually declines.[88] A mean yearly attrition of 0.7% in graft patency[15] with 85% to 90% graft patency at 1 year and 80% to 85% at 5[88] and 6 years[30] (over 95% for internal mammary artery graft)[88] has been reported.

Late symptomatic deterioration following CABS is common and usually reflects a progression of coronary artery disease[81] (particularly in ungrafted coronary arteries).[15,84] Progressive atherosclerotic changes produce symptomatic deteriorations at a rate of 1% to 2% annually.[62] At 2¾ years following CABS, I felt my first chest discomfort, which was emotionally, or stress related. I again felt this discomfort a few months later on exertion in cold weather (this time I resumed medication). Exercise testing reflected a decline in cardiac functional capacity over the years (Figure 18-1).

MULTIFACTORIAL APPROACH TO REHABILITATION OF POSTOPERATIVE REVASCULARIZATION SURGERY PATIENTS

Beginning at age 30 for men and 40 for women, coronary heart disease is the single largest cause of death in the western worlds (actually, the disease probably starts early in life, because fatty streaks are common in the coronary arteries of children by the age of 5 years).*

---

*McArdle, WD, Katch, FL, and Katch, VL: Exercise, aging and cardiovascular disease. In Exercise physiology, ed 2, Philadelphia, 1986, Lea & Febiger.

This chapter is concerned primarily with postsurgical exercise programs; however, it is important to note that a cardiac rehabilitation program that does not consider a multifactorial interventional approach but disproportionally focuses almost solely on exercise will be dissipated by recurrence of patients' symptoms and deterioration in cardiovascular function. Indeed, the impact of exercise appears to be considerably less than that of other risk factors. For example, Finland, despite high levels of occupational and physical activity, has the world's highest coronary mortality.[39] As pointed out by Castelli of the Framingham Heart Study, "much too often cardiac rehabilitation programs that do a splendid job in exercise training fail to assess and properly treat blood cholesterol profiles that did not 'normalize'; and blood pressure, weight, blood sugar or smoking . . .".[17] (See box.) For every 1% fall in cholesterol levels, the coronary heart disease rates fall 2% to 3%.[17]

Psychologic stress has also been linked to the development and progression of cardiovascular disease.[19] Stress could be job related, social, family related, or environmental. Psychologic stress management (relaxation techniques and biofeedback, anxiety, and anger management training) plays an important role in a multidisciplinary cardiac rehabilitation intervention program.[19]

To cope with psychologic stress involves considerable learning. It is important because stress and diet may be the only recognizable factors. During those few weeks before my own surgery, I could identify two risk factors in my life: moderate hypercholesterolemia and stress. There was

RISK APPRAISAL FOR CORONARY HEART DISEASE						
Age (years)	10 to 20 — 1	21 to 30 — 2	31 to 40 — 3	41 to 50 — 4	51 to 60 — 6	61 to 70 and over — 8
Heredity	No known history of heart disease — 1	1 relative with cardiovascular disease; over 60 — 2	2 relatives with cardiovascular disease; over 60 — 3	1 relative with cardiovascular disease; under 60 — 4	2 relatives with cardiovascular disease; under 60 — 6	3 relatives with cardiovascular disease; under 60 — 7
Weight	More than 5 lb below standard weight — 0	−5 to +5 lb standard weight — 1	6-20 lb overweight — 2	21-35 lb overweight — 3	36-50 lb overweight — 5	51-65 lb overweight — 7
Tobacco smoking	Nonuser — 0	Cigar and/or pipe — 1	10 cigarettes or less a day — 2	20 cigarettes a day — 4	30 cigarettes a day — 6	40 cigarettes a day or more — 10
Exercise	Intensive occupational and recreational exertion — 1	Moderate occupational and recreational exertion — 2	Sedentary work and intense recreational exertion — 3	Sedentary occupational and moderate recreational exertion — 5	Sedentary work and light recreational exertion — 6	Complete lack of all exercise — 8
Cholesterol or fat percent in diet	Cholesterol below 180 mg/dl; diet contains no animal or solid fats — 1	Cholesterol 181-205 mg/dl; diet contains 10% animal or solid fats — 2	Cholesterol 206-230 mg/dl; diet contains 20% animal or solid fats — 3	Cholesterol 231-255 mg/dl; diet contains 30% animal or solid fats — 4	Cholesterol 256-280 mg/dl; diet contains 40% animal or solid fats — 5	Cholesterol 281-300 mg/dl; diet contains 50% animal or solid fats — 7
Blood pressure	100 upper reading — 1	120 upper reading — 2	140 upper reading — 3	160 upper reading — 4	180 upper reading — 6	200 or over upper reading — 8
Gender	Female under 40 — 1	Female 40-50 — 2	Female over 50 — 3	Male — 4	Stocky male — 6	Bald stocky male — 7

Score	Relative risk category
6-11	Risk well below average
12-17	Risk below average; OK
18-24	Average risk
25-31	Moderate risk
32-40	High risk
41-62	Very high risk; see your physician

Modified from McArdle, WD, Katch, FI, and Katch, VL: Exercise, aging and cardiovascular disease. In Exercise physiology, Philadelphia, 1986, Lea & Febiger.

no family history of cardiac disease; both parents were living and in their eighties at the time of surgery. I did not smoke, my blood pressure and weight were normal, and I regularly exercised in competitive and recreational sports.

In a carefully organized secondary prevention program, which is the core of a cardiac rehabilitation, psychologic stress management has to be learned under the systematic supervision of a good psychologist. The patient should not rely on unorganized informal advice or home recommendations.

Patient assessment and exercise testing

Evaluation of a patient who has had CABS for a monitored cardiac rehabilitation program includes a medical history, physical examination, coronary risk factor assessment, lipid screening, spirometry, skinfold measurements, psychosocial and personality assessment, and multigraded symptom/sign-limited exercise testing (with the treadmill or cycle ergometer).[60] The functional limits of the patient's cardiovascular system are defined in relation to his symptoms, physical signs, electrocardiographic signs, cardiac imaging, duration of exercise testing, maximal heart rate achieved, systolic blood pressure, and estimation of maximal oxygen intake (VO_2 max). The calculation of the functional aerobic impairment permits an estimation of the left ventricular function impairment and heart rate impairment (the percent difference between observed and predicted values).[10,12,13] Reassessments of the patient provide information for prescribing the level of activity and exercise training and for choosing between a supervised and unsupervised program.

Symptom-limited, graded, low-level exercise treadmill testing before hospital discharge in selected patients following uncomplicated myocardial revascularization surgery is safe and useful in assessing functional capacity.[83] The predischarge low-intensity exercise testing also facilitates a more rapid progression of activity once the patient returns home.[97] Relieving the patient's and family's anxiety, a safe return to daily activities on the patient's return home, and identifying or anticipating potential medical problems[38] (and explaining them to the patient and family) makes the difference between the proper standard care and a potential nightmare following the first few weeks at home for a relatively stable patient without complications.

Exercise testing: low-level graded and multilevel graded symptom/sign limited test

Postoperative treadmill performance is highly dependent on the completeness of revascularization and graft patency.[21,42,43] There is, however, a high incidence of normal exercise test results in patients with residual coronary disease. Thus the usefulness of such tests in estimating the completeness of revascularization in the individual post/operative patient is limited.[56]

A low-level exercise treadmill test in selected patients can be safe and reassures the patient that he or she can safely resume activities at home at the heart rate achieved during exercise at which no adverse signs or symptoms occurred. A low-level exercise test could identify or anticipate medical problems (for instance, arrhythmias) that help to determine the type of exercise program for the patient after discharge (for instance, whether the program should be undertaken at home or be medically supervised).[38] At 4 to 8 weeks following surgery, a multilevel, graded symptom/sign-limited exercise test renders a better assessment of functional capacity.

Maximal functional capacity (also referred to as aerobic capacity, maximal workload, exercise tolerance, cardiovascular endurance capacity, maximal oxygen consumption, or maximal oxygen uptake [VO_2 max]) is the maximal rate at which oxygen can be consumed per minute (at rest, this is approximately 3.5 ml O_2/kg/min; in severe functionally limited patients, 16 ml O_2/kg/min; in symptomatic patients, 22 ml O_2/kg/min[103]; and in the average sedentary male, 35 ml O_2/kg/min). Oxygen uptake may be determined by multiplying the MET value (metabolic equivalent expressed as oxygen consumption per unit of body weight) by 3.5.

Maximal oxygen uptake expressed in METs is estimated from treadmill speed and percentage grade or cycle ergometer power output expressed in kilopondmeter per minute (one MET represents a rate of energy expenditure requiring an oxygen consumption of about 3.5 ml O_2/min/kg body weight while sitting,[5] and it is recommended as the unit energy cost related to workload). A kilopondmeter (kpm/min) is the work done when a mass of 1 k is lifted 1 meter against the force of gravity.[35]

Therefore the activity of an exercise regimen can be quantified in terms of oxygen uptake, MET, or kilopondmeter, as well as in watts and kilocalories per minute.[75] In the opinions of other authors, the assumption that maximal oxygen uptake (VO_2 max) is equivalent to the energy cost of the terminal treadmill stage limits the accuracy of predicted VO_2 max to ± 1 MET.[27] The exercise capacity data may be expressed in a variety of units: New York Heart Association Class, aerobic impairment, treadmill time, kilopondmeter, watt, and MET.[32]

The ideal level of exercise training based on oxygen uptake is between 57% to 78% of maximal aerobic capacity, which is reflected by a training heart rate of 70% to 80% of maximal heart rate.[102] If the test is terminated before maximal work capacity is reached, for clinical reasons (for instance, angina, ST segment depression, or excessive fatigue), the level attained is considered the maximal functional capacity for that particular patient and is used as the basis for the exercise prescription.[33] Standards must be observed and contraindications for tests determining the level of participation in exercise programs must be watched for in postoperative patients.[4,20,24]

Exercise training for patients who have had CABS

Raising the activity threshold at which angina occurs, improving the exercise tolerance and the patient's confidence, and achieving general well-being are the chief benefits of an exercise cardiac rehabilitation program.[39a] During his "armchair treatment" of patients with myocardial infarction, Levin described the beneficial effects on the psychologic state of patients.[48] The psychologic changes, including decreased anxiety and depression and increased emotional stability and self-esteem, may be some of the most striking aspects of a supervised exercise program for postoperative CABS patients.[62,66] There are a number of mechanisms by which exercise enhances the psychologic state of patients. For instance, lactate plays a key role in producing anxiety symptoms and is caused by chronic overproduction of adrenaline. Aerobic training reduces the amount of lactate in the body.[80] In addition, norepinephrine levels are notably low in depressed patients, and exercise dramatically increases them.[80]

Heart rate and blood pressure are important determinants of myocardial oxygen demand,[35] and the double product (heart rate times systolic blood pressure) correlates with measured myocardial oxygen consumption and permits an estimate of the maximal workload of the left ventricle.[103] The ejection fraction of the left ventricle also is improved after successful myocardial revascularization in patients who have had CABS.[96]

Physical conditioning may result in an increase in exercise tolerance with little or no ability to increase myocardial blood flow.[28] Properly administered physical training increases maximal oxygen uptake primarily by peripheral or noncardiac adaptations.[11] In most patients with cardiovascular disease, the restriction of maximal oxygen intake reflects limitations in maximal cardiac output because of a reduction in stroke volume as well as in heart rate.[12] During exercise training, there is an increase in maximal oxygen uptake caused by the increased blood supply to exercising muscle and increased extraction of oxygen from circulating blood.[95]

Oldridge and associates reported an increase in functional capacity of 28% in patients who have had CABS with 32 months of physical conditioning (an increase of from 7 to 9 METs) as compared to the 3% increase observed in matched controls who did not participate in a conditioning program.[67] An average, apparently healthy, 40-year-old man in the United States can function at 10 METs at his maximum capacity; a peak functional capacity of about 8 METs is more than adequate for most occupations.[5] A 5 METs capacity allows a safe range of metabolic reserve for most necessary daily activities.[2] An improvement from 3 to 5 METs means a dramatic change in the performance of daily activities, whereas an improvement of 2 METs in a person with a work capacity of 10 METs would be imperceptible unless he was engaged in fairly strenuous activities.[98]

Periodic assessment to detect a decrease in functional capacity is an important aspect of the cardiac rehabilitation program and requires a careful reevaluation of factors such as graft patency, progression of underlying coronary disease, and left ventricular dysfunction. A continuous exercise program is of the utmost importance in signaling a change, expressed by a lowered threshold of symptom/sign-limited capacity to a given workload. To maintain functional capacity at or close to the postsurgical level is the main goal of an exercise program that is part of a multidisciplinary intervention program. The ''battle for METs'' to keep the patient at a comfortable functional level during daily routine work and leisure activities should be a main task.

An increased threshold for angina is clearly the best documentation of training-induced benefits in patients with coronary artery disease.[52] Generally, 60% to 70% of functional capacity (maximal METs) is an appropriate conditioning intensity for persons with a functional capacity ranging from 3 to 20 METs.[4] The target training zone of 57% to 78% of the maximal aerobic power (VO_2 max) corresponds to approximately 70% to 85% of the maximal heart rate, regardless of age, sex, presence or absence of coronary heart disease, body weight, exercise mode, or drug therapy.[26,35]

Heart rate during exercise increases linearly with workload and oxygen uptake, and this relationship is useful in writing an individualized exercise prescription.[103] But the double product (heart rate times the systolic blood pressure) correlates even better with myocardial work and oxygen consumption.[68] As conditioning proceeds, the double product provoked by a given body exercise intensity declines. Over time, however, it levels off.[70]

When my own symptoms reoccurred and I resumed medication, I also began a new home program of periodically monitored exercise training. In the 2 months that followed, the variables monitored for me (double product and conditioning index) showed a constant improvement (Figure 18-2, *A*).[68] After another 3 months, there was an upward trend (Figure 18-2, *B*), and in the last 3 months, there was no further increase in the conditioning index at a constant workload of 640 kpm/min per session (slightly over 6 METs) 3 times a week (Figure 18-2, *C*).

In addition to heart rate, which is an important indicator of exercise intensity, systolic blood pressure during exercise training is important because the double product during exercise correlates with the oxygen demand of the myocardium and reflects more accurately the level of beginning ischemia (with or without symptoms) than does heart rate alone. Therefore measuring the systolic blood pressure in addition to heart rate during aerobic exercising (for example, after 15 minutes of exercise at a prescribed exercise intensity) is a valuable parameter. The patient should stay under the threshold of myocardial ischemia but within target zone to achieve the training effect. Often, patients have to be taught how to take their own blood pressure during exercise. Adaptive devices are available.

When chest pain or discomfort is experienced during the exercise, the heart rate should be lowered by 5 to 10 beats below the rate at the onset of the angina, even though the exercise training is performed within the prescribed target heart rate. At that exercise session the systolic blood pressure may have been higher or an associated coronary spasm may have occurred. Lowering the heart rate is a safe way to cope with occasionally unusual exercise conditions (for example, increased fatigue, changes in temperature and humidity, or recent emotional upset).

If the beneficial effects of exercise training are to take place, each session of training must be of sufficient intensity (between 70% to 80% of the maximal heart rate attained on the symptom/sign-limited exercise testing), sufficient duration (20 to 30 minutes of aerobic activity), and regularity (three times a week) for an indefinite time.[34] Too little exercise is ineffective, and too much is harmful (Figures 18-3 to 18-5).[68]

Figure 18-2. A, Double product gradually decreasing at given constant workload of 450 kg/min (bicycle ergometer), and conditioning index steadily rising. **B,** Conditioning index continues to have upward trend at 500 kg/min workload. **C,** No further significant increase in conditioning index at constant workload of 640 kg/min exercise training. *Beaded line,* Double product (heart rate times systolic blood pressure; *solid line,* conditioning index (external workload in kg/min − 1 divided by cardiac workload) (double product); *broken line,* external workload level (see reference 69). (From Houston Cardiovascular Rehabilitation Center.)

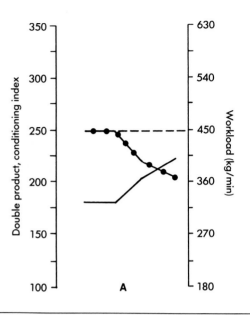

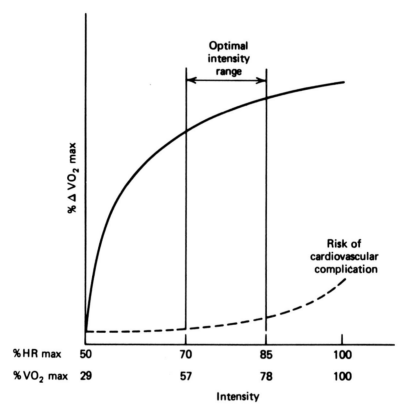

Figure 18-3. Relationship between gain in aerobic capacity (expressed as Vo_2 max, %Δ) and intensity of exercise (expressed as % HR max or % Vo_2 max). As intensity of exercise exceeds 85% maximal heart rate, relative risks of dysrhythmias, angina pectoris, and other ischemic manifestations increases abruptly, whereas improvement in aerobic capacity levels off. (Modified from Dehn, MM, and Mullins, CB: Cardiovasc Med 2:365, 1977. In Hellerstein, HK, and Franklin, BA: Exercise testing and prescription. In Wenger, NK, and Hellerstein, HK, editors: Rehabilitation of the coronary patient, ed 2, New York, 1984, John Wiley & Sons, Inc.)

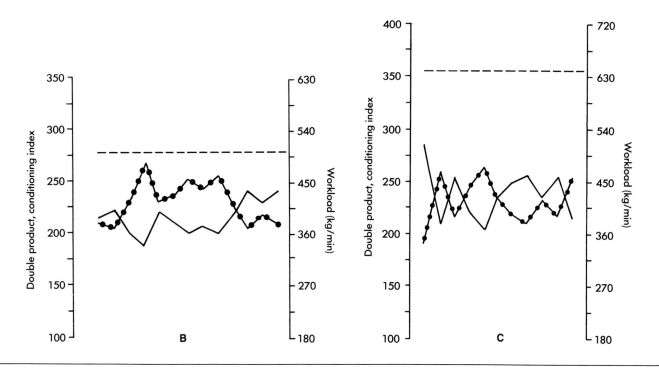

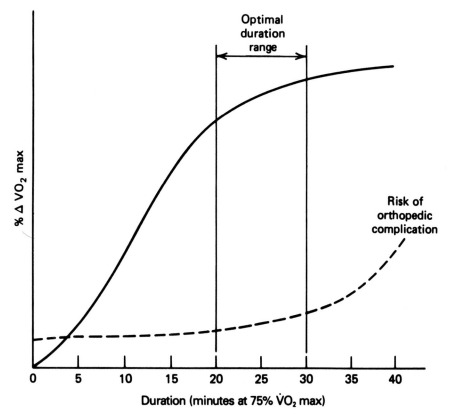

Figure 18-4. Relationship between exercise duration (minutes at 75% Vo_2 max) and increase in aerobic capacity (Vo_2 max, %Δ). Prolonged exercise beyond 30 minutes increases risk of orthopedic complications, with slight additional improvement in aerobic capacity. (Modified from Dehn, MM, and Mullins, CB: Cardiovasc Med 2:365, 1977. In Hellerstein, HK, and Franklin, BA: Exercise testing and prescription. In Wenger, NK, and Hellerstein, HK, editors: Rehabilitation of the coronary patient, ed 2, New York, 1984, John Wiley & Sons, Inc.)

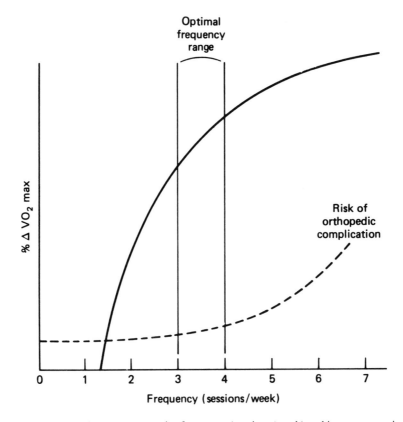

Figure 18-5. Relationship between exercise frequency (sessions/week) and improvement in aerobic capacity (Vo₂ max, %Δ). Risk of orthopedic injury increases markedly for high-frequency training (no more than five sessions/week) with slight additional improvement in aerobic capacity. (Modified from Dehn, MM, and Mullins, CB: Cardiovasc Med 2:365, 1977. In Hellerstein, HK, and Franklin, BA: Exercise testing and prescription. In Wenger, NK, and Hellerstein, HK, editors: Rehabilitation of the coronary patient, ed 2, New York, 1984, John Wiley & Sons, Inc.)

Among the three basic components of an exercise prescription, the intensity of the exercise is the most important determinant of the program's safety. Longer duration and more frequent sessions can compensate for a lower intensity, but a higher intensity is never to be used to compensate for shorter duration or lower frequency.

The subject's perception of exertion during exercise may be used to indicate the relative work intensity.[9] The Rating Perceived Exertion (RPE) Borg Scale is a subjective estimate of effort intensity and correlates well with the physiologic response to exercise (oxygen uptake, heart rate, minute ventilate, and blood lactate).[83] RPE is used extensively as an adjunct to signs and symptoms and heart rate. Studies have shown that the 12 to 13 level on the RPE Borg Scale (the "somewhat hard" level) correlates with 60% to 70% of heart rate reserve.[4,72] The RPE Borg Scale, however, does not assess angina discomfort in a satisfactory manner, so the angina scale should be used in addition because general fatigue symptoms are relatively independent of the sensation of angina pectoris.[51] (See boxes.)

In a home program the patient should have a chart with perceived exertion scale and another with angina scale discomfort; he should be instructed on how to use them properly. During exercise the charts should be placed in front of him within easy view, and the patient should be asked periodically about the level of perceived exertion.[3]

The beneficial effects of exercise training (that is, heart rate, systolic blood pressure, ST segment depression decreases, and maximal exercise capacity increases) were equally effective in patients receiving beta-blockers.[53] The exercise test must be carried out on patients receiving beta-blockers, so the target heart rate prescription of 70% to 85% is calculated from a maximal heart rate under this condition.[105] Any addition or change in medication (for instance, beta-blockers, calcium channel blockers, or long-acting nitrates) requires a new exercise test and a newly adapted exercise prescription.

A significant decrease in the percentage of body fat without a significant decrease in body weight is another training phenomenon resulting from increased muscle mass caused by exercise training.[34] In a cardiac rehabilitation program for overweight patients who have had CABS, the significance of an exercise training program is not to "burn calories." That should be achieved strictly by diet.

RPE AND RATING SCALES

The original rating of perceived exertion scale and the revised ratio scale may be used in exercise testing or exercise programs.

RPE		New rating scale	
6		0	Nothing at all
7	Very, very light	0.5	Very, very weak
8		1	Very weak
9	Very light	2	Weak
10		3	Moderate
11	Fairly light	4	Somewhat strong
12		5	Strong
13	Somewhat hard	6	
14		7	Very strong
15	Hard	8	
16		9	
17	Very hard	10	Very, very strong
18			Maximal
19	Very, very hard		

From American College of Sports Medicine: Guidelines for exercise test administration. In Guidelines for exercise testing and prescription, ed 3, Philadelphia, 1986, Lea & Febiger.

ANGINA SCALE

1 None at all
2 Extremely light
3 Very light
4 Quite light
5 Not so light, rather strong
6 Strong
7 Very strong
8 Extremely strong
9 Maximum, unbearable

From Maresh, CM, and Noble, GJ: Utilization of perceived exertion ratings during exercise testing and training. In Hall, LK, Meyer, GC, and Hellerstein, HK, editors: Cardiac rehabilitation: exercise testing and prescription, New York, 1984, SP Medical & Scientific Books.

When training ceases, a significant decrement in working capacity occurs within 2 weeks. After 12 weeks, almost all of the training adaptations, or functional improvements, return to the pretraining level.[55] On one occasion I changed my exercise program from an indoor cycle ergometer (6 METs steady intensity) to a program of brisk walking of less or variable intensity. After 3 months, when I resumed indoor cycle ergometer exercising because of changed weather conditions, I had to start with a 5 METs workload. Only after several weeks did I reach my previous training level.

Exercise programs

A four-phase cardiac rehabilitation program is practical. Phase I is inpatient rehabilitation; phase II is outpatient rehabilitation (either supervised or unsupervised and monitored or unmonitored); phase III is also outpatient (community or individual) rehabilitation; and phase IV is an advanced maintenance program. Patients should undergo periodic assessment to detect any changes in their functional status that could require a change in the program sequence. For example, a patient could step down from a phase III individual, unmonitored program at home to a phase II hospital-supervised, monitored program if such a change is indicated by test results.

Phase I: inpatient program

An immediate postoperative exercise program for the patient who has had CABS can be safe and helpful in identifying medical problem such as graft failure, postpericardiotomy pain that mimics angina, constrictive pericarditis that mimics congestive failure, ventricular dysrhythmias, dyspnea, hypotension, sternal malunion, and angina pectoris.[82]

The program starts 12 to 48 hours after surgery with deep breathing exercises,[97] followed by an incremental progression of joint range of motion, walking, and climbing one flight of stairs.[1,76] This low-level exercise intensity involves between 1.5 and 3.5 METs.[47] Walking begins with gradual floor ambulation with electrocardiographic telemetry and blood pressure monitoring. Patients who have had uncomplicated cardiac surgery and participated in an early low-level exercise program 12 to 24 hours after surgery have a shorter hospitalization as compared to those who were not exposed to such a program.[93]

In 5 to 7 days, if there are no complications, patients advance to treadmill walking at an exercise intensity of 2.5 to 3.5 METs and a heart rate of 20 to 25 beats per minute above a standing rest and 10 to 15 beats per minute for patients receiving beta-blockers.[31] The participant's progression to an advanced phase I program could be perceived and recorded in an inpatient rehabilitation unit by electrocardiographic telemetry–monitored activity, using treadmills or stationary bicycles at an intensity of approximately 3 METs.[47]

If vital signs are stable and exercise is well tolerated, a predischarge exercise evaluation (low-intensity or symptom-limited exercise) is performed.[47] The home exercise prescription is based on the patient's response to monitored treadmill walking or bicycle exercise with a training heart rate maintained at 20 to 25 beats above a standing rest and a perceived exertion level of "somewhat hard" using the RPE Borg Scale.[31] The duration of this program should be 4 to 6 weeks.

Ventricular dysrhythmias are not rare events following CABS but occur in 70% of patients.[82] In an unprepared patient they could have a detrimental psychologic effect, with a reflection of the "imminence of death" with each event. Thorough explanation of these possibly frequent dysrhythmias before hospital discharge alleviates much of the patient's uncertainty.

When the patient is at home, there are a few important medical problems that may inhibit his activity.[100] Thoracotomy creates incisional and sternal tenderness that may simulate angina and thereby discourage exercise. The pain, paresthesias, and edema at the site of saphenous vein removal may also interfere with the patient's exercise conditioning.[62] The patient's anxiety increases if he confuses incisional discomfort with cardiovascular symptoms.[50] This can happen to both layperson and physician. Incisional discomfort does not respond to nitroglycerin, lasts longer, has no specific precipitating event,[50] and changes occasionally with changing body posture (especially while walking). Selective calisthenic exercises and special exercises performed with a cane are recommended to prevent chest wall adhesions, stiffness, and foreshortening of chest wall musculature.[62,76]

Sometimes for up to 1 year postoperatively, patients find it difficult to sneeze, cough, lie flat, have sex, sit up in bed, drive, bend over, climb stairs, lift things, walk outside, or garden.[100] These problems must be explained to the patient before discharge or during immediate follow-up visits because knowing and anticipating the event for uncomplicated postsurgical patients improves their motivation and compliance with the predischarge recommendations. This is particularly true during physical therapy.

Phase II: supervised versus unsupervised rehabilitation programs

An unsupervised exercise program is frequently the only available alternative for many patients who have had CABS; it can be performed safely with functional improvements similar to those obtained with supervised exercise after uncomplicated CABS.[32,90]

The predischarge low-level graded exercise test is becoming a standard for diagnostic purposes and as an aid in prescribing exercise for both phase II unsupervised home and monitored outpatient exercise sessions. There are diverse opinions as to how long and to what extent sophisticated monitoring is needed. For patients at high risk and with dangerous rhythm disturbances, longer periods of monitoring are recommended.[60,76] Predischarge exercise testing provides the data for a home exercise program; however, the possibility of malignant arrhythmias at peak levels of exercise still exists. A telephonically monitored home exercise program after short walks or bicycle ergometry is suggested to detect new arrhythmias or conduction disturbances.[25]

Beginning the phase II exercise program. Because the programs and opinions about timing differ, several programs are reviewed in the following paragraphs:

Pollack and associates[73] recommend beginning the program 2 to 3 days after the patient is discharged from the hospital. They recommend a supervised, telemetry-monitored program consisting of exercises to condition the upper and lower extremities 3 times a week. Along with exercise, the patient receives an education program emphasizing risk factor reduction, proper health habits, and weight reduction.

Meyer and Hensel[58] begin phase II with a low-level training program (with a heart rate of 20 to 30 beats per minute above a standing rest) that lasts 6 weeks. The patients are supervised and monitored via telemetry during an interval of alternating exercise and rest for both upper and lower extremities using treadmill, bicycle ergometer, free weights, wall pulley, and arm ergometer. After 6 weeks the participants undergo a symptom-limited exercise test and start on a program at an intensity of 65% to 75% of the patient's achieved maximal heart rate attained during the test. The program includes education about coronary artery disease, risk factors, nutrition, sexual activity, and medication.

A program that is designed for patients who are recently discharged from the hospital and that is located in their physical medicine department is described by Milesis and Harville.[59] The patient is monitored while using treadmill or bicycle exercise therapy to improve physical work capacity (attaining a level of aerobic capacity of 6 METs). The program also includes risk factor assessment, health education, and identification of undesirable signs or symptoms during exercise.

The program described by Keteyian and associates[41] starts as early as 2 weeks after CABS, and before hospital discharge patients are given a low-level graded exercise tolerance test that is electrocardiographically monitored. The exercise regimen consists of circuit training of both upper and lower extremities with an exercise intensity of 70% to 85% of the symptom-free peak heart rate from the graded exercise tolerance test.

Murray and Beller's program[62] starts in the first 8 weeks following hospital discharge with a target heart rate range of 70% to 80% of the maximum achieved during the first postoperative exercise stress test.

Based on personal experience, I believe that a patient with uncomplicated CABS, following a predischarge low-level exercise tolerance test, can start a gradual home program immediately following hospital discharge, provided appropriate home guidelines and follow-up monitoring are observed. The program should be low-level training, consisting of walking (or cycle ergometer when weather conditions change) at a heart rate intensity of 20 to 30 beats per minute over standing resting level. The program is set at a lower level if the patient is receiving beta-blockers. After 4 to 6 weeks a symptom/sign-limited exercise test should be performed and a new exercise prescription written. The first one or two sessions should be carried out in a supervised setting to confirm that the data from the stress testing (the 70% to 85% of heart rate levels) is safe and corresponds to the data of exercise training (particularly because training is a longer submaximal stress test 3 times a week).

Phase II: length and cessation. In general, phase II may be terminated when maximal functional capacity is greater than 10 METs for patients less than 55 years old and 8 METs for patients greater than 55 years old who show normal hemodynamic responses to exercise and in whom no potentially dangerous arrhythmias are precipitated by the exercise.[14] Not all patients are able to complete 9 to 11 METs at the conclusion of phase II.

Phase III: outpatient maintenance program

The phase III program may be supervised, monitored, community based, or unsupervised at home.[64] Its emphasis is on maintenance. The intensity of training is based on the patient's medical and physical state as indicated by the symptom/sign-limited graded exercise test.

This interval consists of a 3- to 6-month medically supervised exercise conditioning program that begins 4 to 6 weeks after phase II.[44] The patient works out three times a week with a warm-up and cool-down period for each exercise session. Endurance training—consisting of either walking, jogging, cycling, or swimming for 30 minutes—is preceded by a 10-minute warm-up. The exercise intensity is between 3 and 15 METs; for example, slow long-distance walking is graduated to fast long-distance walking and then to walking-jogging intervals. All sessions are conducted and closely observed by basic cardiac life support certified personnel.[44] The patient jogs with a radiotelemetry ECG once each month.[44] After 3 months a graded exercise test is performed and the program reevaluated.[64]

Phase IV: indefinitely provided cardiac status remains unchanged

Phase IV programs are for those with a functional capacity of at least 9 METs for as long as periodic symptom/sign-limited graded exercise tests reveal no changes.

Participation time in one program varied from 6 months to 5 years.[94] The patients function independently with rehabilitation staff offering guidance and supervision. Exercise tests and lipid profiles are performed every 6 months, and patient education encourages participants to assume responsibility for their own health through independent exercise and modification of life-style.[94]

Another program follows a more traditional format, with objectives of assisting with patient compliance, increasing patient self-confidence and self-awareness so that the participant is able to pursue physical activities in community-based programs or at home with peace of mind, educating the patient about risk factor reduction, and providing periodic medical follow-up evaluation.[47] Patients may choose to exercise in phase IV indefinitely.

Serial testing helps individualize the length of the exercise program.[20] Heart rate used in combination with signs and symptoms is one of the best indicators of when to advance the participant to the next level.[4] Exercise testing from 1 to 5 years after CABS reveals that maximal benefit is reached at 1 year after surgery. My personal experience confirms this view. The serial exercise tests show a slow and gradual loss of improvement in exercise parameters, reflecting ischemia perhaps resulting from graft occlusion, progression of the underlying disease process, or a combination of the two.[29]

Warm-up must precede and cool-down must follow aerobic exercise training. Warm-up can reduce the risk of ischemic ST segment depression and ventricular ectopy, and cool-down permits a return of the heart rate and blood pressure to near resting values, reducing the potential for hypotension and dizziness after exercise.[26] The danger from arrhythmias during cool-down may be considerable, and the drop in blood pressure during recovery appears to trigger the response.[23] I found it safe to rest for another 15 minutes after cool-down, to do only light activities for the following half hour to an hour, and to avoid heavy meals, alcohol, and hot showers for at least 1 hour following the exercise session.

The exercise heart rate is a useful method of adjusting the intensity of exercise for varying environmental conditions,[4] but a cold environment and isometric work may cause stress to the cardiovascular system that is not accurately reflected by heart rate.[98] Low temperatures increase peripheral systemic resistance and arterial blood pressure, causing an increase in myocardial demand.[92] The ideal environment is between 40° and 75° F and below 65% relative humidity.[101] The setting should be indoors during cold weather (using the cycle ergometer) and outdoors (brisk walking at 3 to 4 miles per hour) during warm weather, which satisfies the temperature-humidity requirements and is an appropriate combination for an individual's unsupervised home program. My own program consisted of this regimen.

EXERCISE MODALITIES

A variety of exercise modalities are available for patients. As a general rule, an exercise of constant intensity is safest.[24]

Walking

Walking is easily tolerated and is the best activity, provided that the intensity is within the range of training effect. The patient must understand what it means to pace 2, 3, or 4 miles per hour. This can be learned when using the treadmill during exercise testing. A treadmill may be used for an indoor walking program.

Jogging

During jogging, the MET capacity has to be above 8 METs.[72] However, many patients experience orthopedic and musculoskeletal problems.

Swimming

Swimming, which involves the upper and lower extremities and is a non-weight-bearing exercise, is not recommended until 6 to 8 weeks postoperatively to allow healing of the sternum. It is adequate for patients who are very obese, amputees, or those with orthopedic problems. The energy expenditure can be very high, depending on the individual patient's skills: a 4 METs energy expenditure for a skilled patient may be the same as an 8 METs expenditure for a less skilled patient over the same exercise period. For patients with good skills,[35] swimming is a complex exercise modality.

Bicycling

Bicycling can be done indoors on a cycle ergometer (Figure 18-6) or outdoors. A constant intensity of effort should be maintained. It has been shown that bicycle exercise constitutes a greater stress on the cardiovascular system than does treadmill exercise in terms of double product at any given oxygen uptake.[104] Bicycling is a useful modality. Unfortunately the average American does not bike after his or her adolescent years.[52]

Rope skipping

Rope skipping is a non-weight-bearing exercise requiring high energy[35] and is not indicated for those with lower functional capacity.

Calisthenics

When properly done, calisthenics can elicit a training effect[35]; it is especially valuable during warm-up and cooldown periods.

Stair climbing

The average effort for stair climbing requires a capacity of 4 to 6 METs and is a good adjunct to other exercise modalities, especially during work activities. During my own daily activities, I use the stairs between three floors rather than the elevator.

Aerobic dance

Aerobic dancing is close to calisthenic exercises.

Cross-country skiing

Cross-country skiing requires a higher METs capacity, good endurance, and good weather.

Other modalities

Many recreational and vocational activities rely on arm work more than leg work, and few occupations require sustained walking or jogging.[26] In some exercise programs[35] arm and leg exercises are alternated to achieve total body training: arm cycle ergometer (Figure 18-7), leg cycle ergometer, rowing machine, arm wall wheel, steps, and treadmill (Figure 18-8). Heart rates are monitored and workloads are adjusted to achieve the prescribed training heart rate.[35] Limited upper body exercises as well as upper body training (for instance, arm ergometer, rowing machine, wall pulley,

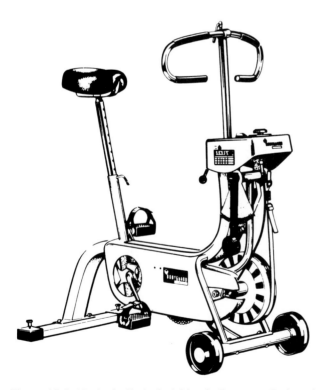

Figure 18-6. Mechanically braked Bicycle Ergometer Bodygard 990 may be used in unsupervised home exercise training program.

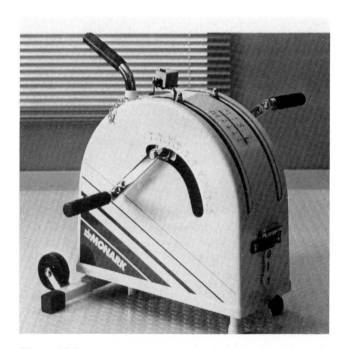

Figure 18-7. Arm ergometer, Monark 881. (Courtesy Monark-Crescent A.B., Varberg, Sweden.)

or light dumbbells exercise) are offered to participants whose occupational or recreational activities (for instance, volleyball, tennis, canoeing, kayaking, or swimming) primarily involve the arms.[99] Repetitive weight lifting has a smaller pressor response[87] in a patient using 1-, 2-, or 3-pound dumbbells exercise while walking.[94]

ABNORMAL RESPONSES DURING AN EXERCISE PROGRAM

The usual accepted criteria for exercise testing and exercise training termination because of abnormal symptoms, signs, or dysrhythmias must be observed.[3]

Angina pectoris

Anginal symptoms are a poor indicator of myocardial ischemia. Patients may have myocardial ischemia without chest pain (70% to 75% of ischemic episodes in patients with typical angina are silent).[6,89] It is misleading to rely on absence of angina during exercise training as an indicator of appropriate exercise intensity. One day during a personal exercise session at home, a 24-hour Holter monitor revealed an ST segment depression of −1.9 mm while I was exercising to a heart rate of 120 beats per minute with no chest discomfort.

Hypotension

Hypotension resulting from exertion (systolic blood pressure decreases more than 10 mm Hg while exercising) is believed to be due to acute severe ischemic left ventricular dysfunction.[78]

Hypertension

Systolic blood pressure increases above 200 mg Hg and diastolic blood pressure above 110 mm Hg during exercise.[22] The systolic hypertensive response is associated with an

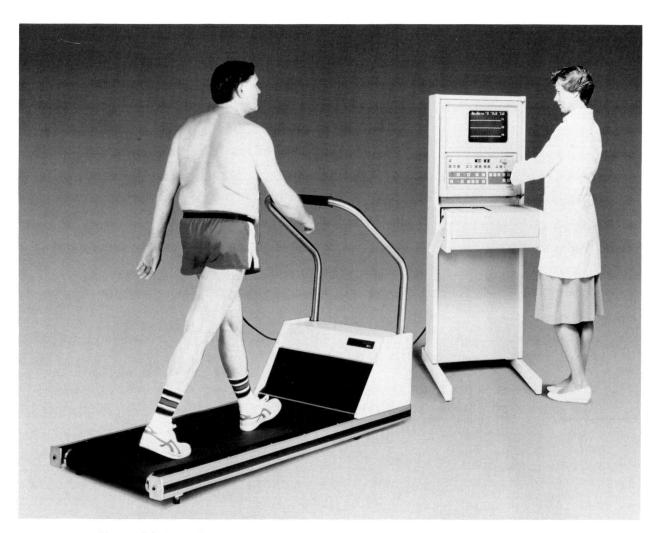

Figure 18-8. Treadmill as exercise device used in cardiac conditioning, especially for patients who should be closely supervised and monitored. Quinton Q55 Treadmill and Q3000 Monitor. (Courtesy Medical Instruments Division, A.H. Robins Co.)

early shift from an aerobic to an anaerobic response to exercise.[70] (Blood pressure of 200 mm Hg and over during exercise training should be avoided.)

Heart rate

A higher than expected heart rate in response to a low workload (during exercise training) might signal the presence of latent left ventricular dysfunction.[63]

Exercise-induced ST segment changes (depression or elevation of >1 mm above isoelectric line)[22]

On ambulatory ECG monitoring, most ST segment deviation does not occur with an increased heart rate and can be due to coronary artery spasm.

Serious dysrhythmias

Serious dysrhythmias include unifocal premature ventricular contractions (more than 10 per minute), multifocal premature ventricular contractions (more than 6 per minute),

ventricular couplets (more than 2 per minute), R on T extrasystole, ventricular and supraventricular tachycardia, and third-degree heart block.[22] These can occur before and during exercising and into cool-down. To assess the influence of environmental and emotional stress on arrhythmias and heart rate or to assess ST segment changes during a home program, ambulatory monitoring for 24 to 72 hours is recommended (Figure 18-9).[86]

Rapid progression of underlying coronary artery disease during a training program is a major contraindication to exercise training. There is approximately one episode of cardiac arrest for every 33,000 patient hours of exercise (most are due to ventricular fibrillation) and one death for every 120,000 patient hours of exercise (most of the complications occur during warm-up and after training periods). The patients who are most prone to cardiac arrest are those who exceed their prescribed training heart rate, those with ST segment depression persisting for more than 1 minute into recovery or greater than 3 mm persisting into recovery.[36]

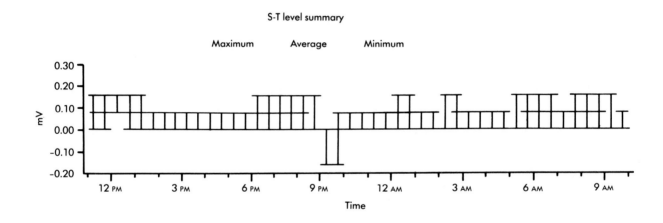

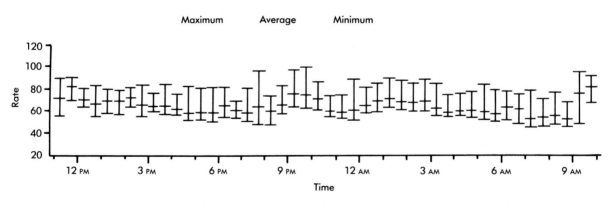

Figure 18-9. Ambulatory 24-hour electrocardiographic monitoring does not reveal ST segment significantly changed during 45 minutes of exercise (brisk walking between 11 AM and 12 PM) but shows ST segment depression of >1 mm between 9 and 10 PM with minimal activity and no symptoms (self-monitoring).

Fatal cases have been reported in marathon runners. Two veteran long-distance runners with 20 years of experience died as a result of severe coronary artery disease.[65]

FURTHER ASSESSMENT OF THE PATIENT WHO HAS HAD CABS ON AN EXERCISE PROGRAM

If symptoms return 6 months following CABS, they are more likely to occur in patients with occluded grafts.[37] Further assessment is advised before continuing the exercise training.

The inability of the patient to perform an exercise that he previously performed should warn the patient and his physician that further evaluation and treatment may be required. Under such circumstances, continuing the same exercise program is of no benefit and could be dangerous. Functional capacity, myocardial perfusion (thallium scintigraphy), left ventricular function (radionuclide angiography at rest and during exercise), and coronary vessel anatomy should be reassessed. This identifies patients at increased risk for cardiovascular complications during exercise training, such as those with new perfusion abnormalities or deteriorating myocardial function.[71] Exercise training thus provides a regular check of continued well-being.[79] Exercise training with serial symptoms/sign-limited exercise testing can reflect, by cardiovascular responses to exercise, improvement, maintenance, or deterioration of cardiovascular status and aerobic capacity (VO_2 max).

CONCLUSION

Successful and complete myocardial revascularization following coronary artery bypass surgery (CABS) is a palliative procedure. Late symptomatic deterioration following CABS is common and usually reflects the progression of coronary artery disease in both grafted and ungrafted vessels.

Cardiac rehabilitation in a CABS patient requires a multifactorial approach to a disease with a multifaceted etiology. Some risk factors are modifiable; others are less amenable to treatment. To modify the least amenable risk factors, prevention has to be initiated early in life, and to modify the most amenable (for instance, hypercholesterolemia, smoking, hypertension, obesity, lack of exercise, and stress), it has to be aggressive. Exercise plays an important role in primary prevention but is not the most important in secondary prevention.

A cardiac rehabilitation program in a patient who has had uncomplicated CABS can be started on the first day after surgery and continue indefinitely with exercise conditioning as the permanent monitoring of the patient's well-being. Predischarge low-intensity exercise testing in patients who have had uncomplicated CABS should become a standard procedure despite controversy over the significance of symptom-limited versus heart rate–limited test results.

The physician should routinely relieve the patient's and family's anxiety on hospital discharge following uncomplicated CABS by explaining, identifying, and anticipating potential medical problems and by formulating a concrete individualized plan of physical activity. Patients should never only be casually told, "Take it easy; in 2 to 3 months you can do everything."

An exercise program's main goal (as part of the multidisciplinary intervention for a patient's secondary prevention program) is to keep the patient at a comfortable functional level during daily routine work and leisure activities. This can also have a great impact on the patient's psychologic status.

In selected patients who have had uncomplicated CABS, a home cardiac rehabilitation program with periodic hospital or medical center follow-up evaluation is a safe alternative to monitored and supervised hospital- or community-based programs. Patients with functional capacity impairments (6 METs and less), myocardial perfusions, and left ventricular impairments, (especially at rest) and those with abnormal cardiovascular responses to exercise, especially at a low level of workload intensity, should be in a structured, supervised, monitored, hospital-based or medical center–based outpatient program. Objective periodic cardiac status assessment (for instance, studies of functional aerobic capacity, myocardial perfusion, left ventricular function, and coronary vessel anatomy when warranted) more accurately delineate low-risk profile cardiac patients versus those with high-risk profiles, enabling physicians and patients to appropriately change the cardiac rehabilitation program.

REFERENCES

1. Ades, PA, et al: The cardiac rehabilitation program of the University of Vermont Medical Center, J Cardiac Rehabil 6:265, 1986.
2. American College of Sports Medicine: Exercise prescription for cardiac patients. In Guidelines for exercise testing and prescription, ed 3, Philadelphia, 1986, Lea & Febiger.
3. American College of Sports Medicine: Guidelines for exercise test administration. In Guidelines for exercise testing and prescription, ed 3, Philadelphia, 1986, Lea & Febiger.
4. American College of Sports Medicine: Principles of exercise prescription. In Guidelines for exercise testing and prescription, ed 3, Philadelphia, 1986, Lea & Febiger.
5. American Heart Association Subcommittee on Rehabilitation Target Activity Group: Standards for cardiovascular exercise treatment programs, Circulation 59:1084A, 1979.
6. Armstrong, WF, and Morris, SN: The ST-segment during continuous ambulatory electrocardiographic monitoring (editorial), Ann Intern Med 98:249, 1983.
7. Bartel, AG, et al: Exercise stress testing in evaluation of aortocoronary bypass surgery, Circulation 48:141, 1973.
8. Block, TA, Murray, JA, and English, MT: Improvement in exercise performance after unsuccessful myocardial revascularization, Am J Cardiol 40:673, 1977.
9. Borg, G, and Linderholm, H: Perceived exertion and pulse rate during graded exercise in various age groups, Acta Med Scand 472:194, 1967.
10. Bruce, RA, Hossack, KR, and DeRouen, TA: Prognostic value of exercise testing, Adv Cardiol 31:7, 1982.

11. Bruce, RA, Kusumi, F, and Frederick, R: Differences in cardiac function with prolonged physical training for cardiac rehabilitation, Am J Cardiol 40:597, 1977.

12. Bruce, RA, Kusumi, F, and Mosmer, D: Maximal oxygen intake and nomographic assessment of functional aerobic impairment in cardiovascular disease, Am Heart J 85:546, 1973.

13. Bruce, RA, et al: Noninvasive predictors of sudden cardiac death in man with coronary heart disease: predictive value of maximal stress testing, Am J Cardiol 39:833, 1977.

14. Byrne-Meyer, A: Nursing assessment of the patient in an out-patient cardiac rehabilitation center. In Hall, KL, Meyer, GC, and Hellerstein, MK, editors: Cardiac rehabilitation: exercise testing and prescription, New York, 1984, SP Medical & Scientific Books.

15. Campeau, L, et al: Aortocoronary saphaenous vein bypass graft changes 5 to 7 years after surgery, Circulation 58(suppl 1):I-170, 1978.

16. Campeau, L, et al: Loss of the improvement of angina between 1 and 7 years after aortocoronary bypass surgery: correlations with changes in vein grafts and in coronary arteries, Circulation 60(suppl 1):I-1, 1979.

17. Castelli, WP: Categorical issues in therapy for coronary heart disease, Cardiol Practice, p. 267, 1985.

18. Castelli, WP: Cardiovascular and pulmonary diseases—risk factor management and Framingham, the Year 2001, Communication, 1st Annual National Convention of American Association of Cardiovascular and Pulmonary Rehabilitation, Dallas, Nov. 15-16, 1986.

19. Chesney, MA, and Ward, MM: Biobehavioral treatment approaches for cardiovascular disorders, J Cardiac Rehabil 5:226, 1985.

20. Council on Scientific Affairs: Physician-supervised exercise programs in rehabilitation of patients with coronary heart disease, JAMA 245:1463, 1981.

21. Cukingham, RA, Jr, Carey, JS, and Brown, GG: Postoperative treadmill performance and graft patency after myocardial revascularization, Ann Thorac Surg 35:24, 1983.

22. Dion, WF, et al: Medical problems and physiologic responses during supervised in-patient cardiac rehabilitation: the patient after coronary artery bypass grafting, Heart Lung 11:248, 1982.

23. Ellestad, MH: Rhythm and conduction disturbances in stress testing. In Ellestad, MH: Stress testing: principles and practice, ed 3, Philadelphia, 1986, FA Davis Co.

24. Erb, BC, Fletcher, FG, and Sheffield, TL: Standards for cardiovascular exercise treatment programs: American Heart Association Subcommittee on Rehabilitation Target Activity Group, Circulation 59:1084A, 1979.

25. Fletcher, GF, et al: Telephonically-monitored home exercise early after coronary artery bypass surgery, Chest 2:198, 1984.

26. Franklin, BA, et al: Exercise prescription for the myocardial infarction patient, J Cardiac Rehabil 6:62, 1986.

27. Froelicher, VF, et al: Prediction of maximal oxygen consumption: comparison of the Bruce and Balke treadmill protocols, Chest 68:331, 1975.

28. Gobel, FL, et al: The rate-pressure product as an index of myocardial oxygen consumption during exercise in patients with angina pectoris, Circulation 57:549, 1978.

29. Gohlke, H, et al: Long-term improvement of exercise tolerance and vocational rehabilitation after bypass surgery: a five-year follow-up, J Cardiac Rehabil 2:531, 1982.

30. Grondin, CM, et al: Atherosclerotic changes in coronary vein grafts six years after operation, J Thorac Cardiovasc Surg 77:24, 1979.

31. Hanson, P, Christoferson, MS, and Giese, M: Cardiac rehabilitation at University Hospital and Clinics, University of Wisconsin, Madison, J Cardiac Rehabil 2:438, 1982.

32. Hanson, P, et al: Exercise capacity and cardiovascular responses to serial exercise testing in men and women after coronary artery bypass graft surgery, J Cardiac Rehabil 5:389, 1985.

33. Hartung, GM: Prescription for cardiac rehabilitation reconditioning program. In Blocker, WD, Jr, and Cardus, DC, editors: Rehabilitation in ischemic heart disease, New York, 1983, SP Medical & Scientific Books.

34. Hartung, GM, and Remberto, R: Exercise training in post-myocardial infarction patients: comparison of results with high risk coronary and post-bypass patients, Arch Phys Med Rehabil 62:147, 1981.

35. Hellerstein, HK, and Franklin, BA: Exercise testing and prescription. In Wenger, NK, and Hellerstein, HK, editors: Rehabilitation of the coronary patient, New York, 1984, John Wiley & Sons.

36. Hossack, KF, and Hartwig, R: Cardiac arrest with supervised cardiac rehabilitation, J Cardiac Rehabil 2:402, 1982.

37. Jensen, RL, Clayton, PD, and Liddle, HV: Relationship between graft patency, post-operative work status and symptomatic relief, J Thorac Cardiovasc Surg 85:503, 1982.

38. Johnston, BL: Exercise testing for patients after myocardial infarction and coronary bypass surgery: emphasis on predischarge phase, Heart Lung 13:18, 1984.

39. Kannel, WB: Epidemiologic insights into atherosclerotic cardiovascular disease from the Framingham study. In Pollock, ML, Schmidt, DH, and Mason, DT, editors: Heart disease and rehabilitation, ed 2, New York, 1986, John Wiley & Sons.

39a. Kannel, WB: Potential for prevention of myocardial reinfarction and cardiac death. In Wenger, NK, and Hellerstein, K, editors: Rehabilitation of the coronary patient, New York, 1984, John Wiley & Sons.

40. Kent, KM, et al: Effects of coronary artery bypass on global and regional left ventricular function during exercise, N Engl J Med 298:1434, 1978.

41. Keteyian, S, et al: The design and philosophy of a hospital and community-based comprehensive cardiac rehabilitation program, J Cardiac Rehabil 5:492, 1985.

42. Kolibash, AJ, et al: Improvement of myocardial perfusion and left ventricular function after coronary artery bypass grafting in patients with unstable angina, Circulation 59:66, 1979.

43. Kolibash, AJ, et al: Myocardial perfusion as an indicator of graft patency after coronary artery bypass surgery, Circulation 61:882, 1980.

44. LaForge, R, et al: The Sharp Memorial Hospital Cardiac Rehabilitation Program, San Diego, California, J Cardiac Rehabil 4:6, 1984.

45. Lawrie, GM, et al: Patterns of patency of 596 vein grafts up to seven years after aorto-coronary bypass, J Thorac Cardiovasc Surg 73:443, 1977.

46. Lawrie, GM, et al: Results of coronary bypass more than five years after operation in 434 patients, Am J Cardiol 40:665, 1977.

47. Leguizamon, EE, et al: Borgess Medical Center's Institute for Cardiovascular Health and Rehabilitation, J Cardiac Rehabil 8:398, 1985.

48. Levine, SA, and Lown, B: "Armchair" treatment of acute coronary thrombosis, JAMA 148:1365, 1952.

49. Loop, FD, et al: An 11 year evolution of coronary arterial surgery (1967-1978), Ann Surg 190:444, 1979.

50. Lovvorn, J: Coronary artery bypass surgery: helping patients cope with post-op problems, Am J Nurs July 1982, p 1073.

51. Maresh, CM, and Bruce, JN: Utilization of perceived exertion ratings during exercise testing and training. In Hall, LK, Meyer, GC, and Hellerstein, HK, editors: Cardiac rehabilitation: exercise testing and prescription, New York, 1984, SP Medical & Scientific Books.

52. Maskin, CS: Aerobic exercise training in cardiopulmonary disease. In Weber, KT, and Janicki, JS: Cardiopulmonary exercise testing, physiologic principles and clinical applications, Philadelphia, 1986, WB Saunders Co.

53. McAllister, RM, and Lee, SJK: The effect of exercise training in patients with coronary artery disease taking beta-blockers, J Cardiopulmonary Rehabil 6:245, 1986.

54. McArdle, WD, Katch, FI, and Katch, VL: Exercise, aging and cardiovascular disease. In Exercise physiology, ed 2, Philadelphia, 1986, Lea & Febiger.

55. McArdle, WD, Katch, FI, and Katch, VL: Training for anaerobic and aerobic power. In Exercise physiology, ed 2, Philadelphia, 1986, Lea & Febiger.

56. McConahay, R, et al: Accuracy of treadmill testing in assessment of direct myocardial revascularization, Circulation 56:548, 1977.

57. McIntosh, HD, and Garcia, JA: The first decade of aortocoronary bypass grafting, 1967-1977, Circulation 57:405, 1978.

58. Meyer, GC, and Hensel, PK: Cardiac rehabilitation: state of the art cardiac treatment centers, J Cardiac Rehabil 3:130, 1983.

59. Milesis, CA, and Harville, GH: Cardiac rehabilitation at University Hospital, Augusta, Georgia, J Cardiac Rehabil 3:624, 1983.

60. Mitchel, M, et al: Cardiac exercise program: role of continuous electrocardiographic monitoring, Arch Phys Med Rehabil 65:463, 1984.

61. Morton, JR, and Tolan, KM: Activity level and employment status after coronary bypass surgery, Am J Surg 143:417, 1981.

62. Murray, GC, and Beller, GA: Cardiac rehabilitation following coronary artery bypass surgery, Am Heart J 105:1009, 1983.

63. Naughton, J: Cardiac rehabilitation: current status and future possibilities. In Wenger, NK, and Brest, AN, editors: Exercise and the heart, ed 2, Philadelphia, 1985, FA Davis Co.

64. Nequin, ND: Cardiac rehabilitation and health enhancement center at Swedish Covenant Hospital, Chicago, J Cardiac Rehabil 2:488, 1982.

65. Noakes, TD, Gillmer, D, and Pittaway, D: Severe incapacitating coronary artery disease in two veteran ultramarathon runners, J Cardiac Rehabil 4:238, 1984.

66. Oberman, A, and Kouchoukos, NT: Role of exercise after coronary artery bypass surgery, Cardiovasc Clin 9:155, 1978.

67. Oldridge, NB, et al: Aortocoronary bypass surgery: effects of surgery and 32 months of physical conditioning on treadmill performance, Arch Phys Med Rehabil 59:268, 1978.

68. Peterson, LH: Exercise in cardiovascular rehabilitation: principles. In Peterson, LH, editor: Cardiovascular rehabilitation: a comprehensive approach, New York, 1983, Macmillan, Inc.

69. Peterson, LH: Introduction: philosophy and scope. In Peterson, LH, editor: Cardiovascular rehabilitation: a comprehensive approach, New York, 1983, Macmillan, Inc.

70. Peterson, LH: Summary and Conclusions. In Peterson, LH, editor: Cardiovascular rehabilitation: a comprehensive approach, New York, 1983, Macmillan, Inc.

71. Pfisterer, M: The role of nuclear cardiology in evaluating patients for cardiac rehabilitation, J Cardiac Rehabil 3:435, 1983.

72. Pollock, ML: Exercise regimens after myocardial revascularization surgery: rationale and results. In Wenger, NK, and Brest, AN, editors: Exercise and the heart, ed 2, Philadelphia, 1985, FA Davis Co.

73. Pollock, ML, Foster, C, and Schmidt, DH: Cardiac rehabilitation program at Mount Sinai Medical Center, Milwaukee, J Cardiac Rehabil 2:458, 1982.

74. Pollock, ML, Wilmore, JH, and Fox, SM, III: Obesity and weight control. In Exercise in health and disease: evaluation and prescription for prevention and rehabilitation, Philadelphia, 1984, WB Saunders Co.

75. Pollock, ML, Wilmore, JH, and Fox, SM, III: Prescribing exercises for the apparently healthy. In Exercise in health and disease, Philadelphia, 1984, WB Saunders Co.

76. Pollock, ML, et al: Exercise prescription for rehabilitation of the cardiac patient. In Pollock, ML, Schmidt, DH, and Mason, DT: Heart disease and rehabilitation, ed 2, New York, 1986, John Wiley & Sons.

77. Rahimtoola, SH: Coronary bypass surgery for chronic angina: 1981—a perspective, Circulation 65:225, 1982.

78. Rahimtoola, SH: Postoperative exercise response in the evaluation of the physiologic status after coronary bypass surgery, Circulation 65(suppl 2):II-106, 1982.

79. Reeves, TJ: Medical management of the patient with angina pectoris: an overview of the problem, Circulation 65(suppl 2):II-3, 1982.

80. Reith, CA: Avoiding posthospital adjustment problems. In Hall, LK, Meyer, GC, and Hellerstein, HK, editors: Cardiac rehabilitation: exercise testing and prescription, New York, 1984, SP Medical & Scientific Books.

81. Robert, EW, et al: Six-year clinical and angiographic follow-up of patients with previously documented complete revascularization, Circulation 58(suppl 1):I-194, 1978.

82. Robinson, G, Froelicher, VF, and Utley, JR: Rehabilitation of the coronary artery bypass graft surgery patient, J Cardiac Rehabil 4:74, 1984.

83. Rod, JL, et al: Symptom-limited graded exercise testing soon after myocardial revascularization surgery, J Cardiac Rehabil 2:199, 1982.

84. Seides, SF, et al: Long-term anatomic fate of coronary-artery bypass grafts and functional status of patients five years after operation, N Engl J Med 298:1213, 1978.

85. Siegel, W, et al: The spectrum of exercise test and angiographic correlations in myocardial revascularization surgery, Circulation (suppl 1):I-156, 1975.

86. Sheldahl, LM, Wilke, NA, and Tristani, FE: Exercise prescription for return to work, J Cardiac Rehabil 5:567, 1985.

87. Sheldahl, LM, et al: Response to repetitive static-dynamic exercise in patients with coronary artery disease, J Cardiac Rehabil 5:139, 1985.

88. Sheldon, WC, and Loop, FD: Coronary artery bypass graft surgery: assessment of current status, Cardiovasc Clin 12:9, 1981.

89. Spodick, DM: Indications for coronary bypass surgery, 1982, Adv Cardiol 31:45, 1982.

90. Stevens, R, and Manson, P: Comparison of supervised and unsupervised exercise training after coronary bypass surgery, Am J Cardiol 53:1524, 1984.

91. Thompson, PD: The cardiovascular risks of cardiac rehabilitation, J Cardiac Rehabil 5:321, 1985.

92. Tommaso, CL, Lesch, M, and Sonnenblick, EH: Alterations in cardiac function in coronary heart disease, myocardial infarction and coronary bypass surgery. In Wenger, NK, and Hellerstein, HK, editors: Rehabilitation of the coronary patient, ed 2, New York, 1984, John Wiley & Sons.

93. Ungerman-deMent, P, Bemis, P, and Siebens, A: Exercise program for patients after cardiac surgery, Arch Phys Med Rehabil 67:463, 1986.

94. Vacek, JL, et al: The cardiac rehabilitation program at U.S.A.F. Medical Center, Keesler, J Cardiac Rehabil 5:241, 1985.

95. Wenger, NK: Research related to rehabilitation, Circulation 60:1636, 1979.

96. Wenger, NK: Coronary bypass surgery as a rehabilitative procedure, Adv Cardiol 31:80, 1982.

97. Wenger, KN: Early ambulation physical activity: myocardial infarction and coronary artery bypass surgery, Heart Lung 13:14, 1984.

98. Williams, RS: Exercise training of patients with ventricular dysfunction and heart failure. In Wenger, NK, and Brest, AN, editors: Exercise and the heart, Philadelphia, 1985, FA Davis Co.

99. Williams, RS, et al: Duke University's preventive approach to cardiology-dupac, J Cardiac Rehabil 2:509, 1982.

100. Wilson-Barnett, J: Assessment of recovery: with special reference to a study with post-operative cardiac patients, J Adv Nurs 6:435, 1981.

101. Wilson, PK, Fardy, PS, and Froelicher, VF: The exercise training session. In Cardiac rehabilitation: adult fitness and exercise training, Philadelphia, 1981, Lea & Febiger.

102. Wilson, PK, Fardy, PS, and Froelicher, VF: Formulating the exercise prescription. In Cardiac rehabilitation: adult fitness and exercise testing, Philadelphia, 1981, Lea & Febiger.

103. Wilson, PK, Fardy, PS, and Froelicher, VF: Interpretation of the exercise test. In Cardiac rehabilitation: adult fitness and exercise testing, Philadelphia, 1981, Lea & Febiger.

104. Wilson, PK, Fardy, PS, and Froelicher, VF: Methodology of exercise testing. In Cardiac rehabilitation: adult fitness and exercise training, Philadelphia, 1981, Lea & Febiger.

105. Zohman, LR: Practical aspects of vigorous exercise programming for coronary patients, Adv Cardiol 31:205, 1982.

CHAPTER 19

Behavioral aspects of cardiac rehabilitation

MERRILL P. ANDERSON

Cardiovascular rehabilitation is essentially a behavioral treatment. In the typical cardiovascular rehabilitation program, participants are expected to change their behavior in the areas of exercise, diet, smoking, and psychologic coping. The hope is that in making such changes they will enjoy short-term benefits of a more rapid physical and psychologic recovery from myocardial infarction (MI) or cardiac surgery and long-term benefits of reduced future risk for recurrent cardiac problems—benefits they would not have realized had they not undertaken the rehabilitation program. Maximization of the long term benefits requires that the behavioral changes initiated during a structured program be maintained following completion of the program. Thus an important aspect of cardiovascular rehabilitation is structuring behavior change programs that will foster long-term compliance. This concern has implications for the structure, content, and staffing of cardiovascular rehabilitation programs.

RISK FACTOR BEHAVIOR CHANGE
Smoking cessation

Cigarette smoking is one of the three greatest risk factors for cardiovascular disease. The amount of risk is directly proportional to the number of cigarettes smoked (indexed as pack-years).[46] Cessation of smoking significantly reduces future risk for cardiac events. Post-MI patients who continue to smoke experience at least twice the reinfarction or death rate of post-MI quitters.[6,46] Smoking status is also one of the few significant predictors of compliance with cardiovascular rehabilitation programs, with smokers more likely to drop out than nonsmokers.[34,35] Considering the risks of smoking and the benefits of cessation, the only proper goal for cardiovascular rehabilitation programs with respect to this risk factor is total and permanent cessation of cigarette smoking.

Heart attack patients who smoke are more successful at quitting than other smokers. Various studies report that approximately 50% of smokers successfully quit after an MI.[6] This compares with the typical long-term quit rates of 20% to 30% for participants in formal smoking cessation programs. Most MI patients achieve cessation without the assistance of formal stop smoking programs. Instead they may be responding to clear, forceful, and timely messages from their physicians about the importance of quitting. The improved quit rate among post-MI patients can reasonably be attributed to increased motivation based on fear and on the immediately present belief that smoking was and is a contributing factor to their cardiac problems.[41] Despite these impressive statistics, 50% of the post-MI smoking population continues to smoke. These people are the prime candidates for formal smoking cessation interventions in cardiovascular rehabilitation programs. Because of the importance of ensuring long-term cessation, recent quitters should also be considered candidates for intervention to reinforce abstinence. The following paragraphs summarize basic treatment strategies for smoking cessation that reflect state of the art knowledge.

Self-management approach

The most widely used treatment strategy for smoking cessation is the broad-spectrum self-management approach. This approach includes a mixture of behavioral and cognitive change techniques and emphasizes developing strategies for long-term maintenance. The maintenance emphasis reflects the work on "relapse prevention training" developed by Marlatt and associates.[32] The typical self-management approach involves three stages: education-preparation, cessation, and maintenance.

The education-preparation phase begins with unequivocal information about smoking and health (especially cardiovascular disease), about quitting strategies, and about the quitting process. Participants typically collect data on the topography of their smoking behavior (self-monitoring) and from this data identify patterns and routines associated with their smoking behavior. Plans for a cessation strategy are developed, a target date for cessation is selected, and strategies for coping with urges to smoke are identified and practiced.

During this preparatory period the thrust of the intervention is toward increasing participants' confidence about their ability to follow their cessation plan. Bandura[1,2] has demonstrated that "self-efficacy," the confidence about one's ability to implement a behavioral change program, is a critical cognitive determinant of persistence. Cessation strategies include nicotine fading, phased withdrawal from cigarettes, and quitting cold turkey.

Nicotine fading involves switching from the preferred brand of cigarettes to brands lower in nicotine on a preplanned schedule. When the lowest level is reached, the person either reduces the number of daily cigarettes until cessation is achieved or quits cold turkey. Phased withdrawal consists of reducing daily cigarette intake until cessation is reached. With both of these strategies, the period of fading or of withdrawal should be kept relatively brief (within 1 month) to maximize motivation and involvement. Typically these approaches are considered when the person enters the treatment with a low sense of self-efficacy about achieving cessation. Through the more gradual approach and the achievement of subgoals along the way to cessation, self-efficacy is gradually improved.

The cold turkey or "designated quitting day" strategy is straightforward. A quit day is selected, coping strategies are identified and practiced, and the plan is implemented.

The maintenance phase involves implementing the strategies for coping with urges after cessation. Counseling during this phase focuses on anticipating high-risk situations for relapse, reviewing successful and unsuccessful coping episodes, modifying coping strategies based on experience, and encouraging other behavioral changes (dietary, exercise, stress-reducing) that support a nonsmoking life-style.[45] The relapse prevention model places special emphasis on minimizing the "abstinence violation effect,"[32] which refers to a cognitive and emotional reaction to violation of an all or none abstinence standard. The person who succumbs to this reaction after one "slip" is considered more vulnerable to a full-blown relapse.

Nicotine chewing gum

Nicotine chewing gum (nicotine polacrilex, or Nicorette) became available through prescription in the United States in 1983. It has become an increasingly popular aid for smoking cessation, especially when the cessation effort is managed from a physician's office. Unfortunately, the effectiveness of the gum as an aid in smoking cessation is frequently reduced by failure of prescribing physicians and of patients to appreciate how the gum is optimally used.

Nicotine chewing gum is most effective when used as one component of a broad-spectrum smoking cessation program that also addresses cognitive and behavioral issues. The current recommendation is that the gum be included as an option within the self-management approach described previously. Even with the help of the gum, there is still need for education and preparation for quitting, for cognitive and behavioral strategies for coping with urges, and for support and planning for long-term maintenance.

Instruction on proper use of the gum is essential. Common misperceptions are that it will make smoking cessation a painless, effortless process and that it will function as a stand-alone treatment. Many patients use the gum sparingly, much as they would if they were trying to limit the number of cigarettes they smoke. In so doing, they may not be maintaining a sufficient nicotine level in their system to minimize the occurrence of withdrawal effects and of urges to smoke. Patients should be encouraged to use the gum freely during the first several weeks of a cessation effort to obtain maximum protection from withdrawal effects and from unexpected urges.

Aversion methods

Aversion methods are the final category of smoking cessation strategies. The most widely researched aversion method is the rapid smoking procedure.[10,30] The patient smokes cigarettes at a prescribed rate (for example, 10 puffs per minute) until unable to continue. The aversive stimuli in this conditioning paradigm are the smoke and unpleasant physiologic responses (nausea, lightheadedness) to the smoke. Typically several trials are held in each treatment session. The first several treatments are held on consecutive days. Subsequent sessions are scheduled according to the subject's perceived ability to maintain abstinence between sessions.

Hall and others[20] report that 50% of a group of cardiopulmonary patients in one study were still abstaining 2 years after treatment. These researchers also found no evidence of cardiac symptoms (ischemia, arrhythmia) following treatment sessions and assert that the method is safe for patients with mild to moderate cardiopulmonary disease. They suggest that candidates for the procedure should be screened for the presence of certain cardiac medications. Among these are the most commonly prescribed medications for cardiac patients (beta-blockers such as propranolol, as well as several commonly prescribed antiarrhythmics). Patients who are using any of these drugs are advised to undergo a medical evaluation before using the rapid smoking procedure. Because these medications are so commonly prescribed, this guideline would seem to limit sharply the number of cardiac patients for whom rapid smoking would be medically appropriate. In fact many clinicians involved in the care of cardiac patients are reluctant to recommend the procedure, especially when alternative (and more appealing) treatments are available. Among cardiac patients, rapid smoking may find its best use with patients who are not successful with the alternative methods.

Dietary factors

Treatment of diet-related risk factors is primarily behavioral and takes the form of a low-fat, low-cholesterol, sodium-restricted diet that emphasizes complex carbohydrates. When weight loss is also a goal, restriction to an intake of 1200 to 1500 calories per day, which is within the guidelines of the American Heart Association's general dietary recommendations, is usually prescribed. For more extreme elevations of cholesterol, drug therapy is necessary.[19] Even for patients receiving cholesterol-reducing medication, dietary change is still an essential component of treatment.[19]

The most common treatment for mild to moderate obesity is behavioral intervention. For medically significant obesity (40 pounds or more overweight), medically supervised very-low-calorie diets are receiving considerable attention. However, a major component of these programs is behavior modification of former eating habits in preparation for long-term maintenance of weight loss. The following discussion focuses on the behavioral aspects of treatment of diet-related risk factors and does not detail the nutritional considerations.

Dietary change when weight loss is not an issue is a less complicated intervention than when weight loss is involved. When the goal is to conform to the American Heart Association's dietary guidelines, proper nutritional education is the major issue. The principal concern is to include sufficient practical advice about shopping and food preparation and about making exchanges within the guidelines to assist patients in making the behavioral changes. A common mistake of such interventions is a failure to appreciate the time and energy required to establish new eating habits. These changes should be made over a period of time (for example, 1 or 2 months) with repeated consultations with the nutritionist, during which time the details of incorporating the new pattern into daily life can be reviewed and problems solved. Attention must be given to individualizing the diet so patients experience minimal frustration concerning the restriction of favorite foods.

When weight loss is a goal, the most widely used approach along with compliance with AHA dietary guidelines, is behavioral treatment. Typically the intervention is delivered by a nutritionist or by a nutritionist-psychologist team. If the treatment is provided by a dietician or nutritionist, it is essential that the service provider be knowledgeable of and clinically skilled with the psychologic (behavioral and cognitive) aspects of treatment.

Brownell and Wadden[5] identify five components of a comprehensive behavioral weight loss program: behavioral techniques, exercise, cognitive change, social support, and nutrition education. Behavioral techniques include such activities as self-monitoring of food intake and calories (food records), stimulus control of food cues, and preplanning. Exercise is increasingly viewed as an important component

of weight loss programming and as essential for the maintenance period after weight loss goals have been achieved. Again, careful attention must be paid to individualizing the exercise prescription according to the person's physical condition and preferences for exercise activity in order that compliance be maximized. Many cardiovascular rehabilitation patients will already be involved in exercise programs, and it is doubtful that they will need to do more than their previously prescribed regimen. Cognitive interventions focus on goal setting, awareness and modification of thought patterns involved with overeating, cognitive skills for coping with mistakes, and general attitude changes to support long-term maintenance.[31] Interventions to encourage social support of new dietary habits should recognize the important social functions of eating and the fact that dietary change is best maintained when it is a family affair. Finally, nutrition education is essential so that patients may choose intelligently within the guidelines and are not made to feel rigidly bound to a list of sanctioned foods.

Much has been learned about what works and what does not work in behavioral weight loss programs over the past 15 years.[5] Expectations for what can be achieved through given amounts of intervention have changed over the years. Current understanding of the critical elements of these programs emphasizes the following aspects of treatment: treatment should be longer than the 8 to 10 weeks of intervention that was the norm in the 1970s; obesity is a chronic, deeply entrenched biologic and psychologic condition, and long-term, clinically significant results are unlikely to be achieved with minimal interventions; emphasis should be placed on exercise, on emotional and cognitive factors that may undermine weight loss and maintenance of weight loss, and on differentiating the weight loss period from the maintenance period in terms of the behavioral and cognitive skills required and the motivational issues unique to each.

For obesity greater than 40 to 50 pounds over ideal weight, the behavioral program described previously may not be the treatment of choice.[4] The reasons for the lack of success are probably varied but may relate to the relatively slow rate of weight loss (1 to 2 pounds per week) and corresponding difficulties in maintaining motivation. Very-low-calorie diets, or protein-sparing modified fasts, are increasingly recommended as the preferred treatment for rapid weight loss. As with any weight loss program, the issue with these diets is long-term maintenance of weight loss. Most treatment programs combine the diet with a comprehensive behavioral program of the type described above. Straight behavioral programs are rarely successful with this degree of obesity.

Exercise

Exercise therapy is the core component of most cardiovascular rehabilitation programs. The importance of exercise to rehabilitation lies primarily in its value in reversing the deconditioning that occurs after acute events and subsequent hospitalization and recuperation. Exercise also confers myriad other benefits, some well established and some fervently claimed. There is little doubt that exercise can produce psychologic benefits, that it is a critical component of weight control, and that it has a positive effect on the so-called good cholesterol or high-density lipoproteins. Questions about the therapeutic benefits of exercise on the myocardium and on risk for recurrent cardiac events are more complicated and controversial. See Chapters 16 and 18 by Shepard and Wenger, respectively, for a discussion of these issues. The discussion in these chapters focuses on the behavioral and psychologic considerations in exercise therapy in cardiovascular rehabilitation.

Exercise prescriptions are typically given in terms of frequency, intensity, and duration. Frequency is usually prescribed at three times per week, or every other day. Intensity is gauged in terms of a target heart rate zone sufficient to produce a conditioning effect. Duration of each exercise session is determined by the total exercise time required to elicit approximately 20 minutes of sustained heart rate in the prescribed target zone. Allowing for warm-up and cool-down periods (during which heart rate gradually increases and then decreases), this usually results in a total duration of between 30 and 35 minutes. Common exercise modalities used in rehabilitation include bicycle ergometers, treadmills, walking, jogging, and swimming. First priority is given to aerobic activities because these are most effective in improving cardiovascular conditioning.

The core behavioral issue with exercise therapy is compliance with the exercise prescription. Patients must do the exercise on a sufficiently regular basis and at sufficient intensity and duration to achieve positive benefits. General considerations for enhancing compliance can be grouped under the headings of minimizing unpleasant or aversive aspects of exercise, convenience, education, social support, and follow-up. Common sense and psychologic theory tell us that people will not persist at activities that are unpleasant. Thus care must be taken in structuring exercise programs to minimize unpleasantness, and conversely, to maximize immediate pleasures, of the exercise activity itself, of concurrent activities, or of the exercise environment. For example, exercise prescriptions that are too demanding in either intensity or frequency (for example, five to seven times per week) run a higher risk of accentuating the unpleasant aspects of exercise in terms of physical discomfort and excessive time away from other activities. Few people are likely to persist at this type of exercise program. The exercise environment should be pleasant and should provide some distraction from the monotony of the kind of repetitive activity usually recommended (ergometry or treadmill, for example). The group support available in structured programs serves a powerful function in providing encouragement, distraction, and camaraderie—all of which enhance compliance.

Convenience is listed as a separate compliance consid-

eration but is closely related to the unpleasantness factor. The more time and effort people must devote to getting their exercise done, the less likely their compliance. This is a problem for structured programs in that patients usually have to travel to the rehabilitation center for their exercise. Because exercise therapy should occur approximately three times per week, a considerable amount of travel can be required to complete the usual 12- to 16-week structured exercise program. Programs that are community or worksite based have an advantage over programs housed in major medical centers. After patients are discharged from structured programs, exercise activities that can be accomplished at home are preferred over activities that require travel (health spa, swimming pool) unless there are offsetting benefits such as group support. Home exercises that are convenient for most patients include walking, jogging, and bicycle ergometry.

Adequate education about the rationale for exercise therapy and about how to do it properly is another compliance-enhancing factor. Leventhal and associates[29] have written extensively about the importance of patients having a clear understanding (at their own levels) of why a therapy is prescribed and how it is to be conducted. A good part of the staff effort during structured exercise sessions should be focused on educating patients about the how and why of the prescribed exercise therapy.

Social support, especially family support, for an exercise program is also a factor that enhances exercise compliance, as well as compliance with any aspect of life-style change. Family support can be facilitated by educating spouses and other family members about the rationale for the program and about the basics of the exercise prescription. Ideally, the exercise program (especially the home program) should disrupt as few of the normal routines of other family members as possible to minimize conflict associated with the exercise.

Long-term follow-up is valuable for patients on home programs. The follow-up visit can be structured in several ways. From a behavioral-psychologic perspective, it should provide feedback about what has been accomplished during the follow-up interval, should offer an opportunity to troubleshoot problems that may have developed, and should provide encouragement. To fully appreciate the importance of follow-up, it is helpful to contrast the exercise therapy in a structured program with home exercise programs. Structured programs can be viewed more as acute care, while home programs are long-term maintenance. Most patients enter structured programs when they are significantly deconditioned, psychologically vulnerable, and experiencing symptoms (chest pain, shortness of breath, arrhythmia). Progress is relatively rapid and is psychologically gratifying. Patients perceive their progress through improved stamina in daily activity, an increasing exercise load, reduced symptoms, and an increased sense of well-being. All of this reinforcement enhances their interest, and involvement, and motivation. Patients are usually discharged to home programs when they have attained a sufficient level of conditioning to pursue their desired set of daily activities. Home exercise programs focus largely on maintenance of conditioning levels achieved in the structured program rather than on further improvement in conditioning. Motivation can be harder to sustain during a maintenance period. Since there are few if any of the positive signs of progress that characterized the structured program, interest and involvement can suffer. To maintain motivation during this period, people need goals. Formal follow-ups serve a valuable function in letting patients know whether they have achieved or are achieving the goal of maintaining the physical conditioning reached in the program. The principal behavior that contributes to achieving the maintenance goal is regularity of exercise. Thus maintenance patients in particular should be encouraged to set goals for their exercise in terms of frequency of exercise rather than intensity. Because the period of greatest attrition in exercise programs is the first 6 to 12 months after exit from a structured program,[7,14,34,35] follow-up monitoring should be scheduled more frequently during this period than later. After the patient has achieved between 1½ and 2 years of regular exercise at home, follow-ups can be done annually. The rationale for recommending this schedule of follow-up is not based on medical necessity. The sole purpose is to enhance long-term compliance with the exercise prescription.

A properly conducted exercise program can be a powerful form of psychologic therapy for cardiac patients. Progress in exercise conditioning is a strong antidote to feelings of helplessness that contribute to depression, excessive anxiety, and avoidance of activity. Progress in exercise produces experiential information about the degree of physical activity the patient can safely undertake. This information is critical to reducing exaggerated fears that, in extreme form, can create the well-known "cardiac cripple." Bandura[1,2] has noted the importance of actual performance accomplishments in improving patients' self-efficacy about their ability to successfully undertake feared activities. Improved confidence should result in increased activity levels. To the extent that exercise improves the patient's sense of physical well-being, it can reduce depression. Participation in an organized exercise program structures patients' weekly schedules during their convalescence and helps minimize the amount of unstructured "down" time. Some patients find large blocks of unstructured time with reduced physical activity to be psychologically difficult and also to be fertile ground for depression. Structured exercise programs provide an occasion to bring together a group of individuals in similar circumstances. The psychologic benefits of group support readily follow.

Emotional stress and coronary-prone behavior

Perhaps none of the risk factors for coronary heart disease is as controversial as the claim that emotional-behavioral

reaction patterns contribute to heart disease. The coronary-prone (type A) behavior pattern (CPBP) is the most widely accepted psychologic risk factor for coronary heart disease.[9] Another characteristic that has received major research attention is acute physiologic reactivity to psychologic stress situations, although this has not been demonstrated empirically to be associated with increased risk.[27]

Coronary-prone behavior pattern

The CPBP refers to a behavioral syndrome found in some people when they perceive challenges or other pressures. The principal characteristics are hurried and impatient behavior, competitiveness, and easily aroused hostility or anger that is often expressed as a critical and distrusting attitude toward others. When these behaviors occur, the individual is assumed to be experiencing elevated levels of neuroendocrine arousal (catecholamines) as the physiologic component of the emotional reaction. The mechanism of risk for coronary-prone behavior is thought to be the elevated hormone levels present if the behavior pattern extends for a period of years. Excessive levels of catecholamines are thought to increase the rate of atherosclerosis through their effect on serum cholesterol and platelet function. Research to document a connection between the behavior pattern and the hypothesized physiologic concomitants of the pattern has been highly suggestive but not definitive.[27]

The status of the CPBP as a risk factor rests largely on the results of the Western Collaborative Group Study (WCGS).[38,39] The WCGS was a prospective study in which groups of men who were identified as coronary prone or as not coronary prone and who showed no signs of cardiovascular disease were followed for 8 years. The coronary-prone group had twice the risk of developing some manifestation of cardiovascular disease over the study period. That finding has been replicated in other studies.[21,26,36] Reviews of the empiric literature have supported the CPBP's risk factor status.[9,22,23]

In recent years there has been increased debate about the importance of the CPBP as a risk factor. Studies have reported no association between the pattern and the extent of angiographically documented atherosclerosis.[11-13] A major multicenter prospective study of the effects of modifying risk factor behaviors in a group of high-risk men who were initially free of coronary heart disease showed no association between the CPBP and disease endpoints.[44] The status of the global type A pattern as the psychologic coronary risk factor has been challenged by research results that implicate hostility, anger, and anger expression as components of the global pattern that account for most of the statistical association between the global pattern and disease endpoints.[43,48] The status of the behavior pattern as a risk factor for recurrent heart attack has also been questioned because of the results of two recent studies.[8,42]

The significance of these negative results is moderated somewhat by methodologic considerations that limit their generality. Especially important are differences in the measurement procedure used in defining the CPBP. The most widely used approaches are a structured clinical interview[15,37] and various self-report questionnaires, of which the Jenkins Activity Survey (JAS)[25] is the most important. The interview was used in the original prospective study. The JAS was derived from the interview questions and was validated as a predictor in early studies.[24] The debate is whether the methods are equivalent. If they are, negative results obtained with one procedure cast doubt on the entire body of research. If one is the "true" or superior measure, negative results with the lesser measure can be dismissed. Supporters of the interview method[15] argue that the interview scores the behavioral characteristics of the subject during the interview (for example, rate of speech, interruptions, voice modulation, motor behavior) that are direct examples of the pattern, whereas the questionnaire only assesses attitudes as the subject is able to report them. The correlations between the two methods are modest, suggesting differences in the characteristics measured.[33] Many of the recent negative results[8,42] have come from studies that used the questionnaire rather than the interview method. They have been criticized on those and other methodologic grounds.

The issue of the degree of risk for recurrent infarction posed by coronary-prone behavior is especially relevant for cardiovascular rehabilitation. If it is a risk, it should be a target for intervention, along with smoking and cholesterol. The best evidence for the value of intervening and for the behavior pattern as a risk factor for recurrent MI comes from the Recurrent Coronary Prevention Project.[16] Recurrence rates over 5 years were evaluated in three groups. The treatment group received a comprehensive 5-year intervention designed to reduce type A behavior. One control group was seen an equal number of times but received only information about cardiovascular disease and risk factors other than coronary-prone behavior. Members of the third group were seen annually by their cardiologists. The result has been a significantly lower recurrence rate for nonfatal infarctions for the type A treatment group. A strong relationship was found between the degree of change in coronary-prone behavior and reduction in recurrence. The primary measure of coronary-prone behavior used in the study was a version of the structured interview.[15]

The significance of the study is clear. First, coronary-prone behavior can be reduced in postinfarction men. Second, reducing coronary-prone behavior is associated with reduced risk of recurrent MI. And third, by inference, type A behavior is a risk factor for recurrent MI.

Further support for the modifiability of coronary-prone behavior, although not for the effects of such modification on disease endpoints, is found in two studies in which coronary-prone behavior was modified in healthy men.[17,40] Type A military officers attending the U.S. Army War College volunteered to participate in a 9-month intervention study.

Participants in the type A treatment group received substantially the same intervention as those in the Recurrent Coronary Prevention Project (RCCP). The degree of change in type A behavior was comparable to that achieved with postinfarction men in the other project and was accomplished in 9 months rather than 5 years. A Canadian study suggests that the amount of time required to modify the pattern may be even less.[40] Healthy managers who volunteered to participate in a type A modification project showed a degree of change in type A behavior after 14 weeks comparable to that achieved by the Friedman group studies. However, the relative durability of the changes achieved in the shorter intervention period compared with the longer intervention period has not been evaluated.

Modification of coronary-prone behavior

The treatments used in the intervention studies can best be described as broad-spectrum cognitive-behavioral therapies. The RCCP project helped participants learn to make environmental, behavioral, cognitive, and physiologic changes to reduce their coronary-prone behavior.[47] For example, they were taught to engineer their environments in ways that reduced the triggers for type A behaviors through better delegation, judicious avoidance of some triggers, and the elimination of nonessential volunteering. Behaviorally, they practiced the opposite of type A behaviors by doing such things as standing in lines, losing games, smiling at strangers, and walking slowly according to weekly assignments in a "drill" book. Cognitively, participants learned ways of restructuring attitudes and beliefs underlying hostility and reactions of anger. In this area special attention was paid to beliefs about the amount of control it is possible and necessary to have over themselves and their environments and also about strong feelings of lacking valued resources (for example, time, love, money, status, attention). Physiologically, they learned deep muscle relaxation procedures and practiced application of relaxation skills to daily situations.

The Montreal Type A intervention was designed to "reduce 'coping costs' by teaching the individual to perceive and respond to potential stressors in a more differentiated fashion, increasing both the number of coping strategies and the flexibility with which they were used" (p. 49).[40] Participants increased their awareness of coronary-prone reactions, learned to anticipate triggers for stress reactions and how to regain control when confronted with unpredictable triggers, practiced new (more adaptive) coping strategies in daily situations, and learned to plan for rest and recuperation periods. As with the RCCP, specific homework assignments for practicing new coping skills in daily life were an integral part of the intervention.

Acute psychophysiologic reactivity

Acute psychophysiologic reactivity to stress and challenge situations has been receiving considerable attention as a factor in cardiovascular risk. The entire area is thoroughly reviewed elsewhere.[27] The theoretic work on the coronary-prone pattern assumed that chronic overactivation of the neuroendocrine system was the link between the behavior pattern and coronary heart disease.

A new research paradigm is developing that allows evaluation of psychophysiologic reactivity and therefore opens the possibility of relating reactivity to disease endpoints and of evaluating the effect of treatments (type A modification programs) on reactivity. The paradigm involves monitoring physiologic reactions (heart rate, blood pressure, catecholamines, respiration, sweating response) while a subject is confronted with any of several laboratory stress situations. One of the problems in this area of research is that there is little standardization of the stimulus situations, and thus it is difficult to generalize results from one study to the next. Stimuli that are commonly used include mental arithmetic, ice water pain, challenging video games, and timed mental arithmetic tests. Reactivity appears to be a stable individual difference variable,[18] but one that is only weakly related to differences in coronary-prone behavior. This is contrary to expectation derived from the theoretic understanding of coronary-prone behavior and may be accounted for by a variety of considerations (methodologic, conceptual).

Acute reactivity has not been demonstrated to be a risk factor for cardiovascular disease. Thus treatment for reactivity per se is not warranted. However, one of the goals of the type A treatments described previously is to reduce this type of reactivity because it is the presumed mechanism of risk for coronary-prone behavior. The Montreal Type A Project attempted to incorporate the reactivity dimension into its design as a selection and outcome variable. The treatment had no significant effect on reactivity (in spite of large changes in the behavior pattern), and the researchers were unable to explain the lack of results. The lack of conclusive data in this exceptionally well-designed study underscores the fact that this research paradigm requires further development before all of the methodologic problems can be solved. The complicated interactions between physiology, cognitions, behavior, and environment make this a challenging research area.

A strict interpretation of the research data would conclude that intervention for moderation of coronary-prone behavior in the cardiac rehabilitation setting is warranted as a secondary prevention measure, but that intervention for psychophysiologic reactivity in the absence of coronary-prone behavior is not. It is likely that the reactivity research paradigm will continue to develop and that new insights into cardiovascular risk from psychologic factors and effective treatments will follow.

REACTIVE EMOTIONAL STATES

Survivors of acute cardiovascular events or cardiac surgery who enter the rehabilitation process will have some kind of emotional reaction. Their reactions should be viewed as normal, and in the majority of cases they are situational rather than indicative of a history of psychopathology. To say that emotional reactions to these events are the norm is not to minimize their significance or imply that a rehabilitation program should not attend to them. If anything, rehabilitation programs should offer an opportunity for participants to express their reactions and should convey an understanding of and respect for the very real basis for fears, anger, frustration, depression, and other reactions after these events.[28] At the same time the well-designed rehabilitation program offers a welcome structure through which most patients can move through their emotional reaction in the most adaptive way.

The issues involved in the emotional reactions of cardiac rehabilitation patients are similar to those faced by other rehabilitation patients. Depression, frustration, and anger in response to having to adjust to limitation, learn new habits, change self-concepts, cope with physical discomfort and pain, and overcome feelings of helplessness are common to many rehabilitation patients. The fears and anxieties of cardiac patients tend to be focused on a sense of vulnerability or threat from the disease. Cardiac patients may be somewhat different from other rehabilitation patients in that cardiac disease carries the risk of a sudden and dramatic death that seemingly can strike without warning. Uncertainties about the safe limits of physical activity or emotional arousal are common expressions of this sense of vulnerability.

Common psychologic-emotional presentations of patients entering rehabilitation can be placed on a continuum, with extreme denial of their disease at one end and morbid absorption in the disease at the other. A particular patient's location on the continuum is determined by many factors, including premorbid psychologic adjustment, stability or instability in the other spheres of the patient's psychosocial environment, and severity of disease.

Absolute denial is repudiation of one's cardiac condition, typified most clearly by the patient who asserts that he or she has not had a heart attack even after experiencing the classic symptoms, being hospitalized, and receiving a formal diagnosis. Denial is one of the basic defense mechanisms of the ego identified by Freud. As with all defense mechanisms, denial protects the ego by reducing distress. In denial this is accomplished by repudiating unpleasant objective realities, or at least the significance of such realities. Denial is traditionally considered a fragile and rigid psychologic defense because of the extent of reality distortion involved. In the case of cardiac patients, absolute denial of the objective facts is more common at earlier stages in the disease process than in the rehabilitation phase. Much has been written about the adaptive value of moderate levels of denial during hospitalization, where denial is associated with shorter hospital stays and fewer complications. This may be related to the lower distress and vulnerability experienced by a denying patient. These patients do not see any cause for fear. However, in rehabilitation extreme denial is almost always predictive of early dropout. In 6 years of counseling with cardiac rehabilitation patients, I have met two patients who flatly asserted that they had not had an MI despite their bulging medical records attesting otherwise. Both of these patients dropped out of the program at early points. The reason for the dropout is relatively simple. Continuing in the program challenged the denial-based premise that they did not have a cardiac condition that warranted such a program. Acknowledging the condition meant increased distress.

Much more common in the rehabilitation setting than absolute denial is a milder form of denial—minimization. Patients who minimize acknowledge their disease but downplay its significance or seriousness. Minimization is reflected in statements such as "My heart attack was only a small one, and there really has not been any damage." Keeping in mind that the function of defense mechanisms is to control the amount of distress, it is important that the rehabilitation team not attempt to strip the patient of the minimization defense. The only reason for attempting to break through the defense is if the minimization is interfering with compliance with the program. Frequently these patients are so successful at minimizing the significance of their disease, and thus their fear, that the recommended secondary prevention activities (exercise, smoking cessation, dietary changes) become less necessary. From the patients' point of view, there is not that much to fear. These patients are best approached with clear—but not exaggerated—information about their condition and at the same time with guidance about what actions they can take to improve the situation. Often minimization or denial is a response to feelings of helplessness. Clear information and guidance can reduce that sense of vulnerability and thus reduce the need to rely on the defense mechanism. The minimization defense needs to be reduced only enough to ensure compliance with the basic recommendations of the rehabilitation program.

The second intermediate quadrant along the continuum is optimism. Optimism can be thought of as a mild form of denial, although this stretches the use of that term. Patients in this category acknowledge their disease and its significance but remain optimistic about their outcome or recovery. They tend to be compliant with the treatment program—with that compliance based on pragmatic concern rather than fear. These patients are relatively protected from overt anxiety and depression. From a psychologic and behavioral perspective, optimistic patients are the least complicated patients to work with for the rehabilitation staff.

On the other side of the midpoint of the continuum is the pessimism quadrant. Pessimistic patients acknowledge their disease and its significance but are uncertain about a satisfactory recovery. They are more vulnerable to episodes of anxiety and depression, which tend to be focused on disease-related themes. These patients are usually highly compliant with recommended treatments. Compliance is initially based on fear because it is seen as a means of protection from the threatening aspects of the disease. The major therapeutic issue with these patients is managing the episodes of anxiety or depression.

The fourth quadrant on the continuum, just before the morbid absorption pole, is preoccupation. Rather than minimizing their disease, these patients exaggerate its seriousness and significance. Accordingly, they are more chronically anxious and depressed, more vulnerable, and more helpless. Frequently problems with anxiety or affective disorders were present before the acute cardiovascular event. The acute event disrupts an already fragile psychological state, and these patients have a hard time reestablishing equilibrium and perspective. Patients whose other life spheres (work, family, finances) have also been seriously disrupted by the acute event are more likely to be in this quadrant. The therapeutic objective with preoccupied patients is to reduce the anxiety or depression to more modest levels in order that the patient can organize himself to participate effectively in the rehabilitation program. A chronically depressed or anxious patient is a poor candidate for compliance with a vigorous program of secondary prevention. Changing health habits requires effort, persistence, and organization and can appear overwhelming at times to better-functioning patients because of the breadth of adjustments required. Many of these patients require individual psychologic counseling to deal effectively with their problems.

The morbid absorption pole is an exaggeration of the preoccupation quadrant, sometimes to the point of paranoid obsession with the disease. Morbid absorption implies more severe disruption to daily activity in multiple life spheres and poses a major threat to productive involvement in rehabilitation. Successful compliance with the rehabilitation program is unlikely without the careful coordination of the mental health specialist and other members of the rehabilitation team. Often the program must be individualized for a period of time to accommodate the patient's emotional reaction. Some of these patients drop out despite the best efforts of the rehabilitation team. A referral to a psychologist or a psychiatrist is usually in order because the psychologic disorder is the primary problem.

Treatment for the reactive emotional-psychologic states can occur through several modalities. At the most general level, participation in a structured cardiovascular rehabilitation program is psychologically therapeutic. Patients learn useful information about their disease and about appropriate and reasonable guidelines for physical activity, and they receive guidance and support for undertaking risk factor modification programs. All of this reduces uncertainty and vulnerability. Tasks appear more achievable, and patients find a realistic basis for hope about achieving a satisfactory recovery, both physically and psychologically. The exercise program has major potential psychologic benefits in that physical activity can be safely undertaken. Bandura[1] asserts that actual performance accomplishment (that is, progress in exercise therapy) is the most powerful means of increasing self-efficacy with respect to feared activities. Exercise also works against depression by reducing the sense of hopelessness, helplessness, and diminished capacity that plagues so many of these patients.

Most rehabilitation programs have patients working in groups, and the group format also has potential psychologic benefits. The companionship of the group is an effective antidote to the isolation experienced by many patients and offers a forum in which perspective on one's experience can be reestablished through interaction with others in similar circumstances. To some degree these benefits of the group format accrue simply from being in an exercise group. They can be enhanced by incorporating a devoted psychologically oriented group meeting into the rehabilitation program. In such a group therapy setting, the emotional issues can be more fully explored, and practical information about improved coping and stress management can be presented.

Individual psychologic counseling should always be available for the more complicated emotional reactions, especially for patients who are experiencing higher levels of stress because of disruption in multiple life spheres. Individual counseling can also be helpful for patients who are struggling with some of the deeper, more existential issues that are raised by exposure to a life-threatening condition. Insofar as the individual counseling is done in the context of a cardiac rehabilitation program, it should remain focused on achieving the goals of that program. Long-term psychotherapy may be appropriate for some patients, but this should not be seen as integral to the rehabilitation program.

In summation, most patients experience some degree of emotional disruption in response to acute cardiac events or surgery. These reactions can complicate recovery and hinder compliance with risk factor reduction programs. Rehabilitation programs are psychologically therapeutic with respect to these situational emotional reactions and can be made more so through the incorporation of a structured psychologic component in the program.

THE PSYCHOLOGIST AS A MEMBER OF THE TREATMENT TEAM

This chapter began with the assertion that cardiovascular rehabilitation is essentially a behavioral treatment program. That statement can be expanded to the assertion that cardiovascular rehabilitation programs are potentially highly therapeutic with respect to the emotional and psychologic disruptions of patients who enter them. Psychology is ideally suited to ensure that the behavioral aspects of the program are effectively structured and delivered and that the therapeutic potential of the setting is realized. A psychologist can thus be a valuable consultant to the other members of

the rehabilitation team (nursing, nutrition, cardiology, exercise physiology).

A common failure in rehabilitation is to assume that providing instruction and information is all that is necessary to elicit behavior change. Contemporary behavior theory recognizes that long-term change in health-relevant behaviors is a complicated endeavor that involves emotional, cognitive (beliefs), informational, social, and motivational factors. Psychologists are able to design and deliver comprehensive behavior change programs that, although more expensive initially, are more likely to achieve higher rates of success in the long term. The emotional-psychologic reactions patients exhibit are mostly situational and are not major psychiatric disorders. Typically only a minority of patients in cardiac rehabilitation require psychotropic medicine, primarily because the programs are so effective at reducing the distress. Much of the instruction in this area is focused on improving stress management and coping—areas in which psychologists have the expertise. Psychologists are also capable of providing the individual, family, and group therapy that may be required to supplement the program. The psychologist has a key role to play on the rehabilitation team because of the importance of behavioral and psychologic issues to the goals of cardiovascular rehabilitation.

REFERENCES

1. Bandura, A: Self-efficacy: toward a unifying theory of behavior change, Psychol Rev 84:191, 1977.
2. Bandura, A: Self-efficacy mechanisms in human agency, Am Psychol 37:122, 1982.
3. Barefoot, J, Dahlstrom, W, and Williams, R: Hostility, CHD incidence, and total mortality: a 25 year follow-up study of 255 physicians, Psychosom Med 45:59, 1983.
4. Blackburn, G, Lynch, M, and Wong, S: The very-low-calorie diet: a weight reduction technique. In Brownell, K, and Foreyt, J, editors: Handbook of eating disorders, New York, 1986, Basic Books.
5. Brownell, K, and Wadden, T: Behavior therapy for obesity: modern approaches and better results. In Brownell, K, and Forety, J, editors: Handbook of eating disorders, New York, 1986, Basic Books.
6. Burling, T, et al: Smoking following myocardial infarction, Health Psychol 3:83, 1984.
7. Carmody, T, et al: Physical exercise rehabilitation: long term dropout rate in cardiac patients, J Behav Med 3:113, 1980.
8. Case, R, et al: Type A behavior and survival after acute myocardial infarction, N Engl J Med 312:737, 1985.
9. Cooper, T, Detre, T, and Weiss, S: Review Panel of Coronary Prone Behavior and Coronary Heart Disease: a critical review, Circulation 63:1199, 1981.
10. Danaher, B: Research on rapid smoking: interim summary and recommendations, Addict Behav 2:151, 1977.
11. Dimsdale, J, et al: Type A personality and the extent of coronary atherosclerosis, Am J Cardiol 42:583, 1978.
12. Dimsdale, J, et al: The relationship between diverse measures for type A personality and coronary angiographic findings, J Psychosom Res 23:289, 1979.
13. Dimsdale, J, et al: Type A behavior and angiographic findings, J Psychosom Res 23:273, 1979.
14. Dishman, R: Compliance/adherence in health related exercise, Health Psychol 1:232, 1982.
15. Friedman, M, and Powell, L: The diagnosis and quantitative assessment of type A behavior: introduction and description of the videotaped structured interview, Integrative Psychiatry, 2:123, 1984.

16. Friedman, M, et al: Alteration of type A behavior and reduction in cardiac recurrences in post-myocardial infarction patients, Am Heart J 109:237, 1984.

17. Gill, J, et al: Reduction in type A behavior in healthy middle-aged American military officers, Am Heart J 110:503, 1985.

18. Glass, D, et al: Stability of individual differences in physiological responses to stress, Health Psychol 2:312, 1983.

19. Gotto, A, et al: Recommendations for treatment of hyperlipidemia in adults, Circulation 69:1067, 1984.

20. Hall, R, et al: Two year efficacy and safety of rapid smoking therapy in patients with cardiac and pulmonary disease, J Consult Clin Psychol 52:574, 1984.

21. Haynes, S, et al: The relationship of psychosocial factors to coronary heart disease in the Framingham study. I Methods and risk factors, Am J Epidemiol 107:362, 1978.

22. Jenkins, C: Recent evidence supporting psychologic and social risk factors for coronary disease. I, N Engl J Med 294:987, 1976.

23. Jenkins, C: Recent evidence supporting psychologic and social risk factors for coronary disease. II, N Engl J Med 294:1033, 1976.

24. Jenkins, C: A comparative review of the interview and questionnaire methods in the assessment of the coronary-prone behavior pattern. In Dembrowski, T, et al, editors: Coronary-prone behavior, New York, 1978, Springer-Verlag.

25. Jenkins, C, Rosenman, R, and Zyzanski, S: Prediction of clinical coronary heart disease by a test for the coronary prone behavior pattern, N Engl J Med 23:1271, 1974.

26. Kornitzer, M, et al: The Belgian Heart Disease Prevention Project: type A behavior pattern and the prevalence of coronary heart disease, Psychosom Med 43:133, 1981.

27. Krantz, D, and Manuck, S: Acute psychophysiologic reactivity and risk of cardiovascular disease: a review and methodologic critique, Psychol Bull 96:435, 1984.

28. Lazarus, R: The trivialization of distress. In Rosen, J, and Solomon, L, editors: Prevention in health psychology, Hanover, NH, 1985, University Press of New England.

29. Leventhal, H, Zimmerman, R, and Guttman, M: Compliance: a self-regulation perspective. In Gentry, W, editor: Handbook of behavioral medicine, New York, 1984, Guilford.

30. Lichtenstein, E, et al: Comparison of rapid smoking, warm smokey air, and attention placebo in the modification of smoking behavior, Consult Clin Psychol 40:92, 1973.

31. Mahoney, M, and Mahoney, K: Permanent weight control: a total solution to the dieter's dilemma, New York, 1976, W.W. Norton.

32. Marlatt, G, and Gordon, J: Relapse prevention: maintenance strategies in the addictive behaviors, New York, 1985, Guilford.

33. Matthews, K, et al: Unique and common variance in the structured interview and Jenkins Activity Survey measures of the type A behavior pattern, J Personality Soc Psychol 42:303, 1982.

34. Oldridge, N, and Spencer, J: Exercise habits and perceptions before and after graduation of dropout from supervised cardiac exercise rehabilitation, Cardiopul Rehabil 5:313, 1985.

35. Oldridge, N, et al: Noncompliance in an exercise rehabilitation program for men who have suffered a myocardial infarction, Can Med Assoc J 118:341, 1978.

36. Quinlan, C, Barrow, J, and Hayes, C: The association of risk factors and CHD in Trappist and Benedictine monks, presented at the 42nd American Heart Association Conference on Cardiovascular Epidemiology, New Orleans, 1969.

37. Rosenman, R: The interview method of assessment of the coronary prone behavior pattern. In Dembrowski, T, et al, editors: Coronary prone behavior, New York, 1978, Springer-Verlag.

38. Rosenman, R, et al: Coronary heart disease in the Western Collaborative Group Study: final follow-up experience of 8½ years, JAMA 233:872, 1975.

39. Rosenman, R, et al: A predictive study of coronary heart disease: the Western Collaborative Group Study, JAMA 189:15, 1964.

40. Roskies, E, et al: The Montreal Type A intervention project: major findings, Health Psychol 5:45, 1986.

41. Scott, R, and Lamparski, D: Variables related to long term smoking status following cardiac events, Addict Behav 10:257, 1985.

42. Shekelle, R, Gale, M, and Norusis, M: Type A score (Jenkins Activity Survey) and the risk of recurrent coronary heart disease in the aspirin myocardial infarction study, Am J Cardiol 56:221, 1985.

43. Shekelle, R, et al: Hostility, risk of coronary heart disease, and mortality, Psychosom Med 45:109, 1983.

44. Shekelle, R, et al: Type A behavior and risk of coronary death in Multiple Risk Factor Trial (MRFIT), presented at the 23rd Annual Conference on Cardiovascular Disease Epidemiology, San Diego, 1983.

45. Shiffman, S, et al: Preventing relapse in ex-smokers: a self-management project. In Marlatt, G, and Gordon, J, editors: Relapse prevention, New York, 1985, Guilford.

46. Surgeon General: The health consequences of smoking: cardiovascular disease, Rockville, Md, 1983, U.S. Department of Health and Human Services.

47. Thoresen, C, et al: Altering the type A pattern in post-infarction patients, J Cardiopul Rehabil 5:258, 1985.

48. Williams, R, et al: Type A behavior, hostility, and coronary atherosclerosis, Psychosom Med 42:539, 1980.

CHAPTER 20

Pritikin approach to cardiac rehabilitation

R. JAMES BARNARD, ROBERT PRITIKIN, MONROE B. ROSENTHAL,
AND STEPHEN INKELES

PRITIKIN PROGRAM

In 1974 Nathan Pritikin published his first book, *Live Longer Now*. In this book he expressed his feeling that coronary artery and other degenerative diseases—including hypertension, non-insulin-dependent diabetes mellitus, and certain forms of cancer—could be controlled or prevented by a radical change in the typical American diet combined with daily exercise. The dietary program outlined by Pritikin called for less than 10% of the total intake of calories to be derived from fat, less than 100 mg of cholesterol per day, and less than 4 g NaCl per day. The diet focused on complex carbohydrates high in fiber. This was a radical change from the typical American high–refined sugar diet consisting of 45% of calories from fat, 600 mg of cholesterol, and 8 to 10 g of NaCl per day.

During the 1970s, Pritikin was highly criticized for his program and the claims he made regarding its success. However, it is interesting to note that in more recent times many groups, including the American Heart Association, the American Diabetes Association, and the American Cancer Association, have adopted dietary guidelines approaching those proposed by Pritikin in the 1970s. For example, in 1984 the American Heart Association adopted a three-stage dietary program for the control of hyperlipidemia.[1] The stage-three diet recommends that Americans reduce their fat consumption to 20% of calories, and their cholesterol consumption to 100 to 150 mg per day.

Pritikin believed that it was important to educate people about their diseases and about how diet and exercise can be effective, in many cases, for controlling them. In five popular books, he did so and provided scientific references to support his concepts. He also established the Pritikin Longevity Center as a residential program where people could learn the Pritikin Program at first hand. Although the Center provided an excellent source for research data and the opportunity for many people to change their life-styles, far more have experienced the Pritikin program by following the guidelines published in the books.

Pritikin diet

The Pritikin diet has been described in several publications.[33,35,36] It actually consists of two diets: the Pritikin Lifetime Eating Plan and the therapeutic modification. In both diets less than 10% of total calories is derived from fat (the ratio of polyunsaturated to saturated is 2:4), 10% to 15% from protein, and the remainder from carbohydrate (90% unrefined). The diet provides 35 to 40 g of dietary fiber per 1000 kcal and only 4 g of sodium chloride. The difference between the two diets is the amount of cholesterol. For the therapeutic modification, cholesterol consumption is limited to 25 mg per day, whereas on the Lifetime Eating Plan the limit is increased to 100 mg per day.

The diets consist primarily of whole grains, beans, peas, other vegetables, and fresh fruits. On the therapeutic plan, protein is derived primarily from vegetable sources except for nonfat milk and limited amounts of nonfat cheese. Table 20-1 gives guidelines on foods to consume and foods to avoid for the maintenance diet. In the therapeutic plan the consumption of meat, fish, or poultry is limited to 3 ounces per week and shellfish* to 1½ ounces per week. The therapeutic plan is served at the Longevity Center. On leaving the Center, patients with severe atherosclerotic disease or suboptimal cholesterol values are encouraged to continue

---

*Only low-cholesterol shellfish—shrimp, crab, and lobster—are permitted.

Table 20-1. Foods to use and to avoid on the Pritikin diet

Category	Foods to use	Quantity permitted	Foods to avoid
Fats, oils	None		All fats and oils, including butter, margarine, shortening, lard, meat fat, all oils, lecithin (as in vegetable spray)
Sugars	None		All extracted sugars, including syrups, molasses, fructose, dextrose, sucrose, and honey
Poultry, fish, shellfish, meat, and soybeans	Chicken, turkey, Cornish game hen (white meat preferred; remove skin)	Limit acceptable poultry, fish, and meat to 3½ oz /day; maximum 1½ lb/week	Fatty poultry: duck, goose, etc.
	Lean round or flank steak, all visible fat removed	Lobster, oysters, clams, scallops, squid, and mussels: 3½ oz/day	Fatty fish: sardines, fish canned in oil, mackerel, etc.
	Lean fish, squid and shellfish	Shrimp and crab: 1¾ oz/day (replaces entire daily allotment of poultry, fish or meat)	Fatty meats: marbled steaks, fatty hamburger and other fatty ground meat, bacon, spareribs, sausage, frankfurters, luncheon meat, etc.
	Soybeans and tofu (soybean curd)	Soybeans and tofu: 3½ oz/day (replaces entire daily allotment of poultry, fish, or meat).	Organ meats: liver, kidneys, hearts, sweetbreads. Smoked, charbroiled or barbecued foods.
Eggs	Egg whites	7/week max. (Raw: 2/week maximum)	Egg yolks. Fish eggs: caviar, shad roe, etc.
Dairy foods	Nonfat (skim) milk, nonfat buttermilk (up to 1% fat by weight) (8 oz = 1 serving)		Cream, half-and-half, whole milk, and lowfat milk or products, containing or made from them, such as sour cream, lowfat yogurt, etc.
	Nonfat yogurt (6 oz = 1 serving)		
	Nonfat (skim) powdered milk (5T = 1 serving)	2 servings/day	Nondairy substitutes: creamers, whipped toppings, etc.
	Evaporated skim milk (4 oz = 1 serving)		Cheeses containing over 1% fat by weight
	100% skim milk cheese, primarily uncreamed cottage cheese such as hoop cheese or dry curd cottage cheese, or cheeses up to 1% fat by weight (2 oz = 1 serving)		

From Pritikin Programs International.

Table 20-1, cont'd. Foods to use and to avoid on the Pritikin diet

Category	Foods to use	Quantity permitted	Foods to avoid
Beans, peas	Sap Sago (green) cheese All beans and peas (except soybeans)	1-2 oz/week maximum Limit to 8 oz cooked beans on days when poultry, fish or meat is not eaten. Avoid on other days except for small amounts in soups, salads, or other dishes.	Soybeans and tofu (unless substituted) (1 oz soybeans or tofu = 1 oz poultry, fish, shellfish, or meat allotment)
Nuts, seeds	Chestnuts	Not limited	All nuts (except chestnuts) All seeds (except in small quantities for seasoning with spices)
Vegetables	All vegetables except avocadoes and olives	Limit vegetables high in oxalic acid such as spinach, beet leaves, rhubarb, and swiss chard	Avocadoes Olives
Fruits	All fresh fruits	5 servings/day maximum	Cooked, canned, or frozen fruit with added sugars
	Unsweetened cooked, canned pureed, or frozen fruit	24 oz/week maximum	Products containing added sugars such as jams, jellies, fruit spreads, and syrups
	Dried fruit	1 oz/day maximum	
	Unsweetened fruit juices	4 oz/day maximum (28 oz/week)	Fruit juices with added sugar
	Frozen concentrates, undiluted	or 1 oz/day maximum (7 oz/week)	
Grains	All whole or lightly milled grains: rice, barley, buckwheat, millet, etc.	Not limited	Extracted wheat germ
	Breads, cereals, crackers, pasta, tortillas, baked goods and other grain products without added fats, oils, sugars or egg yolks	Limit refined grains and grain products (i.e., with bran and germ removed) such as white flour, white rice, white pasta, etc.	Grain products made with added fats, oils, sugars, or egg yolks Bleached white flour; soy flour
Salt	Salt	Limit salt intake to 4 g (1600 mg sodium) or less/day; eliminate table salt and restrict the use of high salt or sodium (Na) foods such as, soy sauce, pickles, most condiments, prepared sauces, dressings, canned vegetables and MSG (monosodium glutamate)	Salt from all sources in excess of permitted amount; eliminate table salt
Condiments, salad dressings, sauces, gravies and spreads	Wines for cooking Natural flavoring extracts Products without fats, oils, sugars, or egg yolks	Dry white wine preferable; moderate use	Products containing fats, oils, sugars or egg yolks such as mayonnaise, prepared sandwich spreads, prepared gravies and sauces and most seasoning mixes, salad dressings, catsups, pickle relish, chutney

Continued.

Table 20-1, cont'd. Foods to use and to avoid on the Pritikin diet

Category	Foods to use	Quantity permitted	Foods to avoid
Desserts or snacks	Dessert and snack items without fats, oils, sugars, or egg yolks	Plain gelatin (unflavored): 1 oz/week maximum	Desserts and snack items containing fats, oils, sugars, or egg yolks such as most bakery goods, package gelatin desserts and puddings, candy, chocolate and gum
Beverages	Mineral water, carbonated water	Limit varieties with added sodium	Alcoholic beverages
	Nonfat (skim) milk or nonfat buttermilk	See restrictions under *Dairy foods* above	Beverages with caffeine: coffee, tea, cola drinks, etc.
	Unsweetened fruit juices	See restrictions under *Fruit* above	Decaffeinated coffee
	Vegetable juices		Beverages with added sweeteners, such as soft drinks
	Red Bush or Chamomile tea preferred	2 cups per day	Diet and other soft drinks with artificial sweetener

From Pritikin Programs International.

with the therapeutic plan as long as needed to control the disease and alleviate symptoms or to bring total serum cholesterol down to 160 mg/dl or less or LDL cholesterol to 100 mg/dl or less. The remaining individuals are placed on the Lifetime Eating Plan once they leave the Center. Beverages with caffeine are not permitted. Although not recommended, alcohol consumption in the form of white wine is permitted (1 glass, 3 or 4 days a week).

Computer analyses of the menus used at the Center show that even the therapeutic plan provides the recommended daily allowance (RDA) for nutrients established by the National Academy of Sciences. In a recent study (unpublished data), 20 patients who had complied with the Pritikin diet longer than 4 years were tested for nutritional adequacy and were compared with 20 similar patients of the same age. Serum cholesterol levels for the Pritikin groups were 159.9 ± 5.9 mg/dl, whereas the controls had levels of 226.4 ± 15.0 mg/dl. In over 50 blood tests for iron status, trace minerals, vitamins, and so forth, we found no signs of nutritional inadequacy. The results are similar to those reported by Anderson and co-workers[3] using essentially the same diet.

Exercise training

Daily walking is an important part of the Pritikin program. Pritikin initially believed that walking might stimulate the development of collateral vessels in the heart to increase oxygen delivery. We no longer believe that this is true for the heart, since experimental evidence indicates that ischemia is the stimulus for collateral development. Obviously cardiac patients cannot risk pushing their hearts to the point of ischemia in the hope of developing collateral vessels. We do think, however, that patients with intermittent claudication can stimulate the development of collateral vessels in the legs by walking to the point of severe pain.[4,24,25]

Although Pritikin was an avid jogger himself, he constantly warned people that if they followed the typical American diet, jogging could result in a heart attack. He encouraged individuals who wanted to do activity more strenuous than walking to follow his diet to avoid serious problems. In spite of his own jogging program, he felt that walking was the best form of exercise for most adult Americans and especially for cardiac patients. The results obtained at the Longevity Center confirm his claim that daily walking can significantly increase endurance and maximal work capacity. Even patients receiving beta-blocking agents can significantly improve their work capacity.[6]

Before starting any exercise program, cardiac patients should have an examination by a physician. At the Longevity Center, all patients are assigned to a physician who conducts an initial history, physical examination, and multistage, symptom-limited treadmill test. Immediately following the treadmill test, the results are evaluated by the supervising physician and a training heart rate is assigned to the participant. The participant then meets with an exercise physiologist who writes an exercise prescription for walking 6 days per week. For the first week the prescription generally calls for 30 to 40 minutes of daily walking with every other day just below the training heart rate. At the end of each week a new prescription is given so that each participant's walking is increased. By the fourth week most cardiac patients are walking for an hour or more each day.

In addition to the walking program the participants are assigned to a supervised exercise class according to the metabolic equivalent (MET) level achieved on the initial treadmill test. Cardiac patients with a MET level of 3 or less are assigned to a class for daily treadmill walking with electrocardiographic (ECG) monitoring. The remaining participants are assigned to a 60-minute group class, which consists of flexibility and stretching activities, muscle-conditioning exercises, and aerobic exercises on a treadmill or bicycle ergometer.

On leaving the Center the patients are encouraged to continue with their flexibility and stretching programs and to walk for an hour at least 4 days every week.

Education

Since Pritikin believed that it was important for patients to understand their diseases and the scientific rationale for changing their life-styles, he included a large educational component to the Pritikin Longevity Center program. Each week the participants attend more than 15 hours of educational classes, including cooking school, educational lectures, and group or individual counseling sessions.

The cooking classes demonstrate how to prepare food in compliance with the Pritikin guidelines for a low-fat, low-cholesterol, and low-salt diet. Participants are taught how to prepare food without using oil, butter, and other commonly used fats and how to use meat as a condiment as opposed to being the major source of calories in the main entree. The preparation of soups, salad dressings and deserts is also demonstrated. Recipes for preparing the various dishes are all included in a cookbook, along with a discussion of the use of various herbs and spices for flavoring. Many of the recipes are also contained in Pritikin's publications.

The educational classes have three aspects. One group of lectures deals with the major diseases—hypertension, diabetes, cancer, and coronary disease—and the roles diet and exercise play in their prevention and management. For example, in the coronary heart disease lecture the patients are taught how the disease develops (the lipid infiltration and endothelial injury hypotheses), the role of risk factors in disease development, factors that determine serum cholesterol levels, and primary and secondary intervention studies supporting the value of cholesterol reduction and life-style modification.

Another group of lectures deals with nutrition and is coordinated with the cooking school classes. The participants are taught which foods are high in fat, cholesterol, and sodium and how to avoid them. They learn that cholesterol is produced only by animals, and thus animal products (meat and dairy), must be limited, whereas vegetable and whole-grain products must be emphasized. Another lecture deals with eating in restaurants. Others discuss reading labels and trips to the supermarket.

The third group of lectures deals with life-style management, which includes understanding and coping with stress and designing a winning life-style. Special sessions are also offered for smokers.

RESPONSE OF PATIENTS WITH ATHEROSCLEROSIS
Short-term response of coronary patients

In an initial study the progress of 29 patients with severe coronary heart disease was reported.[6] During the initial treadmill test, maximal work capacity for the onset of myocardial ischemia (1.0 mm or more ST-segment depression) was 3.1 ± 0.2 METs. On a final treadmill test taken 3 weeks later, maximal work capacity for the onset of myocardial ischemia had increased to 4.3 ± 0.3 METs. Five of 19 patients taking propranolol (Inderal) on the initial test had the drug discontinued before the final test and still achieved a 1.0 MET improvement in maximal work capacity. Of 16 patients experiencing angina during the initial treadmill test, 14 still felt it during the final test; the two patients who lost their angina, however, still developed myocardial ischemia on the final treadmill test. For the entire group ST-segment depression developed at the same heart rate and systolic pressure product on the initial and final treadmill tests, indicating no change in arterial disease or oxygen delivery to the myocardium.

Daily walking increased from 0.83 to 9.33 km per day. The patients lost a significant amount of body weight and achieved significant improvements in blood pressure and serum lipids, as can be seen in Table 20-2. These data show that significant improvements in performance capacity and medical status can be achieved in a few weeks with an intensive dietary and exercise program.

Long-term response of coronary patients

Although the short-term effects of the Pritikin program are impressive, the long-term effects are far more important. A follow-up study[9] was designed to answer two questions: Do participants continue to follow the diet and exercise recommendations once they leave the Center? If so, what is the effect on their long-term health status? Of the first 893 participants in the program, 64 patients with coronary artery disease were identified by angiograms and recommendations for coronary bypass surgery. These patients, 44 to 75 years of age were contacted by phone and asked numerous questions about their compliance to the program and their present health status (Table 20-3). They were asked to have their physicians forward recent medical records and a fasting blood sample.

Table 20-4 shows the estimated percentage of time patients complied with the Lifetime Eating Plan (10% fat, less

Table 20-2. Response of 29 patients with coronary heart disease to Pritikin 26-day program

Variable	Before program	After program
Body weight (kg)	71.2 ± 2.1	68.3 ± 1.9*
Systolic pressure (mm Hg)	130.5 ± 3.7	116.0 ± 3.4*
Diastolic pressure (mm Hg)	77.3 ± 2.3	69.9 ± 1.8*
Serum cholesterol level (mg/dl)	236.4 ± 9.2	178.7 ± 5.6*
Serum triglyceride level (mg/dl)	173.5 ± 12.9	147.3 ± 11.4*

From Barnard, RJ, et al: J Cardiac Rehabil 1:99, 1981.
*(mean ± SE) $p < .05$.

Table 20-3. Cardiac status of 64 patients in 5-year follow-up study

	Number of patients	Percentage of group
Prior myocardial infarction	38	59
Single-vessel disease	8	13
Double-vessel disease	18	28
Triple-vessel disease	38	59
Left main artery disease	3	5
Angina	51	80

From Barnard, RJ, et al: J Cardiac Rehabil 3:183, 1983.

than 100 mg cholesterol): 88% of the respondents complied with the diet more than 50% of the time. The cholesterol values obtained at follow-up examinations were significantly correlated with the estimated percentage of compliance to the diet. During the 26-day program many of the patients had their medication discontinued (Table 20-5). At follow-up examinations, although the patients were being treated by their personal physicians, only a small percentage had resumed taking medication.

Mortality and morbidity data are shown in Table 20-6. Over the 5-year period a total of four individuals died, two of them from coronary artery disease. Two patients had reinfarctions, and two had new infarctions. Twelve of the patients eventually underwent coronary artery bypass surgery. Initially 80% of the patients had angina; at follow-up examinations only 32% still had angina. Obviously, the 19% who underwent bypass surgery lost their angina because of the surgery; however, the remainder spontaneously lost their angina. Others have also reported the loss of angina in patients placed on a low-fat and low-cholesterol diet.[18,37]

Exactly why so many of these patients continued to do so well is unknown. Unfortunately, none of them underwent repeat angiograms, so we cannot document whether any of the patients actually decreased their artery disease or simply arrested its progression. Regression of atherosclerosis has been reported in the literature and has been associated with a reduction in serum cholesterol.[21] Pritikin followed his diet himself after a diagnosis of ischemic heart disease in 1958. By 1960 his serum cholesterol was reduced from a high of 280 mg/dl to 120 mg/dl, a level below which it remained until his death at age 69 in 1985. His autopsy revealed an absence of raised plaques and no compromise of the lumen in his coronary system, suggesting that regression had occurred.[27] Even in the absence of regression, reductions in serum lipids and certain hormones as well as the control of other risk factors, including hypertension and diabetes are important aspects for secondary prevention of coronary artery disease.

Response of patients with intermittent claudication

Peripheral vascular disease (PVD) in the form of intermittent claudication afflicts a significant number of people in this country, especially diabetic patients. The effects of the Pritikin program on reducing serum lipids and controlling other risk factors are important for long-term control of PVD, whereas the exercise program is more important for an immediate improvement in performance capacity. Unlike coronary patients, who are told to exercise below the ischemic threshhold, PVD patients are told to walk to the point of severe leg pain, sit down until the pain subsides, then walk again to severe pain. This procedure of repeated walking to the point of severe pain is performed twice daily for 20 to 30 minutes of walking as described in detail previously.[4,24] The rationale for walking to the point of severe pain is to stimulate the formation of collateral vessels to enhance blood flow and oxygen delivery to the muscles.

Table 20-4. Dietary compliance and serum lipid levels at follow-up examination of patients with coronary heart disease

Estimated compliance (%)	Number of patients	Cholesterol (mg/dl)	Triglyceride (mg/dl)
90-100	15	181 ± 10	109 ± 7
50-89	35	197 ± 6	131 ± 9
< 50	3	209	92
0	4	276 ± 48	276 ± 110

From Barnard, RJ, et al: J Cardiac Rehabil 3:183, 1983.

Table 20-5. Medication status of 64 patients with coronary heart disease

Type of medication	Number of patients taking medication		
	Before program	After program	At follow-up examination
Cardiac	47	26	28
Antihypertensive	35	9	11
Cholesterol-lowering	7	1	2
Other	15	4	6

From Barnard, RJ, et al: J Cardiac Rehabil 3:183, 1983.

Table 20-6. Mortality and morbidity among 64 patients with coronary heart disease at 5-year follow-up examination

	Number of patients	Percentage of group
Total deaths	4	6
Coronary deaths	2	3
Coronary bypass	12	19
Angina	19	32
Infarction or reinfarction	4	6

From Barnard, RJ, et al: J Cardiac Rehabil 3: 183, 1983.

In a case report the remarkable progress of one patient with total occlusion of both external femoral arteries at midthigh was reported.[25] At the time of his arteriogram the patient had no palpable pulses at the ankles and suffered from severe claudication pain. On entry into the Pritikin Longevity Center the patient's walking tolerance was 100 yards. During his stay at the Center the patient completed at least two daily walks, walking to the point of severe pain as outlined in his walking prescription. After 26 days his walking tolerance had increased to 3 miles in 1 hour with little leg pain.

After leaving the Center the patient continued with his walking program and slowly started jogging. In the year following his stay at the center he jogged 1230 miles and walked 600 miles. The following year he jogged 1900 miles, including several 10 km road races and the Chicago Marathon, which he completed in less than 6 hours. During this entire time he continued to follow the Pritikin diet and reduced his cholesterol from 407 mg/dl to a low of 130 mg/dl.

A follow-up examination 4 years after he left the Center revealed palpable but slightly diminished pulses in both ankles. Following the Strandness Doppler exercise test, ankle pressure on the left side increased; however, the pressure on the right side decreased, indicating a significant deficit in oxygen delivery to the lower leg. The patient explained that he still experienced leg pain when he started his runs, but as he continued into the run the pain subsided. A second arteriogram showed a massive collateral network extending from the vertebral and deep femoral arteries to the popliteal artery in both legs. This case study supports animal experiments showing that regular exercise to the point of severe ischemia can enhance collateral vessel formation and significantly improve performance capacity.

Following that case report a study was designed to investigate hemodynamic changes in patients with PVD attending the Pritikin Center.[24] Sixteen patients with previously diagnosed PVD were given symptom-limited treadmill

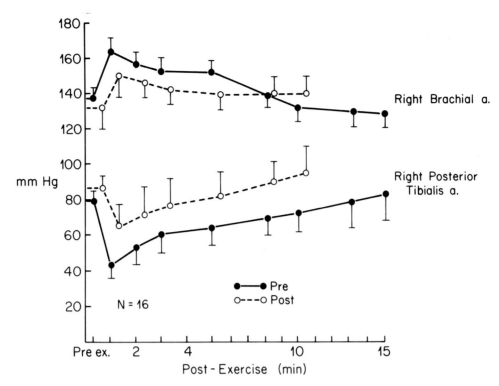

Figure 20-1. Resting and postexercise blood pressure responses in patients with intermittent claudication who completed Pritikin program. (From Hall, JA, and Barnard, RJ: J Cardiac Rehabil 2:569, 1982.)

tests and resting and exercise Doppler examinations at the start and conclusion of the 26-day program. Walking, which was minimal before admission to the program, was increased to 2.3 ± 0.15 hours per day. The maximal symptom-limited work capacity increased from 4.1 ± 0.35 METs to 6.6 +0.4 METs.

Doppler testing (Figure 20-1) showed significant improvements ($p < 0.05$) in the immediate postexercise pressure responses in both legs. The immediate postexercise ankle to arm pressure index increased from 0.26 ± 0.04 to 0.41 ± 0.06 in the right leg and from 0.30 ± 0.04 to 0.45 ± 0.08 in the left leg. The time for ankle pressure to return to resting levels was reduced by 7 minutes for the right leg and by 9 minutes for the left leg. The resting ankle to arm index in the right leg increased significantly from 0.58 ± 0.03 to 0.64 ± 0.04; the slight increase in the left leg was not statistically significant.

Although serial arteriograms were not made on these patients, the improvements in resting and postexercise ankle pressures would suggest collateral vessel development. The fact that the resting pressure improved only in the right leg was to be expected. These patients had a more severe hemodynamic impairment in the right leg, which generally was the leg that limited performance capacity. The ischemic response was ususaly less severe in the left leg, and therefore less adaptation occurred.

SERUM LIPID, HORMONE, AND PLATELET CHANGES
Serum lipids

The relationship between elevated levels of serum cholesterol, especially low-density lipoprotein cholesterol (LDL), and increased risk for coronary artery disease and myocardial infarction has been established in numerous reports.[29] The value of reducing serum cholesterol for both primary and secondary prevention of coronary artery disease has also been documented.[12,26,30,32]

Although cholesterol is produced by humans, primarily in the liver, the excessive dietary consumption of cholesterol and saturated fats appears to be the major factor responsible for the high levels of serum cholesterol currently seen in most industrialized nations. The elegant studies of Brown and Goldstein[13] show that the number of LDL receptors on liver cell membranes is the major factor determining the body's ability to handle dietary cholesterol. Since cholesterol cannot be metabolized by humans, it must be converted to bile or eliminated along with bile via the common bile duct. Some individuals have genetic defects that increase serum cholesterol. One in every million Americans is born without any functional liver LDL receptors. These individuals have serum cholesterol values in excess of 600 mg/dl and develop atherosclerotic problems very early in life. One in every 500 Americans is born with half the normal number

Table 20-7. Effects of the Pritikin program on a patient with severe hyperlipidemia

	Day 1	Day 7	Day 14	Day 21
Cholesterol (mg/dl)	750	544	313	224
Triglyceride (mg/dl)	5260	1461	1068	591
Glucose (mg/dl)	195	161	137	136

of liver LDL receptors, and these individuals generally have serum cholesterol values in excess of 300 mg/dl. These individuals, however, can increase the number of LDL receptors by dietary restriction of cholesterol.[13]

These genetic defects, known as familial hypercholesterolemia, are often diagnosed simply on the basis of elevated serum cholesterol, implying that the patient cannot lower the cholesterol level because of a genetic defect. Table 20-7 gives an example of one such individual, who was told by his personal physician that his elevated lipid levels were caused primarily by a genetic defect. The fact that major reductions were eventually achieved in both cholesterol and triglycerides would suggest that life-style played a major role in determining the very high lipid levels this patient had on entry into the Pritikin Longevity Center.

The typical American consumes between 450 and 600 mg of cholesterol per day. This simply is more cholesterol

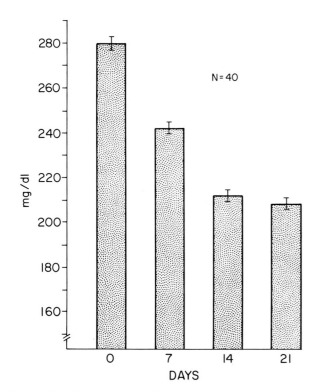

Figure 20-2. Total serum cholesterol changes in participants attending Pritikin Longevity Center.

than the human liver can handle. Reducing cholesterol and saturated fat consumption by following the Pritikin diet has consistently resulted in an average reduction in total serum cholesterol of about 25%. In an analysis of the first 878 participants in the Pritikin Longevity Center, the average reduction in serum cholesterol was 26%.[15] Individuals with cholesterol levels less than 160 mg/dl on entry into the program achieved a 10% reduction; those with levels above 320 mg/dl achieved a 36% reduction over the 26-day program.

In a recent week-by-week study, changes in total serum cholesterol were documented. As can be seen in Figure 20-2, major decreases occurred during the first and second weeks and no significant change thereafter. These results show that the serum pool of cholesterol can be significantly reduced in a relatively short period of time by restricting dietary cholesterol and saturated fats. Long-term compliance with the diet has been shown to be effective for maintaining low levels of cholesterol.[9,10] Table 20-4 shows the relationship between estimated compliance to the Pritikin diet and cholesterol values 3 to 4 years after the patients completed the Pritikin program.

In addition to significantly reducing cholesterol, the Pritikin program is effective in reducing serum triglycerides. Although the relationship between elevated triglycerides and coronary artery disease is not as clear cut as the relationship between elevated cholesterol and coronary artery disease, most physicians feel that it is prudent to reduce elevated levels of triglyceride, particularly when they exceed 250 mg/dl. In the first 873 participants in the Pritikin program, mean serum triglyceride was reduced from 174 to 130 mg/dl (25%).[15] Figure 20-3 shows that most of the reduction in triglycerides occurs during the first week of the program. Both exercise and fat restriction play important roles in reducing triglycerides.

Lipoprotein lipids and apoproteins

The Framingham data have emphasized the relationship between high levels of LDL cholesterol, low levels of high-density lipoprotein (HDL) cholesterol, and the development of coronary artery disease.[23] Most physicians look at the ratio of total cholesterol to HDL to assess the risk for developing coronary artery disease. Table 20-8 gives lipoprotein data from 20 individuals attending the Pritikin Longevity Center. Total cholesterol was reduced by 25% and

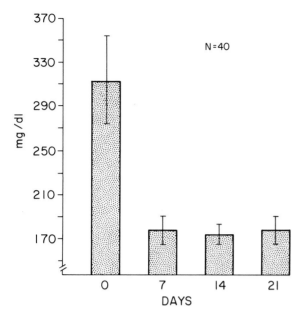

Figure 20-3. Serum triglyceride changes in response to Pritikin program.

LDL cholesterol by 28%. HDL cholesterol was also reduced (by 10%); however, the ratio of total cholesterol to HDL was reduced by 21%, indicating a significant reduction in the risk for coronary artery disease. More recently, research has focused on the specific apoproteins of the lipoproteins, since this portion of the molecule binds to the lipoprotein receptors. Whether apoprotein measurements are more specific than lipoprotein measurements for predicting risk for coronary artery disease has not been established. However, data show that restricting dietary cholesterol and fat reduces serum apoproteins as well as lipoproteins (Table 20-8).

Estradiol

Several recent studies have suggested that hyperestrogenemia in men may be the major predisposing factor for myocardial infarction, with hypercholesterolemia playing a secondary role.[20,34] The effects of the Pritikin program on serum lipids, estradiol, and testosterone were examined in 21 men, age 57 ± 1 year.[38] Total serum cholesterol was reduced by 21%, estradiol was reduced by 50%, and testosterone was unchanged. If estradiol is confirmed as a major predisposing factor for myocardial infarction, our data indicate that a major reduction in risk can be achieved by following the Pritikin program. This may have been a factor responsible for the low mortality and morbidity observed in our 5-year follow-up study of coronary heart disease patients. If this same reduction in estradiol is achieved in women, it has major implications for the prevention of breast and endometrial cancer.[40]

Platelet aggregation

Platelet aggregation is thought to play an important role in the initial stage of atherosclerosis development, as well as in the complications of atherosclerosis, namely myocardial infarction and stroke.[19,39] Diet's important role in reducing platelet reactivity has been demonstrated in several studies in which patients were given supplements of polyunsaturated fatty acids.[22,31] Although supplementing the typical American diet with more polyunsaturated fat may reduce the risk of atherosclerosis, the risk for certain forms of cancer and non-insulin-dependent diabetes mellitus may increase. In an initial study of hypertensive patients, Iacono and Dougherty[28] reported that reducing total fat consumption and increasing the ratio of polyunsaturated to saturated fats reduced platelet aggregation.

Blood samples were obtained from 15 hyperlipidemic men at the beginning and end of the Pritikin Longevity Center's 13-day program to study platelet aggregation in the presence of adenosine diphosphate (ADP) and collagen.[11] Table 20-9 gives the aggregation results and shows that the Pritikin program reduces platelet reactivity. Whether the reduction in platelet aggregation was caused by changes in the biochemical structure of the platelets or by changes in the biochemical composition of the plasma is unknown. In

Table 20-8. Effects of the Pritikin program on serum lipoprotein lipids and apoproteins (in 20 patients)

	Levels before program	Levels after program
Total cholesterol (mg/dl)	250.1 ± 11.9	187.4 ± 10.8*
LDL (mg/dl)	174.9 ± 10.5	125.9 ± 10.3*
HDL (mg/dl)	40.0 ± 1.9	35.9 ± 1.9*
Total cholesterol/HDL	6.6 ± 0.6	5.5 ± 0.5*
Triglycerides (mg/dl)	176.2 ± 19.0	127.6 ± 9.0*
APO B-100 (mg/dl)	105.2 ± 8.2	78.5 ± 5.7*
APO A-1 (mg/dl)	145.9 ± 5.6	119.1 ± 5.5*
APO A-1/APO B-100	1.5 ± 0.2	1.6 ± 0.1

*$p < .01$.

Table 20-9. Platelet aggregation responses to the 2-week Pritikin program (in 15 patients)

	Levels before program (mg/dl)	Levels after program (mg/dl)
Maximum aggregation		
6.6 μM ADP	32.8 ± 5.9	18.7 ± 4.3*
20 μM ADP	52.1 ± 4.9	42.6 ± 4.4*
100 μg/ml collagen	49.3 ± 7.9	36.9 ± 9.0*
200 μg/ml collagen	77.0 ± 5.2	62.9 ± 6.8*
Maximum velocity of aggregation (%/min)		
6.6 μM ADP	39.5 ± 3.4	27.7 ± 4.6*
20 μM ADP	53.7 ± 4.1	46.9 ± 4.0*
100 μg/ml collagen	34.2 ± 7.2	18.2 ± 4.9*
200 μg/ml collagen	59.1 ± 5.9	41.1 ± 6.4*

From Barnard, RJ, et al: Prostaglandins Leukotrienes Med 26:241, 1987.
*$p < .05$ for postintervention versus preintervention values.

addition to reducing platelet aggregation, these patients reduced their serum cholesterol from 266 ± 7 to 210 ± 9mg/dl and their triglycerides from 188 ± 19 to 105 ± 9 mg/dl. Thus the Pritikin program appears to be more effective than supplementation of the American diet with more fat for the overall control of atherosclerosis and other degenerative disease.

RESPONSE OF PATIENTS WITH HYPERTENSION

Hypertension is the most common cardiovascular disease in the United States. The American Heart Association's data indicate that approximately 20% of adult whites and 30% of adult blacks in this country are hypertensive. Most of these individuals have essential hypertension, since the cause is unknown. Data suggest that in a majority of cases essential hypertension is associated with life-style factors and can in most cases be controlled by following the Pritikin program.

Short-term response to the Pritikin program

Of the first 893 participants in the Pritikin Longevity Center program, a total of 268 hypertensive individuals, 38 to 67 years of age, were identified.[8] On entry into the program, 216 were taking antihypertensive medication and had been for more than a year. Of the 52 with a history of hypertension but not receiving medication, 2 were severely hypertensive and were immediately started on a regimen of antihypertensive drugs that continued throughout the program. Resting blood pressure was measured every morning before breakfast with a sphygmetric automated blood pressure recorder. Readings obtained on days 2 through 5 and 22 through 25 were averaged and recorded as before and after values, respectively.

Of the 216 patients initially taking antihypertensive medication, 180 had their medication discontinued and still achieved a small but statistically significant reduction in blood pressure. Blood pressure changes for all groups are shown in Figures 20-4 and 20-5. As can be seen, the biggest change occurred in the group of people who had never received antihypertensive drugs. Thirty-six (13%) of the patients did not respond well to the program. They had no change in their blood pressure and were unable to stop taking medication. The exact reason why this small percentage did not respond to the program is unknown. Possibly the cause for their hypertension simply could not be treated with this nonpharmacologic approach. However, the majority, including the 83% who discontinued medication, responded well.

In a smaller study of 23 hypertensive patients, blood pressure responses during exercise and during rest were studied.[5] Of the 17 patients initially taking antihypertensive medication, nine had their medication discontinued, and the remaining eight had the dosage reduced. Table 20-10 shows the blood pressure changes in these patients. As can be seen, blood pressures were reduced at rest and during exercise, both at the same workload and same heart rate.

Long-term response to the Pritikin program

In an attempt to assess the long-term effects of the Pritikin program on the control of hypertension, follow-up data were obtained from 40 patients 3 to 4 years after they left the Longevity Center.[8] The patients were asked to have their personal physicians send medical records from their most recent medical examinations. At the follow-up examinations, at which the patients were treated by their personal physicians, blood pressure did increase somewhat, but only two patients had returned to medication. Thus over the long

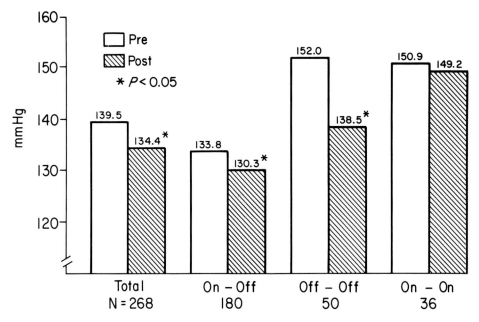

Figure 20-4. Systolic blood pressure responses to Pritikin program. *On-off* refers to medication status at entry and completion of program. (From Barnard, RJ, et al: J Cardiac Rehabil 3:839, 1983.)

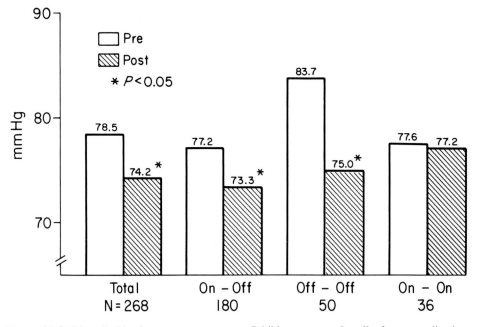

Figure 20-5. Diastolic blood pressure responses to Pritikin program. *On-off* refers to medication status at entry and completion of program. (From Barnard, RJ, et al: J Cardiac Rehabil 3:839, 1983.)

Table 20-10. Resting and exercise blood pressure responses to the Pritikin program (in 23 patients)*

	Levels before program	Levels after program
Resting blood pressure (mm Hg)*	143/83	133/75
Exercise blood pressure (mm Hg)		
Same workload	189/86	167/76
Same heart rate	188/85	170/78

From Barnard, RJ, et al: J Cardiac Rehabil 5:185, 1985.
*All after values were significantly lower than before values; $p < 0.05$; nine of 17 patients had their antihypertensive medication discontinued.

Table 20-11. Three- to four-year follow-up data on 40 hypertensive patients

	Levels before program	Levels after program	Follow-up levels
Blood pressure (mm Hg)	130/79	116/68	130/76
Patients on medication	33	10	12

From Barnard, RJ, et al: J Cardiac Rehabil 3:839, 1983.

term the Pritikin program is very effective for controlling hypertension.

Salt versus fat

The Pritikin program controls elevated blood pressure in several ways, including the diet, daily exercise, and weight loss. In addition, a "spa effect" may be associated with attending the Center; that is, the Center's good results may be influenced by the fact that its patients are away from their routine pressures of job and family. In an attempt to assess which of these factors might be the most important, an outpatient program was conducted in which the patients modified their diet to follow the Pritikin guidelines but did not modify their exercise habits.[8] Figure 20-6 shows that during the 4-week period both systolic and diastolic pressures were reduced, and six of 12 patients had their medication discontinued. The group lost weight only during the first week of the program. Thus the most important aspect of the Pritikin program for controlling hypertension is the diet.

The focus was then narrowed to the two aspects of the diet: the decreases in fat and in salt. The patients were all given 5 g per day of sodium chloride to take with their meals. During the 2-week period both systolic and diastolic pressures rose. Figure 20-7 shows that the rises were caused primarily by the responses of three very salt-sensitive individuals. For a majority of the patients (10 of 13), adding salt back to the diet had no significant effect on blood pressure over the 2-week period. These results suggest that fat or some aspect of the diet other than NaCl may be playing a major role in the hypertension seen in this country.

Others, including Dintenfass,[16] have also implicated fat as a major factor in the etiology of hypertension. According to Dintenfass, fat in the diet increases blood viscosity and red blood cell aggregation, which leads to hypertension. This same concept was espoused by Pritikin and McGrady.[36] In a study conducted by Dintenfass[17] on blood samples obtained from patients attending the Longevity Center, he was able to demonstrate a reduction in viscosity factors, as can be seen in Table 20-12. Viscosity was measured at a high shear rate, and both whole blood and plasma viscosities were significantly reduced. In addition, there was a significant reduction in red blood cell aggregation, which would result in less sludging in the microcirculation. In a subsequent study[5] whole blood and plasma viscosities were measured at very low shear rates, and again viscosity reductions in patients attending the Longevity Center were found.

Another mechanism by which fat in the diet may play an important role in hypertension is through the production of thromboxane, a powerful vasoconstrictor. Tremoli and co-workers[41] reported a reduction in thromboxane formation in isolated blood platelets when total fat in the diet was reduced by 40% and the ratio of polyunsaturated to saturated fat was increased in men but not women. Similar results were found in platelet aggregation studies using male participants at the Center.[11] Thromboxane formation during platelet aggregation in the presence of 6.6 μM ADP was reduced from 3373 ± 842 to 2366 ± 320 pg/ml/5 min. During aggregation in the presence of 100 μg/ml collagen, thromboxane formation was reduced from 3237 ± 662 to 1883 ± 418 pg/ml/5 min. If these same effects occur in vivo, they could be important in the control of hypertension.

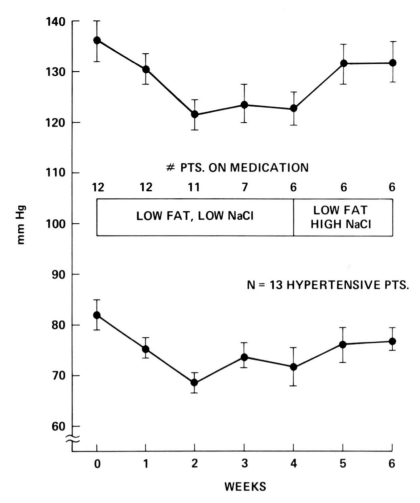

Figure 20-6. Blood pressure responses of 13 hypertensive patients. During first 4 weeks, patients were following Pritikin diet without any other change in life-style. During last 2 weeks, they supplemented Pritikin diet with 5 g NaCl per day. (From Barnard, RJ, et al: J Cardiac Rehabil 3:839, 1983.)

Table 20-12. Effects of the Pritikin program on blood viscosity factors (in 38 patients)*

	Levels before program	Levels after program
Hematocrit (%)	50.1 ± 0.5	46.6 ± 0.6
Whole blood viscosity (mPa.S)	5.52 ± 0.11	5.04 ± 0.12
Plasma viscosity (mPa.S)	1.29 ± 0.01	1.25 ± 0.01
Red cell aggregation (mm/hr)	208 ± 188 a	104 ± 125

Data from Dintenfass, L: Med J Aust 1:543, 1982.

*All after values were significantly less than before values; $p < .05$.

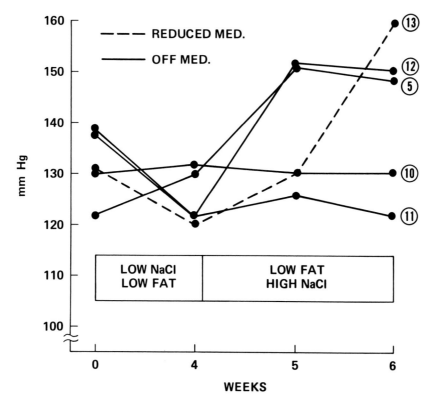

Figure 20-7. Response of five hypertensive patients to addition of NaCl to Pritikin diet. Ten patients in study had responses similar to patients 10 and 11, whereas three patients (5, 12, and 13) were salt sensitive. *MED.*, Medication. (From Barnard, RJ, et al: J Cardiac Rehabil 3:839, 1983.)

RESPONSE OF PATIENTS WITH DIABETES MELLITUS

There are an estimated 10 million diabetic patients in the United States, and a similar number whose disease remains undiagnosed. The incidence of diabetes is increasing at a rate of almost 6% every year, which will result in a doubling of the diabetic population in the next 15 years. The majority of these patients (more than 80%) have non-insulin-dependent diabetes mellitus (NIDDM), which is generally an adult-onset disease.[14] Diabetes is a well-recognized risk factor for the development of both coronary and peripheral vascular atherosclerosis. In fact, the most common cause of death in patients with diabetes mellitus is myocardial infarction.

Short-term response

Data from 60 NIDDM patients attending the Pritikin Longevity Center were analyzed.[7] Forty of these patients were initially taking medication to control their hyperglycemia. Serum lipid and blood glucose levels were significantly reduced, as can be seen in Figure 20-8. The fasting glucose level was reduced from 195 to 145 mg/dl for the total group. In addition, most of these patients were able to discontinue medication. Figure 20-9 shows that 21 of 23 patients discontinued oral hypoglycemic agents, and in these patients fasting glucose level was reduced from 192 to 156 mg/dl. Of the 17 patients initially receiving insulin injections, 13 discontinued the injections, and fasting glucose for the group fell from 211 to 148 mg/dl (Figure 20-10). The average weight loss for the total group was 4.3 kg. However, the decrease in fasting glucose level was not correlated with weight loss, increase in walking time, or increase in MET capacity. The fact that weight loss was not correlated with the improvement in fasting glucose level is not surprising, since seven patients had minimal weight loss but significant reductions in fasting glucose. These observations agree with the data of Anderson and Ward,[2] who placed 20 NIDDM patients on an isocaloric, high–complex carbohydrate, high-fiber diet. Without any significant weight change, the 20 patients reduced their insulin medication from 32 to 3 units/day in 18 days, and fasting glucose fell from 165 to 151 mg/dl.

These data indicate that a high–complex carbohydrate, high-fiber, low-fat diet combined with daily walking can control hyperglycemia and eliminate the need for medication in most NIDDM patients at least for the short term. Diet

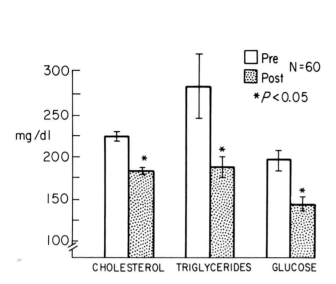

Figure 20-8. Fasting serum lipid and glucose changes in 60 patients with non-insulin-dependent diabetes mellitus attending Pritikin Longevity Center. (From Barnard, RJ, et al: Diabetes Care 5:370, 1982.)

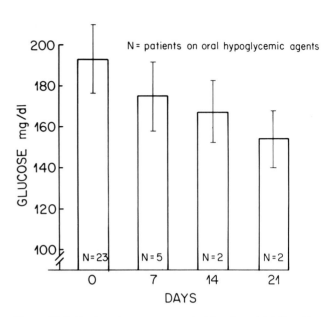

Figure 20-9. Fasting glucose response in 23 patients initially taking oral hypoglycemic agents on entry into Pritikin program. (From Barnard, RJ, et al: Diabetes Care 5:370, 1982.)

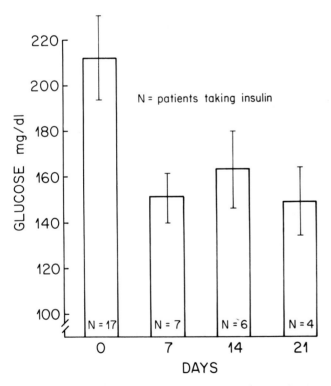

Figure 20-10. Fasting glucose response in 17 patients with non-insulin-dependent diabetes mellitus who were taking insulin when they entered Pritikin program. (From Barnard, RJ, et al: Diabetes Care 5:370, 1982.)

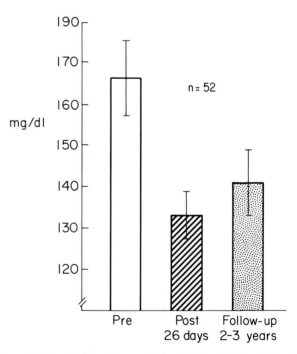

Figure 20-11. Fasting glucose values in 52 patients with non-insulin-dependent diabetes mellitus before *(pre)* and end *(post)* of Pritikin program and 2 to 3 years later. (From Barnard, RJ, et al: Diabetes Care 6:268, 1983.)

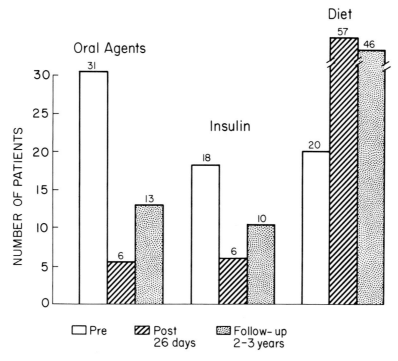

Figure 20-12. Medication status of 69 patients with non-insulin-dependent diabetes mellitus at end *(post)* of Pritikin program and 2 to 3 years later. (From Barnard, RJ, et al: Diabetes Care 6:268, 1983.)

appears to be the most important factor; the results achieved by Anderson and Ward relied not on the use of an intensive walking program but only on dietary modification.[2]

Long-term response

In an attempt to ascertain long-term effects of the Pritikin program for controlling NIDDM, 69 patients were contacted 2 to 3 years after they left the Longevity Center.[10] They were asked numerous questions about their diet, exercise habits, and present health status. They were also asked to have their physicians send recent medical records and a fasting blood sample. The cholesterol and triglyceride values obtained at follow-up were similar to those obtained from the cardiac patients at the 5-year follow-up examination. Although the values had increased over those recorded at the end of the residential program, they were still significantly below the initial values. Figure 20-11 shows the mean fasting glucose values for the 52 patients who provided fasting blood samples; the levels before the program, at the end of the residential program, and 2 to 3 years later were 167, 134, and 142 mg/dl, respectively. The value at the follow-up examination was not statistically different from the value recorded at the end of the program. The medication status of this group of 69 NIDDM patients is shown in Figure 20-12.

In a majority of these patients diabetes was adequately controlled by the Pritikin program, and they were able to discontinue medication. In an attempt to determine why

some patients resumed taking medication, a detailed analysis of food recall data was made. The results indicated no substantial difference in the consumption of dietary fiber or total calories between the seven patients who resumed taking oral medication and those who remained off drugs. The only significant difference was in the percentage of calories derived from fat. Those who continue to follow the Pritikin guidelines for 10% of the calories from fat remained off medication. These data indicate that fat may play a major role in regulating peripheral tissue sensitivity to insulin.

SUMMARY

The studies described in this chapter involved principally patients in their mid- to late fifties. Results from a group of participants 70 years of age and older have also been published.[42] Improvements made in performance capacity and health status in the older individuals were significant but not as great as changes observed in younger patients.

The overall results indicate that the Pritikin intensive dietary and exercise program can lead to significant improvements in performance capacity and the discontinuation of medication in a majority of cases. The limited long-term follow-up data indicate that continued compliance to the program results in effective control of atherosclerotic diseases and the associated risk factors including hyperlipidemia, hypertension, and diabetes.

REFERENCES

1. American Heart Association: Recommendations for the treatment of hyperlipidemia in adults, Arteriosclerosis 4:455A, 1984.
2. Anderson, JW, and Ward, K: High-carbohydrate, high-fiber diets for insulin-treated men with diabetes mellitus, Am J Clin Nutr 32:2312, 1979.
3. Anderson, JW, et al: Mineral and vitamin status on high-fiber diets: long-term studies of diabetic patients, Diabetes Care 3:38, 1980.
4. Barnard, RJ, and Hall, JA: The role of exercise in the detection, treatment and evaluation of patients with peripheral vascular disease. In Franklin, BA, Gordon, S, and Timmis, GG, editors: Exercise in modern medicine: testing and prescription in health and disease, Baltimore, 1987, Williams & Wilkins.
5. Barnard, RJ, Hall, JA, and Pritikin, N: Effects of diet and exercise on blood pressure and viscosity in hypertensive patients, J Cardiac Rehabil 5:185, 1985.
6. Barnard, RJ, et al: Effects of an intensive, short-term exercise and nutrition program on patients with coronary heart disease, J Cardiac Rehabil 1:99, 1981.
7. Barnard, RJ, et al: Response of non-insulin-dependent diabetic patients to an intensive program of diet and exercise, Diabetes Care 5:370, 1982.
8. Barnard, RJ, et al: Effects of a high-complex-carbohydrate diet and daily walking on blood pressure and medication status of hypertensive patients, J Cardiac Rehabil 3:839, 1983.
9. Barnard RJ, et al: Effects of an intensive exercise and nutrition program on patients with coronary artery disease: five-year follow-up, J Cardiac Rehabil 3:183, 1983.
10. Barnard, RJ, et al: Long-term use of a high-complex-carbohydrate, high-fiber, low-fat diet and exercise in the treatment of NIDDM patients, Diabetes Care 6:268, 1983.
11. Barnard, RJ, et al: Effects of a low-fat, low-cholesterol diet on serum lipids, platelet aggregation and thromboxane formation, Prostaglandins Leukotrienes Med 26:241, 1987.
12. Brensike, JF, et al: Effects of therapy with cholestyramine on progression of coronary arteriosclerosis: results of the NHLBI type II coronary intervention study, Circulation 69:313, 1984.
13. Brown, MS, and Goldstein, JL: A receptor-mediated pathway for cholesterol homeostasis, Science 232:34, 1986.
14. Davidson, MB: Diabetes mellitus: diagnosis and treatment, New York, 1986, John Wiley & Sons, Inc.
15. Diehl, H, and Mannerberg, D: Hyptertension, hyperlipidaemia, angina and coronary heart disease. In Trowell, HC, and Burkitt, DP, editors: Western diseases: their emergence and prevention, Cambridge, Mass, 1981, Harvard University Press.
16. Dintenfass, L: Hyperviscosity in hypertension, New York, 1981, Pergamon Press.
17. Dintenfass, L: Effect of low-fat, low-protein diet on blood viscosity, Med J Aust 1:543, 1982.
18. Dodson, P, and Humphreys, D: Hypertension and angina. In Trowell, HC, and Burkitt, DP, editors: Western diseases: their emergence and prevention, Cambridge, Mass, 1981, Harvard University Press.
19. Eichner, ER: Platelets, carotids and coronaries: critique on antiplatelet agents, exercise, and certain diets, Am J Med 77:513, 1984.
20. Entrican, JS, et al: Raised plasma oestrodiol and oestrone levels in young survivors of myocardial infarction, Lancet 2:487, 1978.
21. Gluck, CJ: Role of risk factor management in progression and regression of coronary and femoral artery atherosclerosis, Am J Cardiol 57:35G, 1986.
22. Goodnight, SH, Harris, WS, Jr, and Connor, WE: The effect of W3 fatty acids on platelet composition and function in man: a prospective controlled study, Blood 58:880, 1981.
23. Gordon, T, et al: Lipoproteins, cardiovascular disease, and death: the Framingham study, Arch Intern Med 141:1128, 1981.
24. Hall, JA, and Barnard, RJ: The effects of an intensive 26-day program of diet and exercise on patients with peripheral vascular disease, J Cardiac Rehabil 2:569, 1982.
25. Hall, JA, et al: Effects of diet and exercise on peripheral vascular disease, Physician Sports Med 10:90, 1982.
26. Hjermann, I, et al: Effect of diet and smoking intervention on the incidence of coronary heart disease, Lancet 1:1303, 1981.
27. Hubbard, JD, Inkeles, S, and Barnard, RJ: Nathan Pritikin's heart, N Engl J Med 312:52, 1985.
28. Iacono, JM, and Dougherty, RM: The role of dietary polyunsaturated fatty acids and prostaglandins in reducing blood pressure and improving thrombogenic indices, Prev Med 12:60, 1983.
29. Inkeles, S, and Eisenberg, D: Hyperlipidemia and coronary atherosclerosis: a review, Medicine 60:110, 1981.
30. Lipid Research Clinics Program: The lipid research clinics coronary primary prevention trial results. I. Reduction in incidence of coronary heart disease, JAMA 251:351, 1984.
31. Lorenz, R, et al: Platelet function, thromboxane formation and blood pressure control during supplementation of the western diet with cod liver oil, Circulation 67:504, 1983.
32. Morrison, LM: Diet in coronary atherosclerosis, JAMA 173:884, 1960.
33. O'Brien, LT, et al: Effects of a high-complex-carbohydrate, low-cholesterol diet plus bran supplement on serum lipids, J Appl Nutr 37:26, 1985.
34. Phillips, GB, et al: Association of hyper-estrogenemia and coronary heart disease in men in the Framingham cohort, Am J Med 74:863, 1984.
35. Pritikin, N: The Pritikin promise, New York, 1983, Simon & Schuster, Inc.
36. Pritikin, N, and McGrady, PM, Jr: The Pritikin program for diet and exercise, New York, 1979, Grosset & Dunlap, Inc.
37. Ribeiro, JP, et al: The effectiveness of a low-lipid diet and exercise in the management of coronary artery disease, Am Heart J 108:1183, 1984.
38. Rosenthal, MB, et al: Effects of a high-complex-carbohydrate, low-fat, low-cholesterol diet on levels of serum lipids and estradiol, Am J Med 78:23, 1985.
39. Ross, R: Atherosclerosis: a problem of the biology of arterial wall cells and their interactions with blood components, Arteriosclerosis 1:293, 1981.
40. Simpopulos, AP: Fat intake, obesity, and cancer of the breast and endometrium, Med Oncol Tumor Pharmacother 2:125, 1985.
41. Tremoli, E, et al: North Karelian study: changes in dietary fat reduces thromboxane B2 formation by platelets only in male subjects—preliminary report, Adv Prostaglandins Thromboxane Leukotriene Res 12:203, 1983.
42. Weber, F, Barnard, RJ, and Roy, D: Effects of a high–complex-carbohydrate, low-fat diet and daily exercise on individuals 70 years of age and older, J Gerontol 38:155, 1983.

CHAPTER 21

Cancer rehabilitation

ESIN KAPLAN AND STEPHEN L. GUMPORT

Until recent years patients with the diagnosis of cancer were not considered suitable candidates for rehabilitation, whether the disease was considered cured, controlled, or advanced. The overall outlook was thought to be so poor that such efforts would be a waste of time and money. It was not realized that the very presence of cancer had a profound effect not only on the patient, but also on family, friends, and close contacts. However, the realization has dawned that early death is much more common in such diseases as stroke and heart disease than in malignant disease.

The cancer problem is a staggering one. New major malignancies developed in an estimated 930,000 individuals in the United States in 1986. This large number does not include carcinoma in situ (50,000 cases) nor nonmelanoma skin cancer (more than 400,000 cases).[31]

Figure 21-1 shows the 1986 estimated cancer incidence by site and sex. Note that the breast was the most frequent site in women and the lung in men.

Figure 21-2 shows the 1986 estimated cancer deaths by site and sex. Slightly more women died of lung cancer than of breast cancer. Lung cancer is by far the leading cause of cancer deaths in men.

Figure 21-3 shows the age-adjusted cancer death rates for selected sites in women in the United States from 1930 to 1982. It can be seen that lung cancer is about to overtake

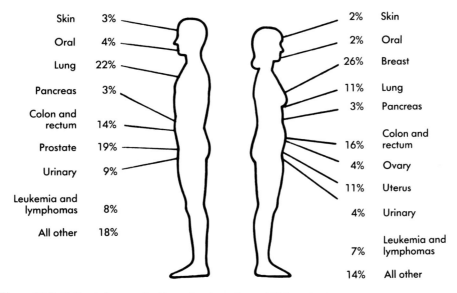

Skin	3%			2%	Skin
Oral	4%			2%	Oral
Lung	22%			26%	Breast
Pancreas	3%			11%	Lung
Colon and rectum	14%			3%	Pancreas
Prostate	19%			16%	Colon and rectum
Urinary	9%			4%	Ovary
Leukemia and lymphomas	8%			11%	Uterus
All other	18%			4%	Urinary
				7%	Leukemia and lymphomas
				14%	All other

Figure 21-1. Estimated cancer incidence by site and sex, 1986, excluding nonmelanoma skin cancer and carcinoma in situ. (From Silverberg, E, and Lubera, J: CA 36:9, 1986.)

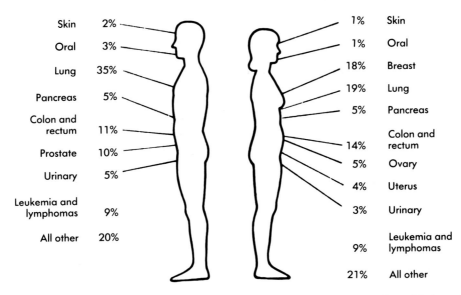

Figure 21-2. Estimated cancer deaths by site and sex, 1986. (From Silverberg, E, and Lubera, J: CA 36:9, 1986.)

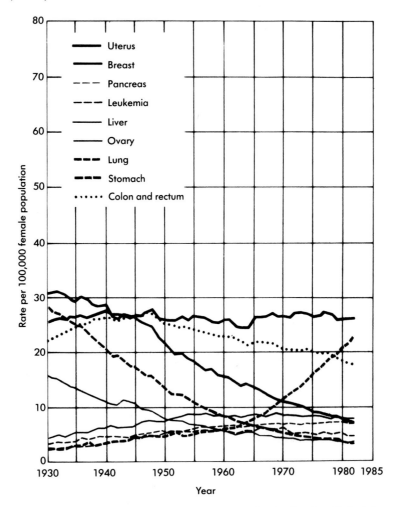

Figure 21-3. Age-adjusted cancer death rates for selected sites in females, United States, 1930-1982. Rates are adjusted to age distribution of 1970 U.S. census population. (Data from U.S. National Center for Health Statistics and U.S. Bureau of the Census. From Silverberg, E, and Lubera, J: Cancer Statistics, 1986, CA 36:9, 1986.)

breast cancer in this group. The rate for uterine cancer has declined, probably related to the routine use of Papanicolaou (Pap) smears.

Figure 21-4 shows the age-adjusted cancer death rates for selected sites in men in the United States from 1930 to 1982. This figure shows how the rate for cancer of the lung began to rise among men about 20 years after World War I ended; at that time smoking had become an accepted and common practice. A similar trend has occurred among women since World War II (Figure 21-3). The rate for cancer of the stomach in both men and women has decreased for reasons still unknown.

Approximately 40% of the 930,000 persons whose major cancers were diagnosed in 1986 will be clinically cured. Of the 60% who are not clinically cured, at least 15% will be alive 15 years from diagnosis. To obtain the best quality of survival possible for very large numbers of individuals, they all should be considered for rehabilitation regardless of the stage of their disease.

Patients who are to undergo a mastectomy or axillary lymph node dissection (or both) should be instructed in arm and shoulder exercises. This is especially true if they have a history of arthritis, bursitis, frozen shoulder, upper extremity weakness, and nerve injuries including congenital brachial plexus involvement.

Instructions in one-handed activities before upper extremity amputations are essential to make these patients independent in daily living activities postoperatively. Partial or non-weight-bearing gait training with an assistive device is important for safety and independence of patients who will undergo extensive lower extremity surgical procedures. Preoperative psychologic counseling is helpful for better understanding of the treatment methods and likely outcome for patients with malignant disease.

Rehabilitation for patients with cancer is not very different from that in other areas of rehabilitation except that the rehabilitation team must be familiar with the various types of tumors and their behavior. Important information about

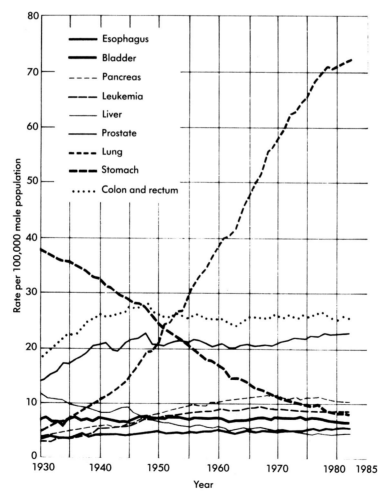

Figure 21-4. Age-adjusted cancer death rates for selected sites in males, United States, 1930-1982. Rates are adjusted to age distribution of 1970 U.S. census population. (Data from U.S. National Center for Health Statistics and U.S. Bureau of the Census. From Silverberg, E, and Lubera, J: CA 36:9, 1986.)

malignancies includes their appearance, their ways of spread, and available methods of treatment, such as surgery, radiation therapy, chemotherapy, hormone treatment, immunotherapy, and laser therapy.[4] Also, a rehabilitation specialist must know the disabilities and complications these treatments can produce, how to avoid them, and how to treat them.

Tissue loss from the tumor and its treatment is not the cancer patient's only problem. Many of the chemotherapeutic treatments result in loss of appetite, loss of a sense of well-being, nausea, vomiting, loss of libido, and partial or complete loss of hair. Fortunately, the hair loss is usually a temporary situation. Among the many other long-term side effects of chemotherapy is sometimes the development of a second and different type of malignancy.

Because these side effects are foreseeable, every effort should be made to lessen the patient's anxiety about them and to reassure the patient concerning their temporary nature (when this is the case). Preparations can be made for some of these problems, such as obtaining a well-made, well-fitted wig before alopecia occurs.

The rehabilitation of a child with cancer is quite different from that of an adult. A child is in the process of physical and psychologic growth and development. The treatments available to treat malignancy, such as surgery, chemotherapy, and radiation therapy, may affect the cancer in a favorable way but produce both short- and long-term ill effects on the child's physical and mental development. These effects may also profoundly trouble the child's family. The aims should be to minimize the negative effects of cancer and its treatment and to integrate the child into the world as an individual who is comfortable and self-confident.

Rehabilitation works best when performed as a team effort. The members of a rehabilitation team may include, among others, a surgical oncologist, medical oncologist, physiatrist, psychiatrist, psychologist, physiotherapist, occupational therapist, social worker, and vocational counselor. A plastic and reconstructive surgeon, speech therapist, stomal therapist, and prosthetist or orthotist should be available for consultation when needed.

Volunteers can be extremely helpful in a cancer rehabilitation program. However, they must be well instructed and supervised. Their tasks should be carefully explained to them and they should be made to feel that they are important members of the team, but they also must understand that they cannot give professional advice. They are particularly useful in directing patients and their families to the appropriate professional members of the cancer rehabilitation team and in making follow-up calls to check on a patient's condition.

A hospital chaplain or the patient's religious advisor may be an important part of the patient's support system. This aspect of assistance should not be neglected. An understanding religious advisor can assist the patient and family in coping with serious problems.

Different problems arise during the treatment of tumors of various areas of the body. This should be kept in mind.

HEAD AND NECK

In treatment of tumors of the head and neck, functional and cosmetic deformities are frequently encountered. They can produce great psychologic trauma and should be corrected or minimized wherever possible. Reconstructive surgeons and prosthetists are helpful.

Unsightly defects from tissue loss can be greatly improved by imaginative plastic surgery. These steps can go far to help the patient cope with the problems produced by cancer.

Prostheses may be made to replace a lost body part. Head and neck prostheses include replacement of facial defects, ears, palatal defects, and even eyes. When well made and carefully fitted, they can be extremely realistic and effective and are a much simpler solution than a surgical procedure would be. They do require replacement from time to time.

Many patients who have been treated for tumors of the head and neck have had neck dissections.[20] These procedures remove the regional cervical lymph nodes that are in the path of the malignancy's lymphatic drainage. The surgery is performed mainly for metastasizing tumors of this region, which include, among others, squamous cell carcinoma and malignant melanoma of the skin, carcinoma of oropharyngeal mucous membranes, and tumors of the salivary glands and thyroid gland. Depending on the type of malignancy and the stage of the disease, the procedures range from simple excision of the primary tumor to a wide and deep resection of soft and bony tissues and to lymph node dissections of varying extent.[16,29]

The rehabilitation specialist must know which structures are at risk and may be injured in these procedures. Among these structures are the facial nerve, the marginal mandibular branch of the facial nerve, the accessory nerve (which innervates the trapezius muscle), the mandible, the eye and its adjoining structures, and the ear. Postoperative rehabilitation programs should include instructions for facial muscle exercises, trials of chewing and swallowing, gentle range-of-motion exercises for the neck, shoulder, and upper trapezius muscle (when this has been approved by the operating surgeon), and speech therapy when required.

The speech therapist plays an important role in the rehabilitation of patients who have had laryngectomies or other extensive head and neck surgery that impairs the ability to speak.

For patients who have had laryngectomies, every effort should be made to restore voice function by mechanical devices, esophageal speech training, or one of the new and quite simple surgical procedures. A high percentage of patients, even those with total laryngectomies, can be taught to use esophageal speech without the need for an external prosthesis. The ability to communicate is of the utmost importance, and specialists in speech therapy should be an integral part of the cancer rehabilitation service.

Unusual problems sometimes arise during reconstructive procedures. Two patients who had partial mandibular resections with bone grafts, which were taken from the iliac crest with attached tensor fascia lata muscle, developed major problems with gait deviation. This was partially corrected by suitable exercises.

BREAST

The treatment of patients with cancer of the breast is in a state of flux. This malignancy is important because of the great number of women in whom it is diagnosed. It is estimated that one white woman in 10 in the United States will have cancer of the breast in her lifetime. This disease is much less common in men; only one man has a malignancy of the breast for every 100 women with the disease.

In the United States 20 years ago, only the Halstead radical mastectomy was considered adequate treatment for a patient with an operable carcinoma of the breast. This required the removal of the entire breast including a wide margin of skin around the tumor site, the resection of the pectoralis major and minor muscles, and a complete axillary lymph node dissection. A skin graft was often required to cover the large residual defect. This radical procedure frequently produces serious functional, cosmetic, and psychologic difficulties.

A number of different types of treatment are available for breast cancer,[14] including the following:
1. Halsted classical radical mastectomy
2. Modified radical mastectomy. This is essentially a total mastectomy and an axillary lymph node dissection. The pectoralis major and minor muscles are not removed, and it is unusual to need a skin graft. Postoperative radiation therapy and chemotherapy may be used depending on whether metastases are found in the axillary lymph nodes.[29]
3. Partial mastectomy. This includes either a partial or a complete axillary lymph node dissection. Postoperative radiation therapy is administered to the remaining breast, and chemotherapy may be given if the axillary lymph nodes are involved.[9,10]
4. Radiation therapy. This may be the sole treatment for breast cancer in selected cases.

All of these treatments are associated with the possibility of lymphedema of the ipsilateral extremity. This may occur in the immediate postoperative period or many years later. This important subject is discussed in detail later in the chapter.

The procedures requiring mastectomy all carry with them the psychologic injury that the loss of a breast inflicts on a woman. Some bear this loss well, but to others it is devastating. Fortunately, breast reconstruction can give an excellent result. It can be done either immediately after mastectomy or as a delayed procedure some time later. In addition, external prostheses are readily available although of varying quality.

Obtaining good function after a mastectomy is important. We suggest a few simple postoperative steps:
1. The patient should leave the operating room with the ipsilateral upper arm abducted 90 degrees from her side and the forearm and hand supported on a pillow.
2. In general, this position is maintained in the early postoperative period except when the patient is up and walking about.
3. On about the second postoperative day the patient is encouraged to use the ipsilateral arm for such tasks as eating, combing her hair, and brushing her teeth.
4. On about the third postoperative day, bedside physical therapy and occupational therapy is begun with instructions in exercises and arm care. The patient is given information and printed literature (see boxes on pp. 290 to 293).

In many hospitals, "Reach to Recovery" members from the American Cancer Society are asked to see the patient postoperatively. These volunteers have all been treated for cancer of the breast and been trained in this work.

Mastectomy procedures frequently leave a residual area of decreased sensation or numbness on the medial aspect of the ipsilateral upper arm. The patient should be informed that this is to be expected and that it decreases with time.

Discomfort or pain in the operated axilla and mastectomy site is not unusual. Occasionally patients even have the sensation of a phantom breast after a mastectomy.[3] These complaints are real and should be treated symptomatically. Use of gentle massage, local desensitization techniques, and transcutaneous electrical nerve stimulation (TENS) may relieve some of the discomfort.

Occasionally a patient has postoperative "winging" of the scapula resulting from trauma to the long thoracic nerve, which innervates the serratus anterior muscle. Specific exercises and the passage of time may improve this problem. Brachial plexus stretch injury also occurs. These conditions can be prevented during surgery by not pulling on the arm and by positioning it carefully on the operating table.

Depending on the degree of involvement, instructions for one-handed activities, careful positioning, splinting of the weak hand, and appropriate exercises are arranged. Sometimes adhesive capsulitis, supraspinatus or biceps tendonitis of the shoulder, or thrombosis and thrombophlebitis of the superficial veins of the upper arm may limit movements and functions.

Patients who have had only axillary dissections performed for such diagnoses as malignant melanoma and squamous cell carcinoma with possible involvement of these nodes are subject to the same sensory and functional changes and lymphedema as mastectomy patients and should be instructed accordingly.[17] Swimming is an excellent exercise for these patients (Figure 21-5).

POST OPERATIVE EXERCISE PROGRAM FOR MASTECTOMY PATIENTS

After a mastectomy it is necessary to begin exercising the shoulder and arm on the affected side(s) to regain strength, mobility, and flexibility of the incisional area.

The following exercises should be done three times a day, beginning first thing in the morning when you feel the most stiff. If pain occurs that radiates down the arm or shoulder blade and is throbbing or shooting in nature, exercise may be continued. This pain is common after surgery and will diminish with time. However, if pain or pulling occurs at the area of incision, stop the exercise. Take several deep breaths for relaxation, and begin again.

Exercise only to the level of your endurance, trying to build up to 10 repetitions of each exercise. Perform each exercise in the order that it is written to progress from simpler to more difficult exercises. Refer to diagrams that follow exercises.

1. Shoulder mobility: Slowly raise shoulders toward ears and then lower them. Roll shoulders gently in and out. (See Figure 1.)
2. Deep breathing: The purpose of this exercise is to promote upper chest wall excursion and ease the feeling of tight skin over the incisional area. Slowly take a deep breath through your nose and exhale through your mouth. As you breathe, place your hand over your upper chest wall, just below your collar bones. Gently roll your shoulders out. You should feel the chest wall expand and relax as you inhale and exhale. (See Figure 2.)
3. Overhead reach: Clasp both hands together, straighten elbows, and slowly lift arms overhead as high as is comfortable. Lower arms slowly. (See Figure 3.)
4. Wall climb (Figure 4)
   a. Stand facing a wall with toes about 12 inches from the wall. Place fingertips against the wall and slowly climb the wall, keeping both arms parallel. If you feel pain at the incisional area, stop at that level; take some deep breaths, and walk your hands back down the wall. Progress to bringing your toes as close to the wall as possible. Climb the wall again.
   b. Now stand sideways so the affected arm is next to the wall. Again, let your fingers slowly climb the wall. The goal of these exercises is to able raise both arms overhead and out to the side without relying on the wall for support.
5. Clasp, reach, and spread: Sit in a straight-back chair and clasp your hands together. Slowly raise clasped hands, moving them toward your forehead. When this becomes comfortable, place clasped hands behind your head with elbows bent. Begin to bring your elbows together in front of you, then spread elbows apart and bring them toward your ears. Lift clasped hands above the head and lower them to the starting position. (See Figure 5.)

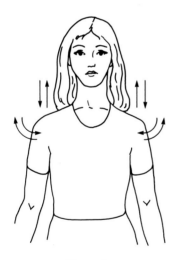

Figure 1

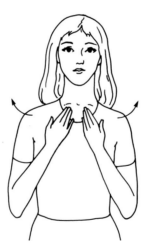

Figure 2

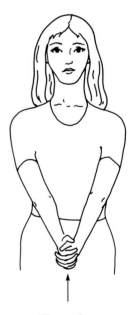

Figure 3

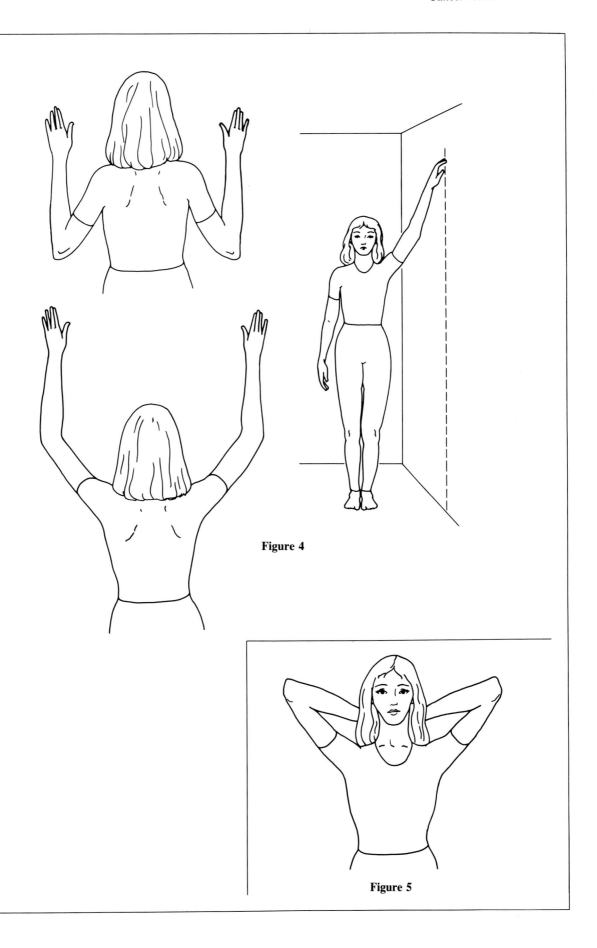

Figure 4

Figure 5

OCCUPATIONAL THERAPY FOR MASTECTOMY PATIENTS

Guidelines of activities for breast cancer patients

This program is to be used only as a guideline to increase the strength and functional use of your arm and hand. The activities listed are *only* suggestions. If an activity is not listed and you have a question about doing it, consider these two points:

1. Is the movement of your arm similar to one of the activities listed, such as raising your arm to shoulder level (90 degrees) or overhead?
2. Is the object lightweight (less than 1 pound), or heavier?

Important factors to consider

1. Use the arm that is normal for you to use in all activities.
2. If the nondominant arm is weaker, remember to include using your arm as an assist in daily activities.
3. Be careful not to substitute your arm movements by using your other hand or by using body motions.
4. Monitor your progress by these three factors:
   a. Pain
   b. Fatigue
   c. Muscle stiffness
   As these three factors decrease, you can increase your activity level.
5. For any activity that you are in doubt of doing, such as sports, please consult your physician.

Activities outline

1. Before discharge from hospital—lightweight activities (less than 1 pound)
   a. Pour liquid into cup.
   b. Apply makeup or shave.
   c. Shake hands.
   d. Pick up phone.
   e. Bathe face, arms, and hands.
   f. Comb hair.
   g. Turn on television.
   h. Turn pages of newspaper.
2. First 2 weeks at home—medium-weight activities (not more than 1 pound)
   a. Brush hair.
   b. Use hair dryer.
   c. Perform light dusting.
   d. Cook.
   e. Reach shelves in market.
   f. Fold laundry.
   g. Carry light clothes to drawers.
   h. Reach arms overhead into sweater.
3. One month at home—medium/heavy activities (not more than 3 pounds)
   a. Hang clothes in closet.
   b. Reach grab handles in bus or subway.
   c. Make bed.
   d. Drive short distances.
   e. Most activities are acceptable now with few exceptions.
4. Two months at home—heavyweight activities (whatever weight is comfortable)
   a. Carry brief case.
   b. Carry purse strap across chest.
   c. Lift child.
   d. Lift shopping bag.
   e. Participate in light sports.
   f. Swimming with OK from physician.

OCCUPATIONAL THERAPY FOR MASTECTOMY PATIENTS—cont'd

Occupational therapy service educational program

After a mastectomy or axillary lymph node dissection, the arm may swell. This is frequently due to the removal of the lymph nodes and the lymph vessels, which makes it more difficult for lymph to return to the rest of the body. Every effort should be made to avoid even trivial injuries, such as cuts, scratches, pinpricks, insect bites, burns, and sunburn, since these can lead to infection and the reduction in the number of remaining lymphatics available to carry fluid back to the rest of the body.

1. Avoid injuries to the arm.
   a. Avoid injections, the taking of blood tests, and the giving of vaccinations in the operated arm.
   b. Do not cut cuticles during a manicure; just push them back gently after a shower or bath.
   c. Wear rubber gloves when using steel wool or other abrasive cleaners.
   d. Wear canvas gloves when gardening or doing other heavy work.
   e. Wear warm gloves in cold weather.
   f. Wear a thimble when sewing to avoid needle pricks.
   g. Avoid harsh detergents that can cause chapped hands.
   h. Use hand cream regularly, especially during winter months.
   i. Use insect repellent to avoid insect bites.
   j. Use an electric razor or depilatory cream to remove hair from under the arms.
2. Avoid constrictions of the arm that may cause swelling.
   a. Blood pressure should not be taken on the affected side but rather on the opposite arm.
   b. Do not wear clothing with elastic or constricting bands; keep sleeves and underclothing straps loose.
   c. Do not wear constricting watches or jewelry.
   d. Do not carry a heavy purse handle over the forearm or carry a heavy shoulder bag.
   e. Avoid carrying heavy objects too long a distance using the affected arm.
   f. Check that bra is not worn too tightly.
3. Avoid burns.
   a. Do not hold cigarettes with the operated arm. Better yet, do not smoke.
   b. Do not reach into the oven with the affected arm; use a padded glove.
   c. Avoid sunburn and use sunscreen. Tan slowly; wear long-sleeved shirt to protect the arm from the sun.
4. Call your physician if you notice a change in your arm.
   a. Sudden swelling, redness, or tenderness
   b. Cuts, burns, bruises, or insect bites that become inflamed and do not heal normally
   c. Any sign of infection in the affected arm
5. Examine your remaining breast and skin over your chest area at monthly intervals. Report any changes to your physician promptly.
6. Keep regular appointments for your medical follow-up examination.

GROIN

When patients have had groin dissections performed because of possibly involved inguinal and iliac lymph nodes,[15] every effort is made to have the patient walk early, usually on the third or fourth postoperative day. A trapeze over the bed can be helpful for bed mobility, particularly for a heavy patient. Lymphedema is an occasional complication of groin dissection. To prevent this, patients are advised not to become overweight, to elevate the lower extremity whenever possible, and not to stand or sit in one position for long periods. For example, when patients go to a theater or take an airplane trip, they should take an aisle seat and get up and move around frequently. Any cellulitis of the extremity should be treated promptly with antibiotics to prevent subsequent lymphedema.

When a skin graft has been placed on the lower extremity, applying a posterior molded-plaster splint to the foot and lower leg helps maintain a neutral position. This prevents the occurrence of an equinus-type deformity from shortening of the Achilles tendon, which can occur quickly and may take many weeks to correct, and also keeps the graft immobile and encourages it to "take."

GASTROINTESTINAL TRACT

The rehabilitation of a cancer patient who has an ostomy opening into the gastrointestinal tract is essentially no different than that of any other patient who has had this procedure done. The exception is that the patient's overall general condition may affect the ability to attend to the care of the ostomy without assistance. It is important that a

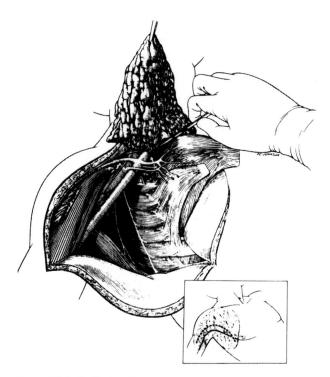

Figure 21-5. Radical axillary lymph node dissection. (From Gumport, SL, Lyall, D, and Zimany, A: Arch Surg 83:227, 1961. Copyright 1961, American Medical Association.)

patient who is going to have such an opening be prepared psychologically beforehand. The patient should be informed as to whether it is temporary or permanent. The site of the stoma should be carefully selected, keeping in mind the patient's occupation and usual physical position during the day. The farther distal from the cecum and the nearer the rectum the colostomy can be placed, the more solid and readily controllable the fecal matter will be without the need for an external appliance, such as a colostomy bag. The regulation of bowel movement by means of diet, daily irrigations, or other methods is another matter for consideration. An enterostomal specialist can teach patients how to handle situations related to the ostomy. The time and effort spent on this instruction is worthwhile, not only for the peace of mind it brings to the patient, but also for the patient's increased ability to cope with the many large and small difficulties in efficiently managing the stoma. The aim should be to make the patient feel as independent and secure as possible. A well-constructed colostomy in the distal colon may require little or no attention from the patient. Once maintenance procedures have been carefully taught, there may be little more difficulty.[5,7]

SOFT TISSUE

Soft tissue malignant tumors include those of connective tissue, blood and lymphatic vessels, smooth and striated muscles, fat, fascia, and synovial structures.[23]

Treatment depends on the lesion's size, extent, and anatomic location. It may range from a simple excision to amputation. A biopsy is important to confirm the diagnosis before definitive surgery. The biopsy should be followed by a metastatic workup. A wide and deep excision should be performed to ensure that wide margins surround the tumor. Cosmetic considerations should be kept in mind when performing these extensive excisions but are secondary. Essential structures should be preserved if possible without jeopardizing the efficacy of the operation in removing the tumor. A tumor that is not completely excised can be expected to reappear, with disastrous results.[6] Some sarcomas, such as fibrosarcomas, spread only by local extension; others, such as osteogenic sarcoma, also spread in this manner but by the bloodstream and lymphatics as well.

Postoperatively, careful long-term follow-up is essential. Periodic chest radiographs should be part of the follow-up monitoring.

The rehabilitation of patients who have had removal of soft tissue tumors depends on the extent of the operative procedure, as well as whether chemotherapy or radiation therapy is required.

Obtaining optimum function and cosmesis requires careful preoperative planning. For example, if a graft is needed on the posterior aspect of the lower leg, it should be kept in mind that a posterior molded splint with the foot in 90 degrees of dorsiflexion is helpful to prevent shortening of the Achilles tendon. This type of deformity can be time consuming to overcome if it is allowed to happen. If the graft is on the upper arm, proper shoulder support and elbow positioning are essential. If the graft is over the forearm, appropriate wrist, hand, and finger positioning is necessary.

Adequate treatment of soft tissue tumors may require removal of a large amount of muscle tissue. Splinting or supporting of major joints might be necessary to permit early resumption of daily living activities and ambulation.

Sometimes the surgical treatment requires the transfer of uninvolved muscle by means of a flap over the defect to improve cosmesis and function. These parts often require retraining of the transferred muscles.

If amputation is going to be done, preoperative consideration should be given to the level of amputation, type of prosthesis, and type of training that will make the postoperative transition easier.

SKELETON

Primary malignant tumors of the skeleton account for less than 1% of all tumors. Their incidence is greatest in children and young adults. The most common primary malignant bone tumors are osteosarcoma, fibrosarcoma, chondrosarcoma, chordoma, Ewing's sarcoma, and multiple myeloma. The last is the most frequently seen and represents approximately 50% of all bone tumors.

Treatment of primary bone tumors may require amputation, although limb-sparing procedures using prostheses are being used more frequently and with good results.[27] Chemotherapy and radiation therapy have increased in importance, and they are considered to be the reasons for the improved prognosis of some tumors, such as Ewing's sarcoma, in recent years. The rehabilitation program depends on the patient's disability, general condition, and motivation.

Metastatic bone tumors are the most common malignancy affecting bones. The common primary sites of these tumors are lung, breast, prostate, kidney, and thyroid gland. The spine, pelvis, and long bones are the most common metastatic sites, but other sites are not uncommon.[8,23,26]

In the spine the vertebral body is the most common site of involvement. Compression of the neural structures is due to direct extension of the tumor or pathologic collapse of bone. The most common early sign of metastatic disease is pain that is usually persistent, dull, not relieved by rest, and often worse at night. Neurologic deficits depend on the level of involvement of the spine, and onset can be gradual or sudden. Diagnosis of bony metastatic disease by routine radiography is possible only if 30% to 35% of the bone is destroyed. A bone scan is a much more sensitive testing method, with 95% to 97% accuracy. Findings on bone scans should be correlated with radiographs.

General management of metastatic disease of the spine includes steroids in high doses, radiation, decompression, and stabilization.[30] Appropriate external support is provided with braces and assistive devices to improve the patient's mobility, safety, and independence.

Metastatic disease of the long bones usually requires open reduction and internal fixation (ORIF). For example, femoral shaft involvement may be treated with intramedullary rod placement. Subtrochanteric and intertrochanteric fractures may require fixation with nail and plate. Femoral head and neck involvement may require hemiarthroplasty.[26] Similar surgical procedures are used for upper extremity long bone involvement. A postoperative rehabilitation program should be arranged depending on the patient's needs and general medical condition. The surgical procedures that have been done previously, as described above, must be considered.

CENTRAL NERVOUS SYSTEM

The most common primary malignant tumors of the central nervous system are gliomas, which represent 45% of intracranial tumors. In the adult population the most common glioma is glioblastoma multiforme, followed by oligodendroglioma, mixed glioma, ependymoma, medulloblastoma, and astrocytoma.

Malignant tumors of the central nervous system do not metastasize to the other organ systems of the body, but they do spread within the central nervous system itself. Ten percent of central nervous system tumors are metastatic from

other parts of the body. The most common site of the primary neoplasm is the lung, which is the source of 65% of metastatic tumors of the central nervous system. Breast, kidney, colon, pancreas, testis, and malignant melanoma are also frequent sites of the primary tumor.

Almost any part of the brain may be involved in a metastatic process. The cerebellum is a common site, but these metastases may involve the central nervous system membranes and scalp as well.

SPINAL CORD

Spinal tumors are classified as epidural, intradural-extramedullary, and intradural-intramedullary. Epidural tumors are most commonly metastatic. Intradural-extramedullary tumors are meningiomas and schwannomas, which are benign in nature. Intradural-intramedullary tumors are ependymomas, astrocytomas, and hemangioblastomas, which are malignant.[23]

Neurologic deficits depend on the location and extent of the tumor and surgery involved. The rehabilitation program is arranged according to the patient's individual needs. Detailed rehabilitation programs for central nervous system involvement are covered elsewhere in the text in sections on brain injury, stroke, and spinal cord lesions.

COMPLICATIONS IN CANCER REHABILITATION
Lymphedema

Lymphedema of an extremity is no trivial matter. Although it causes serious problems in less than 10% of the patients, it can be distressing and disabling. Prevention is more effective than treatment. Lymphedema not only can be progressive, but also can lead to the development of a usually fatal malignancy known as lymphangiosarcoma (Treve's disease).[2,33,34]

The mechanism of lymphedema is essentially the same regardless of the cause. Predisposing factors are lymphatic obstruction owing to the excision or destruction of the lymphatics, or venous obstruction owing to phlebitis with previous lymphangitis. Lymphedema develops when the lymph flow from the extremity is blocked and hydrostatic pressure increases. The protein content of lymph and the proliferation of fibroblasts in the tissue also increase. Lymph is an excellent medium for the growth of bacteria. Infection and cellulitis may lead to thrombosis of the lymph vessels and further blocking of the lymphatics. Increased stasis of the lymph occurs as the fibrosis progresses and the connective tissue proliferates. In summary, edema leads to infections, fibrosis, and on rare occasions sarcoma.[18,32]

The onset of lymphedema may be acute or insidious. Acute lymphedema may occur in a transient, mild form that appears in the immediate postoperative area and usually subsides rapidly, spontaneously, and completely. Another acute form is a painful lymphedema that may be erysipeloid and results in chronic edema of the extremity. This form can occur anytime, even years after the original operation or administration of radiation therapy. Insidious lymphedema may be painless and accompanied by persistent edema. It too can occur weeks and even years after the operation.[19]

Postsurgical lymphedema may occur after simple and radical mastectomies, axillary lymph node dissections, and radical groin dissections. The predisposing factors include obesity, trauma, infection, sunburn, and radiation therapy.

The prevention of lymphedema includes particularly the avoidance of obesity and minimizing any trauma, infection, and sunburn to the part. This prevention should begin at the time of surgery, and care should include elevation of the part, diuretics, weight loss, and exercises of gentle, active, and isometric types. Elastic compression bandages, intermittent pressure, pneumatic devices, and antibiotics are also used.[22,24]

Operative procedures are available for the treatment of lymphedema, but they are used infrequently. They include a lymphangioplasty described by Handley,[13] the building of a pedicle flap to bridge the obstruction to lymphatic flow, the excision of lymphedematous tissue, omental transposition as described by Goldsmith,[12] and, more recently, anastomosis of lymphatics to venous system or proximal lymphatics. This last procedure appears promising but requires microsurgical techniques.[35]

In conclusion, lymphedema is a difficult problem to handle and is much better prevented than treated. It is not just a cosmetic problem but may be physically disabling and over a long period may predispose the patient to the development of lymphangiosarcoma.

Lymphangiosarcoma

The lymphangiosarcoma that develops on the basis of a preexisting lymphedema is a rare type of malignant tumor that arises from the lymphatic endothelium. The majority of the cases have occurred in association with postmastectomy lymphedema, often in patients who have received radiation therapy. The tumor may occur as single or multiple vesicles or multiple bluish red hemorrhagic nodules on the edematous limb. It spreads progressively both proximally and distally and may rapidly metastasize. Treatment responses are usually brief. Even when amputation is performed, the overall prognosis is poor.[1,21]

Pain

The control of pain in a patient with cancer is important. The pain may be acute, temporary, and postoperative in nature, such as phantom limb syndrome or pain following thoracotomy, mastectomy, or a radical neck dissection. On the other hand, it may be chronic and become all pervasive. Invasion of bone and peripheral nerves by the primary disease process may be responsible. Also, postchemotherapy pain syndrome (such as peripheral neuropathy, aseptic ne-

crosis of the femoral head, and steroid pseudorheumatism), postherpetic neuralgia, and postradiation syndromes (such as radiation fibrosis of brachial and lumbar plexus, radiation myelopathy, radiation-induced second primary tumors, and radiation necrosis of bone) may occur.

Careful thought must be given to the cause of the pain and the selection of the appropriate modalities to relieve it. Therapy depends in great part on the nature of the tumor, the prognosis, how advanced the disease process is, and the treatments that have been used previously.

Many drugs alleviate pain when used properly, and psychotherapeutic and neurosurgical procedures are available as well. Behavioral approaches such as hypnosis, visual imagery, relaxation, biofeedback, and acupuncture have been used with some success. When medications are used, they should be given before the pain builds to great heights. They should be administered in sufficient dosage and frequency to keep the patient comfortable. Cooperation of the physician, psychologist, neurosurgeon, and nursing staff is needed for this. The most frequent error in treating patients with malignancy is to give the medication in insufficient dosage and too infrequently to control the pain. It is heartless and cruel to allow a patient to suffer needless pain when it can be relieved or lessened.

Depending on the stage of the disease, physical medicine approaches such as physical therapy, splinting, bracing, and application of TENS might be helpful in pain control.[11,25,36]

Paraneoplastic syndrome

Patients with neoplasms may have subtle symptoms with no obvious tumor. Tumors can produce nonmetastatic changes in the metabolism and functions of all body systems. These systemic effects of cancer are called the paraneoplastic syndrome. In 75% of cancer patients at least one of the paraneoplastic syndrome signs occurs during the course of the illness or as a first symptom of occult malignancy. The signs include fatigue, weight loss, anemia, arthritis, acanthosis nigricans, thrombophlebitis, hypercalcemia, myopathies, neuropathies, myasthenic syndrome, nephrotic syndrome, and many other unusual findings.[37]

CONCLUSION

Cancer carries risks to the patient that extend over many years. In addition, the various treatments available for it, such as surgery, radiation therapy, hormone therapy, laser therapy, chemotherapy, and immunotherapy, pose long-term dangers and are associated with their own complications. It is the task of a rehabilitation specialist to make living with these complications and worries tolerable and to help the patient attain a bearable life-style. This can be done if the specialist always remembers that all the physical and psychosocial rehabilitation in the world is of little value unless it is delivered with understanding, sensitivity, and compassion.

ACKNOWLEDGMENT

Acknowledgment is made and appreciation is extended to the Gladys Houx Rusk Fund and the Fan Fox/Leslie R. Samuels Foundation for their support of this work.

REFERENCES

1. Bart, RS, and Kopf, A: Ulcerated tumor developing a lymphedematous leg, J Dermatol Surg 1:18, 1975.
2. Britton, RC, and Nelson, PA: Causes and treatment of post mastectomy lymphedema of the arm, JAMA 180:95, 1962.
3. Christensen, K, et al: Phantom breast syndrome in young women after mastectomy for breast cancer, Acta Chir Scand 148:351, 1982.
4. DeVita, VT, Jr: Principles of chemotherapy. In De Vita, VT, Jr, et al, editors: Cancer, ed 2, vol 1, Philadelphia, 1985, JB Lippincott Co.
5. Dietz, HJ, Jr: Rehabilitation oncology, Toronto, 1981, John Wiley & Sons, Inc.
6. Enzinger, FM, and Weiss, SW: Soft tissue tumors, St. Louis, 1983, CV Mosby Co.
7. Gunn, AE: Cancer rehabilitation, New York, 1984, Raven Press.
8. Errico, TJ, and Kostnick, JP: Diagnosis and treatment of metastatic disease of the spinal column, Contemp Orthop 13:15, 1986.
9. Fisher, B, et al: Five year results of a randomized clinical trial comparing a total mastectomy with or without radiation in the treatment of breast cancer, N Engl J Med 312:665, 1985.
10. Fisher, B, et al: Ten year results of a randomized clinical trial comparing radical mastectomy and total mastectomy with or without radiation, N Engl J Med 312:674, 1985.
11. Foley, KM: The treatment of pain in the patient with cancer, CA 36:194, 1986.
12. Goldsmith, DS, and Beattie: Relief of chronic lymphedema by omental transposition, Ann Surg 166:567, 1967.
13. Handley, WS: Lymphangioplasty: new method for relief of brawny arm of breast-cancer, and for similar conditions of lymphatic oedema, Lancet 1:783, 1908.
14. Harris, J, et al: Cancer of the breast. In DeVita, VT, Jr, editor: Cancer, vol 2, ed 2, Philadelphia, 1985, JB Lippincott Co.
15. Harris, M, et al: Ilio inguinal lymph node dissection for melanoma, Surg Gynecol Obstet 136:33, 1973.
16. Harris, M, et al: Melanoma of the head and neck, Am Surg 182:86, 1975.
17. Harris, MN, and Gumport, SL: Radical axillary dissection. In Malt, RA, editor: Surgical techniques illustrated, Philadelphia, 1985, WB Saunders Co.
18. Kinmouth, JB, and Taylor, GW: The lymphatic circulation in lymphedema, Ann Surg 139:129, 1954.
19. Leis, HP, Jr, Bowers, WF, and Dursi, J: Postmastectomy edema of the arm, NY State J Med 66:618, 1966.
20. MacComb, WS, and Fletcher, GH: Cancer of the head and neck, Baltimore, 1969, Williams & Wilkins.
21. Maddox, J: Angiosarcoma of skin and soft tissue, Cancer 48:1907, 1981.
22. Markowski, J, Wilcox, JP, and Helm, PA: Lymphedema incidence after specific post mastectomy therapy, Arch Phys Med Rehabil 62:449, 1981.
23. Nealon, TF, Jr: Management of the patients with cancer, ed 3, Philadelphia, 1986, WB Saunders Co.
24. Nelson, PA: Recent advances in treatment of lymphedema of extremities, Geriatrics 21:162, 1966.
25. Pain relief in cancer, Clin Oncol 1984.
26. Radiologic contributions to cancer management, AJR 147:305, 1986.
27. Ragnar, J, et al: Function following mega total hip arthroplasty compared with conventional total hip arthroplasty and healthy matched controls, Clin Orthop Rel Res 192:159, 1985.
28. Roses, DF, et al: Selective surgical management of cutaneous melanoma of the head and neck, Ann Surg 182:86, 1975.
29. Roses, DF, et al: Total mastectomy with complete axillary dissection, Ann Surg 194:4, 1980.
30. Roy-Camille, R, et al: Internal fixation of the lumbar spine with pedicle screw plating, Clin Orthop 203:7, 1986.
31. Silverberg, E, and Lubera, J: Cancer statistics, 1986, CA 36:9, 1986.
32. Smedal, MF, and Evans, JA: The cause and treatment of edema of the arm following radical mastectomy, Surg Gynecol Obstet 111:29, 1960.
33. Sordillo, P, et al: Lymphangiosarcoma, Cancer 48:1674, 1981.
34. Stewart and Treves: Lymphangiosarcoma on post mastectomy lymphedema, Cancer 1:64, 1948.
35. Thompson, N: Surgical treatment of advanced post mastectomy lymphedema of the upper limb, Scand J Plast Reconstr Surg 3:54, 1969.
36. Wiernik, PH: Current concepts of the treatment of cancer: recent advances in solid tumor management derived from lessons learned from the treatment of hematologic malignancies, Med Clin North Am 61:945, 1977.
37. Wyngaarden, JB, and Smith, LH, Jr: Textbook of medicine, ed 16, Philadelphia, 1982, WB Saunders Co.

CHAPTER 22

Rehabilitation management of neuromuscular diseases

WILLIAM M. FOWLER, JR., AND JOSEPH GOODGOLD

There has been a change in philosophy during the last decade toward more aggressive rehabilitative management of patients with neuromuscular diseases and acquired and hereditary disorders of the anterior horn cells, peripheral nerves, and muscles. Recently comprehensive and extensive research has attempted to discover specific therapeutic treatments for some of the more rapidly progressive and early terminal diseases, such as Duchenne muscular dystrophy and amyotrophic lateral sclerosis. An incurable disease, it has been realized, is not an untreatable disease.

With the increasing possibility of specific treatment becoming available in the coming decade, most physicians and therapists believe that it is important to preserve maximal physical capacity and thereby maintain useful function as long as possible; optimal function would thus be present when a specific treatment becomes available. As pointed out by Siegel,[204,208] treatment is not necessarily limited to palliation. It should be prospective to inhibit deformity, prolong independent ambulation, and maximize functional capabilities.

This chapter stresses the management of Duchenne muscular dystrophy, especially management of the musculoskeletal findings and complications, since this disease is one of the more rapidly progressive neuromuscular disorders with many severe musculoskeletal and medical complications.

GENERAL PRINCIPLES OF MANAGEMENT

The general principles of management of patients with neuromuscular disease has been the subject of several comprehensive reviews.* For most of these disorders the mul-

---

*References 42, 49, 65, 66, 75, 76, 122, 125, 127, 140, 204, 208, 211, 222, 227, 229, 232.

tidisciplinary approach to comprehensive care is desirable, since the constantly changing physical, psychologic, and medical problems require frequent consultation with representatives of several specialties. The overall management, however, should be assumed by one physician knowledgeable in neuromuscular diseases.

Rehabilitation should consider the patient's entire needs, and attention to the psychosocial, educational, and vocational aspects is as critical as treatment of the physical complications. Early diagnosis is important, and rehabilitation goals should be established as early as possible. Management is usually divided into prospective and expectant care.[125] Prospective care is the medical attention given to all individuals irrespective of their disease and includes such areas as dental hygiene, vaccinations, and education. Regardless of the disease, expectant care can usually be considered as early (or ambulatory), middle (or wheelchair), or late (when the patient is often totally dependent). Specific treatment of the musculoskeletal system is symptomatic and directed toward weakness, contractures, deformity, and functional ability.[125] Major overall goals are early diagnosis, establishment of a rehabilitation plan based on careful evaluation, maintenance of activities of daily living and ambulation as long as possible, anticipation of complications and development of a program of prevention, supportive counseling to patient and family, and assistance for the patient to lead as normal a life as possible.

Specific objectives of early care include genetic counseling and family planning, instruction in and explanation for the procedures that can delay the onset of functional loss, and advice concerning the prevention or minimization of complications. Objectives of middle-stage care are to maintain activities of daily living, prevent spinal deformity, and achieve wheelchair mobility. During the late stage, objectives are primarily limited to symptomatic management of nonmusculoskeletal complications and facilitation of nursing care.

EVALUATION

The first phase in rehabilitation management is evaluation, since treatment based on function and prognosis is required in any goal-oriented program. With this approach, diseases may be classified as rapidly progressive, slowly progressive (or static), and temporary.[125] The goals and objectives of a rehabilitation program depend primarily on the natural history of the disease. The major musculoskeletal complications of most neuromuscular diseases are weakness, limb contractures, and spinal deformities, usually progressive. These result in diminished physical capacity and function, manifested by a decrease or loss of mobility, upper extremity function, and quality of life. The primary medical complication is restrictive lung disease, especially in individuals with rapidly progressive weakness and spinal deformity. In most disabled persons the components of musculoskeletal and metabolic function can be evaluated by both subjective and quantitative measurements. Such measurements are, of course, critical as a reference base for assessment at varying ages and durations of both the disease process and the patient's response to therapy and management.

Criteria for evaluation protocols

Until recently there were few investigations designed to describe the complications of neuromuscular diseases and their natural course. However, comprehensive studies and reviews regarding evaluation are currently available in the areas of general evaluation design criteria[24,25,51,61,63] and specific studies of measurements of strength, muscle endurance and fatigue,* physiologic and metabolic performance,[30,54,92,137,212] range of joint motion and joint contractures,[10,163,174,193,229] functional ability classification and physical performance,[6,7,36,194] and mobility and pathomechanics of gait.[124,200,220]

Pathokinetics

Musculoskeletal management is based on an understanding of the natural evolution of patterns of weakness, contractures, and deformity. A knowledge of pathokinetics is essential to the proper timing of therapy, bracing, and surgery so measures can be appropriately staged to ensure full use of available strength and function.[204,208]

Ambulatory phase

In patients with anterior horn cell or peripheral nerve disease, weakness is usually distal or generalized. Contractures and deformity, less frequent than in myopathies, are also usually limited to the feet and hands. In the mus-

cle diseases, especially in Duchenne dystrophy, weakness first occurs and is most severe in the musculature of the limb girdles.[68] The most severe contractures occur in muscles that span two joints and in those having a postural function. A detailed chronology of contracture development, incidence and frequency, and relationship to the dominant side of the body has been reported by several investigators.[10,52,174,229]

The rather specific but complex biomechanical sequence leading to the typical posture of lumbar lordosis, hip abduction and flexion, knee flexion, ankle equinus, and calcaneovalgocavus of the feet has been described in detail.[124,200,220] Pes planus secondary to tightness of the plantar flexors is often the first deformity to appear, along with weakness of the hip girdle muscles. As axial and proximal muscles weaken further, it becomes increasingly difficult to maintain torsopelvic alignment by maintaining the line of gravity behind the hips and anterior to the knees. As the knee extensors continue to weaken at the same time that contractures advance in the hip flexors, the triceps surae, and especially the tensor fasciae latae, the support base decreases. In attempting to maintain balance, the patient walks with a wide-based gait characterized by equinus, heel varus, and hip flexion and abduction. Lumbar lordosis increases, and loss of strength in the shoulder depressors leads to instability in torso balance. Increases in abdominal and lumbar extensor weakness result in an inefficient stance and gait. Finally, wasting of the foot musculature produces an equinovarus deformity that prevents the upright posture.

Postambulatory phase

At some point in time, despite even aggressive management, most paralytic patients cease ambulation and a new set of complications arises, especially those associated with an unstable spine in a patient sitting upright for prolonged periods in a wheelchair. Scoliosis is one of the most serious complications of paralytic patients, especially those with rapidly progressive weakness.

Spinal curvature occurs with advancing disability, and its progress is related to the severity of the disease. Studies indicate that paralytic scoliosis is initiated by an increasing kyphotic sitting posture, and that the kyphosis is secondary to the weakening erector spinal muscles.[81,237] The major effect of the kyphosis is to unlock the lumbar posterior facets that normally help to stabilize the spine in the lateral direction. In a kyphotic posture the lumbar spine with its weakened supporting muscles becomes an unstable vertical column that becomes deformed by lateral displacement of the rigid vertebral bodies and that rotates axially by bending and shear deformation of the intervertebral discs. As deformation increases, the eccentricity of the vertical load on the lumbar spine increases. Since this is a relationship between applied movement and axial rotation, even small axial rotations produce failure in a lumbar disc. Relatively small deformations are quite capable of producing irreversible

---

*References 7, 25, 53, 54, 68, 87, 110, 147, 194, 212, 225, 236, 243.

strains that make corrective bracing futile in the late stages of the disease.

Analysis of spinal biomechanics suggests that the evolution of scoliosis in Duchenne muscular dystrophy may follow two paths.[237] Patients with hyperextended spines and rigid paraspinal contracture show comparatively little lateral curvature; those whose spines remain slightly lordotic show modest or late development of scoliosis. Patients with a kyphotic posture almost always have progressive and severe deformity. Although it has been reported that the convexity of the curve is usually toward the dominant hand,[128] a recent study was unable to confirm this observation.[67]

MANAGEMENT OF MUSCULOSKELETAL COMPLICATIONS

A management classification based on function and prognosis is desirable since treatment is goal oriented. Hence, diseases may be classified as rapidly progressive, slowly progressive, static, or temporary.[125]

In rapidly progressive diseases, such as Duchenne dystrophy or amyotrophic lateral sclerosis, the patient's overall objectives are to maintain independent ambulation and to be able to perform normal activities of daily living for as long a time as possible. Methods for achieving these objectives include maintenance of maximal muscle strength within the limitations imposed by the disease process and prevention or slowing of complications, such as disuse atrophy and the development of contractures around the weight-bearing joints.[51,65,229]

In nonprogressive or very slowly progressive disorders—such as some of the congenital myopathies, facioscapulohumeral dystrophy, Charcot-Marie-Tooth syndrome, and some of the spinal muscular atrophies—the objectives are maintenance of strength and function and prevention of contractures. The objectives in diseases such as polymyositis are symptomatic treatment, relief of tenderness, prevention of contractures, and facilitation of return to function during the convalescent phase.

Implementation of these objectives is carried out by use of the various therapeutic modalities, bracing, assistive devices, and surgery. The major therapeutic modalities are stretching and exercise. Orthotic and assistive devices include braces and mechanical aids for the extremities and back, mobility equipment such as wheelchairs, and home use assist devices such as walkers.

Treatment intervenes at various points in the natural evolution of the disease to maintain function, especially ambulation, for as long as possible. Muscle weakness, imbalance, and contractures concurrently contribute to deformity.

The objectives of all modalities are to reduce pain, prevent or reduce the development of contractures, increase strength, and maintain function for as long as possible. Bracing or splinting is indicated for rest or support of weakened muscles, prevention of contractures, joint stability, body alignment, and functional improvement. Assistive devices are used to maintain mobility and the activities of daily living.

Weakness and role of exercise

Since weakness is the predominant finding in neuromuscular diseases, most studies have dealt primarily with evaluations of strength, muscle endurance, and fatigue—usually in individuals with Duchenne dystrophy. Manual muscle tests measuring maximal static voluntary force have usually been used.* However, there has been increasing use of mechanical devices, such as cable tensiometers or muscle dynamometers, to obtain quantitative measurements of strength: static isometric force,† dynamic isokinetic force,[3,87] fatigue and endurance,[3,53,54,87,147] and mechanical and contractile muscle properties.[224,225]

Reliability of the various types of strength measurements used and comparisons between manual muscle testing and quantitative measurements have also been reported. Both manual muscle testing and quantitative measurements of strength have high intraobserver and interobserver reliability.[61,68,236] However, although manual muscle tests may adequately provide a rough profile of the natural course of weakness progression in some diseases, it is doubtful that nonquantitative measurements are sufficiently sensitive to permit a valid assessment of the results of therapeutic interventions, especially in patients with mild weakness or minimal changes in strength. For example, both quantitative static and dynamic force testing of individuals with neuromuscular diseases have shown that widely variant quantitative muscle strength values occur in persons who were graded normal or near normal by manual muscle testing,[3,87] children given manual muscle test grades of normal have demonstrated a 50% mean deficit by quantitative strength tests,[13] and in patients who exhibited the most clinical improvement, manual muscle test grades remained at relatively normal values.[87] In patients who had weakness clearly detectable by manual muscle tests and whose course was rapidly deteriorating, quantitative testing apparently did not add clinically significant information.[87]

In addition, manual muscle testing does not measure muscle endurance or fatigue, and it is becoming apparent that the measurement of dynamic force and fatigue is just as important as the evaluation of static force. Preliminary data from a current study of individuals with slowly progressive weakness indicate that isokinetic testing yields the most information on the measurement of dynamic functional strength. Moreover, patients subjected to endurance testing demonstrated greater fatigability than age- and sex-matched normal controls, with the exception of individuals with myotonic dystrophy, who showed fatigue resistance.[67]

---

*References 7, 25, 35, 87, 194, 243.
†References 68, 87, 110, 147, 194, 236.

Considered elsewhere in this review are linkage between loss of strength and both loss of ambulation* or contractures†; the relationship of strength measurements to functional evaluations‡ or motor performance tests[6,7,25,194]; the correlation between different muscle groups; and the relationship of strength to weight, height, and age.[68,194]

In general, the results from studies regarding the natural history of weakness in Duchenne dystrophy are quite similar regardless of the methodology employed. The least involved muscles were the foot invertors and plantar flexors, and the most involved muscles were the neck flexors, knee extensors, hip muscles, and external shoulder rotators. The first muscle group to become weak is usually the gluteus maximus.[124] Controversy, however, still exists regarding asymmetric involvement.[68,194] Weakness (60% to 85% of normal strength) was found in children by the age of 5 years. There was a linear decline of strength with age for each individual, but considerable variation in the severity of weakness for the overall group, especially when a 50% loss of strength was reached. This variation occurred by the age of 7 years and appeared to be related to different ages of onset. Boys with early severe weakness had a more rapid rate of decline. Decreases in strength ranged from 5% to 15% per year. The tempo of the progression of weakness was not altered during growth spurts, bracing, or loss of ambulation.[25]

In a current study of 28 boys with Duchenne dystrophy, mean longitudinal manual muscle test scores were found to be related to age in a logarithmic fashion; a 1% increase in age led to a 0.9% decrease in strength. Overall, functional deterioration appeared to begin at the age of 8 years in the lower extremities and 10 years in the upper extremities. The lower extremity's functional deterioration plateaued about 2½ years later; there was a similar pattern in the upper extremities, again with a 2-year time lag between lower and upper extremities.[67]

There have been only a few studies of the natural history of loss of strength in other neuromuscular diseases.[68,87] Although there was predominantly proximal involvement in facioscapulohumeral and limb girdle dystrophy, the differences between proximal and distal weakness were relative, the distal muscles were also severely involved as the disease progressed, and there were considerable interpatient differences in strength. There was also a marked difference in strength between muscle groups—with hand grip, shoulder abductor, and elbow extensor strength remaining remarkably stable in most individuals. Trunk flexion-extension, knee flexion-extension, and elbow flexion showed the greatest decreases in strength, and hip flexion was the most variable. Strength in normal individuals showed an increase between childhood and the ages 15 to 24 years, depending on the muscle groups; then it tended to stabilize. In patients with faocioscapulohumeral and limb girdle dystrophy, strength measurements followed the same pattern but peaked at a lower level, and decreased to a far greater degree (at ages 25 to 34 years) before stabilizing. Individuals with myotonic dystrophy also had severe proximal weakness, but there was greater weakness in the distal muscle groups. In all three types of slowly progressive muscular dystrophy, there were marked fluctuations in the progression of weakness, and some individuals had essentially no change in strength during a 3-year period. Because of wide variation in ages at onset, the distribution of weakness, and the durations of the slowly progressive neuromuscular diseases, evaluation of the natural course of each disorder is extremely difficult.

There have also been several investigations of cardiorespiratory and metabolic function. In young boys with Duchenne dystrophy, exercise performance was limited by reduced cardiorespiratory capacity and peripheral oxygen utilization, with marked differences in response to submaximal and maximal exercise testing.[212] During both maximal and submaximal exercise testing, V_{O_2}, stroke volume, cardiac output, and pulmonary ventilation were lower than in normal controls. In addition, during maximal exercise testing, work rate, endurance, heart rate, and respiratory exchange ratio were also reduced. Even a few minutes of passive exercise testing resulted in an increase in cardiac cost.[56] In a wide variety of various nonprogressive or slowly progressive muscle diseases, significantly reduced maximal work capacities and oxygen consumptions were also found.[30,60,62] Diseases of skeletal muscle apparently produce two major patterns of exercise intolerance.[92,137] In the muscular dystrophies there is a progressive loss of muscle fibers, which results in increasing muscle weakness and reduced V_{O_2} owing to loss of functional muscle mass. In disorders of muscle energy metabolism, muscle bulk and resting strength are preserved, but an imbalance in muscle energy production and utilization during exercise results in exertional muscle pain, cramping, weakness, or fatigue. Dynamic exercise is limited in disorders of oxidative metabolism, and static exercise is impaired by disorders of anaerobic glycolysis. In individuals with anterior horn cell and peripheral nerve diseases, an impairment of cardiovascular and metabolic responses has also been reported, including regional ischemia of muscles.[103,132] The results of these studies should be considered when evaluating the effect of exercise training, especially the differences between maximal and submaximal exercise programs.

There has been considerable controversy for many years regarding the use of exercise, especially maximal strengthening exercise programs, for individuals with neuromuscular diseases. Opposing viewpoints have been reviewed in detail.[64,65,71,229,230] A review of the physical tolerance and exercise performance of humans and animals with neuromuscular disorders is critical in understanding the effects of long-term exercise training. It has shown the need to take several factors into account when evaluating the effect of

---

*References 7, 36, 116, 194, 204, 209.
†References 6, 10, 25, 124, 193, 204, 207, 208, 209, 228, 232.
‡References 6, 7, 25, 68, 138, 139, 243.

any modality: (1) maturation, which also occurs in neuromuscular diseases, (2) the natural course of each disease, especially the rate of progression, which can significantly vary from disorder to disorder, (3) the degree of weakness and thus the extent of muscle fiber degeneration, (4) the type of exercise training (highly repetitive or highly resistive), and (5) the intensity and duration of the exercise period: submaximal (aerobic) or maximal (anaerobic).

A review of exercise training in normal animals and humans is also important in understanding the possible effects of exercise on diseased muscle. In high-repetition, low-resistance exercise training, such as running or swimming, which can be either aerobic (submaximal) or anaerobic (maximal), adaptations occur primarily in the cardiopulmonary system, slow-twitch muscle, and type I muscle fibers. In high-resistive, low-repetitive exercise training, such as maximal strengthening exercise, primarily anaerobic, the adaptations appear to be toward a shift to greater usage of fast-twitch muscle and type II fibers. The type of exercise training might be a significant factor to consider in evaluating the effect of exercise on diseased muscle, since many neuromuscular diseases have specific fiber type abnormalities. In Duchenne dystrophy, for example, there is greater type II fiber involvement.[23]

The possibility that exercise training under certain circumstances might lead to weakness and accelerated muscle fiber degeneration should not be surprising. Even in normal animals[134,143,189] and humans,[74,90,157] relatively mild as well as strenuous exercise, especially eccentric contractions, causes fiber splitting and necrosis as well as fiber hypertrophy.

In animal studies normal mice adapted to swimming stress by increasing their resistance to fatigue, but in two of three investigations dystrophic mice did not.[79,214,238] A strenuous treadmill exercise program in dystrophic mice resulted in both markedly reduced muscle isometric tension values in slow-twitch muscle and increased mortality.[223] A lower-intensity mild program, however, had a slightly beneficial effect on slow-twitch muscle and a slightly deleterious effect on fast-twitch muscle.[67]

In adult dystrophic hamsters, vigorous swimming exercise[108] and weight lifting[112] increased cardiac and skeletal muscle degeneration. Weight lifting did not, however, increase muscle degeneration in young hamsters, and relatively mild but long-duration treadmill exercise did not change the severity of lesions of either the heart or skeletal muscle.[199] Furthermore, a training effect was evidenced by increased skeletal muscle respiratory capacity and less severely depressed cardiac contractility, although skeletal muscle myoglobin concentration did not increase.[18,199] Dystrophic chickens had improved muscle performance after repeated righting tests or rotating cage exercise.[11,169]

Decreases in strength associated with increased muscle activity following recovery of strength (after an initial severe loss of strength) were clearly documented in poliomyelitic

patients many years ago.[14,48,109,185,186] This overwork weakness is probably caused by degeneration of the muscle fibers. This is also a possible mechanism for the recently described syndrome of late-onset postpoliomyelitis muscular atrophy.[59,93] About 30 years after the acute episode of the disease these individuals experienced significant reduction in strength in muscles that were previously capable of reduced but adequate function. Overwork weakness has also been reported in partially denervated and reinnervated rat muscle,[101,133] and in humans with peripheral nerve lesions[102] and amyotrophic lateral sclerosis.[122,136,211]

The possibility of overwork weakness in muscle diseases was first suggested by histologic studies of an individual with Duchenne dystrophy in whom muscles assuming the greatest degree of sustained physical activity had the most degeneration.[17] These were predominantly proximal muscles. As pointed out by Edwards and co-workers,[55] because of their postural antigravity role, potentially damaging eccentric activity occurs more often in proximal than in distal muscles. Clinical anecdotal follow-up reports of asymmetric weakness observed in several members of a family with facioscapulohumeral dystrophy suggested that even the usual daily occupations might accelerate the progression of muscle weakness.[126] Muscle-derived enzymes, an indirect indication of muscle tissue breakdown, were found to be reduced after bed rest—and elevated to a greater degree after a vigorous strengthening exercise program in dystrophic patients than in normal controls.[73,154] A mild exercise program failed to result in significant enzyme increases.[70]

Most human studies have dealt with Duchenne dystrophy, and the results are difficult to interpret. Subjective measurements were usually used, there were rarely any controls, and normal growth patterns or the natural course of the disease was usually ignored. Different periods and types of exercise (including home exercise programs, which are limited by patient compliance and documentation of the exercise actually received) were usually used. One report indicated a loss of strength,[105] whereas other reports suggested either maintained strength[41,72,192,240] or modest gains in strength.[1,233]

In our opinion only three studies are worthy of consideration, and even these are subject to different interpretations. One study took age, progression, severity, and preexercise status into account but primarily used manual muscle tests to measure strength.[233] Exercised patients showed slight increases in strength, whereas nonexercised patients had decreased strength. Scott and co-workers,[192] using objective measurements of strength, also considered age, progression, severity, and preexercise status in a study of young Duchenne patients. Since muscle strength deteriorated in the exercised patients and there was no nontreatment group, it is difficult to accept their conclusion that exercise did not cause physical deterioration. The third study[41] avoided use of a nontreated group by using the opposite, nonexercised limb as a control. There was no evidence of any overwork weakness using a submaximal resistive exercise program and objective measurements of strength, but one cannot conclude too much from this because the sample size was very small and had a wide age range.

Other major difficulties in interpretation relate to different periods and types of exercise and the use of home exercise programs. In a 12-month exercise period the greatest gains in strength reportedly occurred in the first 4 months, and only maximal resistive exercise programs were effective.[229,233] The other two studies used 6-month treatment periods.[41,192] One found less-marked deterioration of strength at the end of the program and no difference between resistive and nonresistive exercise programs.[192] Home exercise programs were used in two of the studies.[192,233]

The effect of a submaximal high-repetition aerobic exercise program on patients with various nonprogressive or slowly progressive neuromuscular diseases has also been evaluated.[30,60,62] Cardiovascular training adaptations were not significantly different from those in normal subjects.

In reviewing these studies, five major factors appear to be critical. The first is the degree of weakness at the time the exercise program was started. The second is the rate of the weakness's progression; this was clearly apparent in the animal studies. In dystrophic hamsters, exercise training at an early age did not appear to accelerate the muscle fiber degeneration, and essentially normal fiber hypertrophy occurred in both fast- and slow-twitch muscles. In older hamsters with greater fiber degeneration, weight lifting hastened the fiber degeneration. In dystrophic mice in which the disease is more severe and rapidly progressive than in the dystrophic hamster, exercise training was also more deleterious regardless of type. In chickens, whose performance slightly improved with exercise, the dystrophic process is quite mild and slowly progressive. A maximal resistive exercise program has also been reported to increase strength and muscle work capacity significantly and to reduce the fatigue index in humans with slowly progressive muscular dystrophy even when the muscles were reduced to 20% of normal strength.[147]

A third factor is the type of muscle. In adult dystrophic hamsters the fast-twitch muscle was more severely affected by weight lifting, and in dystrophic mice low-intensity treadmill exercise had a slightly deleterious effect on fast-twitch muscle and a slightly beneficial effect on slow-twitch muscle. The fourth and fifth factors are the type and intensity of the exercise training period. Dystrophic mice subjected to strenuous treadmill exercise had markedly reduced muscle tensions and increased mortality, but a lower-intensity mild program had a slightly beneficial effect. In adult dystrophic hamsters, weight lifting increased cardiac and muscle degeneration, and treadmill exercise did not change the severity of the lesions and increased muscle respiratory capacity and cardiac contractility. In humans with dystrophy, serum enzyme increases produced by exercise were greater during a strengthening exercise program than after single-

bout bicycle exercise, and in other slowly progressive neuromuscular disorders, cardiovascular training adaptations were essentially normal after a high-repetition aerobic exercise program.

It appears that exercise training programs in patients with neuromuscular diseases can be beneficial or at least not result in further muscle fiber degeneration if (1) the exercise program is started early in the course of the disease, (2) it is restricted to individuals with slowly progressive or static disorders, and (3) submaximal resistive or high-repetition aerobic exercise is used. Overwork weakness and further muscle fiber degeneration are, however, a potential danger in patients with rapidly progressive or far-advanced weakness, with maximal high resistive anaerobic exercise, and with eccentric exercise, especially of the proximal muscles.

Electrical stimulation, used for many years on denervated muscle, is a second modality recently advocated for increasing strength. Nix and Vrbova[160] extensively reviewed the structural and functional responses of normal and diseased skeletal muscle to this modality and its effect on increasing strength and resistance to fatigue. In dystrophic animals continuous low-frequency electrical stimulation was shown to reduce or even prevent the degeneration of muscle fibers and increase isometric tension, fatigue resistance, and the percentage of oxidative fibers. Preliminary studies also indicated increased fatigue resistance in humans with dystrophy.

Limb contractures and role of stretching, braces, and surgery

Limb contractures are common in disorders such as Duchenne muscular dystrophy and infantile-onset chronic proximal spinal muscular atrophy but quite rare in other neuromuscular diseases. The presence or absence of contractures in these diseases and the degree of progression are extremely variable, since development of contractures and spinal deformity are directly related to the distribution, duration, and severity of the weakness.[69]

The biomechanical sequence of events leading to limb contractures in Duchenne dystrophy has been extensively described,* as has the natural history of the development of contractures.† Measurements of range of motion were usually obtained with a manual goniometer. With this device, intratester reliability was quite high but intertester reliability showed a wide variation, indicating the need to use the same examiner for longitudinal evaluations.[61,163] In addition, reliability was not the same for all joints and was better for upper extremity movements.[163]

Contractures develop because of a number of mutually reinforcing factors and result in fixed joint deformities. These factors are (1) muscle imbalance caused by the specific pattern of developing weakness, which shows greater

---

*References 124, 204, 207, 208, 220, 229.
†References 7, 10, 25, 174, 193, 195.

early involvement of the extensor muscles than of the flexor muscles; (2) chronic postural adjustments secondary to the attempt to maintain standing and associated with compensatory substitution patterns; and (3) habitual positioning of the knee and hip joints in a flexed position during nonambulation.[229]

The linkage between contractures and loss of strength, dominance, functional level, and loss of ambulation has been described for boys with Duchenne dystrophy in several studies.* In both lower and upper extremities, there is a high correlation between joint contractures and the strength of the antagonist muscles, and when contractures are correlated with hip and leg function, there is a worsening with decreasing ambulation. An unstable standing posture associated with secondary flexion contractures at the knees and hips and plantar flexion contractures accelerates the loss of walking ability. Few boys developed hip or knee contractures while still ambulant. The development of contractures was delayed if they continued to walk with the aid of braces, and there was a linear relationship between the loss of ankle dorsiflexion and functional level. With few exceptions, walking ends with equinovarus deformity and a combined knee and hip antigravity extension lag greater than 90 degrees, since the line of gravity can no longer be maintained.

In the upper extremities, contractures occur relatively late in the course of the disease, at about 8 years of age. Interference with arm and hand function is less than the problems associated with lower extremity contractures. The sequence of contracture development first involves the pronators, then the elbow flexors, and finally the wrist and finger flexors. In the lower extremities at about 6 years of age, the first muscle to become tight, causing alteration in body mechanics, is the tensor fascia lata and the iliotibial tract. This is rapidly followed by contractures of the hip extensors and tightness of the calf muscles. When the patient is about 8 years of age, contractures of the iliotibial bands and plantar flexors become worse, and the associated knee flexion and hip flexion contractures develop as the child spends less time on his feet. The rate of progression of the contractures starts to accelerate at about 9 years of age. As seen with measurements of strength, patients of the same age differ widely in the severity of their contractures. The dominant, more active side of the body often shows a decreased amount of contracture.

The objectives of contracture management have been described in detail.[50,208,227] Vignos recently reviewed studies of the efficacy of stretching, bracing, and surgery.[229] Early in the course of the disease, contracted muscles should be stretched and weak muscles strengthened. Maintenance of body alignment is critical, and preventing contractures is vital to continued ambulation. Standing, especially alternate standing and walking, remain the best functional stretching

activities, and patients should be encouraged to be upright as much as possible. Positioning to promote stretching—for example, having the patient lie prone—is desirable. Areas to be stressed are the tensor fasciae latae, plantar flexors, knee and hip flexors, and elbow and hand flexors.

Although contractures cannot be prevented in diseases such as Duchenne dystrophy, it is generally agreed that positioning and stretching can retard the development of contractures occurring secondary to gravity and compensatory postural habitus.[10,96,127] Although splints or braces are often poorly accepted by patients, especially children, early and persistent splinting has been shown to retard the development of contractures and enhance the ability to walk.[193,195]

Therapeutic heat is often used in conjunction with stretching, as well as for the relief of pain and tenderness in diseases such as polymyositis and poliomyelitis. Some clinicians advocate using heat in conjunction with vasodilatory drugs in muscular dystrophy, apparently because early studies showed that blood flow was reduced in dystrophy.[44,45] However, tissue clearance studies have shown that blood flow and capillary diffusion capacity are normal in the dystrophies.[164] Moreover, heat increases tissue oxygen consumption, vascular permeability, and blood flow and depresses the tension output of skeletal muscle. Since there is already increased vascular permeability and reduced tension output in dystrophic muscle, the possible gains brought about by increased circulation would probably be outweighed by the disadvantages of edema and reduced contractile tension.

Passive stretching has been the principal method used for combating contractures. Despite the advocacy of such stretching by many authorities, there is little agreement on its efficacy. Part of the problem is that there have only been two reports in which stretching alone was used, and in both studies the results were rather vague. In the study by Scott and co-workers,[193] boys with Duchenne dystrophy were divided into three compliance groups after a 3-year program of home stretching exercises and below-knee night splints. Stretching alone (in those with good compliance with the stretching program but who did not wear splints) did not appear to have a significant effect. In earlier reports, children with Duchenne dystrophy who were instructed in a home program of passive stretching were divided into two groups: good and poor care.[10,227] In the good-care group the development of contractures at the ankle and knee only progressed by 12 degrees in 7 years, as compared with an increase of 110 degrees in the poor-care group.

Other studies, including the comparison group in the report by Scott and co-workers,[193] used both a stretching exercise program and splints, braces, or surgery. Four reports indicated a reduction in the progression of the contractures and/or a prolonged period of ambulation,[1,96,193,195] and one study showed only slight improvement in reducing contractures.[105] In these studies and in those on the efficacy of strengthening exercises, population samples were small,

---

*References 7, 25, 52, 124, 193, 204, 207, 208, 229.

there were no control subjects for comparison, and therapy sessions were usually not supervised or documented.

Spinal deformity and role of bracing and surgery

Scoliosis is the most serious complication in persons with rapidly progressive weakness. In addition to marked deformity, scoliosis leads to restrictive lung disease. Even without spinal deformity, severe and progressive restrictive lung disease occurs in many neuromuscular disorders. The two complications occur relatively early and reduce physical capacity and quality of life. In the advanced stages of these diseases, pulmonary complications secondary to the restrictive lung disease contribute significantly to death.

Scoliosis frequently occurs in diseases such as Duchenne dystrophy and infantile-onset proximal spinal muscular atrophy but is an unusual complication in most slowly progressive muscle diseases. As with limb contractures, the presence of scoliosis in these disorders and the degree of progression are variable, depending on the distribution, duration, severity and rate of progression of the weakness. For example, the incidence of scoliosis has been reported to be low in persons with juvenile- and adult-onset chronic proximal spinal muscular atrophy, but as high as 70% in those with the infantile-onset form.[156,175,191] Preliminary data from a current longitudinal study indicates that only 16% of patients with Becker, facioscapulohumeral, and limb-girdle dystrophies and Charcot-Marie-Tooth syndrome had significant scoliosis; 55% of the patients with chronic spinal muscular atrophy had spinal deformity.[67]

Although most reviews state that children with Duchenne dystrophy develop scoliosis rapidly after they can no longer ambulate, a review of published studies indicates considerable variability, caused at least in part by retrospective selection for spinal deformity and dissimilar age groups. Reports in which cases appeared to be selected for spinal deformity implied an incidence of 92% to 100% scoliosis.[114,128,135,198,237] In two studies of 44 nonambulatory patients, the average percentage of those having scoliosis was 66%,[28,115] and in three reports of 108 ambulatory and nonambulatory cases the incidence of scoliosis was only 46%.[94,165,181] In studies in which the patients were still ambulatory, the incidence of scoliosis ranged from 23% to 72%.[94,165,188] Reports of the progression rate of nontreated spinal deformity in Duchenne dystrophy varied from 10 to 18 degrees per year.[81,114,198]

In a current study, clinically diagnosed scoliosis was found in 58% of 109 individuals with Duchenne dystrophy.[67] In patients under the age of 10 scoliosis was relatively rare, with an increasing occurrence between 10 and 13 years of age. After the age of 14 the incidence remained relatively stable. The relationship between the onset of scoliosis and ambulatory status was clearly defined. The patients' average age during onset of wheelchair dependence was 10 years, and 71% of those with spinal deformity developed it after becoming wheelchair dependent. Scoliosis was first noted

3½ years after discontinuing ambulation. Only 9.5% were still walking at the time scoliosis was first noted, with an onset 2 years before the loss of ambulation. During the same periods, at an average age of 13 years, 19% stopped walking and developed scoliosis. In 44 of the 109 patients followed for 3 or more years, there was no correlation between scoliosis and obesity or hand dominance. Depending on pelvic obliquity, the progression of the spinal deformity ranged from 3.8 to 5.5 degrees per year.

The pathokinetics and natural history of spine curvature has been the subject of several reviews.* Most clinicians attribute the development of scoliosis in neuromuscular diseases with symmetric weakness to "gravity collapse" secondary to extreme and progressive weakness of the trunk muscles. Some studies, however, indicate that the incidence of scoliosis may not be related to the duration or degree of clinical weakness[165,188] and that side, type, or site of the curvature is not necessarily related to the distribution or degree of trunk muscle weakness. Some persons develop scoliosis very early in the course of the disease, when weakness is still slight. In ambulatory persons with Charcot-Marie-Tooth syndrome, who have predominately distal limb weakness, the incidence of scoliosis has been reported to be as high as 58%.[165]

Why some children with Duchenne dystrophy develop spinal deformity and others do not remains unresolved. A current explanation is that scoliosis in the nonambulatory patient is initiated by an increasing kyphotic sitting posture, and that the kyphosis is secondary to the weakening erector spinal muscles. Children with hyperextended spines and rigid paraspinal muscle contractures show comparatively little lateral curvature. Those whose spines have become fixed in lordosis have modest or late development of scoliosis, whereas patients with a kyphotic posture usually have progressive and severe deformity. This tendency toward kyphosis is assumed to unlock the posterior facets that would normally help stabilize the spine in the lateral direction.[81,181,237] Based on this observation, management systems have been designed to guide the early straight spine toward the later hyperextended pattern by attempting to prevent kyphosis and pelvic obliquity. They have gained widespread acceptance. These systems include total wheelchair spinal-support systems, lumbar pads, and hyperextension braces, all designed to encourage the extended lordotic position of the spine.† More recent studies, however, have shown that wearing hyperextension braces does not prevent scoliosis but may retard its progress for a limited period of time if worn consistently.[37] Moreover, lumbar hyperextension produced by lumbar pads, although increasing lumbar extension, did not provide resistance to lateral flexion in the supine position.[197]

Intervention strategies to prevent or reduce the progres-

---

*References 81, 114, 128, 165, 181, 188, 201, 237.
†References 16, 80, 81, 152, 210, 241.

sion of scoliosis are primarily limited to bracing or surgery. Early management is directed toward keeping the spine extended and the pelvis level. Wheelchairs should have a firm, level pelvic seat with a top cushion. Because an erect spine is necessary for proper sitting balance, many different types of external spinal containment systems* or trunk supports[144,201] have been advocated to retard the rate of scoliotic progression.

In patients with spinal muscular atrophy, Reddick and co-workers[175] reported that spinal bracing slowed the progression of the deformity most of the time. Most other investigators, however, report that bracing failed to retard the curve progression, but that spinal fusion either corrected or arrested the progression of the scoliosis.[9,100,191] With Duchenne dystrophy, wheelchair spinal-support systems were also reported to prevent significant spinal deformity and the rate of progression of the scoliotic curve.[81] The most comprehensive studies to date of the orthotic management of scoliosis in Duchenne dystrophy, however, clearly show that modular seats, spinal jackets, and custom-molded seats were, at best, capable only of delaying the progression of curvatures less than 25 degrees, and that spinal fusion arrested the progression of the curvature.† As with spinal muscular atrophy, neither bracing nor surgery had any significant effect on pulmonary function tests, and thoracolumbar curves were found to be insignificant in the adverse affecting of pulmonary function.[135]

Surgical stabilization of the spine, used successfully for many years in patients with slowly progressive dystrophy[40,201] and other neuromuscular diseases,[100] is therefore the currently accepted management of spinal deformity in children with Duchenne dystrophy.[114,188,219] Here again, timing of treatment and a knowledge of the natural course of the disease is important. Scoliosis is unusual in the ambulatory boy with Duchenne dystrophy. Moreover, attempting to straighten and stabilize the spine of the ambulatory dystrophic child, either surgically or with a brace, can be harmful. These individuals require torso shift for balance, and spinal rigidity can inhibit ambulation. On the other hand, progressive scoliosis in Duchenne dystrophy adversely affects sitting balance, comfort, and quality of life. Orthotic devices unfortunately have the disadvantage of slowing the development of scoliosis until the pulmonary function levels have declined so low that future spinal surgery is risky. By the time the patient is about 14 years of age, the functional vital capacity (FVC) is usually below 50%. Early spinal instrumentation and fusion is therefore indicated if the thoracic curve is greater than 25 degrees at a time when the FVC is usually greater than 50%.[135]

Role of bracing and surgery in enhancing mobility

There are two management periods related to mobility: wheelchair mobility and maintenance of ambulation by bracing and surgery. In Duchenne dystrophy the extreme variability in the loss of ambulation makes it very difficult to evaluate bracing's or surgery's success of maintaining ambulation. In the most comprehensive study to date, all boys were able to walk and climb until the age of 8 years, and the average age of those who became dependent on leg braces was 10.3 years.[25] The loss of ability to stand occurred between 9.8 and 17.1 years, but most patients between 12 and 16 years of age were able to stand in braces at least.

Attempts have been made to predict loss of ambulation by linkage with the degree of weakness* and contractures.† Most authorities appear to agree that walking ends when lower extremity strength is about 50% to 60% of normal levels and equinovarus deformity is present. Recent studies indicate that timed motor performance tests have a high correlation with lower extremity strength and may also be a good predictor of loss of ambulation.[25,36,61,194] In view of the many studies attempting to link multiple variables—such as age, weight, functional level, motor ability, contractures, and strength—with loss of ambulation, it is interesting to note that (1) the strength of the knee extensors is closely associated with overall muscle strength, (2) the addition of the other variables does not statistically enhance this relationship, and (3) loss of independent ambulation usually occurs at a total muscle strength of about 50%.[194]

In the rapidly progressive diseases such as Duchenne dystrophy, there are as many opponents as enthusiastic advocates of combined surgical-orthotic intervention. General management principles, factors determining success, and outcomes with bracing and surgery have been the subject of many reports.‡ The most effective long-leg brace appears to be a lightweight plastic-molded knee-ankle-foot orthosis with ischial seating.[202,207,208,242] Proper timing is usually of prime importance when there is little useful independent walking, although earlier surgical correction has been advocated.[58,184] Suitability depends on adequate hip-girdle strength, especially hip-abductor strength and minimal hip and knee contractures. Before bracing and while the patient is still fully ambulant, an intensive program of regular passive stretching of the hips, knees, and ankles to prevent contractures, and in particular to try to arrest the development of any asymmetry, is recommended. Severe asymmetry, with greater than 20-degree hip and knee contractures affecting one side, is almost always accompanied by early fixed scoliosis and hampers successful rehabilitation.[97] As with spinal deformity, the window of opportunity is very narrow. Operative techniques should permit early mobilization, and lightweight appliances should be used. Interference, surgical or otherwise, with passive stabilization of the hip or the knee should be avoided, since it often results in loss of ambulation.[124,127] Short-leg braces are rarely used

---

*References 16, 50, 80, 81, 152, 210, 227, 241.
†References 114, 135, 180, 196, 198, 221.

*References 7, 35, 116, 194, 204, 207.
†References 7, 25, 124, 193, 204, 207.
‡References 20, 51, 58, 77, 96, 97, 113, 116, 145, 148, 184, 206, 208, 209, 215, 231, 232, 242.

anymore by the ambulatory patient with Duchenne dystrophy, but they may be of value in reducing the rapid progression of foot deformity after ambulation is lost. Lateral sole and heel wedging, outer T-strap, and corrective shoe inserts may be temporarily successful in forestalling equinocavovarus deformity, but surgical correction eventually becomes necessary.[204]

Most studies regarding outcomes from surgery and/or bracing showed that wheelchair dependence could be delayed in boys with Duchenne dystrophy by an average of 2 to 4 years. Reports, however, are difficult to interpret because of the absence of nontreated control groups, smallness of treatment groups, different severities or durations of disease groups, mixing of treatment interventions, or lack of specific criteria for ambulation. In most studies standing time was considered as ambulation, and there was no distinction made between useful ambulation and nonfunctional ambulation. There is no doubt that the upright position can be maintained with braces, and that bracing delays the onset of scoliosis and lower extremity contractures, but the continuation of useful ambulation remains questionable. Advocates of bracing also claim that it seems to benefit the patient and parents psychologically, although there are no studies documenting this. However, surgery and bracing should be offered as an option to patients, especially if continued walking is a major objective. This should be discussed with the parents at an early age, but other management objectives should also be considered.[77] In our experience, a wheelchair gives the child much more practical, independent mobility than does bracing, and most of the children appeared to take to wheelchairs with relief and even enthusiasm.

In the slowly progressive or static disorders, lower extremity bracing may often be of value. Dorsiflexor weakness and foot drop in facioscapulohumeral, myotonic, and limbgirdle dystrophies and Charcot-Marie-Tooth syndrome can usually be managed with plastic ankle-foot orthoses. Longleg bracing can also be useful in some of the spinal muscular atrophies.

Even with lower-extremity bracing, ambulation eventually ceases in the rapidly progressive neuromuscular disorders, and the primary mobility device becomes the wheelchair. General criteria for successful and comfortable wheelchair mobility have been reviewed by several authors.[32,75,80,227] When the decision regarding wheelchair confinement is reached, the goal should be to make the wheelchair the passport to more rather than less activity.[75] Electrically powered chairs are eventually required for most individuals, although high-mobility wheelchairs can delay the need for powered chairs for several years.

Special wheelchair adaptations are often necessary. These may be provided either through a combination of assistive devices attached to the chair or the patient[32,76,120,222] or through a self-contained total-support system.[80] Objectives of orthotic and assistive devices are to maintain a stable spine, reduce the progression of contractures in the legs,

maintain functional use of the arms, and increase comfort. The progressive development of equinocavovarus foot deformity can be retarded by proper positioning of the feet on the foot pedals and ankle-foot orthoses with lateral Y-straps. Lightweight resting splints keeping the knees in extension and the feet in the neutral position are helpful in retarding contractures of the knees and ankles. Lateral pads or cushions can relieve thigh pressure and prevent hip abduction contractures.[148]

Because of weakness of the shoulder depressor muscles, relatively few patients with muscle disease profit from crutch assistance. In some of the other neuromuscular disorders, characterized by distal weakness and a slower progression, crutches may be beneficial.

Enhancing activities of daily living and self-care

Programs designed to improve or maintain self-care and upper extremity use in patients with Duchenne dystrophy have been reviewed.[32,91,120,150] For these patients, as for all paralyzed patients, a wide variety of home, workplace, and self-care assistive devices are available. Development of techniques and equipment is desirable, so the family can care for and assist the patient. Self-care activities can be related to each progressively changing level of physical function. Functional use of the upper extremities can be maintained by a lap board and balanced forearm orthoses. Increased comfort and stability are provided by molded seat, back inserts, and an extended back rest. A soft contoured mattress insert or pad is useful in relieving the discomfort from hip and knee flexion contractures. A crib-sized hospital bed with side rails allows the patient to turn more easily. The bars can be used as an aid in rising, and the additional height permits some patients to get out of bed independently. A raised toilet seat permits easier lifting, and grab bars may be useful. High stools or chairs enable the patient to arise and sit with a minimum of help. At some stage, hydraulic lifts are required. Clothing adaptations may be necessary.

The only studies evaluating the effect of a comprehensive rehabilitation program on activities of daily living are conflicting. Hoberman[105] reported that 71% improved, whereas Abramson and Rogoff[1] found improvement in only 33%. There have been no studies regarding the impact of rehabilitation programs on quality of life.

With the exception of some disorders such as Charcot-Marie-Tooth syndrome, weakness and contractures in the upper extremities are usually not severe enough to interfere with function until the patient is confined to a wheelchair.[208] Indeed, elbow flexion contractures of up to 15 degrees may even help initiate further flexion. At this stage, assistive appliances such as overhead slings and balanced forearm orthoses (balanced to enable weakened musculature to operate across rather than against gravity) can be beneficial.

In ambulatory patients with facioscapulohumeral dystrophy, early shoulder weakness and lack of scapular stability can significantly interfere with upper extremity function. Special bracing designed to force the scapula to the chest wall can, on occasion, assist in decreasing winging of the scapula and increase shoulder stability.[204] In patients with distal weakness, such as chronic peripheral nerve diseases, hand and finger orthoses may be tried, although they are not frequently used and are rarely accepted by patients. Clinicians are turning more toward surgery in the slowly progressive disorders.

Although functional evaluation scales and classifications are in wide usage in neuromuscular disease clinics, their usefulness as a measure of disease progression and a criterion against which to evaluate treatment has been recently questioned. Several studies have shown that there is little or no correlation between functional evaluations and pulmonary function, metabolic performance, strength, and other musculoskeletal factors.* There is, however, good intraobserver and interobserver reliability.[61] These scales may be of some value as a rough clinical index of the overall evaluation of comprehensive rehabilitation programs.

MANAGEMENT OF MEDICAL COMPLICATIONS

The major medical complications in persons with neuromuscular diseases include obesity, restrictive lung disease, cardiomyopathies, and psychosocial problems.

Obesity

Obesity is, of course, common in nonambulatory individuals, regardless of disease, since food intake is usually far in excess of energy demand. Psychic overeating and parental pampering often add to the problem. Obesity should be prevented by a well-balanced, low-calorie, vitamin-supplemented diet as soon as the individual becomes nonambulatory. Once obesity sets in, weight loss is difficult if not impossible.

It is usually stated that there is a substantial weight gain in Duchenne dystrophy, especially around the time of losing independent ambulation, and that this weight gain is a contributing factor to loss of ambulation.[174,229,231] Although there may be an increasing tendency to obesity as the boy grows older, weight is actually quite variable.[7,68,174,193] In one study about 50% of the boys fell within normal limits, 20% were below 1 standard deviation, and only 30% were above 1 standard deviation when compared with normal growth curves. In addition, most of the boys continued along the same channel that had been established at an early age.[68] Similar findings have been reported by others.[7,110,174,243] Height has usually been reported to be within normal limits in boys with Duchenne dystrophy,[68,194] although Allsop and Ziter[7] found that one third fell below the third percentile in both height and weight. Retarded growth in these children may be more frequent than previously recognized.

In patients with slowly progressive muscle diseases and who were usually still ambulatory, weight was reported to be lower than normal.[68] Preliminary data from a current study, however, indicates that individuals with slowly progressive neuromuscular diseases weigh more than age- and sex-matched controls, with a greater percentage of their body weight stored as fat.[67]

In normal children and adults there is a high correlation between strength and height, weight, and surface area, whereas in dystrophic individuals there is no correlation.[68] There is also a disturbance of the normal correlation between different muscle groups, especially between antagonists and synergists and muscle groups belonging to the same region.[68,194]

Restrictive lung disease and pulmonary complications

Restrictive lung disease—secondary to weakness of the respiratory musculature and often compounded by scoliosis—occurs in most neuromuscular diseases, especially in those that are rapidly progressive. This decrease in respiratory function can lead to cor pulmonale with right-sided heart failure, cardiomyopathy, chronic alveolar hypoventilation, and pulmonary infection secondary to inanition, reduced ability to cough, and poor respiratory toilet. A major cause of death is acute respiratory distress.

When indicated, a vigorous pulmonary rehabilitation program should be maintained. The objectives are to strengthen respiratory muscles, develop pulmonary endurance, maintain an efficient breathing pattern, and learn the principles of pulmonary hygiene. Humidification, intermittent positive-pressure breathing therapy, and the use of a suction apparatus and mechanical respirators may be indicated, in addition to postural drainage, diaphragmatic breathing, and chest percussion.

Most of the neuromuscular diseases show pulmonary function evidence of restrictive lung disease at some point in time, although there may not be any clinical findings. This includes amyotrophic lateral sclerosis,[89,155] myotonic dystrophy,[29,89,95,121] facioscapulohumeral dystrophy and limb-girdle dystrophy,[179] Becker dystrophy,[28,187] polymyositis,[26,46] and Duchenne dystrophy.* Serious respiratory dysfunction usually does not occur in facioscapulohumeral dystrophy, Becker dystrophy, myasthenia gravis, the congenital myopathies, or Charcot-Marie-Tooth syndrome. Marked restrictive lung disease is always present in amyotrophic lateral sclerosis and Duchenne dystrophy, often present in myotonic dystrophy and spinal muscular atrophy, and occasionally present in limb-girdle dystrophy. Several detailed reviews of the pathophysiology of the respiratory system in neuromuscular diseases and general pulmonary management are available.[82,86,158,176,179]

Most studies have been restricted to individuals with Duchenne dystrophy, in whom restrictive lung disease usually becomes rapidly progressive shortly after ambulation ceases. By about 14 years of age the FVC is usually below

---

*References 6, 7, 25, 68, 94, 138, 139, 179, 243.

*References 25, 28, 83, 89, 94, 117, 123, 142, 179, 187.

50%. In a current study of 50 boys with Duchenne dystrophy with an average duration of 13 years, mean vital capacity (VC) was 48% of predicted normal values. Longitudinal testing also revealed moderate to severe impairment of total lung capacity (TLC) and maximal voluntary ventilation (MVV), with residual volume (RV) moderately increased. MVV decreased with disease duration, RV increased, and VC dropped to levels consistent with severe impairment between the ages of 12 and 14 years. In 10 patients with amyotrophic lateral sclerosis with an average duration of 5 years, mean VC was 78% of predicted normal values. Longitudinal testing also showed moderate to severe impairment of MVV and RV but normal total lung volume (TLV). VC, TLC, and MVV decreased, and RV increased with disease duration. In 15 patients with chronic spinal muscular atrophy with an average duration of 21 years, mean VC was 58% of predicted normal values. Longitudinal testing also revealed moderate to severe impairment of TLV, MVV, and RV. There was no relationship between pulmonary function test values and disease duration. In 64 patients with slowly progressive weakness of a 22-year average duration, mean VC was 74% of predicted normal values. Longitudinal testing showed either normal or mild impairment of TLV, MVV, and RV, with no relationship between test values and disease duration.[67]

Although alluded to in some reports, the possible relationship between the degree and rate of progression of pulmonary involvement and other factors, such as trunk muscle weakness, obesity, and scoliosis, is not well established. A major reason for the difficulty in establishing correlations between these factors is that most of the studies in the past have not included longitudinal analysis of pulmonary function and other variables in the same group of individuals.

Incidence, rate, and severity of restrictive lung disease and the incidence of pulmonary infections, acute respiratory failure, and concurrent obstructive lung disease are difficult to evaluate from the literature. Most studies were limited to only a few individuals and not correlated with the stage of the disease, and selection criteria were rarely precise. In addition, some pulmonary function measurements, such as maximal expiratory pressure (often abnormal early in spite of normal spirometric values) were not used. Most studies have shown, however, significant reductions in mean percentages of forced vital capacity (FVC), peak flow rate (PFR), and MVV, and no change in the percentage of forced expiratory volume (FEV_1)/FVC.* FVC is the parameter most strongly correlated with age and scoliosis measurements.[135]

There still remains considerable confusion regarding the rate of progression of restrictive lung disease in Duchenne dystrophy. Part of the problem is that only one long-term longitudinal study has been reported, and it showed a progressive deterioration of pulmonary function.[94] Over a short-term period of 1 year, however, a consistent improvement of the absolute FVC and MVV in 50% of the individuals was observed. Such improvement occurred at any age between 5 and 12 years.[25]

All textbooks and major review articles state that respiratory infections are common in Duchenne dystrophy. Yet only three studies have been reported with actual data, and two of them reported a low incidence.[28,83] Several studies have attempted to relate the level of pulmonary function involvement, the number of respiratory infections, and the incidence of acute respiratory failure to the stage of the disease or the degree of muscle weakness.* The results are contradictory and need further evaluation.

Since scoliosis alone causes restrictive lung disease and reduced pulmonary volumes, the relationship between spinal deformity and the restrictive lung disease syndrome has been investigated. Some reports have indicated that scoliosis in children with Duchenne dystrophy did not play a significant role in the development of pulmonary function changes,† whereas other studies have shown a high correlation.[28,179,187,235] This is an area that needs clarification, since the precise role of progressive weakness of the respiratory muscles in the etiology of the restrictive respiratory syndrome has not been proven.[179]

Early-intervention management has included programs of respiratory therapy (breathing exercise, incentive spirometers, and so on) and spinal bracing. Although bracing appears to have little effect on the progression of scoliosis, Rideau[178] has reported that early bracing to prevent scoliosis helps to maintain lung compliance and higher VC in patients with Duchenne dystrophy. Five studies have been reported regarding the effect of an early program of respiratory therapy. The results in four indicated that this early intervention either improved or maintained pulmonary function.[2,47,105,203] In these studies, however, there were no control subjects, and the number of patients in each study were limited; intermittent positive-pressure therapy was also used in two studies. Howser and Johnson,[111] in a reasonably well-designed 3-month supervised therapy program with an age-matched control group, reported that pulmonary function values continued to decline in both groups, although the treated group showed less decline. Positive pressure breathing and abdominal binders were used in addition to breathing exercises. DiMarco and co-workers[47] reported significant increases in the maximal resistance that could be tolerated and in the maximal duration that ventilations could be sustained after a 6-week program of respiratory resistance training. Not affected by training were spirometry, functional residual capacity (FRC), and maximal inspiratory and expiratory pressures. What is needed is a long-term longitudinal study starting early in the course of the disease.

Late-intervention measures, including body respirators and cuirass ventilation, have been the subject of several

---

*References 28, 135, 142, 179, 187, 235.

---

*References 28, 83, 94, 117, 179, 228.
†References 82, 83, 94, 117, 135, 228.

reviews.[4,86,158] Reports concerning the effects of late intervention on cost-benefit ratios, longevity, quality of life, or pulmonary function are few in number and difficult to interpret. Vignos[228] reported that a comprehensive pulmonary management approach was successful in 79% of boys with Duchenne dystrophy admitted for severe respiratory infections. Curran[39] observed that night ventilation with body respirators in late-stage Duchenne dystrophy resulted in a constant significant improvement in daytime gas exchange, with prolonged survival. Others reported similar results.[12,161] DeTroyer and Deisser,[43] however, found that persons with long-standing neuromuscular disease did not benefit from brief daily periods of intermittent positive breathing. The number of subjects in each study was limited, and there were no control groups. Splaingard and co-workers,[216] in the most well-documented review to date, reported that home negative pressure ventilation initiated on an elective rather than an emergent basis saved an average of $12,000 during initial hospitalization. There was a 5-year survival of 76% and a 10-year survival of 61%. According to a recent survey, aggressive late intervention management was only routinely advocated by 33% of the Muscular Dystrophy Clinics, indicating that respiratory device usage has not received wide acceptance.[38]

Cardiac complications

There is a high frequency of cardiac involvement in Duchenne dystrophy,[84,159,166-168,177] Becker and Emery-Dreifuss dystrophies,[21,69,159,183] and myotonic muscular dystrophy*; there is less frequent involvement in facioscapulohumeral dystrophy,[166,167] limb-girdle dystrophy,[166,167] congenital myopathies,[162] myasthenia gravis,[106] and polymyositis[88,98,217,218]; and infrequent involvement exists in Charcot-Marie-Tooth syndrome[118] and chronic spinal muscular atrophy.[69,156]

In a current study of 65 patients with Duchenne dystrophy, and an average age of 14 years, 92% had abnormal electrocardiograms (ECGs), whereas only 18% had clinical evidence of cardiac disease. There was no correlation between ECG abnormality and age, disease duration, or severity of weakness.[67] Of 62 patients with myotonic muscular dystrophy and an average age of 39 years, 92% had abnormal ECGs, and only 8% had clinical evidence of cardiac disease. There was a significant correlation between ECG abnormality and age, duration of the disease, and severity of weakness. Through age 36 years, the older the patient and the longer the duration of the disease, the higher the percentage of ECG abnormality.[67] Of 81 patients with Becker, facioscapulohumeral, and limb-girdle dystrophies and congenital myopathies (average age 30 years), 65% had abnormal ECGs, and only 6% had clinical evidence of cardiac disease. There was no correlation between ECG abnormality and age, disease duration, and severity of weakness.[67]

The involvement is usually a cardiomyopathy, but there is also a high incidence of conduction defects in myotonic, Emery-Dreifuss, and Duchenne dystrophies. In spite of severely abnormal ECGs and echocardiograms, most patients do not show clinical evidence of heart disease before the preterminal stage of their disorder. Management of conduction defects and heart failure is the same as for the individual without neuromuscular disease.

Neuropsychologic function

A higher incidence of cognitive and intellectual impairment in individuals with Duchenne and myotonic dystrophy has been well documented. In Duchenne dystrophy there appears to be general, early, and nonprogressive impairment of verbal intelligence, and in some children nonverbal deficits also occur at an early age.[129,130,141] Verbal scale intelligence quotients (IQs) in patients 20 years or older are within normal limits, indicating that the low cognitive skills in younger boys are not fixed or global but reflect selective defects.[146,213] Genetic factors may play an important role in determining mental status, showing high concordance with the intellectual ability in affected siblings.[34]

Cognitive dysfunction has been reported in individuals with myotonic dystrophy for many years.[95] Significant defects occurred in every neuropsychologic measure, even when tests of motor skills were excluded, with the greatest involvement in immediate recall, abstraction, orientation, and spatial manipulation.[15,170,239] Females have been reported to be more affected than males,[15] and limited cognitive ability has been shown to be correlated with maternal inheritance of the gene.[15,171,172] There is some deterioration with time if the interval is greater than 3 years, and no correlation exists with the degree of weakness or myotonia.[172,239]

Karagan and Sorensen[131] also reported that a high proportion of individuals with Becker, limb-girdle, and facioscapulohumeral dystrophy had significant impairment of verbal scale IQs in relation to nonverbal scale IQs, and a relationship between the IQ level and the severity of the disease. Others, however, did not find any difference between patients with limb-girdle and facioscapulohumeral dystrophy and normal controls or individuals with spinal cord injury.[67,173]

Recent studies have shown a high level of personality abnormalities,[15] especially depression in individuals with myotonic, limb-girdle, and facioscapulohumeral dystrophy.[67,173] Measures of depressive maladjustment had significant negative correlations with measures of positive mental health, but depression was not correlated with gender, age, duration of illness, severity of disability, and employment status.

Psychosocial, educational, and vocational considerations

The management of the patient with neuromuscular disorders also requires attention to psychosocial problems and

---

*References 29, 85, 88, 95, 149, 166, 167, 177.

educational or vocational needs. Total management includes the family, and consideration of social and psychologic factors may make the difference between inactivity and future well-being.[208]

Several articles, based primarily on clinical observations, have reviewed the fairly characteristic psychologic and social problems of patients and families with Duchenne dystrophy.* A comprehensive guide providing information about sexuality has also been published.[8] There have been, however, very few studies of evaluations of psychologic reactions or intervention measures.[19,22,27,190,226] Detailed recommendations for management of these social and psychologic problems have been made by Siegel.[204]

Scholastic performance[227] and vocational rehabilitation[119] are complicated by the associated deficits in cognitive function as well as by various psychologic and musculoskeletal factors. Since psychosocial and intellectual factors have a marked implication for educational and vocational planning, this area should be a high priority for future research.

Other complications

Osteoporosis is a late change in most patients with advanced neuromuscular disease caused by disuse, and there is usually marked demineralization.[57] Fractures are common, since patients tend to fall more frequently as muscle weakness increases. Fortunately, dystrophic bones heal satisfactorily with minimal displacement of bone fragments and little pain, since there is minimal muscle spasm.[104,205] Fractures, like all surgical procedures, must be treated with minimal splintage to encourage early and continued ambulation. Deterioration in muscle strength inevitably follows long periods of immobilization, and fractures should be treated for ambulation whenever feasible.

Other complications occurring in some of the neuromuscular disorders are acute gastric dilatation and acute megacolon,[182] other dysfunctions of smooth muscle,[78] dysphagia,[153] and hearing acuity.[5,234] Rectal prolapse secondary to sphincter weakness can occur, and fecal impaction is a common complication of terminal motor unit disease. The outcome of prolonged immobilization or even brief restraint in some diseases, such as Duchenne dystrophy, is well known and should be avoided. Risks from anesthesia and malignant hyperthermia have been well documented.[33]

SUMMARY

Management of patients with neuromuscular disorders is more aggressive than it was in the past, and most physicians and therapists currently believe that it is important to preserve maximal function for as long as possible. Treatment should be prospective to inhibit deformity, prolong independent ambulation, and maximize functional capabilities.

Management is best carried out by a multidisciplinary

*References 31, 99, 107, 151, 204, 227.

approach to comprehensive care that considers the entire needs of the patients. Major goals are early diagnosis and establishment of a rehabilitation plan, maintenance of activities of daily living and ambulation for as long as possible, anticipation of complications, and development of a program of prevention and supportive counseling to the patient and family.

Management of musculoskeletal complications is based on an understanding of the natural evolution of patterns of weakness, contractures, and deformity. A knowledge of pathokinetics is essential to the proper timing of therapy, bracing, and surgery. Treatment is goal oriented for disorders that are rapidly progressive, static, or temporary. Implementation of these goals is carried out in various therapeutic modalities, bracing, assistive devices, and surgery. The total management of the patient also requires attention to cardiovascular, pulmonary, and other complications, as well as psychosocial care.

Advances in clinical research have occurred primarily in the management of musculoskeletal complications and in descriptive studies of the natural course of Duchenne dystrophy. The efficacy of exercise in progressive neuromuscular diseases remains controversial. Exercise therapy does not appear to have a short-term deleterious effect if started early in the course of the disease and carried out at submaximal levels. Although stretching alone has not been found to be very effective, the combined use of stretching and braces has been shown to result in a significant reduction in the progression of lower extremity contractures. There is no question that lower extremity bracing and surgery reduce the progression of contractures and spinal deformity and prolong mobility, but there remains considerable doubt that the mobility is functional. Spinal orthosis may slow the progression of minor curvatures, but bracing has little or no effect on severe scoliosis. Early surgical spinal stabilization is the only effective means of controlling scoliosis in rapidly progressive neuromuscular diseases.

Rehabilitation management of individuals with neuromuscular disorders has been based primarily on clinical observations in the past. Most investigations of treatment failed to follow sound clinical research techniques and were retrospective. In addition to appropriate clinical research methodology, two parallel categories of research are desirable: investigations of the natural history of each disease, preferably using longitudinal measurements, and studies of treatment outcomes. Prospective studies of treatment interventions are needed, designed to include an adequate treatment group sample, control subjects matched for duration or severity of disease, supervised therapy sessions, and an appropriate, objective, valid, and reliable measurement criterion against which to assess outcomes.

REFERENCES

1. Abramson, AS, and Rogoff, J: Approach to rehabilitation of children with muscular dystrophy, Proceedings of the first and second medical

conferences of MDAA, Inc., New York, 1952, Muscular Dystrophy Associations of America, Inc.

2. Adams, MA, and Chandler, LS: Effects of physical therapy program on vital capacity of patients with muscular dystrophy, Phys Ther 54:494, 1974.

3. Aitkens, SG, et al: Relationship between manual muscle testing and objective strength measurements, Muscle Nerve 9:255, 1986.

4. Alexander, MA, et al: Mechanical ventilation of patients with late stage Duchenne muscular dystrophy: management in home, Arch Phys Med Rehabil 60:289, 1979.

5. Allen, NR: Hearing acuity in patients with muscular dystrophy, Dev Med Child Neurol 15:500, 1973.

6. Allsop, KG, and Ziter, FA: Effectiveness of timed functional activities in Duchenne muscular dystrophy, Phys Ther 60:584, 1980.

7. Allsop, KG, and Ziter, FA: Loss of strength and functional decline in Duchenne's dystrophy, Arch Neurol 38:406, 1981.

8. Anderson, F, Bardach, J, and Goodgold, J: Sexuality and neuromuscular disease (Rehabilitation monograph no. 56), New York, 1979, Institute of Rehabilitation Medicine and the Muscular Dystrophy Association.

9. Aprin, H, et al: Spine fusion in patients with spinal muscular atrophy, J Bone Joint Surg 64:1179, 1982.

10. Archibald, KC, and Vignos, PJ, Jr: Study of contractures in muscular dystrophy, Arch Phys Med Rehabil 40:150, 1959.

11. Asmundson, VS, Kratzer, FH, and Julian, LM: Inherited myopathy in chicken, Ann NY Acad Sci 138:49, 1966.

12. Bach, J, et al: Long-term rehabilitation in advanced stage of childhood onset, rapidly progressive muscular dystrophy, Arch Phys Med Rehabil 62:328, 1981.

13. Beasley, WC: Quantitative muscle testing: principles and applications to research and clinical services, Arch Phys Med Rehabil 42:398, 1961.

14. Bennett, RL, and Knowlton, GC: Overwork weakness in partially denervated skeletal muscle, Clin Orthop 12:22, 1958.

15. Bird, TD, Follett, C, and Griep, E: Cognitive and personality function in myotonic muscular dystrophy, J Neurol Neurosurg Psychiatry 46:971, 1983.

16. Bleck, EE: Mobility of patients with Duchenne muscular dystrophy, Dev Med Child Neurol 21:823, 1979.

17. Bonsett, CA: Pseudohypertrophic muscular dystrophy: distribution of degenerative features as revealed by anatomical study, Neurology 13:728, 1963.

18. Booth, FW: Inability of myoglobin to increase in dystrophic skeletal muscle during daily exercise, Pflugers Arch 373:175, 1978.

19. Botvin-Madorsky, JG, Radford, LM, and Neumann, EM: Psychosocial aspects of death and dying in Duchenne muscular dystrophy, Arch Phys Med Rehabil 65:79, 1984.

20. Bowker, JH, and Halpin, PH: Factors determining success in reambulation of child with progressive muscular dystrophy, Orthop Clin North Am 9:431, 1978.

21. Bradley, WG, et al: Becker-type muscular dystrophy, Muscle Nerve 1:111, 1978.

22. Bregman, AM: Living with progressive childhood illness: parental management of neuromuscular disease, Soc Work Health Care 5:387, 1980.

23. Brooke, MH: Pathologic interpretation of muscle histochemistry. In Pearson, CM, and Mostofi, FK, editors: The striated muscle, Baltimore, 1973, Williams & Wilkins Co.

24. Brooke, MH, et al: Clinical trial in Duchenne dystrophy. I. Design of protocol, Muscle Nerve 4:186, 1981.

25. Brooke, MH, et al: Clinical investigation in Duchenne dystrophy. II. Determination of the "power" of therapeutic trials based on the natural history, Muscle Nerve 6:91, 1983.

26. Brown, NMT, Arora, NS, and Rochester, DF: Respiratory muscle and pulmonary function in polymyositis and other proximal myopathies, Thorax 38:616, 1983.

27. Buchanan, DC, et al: Reactions of families to children with Duchenne muscular dystrophy, Gen Hosp Psychiatry 1:262, 1979.

28. Burke, SS, et al: Respiratory aspects of pseudohypertrophic muscular dystrophy, Am J Dis Child 121:230, 1971.

29. Cannon, PJ: The heart and lungs in myotonic muscular dystrophy, Am J Med 32:765, 1962.

30. Carroll, JE, et al: Bicycle ergometry and gas exchange measurements in neuromuscular diseases, Arch Neurol 36:457, 1979.

31. Charash, LI, et al, editors: Psychosocial aspects of muscular dystrophy and allied diseases, Springfield, Ill, 1983, Charles C Thomas, Publishers, Inc.

32. Chyatte, SB, Long, C, II, and Vignos, PJ, Jr: Balanced forearm orthosis in muscular dystrophy, Arch Phys Med Rehabil 46:633, 1965.

33. Cobham, IG, and Davis, HS: Anesthesia for muscular dystrophy patients, Anesth Analg 43:22, 1964.

34. Cohen, HJ, Molnar, GE, and Taft, LT: Genetic relationship of progressive muscular dystrophy (Duchenne type) and mental retardation, Dev Med Child Neurol 10:754, 1968.

35. Cohen, L, et al: Statistical analysis of loss of muscle strength in Duchenne's muscular dystrophy, Res Commun Chem Pathol Pharmacol 37:123, 1982.

36. Cohen, L, et al: Fast walking velocity in health and Duchenne muscular dystrophy: a statistical analysis, Arch Phys Med Rehabil 65:573, 1984.

37. Colbert, AP, and Craig, C: Scoliosis management in Duchenne muscular dystrophy: prospective study of modified Jewett hyperextension brace, Arch Phys Med Rehabil 68:302, 1987.

38. Colbert, AP, and Schock, NC: Respirator use in progressive neuromuscular diseases, Arch Phys Med Rehabil 66:760, 1985.

39. Curran, FJ: Night ventilation by body respirators for patients in chronic respiratory failure due to late stage Duchenne muscular dystrophy, Arch Phys Med Rehabil 62:270, 1981.

40. Daher, YH, et al: Spinal deformities in patients with muscular dystrophy other than Duchenne: a review of 11 patients having surgical treatment, Spine 10:614, 1985.

41. DeLateur, BJ, and Giaconi, RM: Effect on maximal strength of submaximal exercise in Duchenne muscular dystrophy, Am J Phys Med 58:26, 1979.

42. DeLisa, JA, et al: Amyotrophic lateral sclerosis: comprehensive management, Am Fam Physician 19:137, 1979.

43. DeTroyer, A, and Deisser, P: The effects of intermittent positive pressure breathing on patients with respiratory muscle weakness, Am Rev Respir Dis 124:132, 1981.

44. Demos, J: Early diagnosis and treatment of rapidly developing Duchenne de Boulogne type myopathy (type DDB I), Am J Phys Med 50:271, 1971.

45. Demos, J, Treumann, F, and Schroeder, W: Anomalies de régulation de la micro-circulation musculaire chez les enfants atteints de dystrophie musculaire progressive par rapport a des enfants normaux du meme age, Rev Franc Etud Clin Biol 13:467, 1968.

46. Dickey, BF, and Myers, AR: Pulmonary disease in polymyositis/dermatomyositis, Semin Arthritis Rheum 14:60, 1984.

47. DiMarco, AF, et al: The effects of inspiratory resistive training on respiratory muscle functions in patients with muscular dystrophy, Muscle Nerve 8:284, 1985.

48. Drachman, DB, et al: "Myopathic" changes in chronically denervated muscle, Arch Neurol 16:14, 1967.

49. Drennan, JC: Orthopaedic management of neuromuscular disorders, Philadelphia, 1983, JB Lippincott Co.

50. Dubowitz, V: Prevention of deformities, Isr J Med Sci 13:183, 1977.

51. Dubowitz, V, and Heckmatt, J: Management of muscular dystrophy: pharmacological and physical aspects, Br Med Bull 36:139, 1980.

52. Edelstein, G: Correlation of handedness and degree of joint contracture in bilateral muscle and joint diseases, Am J Phys Med 38:45, 1959.

53. Edwards, RHT: Studies of muscular performance in normal and dystrophic subjects, Br Med Bull 36:159, 1980.

54. Edwards, RHT: New techniques for studying human muscle function, metabolism, and fatigue, Muscle Nerve 7:599, 1984.

55. Edwards, RHT, et al: Role of mechanical damage in pathogenesis of proximal myopathy in man, Lancet 1:548, 1984.

56. Eickelberg, WWB, and Less, M: Effects of passive exercise of skeletal muscles on cardiac cost, respiratory function and associative learning in severe myopathic children, J Hum Ergol 3:157, 1975.

57. Epstein, BS, and Abramson, JL: Roentgenologic changes in bones in cases of pseudohypertrophic muscular dystrophy, Arch Neurol Psychiatry 46:868, 1941.

58. Eyring, EJ, Johnson, EW, and Burnett, C: Surgery in muscular dystrophy, JAMA 222:1056, 1972.

59. Feldman, RM: The use of strengthening exercises in post-polio sequelae, Orthopedics 8:889, 1985.

60. Florence, JM, and Hagberg, JM: Effect of training on the exercise responses of neuromuscular disease patients, Med Sci Sports Exerc 16:460, 1984.

61. Florence, JM, et al: Clinical trials in Duchenne dystrophy: standardization and reliability of evaluation procedures, Phys Ther 64:41, 1984.

62. Florence, JM, et al: Endurance exercise in neuromuscular disease. In Serratrice, G, editor: Neuromuscular diseases, New York, 1984, Raven Press.

63. Fowler, WM, Jr: Treatment of muscular dystrophy, Arch Phys Med Rehabil 54:281, 1973.

64. Fowler, WM, Jr: Importance of overwork weakness (letter), Muscle Nerve 7:496, 1984.

65. Fowler, WM, Jr: Rehabilitation management of muscular dystrophy and related disorders. II. Comprehensive care, Arch Phys Med Rehabil 63:322, 1982.

66. Fowler, WM, Jr: Medical rehabilitation of persons with muscular dystrophy and other neuromuscular disorders (Rehabilitation research review series, National Rehabilitation Information Center), Washington, DC, 1985, Catholic University of America.

67. Fowler, WM, Jr: Comprehensive rehabilitation management of neuromuscular diseases, project no. 133 JH60015, National Institute on Disability and Rehabilitation Research, progress report, Yr 04, Nov 1986.

68. Fowler, WM, Jr, and Gardner, GW: Quantitative strength measurements in muscular dystrophy, Arch Phys Med Rehabil 48:629, 1967.

69. Fowler, WM, Jr, and Nayak, NN: Slowly progressive proximal weakness: limb-girdle syndromes, Arch Phys Med Rehabil 64:527, 1983.

70. Fowler, WM, Jr, and Pearson, CM: Diagnostic and prognostic significance of serum enzymes. I. Muscular dystrophy, Arch Phys Med Rehabil 45:117, 1964.

71. Fowler, WM, Jr, and Taylor, M: Rehabilitation management of muscular dystrophy and related disorders. I. The role of exercise, Arch Phys Med Rehabil 63:319, 1982.

72. Fowler, WM, Jr, et al: Ineffective treatment of muscular dystrophy with anabolic steroid and other measures, N Engl J Med 272:875, 1965.

73. Fowler, WM, Jr, et al: Effect of exercise on serum enzymes, Arch Phys Med Rehabil 49:554, 1968.

74. Fridén, J, Sjöström, M, and Ekblom, B: Myofibrillar damage following intensive eccentric exercise in man, Int J Sports Med 4:170, 1983.

75. Gardner-Medwin, D: Management of muscular dystrophy, Physiotherapy 63:46, 1977.

76. Gardner-Medwin, D: Objectives in management of Duchenne muscular dystrophy, Isr J Med Sci 13:229, 1977.

77. Gardner-Medwin, D: Controversies about Duchenne muscular dystrophy. II. Bracing for ambulation, Dev Med Child Neurol 21:659, 1979.

78. Garrett, JM, et al: Esophageal and pulmonary disturbances in myotonia dystrophica, Arch Intern Med 123:26, 1969.

79. Gey, GO, and Kennard, DW: Work and power capacity of normal mice and those suffering from muscular dystrophy, measured during stationary swimming, Nature 202:264, 1964.

80. Gibson, DA, Albisser, AM, and Koreska, J: Role of wheelchair in management of muscular dystrophy patient, Can Med Assoc J 113:964, 1975.

81. Gibson, DA, et al: Management of spinal deformity in Duchenne's muscular dystrophy, Orthop Clin North Am 9:437, 1978.

82. Gibson, GJ, et al: Pulmonary medicine in patients with respiratory muscle weakness, Am Rev Respir Dis 115:389, 1977.

83. Gilroy, J, et al: Cardiac and pulmonary complications in Duchenne's progressive muscular dystrophy, Circulation 27:484, 1963.

84. Goldberg, S, et al: Serial two-dimensional echocardiography in Duchenne muscular dystrophy, Neurology 32:1101, 1982.

85. Gottdiener, JS, et al: Left ventricular relaxation, mitral valve prolapse, and intracardiac conduction in myotonia atrophica: assessment by digitized echocardiography and noninvasive His bundle recording, Am Heart J 104:77, 1982.

86. Greenberg, M, and Edmonds, J: Chronic respiratory problems in neuromyopathic disorders: their nature and management, Pediatr Clin North Am 21:927, 1974.

87. Griffin, JW, McClure, MH, and Bertorini, TE: Sequential isokinetic and manual muscle testing in patients with neuromuscular disease, Phys Ther 66:32, 1986.

88. Griggs, RC: Hypertrophy and cardiomyopathy in the neuromuscular diseases, Circ Res 35:145, 1974.

89. Griggs, RC, et al: Evaluation of pulmonary function in neuromuscular disease, Arch Neurol 38:9, 1981.

90. Hagerman, FC, et al: Muscle damage in marathon runners, Phys Sports Med 12:39, 1984.

91. Hall, DS, and Vignos, PJ, Jr: Clothing adaptations for child with progressive muscular dystrophy, Am J Occup Ther 18:108, 1964.

92. Haller, RG, and Lewis, SF: Pathophysiology of exercise performance in muscle disease, Med Sci Sports Exerc 16:456, 1984.

93. Halstead, L, and Wiechers, DO, editors: Late effects of poliomyelitis, Miami, 1985, Symposia Foundation.

94. Hapke, EJ, Meek, JC, and Jacobs, J: Pulmonary function in progressive muscular dystrophy, Chest 61:41, 1972.

95. Harper, PS: Myotonic dystrophy. In Major problems in neurology, vol 9, Philadelphia, 1979, WB Saunders Co.

96. Harris, SE, and Cherry, DB: Childhood progressive muscular dystrophy and the role of physical therapy, Phys Ther 54:4, 1974.

97. Heckmatt, JZ, et al: Prolongation of walking in Duchenne muscular dystrophy with lightweight orthoses: review of 57 cases, Dev Med Child Neurol 27:149, 1985.

98. Henderson, A, et al: Cardiac complications of polymyositis, J Neurol Sci 47:425, 1980.

99. Henley, TF, and Albam, BA: Psychiatric study of muscular dystrophy: the role of the social worker, Am J Phys Med 34:258, 1955.

100. Hensinger, RN, and MacEwen, GD: Spinal deformity associated with heritable neurological conditions: spinal muscular atrophy, Friedreich's ataxia, familial dysautonomia, and Charcot-Marie-Tooth disease, J Bone Joint Surg 58:13, 1976.

101. Herbison, GJ, et al: Effects of overwork during reinnervation of rat muscle, Exp Neurol 54:511, 1973.

102. Hickok, RJ: Physical therapy as related to peripheral nerve lesions, Phys Ther Rev 41:113, 1961.

103. Hilsted, J, Galbo, H, and Christensen, NJ: Impaired cardiovascular responses to graded exercise in diabetic autonomic neuropathy, Diabetes 28:313, 1979.

104. Hirotani, H, et al: Fractures in patients with myopathies, Arch Phys Med Rehabil 60:178, 1979.

105. Hoberman, M: Physical medicine and rehabilitation: its value and limitations in progressive muscular dystrophy, Am J Phys Med 34:109, 1955.

106. Hofstad, H, et al: Heart disease in myasthenia gravis, Acta Neurol Scand 70:176, 1984.

107. Holroyd, J, and Guthrie, D: Stress in families of children with neuromuscular disease, J Clin Psychol 35:734, 1979.

108. Homburger, F, et al: Hereditary myopathy in Syrian hamster: studies on pathogenesis, Ann NY Acad Sci 138:14, 1966.

109. Horstmann, DM: Acute poliomyelitis: relation of physical activity at the time of onset to the course of the disease, JAMA 142:236, 1950.

110. Hosking, GP, et al: Measurements of muscle strength and performance in children with normal and diseased muscle, Arch Dis Child 51:957, 1976.

111. Houser, CR, and Johnson, DM: Breathing exercises for children with pseudohypertrophic muscular dystrophy, Phys Ther 51:751, 1971.

112. Howells, KF, and Goldspink, G: Effect of exercise on progress of myopathy in dystrophic hamster muscle fibres, J Anat 117:385, 1974.

113. Hsu, JD: Management of foot deformity in Duchenne's pseudohypertropic muscular dystrophy, Orthop Clin North Am 7:979, 1976.

114. Hsu, JD: The natural history of spine curvature progression in the nonambulatory Duchenne muscular dystrophy patient, Spine 8:771, 1983.

115. Hsu, JD, et al: Control of spine curvature in the Duchenne muscular dystrophy (DMD) patient, Orthop Trans 7:24, 1983.

116. Hyde, SA, et al: Prolongation of ambulation in Duchenne muscular dystrophy by appropriate orthoses, Physiotherapy 68:105, 1982.

117. Inkley, SR, Oldenburg, FC, and Vignos, PJ, Jr: Pulmonary function in Duchenne muscular dystrophy related to stage of disease, Am J Med 56:297, 1974.

118. Isner, JM, et al: Cardiac findings in Charcot-Marie-Tooth disease: a prospective study of 67 patients, Arch Intern Med 139:1161, 1979.

119. Jamero, PM, and Dundore, DE: Three common neuromuscular diseases: considerations for vocational rehabilitation counselors, J Rehabil 48:43, 1982.

120. James, WV, and Orr, JF: Upper limb weakness in children with Duchenne muscular dystrophy—a neglected problem, Prosthet Orthot Int 8:111, 1984.

121. Jammes, Y, et al: Pulmonary function and electromyographic study of respiratory muscles in myotonic dystrophy, Muscle Nerve 8:586, 1985.

122. Janiszewski, DW, Caroscio, JT, and Wisham, LH: Amyotrophic lateral sclerosis: a comprehensive rehabilitation approach, Arch Phys Med Rehabil 64:304, 1983.

123. Jenkins, J, et al: Evaluation of pulmonary function in muscular dystrophy patients requiring spinal surgery, Crit Care Med 10:645, 1982.

124. Johnson, EW: Walter J Zieter lecture: pathokinesiology of Duchenne muscular dystrophy—implications for management, Arch Phys Med Rehabil 58:4, 1977.

125. Johnson, EW, and Alexander, MA: Management of motor unit diseases. In Kottke, FJ, Stillwell, GK, and Lehman, JF, editors: Krusen's handbook of physical medicine and rehabilitation, Philadelphia, 1982, WB Saunders Co.

126. Johnson, EW, and Braddom, R: Over-work weakness in facioscapulohumeral muscular dystrophy, Arch Phys Med Rehabil 52:333, 1971.

127. Johnson, EW, and Kennedy, JH: Comprehensive management of Duchenne muscular dystrophy, Arch Phys Med Rehabil 52:110, 1971.

128. Johnson, EW, and Yarnell, SK: Hand dominance and scoliosis in Duchenne muscular dystrophy, Arch Phys Med Rehabil 57:462, 1976.

129. Karagan, NJ: Intellectual functioning in Duchenne muscular dystrophy: a review, Psychol Bull 86:250, 1979.

130. Karagan, NJ, Richman, LC, and Sorensen, JP: Analysis of verbal disability in Duchenne muscular dystrophy, J Nerv Ment Dis 168:419, 1980.

131. Karagan, NJ, and Sorensen, JP: Intellectual function in non-Duchenne muscular dystrophy, Neurology 31:448, 1981.

132. Karpati, G, Klassen, G, and Tanser, P: Effects of partial chronic denervation on forearm metabolism, Can J Neurol Sci 6:105, 1979.

133. Kinney, CL, et al: Overwork effect on partially denervated rat soleus muscle, Arch Phys Med Rehabil 67:286, 1986.

134. Kuipers, H, et al: Muscle degeneration after exercise in rats, Int J Sports Med 4:45, 1983.

135. Kurz, LT, et al: Correlation of scoliosis and pulmonary function in Duchenne muscular dystrophy, J Pediatr Orthop 3:347, 1983.

136. Lenman, JA: A clinical and experimental study of the effects of exercise on motor weakness in neurological disease, J Neurol Neurosurg Psychiatry 22:182, 1959.

137. Lewis, SF, Haller, RG, and Blomqvist, CG: Neuromuscular diseases as models of cardiovascular regulation during exercise, Med Sci Sports Exerc 16:466, 1984.

138. Lord, JP, et al: Upper extremity functional rating for patients with Duchenne muscular dystrophy, Arch Phys Med Rehabil 68:151, 1987.

139. Lord, JP, et al: Upper vs lower extremity functional loss in neuromuscular disease, Arch Phys Med Rehabil 68:8, 1987.

140. Maloney, FP, Burks, JS, and Ringel, SP, editors: Interdisciplinary rehabilitation of multiple sclerosis and neuromuscular disorders, New York, 1985, JB Lippincott Co.

141. Marsh, GG, and Munsat, TL: Evidence for early impairment of verbal intelligence in Duchenne muscular dystrophy, Arch Dis Child 49:118, 1974.

142. Matsuka, Y, Toyoshima, Y, and Wada, N: Spinal deformity and pulmonary function in Duchenne muscular dystrophy, Therapeutics (Tokyo) 27:692, 1973.

143. McCully, KK, and Faulkner, JA: Injury to skeletal muscle fibers of mice following lengthening contractions, J Appl Physiol 59:119, 1985.

144. McKenzie, MW, and Rogers, JE: Use of trunk supports for severely paralyzed people, Am J Occup Ther 27:147, 1973.

145. Miller, G, and Dunne, N: An outline of the management and prognosis of Duchenne muscular dystrophy in western Australia, Aust Paediatr J 18:277, 1982.

146. Miller, G, Tunnecliffe, M, and Douglas, PS: IQ, prognosis and Duchenne muscular dystrophy, Brain Dev 7:7, 1985.

147. Milner-Brown, HS, Mellenthin, M, and Miller, RG: Quantifying human muscle strength, endurance and fatigue, Arch Phys Med Rehabil 67:530, 1986.

148. Molnar, GE: Orthotic management of children. In Redford, JB, editor: Orthotics etcetera, ed 2, Baltimore, 1980, Williams & Wilkins Co.

149. Moorman, JR, et al: Cardiac involvement in myotonic muscular dystrophy, Medicine 64:371, 1985.

150. Morris, AG, and Vignos, PJ, Jr: Self-care program for child with progressive muscular dystrophy, Am J Occup Ther 14:301, 1960.

151. Morrow, RS, and Cohen, J: Psycho-social factors in muscular dystrophy, J Child Psychiatry 3:70, 1954.

152. Motloch, WM: Seating and positioning for the physically impaired, Orthop Prosthet 31:11, 1977.

153. Mullendore, JM, and Stoudt, RJ, Jr: Speech patterns of muscular dystrophic individuals, J Speech Hear Disord 26:252, 1961.

154. Nakane, K: Change of serum creatine phosphokinase activity after exercise in Duchenne type of progressive muscular dystrophy, Nagoya Med J 17:203, 1972.

155. Nakano, KK, et al: Amyotrophic lateral sclerosis: a study of pulmonary function, Dis Nerv Sys 37:32, 1976.

156. Namba, T, Aberfeld, DC, and Grob, D: Chronic proximal spinal muscular atrophy, J Neurol Sci 11:401, 1970.

157. Newham, DJ, et al: Ultrastructural changes after concentric and eccentric contractions of human muscle, J Neurol Sci 61:109, 1983.

158. Newson-Davis, J: The respiratory system in muscular dystrophy, Br Med J 36:135, 1980.

159. Nigro, G, et al: Prospective study of X-linked progressive dystrophy in Campania, Muscle Nerve 6:253, 1983.

160. Nix, WA, and Vrbova, G: Electrical stimulation and neuromuscular disorders, Berlin, 1986, Springer-Verlag.

161. O'Leary, J, et al: Cuirass ventilation in childhood neuromuscular disease, J Pediatr 94:419, 1979.

162. Otsuji, Y, et al: Cardiac involvement in congenital myopathy, Int J Cardiol 9:311, 1985.

163. Pandya, S, et al: Reliability of goniometric measurements in patients with Duchenne muscular dystrophy, Phys Ther 65:1339, 1985.

164. Paulson, OB, Engel, AG, and Gomez, MR: Muscle blood flow in Duchenne type muscular dystrophy, limb-girdle dystrophy, polymyositis, and in normal controls, J Neurol Neurosurg Psychiatry 37:685, 1974.

165. Pecak, F, Trontelj, JV, and Dimitrijevic, MR: Scoliosis in neuromuscular disorders, Int Orthop 3:323, 1980.

166. Perloff, JK: Cardiomyopathy associated with heredofamilial neuromyopathic diseases, Mod Concepts Cardiovasc Dis 40:23, 1971.

167. Perloff, JK: Cardiac involvement in heredofamilial neuromyopathic diseases, Cardiovasc Clin 4:333, 1972.

168. Perloff, JK: Cardiac rhythm and conduction in Duchenne's muscular dystrophy: a prospective study of 20 patients, J Am Coll Cardiol 3:1263, 1984.

169. Peterson, DW, Hamilton, WM, and Lilyblade, AL: Retardation of fatty infiltration in atrophic muscle of genetically dystrophic chickens by diet or exercise, J Nutr 101:453, 1971.

170. Portwood, MM, et al: Psychometric evaluation in myotonic muscular dystrophy, Arch Phys Med Rehabil 65:533, 1984.

171. Portwood, MM, et al: Intellectual and cognitive function in adults with myotonic muscular dystrophy, Arch Phys Med Rehabil 67:299, 1986.

172. Portwood, MM, et al: Longitudinal study of intellectual function in myotonic muscular dystrophy, Muscle Nerve 9:199, 1986.

173. Portwood, MM, et al: Psychometric evaluation in facioscapulohumeral dystrophy and limb-girdle syndrome, Arch Phys Med Rehabil 67:621, 1986.

174. Price, A: Regression of function in pseudo-hypertrophic muscular dystrophy (American Occupational Therapy Association Monograph no 1), Milwaukee, 1965, North Shore Publishing Co.

175. Reddick, MF, Winter, RB, and Lutter, LD: Spinal deformities in patients with muscle atrophy: a review of 36 patients, Spine 7:476, 1982.

176. Redding, GJ, et al: Sleep patterns in nonambulatory boys with Duchenne muscular dystrophy, Arch Phys Med Rehabil 66:818, 1985.

177. Reeves, WC, et al: Echocardiographic evaluation of cardiac abnormalities in Duchenne's dystrophy and myotonic muscular dystrophy, Arch Neurol 37:273, 1980.

178. Rideau, Y: Le traitement des dystrophies musculaires progressives: espoir ou realite? Quest-Medical 28:1777, 1975.

179. Rideau, Y, Jankowski, LW, and Grellet, J: Respiratory function in muscular dystrophies, Muscle Nerve 4:155, 1981.

180. Rideau, Y, et al: The treatment of scoliosis in Duchenne muscular dystrophy, Muscle Nerve 7:281, 1984.

181. Robin, GC: Scoliosis in Duchenne muscular dystrophy, Isr J Med Sci 13:203, 1977.

182. Robin, GC, and Falewski, G de L: Acute gastric dilation in progressive muscular dystrophy, Lancet 2:171, 1963.

183. Rowland, LP, et al: Emery-Dreifuss muscular dystrophy, Ann Neurol 5:111, 1979.

184. Roy, L, and Gibson, DA: Pseudohypertrophic muscular dystrophy and its surgical management: review of 30 patients, Can J Surg 13:13, 1970.

185. Russell, WR: Poliomyelitis: the pre-paralytic stage, and the effect of physical activity on the severity of paralysis, Br Med J 2:1023, 1947.

186. Russell, WR, and Fischer-Williams, M: Recovery of muscular strength after poliomyelitis, Lancet 1:330, 1954.

187. Saheki, B, Fukyama, K, and Miyoski, M: Studies on the pulmonary function of the patients of progressive muscular dystrophy, Iryo (Tokyo) 21:794, 1967.

188. Sakai, DN, et al: Stabilization of collapsing spine in Duchenne muscular dystrophy, Clin Orthop 128:256, 1977.

189. Salminen, A, and Vikko, V: Susceptibility of mouse skeletal muscles to exercise injuries, Muscle Nerve 6:596, 1983.

190. Schoelly, M-L, and Fraser, AW: Emotional reactions in muscular dystrophy, Am J Phys Med 34:119, 1955.

191. Schwentker, EP, and Gibson, DA: Orthopaedic aspects of spinal muscular atrophy, J Bone Joint Surg 58:32, 1976.

192. Scott, OM, et al: Effect of exercise in Duchenne muscular dystrophy: controlled six-month feasibility study of effects of two different regimes of exercises in children with Duchenne dystrophy, Physiotherapy 67:174, 1981.

193. Scott, OM, et al: Prevention of deformity in Duchenne muscular dystrophy: a prospective study of passive stretching and splintage, Physiotherapy 67:177, 1981.

194. Scott, OM, et al: Quantitation of muscle function in children: a prospective study in Duchenne muscular dystrophy, Muscle Nerve 5:291, 1982.

195. Seeger, BR, Caudrey, DJ, and Little, JD: Progression of equinus deformity in Duchenne muscular dystrophy, Arch Phys Med Rehabil 66:286, 1985.

196. Seeger, BR, and Sutherland, A D'A: Modular seating for paralytic scoliosis: design and initial experience, Prosthet Orthot Int 5:121, 1981.

197. Seeger, BR, and Sutherland, A D'A: Lumbar extension in Duchenne muscular dystrophy: effect on lateral curvature, Arch Phys Med Rehabil 66:236, 1985.

198. Seeger, BR, Sutherland, A D'A, and Clarke, MS: Orthotic management of scoliosis in Duchenne muscular dystrophy, Arch Phys Med Rehabil 65:83, 1984.

199. Sembrowich, WL, Knudson, MB, and Gollnick, PD: Muscle metabolism and cardiac function of the myopathic hamster following training, J Appl Physiol 43:936, 1977.

200. Siegel, IM: Pathomechanics of stance in Duchenne muscular dystrophy, Arch Phys Med Rehabil 53:403, 1972.

201. Siegel, IM: Scoliosis in muscular dystrophy: some comments about diagnosis, observations on prognosis, and suggestions for therapy, Clin Orthop 93:235, 1973.

202. Siegel, IM: Plastic-molded knee-ankle-foot orthosis in the management of Duchenne muscular dystrophy, Arch Phys Med Rehabil 56:322, 1975.

203. Siegel, IM: Pulmonary problems in Duchenne muscular dystrophy: diagnosis, prophylaxis and treatment, Phys Ther 55:160, 1975.

204. Siegel, IM: Clinical management of muscle disease: practical manual of diagnosis and treatment, Philadelphia, 1977, JB Lippincott Co.

205. Siegel, IM: Fractures of long bones in Duchenne muscular dystrophy, J Trauma 17:219, 1977.

206. Siegel, IM: Orthopaedic correction of musculoskeletal deformity in muscular dystrophy, Adv Neurol 17:343, 1977.

207. Siegel, IM: Prolongation of ambulation through early percutaneous tenotomy and bracing with plastic orthosis, Isr J Med Sci 13:192, 1977.

208. Siegel, IM: The management of muscular dystrophy: a clinical review, Muscle Nerve 1:453, 1978.

209. Siegel, IM: Maintenance of ambulation in Duchenne muscular dystrophy, Clin Pediatr 19:383, 1980.

210. Siegel, IM, Silverman, O, and Silverman, M: The Chicago insert: an approach to wheelchair seating for the maintenance of spinal posture in Duchenne muscular dystrophy, Orthot Prosthet 35:27, 1981.

211. Sinaki, M, and Mulder, DW: Rehabilitation techniques for patients with amyotrophic lateral sclerosis, Mayo Clin Proc 53:173, 1978.

212. Sockolov, R, et al: Exercise performance in 6- to 11-year-old boys with Duchenne muscular dystrophy, Arch Phys Med Rehabil 58:195, 1977.

213. Sollee, ND, et al: Neuropsychological impairment in Duchenne muscular dystrophy, J Clin Exp Neuropsych 7:486, 1985.

214. Soltan, HC: Swimming stress and adaptation by dystrophic and normal mice, Am J Physiol 203:91, 1962.

215. Spencer, GE, Jr, and Vignos, PJ, Jr: Bracing for ambulation in childhood progressive muscular dystrophy, J Bone Joint Surg 44:234, 1962.

216. Splaingard, ML, et al: Home negative pressure ventilation: report of 20 years of experience in patients with neuromuscular disease, Arch Phys Med Rehabil 66:239, 1985.

217. Stern, M, et al: ECG abnormalities in polymyositis, Arch Intern Med 144:2185, 1984.

218. Strongwater, S, Annesley, T, and Schnitzer, TJ: Myocardial involvement in polymyositis, J Rheumatol 10:459, 1983.

219. Sussman, MD: Advantage of early spinal stabilization and fusion in patients with Duchenne muscular dystrophy, J Pediatr Orthop 4:532, 1984.

220. Sutherland, DH, et al: The pathomechanics of gait in Duchenne muscular dystrophy, Dev Med Child Neurol 23:3, 1981.

221. Swank, SM, Brown, JC, and Perry, RE: Spinal fusion in Duchenne's muscular dystrophy, Spine 7:484, 1982.

222. Taft, LT: Care and management of child with muscular dystrophy, Dev Med Child Neurol 15:510, 1973.

223. Taylor, RG, Fowler, WM, Jr, and Doerr, L: Exercise effect on contractile properties of skeletal muscle in mouse muscular dystrophy, Arch Phys Med Rehabil 57:174, 1976.

224. Taylor, RG, et al: In vivo quantification of muscle contractility in humans: normal subjects and patients with myotonic muscular dystrophy, Muscle Nerve 9:246, 1986.

225. Torres, C, Moxley, RT, and Griggs, RC: Quantitative testing of hand grip strength, myotonia, and fatigue in myotonic dystrophy, J Neurol Sci 60:157, 1983.

226. Truitt, CH: Personal and social adjustments of children with muscular dystrophy, Am J Phys Med 34:124, 1955.

227. Vignos, PJ, Jr: Rehabilitation in progressive muscular dystrophy. In Licht, S, editor: Rehabilitation and medicine, New Haven, Conn, 1968, E Licht.

228. Vignos, PJ, Jr: Respiratory function and pulmonary infection in Duchenne muscular dystrophy, Isr J Med Sci 13:207, 1977.

229. Vignos, PJ, Jr: Physical models of rehabilitation in neuromuscular disease, Muscle Nerve 6:323, 1983.

230. Vignos, PJ, Jr: Importance of overwork weakness (letter), Muscle Nerve 7:498, 1984.

231. Vignos, PJ, Jr, and Archibald, KC: Maintenance of ambulation in childhood muscular dystrophy, J Chron Dis 12:273, 1960.

232. Vignos, PJ, Jr, Spencer, GE, Jr, and Archibald, KC: Management of progressive muscular dystrophy of childhood, JAMA 184:89, 1963.

233. Vignos, PJ, Jr, and Watkins, MP: Effect of exercise in muscular dystrophy, JAMA 197:843, 1966.

234. Voit, T, et al: Hearing loss in facioscapulohumeral dystrophy, Eur J Pediatr 145:280, 1986.

235. Wada, N: Study on spinal deformities in patients with progressive muscular dystrophy, Skikoku Acta Med 32:185, 1976.

236. Wiles, OM, and Karni, Y: The measurement of muscle strength in patients with peripheral neuromuscular disorders, J Neurol Neurosurg Psychiatry 46:1006, 1983.

237. Wilkins, KE, and Gibson, DA: Patterns of spinal deformity in Duchenne muscular dystrophy, J Bone Joint Surg 58:24, 1976.

238. Wilson, R, Carrow, R, and Walker, BE: Effects of forced swimming exercise on dystrophic mice, Arch Phys Med Rehabil 52:216, 1971.

239. Woodward, JB, III, et al: Neuropsychological findings in myotonic dystrophy, J Clin Neuropsychol 4:335, 1982.

240. Wratney, MJ: Physical therapy for muscular dystrophy children, Phys Ther Rev 38:26, 1958.

241. Young, A, et al: A new spinal brace for use in Duchenne muscular dystrophy, Dev Med Child Neurol 26:808, 1984.

242. Ziter, FA, and Allsop, KG: The value of orthosis for patients with Duchenne muscular dystrophy, Phys Ther 59:1361, 1979.

243. Ziter, FA, Allsop, KG, and Tyler, FH: Assessment of muscle strength in Duchenne muscular dystrophy, Neurology 27:981, 1977.

CHAPTER 23

Biofeedback

JOSEPH BRUDNY

The role of feedback in information and control theories is based on Ashby's truism that "a variable cannot be controlled, unless information about the variable is provided to the controller."[4] It then followed that feedback principles and regulatory mechanisms could be applied in medicine. Biofeedback is the technique that allows instrumental measuring and displaying of quantifiable variables of disturbed physiologic activities that are otherwise covert, so patients may learn to regulate them by gaining control over their own responses. This concept is founded on theoretic issues of volitional neural control over some autonomic and somatic motor portions of the nervous system. It requires the use of recording and monitoring devices and the participation of professional personnel in the learning process.

This chapter makes a distinction between the general use of biofeedback in clinical psychology and the specific use of electromyographic (EMG) feedback in rehabilitation medicine, so only a brief review of biofeedback is presented. Details may be found in texts by Gaarder and Montgomery[34] and Basmajian.[9]

ORIGIN AND EVOLUTION

The term "biofeedback" was coined in 1969 to describe the findings of experimental animal laboratory studies reported by Miller[54] and preliminary clinical trials described by Kamiya.[46] With the aid of operant conditioning techniques, various physiologic functions—such as heart rate and rhythm, intestinal motility, blood pressure, skin temperature, and brain wave patterns—were reportedly brought under voluntary control. This challenged traditional views in anatomy and the behavioral sciences and created a notion of unlimited therapeutic potentials based on the involuntary becoming voluntary.

These excessive expectations were soon tempered. An extensive, decade-long examination of the dual issues of mechanisms and efficacy of biofeedback took place in laboratory and clinical studies, and the collected data of these investigations[74] provided the following realistic appraisal of biofeedback status:

1. The use of biofeedback in stress-related disorders is helpful but nonspecific in the sense that other behavioral noninstrumental techniques may be equally efficacious.

2. The specificity of biofeedback is recognized in treatment of certain disorders of the central nervous system (CNS), of which EMG feedback in restoration of neuromotor control is the soundest and most widely practiced, whereas operant conditioning of the electroencephalogram (EEG) in intractable epilepsy and operant conditioning of sphincteric responses in control of bowel and bladder incontinence are just emerging from research laboratories.

3. The theoretic mechanisms of biofeedback, although not entirely clear, apparently reflect in stress-related disorders the restoration of homeostatic controls, since the cognitive aspects of the training process sharpen the patient's awareness.[55] This hypothesis conforms with findings by Noback and Demarest[58] that a vague cortical awareness of homeostatic mechanism is normally acting below the conscious level.

The alternative theoretic mechanism of biofeedback, particularly in learning motor control, is the stimulus-response-control hypothesis advanced by Brener.[15] The feedback signal represents a stimulus that is centrally processed, to be followed by a response. While the response occurs, response programming takes place, and central cerebral feedback loops are involved in learning greater response discrimination and in storing strategies of response that will remain effective in controlling the given physiologic activity after withdrawal of feedback.

USE IN BEHAVIORAL MEDICINE

Biofeedback has helped to focus the attention of the therapeutic community on the importance of modes of disease treatment that are alternatives to the conventional ones of pharmacotherapy, surgery, and psychiatry. This has contributed to the emergence of behavioral medicine, the appeal of which is based on discovering ways to manipulate the relationship between observable signs of disease and the underlying dysfunctions of the CNS governing all behavior, with a potential for long-term effective prevention and control of chronic illness.

In controlled studies on the treatment of hypertension[73] and migraine,[13] behavioral medicine—although often using biofeedback—demonstrated that equally successful outcomes can be achieved using noninstrumental approaches. Such approaches include the progressive muscle relaxation developed by Jacobson[44] and intended to sharpen the proprioceptive differentiation between tense and relaxed muscles, the autogenic training described by Schultz and Luthe[64] and based on use of autosuggestive sentences focusing in feelings of relaxation, warmth, and heaviness of muscles, and various transcendental meditation techniques, of which the relaxation response by Benson[11] is the simplest, focusing the attention on relaxation and on avoidance of conceptual thinking and worrying.

USE IN STRESS-RELATED DISORDERS

Repeated and sustained stress episodes, especially the classic "fight, fright, and flight" activities, are accompanied by acceleration of the rate and force of heartbeat, increase in blood pressure, concentration of blood glucose, and redirection of blood flow to the muscles at the expense of flow to the viscera and the skin. These episodes are the most common reasons for the failure of homeostatic controls, which results in a number of functional disorders, leading to states of disease including hypertension, cardiovascular disease, cardiac arrhythmias, peptic ulcers, peripheral blood flow disorders (such as Raynaud's disease), migraine headaches, and sustained muscular tension, producing head and neck pain.

Biofeedback techniques have been most successful with these functional disorders, providing instrumental indications of any of the various altered physiologic activities that are otherwise covert, such as the variables of blood pressure, blood flow, cardiac rate and rhythm, EMG activity, patterns of EEG activity, and electrodermal response reflecting activity of sweat glands.

Instruments have various levels of complexity and sophistication. They range from simple analog devices indicating the changes in measured activity by dial movements or proportional change in intensity or pitch of sound to complex multichannel digital computers supported by video displays of software capable of storage, reduction, and retrieval of monitored data.

Regardless of the biofeedback instrument used, the most important elements in the process are the clinical background, competence, and educational level of the professional (usually a physiologic or clinical psychologist) and the nature of paradigm used to instruct the patient. The prevailing tendency is to use instructional effects and relaxation training to help the patient alter the feedback displays and thus direct the underlying physiologic activity toward a more healthy level.

During a typical biofeedback session the skin temperature of a finger, for example, is monitored to provide a signal whose intensity reflects the degree of arousal of the sympathetic nervous system and whose step-by-step alteration, produced by the patient's responses with the therapist's aid, lessens the arousal. Constriction of skin blood vessels is mediated by increased sympathetic activity, and increased blood flow is the result of the decrease in sympathetic input. The therapist controls the sensitivity gains of biofeedback equipment to achieve the initial response, interprets changes in the signal, and encourages a "passive volition" attitude rather than an attitude of trying too hard. In the course of several sessions the patient may learn to increase skin temperature of a finger by 5° to 10° F. This is invariably accompanied by a lessening of sympathetic nervous system arousal and a corresponding feeling of relaxation. With repeated biofeedback sessions, patients learn to "warm" their hands regularly in real life situations and often report absence or lessening of stress-related symptoms and signs.

The use of biofeedback in stress-related disorders, although nonspecific, can modulate symptoms of stress; it focuses on cognitive, perceptual, and emotional factors, with resulting change in patients' attitudes and life-styles.

USE IN CONTROL OF INTRACTABLE EPILEPSY

A behavioral alternative to surgery has evolved over the past 10 years for patients resistant to anticonvulsant medication. It is based on operant conditioning of a particular EEG pattern of 12 to 14 Hz, known as sensory motor rhythm (SMR). Experimental work in animals trained to suppress the learned motor response for food acquisition demonstrated the presence of SMR.[72] These animals also became resistant to drug-induced convulsions.

Further research indicated that most anticonvulsant drugs produce the same SMR effects.[47,50,71] In time it became clear that therapeutic benefits could result from facilitation of normal SMR activity in epileptic patients who typically demonstrate abnormal patterns of SMR. The operant conditioning of SMR enhancement was routinely established with the aid of modified encephalographic equipment in the clinic as well as in the patient's home. Learning to produce normal patterns of SMR activity is a lengthy process, but for most patients such conditioning is rewarded by a seizure-free status.

SMR effectiveness in preventing epileptic seizures is thought to be caused by its contributions to the thalamic pacemaker's role as a gate mechanism regulating afferent and efferent aspects of sensorimotor activity.[70] The integrity of this gate mechanism appears to be essential for the filtering of incoming somatosensory signals and the control of corresponding motor responses. Damage to this gate (reduced or disordered rhythmic patterns) could presumably reflect aberrant input-output characteristics, one manifestation of which could be the development of seizures.

USE IN CONTROL OF BLADDER AND BOWEL INCONTINENCE

Urinary incontinence in the elderly is a major medical, psychologic, and social problem that affects approximately 50% of those in institutions.

Fecal incontinence is common in both the young and elderly population. Some 40% of children born with spina bifida are incontinent. The cause of incontinence in the elderly is multifaceted, frequently requiring institutional placement.

The biofeedback treatment of urinary and fecal incontinence has been studied extensively.[25,26,32,75] The convincing results warranted the extension of such treatment to clinics and offices.

It has been known since the nineteenth century that distention of the rectum produces a reflex relaxation of the internal anal sphincter and a reflex contraction of the external anal sphincter. This observation has been used therapeutically in patients with loss of external sphincter tone. Insertion of a distensible three-balloon probe into the rectum allows one balloon to distend the rectum, while the other two measure and monitor the muscles' responses in both the internal and external rectal sphincters.

With feedback from this polygraph recording of the external rectal sphincter and proper instructions, and over a relatively short time period (4 to 6 hours of training), patients have been able to learn and practice increasingly strong voluntary contractions of the external sphincter, with a resultant decrease in incontinence in over 75% of treated patients.

Crucial to long-term retention of control was the increased discrimination of rectal distention and learned avoidance of increased intraabdominal pressure during voluntary contraction of the external sphincter.

In a patient with meningomyelocele who had no control over the internal sphincter, innervated by sympathetic and parasympathetic nerves, nor over the external sphincter, innervated by the somatic peripheral nerves, similar training resulted in learning to relax the internal sphincter, to elim-inate fecal impaction, to contract the external sphincter—and thus to establish control over incontinence.[31]

Urinary stress incontinence, especially in older women, is often caused by weak pelvic floor muscles and weak external sphincter contractions. It can be similarly modified by training the patient to be aware of bladder volume and to increase voluntary contractions of the pelvic floor muscles and the external sphincter, the latter having a common somatic innervation (the pudendal nerve) with the external rectal sphincter.

Recently, rectal and vaginal probes containing EMG surface electrodes were successfully used to reflect the degree of striated muscles' contractions during training sessions.[59a]

NEUROMOTOR CONTROL ISSUES

Neuromotor control, or the way the CNS efficiently interacts with effectors of movement—the muscles—is of utmost importance to self-care, manipulation of the environment, and survival of the species. Although this system of interaction is complex and not yet fully understood, a great deal has been learned since Lord Adrian's 1935 observation that "the chief function of the nervous system is to send messages to the muscles which will make the body more effective."[2] Granit[39] defined neuromotor control as constant interaction within the triad that consists of muscles, their sensory organs, and motor neurons, all carrying out automatic and volitional commands emanating from supraspinal centers concerned with movement. Implied in such interaction are sensorimotor integration, cortical control, and reflexive phenomena, as well as multiple servosystems and negative feedback loops operating on all levels of the CNS.

No consensus has been reached regarding the role of feedback in motor control. Adams[1] proposed the closed-loop theory as a self-regulating system that has feedback, error detection, and error correction as main elements. Lashley[49] argued for the open-loop theory, according to which central mechanisms, or programs, contain all the information needed to specify the temporal and quantitative aspects of movement. Schmidt[62] advanced the schema notion, in which movements are constructed by means of rules contained in memory and concerned with general characteristics about a class of movements. More recently the action theory described by Whiting[76] and by Newell[57] has been gaining recognition; it states that movements do not need to be specified in an action plan and can be performed by using movement combinations.

However, when it comes to learning motor control, there is universal agreement that feedback is essential for acquisition of a motor program. To this end Numan[59] and Schmidt[63] have provided a model for understanding the role of feedback and error detection and error correction mechanisms in motor learning and motor programming. Based on feedback information from evolving movement, muscles' afferents, and environmental changes, and aided by the motivational drive, cortical sensorimotor integration takes place. It is followed by formation of motor programs in terms of spatiotemporal coordinated outflow of neuronal stimuli to the muscles. A copy of this initial program is stored in the memory of the system, the hippocampus, and the efferent copy of the pyramidal tract outflow is also stored in the cerebellum.[30]

On consecutive attempts at refining the movement, a reafferent feedback copy is compared with the stored program, and if error is found, adjustments take place and a new program is designed and compared again with reafference until the error is eliminated. Then patterning of the motor program is initiated and is continually reinforced by successful repetitive performances of the motor act.

The kinesthetic feedback from muscles' afferents is especially important and can suffice when joint and cutaneous afferents are not functional.[38] Phillips[60] points to the known alpha-gamma coactivation in the motor output as a mechanism to allow signaling to the higher cerebral levels from the muscle spindles concerning the length of the muscle and the rate of its change during movements.

The transcortical servomechanism of Miles and Evarts[53] also views the gamma-motor neuron discharge as an afference copy needed for the error detection and error correction mechanism of the brain.

The foregoing indicates that the information provided by muscles' afferents informs the higher-level brain centers about the degree and rate of muscular contractions, knowledge of which is essential for sensorimotor integration and for cortical control over spatial distribution and temporal sequencing of a selected motor program output. Because the kinesthetic data rarely reach awareness (being processed mainly subcortically), the disruption or distortion of cerebral levels' processing of the muscles' afferent feedback is overlooked clinically, although it is often the cause of neuromotor control breakdown.

When brain insults interrupt the orderly flow and processing of intrinsic feedback pertaining to movement, neuromotor control is disrupted, leaving only a residual degree of movement. The objective of rehabilitating motor deficits in such cases is to improve coordinated muscular activity, leading to restoration of function. The need to compensate for inadequate intrinsic sensory feedback is well appreciated by proponents of various physical therapy techniques. But alone these techniques fail to provide the unambiguous, continuous, immediate, and quantifiable feedback information that is essential for enhancement of sensorimotor integration, for "recalibration" of residual intrinsic feedback, and for cortical control over the reorganization of surviving neural substrate.[41,61]

Basic to functional reorganization of the neural substrate is cerebral plasticity—that is, the neural substrate's adaptive response to functional demand, which renders the brain capable of interpreting and using different sensory cues according to need and requires immediate and pertinent feedback concerning fulfillment of demand.[40] If such demand is repeatedly met, lasting functional changes are known to occur.

Such sensory plasticity is fundamental to intersensory translation of visual and kinesthetic information,[28] and to sensory substitution (for instance, the tactile-visual substitution system in the blind[5]). Vision seems to be the dominant modality in strengthening the "perceptual trace" during the development of motor skills.[65] Against this theoretic background of motor control and cerebral plasticity issues, the rationale for therapeutic use of video monitor feedback displays of EMG is discussed in the following section.

ELECTROMYOGRAPHIC FEEDBACK IN RESTORATION OF NEUROMOTOR CONTROL OR SENSORY FEEDBACK THERAPY
Diagnostic versus therapeutic electromyography

Visual-motor loops connect the visual and motor cortices and participate in guiding body and limb movement; the development of therapeutic techniques that facilitate the links between the visual input and the motor output therefore seems to be a logical approach. The first evidence of therapeutic usefulness of audiovisual displays of needle electrode transduced EMG was observed in 1960 by Marinacci and Horande,[51] Los Angeles neurologists and electromyographers, during examination of patients with stroke and peripheral nerve injuries. Since then many clinicians have tested the therapeutic applications of EMG, and in the past decade a substantial body of evidence has accumulated, confirming these original, albeit anecdotal, observations.

The "raw" EMG signals used for diagnostic purpose lacked sufficient quantification of overall muscle activity, and the use of needle electrodes could hardly be practical in long-term therapy. Therefore the therapeutic potential of EMG was strongly enhanced by use of computer technology for control and video display of signals. It was also enhanced by the recognition that, when transduced by surface electrodes and integrated digitally during short time periods, the integrated EMG (iEMG) adequately reflects the ongoing muscle activity—that is, the degree of muscle contraction (or its length) and the rate of changes of such contraction.[29,35]

Several reviews of the subject are contained in the literature. The most recent was put out by the American College of Physicians.[3] The most comprehensive contribution—in terms of numbers of patients treated, clinical entities tested, therapeutic systems and methods developed, and hypothetic reasoning concerning the outcome mechanisms—was the New York University Medical Center–supported study of EMG feedback therapy, or sensory feedback therapy (SFT), as the modality of treatment of nervous system disorders of movement. It was initiated in 1972.[20] This chapter describes the experience obtained over the past 15 years with SFT, supplemented with results and conclusions of other clinical researchers.

Equipment

The EMG system developed for the NYU Medical Center study established the state-of-the-art requirements. Its description can therefore serve as a guide in the selection of equipment, either commercially available or custom designed for clinical use. Such a microprocessor-based system permits detection, measurement, and display of two channels of EMG activity on a video monitor and also contains augmented feedback capabilities for training purposes.

The system provides potential for both analysis and therapy. On-line real-time computation of EMG permits the measurement and recording of digitally integrated muscle potentials in units of microvolt-seconds, a concept derived from computation of the raw EMG.[19] The recording of microvolt-seconds as an indication of muscle activity during movement provides a means of verifying the altered status of motor control.

Recording devices such as polygraphs, tapes, discs, and printers should be able to accept and store data. A capacity for storage and retrieval of various discriminative traces derived from an iEMG recorded during movement, serving as models for replication by the patient, is also essential.

Plotted by a microprocessor over time, iEMG appears instantaneously on a video monitor in the form of amplitude-varying traces. The displacement of the trace along the vertical axis reflects the *magnitude* of activity generated in the muscle; the *rate* of such activity is reflected in the vertical displacement over time (horizontal axis). This visual display thus reflects in a continuous manner the information regarding the spatiotemporal events occurring in the monitored muscle during attempted or ongoing movement, which is correlated with the intrinsic muscles' afferent feedback information. Such a display provides knowledge of the occurrence, as well as the outcome of one's own response, instantaneously and while performance is still ongoing. Scheduling and presentation of auditory signals are used mainly as reinforcement for successful matching or approximating the iEMG response to various model displays on the video screen.

Analytic procedures

The analysis of a patient's iEMG response helps to establish specific training goals. In normal subjects the patterns of the iEMG in response to command or volition are quite constant, reproducible, and clearly reflective of cerebral control of response both spatially and temporally. The coordinated nature of facilitation and inhibition of agonist and antagonist activities is apparent. With such displays of iEMG, the monitored muscles truly "come alive," to paraphrase Basmajian.[8] Their interplay becomes clearly expressed in the visually organized form of peaks, valleys, and plateaus, which can be clearly recognized and interpreted (Figure 23-1, *A*).

In contrast, the iEMG patterns derived from monitoring the muscles in a patient with a spastic, paretic, or dyskinetic disorder of voluntary movement show typical abnormalities of cerebral response, reflecting some of the underlying cerebral dysfunction—if one accepts the premise of Sokolov[68]

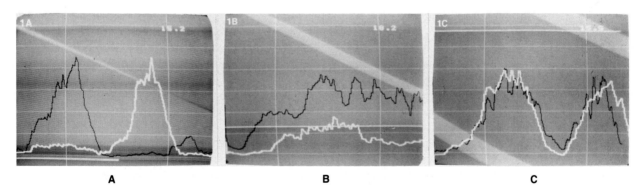

| A | B | C |

Figure 23-1. Various patterns of video monitor displays of iEMG. **A,** Coordinated facilitation and inhibition of agonist-antagonist interaction in normal subject during forearm extension and flexion. Black trace reflects activity of triceps muscle, white trace of biceps. **B,** Training inhibition of spastic biceps muscle activity *(white trace)* during facilitation of paretic triceps *(black trace)* for extension of forearm. Horizontal white line is sound coupled to alert patient by tone, whenever biceps activity (amplitude of iEMG) exceeds selected level. **C,** Training spatiotemporal control of performance. White trace represents iEMG pattern derived from monitoring and storing activity of wrist dorsiflexors in unaffected limb during wrist extension and return to neutral position. When black trace, reflecting activity of homologous paretic muscles, approximates or matches sample, tone is produced to inform patient regarding accuracy of performance.

that the EMG actually reflects a chain of neural events up to the highest level of the neuraxis, the cortex. Similar observations were made recently that disruption of central motor programs produces specific patterns of EMG when such is recorded from a pair of antagonists muscles.[66]

Paretic muscles show temporal delay in iEMG response and an inability to reach and sustain the steady levels of response needed for function. Muscles with clinically observed excessive tone (spasticity or spasmodic activity) demonstrate a loss of temporal and spatial control, as shown by an excessive and uncontrollable rise of iEMG levels as well as an inability to reduce such levels quickly, if at all.

When agonist and antagonist muscles are monitored simultaneously, a pattern of co-contraction is frequently seen. This pattern may completely restrict movement or prevent it from becoming functional as a result of excessive effort followed by ensuing fatigability. The patient is usually unaware of the interfering factors and can rarely identify or suppress the undesired muscle activity. Overflow to other muscle groups occurring during excessive effort further complicates attempts at movement.

Training procedures

Following the clinical evaluation and analysis of major abnormalities of iEMG response, the physician should establish treatment procedures for each patient individually, and the therapist can train the patient to make volitional alterations of any existing abnormal activity in muscles involved in the production of an active functional movement.

The techniques used in EMG feedback training entail the formulation of appropriate motor programs that can be visually defined on the video monitor either by artificially creating a graphic representation of desired iEMG response (Figure 23-1, *B*) or by using the "stored" iEMG traceform response from homologous contralateral normal muscle during execution of a requested motor task (Figure 23-1, *C*).

The essence of training is progressive altering or shaping of patient's iEMG response during attempted motion toward an approximation of the video monitor–outlined patterns. This task, not unlike learning written language, is aided by the immediacy of displayed information regarding the occurrence of iEMG response and its adequacy (performance to sample training). This immediacy and pertinence of information helps to define the effort that is needed and allows the spatiotemporal modification of motor response to take place during response evolution, so that error gap between the actual and intended performance can be gradually bridged. When the patient is able to carry out the specific motion with no feedback, the strategy established in training has apparently become "internalized," or patterned. At this stage some patients may require just a few, infrequent reinforcement sessions to retain the new patterns of motor control.

The frequency of training is usually three times a week with duration of each treatment approximately 30 minutes, and the length of training varies from 3 months up to 2 years. Between training sessions the patients should routinely be given detailed instructions to carry out a program of repetitive, daily, self-administered exercises at home that are directed toward extending control over primary movers that had previously been trained.

Evaluation procedures

EMG measures can be obtained by recording microvolt-second values before, during, and after treatment. The systematic recording of microvolt-seconds was described in a single-subject methodology by Gianutsos and co-workers.[36]

In addition to iEMG measures, results must be evaluated in relation to changes in functional capacity, since the major concern is to improve the patient's functional status for activities of daily living. Functional capacity should be assessed at varying intervals with various grading scales available in the literature.

Patient selection

Over 400 patients with a variety of chronic neurologic disorders were studied and treated. These included small numbers of patients with incomplete spinal cord injuries,[21] as well as peripheral nerve injuries,[24] and the response was encouraging. The majority of patients had suffered brain insult, and their conditions fell into three groups: hemiparetic-spastic syndromes, focal-dystonic syndromes, and hypoglossal-facial nerve anastomoses. The selection of these three groups was prompted by their low recovery rate with conventional therapies.

Hemiparesis

Most clinical studies were primarily directed toward treatment of the upper extremity, in which the recovery of function is very low. Several reports in literature describe their findings.*

In my experience a group of 70 patients, aged 12 to 78 and with a mean duration of illness of 2½ years, received a 9-month course of SFT for nonfunctional hemiparetic upper extremity.[23] The results showed that 10% of patients attained prehensile capacity and 60% attained assistive capacity of the limb (control over shoulder, elbow, and wrist only).

The hemiparetic patients who responded well to SFT demonstrated the ability to break up the pathologic synergies present and were able to plan and execute patterned movement in a functional manner. The greatest significance seemed to be the knowledge of a strategy to identify and suppress the undesirable motor activity. Although most patients markedly increased the speed and accuracy of executing the intended movement, their performance still rarely resembled the rapid, easily produced type of patterned movement characteristic of health. There was often a need for planning the intended movement and for constant visual observation to facilitate its execution. Some patients even-

---

*References 10, 36, 43, 67, 77, 78.

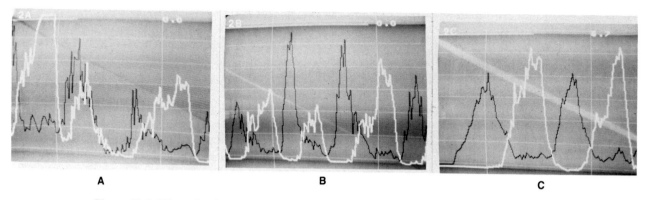

Figure 23-2. "Normalization" of iEMG response following training of patient with 2 years' duration of right hemiparesis. **A,** Before training. Attempt at extension of forearm is short-lasting and futile because of biceps muscle co-contraction *(white trace)* preventing facilitation of triceps *(black trace)*. **B,** Following 4 weeks of training, with evidence of voluntary inhibition of undesired biceps co-contraction and greater responsiveness of triceps. **C,** After 8 weeks of training. Flexion and extension of the forearm are carried out efficiently, fully, and without feedback information. Performance of same task by a normal subject (see Figure 23-1, *A*) shows similarity of iEMG response. (From White, L, and Tursky, B, editors: Clinical biofeedback: efficacy and mechanics New York, 1982, Guilford Press.)

tually became capable of carrying out the intended movement and actions automatically, smoothly, accurately, and repeatedly, but others showed a lasting need for awareness and "attuning" to motor activity in the muscles.

Whenever the patient succeeded in learning adequate motor control of a specific action, normalization of iEMG response was always demonstrated in the primary movers responsible for this task.[16] "Normalization" can be defined as a progressive decrease in pathologic reflexive components of movement with a simultaneous increase in its volitional, supraspinal components (Figure 23-2).

More extended duration of treatment adds materially to the degree of functional recovery. It allowed more of these patients to attain prehension. Recovery of motor function after brain insult may require a long period of time, and one can accordingly observe ongoing degrees of return to skillful use of the arm and hand in patients followed for many years. In this light, extension of SFT beyond the boundaries of hospital and clinic and into the patient's home to overcome the fiscal constraints related to the length of retraining needed seems to be a concept worthy of widespread testing and implementation.

Focal dystonia—spasmodic torticollis

The selection of patients with spasmodic torticollis has long been of interest to investigators.[12,18,27,45] The bizarre nature of the illness—involuntary turning or twisting of the head, spasmodic activity in neck muscles during certain actions, and their increased incidence during mental stress—all led to the belief that this disorder is psychogenic. Only recently has this focal dystonic syndrome been classified as a neurologic entity with a pathophysiology similar to dystonia.[52] The underlying disturbance is caused by an

imbalance in neuronal transmittal agents relating to the extrapyramidal system.[33] The abnormal motor activity in dystonia is considered to be related to disturbances of processing incoming sensory signals in basal ganglia, with resulting excessive input relayed to the motor cortex.[79] If such is the case, the motor manifestations of dystonia imply malfunctioning gating mechanisms.

A group of 80 patients with focal dystonic syndrome was treated and followed for up to 4 years.[48] Patients responding to SFT learned to discriminate the onset of spasmodic activity early and could suppress it for varying time periods. In the initial phases of SFT, constant attention to monitor displays of variables of motor activity was obvious. Later the patients clearly demonstrated automatic, acquired control and were unaware of its mechanism. It is conceivable that, while in SFT, some were also learning to discriminate and integrate other information derived from intact sensory modalities—for example, from receptors in skin, joints, and visual and vestibular systems—and could retain these patterns to aid motor performance after withdrawal of feedback (Figure 23-3).

Patients able to control their movement disorders during activities of daily living for days and weeks were considered therapeutic successes. Of the 80 patients treated, 45 (56%) were considered such successes. Along with learning control over previously spasmodic muscles, they demonstrated significant changes in their daily activities; for example, they resumed some kind of work, drove a car, and renewed social contacts.

Hypoglossal-facial nerve anastomosis

Total unilateral facial paralysis is a devastating illness that causes functional disability and psychologic distress owing

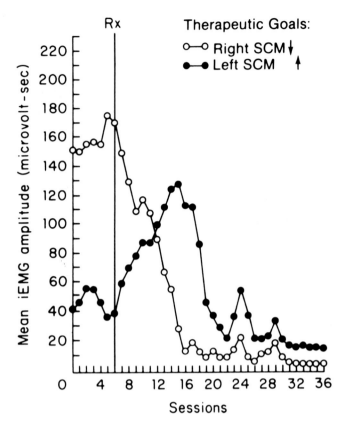

Figure 23-3. Single case study of training response in patient with 5-year duration of spasmodic torticollis to left. Therapeutic goals are outlined. During first 6 baseline sessions, with feedback information withheld, patient is attempting to assume neutral head position without success. Over next 30 sessions, with feedback available, inhibition and facilitation of respective muscles are gradually attained. Neutral head position is maintained with no effort over last six sessions, and subsequently without feedback as well. (From Surwit, RS, et al: Behavioral treatment of disease, New York, 1982, Plenum Publishing Co.)

to the loss of body image and the inability to express emotions visibly. Damage to cranial nerve VII—for example, by an acoustic neuroma—is a frequent complication of cerebellopontine angle tumor surgery. For reanimation and reinnervation of the face, hypoglossal-facial nerve anastomosis is often the surgery of choice, providing a powerful motor supply from cranial nerve XII's system, patterned to perform or behave in an appropriate manner during use of the tongue for speech, mastication, and swallowing—but lacking the programmatic routines (of cranial nerve VII's system) necessary for facial function and expressions. A behavioral dilemma is thus created. Although contractions of facial muscles can result from invoking lingual musculature (activation of cranial nerve XII's motor system), the majority of patients find it difficult to coordinate bilaterally the activities of two different cranial motor systems; they usually obtain only good facial tone but are distressed by the varying degrees of facial spasm involuntarily triggered by

motion of the tongue. Single case histories of EMG feedback training of such patients have been reported.[7,14]

Thirty patients with cranial nerve XII-VII anastomosis received EMG feedback training over a 5-year period.[22] These patients were trained to develop the strategy of selective muscle control (facilitation or inhibition or both) to aid eventually in obtaining symmetry and synchrony of facial function and spontaneity of expression without use of lingual musculature. Over one third of patients fully achieved these goals, including elimination of facial spasms on motion of the tongue. To achieve selective muscle control, the patients had to learn highly specific cerebral control over the facilitation and outflow of neural stimuli from cranial nerve XII's motor nucleus during facial movements or emotional expressions. They also had to learn to gate such outflow while using the tongue during mastication and swallowing. Spontaneity was eventually achieved; the patient could show emotional expressions and demonstrate synchrony and symmetry of facial muscle activity without awareness or need for any tongue motions.

When stressed, fatigued, or startled, patients showed occasional loss of control during the 1-year follow-up period. But thinking about the intended facial motion rapidly recalled the previously learned patterns of control.

HYPOTHETIC MECHANISMS OF SFT EFFICACY

Basic to all existing hypotheses about restoration of neuromotor control after cerebral insult is the plasticity of the brain—that is, its ability to respond adaptively to functional demands, provided that fulfillment of demand is reinforced by immediate, pertinent, continuous, and quantifiable feedback information.

Bach-y-Rita[6] described clinically effective sensory substitution mechanisms and proposed the concept of unmasking the existing but unused neural pathways as the most plausible mechanism of functional reorganization. He considered EMG feedback as another example of sensory substitution.

Mulder and Hulstyn[56] similarly proposed that EMG activity displayed continuously and quantifiably on a video monitor is a form of an artificial sensory (substitution) feedback, which can serve as an external model and thereby help to develop the desired motor planning response. I suggested that the success of iEMG visual feedback may be caused by an existence of visual motor loops within the CNS.[17] The precision of languagelike visual displays, with all vagueness eliminated, can be readily used by brain algorithms concerned with movement patterning and execution.

All of these concepts regarding the efficacy of EMG feedback training, although still hypothetic, are considerably reinforced by the therapeutic outcome of EMG feedback training in patients with cranial nerve XII-VII anastomosis, since the observable changes that followed such training must have reflected functional alterations in well-defined neuroanatomic areas and a well-known pathophysiology of the disorder—which was not always the case with other cerebral insults.

Both cranial nerve XII's and VII's motor nuclei coordinate the execution of their respective motor programs in intricate and synchronized movements of the tongue and lips for speech articulation, food intake, and mastication. To orchestrate such a complex performance, both motor nuclei contain specialized motor zones and are in turn constantly interacting with cortical mechanisms involved in planning and execution of all of those motor tasks.

The existence of intranuclear connections between the facial, hypoglossal, and trigeminal nerves by means of electrophysiologic studies was demonstrated by Stennert and Limberg[69] and confirmed by Holstege, Kuypers, and Decker.[42]

I believe that during training of patients with cranial nerve XII-VII anastomosis, EMG sensory feedback provides immediate, pertinent, continuous, and quantifiable information that, when decoded and translated by cortical structures, aids the formation of cortical feedback loops involved in both facilitory and inhibitory mechanisms of learned motor control. The facilitory loops are capable of therapeutic manipulation of preexisting neural connections between the cranial nerve XII and VII motor nuclei and their "unmasking"; this aids in the eventual formation of a working relay from certain zones of the ipsilateral nerve VII motor nucleus to appropriate zones of the nerve XII motor nucleus. All this occurs simultaneously with the coordinated outflow of neuronal stimuli from the contralateral nerve VII motor nucleus. Such a hypothetic mechanism would explain the occurrence of selective muscle control—needed for symmetry and synchrony of bilateral facial activity and for spontaneity of expressions—without calling on the use of lingual musculature.

The inhibitory negative cortical feedback loops, formed as the result of training, gate the outflow of kinetic neuronal stimuli from cranial nerve XII's motor nucleus on the anastomized side during motions of the tongue. In patients with hypoglossal-facial anastomosis the tongue movement is facilitated only by the single contralateral hypoglossal motor system.

The stimulus-response model of CNS information processing can perhaps be considered as involved in the training process. Control of involuntary spasms (cranial nerve XII's motor nerve system activity) is cued by increased discrimination of visual characteristics of displayed iEMG (stimulus discrimination) and by establishing gating mechanisms (response control).

Lasting control entails an ability, based on learned and stored motor strategies, to discriminate the need to emit the response without the benefit of external feedback. The central feedback loops presumably assume this role. Lasting control also requires extended, relevant, and well-structured training, with a high degree of motivation required for success.

Extending this reasoning to results obtained in patients with hemiparetic-spastic and dystonic syndromes (despite less exact knowledge of neuroanatomy and neuropathology), one can still argue that therapeutic manipulation of cerebral circuits by means of visual displays of iEMG is capable of inducing, similarly, facilitory or inhibitory central responses, which often are of a lasting (learned) nature and which aid in restoration of neuromotor control. Such achieved normalization of central responses accords with the need, noted by Shahani,[66] for development of neurophysiologic therapeutics that modify motor activity by reorganizing the central programs to behave as normally as possible.

CONCLUSION

The role of feedback of pertinent information in normalization of cerebral control over autonomic and somatic portions of the CNS has been reviewed. The conceptual development of computer-based equipment and training procedures for restoration of neuromotor control has also been described.

A video monitor–defined model that is replicated in training by the iEMG output of the patient under a professional's guidance appears to help in the cerebral strategy of motor response planning and execution.

SFT, or EMG feedback therapy, as presented in this chapter, obviously provides only some information regarding the quality of evolving movement and action. However, by creating a working sensory substitution and linking the visual input with motor output, along with error detection and error correction potential provided by digital computers, the first rational step has been taken toward therapeutically influencing the cerebral facilitory and inhibitory mechanisms of disturbed neuromotor control—which will eventually lead to normalization.

The significance of this behavioral training modality in therapeutic manipulation of cerebral neuronal circuitry should not be overlooked by the physiatrists who in the past tended to remove themselves from the therapeutic scene, as commented on by Goodgold.[37] Physiatrists, because of their educational background and clinical role, are most suited to make important contributions toward approaches for treatment of patients with brain insult.

The psychologic community is already using digital computers in the rehabilitation of brain insult–related cognitive function. Digital computers can be of similar use in the rehabilitation of neuromotor control in patients with brain insults and should be used to a greater degree by physiatrists as well.

In the near future one can envision the harnessing of artificial intelligence logic and rules both for programming the digital computer and for developing an "intelligent tutor," which directs and monitors the patient's performance during movement and action, using iEMG and other feedback parameters. Such a development—given interest, supervision, and support by physiatrists at large—would free the therapist from the costly and demanding one-to-one relation with the patient. It would also allow many patients to help themselves beyond the scope of the current therapy (with periodic input by the physiatrist) at a fraction of the ever-rising cost of rehabilitation efforts.

REFERENCES

1. Adams, JA: A closed loop theory of motor learning, J Motor Behav 3:111, 1971.
2. Adrian, ED: The mechanism of nervous action, Philadelphia, 1935, University of Pennsylvania Press.
3. American College of Physicians, Health and Public Policy Committee: Position papers: biofeedback for neuromuscular disorders, Ann Intern Med 101:854, 1985.
4. Ashby, WR: An introduction to cybernetics, New York, 1963, John Wiley & Sons.
5. Bach-y-Rita, P: Brain mechanism in sensory substitution, New York, 1972, Academic Press.
6. Bach-y-Rita, P: Brain plasticity as basis for therapeutic procedures. In Bach-y-Rita, P, editor: Recovery of function: theoretical consideration for brain injury rehabilitation, Baltimore, 1980, University Press.
7. Baillet, R, Shinn, JB, and Bach-y-Rita, P: Facial paralysis rehabilitation: retraining selective muscle control, Int Rehabil Med 4:67, 1982.
8. Basmajian, JV: Muscles alive, Baltimore, 1967, Williams & Wilkins Co.
9. Basmajian, JV, editor: Biofeedback: principles and practice for clinicians, Baltimore, 1983, Williams & Wilkins Co.
10. Basmajian, JV, et al: EMG feedback treatment of the upper limb in hemiparetic stroke patients, Arch Phys Med Rehabil 63:613, 1982.
11. Benson, H: The relaxation response, New York, 1975, William Morrow & Co.
12. Bird, BL, and Cataldo, MF: Experimental analysis of EMG feedback in treating dystonia, Ann Neurol 3:310, 1978.
13. Blanchard, EB, et al: Temperature feedback in the treatment of migraine headaches, Arch Gen Psychiatry 35:581, 1976.
14. Booker, HE, Rubow, RT, and Coleman, PJ: Simplified feedback in neuromuscular retraining: an automated approach using electromyographic signals, Arch Phys Med Rehabil 50:621, 1969.
15. Brener, J: Psychobiological mechanisms in biofeedback. In White, L, and Tursky, B, editors: Clinical biofeedback: efficacy and mechanisms, New York, 1982, Guilford Press.
16. Brudny, J: Biofeedback in chronic neurological cases. In White, L, and Tursky, B, editors: Clinical biofeedback: efficacy and mechanisms, New York, 1982, Guilford Press.
17. Brudny, J: EMG feedback in neuromuscular rehabilitation of spasmodic torticollis: therapeutic electromyography. In Surwit, RS, et al, editors: Behavioral treatment of disease, New York, 1982, Plenum Publishing Corp.
18. Brudny, J, Grynbaum, BB, and Korein, J: Spasmodic torticollis: treatment by feedback display of the EMG, Arch Phys Med Rehabil 55:403, 1974.
19. Brudny, J, Weisinger, M, and Silverman, G: Single system for displaying EMG activity designed for therapy, documentation of results, and analysis of research. In Foulds, R, and Lund, R, editors: 1976 Conference on systems and devices for the disabled, Boston, 1979, Biomedical Engineering Center.
20. Brudny, J, et al: Sensory feedback therapy as a modality of treatment in central nervous system disorders of voluntary movement, Neurology 24:925, 1974.
21. Brudny, J, et al: EMG feedback therapy: review of treatment of 114 patients, Arch Phys Med Rehabil 9:155, 1977.
22. Brudny, J, et al: Electromyographic rehabilitation of facial function and introduction of facial paralysis grading scale for hypoglossal-facial nerve anastomosis laryngoscope, Laryngoscope 98:405, 1988.
23. Brudny, J, et al: Helping hemiparetics to help themselves: sensory feedback therapy, J Am Med Assoc 241:814, 1979.
24. Brudny, J, et al: The role of sensory feedback of integrated EMG in the absence of proprioception: proceedings of the Fourth Congress of the International Society of Electrophysiological Kinesiology, Boston, 1979.
25. Burgio, KL, Robinson, JC, and Engel, BT: The role of biofeedback in Kegel exercise training for stress urinary incontinence, Am J Obstet Gynecol 154:58, 1986.
26. Burgio, KL, Whitehead, WE, and Engel, BT: Urinary incontinence in the elderly: bladder-sphincter biofeedback and toileting skills training, Ann Intern Med 104:507, 1985.
27. Cleeland, C: Behavioral techniques in modification of spasmodic torticollis, Neurology 23:1241, 1973.
28. Connolly, K, and Jones, B: Developmental study of afferent-reafferent integration, Br J Psychol 61:259, 1970.
29. DeVries, HA: Efficiency of electrical activity as a physiological measure of the functional state of muscle tissue, Am J Phys Med 47:10, 1968.
30. Eccles, JC: A reevaluation of cerebral function in man. In Desmedt, JE, editor: New developments in electromyography, vol 3, Basel, 1973, S Karger.
31. Engel, BT: The treatment of fecal incontinence by operant conditioning, Automedica 2:101, London, 1978.
32. Engel, BT, Nikoomanesh, P, and Schuster, MM: Operant conditioning of rectosphincteric responses in the treatment of fecal incontinence, N Engl J Med 290:646, 1974.
33. Fahn, S: Biochemistry of the basal ganglia. In Eldridge, R, and Fahn, S, editors: Advances in neurology: dystonia, New York, 1976, Raven Press.
34. Gaarder, KR, and Montgomery, PS: Clinical biofeedback: a procedural manual, Baltimore, 1977, Williams & Wilkins Co.
35. Gans, BM, and Noordergraaf, A: Voluntary skeletal muscles: a unifying theory on the relationship of their electrical and mechanical activities, Arch Phys Med Rehabil 56:194, 1975.
36. Gianutsos, J, et al: EMG feedback in the rehabilitation of upper extremity function: single case studies of chronic hemiplegics, Int Neuropsychol Soc Bull 1979, p 12.
37. Goodgold, J: Rehabilitation medicine: affirmations and actions, Arch Phys Med Rehabil 61:7, 1980.
38. Goodwin, GM, McCloskey, DI, and Mathews, PBL: The contribution of muscles' afferents to kinesthetics shown by vibration-induced illusions of movement and by the effect of paralyzing afferents, Brain 95:705, 1972.
39. Granit, R: Basis of motor control, New York, 1970, Academic Press.
40. Granit, R: Constant errors in the execution and appreciation of movement, Brain 95:649, 1972.
41. Herman, R: Augmented sensory feedback in control of limb movement. In Field, WS, and Leavitt, LA, editors: Neural organization and its relevance to prosthetics, New York, 1973, Intercontinental Medical Books.
42. Holstege, G, Kuypers, HGJM, and Decker, JJ: The organization of bulbar fiber connections to the trigeminal facial and hypoglossal motor nuclei (anteradiographic study), Brain 100:265, 1977.
43. Inglis, J, et al: Electromyographic feedback and physical therapy of the hemiplegic upper limb, Arch Phys Med Rehabil 65:755, 1984.
44. Jacobson, E: Progressive relaxation, Chicago, 1938, University of Chicago Press.
45. Jankel, WR: Electromyographic feedback in spasmodic torticollis, Am Clin Biofeedback 1:28, 1978.

46. Kamiya, J: Operant conditioning of EEG alpha-rhythm and some of its reported effects on consciousness. In Tart, CT, editor: Altered states of consciousness: a book of readings, New York, 1969, John Wiley & Sons.

47. Kaplan, BJ: Biofeedback in epileptics: equivocal relationship of reinforced EEG frequency to seizure reduction, Epilepsia 16:477, 1975.

48. Korein, J, and Brudny, J: Integrated EMG feedback in the management of spasmodic torticollis and focal dystonia: a prospective study of 80 patients. In Yahr, MD, editor: The basal ganglia, New York, 1976, Raven Press.

49. Lashley, KS: The accuracy of movement in the absence of excitation from the moving organ, Am J Physiol 43:169, 1917.

50. Lubar, JF, et al: EEG operant conditioning in intractable epileptics, Arch Neurol 38:700, 1981.

51. Marinacci, AA, and Horande, M: Electromyogram in neuromuscular reeducation, Bull Los Angeles Neurol Soc 25:57, 1960.

52. Marsden, CD: The problem of adult-onset idiopathic torsion dystonia and other isolated dyskinesias in adult life. In Eldridge, R, and Fahn, S, editors: Advances in neurology, ed 14, New York, 1976, Raven Press.

53. Miles, FA, and Evarts, EV: Concepts of motor organization, Ann Rev Psychol 30:327, 1979.

54. Miller, NE: Learning of visceral and glandular responses, Science 163:434, 1969.

55. Miller, NE, and Dworkin, BR: Homeostasis as goal-directed learned behaviour. In Thomson, RF, Hicks, LH, and Shvyrkov, VB, editors: Neural mechanisms of goal-directed behaviour, New York, 1980, Academic Press.

56. Mulder, T, and Hulstyn, W: Sensory feedback therapy and theoretical knowledge of motor control and learning, Am J Phys Med 65:226, 1984.

57. Newell, KM: Skill learning. In Holding, D, editor: Human skills, London, 1981, John Wiley & Sons.

58. Noback, RC, and Demarest, RJ: The human nervous system, New York, 1975, McGraw-Hill Book Co.

59. Numan, R: Cortical-limbic mechanisms and response control: a theoretical review, Physiol Psychol 6:445, 1978.

59a Perry, JD, Hullett, LT, and Bollinger, JR: Urinary incontinence treated by EMG biofeedback method, Gerontologist 28:209, 1987.

60. Phillips, CG: Changing concepts of the precentral motor area. In Eccles, JC, editor: Brain and conscious experience, New York, 1966, Springer-Verlag.

61. Rosner, BS: Recovery of function and localization of function in historical perspective. In Stein, DG, Rosen, JJ, and Butters, N, editors: Plasticity and recovery of function in the central nervous system, New York, 1974, Academic Press.

62. Schmidt, RA: The schema as a solution to some persistent problems in motor learning theory. In Stelmach, GE, editor: Motor control: issues and trends, New York, 1976, Academic Press.

63. Schmidt, RA: Motor control and learning: a behavioral emphasis, Champaign, Ill, 1982, Human Kinetics Publishing.

64. Schultz, JJ, and Luthe, W: Autogenic training, New York, 1959, Grune & Stratton.

65. Scott, RW, Kelso, JA, and Stelmach, GE: Central and peripheral mechanisms in motor control. In Stelmach, GE, editor: Motor control: issues and trends, New York, 1976, Academic Press.

66. Shahani, BT: Control of voluntary activity in man and physiological principles of biofeedback. In Shahani, BT, editor: Central EMG, Stoneham, Mass, 1984, Butterworth.

67. Shahani, BT, Connors, L, and Mohr, JP: Electromyocgraphic audio-visual effect in the motor performance in patients with lesions of the central nervous system, Arch Phys Med Rehabil 58:519, 1977.

68. Sokolov, AN: Studies of the speech mechanisms of thinking. In Cole, M, and Maltzman, I, editors: A handbook of contemporary Soviet psychology, New York, 1969, Basic Books.

69. Stennert, E, and Limberg, CH: Central connections between fifth, seventh and twelfth cranial nerves and their clinical significance. In Graham, MD, and House, VM, editors: Disorders of the facial nerve, New York, 1982, Raven Press.

70. Sterman, MB, and Bowersox, SS: Sensorimotor electroencephalogram rhythmic activity: a functional gate mechanism, Sleep 4:408, 1981.

71. Sterman, MB, and Friar, L: Suppression of seizures in an epileptic following sensorimotor EEG feedback training, Electroencephalogr Clin Neurophysiol 33:89, 1972.

72. Sterman, MB, Goodman, SJ, and Kovalesky, RA: Effects of sensorimotor EEG feedback training on seizure susceptibility in the Rhesus monkey, Exp Neurol 62:735, 1978.

73. Surwit, RS, Shapiro, D, and Good, MI: A comparison of cardiovascular biofeedback, neuromuscular biofeedback, and meditation in the treatment of borderline essential hypertension, J Consult Clin Psychol 48:252, 1978.

74. White, L, and Tursky, B, editors: Clinical biofeedback: efficacy and mechanisms, New York, 1982, Guilford Press.

75. Whitehead, WE, Burgio, KL, and Engel, BT: Biofeedback treatment of fecal incontinence in geriatric patients, J Am Geriatr Soc 33:320, 1985.

76. Whiting, HTA: Dimensions of control in motor learning. In Stelmach, GE, and Requin, J, editors: Tutorials in motor behaviour, Amsterdam, 1980, North Holland Publishers.

77. Wolf, SL: Essential consideration in the use of EMG biofeedback, Phys Ther 58:25, 1978.

78. Wolf, SL, Baker, MP, and Kelly, JL: EMG biofeedback in stroke: one-year follow-up on effects of patient characteristics, Arch Phys Med Rehabil 61:351, 1980.

79. Zeman, W: Pathology of the torsion dystonias: dystonia musculorum deformans, Neurology 20:79, 1970.

CHAPTER 24

Late complications of poliomyelitis

LAURO S. HALSTEAD

This chapter deals with the late effects of poliomyelitis. Although acute polio is virtually extinct in the United States, a sizable number of adults alive today contracted paralytic polio before the Salk and Sabin vaccines were introduced between 1955 and 1960.

In the past, residual motor loss from polio was generally considered a chronic, stable lesion. Following the acute illness and a period of rehabilitation, patients eventually achieved a plateau of neurologic and functional recovery that was believed to remain essentially static more or less indefinitely. Even within the field of physical medicine and rehabilitation, polio was classified as a *static* disease as recently as 1982.[22] For the majority of persons who had paralytic polio years ago, this may be true. However, it is definitely not true for many others. As many as one fourth of all paralytic polio survivors experience new health problems that appear to be related to their earlier illness. Typically these problems occur 30 to 40 years after the acute episode of polio and include excessive fatigue, progressive weakness, pain, and functional loss. Persons most likely to develop these problems had fairly severe polio at onset with good neurologic recovery that allowed them to lead physically active lives. The cause for the new neurologic changes is unknown, but it appears to be related to a progressive dysfunction of the motor units manifested by a deterioration of individual peripheral axon sprouts.

HISTORICAL BACKGROUND

For more than 100 years it has been recognized that late sequelae of polio occur in some patients many years after their initial illness. The first descriptions appeared in 1875 when three patients were reported in the French literature.[7,9,32] All of the cases involved young men who had had paralytic polio in infancy and developed significant new weakness and atrophy as young adults. The weakness and atrophy occurred not only in previously affected muscles but, in at least two instances, also in previously unaffected muscles. All of the subjects had physically demanding jobs that required strength and repetitive activities. In a commentary on one of the cases,[32] the great nineteenth century French neuropathologist Jean Martin Charcot suggested several hypotheses for these new changes that are still relevant today. He believed that a previous disease of the spinal cord might leave a patient more susceptible to a subsequent spinal disorder and that the new weakness was due to overuse of the involved limbs.

Since those initial reports there has been only sporadic interest in the phenomenon of late sequelae. In the century following Charcot's observations, fewer than 35 published reports, which altogether described fewer than 250 cases, appeared.[36] As with the first subjects, these reports described new problems that included weakness, atrophy, and fasciculations occurring up to 71 years after an acute and generally severe attack of paralytic polio. The neurologic changes were most commonly diagnosed as a form of progressive muscular atrophy, although many other diagnostic terms such as chronic anterior poliomyelitis, late motor neuron degeneration, and forme fruste amyotrophic lateral sclerosis were used.[6,23,26]

Why the late sequelae of polio remained an obscure and largely unexplored area of medicine until recently is not entirely clear. Few diseases are as widely prevalent in the world or have been as intensively investigated. Part of the explanation may be that over the years polio has been viewed as a classic example of an acute viral infectious disease. Therefore most of the energy and resources were directed at early management and prevention. With widespread use of the vaccines, polio quickly became a medical oddity in the industrialized world, and interest and funding in polio-related problems waned. In addition, the big epidemics in this century did not occur until the 1940s and 1950s. Since new neurologic changes tend to appear 30 to 40 years past the onset, many thousands of polio survivors are only now experiencing new problems related to polio. By sheer weight of numbers they are finally attracting attention from the medical and lay communities.

EPIDEMIOLOGIC ASPECTS

Accurate figures about the number of persons who have new polio-related problems are not available and probably never will be. The Household Survey of Disabling Conditions conducted by the National Center for Health Statistics in 1977 found that over 250,000 persons had residual paralysis from polio.[27] Although there are several reasons to believe this figure is low, it provides a rough approximation until a more detailed survey planned for 1987 is completed. In the meantime an unknown number of the polio population have died since the first survey in 1977. However, over the past decade there has also been an unknown—and largely unexpected—increase in the number of polio survivors in the United States resulting from the influx of affected immigrants, refugees, and illegal aliens from Southeast Asia and Latin America.

In 1984, researchers at the Mayo Clinic conducted a population-based study of residents in Rochester, Minnesota. They found that one in four persons who had a history of paralytic polio was experiencing new problems, probably related to the earlier illness. If the Mayo Clinic study is representative of the experience of polio survivors elsewhere in the United States, approximately 60,000 persons in this country are currently experiencing new polio-related problems and may be in need of rehabilitation services.* It is reasonable to assume that the numbers experiencing new problems will increase as the polio population ages.

PATHOPHYSIOLOGY
Acute poliomyelitis

Knowledge of the pathophysiology of acute polio is necessary to understand the possible causes for the new neurologic changes and to provide a rational basis for their management.

Acute polio is caused by RNA viruses of the enterovirus group. Because the three known viruses are antigenically distinct, infection with one does not provide protection against the others. The major route of infection is through the mouth. Following multiplication in the pharynx and intestine, the virus penetrates the intestinal wall and travels in the blood to all parts of the body. The vast majority of infected individuals remain asymptomatic or experience a self-limited illness characterized by fever and gastrointes-

tinal symptoms for several days. In 1% to 5% of persons the virus invades the spinal cord, where it has a predilection for motor neurons in the lateral anterior horns, resulting in a variable amount of paralysis. Regardless of the extent of paralysis, however, the virus is widely disseminated, typically infecting over 95% of the motor neurons. Following this invasion, cells either die or shed the virus and regain a normal morphologic appearance. Whether these recovered motor neurons remain more susceptible to insults later in life is unknown, but if they do, it might provide one explanation for delayed motor neuron dysfunction.

After the virus invades the central nervous system, the extent of neurologic and functional recovery is determined by three major factors: the number of motor neurons that survive unimpaired, the number of motor neurons that recover and resume their normal function, and the number of motor neurons that develop terminal axon sprouts to reinnervate muscle fibers left orphaned by the death of their original motor neurons. The phenomenon of terminal axon sprouting (Figure 24-1) makes it possible for an uninvolved or recovered motor neuron to "adopt" up to five additional muscle fibers for every muscle cell innervated originally.[11] A single motor neuron that originally innervated 100 muscle fibers might eventually innervate 400 to 500 fibers. Thus the size of many motor units increases significantly following acute polio, allowing fewer motor neurons to do the work of many. This mechanism of neurophysiologic compensation is so effective that up to 50% of the original number of motor neurons can be lost without the muscle losing clinically normal strength.[33] After 30 to 40 years these giant motor units appear to lose the ability to sustain so many fibers, and the terminal axon sprouts and individual neuromuscular junctions may gradually deteriorate, so the number of muscle fibers driven by a given motor neuron declines.[37]

Chronic poliomyelitis

The pathologic changes that underlie the late complications of polio are incompletely understood. However, at least three processes, singly or in combination, may play a role in any individual patient: motor unit dysfunction, musculoskeletal overuse, and musculoskeletal disuse. Each may produce the cardinal symptom of progressive weakness. These three etiologic mechanisms and their associated complications and potential interactions are shown schematically in Figure 24-2. Thus far the neurologic or motor unit changes have attracted the most attention, but in the final analysis they may not be more prevalent or damaging than nonneurologic changes. The pathologic mechanism of musculoskeletal *disuse* and the resultant complications of weakness, contractures, atrophy, diminished endurance, and so on are probably similar to the disuse phenomenon, which has been extensively studied and described in other groups of patients who have neuromuscular lesions or lead sedentary lives. The pathologic process of musculoskeletal *overuse* is not as

---

*An update of the Mayo Clinic study suggests that 60,000 may be low. A comprehensive follow-up evaluation of a random sample of the original respondents showed that 66% were experiencing new weakness.[39]

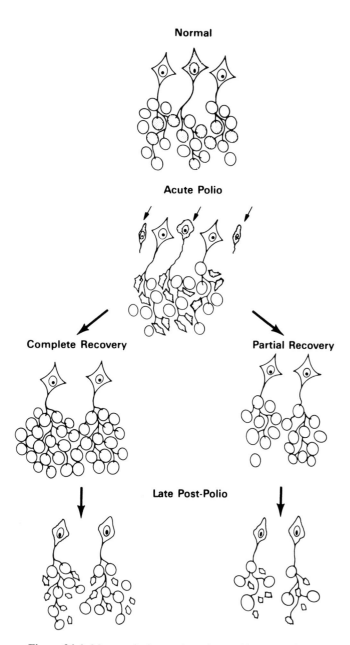

Figure 24-1. Motor unit changes in patients with acute and chronic poliomyelitis. Diagrammatic changes in motor units of patients after acute polio and immediate recovery and many years later (postpolio). Death of anterior horn cells after acute polio is followed by complete or partial recovery by reinnervation and sprouting of terminal axons from neighboring healthy motor neurons, which now supply a larger number of muscle fibers. These "overworking" anterior horn cells may succumb earlier to aging process, resulting in noticeable weakness (late postpolio) because they control a greater than normal percentage of muscle function. (Modified from Dalakas, MC, et al: Neuromuscular symptoms in patients with old poliomyelitis: clinical, virological and immunological studies. In Halstead, LS, and Wiechers, DO: Late complications of poliomyelitis, Miami, 1985, Symposia Foundation.)

well understood. Evidence based on clinical and animal studies with a variety of lesions including polio suggests a relationship between muscle damage, the intensity and duration of exercise, and the number of motor units.[20] The extent to which a primary muscle defect may contribute to late-onset weakness in some polio patients is unknown. Regardless of the cause of weakness, however, many of these patients experience an overuse phenomenon from chronic mechanical strain on joints, ligaments, and soft tissues that have been improperly or inadequately supported for 30 or more years. The consequence of this overuse creates a self-perpetuating chain reaction of symptoms and further complications until effective interventions are implemented.

The cause of apparently new motor unit dysfunction in polio survivors many years after their acute illness is unknown. However, there are a number of possible theories and evidence is accumulating to support several of these. One theory suggests that there may be persistence of the polio virus or viral fragments that have lain dormant and then are reactivated by some unknown trigger mechanism. Although it has been shown that polio virus can cause persistent asymptomatic infection in animals,[25] this phenomenon has not yet been demonstrated in human studies. Another theory suggests that an immunologic mechanism may play a role. Preliminary evidence for this has been described by Dalakas and co-workers, who found a lymphocytic response in muscle biopsy specimens and IgG oligoclonal bands in the cerebrospinal fluid (CSF) of some symptomatic patients. By contrast, no oligoclonal bands were found in the CSF of a group of asymptomatic patients.[12] However, these findings have yet to be confirmed by other investigators, and patients generally have not responded to immunosuppressant therapy. A third possibility concerns changes in the spinal cord that might compromise motor neuron function. A recent report by Pezeshkpour and Dalakas[29] described active inflammatory gliosis, neuronal chromatolysis, and axonal spheroids in the spinal cords of polio patients who died many years later of other causes. Whether these changes represent a primary lesion in the cord or a response to a lesion in the distal axon is unknown.

Another hypothesis is that the new neuromuscular changes are caused by premature aging of the polio patient. Normally, significant attrition of motor neurons does not occur until the seventh decade.[34] However, in polio survivors with a greatly reduced population of anterior horn cells, the loss of a relatively few giant motor units might result in a disproportionate loss of clinical function. Although this hypothesis is intuitively attractive and may in fact explain new weakness in some individuals, muscle biopsy studies for the most part have failed to show significant muscle group atrophy and other changes that would be consistent with new loss of whole motor units. Furthermore, if motor neuron loss with advancing age were a major factor, one would expect a steady increase in new difficulties as the population

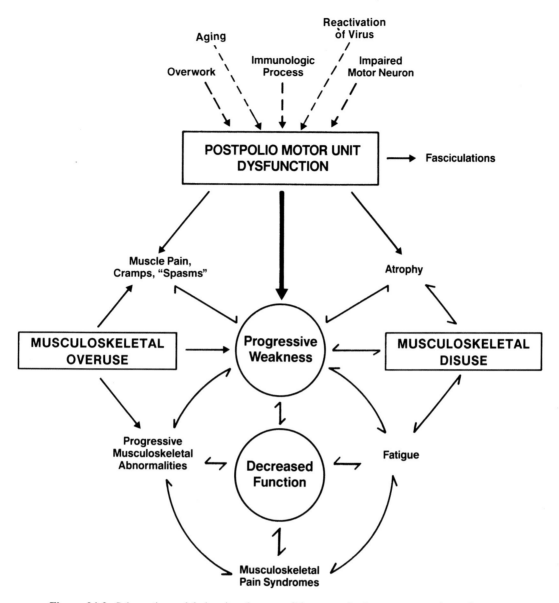

Figure 24-2. Schematic model showing three possible causes for late neuromuscular and musculoskeletal complications of polio and their interactions.

at risk becomes progressively older. In fact, several studies have failed to show a positive relationship between the onset of new weakness and chronologic age.[19,39] To the contrary, these studies suggest that it is the *length* of the interval between onset of polio and the appearance of new symptoms that is a determining variable.

Finally, a fifth theory, and the most plausible in light of the limited information available at this time, suggests that the new clinical changes are a result of motor neuron overwork that eventually produces neuronal dysfunction. This theory is based on several assumptions and observations. The giant motor units characteristic of postpolio reinnervated muscles create an increased metabolic demand on the remaining motor neurons. According to the theory, the in-

creased metabolic load results in neurologic dysfunction after a critical number of years. This concept of overuse is supported indirectly by several clinical studies and electromyographic (EMG) data. In a group of 17 patients evaluated in a postpolio clinic, Maynard[24] observed that new weakness occurred more commonly in the legs than the arms. Similarly, in the Mayo Clinic study, Windebank and co-workers[39] found that, in muscles with similar involvement at onset of polio, new weakness occurred more commonly in the weight-bearing muscles of the legs than the non-weight-bearing muscles of the arms. Further, new weakness was more likely to occur in limbs most affected by the original disease. In another study, Perry and co-workers[28] observed that, in postpolio subjects with approximately the same re-

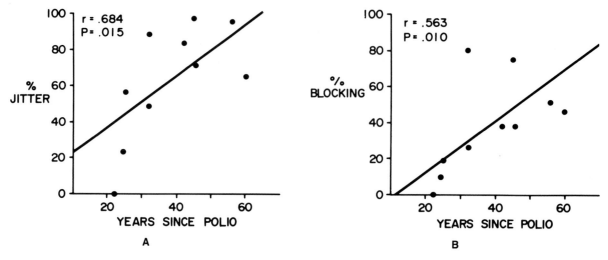

Figure 24-3. A, Relationship between percentage of motor unit recordings with abnormal jitter found in each patient with polio and number of years elapsed since attack of polio. Analysis by product-moment correlation and rank order correlation coefficients showed significant association (r = .684, p = .15) between the percentage of jitter found and number of years since attack of polio. **B,** Relationship between percentage of motor unit recordings demonstrating blocking found in each patient with polio and number of years elapsed since attack of polio. Analysis by product-moment correlation and rank order correlation coefficients showed significant association (r = .563, p = .010) between percentage of blocking and number of years since attack of polio. (From Wiechers, DO, and Hubbell, SL: Muscle Nerve 4:524, 1981.)

sidual loss, symptomatic polio survivors had a less efficient gait with an increase in intensity and in duration of extensor muscle contraction in the legs when compared with those who were asymptomatic.

Electrophysiologic studies by Wiechers, Dalakas, and others[12,38] have shown neuromuscular transmission abnormalities suggesting that the giant motor neurons may be unable to sustain the metabolic demands of all their sprouts indefinitely. This results in a slow deterioration of individual terminals and a dropoff of reinnervated muscle fibers. As more muscle fibers are lost, slowly progressive weakness becomes clinically apparent. Figure 24-3 shows an increase in jitter and blocking on single fiber EMG with increased time after polio in a group of asymptomatic subjects, which is consistent with the theory of a gradual deterioration of individual peripheral nerve terminals. These observations are in contrast to static nerve injuries where electrophysiologic stability is achieved within 12 to 18 months after reinnervation.

Related to the "overwork" theory is the possibility that the original viral attack of the anterior horn cells left some motor neurons functional but impaired and thus more vulnerable to dysfunction with the passage of time. Tomlinson noted many smaller-than-normal neurons in the spinal cords of persons surviving long after a polio attack. Based on this observation and the work of Bodian, he concluded that any cell invaded by the polio virus is likely to be permanently affected, particularly in relation to "protein synthetic mech-

Table 24-1. Most common new health and functional problems for 132 consecutive patients with confirmed polio

Problem	Number	Percent
Health		
Fatigue	117	89
Muscle pain	93	71
Joint pain	93	71
Weakness		
Previously affected muscles	91	69
Previously unaffected muscles	66	50
Cold intolerance	38	29
Atrophy	37	28
Cramps	24	18
Fasciculations	16	12
Activities of daily living		
Walking	84	64
Climbing stairs	80	61
Dressing	23	17

From Halstead, LS, and Rossi, CD: Post-polio syndrome: clinical experience with 132 consecutive outpatients. In Halstead, LS, and Wiechers, DO, editors: Research and clinical aspects of the late effects of poliomyelitis, White Plains, NY, 1987, March of Dimes Birth Defects Foundation BD:OAS 23(4):121-134, 1987, with permission from the copyright holder.

anisms."[35] Thus it seems possible that some motor neurons experienced an injury at the time of the acute infection, which is exacerbated by many years of increased metabolic demand to sustain a greatly enlarged motor unit.

CLINICAL FEATURES

In response to the increased recognition of new health problems in the polio population, a number of postpolio clinics have opened in the United States over the past few years. The observations reported by these clinics and in a number of research studies have clarified the major clinical features presented by postpolio patients. The experience obtained in the Post Polio Clinic at the Institute for Rehabilitation and Research in Houston[18] is fairly typical and is summarized in Tables 24-1 to 24-5. Table 24-1 lists the most common new health and functional problems in 132 consecutive persons seen over a 1-year period. All patients were carefully evaluated to confirm the diagnosis of old polio and rule out nonpolio causes for their new symptoms. The majority of patients were women (66%), white (92%),

and middle-aged (median age 45 years, with a range from 24 to 86 years). Most were married, well educated, working outside the home, and about 35 to 40 years past the onset of acute polio. The median age at onset of polio was 7 years (range 3 months to 44 years) with a median interval of 31 years between onset of polio and onset of new health problems. A similar interval is found in other studies, but the range has been reported to extend from two to eight decades.[12,19]

In general, the patients most at risk for developing new problems are those who experienced more severe polio at onset, although some patients with typical postpolio symptoms had seemingly very mild polio with excellent clinical recovery. The age at onset of polio is also a factor in the development of late-onset problems. Thus persons who were older when they contracted polio appear to be at an increased risk for new neurologic symptoms. The onset of these new problems is most commonly insidious, but in many persons they are precipitated by specific events such as a minor accident, fall, period of bed rest, or weight gain. Patients characteristically say that a similar event several years earlier

Table 24-2. The six most common problem areas for 132 postpolio patients

Number of problems	Number of persons	Percent of persons	New health problems*					
			F	P	W	FL	CI	A
2	11	8	4	7	4	3	2	0
3	22	17	17	15	14	11	1	2
4	51	39	48	46	45	45	4	7
5	36	27	33	32	33	32	18	16
6	12	9	12	12	12	12	12	12
TOTAL	132	100	117	113	110	103	38	37

From Halstead, LS, and Rossi, CD: Post-polio syndrome: clinical experience with 132 consecutive outpatients. In Halstead, LS, and Wiechers, DO, editors: Research and clinical aspects of the late effects of poliomyelitis, White Plains, NY, 1987, March of Dimes Birth Defects Foundation BD:OAS 23(4):121-134, 1987, with permission from the copyright holder.
*F, Fatigue; P, pain in muscles or joints; W, weakness in previously affected or unaffected muscles; FL, functional loss in walking, climbing stairs, dressing, and so on; CI, cold intolerance; A, new atrophy.

Table 24-3. Prevalence of chronic pain by method of locomotion in 114 postpolio patients

Method of locomotion	Number	Number with pain	Percentage with pain
Ambulatory, no brace (independent)	67	56	84
Ambulatory with brace (independent)	12	11	92
Ambulatory with crutches (independent)	21	21	100
Wheelchair locomotion (independent)	7	7	100
Wheelchair locomotion (need personal assistance)	7	7	100
TOTAL	114	102	90

From Smith, LK, and McDermott, K: Pain in post poliomyelitis addressing causes versus treating effects. In Halstead, LS, and Wiechers, DO, editors: Research and clinical aspects of the late effects of poliomyelitis, White Plains, NY, 1987, March of Dimes Birth Defects Foundation BD:OAS 23(4):121-134, 1987, with permission from the copyright holder.

Table 24-4. Location of chronic pain by method of locomotion in 114 postpolio patients

	Number	Percentage
Independent ambulators with or without lower extremity orthoses	79	69
Back	37	47
Hip	19	24
Diffuse lower extremity	18	22
Other (neck, shoulder, knee, ankle)	31	39
Locomotion performance using crutches or wheelchairs	35	31
Neck and shoulder	18	51
Back	13	37
Glenohumeral joint	11	31
Elbow	6	17
Wrist and hand	9	26
Other (lower extremity and head)	15	43

From Smith, LK, and McDermott, K: Pain in post poliomyelitis addressing causes versus treating effects. In Halstead, LS, and Wiechers, DO, editors: Research and clinical aspects of the late effects of poliomyelitis, White Plains, NY, 1987, March of Dimes Birth Defects Foundation BD:OAS 23(4):121-134, 1987, with permission from the copyright holder.

Table 24-5. Clinical and laboratory findings in late postpolio and amyotrophic lateral sclerosis

Finding	Late postpolio	ALS
Clinical		
Weakness	Asymmetric, focal	Often asymmetric, generalized
Bulbar signs-symptoms	Rare	Common
Fasciculations	Occasional	Common
Long tract signs	Very rare	Very common
Sensory changes	Absent	Absent
Prognosis	Slow progression: 1%/yr	Rapid downhill course: death in 3-5 yr
Laboratory		
DNA repair	Normal	Abnormal
CPK	Occasionally elevated	Frequently elevated
EMG		
Fibrillations and positive sharp waves	Increased	Greatly increased
Fasciculations	Increased	Greatly increased
MUP	Often >10 mV	Rarely >10 mV
Fiber density	Greatly increased	Increased
Jitter/blocking	Increased	Increased
Neurogenic jitter	Rare	Often present
Muscle biopsy	Group atrophy uncommon; inflammation in 40%	Group atrophy common; scattered angulated fibers; inflammation rare

Modified from Dalakas, MC: Amyotrophic lateral sclerosis and post-polio: differences and similarities. In Halstead, LS, and Wiechers, DO, editors: Research and clinical aspects of the late effects of poliomyelitis, White Plains, NY, 1987, March of Dimes Birth Defects Foundation BD:OAS 23(4):121-134, 1987, with permission from the copyright holder.

would not have caused the same decline in health and function. Likewise, new problems may begin when coexisting medical problems such as diabetes develop or worsen.

Although the frequency distribution of the problems listed in Table 24-1 may differ from clinic to clinic, there is a common set of complaints quite specific to postpolio patients. Further, as shown in Table 24-2, often a cluster of problems occurs. In the Houston patients the most common cluster (experienced by 39%) was excessive fatigue, pain, weakness, and functional loss. New atrophy was relatively uncommon (28%); it did not occur as an isolated finding but tended to be present when there were four or more other problems.

Fatigue

The fatigue is sometimes focal but more typically generalized and is usually described as overwhelming exhaustion accompanied by a marked change in the level of energy, endurance, and sometimes mental alertness. It is typically brought on by an accumulation of activities that previously had been carried out on a daily basis without special effort or noticeable sequelae. Commonly it occurs in late afternoon or early evening and is described by some people as like hitting a wall. When it occurs, the individuals must stop what they are doing, rest, and if possible take a short nap.

Pain

The pain occurs in the muscles or joints or both. The muscle pain is sometimes described as "close to the surface" and is occasionally associated with hypersensitivity and a crawling or cramping sensation, especially at night. More often, however, it occurs as a deep, aching pain that many patients say is similar to the muscle pain experienced during their acute illness years earlier. These muscle pains are often aggravated by physical activity and cold temperature. The joint pains are also commonly associated with specific physical activities such as weight bearing but are only rarely accompanied by swelling and inflammation. These pains are usually improved by conservative measures such as decreased activity, better support of unstable joints, improved biomechanics of the body during common daily activities, and low doses of anti-inflammatory agents.

Weakness and functional loss

New weakness may appear in muscles previously affected or muscles believed to be previously spared. However, the weakness is usually greatest in the muscles most severely involved in the initial illness. Diminished functional capacity tends to parallel the muscle weakness and can be dramatic if functional reserve was marginal. One of the characteristics of many persons with polio was their ability to appear normal or function at an extraordinarily high level of performance on relatively few good muscle groups. This was possible because of the random, scattered nature of the motor deficits and the body's uncanny ability to compensate with unconventional muscle and joint function. In this situation, then, late-onset weakness of a critical muscle often leads to disruption of a delicate balance that has been maintained for years, leading to a disproportionate amount of functional loss. Persons with involvement of one or both legs may have increased difficulty in walking, standing, climbing stairs, or other endurance activities. Individuals with presumably normal upper extremities who have been using crutches and "walking" on their arms for years may find that ambulating, transfers, driving a car, or even dressing is more taxing and the time to recover takes longer than formerly. Persons with initial respiratory weakness may develop new difficulty with breathing, especially at night or with exertion.

"POLIO PERSONALITY"

Many health-care workers who were involved with large numbers of polio patients during the big epidemics in the 1940s and 1950s have commented on the existence of a "polio personality." Whether this was a function of social circumstances, the individual's response to the disease, or some kind of natural selection also associated with certain behavioral characteristics is unknown. However, a genetic predisposition to polio has been shown.[21] In addition, persons with polio tend to perform at high levels in many areas. For example, they are employed full time at four times the rate of the general disabled population,[8] they have more years of formal education on average than the general able-bodied population,[15] and they take on marriage and family responsibilities at approximately the same rate as persons who are not disabled.[5] Furthermore, all of these individuals overcame a serious and often life-changing illness. Although the behaviors that were learned in dealing with that illness may have varied from individual to individual, they were behaviors that helped each individual survive—which is one of the reasons so many polio patients call themselves survivors. These behaviors include independence, patience, industriousness, detachment, creativity, and denial of limitations. Because they were successful once, these same behaviors are likely to be used later in life in coping with other challenges and illness. As a group, polio survivors tend to be competent, hard-driving, time-conscious overachievers who have high standards for themselves and others. In a questionnaire study of type A behavior by Bruno and Frick,[5] they found that the mean type A score for polio survivors was significantly higher than that reported for a nondisabled control population. What is more, the polio group exhibited a high rate of symptoms associated with chronic stress, which Bruno and Frick believed may have initiated or exacerbated some of the new health problems.

EVALUATION, DIFFERENTIAL DIAGNOSIS, AND DIAGNOSIS
Evaluation

Because of the number and diversity of problems presented by postpolio patients, an interdisciplinary evaluation by several persons is desirable. In addition to the physician, we have found it helpful to include a physical therapist and social worker as part of the initial evaluation team with referral to other disciplines and medical specialists as needed. Because postpolio-related complications are diagnosed by *exclusion,* it is essential that every patient receive a careful history and physical examination, along with appropriate laboratory, x-ray, and diagnostic studies to rule out other medical, orthopedic, or neurologic conditions that might be causing or aggravating the symptoms. A psychosocial evaluation is invariably helpful, together with an assessment of function, gait, and orthotic needs and a baseline measure of strength and endurance of key muscle groups.

For most patients an electromyogram/nerve conduction study (EMG/NCV) is useful to help confirm the presence of polio, identify possible subclinical involvement, establish a baseline, and exclude other neurologic conditions. However, a standard battery of screening tests (SMA 24, thyroid panel, Tensilon test, and so on), used on a routine basis, is generally not helpful or cost effective. Some clinicians monitor serum creatinine phosphokinase (CPK) levels on a regular basis, but the diagnostic and clinical implications, if any, are still not clear. Patients who had respiratory involvement initially and have a history of pulmonary disease should have pulmonary function studies and, if indicated, arterial blood gas studies.

Finally, all attempts to find laboratory tests or diagnostic studies that distinguish the symptomatic from the asymptomatic postpolio patient have been unsuccessful. Despite the growing body of evidence suggesting that the major pathologic process is motor unit dysfunction, there is still no objective method to predict who might become symptomatic in the future or to monitor the progress of the underlying disease in the subject who has already become symptomatic. Specifically, no serologic, enzymatic, or electrodiagnostic test has been helpful to separate the symptomatic from the asymptomatic groups.

Differential diagnosis

Three major criteria should be established to make a diagnosis of a polio-related problem: objective evidence of a prior episode of paralytic polio, a characteristic pattern of recovery and neurologic stability preceding the onset of new problems, and exclusion of other medical, orthopedic, and neurologic conditions that might cause the symptoms. The

first two criteria are usually easier to satisfy than the third. The diagnosis of paralytic polio can almost always be confirmed with the following information: a credible history of an acute, febrile illness resulting in motor loss and no sensory loss; the occurrence of a similar illness in family or neighborhood contacts; the presence of focal, asymmetric weakness or atrophy on examination; EMG changes of chronic denervation compatible with prior anterior horn cell disease; and examination of the original medical records whenever possible. The changes on routine EMG compatible with prior polio include increased amplitude and duration of motor unit action potentials, an increase in the percentage of polyphasic motor units, and a decrease in the number of motor units on maximum recruitment. Positive sharp waves and fibrillations are present occasionally, and less commonly fasciculations may be seen.

In patients with late complications of polio the pattern of events from onset of polio to onset of new problems is so characteristic that when it is absent the diagnosis should be seriously questioned. The pattern generally consists of four stages as shown in Figure 24-4: paralytic polio in childhood or later in life, partial to fairly complete neurologic and functional recovery, a period of functional and neurologic stability lasting many years (usually 20 or more), and the gradual or abrupt onset of one or more of the new health problems listed in Table 24-1. Most students of postpolio syndrome agree that one of the new problems should be *nondisuse weakness*. However, for practical reasons, nondisuse weakness may be difficult to document, although frequently it can be inferred from the onset of diminished function despite maintenance of the usual level and intensity of activity.

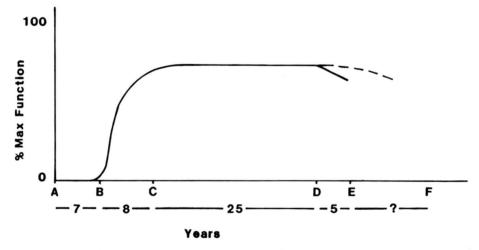

Figure 24-4. Natural history of polio based on data from patients evaluated in the Post Polio Clinic, Houston, Texas. *A,* Birth; *B,* onset of polio; *C,* maximum recovery; *D,* onset of new health problems; *E,* time of evaluation; *F,* death. (From Halstead, LS, and Rossi, CD: Post polio syndrome: clinical experience with 132 consecutive outpatients. In Halstead, LS, and Wiechers, DO, editors: Research and clinical aspects of the late effects of poliomyelitis, White Plains, NY, 1987, March of Dimes Birth Defects Foundation BD:OAS 23[4]:121-134, 1987, with permission from the copyright holder.)

There are several dilemmas in making a diagnosis by exclusion in the postpolio population. First, the symptoms are frequently so general that ruling out all possible causes is impractical and can be prohibitively expensive. Second, coexisting medical, orthopedic, and neurologic conditions may be present and can produce a similar set of overlapping signs and symptoms, as shown in Figure 24-5. Examples of such conditions are compression neuropathies, radiculopathies, degenerative arthritis, disc disease, obesity, anemia, diabetes, thyroid disease, and depression. In addition, as indicated in Figure 24-2, once a problem such as weakness occurs—regardless of the underlying cause—it may initiate a chain reaction of other complications that makes the original problem impossible to identify. Nonetheless, because of the central importance of new weakness in this population and because of its diagnostic and management implications, every effort should be made to *exclude* disuse weakness as a major factor.

Likewise, the role of chronic musculoskeletal wear and tear should be clarified. Many of the problems that appear to be related to "overuse" of weakened muscles, as well as abnormal joint and limb biomechanics, may simply represent the normal consequences of chronic disability and be no more common in postpolio patients than they are in individuals with other neuromuscular diseases. In any event the management of overuse complications is fairly straightforward. Most patients respond favorably to conservative interventions aimed at reducing mechanical stress, supporting weakened muscles, and stabilizing abnormal joint movements. If chronic overuse is the only or major underlying disorder present, such interventions can often slow or prevent further deterioration and possibly lead to a reversal of symptoms and improved function.

Finally, every postpolio patient who develops new symptoms should be carefully evaluated to exclude amyotrophic lateral sclerosis (ALS). Although these diseases have a number of similarities, there are enough dissimilarities that the two can usually be distinguished without great difficulty.[10] Table 24-5 summarizes the major differential features found on clinical and laboratory examination. Over the years there has been considerable speculation that an antecedent infection with polio might be associated with developing ALS later in life.[30,31,40] However, with the recent interest in the late complications of polio and the new understanding about some of the possible pathophysiologic mechanisms, it now seems likely that many of the patients who had polio and later were diagnosed as having a benign form of ALS were misdiagnosed. In a recent reexamination of five patients with a history of both polio and ALS, Brown and Patten[4] concluded that none of the patients would now be classified as having ALS but rather as having postpolio syndrome.

Diagnosis

There is no clear consensus about the most appropriate names or diagnostic labels to use for postpolio patients with new health problems. A number of terms have been proposed, including postpolio syndrome, postpolio muscular atrophy, late effects of polio, and postpolio sequelae. One reason that none of these terms is suitable for all individuals is the lack of specificity in diagnostic criteria. This in turn is related to the absence of any pathognomonic tests and an incomplete understanding of the pathophysiologic factors underlying the presenting complaints. Another reason no single term is suitable for all individuals is that one, two, or more pathologic processes may be present at any one time, producing similar, overlapping symptoms (Figures 24-2 and 24-5). Separating out the origin of each symptom may be not only impractical but impossible, which gives rise to the need for a more general and less precise diagnostic term.

At the present time, postpolio progressive muscular atrophy (PPMA) has the most specific criteria. This term applies to patients who have documented objective evidence of neuromuscular deterioration and have had a muscle biopsy that shows evidence of active denervation in the form of scattered angulated fibers.[12] An alternative term is postpolio motor neuron disease (PPMND), which has the same meaning but has the advantage of being more generic and less restrictive, especially in view of the relative infrequency of new atrophy as part of the clinical picture.

In contrast to PPMA (or PPMND), postpolio syndrome is a more heterogeneous term and therefore more practical in the typical clinical setting. However, it should not be used indiscriminately for every person with a history of paralytic polio and a new complaint. The following are provisional criteria for making this diagnosis:

1. A prior episode of paralytic polio confirmed by history, physical examination, and when possible, EMG
2. A period of neurologic recovery followed by an extended interval of functional stability preceding the onset of new problems; the interval of neurologic and functional stability usually lasts 20 or more years

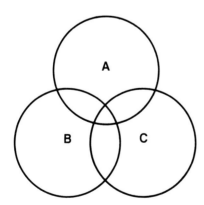

Figure 24-5. Schematic diagram of possible combinations of presenting complaints and their causes found in postpolio patients. *A,* Health problems from neuromuscular dysfunction. *B,* Health problems from orthopedic dysfunction. *C,* Health problems from medical dysfunction.

3. The gradual or abrupt onset of *nondisuse weakness* in previously affected or unaffected muscles, which may or may not be accompanied by other new health problems such as excessive fatigue, muscle pain, joint pain, decreased function, and atrophy

4. Exclusion of medical, orthopedic, and neurologic conditions that might cause the health problems listed above

These criteria are based on the assumption that the major pathologic process involves motor unit dysfunction with a variable contribution from musculoskeletal overuse. For this reason the presence of nondisuse weakness is considered a necessary finding to make this diagnosis. Ideally, then, the diagnosis of postpolio syndrome should be made only after a trial of closely supervised exercise to exclude the possibility of disuse weakness. As new information becomes available about the underlying mechanism(s) that produce late-onset complications, these criteria will undoubtedly change and new terminology be developed to fit the improved understanding.

MANAGEMENT

The proper management of new health problems in polio patients begins with a comprehensive evaluation to exclude other medical, orthopedic, and neurologic diagnoses. The major principles and guidelines for managing the most common problems associated with the late complications of polio are outlined in this section.

Psychologic issues

Everyone who experiences new changes from their polio—no matter how small—is inevitably confronted with a number of psychologic issues. These are often as traumatic and disabling as the physical problems, and they need to be given special attention. Because it is easy to be distracted by more tangible concerns such as a brace or exercise program, the psychologic issues are discussed first with the hope they will be given the same priority in the reader's office. As a rule, postpolio patients experience a wide range of emotions, including denial, anger, frustration, and hopelessness, that need to be identified and dealt with before effective interventions can be implemented. While all of these emotions and others may be present in any one patient, there seem to be three fairly distinct groups representing three different psychologic responses. One group includes patients who simply do not see themselves as handicapped, regardless of the extent of involvement and the presence of obvious deformities. A second group includes those who feel they are experiencing their handicap for the first time. A successful businesswoman and mother of two children summarized this feeling when she said, "I was paralyzed by polio at age 15 but did not feel disabled until 2 years ago at the age of 45." A third group includes people who feel they are experiencing polio for a second time. They believe they have been twice cursed, which gives rise to feelings of anger, frustration, and despair.

Regardless of their feelings about their present health, however, most patients with polio have a common past history. They worked hard to overcome the initial paralysis and often achieved a high level of functional performance and personal fulfillment. They were "mainstreamed" before that term became public policy. The level of integration and acceptance they achieved in society resulted in their disappearing from view both individually and collectively as a disabled group. Because society seldom viewed these individuals as handicapped, their desire to end the long struggle of recovery was reinforced by the belief that they did not have a handicap—that polio had in fact been conquered and was behind them. Even though a disability remained, many believed their polio was over. Now, however, with the onset of new weakness and other changes in their health, the delicate balance of high performance on limited reserves has been disrupted. Unexpectedly, and rather abruptly, new limitations develop and the old remedy "push 'til it hurts" no longer works. Nevertheless, many patients want to hear that there is a simple formula and a universal panacea that will enable them to regain what has been lost and make them feel better again. After all, their own experience years earlier taught them that, if they worked hard and persevered, they could restore their health. Forty years ago the advice was to try harder; now the advice is often to slow down.

The dynamics of this combination of denial and a personal history of successful coping frequently make it difficult to implement effective changes. If patients are reluctant to try something *new*, they may be willing to modify *old* coping mechanisms that are familiar. For example, rather than prescribe a new brace on the first visit, the physician can have the old one repaired. If patients are hesitant to make *major* changes that are clearly necessary, a *minor* intervention may be acceptable. For instance, rather than urging a reluctant patient who has been ambulatory for 35 years to buy a wheelchair, the physician might suggest that he or she use a cane or try using a wheelchair when next at an airport. When the patient realizes that the cane is helpful but not enough, a wheelchair may become more acceptable. Finally, if patients are reluctant to make a change because of the symbolism of suddenly appearing "handicapped" in public or at work, they can be helped to make changes that allow them to maintain control over when and where such situations occur. For example, patients who have never used a handicapped parking permit often find it more acceptable to obtain a placard that can be displayed on the dashboard when desired rather than handicapped license plates. These same strategies can be applied to implementing changes in other areas including exercise, work, avocational interests, and activities inside the home.

Weakness

Because of the importance of weakness as a cardinal symptom of motor neuron dysfunction and postpolio changes in general, it should be addressed early and repeatedly. If new weakness occurs in a patient who has been inactive or relatively sedentary for a period of time, and the rest of the evaluation is consistent with disuse weakness, an initial trial on a carefully supervised program of progressive exercise is indicated. Before a trial of exercise, however, it is essential to obtain objective, quantitative documentation of baseline strength and endurance of key muscle groups.

If new muscle weakness occurs in muscles that have been consistently or maximally used in daily activities, every effort should be made to provide more rest and support for those muscles. In patients who have been pushing themselves and their muscles to a maximum performance on a regular basis (that is, completing the equivalent of a daily marathon), a change in life-style with more rest, less stress, and better support of weakened muscles commonly reduces the loss of strength and may even result in improvement. However, successful interventions usually must occur at several levels. It is not just an isolated muscle that needs rest but a whole life-style that needs to be modified. For this reason, when a new brace or crutch is indicated, it should be prescribed together with an assessment of the impact of recommended changes on family members, friends, and associates at work.

Exercise

Despite the appropriate concern with weakness in this group of patients, it is important that they be encouraged to remain as active as possible within limits of comfort and safety—for both physical and psychologic reasons. A formal exercise program of some kind is desirable for virtually all patients. For some this may be nothing more strenuous than gentle stretching or various types of yoga. For others it may be considerably more vigorous and even include aerobic training. Work capacity testing of 35 postpolio survivors described by Alba and co-workers[1] showed that 66% were able to attain normal cardiopulmonary levels during exercise using a Monarch arm ergometer, Quinton treadmill, or Collins Chair ergometer. The rest of the subjects were unable to obtain a normal range of work capacity owing to focal or generalized fatigue in their extremities or improper biomechanical techniques while exercising.

Regardless of the amount and intensity of exercise, the importance of a regular routine and the feeling of taking positive action cannot be overemphasized. In patients with an element of apparent disuse weakness, several studies have shown improvement in strength in response to carefully supervised exercise programs.[13,16] However, the effects of long-term exercise on such muscles is unknown. If there is clinical or EMG evidence of prior polio involvement of these muscles, there may be a risk over time of accelerating motor unit dysfunction and, paradoxically, producing nondisuse weakness. In view of our uncertainty about the pathologic mechanism of nondisuse weakness in polio patients, we feel it is prudent to recommend long-term maintenance or strengthening-type exercises *only* in muscles that show no clinical or EMG evidence of prior polio involvement. When

prescribing more vigorous exercises, the physician may select any repetitive activity that appeals to the patient and does not cause undue pain or muscle fatigue. A sense of weakness or discomfort that persists for several hours is a useful sign of excessive activity. Many patients find that swimming in a heated pool is the most acceptable exercise because it allows a diversity of activity and avoids the stresses and microtrauma of other exercises.

Pain

As shown in Table 24-3, the location of pain in this population is strongly related to the method of locomotion. Pain is best addressed by looking for the cause. In many postpolio patients, muscle and joint pains appear to be a direct result of abnormal body mechanics. The body has an uncanny capacity to maintain function despite major muscle weakness and skeletal abnormalities. However, this function is maintained at the cost of increased workloads on the remaining innervated muscles. Abnormal and excessive forces on unstable joints and supporting tissues increase the energy expenditure required to perform a given task. These costs accumulate over a period of many years without causing symptoms and then, eventually, appear to cross a critical threshold resulting in painful muscles, joints, and ligaments.

The major principles of pain management in postpolio patients are (1) improve abnormal body mechanics; (2) relieve or support weakened muscles; and (3) promote life-style modifications. Initial management of pain may require that these principles be supplemented with moist heat, transcutaneous electrical nerve stimulation (TENS), or other modalities along with a short-term course of anti-inflammatory agents. However, in our experience the long-term use of even low-dose anti-inflammatory or pain medication is not indicated in the vast majority of patients. Abnormal biomechanics can often be modified with fairly simple and practical interventions, such as cervical pillows, lumbar rolls, gluteal pads, dorsal-lumbar corsets, and heel-lifts. In particular, efforts should be directed at improving musculoskeletal mechanics during routine activities that occur on a daily basis, such as sitting, standing, walking, and sleeping, as well as any repetitive activities at work. Providing adequate support for weakened muscles and unstable joints can often be a difficult challenge; however, the basic orthotic principles are similar to those used in the management of other neuromuscular disorders. Many patients need an orthosis that combines strength and lightness. The new plastics and lightweight metals can often be used alone or in combination, but unfortunately, the most functional solution may not be cosmetically acceptable. Many patients still have their old heavy braces that were well made and have provided years of good support. Frequently they prefer to have these familiar and proven braces repaired rather than begin over with new ones.

Life-style modifications that will help reduce the level of pain are mentioned in other sections of the chapter. The most common changes require stress reduction, activity reduction, and weight reduction. Accomplishing these changes—especially the first two—necessitates altering the pace and intensity of discretionary activities and finding ways to gain control over when and how activities in general are performed. The issue of control is not an easy one, since it often requires developing behaviors that are contrary to the old ways of coping. Assuming more control begins with the patient clarifying and eventually accepting his or her own limitations. Next the patient must acknowledge the need to make these limitations known to others. The final step is for the patient to deal directly with family, friends, and colleagues at work to negotiate when and how various activities will be performed to fit that individual's limitations. The physician's role throughout this process is critical in providing encouragement and support to the patient and information and the rationale to family and colleagues.

Respiratory failure

During the acute phase of polio the most feared complication was respiratory failure. Now, 30 to 40 years later, it appears that the late effects of polio are generally benign with the major exception of respiratory problems. These may be brought on by a number of mechanisms, including increased weakness of respiratory muscles, increased scoliosis, recurrent pulmonary infection, smoking, and decreased compliance of respiratory tissue, which in turn can lead to respiratory insufficiency and, if not properly treated, death.

The persons at greatest risk for serious late-onset pulmonary complications had moderate to severe respiratory involvement initially and usually required ventilatory assistance. The other high-risk group is individuals who developed thoracic spine deformities resulting in severe scoliosis and kyphoscoliosis. Data on the percentage of persons who were successfully weaned from a respirator years ago and have since had to return to a ventilator full or part time are not currently available. However, several preliminary studies suggest that the number may range as high as 18% to 38%.[17,19] In a study by Alcock and co-workers of 113 persons who were never weaned completely from a ventilator, the long-term prognosis appears generally favorable.[2] Patients were interviewed 21 to 30 years after polio, and more than half believed that their respiratory treatment was unchanged from 1 year after onset, while 27% perceived that their impairment was worse and 17% said it had improved. Only four required more respiratory support each day than many years earlier.

A discussion of the management of ventilator-dependent patients and those with chronic respiratory insufficiency is beyond the scope of this chapter. However, the preliminary evaluation and management of nonventilator patients is within the purview of all clinicians who see postpolio patients and begins with a high index of suspicion for anyone who falls in the following groups:

1. Those who had moderate to severe respiratory involvement initially
2. Those who required a ventilator full or part time at onset
3. Those who have developed severe scoliosis or kyphoscoliosis
4. Those who have a history of smoking, recurrent pulmonary infections, or other pulmonary disease
5. Those who have complaints suggestive of respiratory impairment such as shortness of breath, exertional dyspnea, daytime somnolence, early morning headaches, sleep disturbances, or sleep apnea

The initial assessment should include measurement of vital capacity and, in most cases, pulmonary function tests and arterial blood gas studies. Asymptomatic patients whose studies are essentially normal should be reevaluated at regular intervals and at least once yearly. Patients with nighttime sleep disturbances—especially dypnea or apnea—and with elevated PCO_2 should undergo sleep studies, if available, or at a minimum have their nighttime oxygen saturation evaluated with ear oximetry.[14] In addition, if a patient has sleep apnea, an effort should be made to distinguish between central and obstructive apnea. For this and other aspects of respiratory management, referral to a pulmonologist, preferably with experience in neuromuscular diseases, is indicated. If nighttime desaturation is documented, in many patients the symptoms clear with supplemental oxygen alone. In others, however, a trial with ventilatory assistance during the night may be necessary. Patients whose respiratory insufficiency is due largely to fatigue or weakness of the respiratory muscles usually experience a gratifying improvement in both nighttime and daytime symptoms. The most practical means of providing nighttime ventilatory assistance are the pneumo-wrap or "raincoat" and the chest cuirass. Other alternatives, which often are not as practical or available, include intermittent positive pressure with a Bennett mouth seal, nasal continuous positive airway pressure (CPAP), and the iron lung. At one time, many patients who developed respiratory failure were treated with a tracheostomy, but most authorities now believe that a tracheostomy is seldom helpful and should be avoided.[3,14] Finally, all patients with impaired pulmonary function or a history of recurrent respiratory infections should receive influenza vaccines on a regular basis and Pneumovax at least once.

PROGNOSIS

All of the evidence available at this time—both clinical and research—strongly suggests that the pathologic process or processes causing the late complications of polio are benign. The initial fear that the postpolio syndrome was a form of ALS was unfounded. As of this writing, no group has been followed long enough to estimate the mean survival time, and unless there is severe pulmonary involvement or a swallowing disorder, it appears that no aspect of the late complications of polio is directly life threatening.

However, there is a broad spectrum of clinical involvement that makes some of the complications less benign for specific individuals. Many patients experience only minor weakness and associated symptoms that are a mild annoyance; at the other end of the spectrum, many others experience profound weakness with diminished function and associated social and vocational isolation, as well as increased risks for additional disabling conditions such as osteoporosis, fractures, contractures, and depression.

In the only longitudinal study of postpolio subjects, Dalakas and co-workers[12] found in a group of 27 persons who had been followed for a mean of 8.2 years that the average loss of strength per year was approximately 1%. No mention was made of any interventions in this group, so presumably this amount of decline represents the rate of natural progression. If the underlying disorder reflects, in part, an overwork phenomenon of the motor unit and an element of musculoskeletal overuse, interventions designed to reduce the metabolic demand on the overextended motor unit and minimize the stress to the musculoskeletal system may be able to modify the observed rate of decline. While there have not been any long-term studies that document the effects of such interventions, many clinicians have observed anecdotally that patients who conscientiously adjust their life-styles and incorporate the recommended interventions experience an improvement in their symptoms and often an increase in strength and stabilization of function.

THE FUTURE

Although a great deal has been learned about the late complications of polio in recent years, many unanswered questions remain: What are the underlying pathologic mechanisms? What are the best forms of treatment? Are there any medications which might prove helpful? What is the proper role of exercise, and what is the best way to monitor it? What is the long-term prognosis? For those who had paralytic polio and are experiencing new health problems or may in the future, these questions should be investigated as broadly and deeply as possible.

However, the resources to mount a major attack on postpolio are limited and the prospects for significant expansion in the near future are not optimistic. Polio in the United States has become an orphan disease. There is no national organization, as in other countries, available to help raise funds and coordinate research and clinical activities. Because acute polio afflicts so few, chronic polio seems remote to most people. Thus finding room for it on the nation's crowded agenda of health care needs is difficult. Yet there are numerous reasons why it should remain there in a prominent place. Beyond helping the thousands of persons with

paralytic polio who will survive well into the twenty-first century, knowledge acquired about functioning of the postpolio motor unit may be important in our understanding of other neurologic disorders. Similarly, there is much to be learned from postpolio patients about aging with a disability, both physically and psychologically, which will be useful in our understanding of the aging process in other disability groups. Finally, the management of polio provided the first model for the organization and delivery of rehabilitation services to patients in the early stages of disability; now, 40 years later, it appears that polio may provide the opportunity to develop another model for the organization and delivery of rehabilitation services in the late stages of disability. This is an opportunity that neither society nor the field of rehabilitation can afford to lose.

REFERENCES

1. Alba, A, et al: Exercise testing as a useful tool in the physiatric management of the post-polio survivor. In Halstead, LS, and Wiechers, DO, editors: Research and clinical aspects of the late effects of poliomyelitis, White Plains, NY, 1987, March of Dimes.
2. Alcock, AJW, et al: Respiratory poliomyelitis: a follow-up study, Can Med Assoc J 130:1305, 1984.
3. Bach, JR, et al: Glossopharyngeal breathing and non-invasive aids in the management of post-polio respiratory insufficiency. In Halstead, LS, and Wiechers, DO, editors: Research and clinical aspects of the late effects of poliomyelitis, White Plains, NY, 1987, March of Dimes.
4. Brown, S, and Patten, BM: Post-polio syndrome and amyotrophic lateral sclerosis: a relationship more apparent than real. In Halstead, LS, and Wiechers, DO, editors: Research and clinical aspects of the late effects of poliomyelitis, White Plains, NY, 1987, March of Dimes.
5. Bruno, RL, and Frick, NM: Stress and type "A" behavior as precipitants of post-polio sequelae. In Halstead, LS, and Wiechers, DO, editors: Research and clinical aspects of the late effects of poliomyelitis, White Plains, NY, 1987, March of Dimes.
6. Campbell, AMG, Williams, ER, and Pearce, J: Late motor neuron degeneration following poliomyelitis, Neurology (Minneap) 19:1101, 1969.
7. Carriere: Amytrophies secondaire, These de Montpelier, France, 1875.
8. Codd, MB, et al: Poliomyelitis in Rochester, Minnesota, 1935-1955: epidemiology and long-term sequelae; a preliminary report. In Halstead, LS, and Wiechers, DO, editors: Late effects of poliomyelitis, Miami, 1985, Symposia Foundation.
9. Cornil, L: Sur un cas de paralysie generale spinale anterieure subaigue, suivi d'autopsie, Gaz Med (Paris) 4:127, 1875.
10. Dalakas, MC: Amyotrophic lateral sclerosis and post-polio: differences and similarities. In Halstead, LS, and Wiechers, DO, editors: Research and clinical aspects of the late effects of poliomyelitis, White Plains, NY, 1987, March of Dimes.
11. Dalakas, MC, et al: Neuromuscular symptoms in patients with old poliomyelitis: clinical, virological and immunological studies. In Halstead, LS, and Wiechers, DO, editors: Late effects of poliomyelitis, Miami, 1985, Symposia Foundation.
12. Dalakas, MC, et al: A long-term follow-up study of patients with postpoliomyelitis neuromuscular symptoms, N Engl J Med 314:959, 1986.
13. Feldman, RM: The use of strengthening exercises in post-polio syndrome: methods and results, Orthopedics 8:889, 1985.
14. Fischer, DA: Poliomyelitis: late respiratory complications and management, Orthopedics 8:891, 1985.
15. Frick, NM: Demographic and psychological characteristics of the post-polio community, paper presented at the First Annual Conference on the Late Effects of Poliomyelitis, Lansing, Mich, October 1985.

16. Grimby, G, and Einarsson, G: Muscle morphology with special reference to muscle strength in post-polio subjects. In Halstead, LS, and Wiechers, DO, editors: Research and clinical aspects of the late effects of poliomyelitis, White Plains, NY, 1987, March of Dimes.

17. Halstead, LS, and Rossi, CD: New problems in old polio patients: results of a survey of 539 polio survivors, Orthopedics 8:845, 1985.

18. Halstead, LS, and Rossi, CD: Post-polio syndrome: clinical experience with 132 consecutive outpatients. In Halstead, LS, and Wiechers, DO, editors: Research and clinical aspects of the late effects of poliomyelitis, White Plains, NY, 1987, March of Dimes.

19. Halstead, LS, Wiechers, DO, and Rossi, CD: Late effects of poliomyelitis: a national survey. In Halstead, LS, and Wiechers, DO, editors: Late effects of poliomyelitis, Miami, 1985, Symposia Foundation.

20. Herbison, GJ, Jaweed, MM, and Ditunno, JF: Exercise therapies in peripheral neuropathies, Arch Phys Med Rehabil 64:201, 1983.

21. Herndon, CN, and Jennings, RG: A twin-family study of susceptibility to poliomyelitis, Am J Hum Genetics 3:17, 1951.

22. Johnson, EW, and Alexander, MA: Management of motor unit diseases. In Kottke, FJ, Stilwell, GK, and Lehmann, JF, editors: Krusen's handbook of physical medicine and rehabilitation, ed 3, Philadelphia, 1982, WB Saunders Co.

23. Kayser-Gatchalian, MC: Late muscular atrophy after poliomyelitis, Eur Neurol 10:371, 1973.

24. Maynard, FM: Differential diagnosis of pain and weakness in post-polio patients. In Halstead, LS, and Wiechers, DO, editors: Late effects of poliomyelitis, Miami, 1985, Symposia Foundation.

25. Miller, JR: Prolonged intracerebral infection with poliomyelitis in asymptomatic mice, Ann Neurol 9:590, 1981.

26. Mulder, DW, Rosenbaum, RA, and Layton, DD: Late progression of poliomyelitis or forme fruste amyotrophic lateral sclerosis? Mayo Clin Proc 47:756, 1972.

27. National Health Survey: Prevalence of selected impairments, Ser 10, No 134, Washington, DC, 1981, Dept of Health and Human Services.

28. Perry, J, Barnes, G, and Granley, JK: Post polio muscle function. In Halstead, LS, and Wiechers, DO, editors: Research and clinical aspects of the late effects of poliomyelitis, White Plains, NY, 1987, March of Dimes.

29. Pezeshkpour, GH, and Dalakas, MC: Pathology of spinal cord in postpoliomyelitis muscular atrophy. In Halstead, LS, and Wiechers, DO, editors: Research and clinical aspects of the late effects of poliomyelitis, White Plains, NY, 1987, March of Dimes.

30. Pierce-Ruhland, R, and Patten, BM: Repeat study of antecedent events in motor neuron disease, Ann Clin Res 13:102, 1981.

31. Poskanzer, DC, Cantor, HM, and Kaplan, GS: The frequency of preceding poliomyelitis in amyotrophic lateral sclerosis. In Norris, FH, Jr, and Kurland, LT, editors: Motor neuron diseases: research on amyotrophic lateral sclerosis and related disorders, New York, 1969, Grune & Stratton.

32. Raymond, M (with contribution by Charcot, JM): Paralysie essentiele de l'enfance: atrophie musculaire consecutive, Gaz Med (Paris), 1875, p 225.

33. Sharrad, WJW: Correlation between changes in the spinal cord and muscle paralysis in poliomyelitis, Proc Soc Med 40:346, 1953.

34. Tomlinson, BE, and Irving, D: The numbers of limb motor neurons in the human lumbosacral cord throughout life, J Neurol Sci 34:213, 1977.

35. Tomlinson, BE, and Irving, D: Changes in spinal cord motor neurons of possible relevance to the late effects of poliomyelitis. In Halstead, LS, and Wiechers, DO, editors: Late effects of poliomyelitis, Miami, 1985, Symposia Foundation.

36. Wiechers, DO: Late effects of polio: historical perspectives. In Halstead, LS, and Wiechers, DO, editors: Research and clinical aspects of the late effects of poliomyelitis, White Plains, NY, 1987, March of Dimes.

37. Wiechers, DO: Reinnervation after acute poliomyelitis. In Halstead, LS, and Wiechers, DO, editors: Research and clinical aspects of the late effects of poliomyelitis, White Plains, NY, 1987, March of Dimes.

38. Wiechers, DO, and Hubbell, SL: Late changes in the motor unit after acute poliomyelitis, Muscle Nerve 4:524, 1981.

39. Windebank, AJ, et al: Late sequelae of paralytic poliomyelitis in Olmstead County, Minnesota. In Halstead, LS, and Wiechers, DO, editors: Research and clinical aspects of the late effects of poliomyelitis, White Plains, NY, 1987, March of Dimes.

40. Zilkha, KJ: Untitled discussion, Proc R Soc Med 55:1028, 1962.

CHAPTER 25

Rehabilitation of the patient with multiple sclerosis

STANLEY F. WAINAPEL

Multiple sclerosis (MS) is the best known and most frequently encountered member of a group of diseases whose common feature is demyelination in the central nervous system (CNS). It is also one of the most common causes of significant physical disability among young adults; of the currently estimated 250,000 to 500,000 Americans with the disease,[73] 90% had an onset between 15 and 50 years of age.[87] Since the first description of MS by Charcot,[17] many distinguished clinicians and research scientists have studied it intensively and have developed a number of theories about its etiology, but it remains a disease whose cause is unknown and for which there are neither preventive measures nor definitive treatment.

In contrast to the voluminous literature on the epidemiology,[58] etiology,[67] pathogenesis,[70] and diagnosis[90] of MS, rehabilitation has received disproportionately little attention,[9,30,102,103] considering its importance in the overall management of a chronic disabling disease whose prevalence may be double that of spinal cord injury.[56] General texts in rehabilitation medicine have rarely given MS a chapter of its own,[14,15] and it was not until 1985 that a book primarily devoted to MS rehabilitation was published.[73] A review of volumes 62 to 66 (1981-1985) of the *Archives of Physical Medicine and Rehabilitation* confirms this relative neglect; during these 5 years only 10 articles dealt with MS, as compared with 104 on spinal cord injury. This disparity may reflect the common misconception that MS is a relentlessly progressive disease whose downhill course augurs poorly for successful rehabilitation; as discussed subsequently, such therapeutic nihilism is not based on an accurate view of the usual clinical course and prognosis of the disease. This chapter is therefore limited to the rehabilitative management of MS, with only brief mention of relevant aspects pertaining to diagnosis and prognosis. A more general overview can be obtained in other sources.[75,76,86]

DIAGNOSIS

Although most MS patients are referred to rehabilitation professionals after a diagnosis has been established, physicians and therapists sometimes see patients with undiagnosed or misdiagnosed MS because of unexplained symptoms that produce physical disability. Therefore these professionals need some familiarity with the various clinical presentations of MS, the commonly used diagnostic criteria, and tests used to confirm the diagnosis.

MS can masquerade as a number of other CNS disorders such as stroke, brain tumor, spinal cord tumor, and cerebellar degeneration. The most common symptoms at onset are visual disturbances (particularly acute optic neuritis), weakness (particularly in the legs), incoordination, isolated paresthesias, and disturbances in bladder or bowel function.[103] The diagnosis is based primarily on clinical findings, the sine qua non of which is the documentation of neurologic dysfunction that has occurred on more than one occasion and at more than one anatomic site and that cannot be better explained by other disease processes.[38] Over the past 20 years a number of authors have developed criteria for making a diagnosis of MS.[75,89,104] Among the earliest but still most widely used are the Schumacher criteria[104]:

1. Objective clinical evidence of CNS dysfunction
2. Involvement of two or more sites in the CNS based on history or examination or both
3. CNS disease reflecting primarily white matter involvement
4. Involvement in one of two patterns
   a. Two or more episodes of over 24 hours' duration at least 1 month apart
   b. Slow or stepwise progression over at least 6 months
5. Signs and symptoms that cannot be better explained by other disease

Table 25-1. Poser criteria for diagnosis of MS*

Category	Attacks	Clinical evidence		Paraclinical evidence	CSF OB†/IgG
Clinically definite MS					
1	2	2		—	—
2	2	1	and	1	—
Laboratory-supported definite MS					
1	2	1	or	1	+
2	1	2		—	+
3	1	1	and	1	+
Clinically probable MS					
1	2	1		—	—
2	1	2		—	—
3	1	1	and	1	—
Laboratory-supported probable					
1	2	—		—	+

From Poser, CM, et al: Ann Neurol 13:227, 1983. Reprinted by permission of Little, Brown & Co.
*Numbers in table represent number of attacks or of clinical or paraclinical signs. +, Present; −, absent.
†OB, Oligoclonal bands.

In 1983 Poser and co-workers[89] incorporated recent advances in nonclinical diagnostic techniques into a set of criteria outlined in Table 25-1. The "paraclinical evidence" in these criteria include cerebrospinal fluid (CSF) analysis, neuroimaging, evoked potential electrodiagnosis, neuropsychologic testing, and neurourologic evaluation. The first three of these are briefly discussed in this section of the chapter; the latter two of these are discussed separately in subsequent sections dealing with, respectively, cognitive and bladder dysfunction. Taken together, these tests detect CNS lesions in the absence of corroborative neurologic signs.

Abnormalities in cerebrospinal fluid immunoglobulins can be detected in over 90% of MS patients.[34,52] The most common findings are increased levels of immunoglobulin G (IgG), elevated IgG/albumin ratio, and discrete (oligoclonal) bands of IgG seen on immunoglobulin electrophoresis.

Identification of discrete white matter plaques by computerized tomography (CT) scanning is a useful diagnostic procedure,[1,16,93] particularly when combined with contrast enhancement techniques (Figure 25-1). Magnetic resonance imaging (MRI) has provided an even greater degree of diagnostic sensitivity than CT scanning,[69,119] making it invaluable in establishing a diagnosis in questionable cases.[40] Its potential utility in the monitoring of disease progression was recently demonstrated.[108]

Physiatrists may be called on to perform electrodiagnostic studies as part of the evaluation of patients with suspected MS. The most frequently positive results are seen with visual evoked responses (VERs), brainstem auditory evoked responses (BAERs), somatosensory evoked potentials (SEPs), and blink reflex (BR). Over the past decade an extensive literature has established the value of these tests (particularly VER[2,45,46] and BAER[18,94]) in the diagnostic evaluation of MS[31]; Cohen and associates,[23] using the critical frequency of photic driving technique for VER, found abnormalities in 20 (91%) of 22 MS patients; these changes allow physicians to identify subclinical demyelinating lesions involving the visual pathways. Similarly, Stockard and co-workers[109] were able to detect clinically silent brainstem lesions in 53% of 70 patients with suspected MS through the use of BAER testing. The diagnostic yield of these electrophysiologic studies varies depending on whether they are being performed in clinically suspected or clinically definite cases; for example, in reviewing his experience with BR testing in 260 patients, Kimura[53] noted delayed responses in 66% of those with a definite diagnosis, in 56% of probable MS cases, and in only 20% of patients with possible MS.

None of these diagnostic tests are absolutely specific for MS; they are adjuncts to accurate history and careful clinical examination. The frequency of misdiagnosis, even in specialized MS clinics, can be as high as 10%. Rudick and co-

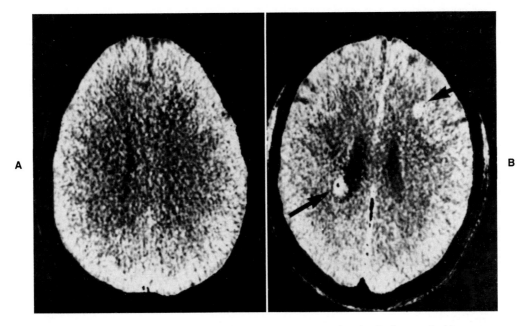

Figure 25-1. A, Normal computerized tomographic (CT) scan of brain. **B,** Scattered white matter lesions in multiple sclerosis. (From Franklin, GM, and Burks, JS: Diagnosis and medical management of multiple sclerosis. In Maloney, FP, Burks, JS, and Ringel, SP, editors: Interdisciplinary rehabilitation of multiple sclerosis and neuromuscular disorders, Philadelphia, 1985, JB Lippincott Co.)

workers[96] have identified the following clinical features that if present make the diagnosis of MS less likely*:

1. Absence of eye findings
    a. Optic nerve involvement
    b. Oculomotor abnormalities
2. Absence of clinical remission (more worrisome in a young patient)
3. Localized disease
    a. Posterior fossa
    b. Craniocervical junction
    c. Spinal cord
4. Atypical clinical features
    a. Absence of sensory findings
    b. Absence of bladder involvement
5. Absence of cerebrospinal fluid abnormalities

CLINICAL COURSE AND OUTCOME PREDICTION

Multiple sclerosis is a disease that often results in major disability or even death, but not invariably; the most consistent aspect of its natural history is its inconsistency. As shown in Table 25-2, more than half the cases follow a benign or nonprogressive remitting and exacerbating course.[56] Kurtzke and co-workers[61] reported a mean survival of 35 years from onset, suggesting that overall life expec-

tancy is only modestly reduced. Perhaps even more significant than mortality figures are those documenting morbidity resulting from MS; a surprising number of patients remain quite functional for many years. Percy and co-workers[82] found that 66% of their patients were still ambulatory 25 years after onset of symptoms. Kraft, Freal, and Coryell,[57] surveying 656 patients, found that 25% had no mobility problem whatsoever, another 16% walked unaided but had slightly reduced endurance, and an additional 29% walked independently with various assistive devices; thus 70% of their patients had maintained the capacity to walk.

Predicting whether patients are likely to experience a benign or a progressively downhill clinical course is highly desirable, and a number of studies have identified predictive factors for future functional outcome. Reviewing 527 men with definite or probable MS of 10 to 15 years' duration, Kurtzke and associates[61] reported that functional status 5 years after diagnosis, particularly in terms of pyramidal or cerebellar dysfunction, was the best predictor of a future benign or malignant clinical course. Liebowitz and Alter[67] observed that older age at onset was associated with greater disability and a more malignant course. This finding is corroborated in a case-control study of 834 patients by Clark and co-workers[19] who also found that visual or sensory symptoms at onset were associated with a more benign subsequent course.

Kraft and associates,[57] after an extensive review of the

*From Rudick, RA, et al: Arch Neurol 43:578, 1986. Reprinted by permission of the American Medical Association.

Table 25-2. Disease course in multiple sclerosis

Type of course	Characteristics	Approximate frequency (%)*
Benign	Sudden onset; one or two mild exacerbations with complete or nearly complete remission; no permanent functional disability	20 or more
Exacerbating/ remitting	Sudden onset; symptoms remit partially or totally after exacerbations; long periods of stability: months, even years	20-30
Remitting/ progressive	Same as exacerbating/remitting in beginning; at some time during course, symptoms no longer remit and disability slowly increases	40
Progressive	Insidious onset; steady progression of symptoms	10-20

From Kraft, GH, et al: Arch Phys Med Rehabil 62:54, 1981.
*Frequencies estimated from McAlpine, D: Br Med J 2:1029, 1964; and Poser, S: Analysis of 812 cases by means of electronic data processing, Berlin, 1978, Springer-Verlag.

available literature, identified the following factors as associated with a more benign future clinical course:

1. Onset before 35 years of age
2. Single symptom at onset
3. Initial visual or sensory symptoms
4. Sudden onset of symptoms
5. No initial motor symptoms
6. No pyramidal or cerebellar signs on initial physical examination
7. Initial remission within 1 month
8. Absent or minimal residual deficits after exacerbations
9. Retained ability to ambulate
10. Minimal pyramidal or cerebellar signs 5 years after onset

MANAGEMENT OF SYMPTOMS AND RESULTING FUNCTIONAL LOSSES

The symptoms produced by MS are protean; their ability to mimic other diseases has already been mentioned. MS is rarely monosymptomatic, and the presence or treatment of one symptom can adversely affect others. Those symptoms with the greatest negative impact on function are the primary concern of rehabilitation professionals. Table 25-3 presents the most common complaints reported by 656 MS patients and specifically identifies the proportion of patients in whom activities of daily living (ADLs) were affected.[56] The dis-

cussion of symptom management that follows uses a classification based on type of dysfunction, as outlined below:

1. Generalized ("invisible") dysfunction
    a. Fatigue
    b. Heat intolerance
2. Sensory dysfunction
    a. Visual
    b. Pain
    c. Sensory loss and paresthesias
3. Motor dysfunction
    a. Weakness
    b. Spasticity
    c. Cerebellar
    d. Dysarthria and dysphagia
4. Bladder dysfunction
5. Bowel dysfunction
6. Sexual dysfunction
7. Cognitive dysfunction
8. Psychosocial dysfunction

Fatigue

Fatigue could be considered as a form of motor dysfunction, but it is so prevalent, characteristic, and significant a symptom that it is considered here as a generalized dysfunction. It is one of the most disabling problems faced by the patient with MS; three out of four report fatigue, and two thirds of those with it have resulting activities of daily living (ADL) problems (see Table 25-3). Surprisingly little literature has been devoted to this subject; the "invisible" disability it produces makes its study particularly difficult. Freal and associates[39] recently conducted a thorough questionnaire survey of 309 MS patients who had reported symptomatic fatigue; it was described as "tiredness . . . a need to rest" by 90%, and as "sleepiness" by 43%. In two thirds of these patients fatigue was a daily occurrence (most frequently in the late afternoon or evening) and usually abated after a few hours, but in 8% the symptom persisted for more than 6 hours. Almost half the patients felt that it exacerbated other MS symptoms. Warm temperature or vigorous exercise increased fatigue in the great majority of cases. As a result of this symptom 22% had to reduce or change the pace of their activity, 14% had to rest more frequently, and 10% had to stop working entirely.

When evaluating the complaint of fatigue, the physician must rule out any contributing factors that might lead to this symptom. The development of fatigue in the late afternoon may be due to an elevation of the core body temperature at that time,[12] and any exposure to warm environmental conditions could potentiate this effect. Depression can also produce a general feeling of tiredness that is exacerbated by associated sleep disturbances. A third potential contributor is drugs, such as baclofen (Lioresal) or diazepam (Valium), that produce sedating side effects. Finally, fatigue can be a reflection of the inefficiency of movement engendered by other problems such as weakness, spasticity, or ataxia.

Table 25-3. Reported symptoms of 656 patients with multiple sclerosis

Symptom present	No ADL* difficulty (%)	With ADL difficulty (%)	Total (%)
Fatigue	21	56	77
Balance problems	24	50	74
Weakness or paralysis	18	45	63
Numbness, tingling, or other sensory disturbance	39	24	63
Bladder problems	25	34	59
Increased muscle tension (spasticity)	23	26	49
Bowel problems	19	20	39
Difficulty remembering	21	16	37
Depression	18	18	36
Pain	15	21	36
Laugh or cry easily (emotional lability)	24	8	32
Double or blurred vision, partial or complete blindness	14	16	30
Shaking (tremor)	14	13	27
Speech and/or communication difficulties	12	11	23
Difficulty solving problems	12	9	21

From Kraft, GH, Freal, MS, and Coryell, JK: Arch Phys Med Rehabil 67:164, 1986.
*ADL, Activity of daily living.

Although CNS stimulants such as caffeine, methylphenidate (Ritalin), and dextroamphetamine (Dexedrine) have been suggested to treat fatigue in MS, as have exercise and anticholinesterase drugs such as pyridostigmine (Mestinon), none of these has been consistently helpful.[38] However, the treatment of spasticity can produce beneficial effects by reducing energy expenditure. A similar effect can be obtained if an appropriate orthotic device produces a more efficient gait pattern.

The most significant aspects of management are pacing and energy conservation. The patient must reorganize time both at home and at work to take maximal advantage of the earlier (and cooler) hours of the day when fatigue is least likely to interfere with function. Regular rest periods need to be scheduled, particularly in late afternoon or evening. Daily activities such as cooking can be made less strenuous by using energy-saving devices (for example, electric can-opener, food processor) and by locating equipment so that it is easy to reach or move, as by use of a rolling cart. If ambulation is contributing to the development of fatigue, judicious use of a wheelchair, sometimes only for outdoor ambulation, may provide the needed respite to allow a patient to continue full-time employment. Such changes in life-style are not always easily accomplished; they can significantly disrupt long-standing behavior patterns, but they can do more to reduce overall disability from MS than sophisticated rehabilitation equipment and techniques.

Heat intolerance

The adverse effect of heat on MS has long been recognized[79] and has even led to the use of heat as a diagnostic maneuver in the hot bath test, which assists in the documentation of previously unwitnessed or unsuspected neurologic symptoms or signs.[29] Elevation of body temperature may block conduction along myelinated nerve tracts in MS patients because the threshold for such blocking is lowered by the demyelinating process. By the time the myelin sheath has been reduced to one fourth of its normal thickness, this threshold has been halved, from 40° to 20° C, a figure already well below normal body temperature.[88] Any process that causes a rise in body temperature (infection, warm environment, hot water) increases this tendency for conduction block. Even the normal diurnal daily fluctuation of temperature, which is maximal in late afternoon and evening, can have an exacerbating influence and may contribute to the development of fatigue at that time of day.[12,79]

Heat intolerance, which worsens symptoms, is extremely common in MS; Clark and co-workers[19] reported that 58.5% of 834 patients experienced it, and the rate was particularly high (70.3%) among those whose disease had a more malignant course. About one third of this latter group also reported symptomatic deterioration associated with fever.

Theoretically, anything that transiently lowers body temperature (local ice pack, cold baths) may have a beneficial effect on symptoms of MS.[14,116] The beneficial effects of cryotherapy on underlying spasticity may contribute to this phenomenon. In the aforementioned case-control study by Clark and associates,[19] 18.4% of the subjects reported some improvement of symptoms when they took cold baths. A related approach to exercise therapy that has been advocated in light of the problem of heat intolerance is the use of a temperature-controlled pool whose water is maintained at 24° to 27.5° C for vigorous underwater exercise.[41] If a patient can tolerate this rather uncomfortably cool medium, it offers a number of advantages, including the buoyancy of water as a medium for exercise of weakened muscles, as well as the ability to avoid the development of excessive heat during vigorous exercise. Such an aquatic fitness program is a promising area for controlled clinical investigation, but it is not readily available in most rehabilitation facilities if they lack a therapeutic pool; in this event immersion in a Hubbard tank may be an alternative, although it precludes underwater ambulation and more vigorous movements.

Prevention is also important in avoiding heat intolerance. Anything that might elevate body temperature must be assiduously avoided. This includes the extensive application of heating modalities, generalized heating with Hubbard tank or infrared therapy, or excessive exposure to a high ambient temperature. Optimal climate control, particularly in terms of adequate air-conditioning, is essential in both the home and the workplace for all patients. Vigorous exercise such as that performed during physical therapy usually does not elevate body temperature, but it can if the therapy area is overheated or underventilated. When traveling or working outdoors, MS patients should avoid protracted periods in direct sunlight and should wear clothing that reflects light.

Visual dysfunction

Visual symptoms are frequently prominent at onset of MS; optic neuritis is one of the classic presentations. Cohen, Lessell, and Wolf[22] carried out a prospective study of 60 patients with optic neuritis over a mean period of 7.1 years and found that definite MS eventually developed in 17 (28%) and probable or possible MS developed in another 4 (7%). Moreover, among those 21 to 40 years of age, one half went on to develop MS during the course of the study. Optic neuritis can be painful and disabling, frequently producing blindness, but fortunately it is most often a transient symptom that resolves completely or in part after several weeks. Persistent monocular blindness or progressive bilateral visual loss is uncommon. When they do occur, they produce a major disability that requires specialized visual rehabilitation services, but the patient's ability to use them may be significantly compromised by motor dysfunction; for example, reading Braille may be impossible in the presence of significant ataxia and incoordination of the upper extremities. The Talking Books program of the Library of Congress or Recorded Periodicals services may be more valuable resources for such patients.[30]

About 30% of patients with an established diagnosis of MS report symptoms related to visual involvement, but only about half of these report that their abilities to perform ADLs are affected by it.[57] The most common problems are diplopia, visual scotomas, and blurred vision; a characteristic clinical sign associated with visual involvement is intranuclear ophthalmoplegia, with impaired horizontal eye movements resulting from involvement of the supranuclear connections to brainstem oculomotor nuclei. Nystagmus also occurs and may be sufficiently severe to affect reading ability.[38] Diplopia may be alleviated by such simple devices as an eye patch or a unilateral frosted lens.[9] Scotomas and visual blurring may be less amenable to remediation but can be compensated for if the patient is aware of their presence.

Pain

Several types of pain problems can occur in patients with MS, including painful spasticity, trigeminal neuralgia, diffuse burning pain, nonspecific limb pain, and Lhermitte's sign. The reported frequency of pain symptoms has varied widely in the literature. Franklin and Burks[38] reported that it occurred in only 10% to 20% of their patients, but Kraft, Freal, and Coryell[57] found a rate of 36% based on the reports of surveyed patients, with negative ADL effects noted by 21%. In a recently published review of 317 patients, Clifford and Trotter[20] found that 28.8% had pain; their distribution among the various syndromes is illustrated in Table 25-4.

Painful spasticity has been reported by patients with traumatic paraplegia and quadriplegia, and its occurrence among MS patients with spasticity is not surprising. The treatment of choice is to reduce spasticity with appropriate medication (see "Spasticity"), but it should be remembered that underlying problems such as urinary tract infection or pressure sores may be contributory factors.

The paroxysmal facial pain described as tic douloureux or trigeminal neuralgia (TN) is definitely associated with MS. Its incidence in the previous literature has varied from 0.75%[78] to 1.05%[97]; Clifford and Trotter's series included five cases, a 1.36% incidence.[20] Compared with idiopathic TN, the TN associated with MS occurs at an earlier age and is more often bilateral.[47] Some neuropathologic studies have demonstrated demyelinating plaques involving the brainstem trigeminal sensory pathways,[113] and a recent case study using evoked potential techniques (BAER) in an MS patient with TN supports this pathophysiologic explanation.[50] As with idiopathic TN, symptoms usually respond well to treatment with carbamazepine (Tegretol).[112]

Diffuse, burning pain in the extremities was the most commonly occurring pain syndrome among Clifford and Trotter's patients[20]; 5.6% of them had this symptom, and they accounted for nearly 20% of all pain complaints. The majority of these patients had complete or partial relief of pain when given tricyclic antidepressants. Nonspecific and

Table 25-4. Nonheadache pain syndrome in 91 patients with multiple sclerosis

Pain syndrome	Number of patients	Useful treatments	Number
Burning extremity pain	18	Codeine sulfate	3
		Tricyclic antidepressant	11
		Baclofen	2
		Phenol spinal block	1
Nonspecific limb pain	15	Tricyclic antidepressant	2
		Balclofen	1
		Corticotropin	4
		Phenytoin sodium	1
Back pain only	7	Muscle relaxants + nonsteroidal anti-inflammatory	2
		Tricyclic antidepressant	2
		Corticotropin	1
Root pain only	7	Surgery (herniated disc)	1
		Tricyclic antidepressant	3
		Intermittent pain, no therapy	3
Joint pain	6	Corticotropin	1
		Nonsteroidal anti-inflammatory	4
Painful extremity spasms	6	Benzodiazepine or baclofen	6
Myalgias and cramps	5	Benzodiazepine	5
Optic neuritis pain	5	Corticotropin	5
Face or head neuralgic pain	5	Carbamazepine	3
Painful Lhermitte's sign	5	Collar	
Thoracic pain	4	Tricyclic antidepressant	2
		Corticotropin	1
		Phenytoin	1
Back pain with nonspecific leg pain	3	Muscle relaxants + nonsteroidal anti-inflammatory	1
		Tricyclic antidepressant	
Back pain with sciatica	2	Surgery	1
		Muscle relaxants + nonsteroidal anti-inflammatory	1
Nonburning dysesthesias	2	Tricyclic antidepressant	1
Electric shock in limbs	2	Tricyclic antidepressant	1
Neck pain	1	Pain intermittent, no therapy	1

Modified from Clifford, DB, and Trotter, JL: Arch Neurol 41:1270, 1984. Copyright 1984, American Medical Association.

often poorly described limb pain was almost as common as the burning pain described previously, but its management was notably less successful, with relatively few patients responding to tricyclic antidepressants or other medications.

Lhermitte's sign—a classic diagnostic symptom characterized by a shocklike sensation in the spine or down the arms provoked by neck flexion—was a distinctly uncommon finding, occurring in only five of 317 cases. No treatment has been suggested other than utilization of a cervical collar to reduce neck flexion.

Prolonged and unresolved pain can have serious psychologic consequences in the MS patient. The development of pain behavior can result in significant secondary disability and problems relating to overuse of analgesic drugs. Depression is also a frequent concomitant of chronic pain and may

warrant a trial of tricyclic antidepressants. Cognitive strategies for pain management, such as those used by Blinchik and Grzesiak[8] in patients with spinal cord injuries, may be applicable to MS patients as well.

Sensory loss and paresthesias

Sensory disturbances are extremely common in MS, but they are less commonly disabling; about two thirds of patients with the disease report them, but less than one fourth experience ADL difficulty resulting from the symptom (Table 25-3).[57] Loss of vibratory sensation in the distal lower extremities is the most frequent physical finding and may not be associated with any functional losses, but more significant proprioceptive loss can significantly jeopardize standing balance. Monosymptomatic paresthesias are a common initial manifestation of MS. Like optic neuritis, they usually resolve, frequently leaving no residual deficits,[55] and are associated with a more benign subsequent clinical course.[56]

There are few definite forms of treatment for persistant sensory dysfunction, although Illis[49] has reported improvement in two patients treated with dorsal column stimulation. Protective and compensatory maneuvers are the primary components of appropriate rehabilitative management and include the following[9]:

1. Avoiding application of local heat or cold to areas with impaired sensation
2. Relieving pressure over bony prominences in areas with impaired sensation
3. Using vision (if unaffected) to compensate for affected peripheral sensation and act as a substitute form of sensory feedback

Muscle weakness

Weakness in multiple sclerosis is a composite symptom that reflects, in varying degrees, several underlying mechanisms: disuse, fatigue, spasticity, ataxia, proprioceptive loss, or pain. Its management entails treating any or all of these associated problems. Three fourths of MS patients report muscle weakness or paralysis, and two thirds of those who do so experience impaired function.[57] Weakness occurs most frequently in the lower extremities and is often combined with spasticity to produce a spastic paraparesis.[38] Upper extremity weakness is less common but can have major consequences on ADL abilities, especially in combination with ataxia. Atrophy and weakness of the intrinsic hand muscles were described in nine (6%) of 150 MS patients by Fisher, Long, and Drachman,[36] who hypothesized that this finding reflects underuse of the hands resulting from impaired central control.

The consequences of untreated weakness can be extremely disabling. Joint contractures develop unless a daily range-of-motion program is instituted promptly. Such secondary contractures may make ambulation or even bed mobility difficult. Pressure sores can also develop when the patient is not strong enough to move and relieve pressure. This is particularly likely in the presence of concomitant joint contractures. The best treatment is prevention, which can be accomplished through maintenance of joint mobility and regular relief of pressure over bony prominences. When spasticity is contributing to joint contractures, it must be treated aggressively (see "Spasticity").

Exercise of weakened muscles must take into account the problems of fatigue and heat intolerance as discussed previously. To increase endurance, exercise can be carried to the point of fatigue, but it should never exceed this point.[12] A cooler environment such as a pool with lower than usual water temperature[41] may allow more vigorous exercise without producing undue fatigue. When weakness of foot, ankle, or knee musculature produces an unsafe or inefficient gait,

an angle-foot orthosis (AFO) or, occasionally, a knee-ankle-foot orthosis (KAFO) may provide sufficient external support and muscular assistance to improve the mechanics of ambulation. Perry, Gronley, and Lunsford[83] recommended the use of a clog-type rocker shoe to improve ambulation in selected MS patients; its elevated heel compensates for plantar flexion of the ankle and the curved sole assists in initiating knee flexion.

Several authors have reported encouraging responses to spinal cord stimulation in MS patients with muscle weakness.[25,49] Recent successes in using muscle stimulation for assisted exercise or ambulation in traumatic paraplegia and quadriplegia[85] suggest that similar techniques hold promise in MS as well. A note of caution must be sounded, however; it is possible to induce muscle fatigue with an electrical exercise program.

Spasticity

Spasticity contributes to weakness, incoordination, and the development of joint contractures in MS patients. Its management in such patients differs significantly from that recommended for patients with spinal cord injuries because MS is an unstable disease with periods of remission and exacerbation and because motor and sensory losses are often partial rather than total. Thus spasticity treatment techniques that produce lasting motor or sensory sequelae, such as subarachnoid block, rhizotomy, or phenol nerve blocks, are to be avoided if at all possible. An exception can be made for patients with a long-standing, nonremitting course or prolonged, stable neurologic deficits. More localized nerve blocks such as obdurator nerve block for hip adductor spasticity or lumbar paravertebral block for hip flexor spasticity may have a place in treatment of some patients,[30] and selective motor point blocks can produce localized effects without compromising sensation.

The mainstay of spasticity management in MS is pharmacologic. The three most commonly prescribed drugs are baclofen, dantrolene sodium (Dantrium), and diazepam; their actions, indications, and side effects have been summarized by Young and Delwaide.[120] Whereas baclofen is the drug of choice in traumatic myelopathy because it is so well tolerated by most patients, the sedative side effects are more problematic in patients with MS. Similarly, the side effects of muscle weakness and drowsiness interfere with the use of dantrolene and diazepam, respectively. The optimal therapeutic effect with the least degree of undesirable side effects can be achieved by using two drugs simultaneously at relatively low dosages; their effects on spasticity are potentiated while side effects are kept to a minimum.

Spasticity is not always undesirable, and any treatment plan must consider whether it is actually assisting the patient's function. Some patients use hypertonicity of the lower extremities during standing and in the stance phase of gait. Eliminating spasticity in such cases can even lead to a loss of ambulatory capacity.[38]

Cerebellar dysfunction

Cerebellar involvement in MS is common and produces considerable disability in self-care activities because of the disease's predilection for the upper extremities with resultant ataxia and intention tremor. Truncal ataxia may also have an adverse effect on sitting balance, transfers, and ambulation, even in the presence of significant degrees of retained muscle strength. Less severe involvement can produce a wide-based gait pattern and moderate truncal instability.[38] Upper extremity symptoms can be so severe that they preclude independent feeding, grooming, dressing, and writing.

Treatment of these disabling symptoms has been notable primarily for its lack of success. No specific antiataxia drug has been consistently successful, although a reduced intention tremor with isoniazid (INH), 800 to 1200 mg daily, has sometimes been reported.[99] Stereotaxic neurosurgical procedures such as ventrolateral thalamotomy have been recommended for some patients who have uncontrollable and progressive cerebellar dysfunction that has rendered them bedridden and totally dependent.[14] This surgery can have major associated morbidity such as a postoperative limb plegia, but in selected cases the loss of muscle strength and tone may be preferable. However, patient selection for such procedures may be difficult.

Rehabilitation techniques for treating cerebellar dysfunction have not been notably successful either, but they can increase independence by limiting the movements produced by these symptoms or by planning for the potential consequences of such movements. Adaptive equipment for the upper extremities includes cuff weights to reduce the excursion of involuntary movements of forearm and hand, large-handled eating utensils, and a plate guard to facilitate self-feeding (Figure 25-2). A well-fitting neck brace is sometimes used to partially control heat tremor, and a weighted walkerette may be helpful for ambulation. Dressing difficulties produced by incoordination may require the substitution of Velcro closures for buttons and shoelaces. Automatic devices such as an electric toothbrush or electric page turner may be useful for severely affected patients.[118]

Dysarthria and dysphagia

Approximately one fourth of MS patients report problems in speech or communication, but only 11% experience ADL difficulties as a result of this symptom.[57] Benkelman, Kraft, and Freal[5] point out that an even smaller proportion of patients are unable to communicate with strangers (4%) or require the use of augmentative communication devices (1%). Nevertheless, for those with significant communication impairment it may be a serious impediment to successful social and vocational adjustment.

Dysarthria is the most common communication impairment among MS patients.[28,32] This term refers to a group of speech disorders characterized by disturbances in muscular control of the speech mechanism as a result of damage

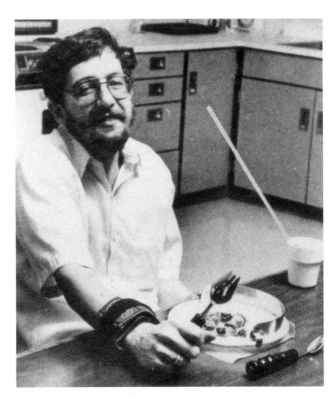

Figure 25-2. Adaptive equipment for multiple sclerosis patient with ataxia: cuff weights, large-handled fork, and plate guard. (From DeLisa, JE, et al: Am Fam Phys 32:152, 1985. Reprinted by permission of American Association of Family Physicians.)

to the central or peripheral nervous system. Darley, Aronson, and Brown[27] distinguish five patterns of dysarthria: flaccid, spastic, ataxic, hypokinetic, and hyperkinetic. Paralysis, weakness, and incoordination of the speech musculature can coexist in the same patient just as they do in the peripheral musculature; thus a mixture of dysarthric syndromes may be encountered rather than one of the "pure" dysarthric types. Characteristic symptoms include weak or harsh vocal quality, reduced rate of speech, inappropriate stress patterns, and imprecise articulation. The last reflects involvement of cranial nerve tracts that innervate the musculature of lips, tongue, and mandible.[98] This pattern of weakness, when combined with weakness of neck, laryngeal, and respiratory muscles, leaves the dysarthric patient at risk for difficulty in swallowing (dysphagia) with an increased incidence of aspiration and subsequent pulmonary infections.

Because dysarthria and dysphagia often coexist and have a similar etiologic basis, their management is usually combined. An appropriate body position (particularly a flexed neck) facilitates swallowing and affords protection of the trachea by the back of the tongue. Dietary selection is also important in symptomatic dysphagia. Thin liquids and pureed foods should be avoided; a semisoft diet is better tolerated and less likely to produce aspiration. Slow, deliberate chewing and maneuvers to increase saliva production are also components of the dysphagia program. The treatment of dysarthria involves an individualized program of exercises to promote greater control of the oral structures, a more appropriate speech rate, and proper phrase lengths. Education and supportive counseling are important; the family and patient should be taught all exercises and techniques, which should be described in writing when appropriate (for example, for a patient with cognitive impairment). The primary treatment goals are maintenance of functional verbal or nonverbal communicative abilities and maximal energy conservation.[98] In view of the progressive, variable nature of the disease, treatment should be reinstituted promptly whenever symptoms develop or change in severity.

Bladder dysfunction

Urinary problems caused by neurogenic vesical dysfunction frequently accompany the sensorimotor symptoms discussed previously, and they can have a profound impact on overall physical and social function. Symptoms are usually irritative (urgency, frequency, nocturia, incontinence) or obstructive (hesitancy, weak stream, urinary retention), with the former usually predominating.[3] Bradley, Logothetis, and Tim[11] found that among 99 MS patients undergoing urologic evaluation the most common complaints were urgency, frequency, and incontinence; the last of these occurred in only 38% of men but was reported by 70% of women. However, Blaivas[6,7] pointed out that correlation between bladder symptoms and the type of neurogenic bladder diagnosed through urodynamic testing is poor, so "symptomatic" treatment without the benefit of objective neurourologic testing is often ineffective because of its lack of specificity. He therefore recommended that cystometric testing with simultaneous EMG recording of sphincter activity be a routine component of the assessment of any MS patient who reports symptoms of voiding dysfunction.

Augspurger[3] recently reviewed the results of urodynamic evaluations of 133 consecutive MS patients with urinary symptoms (Table 25-5). Uninhibited neurogenic bladder (UNB) was the predominant form of dysfunction; one third of all patients had UNB with associated vesicosphincteric dyssynergia (VSD), and another one third had UNB without VSD. The remaining one third of patients were equally divided between normal and flaccid neurogenic bladder categories. Based on these findings, Augspurger developed a useful algorithm summarizing methods of bladder management in MS that have resulted in overall success rates of from 50% to 73% (Figure 25-3), success being defined as subjective improvement or complete elimination of symptoms. Prominently absent from this scheme of management are cholinergic drugs such as bethanechol (Urecholine) and alpha-adrenergic blockers such as phenoxybenzamine (Dibenzyline), both of which have been used frequently for patients with traumatic spinal cord injury and neurogenic bladder. Blaivas[6] has found these drugs to be of limited use

Table 25-5. Urodynamic findings in 133 MS patients

Urodynamic finding	Percentage of patients
Normal	17
Flaccid neurogenic bladder	14
Uninhibited neurogenic bladder	69
Normal sphincter	53
Dyssynergia	47
Tonic-clonic	66
Uninhibited relaxation	33

From Augspurger, RR: Bladder dysfunction in multiple sclerosis. In Maloney, FP, Burks, JS, and Ringel, SP: Interdisciplinary rehabilitation of multiple sclerosis and neuromuscular disorders, Philadelphia, 1985, JB Lippincott Co.

for MS patients. Also not mentioned are antispastic medications such as baclofen (Lioresal), which might be anticipated to have a beneficial effect on those with UNB associated with significant degrees of VSD. The mainstays of Augspurger's approach are anticholinergic drugs, such as propantheline (Pro-Banthine) and oxybutynin (Ditropan), and intermittent catheterization.[3] Several potential problems associated with these methods should be kept in mind when considering their use in individual patients:

1. Anticholinergic drugs can produce troublesome side effects such as dry mouth (a problem when dysphagia is present), sedation, and constipation.
2. Unlike patients with traumatic paraplegia, many MS patients do not have total loss of urethral sensation, so frequent self-catheterization can produce a significant degree of local discomfort.
3. An MS patient with significant cerebellar involvement may not have adequate upper extremity coordination to permit independent, safe, nontraumatic self-catheterization; in this situation an intermittent catheterization program may require the regular participation of family members or other caretakers.

An indwelling catheter may be necessary when conservative management has been unsuccessful, especially in female patients, for whom external incontinence devices are less satisfactory. This is particularly likely when the disease follows a more progressive course. Suprapubic cystotomy may be preferable for long-term indwelling catheterization, especially in men, who are at risk for development of abscesses at the penoscrotal junction. Those with the more benign varieties of MS may experience significant changes in bladder function during periods of disease remission or exacerbation, and repeated neurologic evaluations should be performed to reevaluate the current mode of therapy. A recent report on serial urodynamic studies in MS by Wheeler and co-workers[117] illustrates this principle; 55% of the pa-

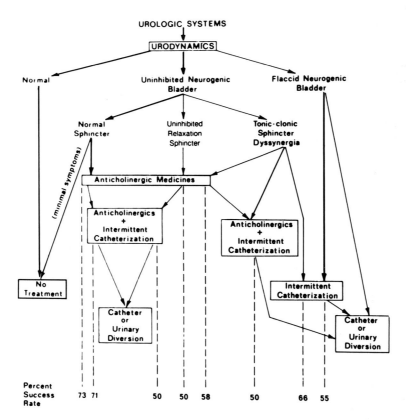

Figure 25-3. Algorithm for management of neurogenic bladder in multiple sclerosis. (From Augspurger, RR: Bladder dysfunction in multiple sclerosis. In Maloney, FP, Burks, JS, and Ringel, SP: Interdisciplinary rehabilitation of multiple sclerosis and neuromuscular disorders, Philadelphia, 1985, JB Lippincott Co.)

tients studied had significant urodynamic changes on repeat evaluations.

Urinary tract infection (UTI) can occur frequently in patients who have significant postvoiding residual urine volumes or indwelling catheters or whose intermittent catheterization technique is incorrect. Long-term low-dose antibiotic therapy may be considered for prophylaxis in these patients. UTI may contribute to the development of excessive spasticity and therefore have an indirect adverse effect on motor function.

Bowel dysfunction

MS patients less frequently report bowel dysfunction than other symptoms, but in up to one fifth of them it can create major disruptions in daily routine.[57] Fear of embarrassing bowel accidents can be a major cause of social isolation and even unemployment of such patients.

The pathophysiologic characteristics of the neurogenic bowel in MS are much less well understood than those of the neurogenic bladder. Glick, Meshkinfoos, and Haldeman[43] recently performed detailed electrophysiologic studies of colonic function in a small group of patients with advanced MS. The colon showed a rapid and pronounced rise in intraluminal pressure after water instillation, a re-

sponse analogous to that of the uninhibited neurogenic bladder mentioned previously. The gastrocolic reflex, a normal response to eating which produces increased colonic motor and myoelectric activity, was usually abnormal or even absent. A final abnormality was the inability of patients to sense the presence of stool in the rectal ampulla. In addition to these physiologic changes, several other factors contribute to abnormal bowel function: reduced overall mobility, abdominal muscle weakness, spasticity of the muscles of the pelvic floor, other medications (for example, anticholinergic agents for UNB), and depression.

The most common symptoms produced by neurogenic bowel dysfunction are constipation, fecal impaction, and bowel incontinence; the latter two are fortunately uncommon among patients with less severe forms of MS. Impaction is the result of unsuccessfully managed chronic constipation and may paradoxically produce unexplained diarrhea. It is also the most common cause of fecal incontinence. Therefore the early and appropriate management of constipation is the best way to prevent these secondary problems.

The goal of treatment is the production of formed bowel movements at regular intervals without resorting to laxatives or enemas. Levine[65] provided a logical outline of management whose components can be summarized as time, mechanical factors, adequate fiber and bulk, and avoidance of laxatives and enemas.

Time refers both to spending adequate amounts of time in the act of defecation and to the timing of this activity. Typically a 30-minute period is set aside immediately after breakfast (to take advantage of the gastrocolic reflex) during which the patient sits on the toilet and attempts to empty the rectum fully. A hurried routine tends to result in incomplete emptying with increased risk of subsequent unexpected bowel movements. Mechanical factors include avoidance of bedpans and the assumption of maximally flexed hip position (which decreases the anal-rectal angle) by using a lowered toilet seat or placing the feet on a footstool when using a normal height toilet or commode. Digital stimulation may help initiate defecation in patients with pelvic muscle spasm, and abdominal massage may increase intra-abdominal pressure during defecation in patients whose abdominal muscles are weak. A diet high in fiber can be supplemented by bulk agents such as psyllium and senna. Adequate water intake (at least eight glasses daily) is recommended to prevent the development of excessively hard stools. Use of laxatives and enemas should be avoided, and if the patient has previously been dependent on them, they should be discontinued gradually as mechanical and dietary interventions are initiated. Underlying problems that may contribute to constipation, such as spasticity and depression, should be treated vigorously as part of a total bowel management program. The patient's premorbid bowel habits may determine the optimal schedule for future bowel function.

Sexual dysfunction

Problems with sexual function contribute greatly to the psychologic and interpersonal difficulties of MS patients. Vas,[115] studying 37 ambulatory, working, male patients, found that 43% complained of impotence and 47% experienced erectile dysfunction. Similarly, among a group of 25 women with the relatively benign variety of MS studied by Lumberg,[71] 52% reported sexual dysfunction, the two most common symptoms being decreased libido (36%) and orgasmic difficulties (36%). Lillus[68] found that sexual function was altered in 91% of the men and 72% of the women among members of the Helsinki MS Society; the most common symptom in men was erectile dysfunction (62%), and the women's most frequent symptoms were orgasmic dysfunction (33%) and decreased libido (27%).

Valleroy and Kraft[114] recently reported on sexual function among 217 patients (149 women and 68 men) from the University of Washington MS Project. The sexual symptoms of these subjects are listed in Table 25-6. Overall, 62% of the subjects (75% of the men and 56% of the women) had sexual difficulties. Fatigue and decreased sensation were the most frequent symptoms among women, and men experienced difficulty in achieving or maintaining an erection and decreased sensation as their most common symptoms. Frequency of sexual intercourse decreased for many subjects,

Table 25-6. Sexual symptoms in 217 MS patients (149 women and 68 men)

Symptom	Absolute frequency	Percentage
In women		
Fatigue	97	68
Decreased sensation	68	48
Decreased libido	58	41
Decreased orgasm	52	37
Anorgasmia	53	37
Difficulty with arousal	50	35
Frequent urinary tract infection	30	21
In men		
Difficulty achieving erection	41	63
Decreased sensation	35	55
Difficulty maintaining erection	34	52
Fatigue	33	51
Decreased libido	31	48
Difficulty with ejaculation or orgasm	28	44
Spontaneous morning or night erections	24	37
Frequent urinary tract infection	7	11

From Valleroy, ML, and Kraft, GH: Arch Phys Med Rehabil 65:125, 1984.

and 26% rated themselves "not now sexually active"; two thirds of this latter group were 50 to 69 years of age. Sexual problems were also related to specific physical symptoms such as weakness (58%), spasticity (24%), joint contractures (12%), indwelling catheter (5%), and urinary incontinence (5%).

Managing sexual dysfunction in MS patients entails both physical and psychologic interventions. Spasticity and joint contractures (which are often interrelated) should be optimally treated with appropriate medications, positioning, and stretching exercises; in selected cases, such as a woman with severe hip adductor spasticity, a local nerve block can be of enormous benefit to sexual functioning. Correct bladder management minimizes the need for a Foley catheter or the likelihood of urinary incontinence. Individualized sexual counseling for the patient and his or her sexual partner must be an integral part of the rehabilitation process. A frank and open attitude from the counseling professional (whether physician or nonphysician) is essential for optimal communication; the participation of rehabilitation professionals, patients, and patients' significant others in sexual attitude reassessment (SAR) seminars[24] should be encouraged as a valuable educational experience. Sexual techniques and approaches developed for spinal cord–injured individuals[77,106] have considerable applicability to many MS patients; however, special problems associated with MS, such as upper extremity ataxia, may make some techniques difficult or impractical. As always, an open attitude on the part of sexual

Table 25-7. Cognitive dysfunction in 52 MS patients

| | | Number of patients | |
| | | Psychologic evaluation | |
Symptom	Neurologic evaluation	Intact function	Impaired function
Cerebral involvement			
Visual problems	22	8	14
Decreased mentation	2	1	1
Visual and mentation problems	5	0	5
TOTAL	29	9 (31.00)*	20 (73.75)
No cerebral involvement	23	15 (35.13)	8 (72.75)
TOTAL	52	24 (33.58)	28 (73.46)

From Peyser, JM, et al: Arch Neurol 37:577, 1980. Copyright 1980, American Medical Association.
*Numbers in parentheses are mean category errors.

partners that encourages mutual exploration of the body's erogenous potential holds the best promise for an optimal sexual adjustment. Sexuality needs to be viewed in its broadest context, encompassing the gamut of human expression associated with the relationship between two individuals.

Studies of male fertility in MS have not been reported, but based on experience with traumatic myelopathy it can be hypothesized that patients with relatively complete and progressive neurologic deficits may have reduced fertility. Electroejaculation with sperm collection for future insemination is a technique used in spinal cord–injured men[13] and its applicability to MS patients remains to be investigated.

The ability to conceive and bear children appears to be unaffected in women with MS. It has been suggested that symptoms of MS may begin during, be accentuated by, or become worse in the weeks following pregnancy, but it is generally believed that pregnancy is nondeleterious in patients who have not had an exacerbation in the preceding 2 years.[103] Poser and Poser,[91] reviewing 512 women with MS who have borne children, reported that the risk of onset, exacerbation, or progression of the disease during the 6 months *after* pregnancy was two to three times as great as *during* pregnancy. However, long-term outcome is not thought to be adversely affected by pregnancy.[111]

Cognitive dysfunction

Impaired intellectual function associated with MS was recognized by early clinicians such as Charcot[17] and Lhermitte[66]; subsequent research has documented the presence of cognitive impairments in a considerable proportion of patients, particularly those with long-standing disease.[51,81,92] Neuropsychologic testing has revealed a higher incidence of these problems than would be expected based on standard clinical testing. In one series of 52 patients studied by Peyser and associates,[84] 28 (53.9%) showed cognitive impairments on neuropsychologic testing (Table 25-

7). Of the 45 patients judged to be normal by neurologic examination, 22 (48.9%) demonstrated cognitive deficits on neuropsychologic testing (Table 25-8). There was no evidence of other potential contributors to cognitive dysfunction such as depression[44] or fatigue.[35] Lyon-Caen and coworkers[72] recently studied a group of MS patients with a relatively recent onset (less than 2 years' duration) and found neuropsychologic evidence of mild to moderate cognitive dysfunction in 57.3%; also, six of a group of nine patients with isolated optic neuritis showed cognitive impairment. Memory problems occurred whether the information was presented in verbal or visual form; temporospatial abilities, calculation, verbal fluency, and naming ability were unaffected.

Patients report cognitive problems considerably less often than the nearly 60% incidence found on neuropsychologic testing. Of Kraft, Freal, and Coryell's patients, 37% reported memory problems and only 21% reported difficulty in problem solving.[57] Since such deficits often go undiagnosed by objective clinical observation, it should come as no surprise that patients themselves are often unaware of the presence of cognitive deficits. Formal neuropsychologic testing is therefore advisable for any patient with an established diagnosis of MS regardless of the presence or absence of clinical evidence or symptoms suggesting cognitive impairment. The documentation of such deficits can aid in the diagnosis of suspected MS; Poser and co-workers[89] consider them a form of "paraclinical evidence" (Table 25-1).

Members of the rehabilitation team must be aware of the presence and severity of cognitive dysfunction to establish realistic goals and appropriate strategies to maximize learning and carryover. This is particularly important when a patient demonstrates subtle subclinical deficits that an unaware physician or therapist might misinterpret as indications of noncompliance or lack of motivation. Patients may forget to take medications, to perform daily exercise pro-

Table 25-8. Comparison of clinical and neuropsychologic tests in the diagnosis of 52 patients with MS

Evaluative method	Intact cognitive function		Impaired cognitive function	
	Number	Percentage	Number	Percentage
Clinical estimation	45		7	
Psychologic testing				
Intact	23	51.1	1	14.3
Impaired	22	48.9	6	85.7

From Peyser, JM, et al: Arch Neurol 37:577, 1980. Copyright 1980, American Medical Association.

grams, or even to attend therapy sessions. Under these circumstances the simple expedient of a written schedule of treatments and detailed instructions may be enough to eliminate the problem. Discussions with patients can also be taped for review at a later time or for a patient with significant visual impairment. Family members should be informed about the presence of cognitive deficits so they do not misinterpret their manifestation.

Primary cognitive impairments must be differentiated from secondary problems resulting from fatigue and depression. The latter are discussed in the next section of this chapter.

Psychosocial dysfunction

MS is often associated with emotional and social problems that reflect the chronic and unpredictable nature of the disease, as well as its propensity for particular anatomic locations in the brain. Such distinctions are clearly important when evaluating disturbances of mood in MS patients. Euphoria and emotional lability are believed to be the result of involvement of the frontal lobes[105] and supranuclear brainstem connections,[38] respectively. The latter, often referred to as "emotional incontinence," is not necessarily indicative of cognitive impairment; its underlying organic basis should be explained to the patient and family, who may be particularly distressed by this symptom because they fear that it implies mental deterioration. The euphoric affect noted in many MS patients can significantly interfere with the rehabilitation process, since these patients tend to minimize or even deny the severity of their disabilities, making realistic goal setting difficult at best. Signs of cognitive impairment may also be found in association with euphoric affect.

In contrast to the organically produced mood disturbances mentioned previously, depression in MS patients is a reactive phenomenon whose pattern is similar to that occurring with other chronic disabling disorders such as rheumatoid arthritis and spinal cord injury.[10] A depressed MS patient is usually reacting to the functional losses produced by the disease, its interference with current or future life plans, and insecurity about the future clinical course engendered

by the remitting and exacerbating nature of the disability.[54] Changing levels of disability require periodic readjustments in life-style at an age when the individual's primary concerns center on establishing a career, forming lasting relationships, and starting a family.[48]

In one study of 30 patients with recent onset of MS, 12 (36.7%) met the DSM-III criteria for a diagnosis of major depression.[72] This figure is in close agreement with the 36% of patients who reported having the symptom of depression on a questionnaire survey (Table 25-3).[57] The presence of depression can have a negative effect on other symptoms of MS such as fatigue and constipation; conversely, symptoms of fatigue or cognitive dysfunction can be mistakenly interpreted as manifestations of an underlying depression.

In evaluating and treating a depressed MS patient, the physician should recognize potential secondary causes such as the effects of steroids and other drug side effects that might mimic depressive symptoms (for example, the lethargy and somnolence associated with high-dose diazepam or baclofen therapy for spasticity). Most patients do not require pharmacologic intervention; this is fortunate, since side effects of the tricyclic antidepressants, such as dry mouth, urinary retention, constipation, and sedation, may be poorly tolerated by patients who already have swallowing, bladder, bowel, or cognitive dysfunction. Individual[62,110] or group[26,48] psychotherapy, in conjunction with a supportive attitude from the entire rehabilitation team, is the treatment of choice. A number of authors have documented the beneficial effects of group psychotherapy in MS patients. Hartings, Pavlou, and Davis[48] have identified six primary issues that frequently surface during these group sessions:

1. Ambiguity of health status—the difficulty of diagnosis
2. Borderline phenomenon—subjective "invisible" disability
3. Uncertainty about future status
4. Dependency
5. Anger and aggression
6. Sexuality

Table 25-9. Employment status of 257 MS patients

Status	Number	Percentage
Employed	50	19.5
Independent homemaker	55	21.4
Semi-independent homemaker	33	12.8
In training	0	0.0
Employed in sheltered workshop	3	1.2
Retired	10	3.9
Student	6	2.3
Unemployed	99	38.5
Other	1	0.4

From Scheinberg, L: NY State J Med 80:1395, 1980. Reprinted by permission of the Medical Society of the State of New York.

Table 25-10. Causes of loss of employment by 182 MS patients

Reason	Number*	Percentage*
Visual difficulty	29	15.9
Physical difficulty	96	52.7
Fatigue	17	9.3
Transportation difficulty	22	12.1
Emotional difficulty	3	1.6
Economic difficulty	1	0.5
Other (mainly marriage and/or pregnancy)	68	37.4

From Scheinberg, L: NY State J Med 80:1395, 1980. Reprinted by permission of the Medical Society of the State of New York.
*Many patients reported more than one difficulty.

The first three of these problems are prominent in patients with recent onset of symptoms and relatively mild disability. The last, sexuality, may warrant the addition of therapy for the couple to allow a more frank and individualized approach to specific problems or conflicts.

Matson and Brooks[74] have reviewed various studies of the social-psychologic adjustments in MS and have outlined a four-stage model of the coping strategies of these patients:

Stage 1. Denial. "It's not true; it can't be happening to me"; concealing symptoms; seeking professional denial of diagnosis; refusing assistance; clinging to prior life-style

Stage 2. Resistance. "It won't get me down!"; searching for cure or definitive treatment; seeking other patients; reluctant to accept help; initial recognition of change in life orientation

Stage 3. Affirmation. "I guess I have to face it"; grieving for loss of former self; learning to accept help; rearranging priorities in life

Stage 4. Integration. "I know it's there but I don't think much about it"; living with disability; spending time and energy on other matters; accepting necessary help; integration of life-style with new values

Not only MS patients must learn to cope with the disease and its resultant disability; the stresses placed on their families are considerable. Social roles are disrupted. Other family members—spouse, children, parents—may have to make major alterations in their daily routines to provide the requisite assistance for the patient. The unexpected demands imposed by the onset of MS-related disabilities may cause family or friends to withdraw from or reject the patient because of their unwillingness to assume the role of caregiver.[54] Feelings of anxiety, anger, depression, and guilt are common and can become overwhelming.[9] Financial insecurity resulting from unemployment and marital tensions

stemming from sexual dysfunction are also major causes of social conflict.

The vocational consequences of MS are particularly serious in view of the relatively young age of the patient population. High rates of unemployment are characteristic, and there is general agreement in the literature that the vocational rehabilitation potential of these patients has been incompletely addressed.[56,57] Rozin and co-workers,[95] reviewing 172 Israeli patients, found that 94 (54.7%) were working, but of those who were unemployed only 41 (23.8%) were severely disabled; almost half the unemployed group had significant vocational potential. Among 1271 MS patients 20 years after onset reported by Bauer,[4] only 30% were still employed. A striking demonstration of the magnitude of the problem is found in a survey of 257 patients (mostly with disease of less than 20 years' duration) by Scheinberg and co-workers.[101] The overall employment rate, excluding the category of independent homemaker, was only 19.5% (Table 25-9). The reasons for unemployment in this study are listed in Table 25-10. Only 46 patients (17.9%) had had any contact with a vocational counselor or vocational rehabilitation agency. More recently, LaRocca and associates[64] reviewed 312 patients with a mean disease duration of 13 years; 23% were still employed. Patients who were older, male, less disabled, and better educated were more likely to be employed.

In light of the social consequences of MS, a detailed assessment of each patient's total life situation, including significant relationships, family structure, educational background, and vocational history, is as essential as a medical assessment. The fears and underlying feelings of family members require the support and sympathetic attention of the rehabilitation professional, and family members need to be actively involved in educational programs concerning proper medical and rehabilitative care. Based on an evaluation of needs at home, provision of nursing, homemaker, or therapist services may reinforce these educational goals and provide much needed respite for family members who are caring for the patient at home. Family groups can be valuable as a vehicle for fostering education and developing mutual support among families. In her discussion of the social worker's role in MS rehabilitation, Geronemus[42] stressed the importance of crisis *prevention* as well as crisis intervention when treating the families of MS patients.

A strong case can be made for a greater degree of involvement by vocational rehabilitation personnel and agencies in MS rehabilitation. Although MS is at least as prevalent as spinal cord injury, affects a similar age group, and has a similar life expectancy, the number of MS patients rehabilitated by state departments of vocational rehabilitation in 1976 was only one-fifth that of patients with spinal cord injury.[56] Scheinberg and associates[101] emphasize the employability of MS patients based on level of education (almost half of their 257 patients had at least some college education, and four fifths had completed high school), presence of family support, and relative freedom from disabling pain (which is only about half as common as after spinal cord injury[80]), and long life expectancy.[61] A patient who is expected to have a relatively benign clinical course is a particularly good candidate for vocational rehabilitation.

RATIONAL APPROACH TO COMPREHENSIVE REHABILITATION

The disability produced by MS is greater than the sum of its symptoms, and successful rehabilitation requires treatment that is individualized, function oriented, flexible, and interdisciplinary. Methods developed for the management of other disorders, such as spinal cord injury, cerebellar disease, blindness, or chronic pain, can be applied in modified form to MS patients, and because these patients usually have more than one symptom, several concurrent strategies may be indicated. Because of its variable clinical course and wide range of disabling sequelae, the comprehensive rehabilitation of MS demands a degree of therapeutic eclecticism rarely required with other diseases. Seven major components of this approach are briefly outlined below; they are easily remembered because, like eclecticism, all begin with the letter "E":

1. Early evaluation
2. Exercise efficiency
3. Energy conservation
4. Equipment prescription
5. Environmental modification
6. Emotional support
7. Education

Functional assessment of a patient with newly diagnosed MS by physician, physical therapist, occupational therapist, speech and language pathologist, psychologist, social worker, rehabilitation counselor, and nurse, with periodic reassessments based on the nature and degree of disability, as well as its pattern of progression, is the first step in the

rehabilitation process. The early identification of functional deficits in the context of the patient's physical and social environment helps to prevent the development of secondary problems (joint contractures, pressure sores, aspiration pneumonia, urinary infection, fecal impaction, and so on), maintains maximal adaptation to a changing disease, and forms the basis for establishing a set of achievable therapeutic goals. A truly interdisciplinary—not merely multidisciplinary—team is an essential ingredient of this type of assessment, and the forging of such a cohesive group is a complex, time-consuming process whose successful operation requires commitment, availability, leadership, good morale, effective conflict management, and a sense of direction and growth in each of its members.[21]

Documentation of functional status at the time of initial evaluation and at subsequent visits is desirable for optimal communication among members of the treatment team, and a number of authors have developed disability rating scales for this purpose.[37,59,63,107] Some, such as the Mobility Level Scale[37] limit themselves to a single functional component and are easily interpreted. Components of the Mobility Level Scale are as follows[57]:

1. The patient has no restrictions on activities of normal employment and/or domestic life but is not necessarily symptom free.
2. The patient can walk on level surfaces using no aids for short distances only (for about 15 minutes) before he or she must stop and rest. The patient can climb stairs.
3. The patient can walk alone but must use aids (walls, furniture, cane, crutches, walker, braces).
4. The patient can walk a few steps but usually uses a wheelchair. The patient can transfer from a chair.
5. Same as number 4 above, but the patient cannot walk at all.
6. The patient uses a wheelchair exclusively but cannot transfer.
7. The patient must be in bed most or all of the time.

More complex scales by Kurtzke[59] (Expanded Disability Status Scale [EDSS]) and by Sipe[107] (Neurologic Rating Scale [NRS]) monitor deficits in motor, cerebellar, brainstem, visual, sensory, bowel and bladder, and mental functions; the EDSS scores range from 0 (normal) to 10 (death), and the NRS composite rating ranges from 0 (death) to 100 (normal).

Prescription of therapeutic exercise is a particularly good example of the eclectic approach called for in MS. Cailliet's discussion of this subject includes forms of exercise for lower motor neuron, upper motor neuron, and cerebellar disorders; the choice of method depends on whether the goal is induction of voluntary motor activity, improvement in sensory feedback, inhibition of unwanted motor patterns, improvement in coordination, or prevention of joint contractures.[15] Since it is not unusual to encounter spasticity, ataxia, and disuse weakness in the same patient, the appropriate exercise regime is a melange of techniques that challenges the ingenuity and creativity of the rehabilitation team. Fatigue and heat intolerance, both of which are common problems, must be taken into account because of their potentially adverse effects. Useful guidelines for the establishment of an exercise program include the following:

1. Treat in a well-ventilated and relatively cool room; an alternative environment would be a pool with water temperature betwen 24° and 27.5° C.[41]
2. Treat in the early morning when body and ambient temperature are lowest and when fatigue is least prominent.
3. Allow frequent rest periods during exercise sessions.
4. Observe energy conservation techniques whenever possible (see below).
5. Teach the patient (in writing when there are memory deficits) and family how to carry out exercise at home or in the hospital room.
6. Never carry exercise past the point of fatigue; however, exercise up to the point of fatigue may increase endurance.[12]
7. Treat underlying spasticity aggressively.

Energy conservation and work simplification are among the most central principles in MS rehabilitation. The selection of adaptive equipment—self-help aids for the upper extremities, lower extremity orthoses, wheelchairs, or other ambulation aids—and the modification of home or work environments are outgrowths of these principles, which have been summarized by Wolf[118] as follows:

1. Preplan and organize activities before initiating them.
2. Allow enough time to avoid rushing.
3. Eliminate all unnecessary tasks and simplify those that remain.
4. Pace all activities, allowing sufficient time for rest.
5. Use both upper extremities.
6. Slide objects rather than lifting or carrying them.
7. Use work surfaces of appropriate height.
8. Sit whenever possible.
9. Take advantage of gravity and momentum.

To these may be added the following, which relate to equipment and environment:

1. Make liberal use of ambulation aids, including wheelchairs, to avoid excessive energy expenditure.
2. For patients with severe neurologic impairment, provide an adjustable-height bed to facilitate bed mobility and transfer activities (for caretakers as well as the patient).
3. Plan the most strenuous aspects of the workday for the early morning hours.
4. Organize the workday to include regularly scheduled periods of rest, particularly in the afternoon.
5. Provide adequate air-conditioning at home, at work, and in any vehicle used for travel between them.
6. Avoid prolonged periods outdoors during the hours when the temperature is maximal.

The psychologic toll of MS is mentioned in a preceding section of this chapter. The needs of patient and family for emotional support must be addressed promptly and with sensitivity by all members of the rehabilitation team. The choice of individual, couple, group, or family therapy (more than one may be indicated) should be made after initial assessments have been completed and team members have discussed their findings among themselves, as well as sharing them with the patient and family. Such patient-team meetings are an opportunity to initiate the educational process that is the final component of the rehabilitation program. A familiarity with the nature of MS and its symptoms allows the patient to assume a greater degree of responsibility in the implementation of rehabilitation therapy and the formulation of life goals. Since 1946 the National Multiple Sclerosis Society has been an excellent information source, providing a wide range of printed material about most aspects of MS. Scheinberg[100] has also contributed a valuable handbook designed for use by patients and families. An often neglected area of education is that required by health care professionals themselves. Commonly held misconceptions about the prognosis of MS (see "Clinical Course and Outcome Prediction") may be partly responsible for the underutilization of vocational rehabilitation services by these patients. Several authors have pointed out that the vocational potential of MS patients is considerable, yet much of it remains untapped.[56,91,101]

Although it is possible to provide adequate care for MS patients individually, the optimal milieu is one in which many patients are being managed concurrently. The advantages of such centralized MS treatment centers include the following:

1. They allow treatment staff to develop particular expertise in the eclectic treatment approach outlined previously.
2. They make it possible to establish and maintain ongoing patient groups for peer support, group psychotherapy, and educational programs.
3. By their specialized function and staff selection, they ensure a treatment team with a high degree of interest in MS patients and their rehabilitation.
4. They facilitate the performance of well-controlled clinical rehabilitation research, which has been a neglected area in the literature on MS.

Since the majority of MS patients do not require hospitalization, MS centers are predominantly outpatient facilities. However, if hospitalization becomes necessary, the potential needs of MS patients for medical specialists in neurology, rehabilitation medicine, urology, infectious disease, psychiatry, gastroenterology, ophthalmology, and otolaryngology, as well as a skilled team of nursing, physical therapy, occupational therapy, speech and language pathology, psychology, and social work professionals, dictate that such MS centers should be affiliated with a large medical center in which all these services are readily available.

Scheinberg and co-workers[102] have outlined the organization of one such facility, the Multiple Sclerosis Comprehensive Care Center at the Albert Einstein College of Medicine (Bronx, New York), which has been in operation since 1974.

SUMMARY

Although MS has neither a clear-cut cause nor a definitive treatment, it does have a major rehabilitation component in its management. Despite its label as the "great crippler of young men,"[102] this enigmatic disease is compatible with a long and productive life for many of those who have it. With appropriate medical management, a comprehensive interdisciplinary team approach to disabling symptoms, and a supportive therapeutic milieu, restoration of maximal function is feasible and can even be cost effective.[33] Since there are no measures to prevent MS and patients survive for many years, its prevalence is likely to increase significantly in the future. Given this growing population and its demonstrated functional potential, more attention should be focused on the role of rehabilitation techniques and technology, and this should be reflected in a greater prominence of MS in the rehabilitation literature.

REFERENCES

1. Aita, JF, et al: CT appearance of multiple sclerosis, Neurology 28:251, 1978.
2. Asselmann, P, Chadwick, DW, and Marsden, CW: Visual evoked responses in the diagnosis and management of patients suspected of multiple sclerosis, Brain 98:261, 1975.
3. Augspurger, RR: Bladder dysfunction in multiple sclerosis. In Maloney, FP, Burks, JS, and Ringel, SP, editors: Interdisciplinary rehabilitation of multiple sclerosis and neuromuscular disorders, Philadelphia, 1985, JB Lippincott Co.
4. Bauer, HF: Problems of symptomatic therapy in multiple sclerosis, Neurology 28(9:Part 2):8, 1978.
5. Benkelman, DR, Kraft, GH, and Freal, J: Expressive communicative disorders in persons with multiple sclerosis, Arch Phys Med Rehabil 66:675, 1985.
6. Blaivas, JG: Management of bladder dysfunction in multiple sclerosis, Neurology 30:12, 1980.
7. Blaivas, JG, Bhimani, G, and Labid, KB: Vesicoureteral dysfunction in multiple sclerosis, J Urol 122:342, 1979.
8. Blinchik, ER, and Grzesiak, RC: Reinterpretive cognitive strategies in chronic pain management, Arch Phys Med Rehabil 60:609, 1979.
9. Block, JM, and Kester, NC: Role of rehabilitation in management of multiple sclerosis, Mod Treatment 7:930, 1970.
10. Bourestom, NC, and Howard, MT: Personality characteristics of three disability groups, Arch Phys Med Rehabil 46:626, 1965.
11. Bradley, WE, Logothetis, JL, and Tim, GW: Cystometric and sphincter abnormalities in multiple sclerosis, Neurology 23:1131, 1973.
12. Brar, SP, and Wangaard, C: Physical therapy for patients with multiple sclerosis. In Maloney, FP, Burks, JS, and Ringel, SP, editors: Interdisciplinary rehabilitation of multiple sclerosis and neuromuscular disorders, Philadelphia, 1985, JB Lippincott Co.
13. Brindley, GS: Electroejaculation: its technique, neurological implications and uses, J Neurol Neurosurg Psychiatry 44:9, 1981.
14. Cailliet, R: Rehabilitation in multiple sclerosis. In Licht, SH, editor: Rehabilitation and medicine, New Haven, Conn, 1968, Elizabeth Licht Publisher.
15. Cailliet, R: Exercise in multiple sclerosis. In Basmajian, JV, editor: Therapeutic exercise, ed 3, Baltimore, 1978, Williams & Wilkins Co.
16. Cala, LA, Mastaglia, FL, and Black, JL: Computerized tomography of the brain and optic nerve in multiple sclerosis, J Neurol Sci 36:411, 1978.
17. Charcot, JM: Lectures on the diseases of the nervous system, London, 1877, New Sydenham Society.
18. Chiappa, KH, et al: Brainstem auditory-evoked potentials in 200 patients with multiple sclerosis, Ann Neurol 7:135, 1980.
19. Clark, VA, et al: Factors associated with a malignant or benign course of multiple sclerosis, JAMA 248:856, 1982.
20. Clifford, DB, and Trotter, JI: Pain in multiple sclerosis, J Neurol 41:1270, 1984.
21. Cobble, ND, and Burks, JS: The team approach to the management of multiple sclerosis. In Maloney, FP, Burks, JS, and Ringel, SP, editors: Interdisciplinary rehabilitation of multiple sclerosis and neuromuscular disorders, Philadelphia, 1985, JB Lippincott Co.
22. Cohen, MM, Lessell, S, and Wolf, PA: Prospective study of risk of developing multiple sclerosis in uncomplicated optic neuritis, Neurology 29:208, 1979.
23. Cohen, SN, et al: Critical frequency of photic driving in the diagnosis of multiple sclerosis: a comparison to the pattern evoked responses, Arch Neurol 37:80, 1980.
24. Cole, TM, Chilgren, R, and Rosenberg, PA: A new programme of sex education and counseling for spinal cord injured adults and health care professionals, Paraplegia 11:111, 1973.
25. Cook, AW: Electrical stimulation in multiple sclerosis, Hosp Pract 11:51, 1976.
26. Crawford, JD, and Melvor, GP: Group psychotherapy: benefits in multiple sclerosis, Arch Phys Med Rehabil 66:810, 1985.
27. Darley, FL, Aronson, AE, and Brown, JR: Differential diagnostic patterns of dysarthria, J Speech Hearing Res 12:246, 1969.
28. Darley, FL, Brown, JR, and Goldstein, NP: Dysarthria in multiple sclerosis, J Speech Hearing Res 15:229, 1972.
29. Davis, F: The hot bath test in the diagnosis of multiple sclerosis, J Mt Sinai Hosp NY 33:280, 1966.
30. DeLisa, JA, et al: Multiple sclerosis. I. Common physical disabilities and rehabilitation, Am Fam Phys 32:157, 1985.
31. Eisen, A: Neurophysiology of multiple sclerosis, Neurol Clin 1:615, 1983.
32. Farmakides, MN, and Boone, DR: Speech problems of patients with multiple sclerosis, J Speech Hearing Disorders 25:385, 1960.
33. Feigenson, JS, et al: Cost-effectiveness of multiple sclerosis rehabilitation: model, Neurology 31:1316, 1981.
34. Fink, H, and Tibbling, G: Principles of albumin and IgG analyses in neurological disorders. III. Evaluations of IgG synthesis within the central nervous system in multiple sclerosis, Scand J Clin Lab Invest 37:397, 1977.
35. Fink, SL, and Houser, HB: An investigation of physical and intellectual changes in multiple sclerosis, Arch Phys Med Rehabil 47:56, 1966.
36. Fisher, M, Long, RR, and Drachman, DA: Hand muscle atrophy in multiple sclerosis, Arch Neurol 40:811, 1983.
37. Frankel, DL, et al: Multiple sclerosis: disability assessment by mobility scale, Arch Phys Med Rehabil 64:505, 1983.
38. Franklin, GM, and Burks, JS: Diagnosis and medical management of multiple sclerosis. In Maloney, FP, Burks, JS, and Ringel, SP, editors: Interdisciplinary rehabilitation of multiple sclerosis and neuromuscular disorders, Philadelphia, 1985, JB Lippincott Co.
39. Freal, JE, Kraft, GH, and Coryell, JF: Symptomatic fatigue in multiple sclerosis, Arch Phys Med Rehabil 65:135, 1984.
40. Gebarski, SS, et al: The initial diagnosis of multiple sclerosis: clinical impact of MRI, Ann Neurol 17:469, 1985.
41. Gehlsen, G, et al: Gait characteristics in multiple sclerosis: progressive changes and effects of exercise on parameters, Arch Phys Med Rehabil 67:536, 1986.

42. Geronemus, DF: The role of the social worker in the comprehensive long-term care of multiple sclerosis patients, Neurology 30:48, 1980.

43. Glick, ME, Meshkinfoos, H, and Haldeman, S: Colonic dysfunction in multiple sclerosis, Gastroenterology 83:1002, 1982.

44. Goldstein, G, and Shelly, CH: Neuropsychological diagnosis of multiple sclerosis in the neuropsychiatric setting, J Nerv Ment Dis 158:280, 1974.

45. Halliday, AM, McDonald, WI, and Mushin, J: Visual evoked responses in diagnosis of multiple sclerosis, Br Med J 4:661, 1973.

46. Halliday, AM, McDonald, WI, and Mushin, J: Visual evoked potentials in patients with demyelinating disease. In Desmedt, JE, editor: Visual evoked potentials in man: new developments, Oxford, Eng, 1977, Clarendon Press.

47. Harris, W: An analysis of 1433 cases of paroxysmal trigeminal neuralgia (trigeminal-tic) and the end-results of gasserian alcohol injection, Brain 63:209, 1940.

48. Hartings, MF, Pavlou, MM, and Davis, FA: Group counseling of MS patients in a program of comprehensive care, J Chron Dis 29:65, 1976.

49. Illis, LS, et al: Dorsal-column stimulation in rehabilitation of patients with multiple sclerosis, Lancet 1:1383, 1976.

50. Iraqui, VJ, et al: Evoked potentials in trigeminal neuralgia associated with multiple sclerosis, Arch Neurol 43:444, 1986.

51. Jambor, RL: Cognitive functioning in multiple sclerosis, Br J Psychiatry 115:765, 1969.

52. Johnson, KP, and Nelson, BJ: Multiple sclerosis: diagnostic usefulness of cerebrospinal fluid, Ann Neurol 2:425, 1977.

53. Kimura, J: Electrically elicited blink reflex in diagnosis of multiple sclerosis: review of 260 patients over a seven-year period, Brain 98:413, 1975.

54. Knutson, LL: Understanding and managing the psychosocial aspects of multiple sclerosis. In Maloney, FP, Burks, JS, and Ringel, SP, editors: Interdisciplinary rehabilitation of multiple sclerosis and neuromuscular disorders, Philadelphia, 1985, JB Lippincott Co.

55. Kostulas, VK, Henriksson, A, and Link, H: Monosymptomatic sensory symptoms and cerebrospinal fluid immunoglobulin levels in relation to multiple sclerosis, Arch Neurol 43:447, 1986.

56. Kraft, GH, Freal, JE, and Coryell, JK: Disability, disease duration, and rehabilitation service needs in multiple sclerosis: patient perspectives, Arch Phys Med Rehabil 67:164, 1986.

57. Kraft, GH, et al: Multiple sclerosis: early prognostic guidelines, Arch Phys Med Rehabil 62:54, 1981.

58. Kurtzke, JF: Epidemiologic contributions to multiple sclerosis: an overview, Neurology 30:61, 1980.

59. Kurtzke, JF: Rating neurologic impairment in multiple sclerosis: an expanded disability status scale, Neurology 33:1444, 1983.

60. Kurtzke, JF, et al: Studies on the natural history of multiple sclerosis. 8. Long-term survival in young men, Arch Neurol 22:215, 1970.

61. Kurtzke, JF, et al: Studies on natural history of multiple sclerosis. 8. Early prognostic features of later course of illness, J Chron Dis 30:819, 1977.

62. Langworthy, G, and LeGrand, D: Personality structure and psychotherapy in multiple sclerosis, Am J Med 12:586, 1952.

63. LaRocca, N, et al: Field testing of a minimal record of disability in multiple sclerosis: the United States and Canada, Acta Neurol Scand 101(suppl):126, 1984.

64. LaRocca, N, et al: Factors associated with unemployment of patients with multiple sclerosis, J Chron Dis 38:203, 1985.

65. Levine, JS; Bowel dysfunction in multiple sclerosis. In Maloney, FP, Burks, JS, and Ringel, SP, editors: Interdisciplinary rehabilitation of multiple sclerosis and neuromuscular disorders, Philadelphia, 1985, JB Lippincott Co.

66. Lhermitte, J: Les troubles psychiques dans la sclerose en plaques, Paris Med 53:307, 1924.

67. Liebowitz, I, and Alter, M: Multiple sclerosis: clues to its cause, New York, 1973, Elsevier Publishing Co.

68. Lillus, HG, Valtoneu, EJ, and Wikstrom, J: Sexual problems in patients suffering from multiple sclerosis, J Chron Dis 29:643, 1976.

69. Lukes, SA, et al: Nuclear magnetic resonance imaging in multiple sclerosis, Ann Neurol 13:592, 1983.

70. Lumsden, CE: The neuropathology of multiple sclerosis. In Vinken, PJ, and Brugn, GW, editors: Handbook of clinical neurology, vol 9, Amsterdam, 1970, North-Holland Publishing Co.

71. Lundberg, PO: Sexual dysfunction in patients with multiple sclerosis, Sexuality Disabil 1:218, 1978.

72. Lyon-Caen, O, et al: Cognitive function in recent-onset demyelating disease, Arch Neurol 43:1138, 1986.

73. Maloney, FP, Burks, JS, and Ringel, SP, editors: Interdisciplinary rehabilitation of multiple sclerosis and neuromuscular disorders, Philadelphia, 1985, JB Lippincott Co.

74. Matson, RR, and Brooks, NA, Adjusting to multiple sclerosis: an exploratory study, Soc Sci Med 11:245, 1977.

75. McAlpin, D, Lumsden, CE, and Acheson, ED: Multiple sclerosis: a reappraisal, ed 2, Baltimore, 1972, Williams & Wilkins Co.

76. McFarlin, DE, and McFarland, HF: Multiple sclerosis, I and II, N Engl J Med 307:1183, 1246, 1982.

77. Money, TO, Cole, TM, and Chilgren, RA: Sexual options for paraplegics and quadriplegics, Boston, 1975, Little, Brown & Co.

78. Muller, R: Studies on disseminated sclerosis—with special reference to symptomatology, course, and prognosis, Acta Med Scand 222(suppl):1, 1949.

79. Namerow, NS: Circadian temperature rhythm and vision in multiple sclerosis, Neurology 18:417, 1968.

80. Nepomuceno, C, et al: Pain in patients with spinal cord injury, Arch Phys Med Rehabil 60:605, 1979.

81. Parsons, OA, Stewart, KD, and Arenberg, D: Impairment of abstracting ability in multiple sclerosis, J Nerv Ment Dis 125:221, 1957.

82. Percy, AK, et al: Multiple sclerosis in Rochester, Minnesota: a 60-year appraisal, Arch Neurol 25:105, 1971.

83. Perry, J, Gronley, J, and Lunsford, T: Rocker shoe as walking aid in multiple sclerosis, Arch Phys Med Rehabil 62:59, 1981.

84. Peyser, Jm, et al: Cognitive function in patients with multiple sclerosis, Arch Neurol 37:577, 1980.

85. Phillips, Ca, et al: Functional electrical exercise: a comprehensive approach for physical conditioning of the spinal cord injured patient, Orthopedics 7:1112, 1984.

86. Poser, CM: Diseases of the myelin sheath. In Baker, AB, and Baker, LH, editors: Clinical neurology, Hagerstown, Md, 1978, Harper & Row Publishers, Inc.

87. Poser, CM: A numerical scoring system for the classification of multiple sclerosis, Acta Neurol Scand 60:100, 1979.

88. Poser, CM: Exacerbations, activity, and progression in multiple sclerosis, Arch Neurol 37:471, 1980.

89. Poser, CM, et al: New diagnostic criteria for multiple sclerosis: guidelines for research protocols, Ann Neurol 13:227, 1983.

90. Poser, CM, et al, editors: The diagnosis of multiple sclerosis, New York, 1984, Thieme Medical Publishers, Inc.

91. Poser, S, and Poser, W: Multiple sclerosis and gestation, Neurology 33:1422, 1983.

92. Rao, SM, et al: Memory disturbances in chronic progressive multiple sclerosis, Arch Neurol 13:573, 1984.

93. Reisner, T, and Maida, E: Computerized tomography in multiple sclerosis, Arch Neurol 37:475, 1980.

94. Robinson, K, and Rudge, P: Abnormalities of the auditory evoked responses in patients with multiple sclerosis, Brain 100:19, 1977.

95. Rozin, R, et al: Vocational status of MS patients in Israel, Arch Phys Med Rehabil 56:300, 1975.

96. Rudick, RA, et al: Multiple sclerosis: the problem of incorrect diagnosis, Arch Neurol 43:578, 1986.

97. Rushton, JG, and Olfason, RA: Trigeminal neuralgia associated with multiple sclerosis, Arch Neurol 13:383, 1965.

98. Ruttenberg, N: Assessment and treatment of speech and swallowing problems in patients with multiple sclerosis. In Maloney, FP, Burks, JS, and Ringle, SP, editors: Interdisciplinary rehabilitation of multiple sclerosis and neuromuscular disorders, Philadelphia, 1985, JB Lippincott Co.

99. Sabra, AF, et al: Treatment of action tremor in multiple sclerosis with isoniazid, Neurology 32:912, 1982.

100. Scheinberg, LC, editor: Multiple sclerosis, a guide for patients and their families, New York, 1983, Raven Press.

101. Scheinberg, L, et al: Multiple sclerosis: earning a living, NY State J Med 80:1395, 1980.

102. Scheinberg, L, et al: Comprehensive long-term care of patients with multiple sclerosis, Neurology 31:1121, 1981.

103. Schneitzer, L: Rehabilitation of patients with multiple sclerosis, Arch Phys Med Rehabil 59:430, 1978.

104. Schumacher, G, et al: Problems of experimental trials of therapy in multiple sclerosis: report by the panel on evaluation of experimental trials of therapy in multiple sclerosis, Ann NY Acad Sci 122:552, 1965.

105. Sedal, L: Management of multiple sclerosis, Patient Management 12:69, 1980.

106. Sha'ked, A: Human sexuality and rehabilitation medicine: sexual functioning following spinal cord injury, Baltimore, 1981, Williams & Wilkins Co.

107. Sipe, JC, et al: A neurological rating scale (NRS) in multiple sclerosis, Neurology 34:1368, 1984.

108. Stevens, JC: Magnetic resonance imaging: clinical correlation in 64 patients, Arch Neurol 43:1145, 1986.

109. Stockard, J, et al: Detection and localization of occult lesions with brainstem auditory responses, Mayo Clin Proc 52:761, 1977.

110. Surridge, D: Investigation into some psychiatric aspects of multiple sclerosis, Br J Psychiatry 115:749, 1969.

111. Thompson, DS, et al: The effects of pregnancy on multiple sclerosis (MS): a retrospective study, Neurology 34(suppl):244, 1984.

112. Twomey, JA, and Espir, LE: Paroxysmal symptoms as the first manifestation of multiple sclerosis, J Neurol Neurosurg Psychiatry 43:295, 1980.

113. Tyndel, FJ, Bilbao, JM, and Tucker, WS: Unsuspected lesions in patients with bilateral tic douloreux, Lancet 1:1418, 1984.

114. Valleroy, MI, and Kraft, GH: Sexual dysfunction in multiple sclerosis, Arch Phys Med Rehabil 65:125, 1984.

115. Vas, CJ: Sexual impotence and some autonomic disturbances in men with multiple sclerosis, Acta Neurol Scand 45:166, 1969.

116. Watson, C: Effects of lowering body temperature on the symptoms and signs of multiple sclerosis, N Engl J Med 261:1253, 1959.

117. Wheeler, JS, et al: The changing neurourologic pattern of multiple sclerosis, J Urol 130:1123, 1983.

118. Wolf, BG: Occupational therapy for patients with multiple sclerosis. In Maloney, FP, Burks, JS, and Ringel, SP, editors: Interdisciplinary rehabilitation of multiple sclerosis and neuromuscular disorders, Philadelphia, 1985, JB Lippincott Co.

119. Young, IR, et al: Nuclear magnetic resonance imaging of the brain in multiple sclerosis, Lancet 2:1063, 1981.

120. Young, RR, and Delwaide PJ: Spasticity, I and II, N Engl J Med 304:28, 96, 1981.

CHAPTER 26

Chronic obstructive pulmonary disease

PATHOGENESIS AND MANAGEMENT

ADAM N. HUREWITZ AND EDWARD H. BERGOFSKY

ETIOLOGY AND PATHOGENESIS

The treatment of chronic obstructive pulmonary disease (COPD) combines the principles of preventive and rehabilitative methods with classic medical and pharmacologic approaches. The most important goals of therapy are to improve functional activity, reduce chronic breathlessness, and prolong survival. A comprehensive program aimed at achieving these goals can best be designed when mechanisms underlying impaired function are addressed. To this end, the pathophysiologic principles of COPD are emphasized in this chapter.

COPD by our usage includes obstructive bronchitis, pulmonary emphysema, or a mixture of the two[7]; bronchial asthma and cystic fibrosis are not discussed at any length, although many of the same management principles are applicable to these conditions.

Etiology

An overwhelmingly important cause of COPD is tobacco smoke inhalation. The effects of the tobacco smoke are found at two distinct sites in the lung. The first is the mucous membrane of the tracheobronchial tree.[3] The clinical syndrome at this site is *bronchitis* and centers on bronchospasm or chronic cough with sputum production for greater than 3 months per year over a 2-year period.[1] Frequent tracheobronchial infections with prolonged convalescence are also typical. The anatomic counterpart of this syndrome consists of surface epithelial metaplasia and submucosal glandular hypertrophy.[19] The physiologic counterpart consists of pulmonary function derangements relating to delayed expiratory flow and impaired mucociliary elimination of particles and mucus.[14]

The other site at which tobacco smoke exerts its effect is the lung parenchyma. The majority of patients with COPD have some degree of parenchymal destruction superimposed on the chronic bronchitis, and in some this effect may be more prominent—or even the sole clinically apparent disease. This clinical syndrome is *pulmonary emphysema*.

Most aspects of pulmonary emphysema can be attributed to the loss of the balance that normally exists between proteases released by migrating scavenger cells and the amount of active tissue antiproteases. The result is persistent connective tissue destruction throughout the lung (Figure 26-1). Oxidants in smoke are capable of inactivating tissue antiproteases. The irritant effects of smoke also induce increased numbers of neutrophils and macrophages to migrate into the lung. Thus the stage is set to increase the protease/antiprotease ratio in the lung, which in turn leads to damage of the connective tissue matrix.[5] This scenario is associated with an insidious loss of nearly 75 ml of vital capacity per year in smokers, compared with only 30 ml per year in nonsmokers.[6] Such losses accumulate to a considerable degree, so that over a 20-year period of smoking, both the slow and the timed vital capacity substantially decrease. Additional loss of lung function occurs in smokers during acute respiratory tract infections. The magnitude of this loss has been attributed to the partial inactivation of alpha-1-antiprotease in smokers, setting the stage for inadequate binding of proteases from infiltrating neutrophils and macrophages during both chronic and acute infection.

Pathologic changes observed in the lung parenchyma are consistent with this pathogenesis. The lung is grossly hyperinflated, often with evidence of bulla formation on the uncut surface and in the lung sections. Histologically the mean diameter of alveoli is greatly increased, air spaces show coalescence, broken alveolar walls appear as clubbed spokes, and the whole lobule or just the center of a lobule may be involved by this loss of alveoli and blood vessels.[20]

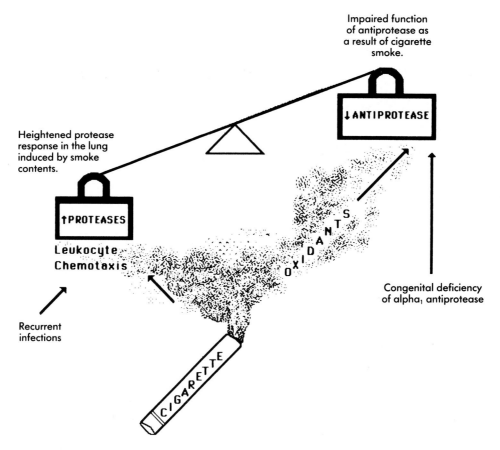

Figure 26-1. Cigarette smoking alters balance between proteases and antiproteases in lung. Products contained in smoke increase lung protease concentrations by recruiting protease-containing white blood cells and macrophages into lung. Cigarette smoke also oxidizes naturally occurring antiproteases, further promoting damage incurred by abundant proteases. Genetic deficiency of antiprotease further intensifies this relationship.

Pathophysiology
Ventilatory dysfunction

Progressive decreases in airway caliber are the hallmark of COPD. From the pathogenetic standpoint, several mechanisms underlie these changes. The first involves *morphologic narrowing* of the airway. Excess secretions from hypertrophied submucous glands, bronchial smooth muscle contraction, and inflammatory edema and cellular infiltration have all been demonstrated morphologically in COPD and have varying degrees of reversibility with treatment. *Functional narrowing* refers to a defect produced by disease outside the airway. This may take two forms: loss of circumferential tethering of small airways owing to a reduction in circumbronchial alveoli and their connective tissue, or reduction of intrabronchial pressure during expiration owing to loss of elastic recoil pressure from disappearing alveoli. Functional narrowing is most strikingly manifest during expiration, when positive pleural pressures tend to cause dynamic compression of flaccid airways.

Airway obstruction in COPD is thus worse during expiration and in fact may be minimal during inspiration. As a result, not all of the inspired volume may be expired. Although the difference between inspired and expired tidal volumes under these conditions is small, hyperinflation of the lung may occur with time because of this effect. The result, in moderation, is not all bad, because the hyperinflated lung improves flow during expiration. This comes about because the hyperinflation places whatever connective tissue remains in these lungs on the stretch, thus enhancing both alveolar elastic recoil and bronchial tethering. Consequently, expiration is enhanced, and a new equilibrium is produced wherein inspired and expired volumes are equal (Figure 26-2).

In addition to air trapping, another cause for hyperinflation when emphysema is present is the loss of elastic tissue and the subsequent increase in lung compliance. These changes elicit large increases in the functional residual capacity, and the increase in lung compliance often permits the vital capacity to at least remain within normal limits during much of the course of this illness. As a result, the total lung capacity is enlarged, but how large it becomes depends on the ability of the thoracic cage (rib cage and

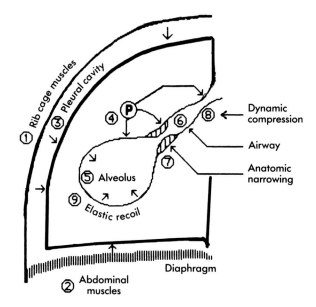

Figure 26-2. Dynamic compression of airways in chronic obstructive pulmonary disease (COPD). Patients with COPD may attempt to augment expiration by using expiratory muscles of rib cage *(1)* and abdomen *(2)*. Resulting increase in pleural *(3)* and pulmonary *(4)* pressures *(P)* is also imposed on alveolus *(5)* and airway *(6)*. Anatomic narrowing in upstream airway *(7)* produces unusually large intraluminal pressure drops in downstream airway *(8)*. Pulmonary pressure *(4)* therefore tends to exceed airway pressure *(8)* and cause dynamic compression during expiration. Airway in COPD thus develops two resistances that impede expiration: anatomic *(7)* and dynamic *(8)*. To alleviate this bind, COPD patient can apply more alveolar elastic recoil pressure *(9)* rather than pleural or pulmonary pressures *(3,4)*; this, however, requires hyperinflation of lung.

diaphragm), which contains the lungs, to undergo the conformational enlargement that will allow the lungs to expand.

Respiratory muscle dysfunction

The work of breathing *(W)* is elevated in COPD—as in other respiratory diseases such as scoliosis or interstitial fibrosis. In addition, depression of the diaphragm in patients with COPD may reduce the efficiency *(E)* of this muscle. As a result, the O_2 consumption ($\dot{V}O_2$) of the diaphragm is unduly high in accord with the standard equation relating muscular work, oxygen consumption, and muscle efficiency: $\dot{V}O_2 = W/E$. These considerations are no doubt applicable to the other inspiratory and expiratory muscles of respiration as well.[8]

In the light of these relationships, the effects of excess work on respiratory muscle fatigue must be considered. This is demonstrated in normal individuals by adding loads (negative tracheal pressures, resistances, and so forth) to breathing and observing decreases in the pressure developed by the diaphragm. This principle of resting a presumably fatigued muscle has also been associated in COPD, scoliosis,

Table 26-1. Typical blood gas derangements in COPD

Clinical stage	Po$_2$ (mm Hg)	Sao$_2$ (%)*	Pco$_2$ (mm Hg)	pH
Moderate	70	94	38	7.40
Advanced				
Chronic	55	86	38	7.40
Acute	42	77	50	7.30
Late	50	80	50	7.36

*Arterial oxygen saturation.

and other diseases with increased respiratory work. Nocturnal mechanical ventilation has a carryover effect into the following day, as manifested by improved arterial blood gas levels, presumably caused by improved respiratory muscle function.[9]

Gas exchange

As COPD advances, abnormalities of gas exchange are commonplace. Arterial Po$_2$ values are lowered by 10 to 20 mm Hg in mild to moderately ill patients and by 40 mm Hg in the more seriously ill. At these levels of lung disease there is little likelihood of concomitant CO_2 retention. When the lung disease becomes sufficiently severe to reduce Pao$_2$ below 50 mm Hg, the emergence of hypercapnia poses an additional threat to the sensorium and the blood acid-base balance. Table 26-1 lists blood gas values typical of, but not confined to, various stages of advancement of COPD. The table indicates the Pao$_2$ tends to fall with advancing disease but also that acute decompensations caused by respiratory infections may produce temporary reductions in Po$_2$ and acute rises in Pco$_2$. Established chronic elevations of Pco$_2$ are usually accompanied by renal compensation (elevated HCO_3^- and base excess) so that the pH change is minimized; when an acute respiratory infection occurs in that setting, only partial compensation of the pH decrease may be seen.

At least four physiologic processes in COPD are capable of contributing to abnormal gas exchange in the lung: ventilation-perfusion imbalance, anatomic shunts, net alveolar hypoventilation, and diffusion limitation (Figure 26-3).

Ventilation-perfusion imbalance. The most important of the processes contributing to abnormal gas exchange in the lung is ventilation perfusion imbalance. The precise anatomic basis of this imbalance in the COPD lung is uncertain, but presumably it stems largely from areas of the lung that are poorly ventilated because of airway obstruction. If these areas are still perfused, venous admixture results. This suggests that venous blood, high in CO_2 and low in O_2 content, passes through the lung unrefreshed and mixes with arterialized blood from the better-preserved and better-ventilated units. These better-preserved units are so well ventilated that both the partial pressure of CO_2 and the CO_2 content

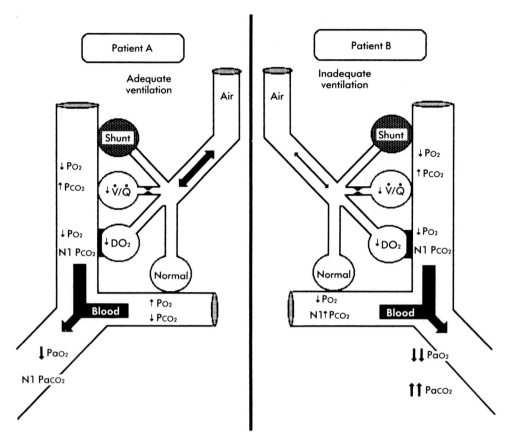

Figure 26-3. Causes of abnormal gas exchange in patients with chronic obstructive pulmonary disease. Reduction of arterial Po_2 can result from airway secretions or alveolar-capillary injury (such as seen with emphysema) through impairment of ventilation-perfusion matching or reduction of oxygen diffusion. If ventilatory reserve is intact *(patient A)*, these processes will produce hypoxemia, but hypercapnia is avoided through increased ventilation of noninjured lung regions. However, when ventilatory reserve is lost *(patient B)*, effects of V/Q mismatch, anatomic shunt, and impaired diffusion combine to produce both severe hypoxemia and hypercapnia with respiratory acidosis.

are greatly reduced. Corresponding increases in oxygen content are not achievable. This is because at high levels of Po_2 the O_2 dissociation curve is flat and O_2 content is not improved with modest rises of alveolar Po_2 achieved in well-ventilated alveoli. In summary, when blood from well-ventilated alveoli mixes with blood from poorly ventilated alveoli, the final arterial blood has a normal Pco_2 and CO_2 content but a reduced Po_2 and O_2 content. This mechanism is the chief cause of hypoxemia in COPD.

Ventilation-perfusion imbalance has an additional physiologic defect: reduced perfusion to some areas, possibly as a result of destruction of portions of the capillary bed. The result is excess ventilation relative to the degree of blood perfusion in some regions of the lung. Since reduced or absent gas exchange can occur in these areas, they have been termed alveolar dead space. The presence of significant dead space implies wasted ventilation and requires COPD

patients to increase their minute ventilation to satisfy normal gas exchange requirements.

Anatomic shunts. In principle, anatomic shunts are similar to ventilation-perfusion imbalance in their effect on gas exchange: venous admixture occurs with arterial hypoxemia but normal arterial Pco_2 levels. The chief characteristic that differentiates anatomic shunts from the usual defect of ventilation-perfusion is the virtually complete lack of any ventilation to these areas. Their anatomic counterparts are areas that are unventilated because of severe airway obstruction, noncompliant parenchyma, or, as may intermittently occur, atelectasis resulting from airway secretions. A major difference between anatomic shunts and the usual ventilation-perfusion imbalance is their response to oxygen breathing. The Po_2 of alveoli involved in the anatomic shunt is not altered by O_2 breathing, since O_2 has no access route; hence arterial Po_2 is little improved by oxygen breathing under these conditions. On the other hand, when alveoli have some ventilation, even though this may be as little as one tenth of the normal level, doubling or tripling the inspired oxygen produces substantial elevations of the Po_2 levels of affected alveoli and thus raises arterial Po_2.

Net alveolar hypoventilation. Unlike the effects of venous admixture and anatomic shunts, the contribution of the net alveolar hypoventilation to arterial hypoxemia in COPD is disputable. The concept of overall alveolar hypoventilation, in which virtually every air space is underventilated to a similar degree, is easiest to conceive of with respect to diseases of the chest wall and pleura or neuromuscular impairment. In COPD, different mechanisms must operate to achieve alveolar hypoventilation or, more accurately, an elevation of arterial Pco_2. As was just described, the straight-line CO_2 dissociation permits a well-ventilated alveolus to impose a low Pco_2 on blood and thus compensate for poorly ventilated regions with high values of Pco_2. On the other hand, the shape of the O_2 dissociation curve prevents oxygen from being added in significant quantities to blood in the well-ventilated alveoli. With progression of the COPD, however, fewer and fewer well-ventilated alveoli are available, and blood Pco_2 inevitably rises. In some instances, an ingredient of overall alveolar hypoventilation may be added to this mechanism because of respiratory muscle weakness or respiratory center depression. However, the distinctions between these factors and simple progression of ventilation-perfusion imbalance to account for the rising Pco_2 is not readily apparent in the clinical setting.

Diffusion limitation. Although reductions in diffusing capacity may occur in COPD and are generally attributed to morphologic emphysema, the degree to which they contribute to arterial hypoxemia is uncertain. Very large reductions in diffusing capacity must exist before disequilibrium between alveolar and pulmonary end-capillary O_2 tensions occurs and these reductions are evident only in far-advanced disease.

PATIENT EVALUATION
History

The first tier of patient evaluation, the history, is the story of the disease as told by the patient. It is of particular value in patients with pulmonary diseases, since much of the information obtained is not available from laboratory tests and other sources.

The history of cigarette smoking is one such example. As noted previously, cigarette smoking is the major cause of most cases of COPD. Several studies have correlated the extent of emphysema, determined at autopsy, with the number of cigarettes smoked.[2,23] In these studies nonsmoking men rarely (less than 10%) were found to have emphysema, and none showed changes of severe emphysema. By contrast, at least some degree of emphysema was found in those

who smoked one pack a day, with some 50% of this group having moderate to severe histologic changes.[2]

The absence of a smoking history in a patient with COPD should raise one's suspicion of a possible occupational etiology. A number of pulmonary irritants found in the workplace induce a clinical disease that is difficult to distinguish from COPD caused by cigarette smoke. Examples include the inhalation of nonfibrous materials, such as coal or silica dust; exposure to gaseous irritants, such as chlorine; or inhalation of aerosolized organisms, such as thermoactinomycetes found in air vents. If the patient also smokes cigarettes, the distinction between symptoms caused by work exposure and those caused by smoking is even more uncertain. An accurate occupational history often takes 15 to 30 minutes to obtain. An attempt should be made to determine specific agents to which the patient was exposed, the duration of exposure, alteration of symptoms during absences from work (such as vacations), and the presence of similar symptoms in fellow workers. Such documentation is important for planning to avoid the offending agent or for certifying that the patient is unable to return to the workplace.

The family history also provides important insights into the pathogenesis of COPD in certain patients. Congenital antiprotease deficiency is probably the most intensely studied example.[4] Individuals homozygous for the PiZ allele have reduced levels of serum alpha-1-antiprotease and develop pulmonary emphysema as early as the second decade of life. Until recently these patients had little hope for leading normal lives; however, exogenous antiproteases are being used in experimental protocols for those with early disease, and attempts at bilateral lung transplants are under way to treat those with already established disease. A second line of evidence in favor of familial predisposition can be found in the unusual clustering of cases of COPD in some families without antiprotease deficiency.[11] These cases are somewhat different from the antiprotease deficiencies in that the pathologic disorder is not primarily emphysema. A third line of evidence in support of familial predisposition to COPD may underlie the apparent resistance of some individuals to the damage of cigarette smoke. Although patterns of resistance within families have not been documented, the numbers of smokers who do not develop clinically apparent obstructive lung disease remains unaccountably high.[16]

Physical examination

Elements of the physical examination form the second tier of patient evaluation. As with the history taking, the time spent during physical examination helps establish a bond between physician and patient and is a source of data that is obtainable without risk.

From the physical appearance of the patient, the clinician can recognize characteristics of various lung diseases. Dorhorst[10] described two distinct appearances of patients

Table 26-2. Clinical presentation in obstructive lung disease

	Emphysema (type A, pink puffer)	Bronchitis (type B, blue bloater)
Clinical features		
Cough, sputum	Minimal	Prominent
Cyanosis	Minimal	Prominent
Weight loss	Prominent	Minimal
Leg edema	Minimal	Prominent
Dyspnea	Prominent	Moderate
Laboratory appearance		
Hypoxemia, hypercapnia	Minimal	Prominent
Polycythemia	Minimal	Prominent
Pulmonary hypertension	Minimal	Prominent
Radiographic appearance		
Hyperinflation	Prominent	Moderate
Hyperlucency	Prominent	Moderate
Parenchymal markings	Minimal	Prominent
Enlarged heart	Minimal	Prominent

with COPD: blue bloaters and pink puffers (Table 26-2). Although "blue bloater" implies a predominance of bronchitic disease and "pink puffer" correlates with changes of emphysema, most patients have a mixture of both elements in the underlying disorder and in their appearance.

Inspection of the chest and auscultation of the lungs provide some separation between emphysematous and bronchitic patterns. Although both types of patient have barrel-shaped chests with hyperresonance on percussion, these findings are often more striking in a patient with emphysema. The emphysema patient also has more distant breath sounds with fewer adventitious sounds—the so-called quiet chest. By contrast, auscultation of the lungs of a bronchitic patient is sure to be anything but quiet, with diffuse rhonchi and wheezes being the rule. As with most other findings, a mixture of these elements is usually found in any one patient.

Laboratory

To evaluate both the structural and functional impairment of patients with COPD, the clinician can call on a variety of laboratory tests to support the suspicions raised during the history and physical examination. Evaluation of structural impairment is based, in large measure, on radiographic and radioisotopic data, since the risks of lung biopsy outweigh any advantage gained from a precise knowledge of lung morphology. On the other hand, an enormous database of functional capacity can be obtained from relatively non-invasive tests. These include measurements of lung volumes, inspiratory and expiratory flows, arterial blood gases, and exercise capacity. A combination of these data can be enlisted to predict the degree of disability in a given patient successfully. The following paragraphs briefly outline the value of some of these tests.

Pulmonary function tests

Pulmonary function tests are an excellent means of guiding the clinician toward a specific diagnosis and a specific treatment regimen. In patients with COPD, they help resolve four important questions: How severe is the airflow obstruction? Does airflow improve with therapy? Is the lung severely overinflated? Has lung parenchyma been lost? The answers to these questions in a given patient may differentiate between bronchial asthma and COPD and between chronic bronchitis and pulmonary emphysema—and also indicate the relative value of bronchodilator therapy.

Spirometry is a simple, sensitive, safe method for evaluating lung function. Most patients can be described as having either restrictive or obstructive lung disease. Although some overlap exists between them, the major elements of this distinction are as follows: Restrictive lung disease is characterized by reduced volumes and normal or increased expiratory flows. The finding of restriction suggests either a parenchymal process, such as interstitial fibrosis, or a chest wall disorder, such as kyphoscoliosis. Obstructive lung disease is characterized by reduced expiratory flows and normal or increased end-expiratory lung volumes (functional residual capacity, or FRC). These changes can be ascribed in almost all cases to asthma, emphysema, or obstructive bronchitis.

Obstruction is characterized by a reduction of the volume of air exhaled in 1 second following a maximal inspiration (FEV_1); the result is usually expressed as a percentage of the entire vital capacity (FVC). This parameter (FEV_1/FVC) can detect relatively mild degrees of obstruction and is reasonably specific, in that a reduction from the normal value of 80% usually correlates with symptomatic dyspnea. A classification of obstructive disease into mild, moderate, and severe categories can be constructed based on the FEV_1/FVC ratio: 60% to 80% is mild obstruction, 40% to 60% is moderate obstruction, and less than 40% is severe obstruction.

Asthma, obstructive bronchitis, and emphysema have in common a reduction of FEV_1/FVC. Distinction between these three diseases requires additional tests. Repetition of the FEV_1/FVC ratio after administration of an inhaled bronchodilator is probably the best clinical method of making this distinction. A rise of FEV_1/FVC by more than 15% is characteristic of bronchial asthma. The response in patients with emphysema is usually negligible, whereas a somewhat intermediate response is typically observed in patients with obstructive bronchitis. Although responses of less than 15% might be clinically important and should not be ignored,

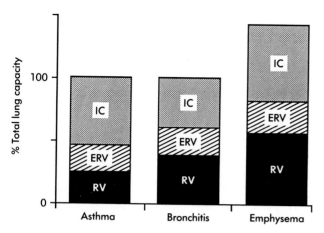

Figure 26-4. Lung volume changes in chronic obstructive pulmonary disease compared with patients in normal studies, patients with chronic bronchitis and emphysema both develop increase of residual volume *(RV)* as result of expiratory obstruction. In bronchitic patient, total lung capacity sets upper limit of lung expansion. Increase of RV thus causes parallel reduction of inspiratory capacity *(IC)* and expiratory reserve volume *(ERV);* their sum, or vital capacity, is also diminished. Patient with emphysema has more marked expansion of RV but, unlike bronchitic patient, is able to expand total lung capacity, preserving relatively normal vital capacity.

the variability of the methodology is such that a small response cannot be ascribed with any certainty to a true physiologic improvement.

Further evaluation of the underlying pathophysiology requires tests that are more complex than simple spirometry and may not be readily available. Measurement of the FRC and other lung volumes during a slow expiration can assist in distinguishing among the various causes of obstructive lung disease. An elevated FRC exists in nearly all instances of COPD and helps distinguish them from other types of lung disease, such as diffuse fibrosis. Some differences do exist between the various categories of COPD as regards the size of the vital capacity and the total lung capacity, as shown in Figure 26-4. Further distinctions can be obtained with the measurement of the carbon monoxide–diffusing capacity. In emphysema the diffusion capacity is markedly reduced as a result of destruction of the alveolar and capillary beds. This contrasts with the preserved diffusing capacity in obstructive bronchitis and the supranormal diffusing capacity in bronchial asthma.

Arterial blood gas analysis

Arterial blood gas interpretation remains the standard method for evaluating gas exchange and acid-base regulation functions of the lung. Its value stands independent of the degree of obstruction found at spirometry, since some patients with relatively moderate obstruction have severe impairment of gas exchange (bronchitic type), whereas others

have surprisingly well-preserved gas exchange despite extraordinarily severe obstruction of expiratory airflow (emphysema type).

Analysis of oxygen carriage by blood can be approached from several perspectives. The arterial oxygen tension (Po_2) and arterial oxygen saturation (Sao_2) estimate the success with which the lungs deliver oxygen to the arterial blood. From these measurements, the clinician can predict not only the degree of impairment of gas exchange in the lung but also the likelihood of developing pulmonary hypertension, which appears to be increased when Pao_2 falls below 60 mm Hg. Indications for supplemental oxygen therapy are usually based on alterations of arterial oxygen saturation. When Sao_2 falls below 90%, supplemental oxygen is warranted, in part to diminish the risk of pulmonary hypertension but also to improve tissue oxygenation. This guideline applied to the COPD patient with either an acute respiratory decompensation or chronic hypoxemia and the need for long-term domiciliary oxygen.

The alveolar-to-arterial oxygen gradient (A-a ΔO_2) is an additional means of estimating oxygen exchange in the lung. This gradient permits a distinction between hypoxemia resulting from parenchymal lung disease and hypoxemia resulting from hypoventilation caused by chest wall or central nervous system disease. The alveolar Po_2 can be estimated as follows:

$$PAo_2 = Fio_2 * (P_B - 47) - \frac{Paco_2}{RQ}$$

PAo_2 is the alveolar Po_2, Fio_2 is the inspired oxygen fraction, P_B is the barometric pressure, and RQ is the respiratory quotient (for which values typically vary between 0.7 and 1, depending on diet).

Breathing room air, the difference between this estimated PAo_2 and the arterial Po_2, should be 5 to 10 mm Hg but may rise to 50 mm Hg or more in patients with severe COPD. The equation permits one to estimate the effects of alteration of alveolar ventilation (using $Paco_2$) or the changes of inspired oxygen tensions (Fio_2) upon alveolar, and thus arterial, oxygen tension.

Calculation of arterial oxygen content (C_aO_2) may be another useful means of estimating oxygen delivery to tissues in patients with chronic lung disease. C_aO_2 is the product of the arterial oxygen saturation (Sao_2) and the binding of oxygen by hemoglobin (Hb): Hb $\times$ 1.34. The oxygen content reflects the *quantity* of oxygen in blood and is affected not only by lung function (Sao_2) but also by alterations of hemoglobin concentrations in blood and by the affinity with which hemoglobin binds oxygen. Patients with severe COPD not uncommonly have hematocrits exceeding 50% (see later), raising the blood's oxygen content despite very low values for oxygen saturation. However, the advantages of this are opposed by a rise in blood viscosity imposed by the increased red cell mass, so that an increase of hematocrit beyond 55% is considered overall to be disadvantageous.

On the other hand, anemia reduces the hemoglobin concentration and reduces O_2 content. The patient with COPD and anemia is thus at severe risk of tissue hypoxia, and correction of both the anemia and the reduced PO_2 must be equally addressed.

A more precise estimate of the amount of oxygen transported in arterial blood to the tissues is calculated from the product of the arterial oxygen content and cardiac output ($C_aO_2 \times CO$) and is referred to as the systemic oxygen transport (SOT). Since the measure of cardiac output requires cardiac catheterization, this value is not routinely obtained in patients with COPD; C_aO_2 is accepted as a reasonable estimate of tissue oxygen delivery.

Carbon dioxide elimination. If changes of the PO_2 or SaO_2 are in many ways the most sensitive measures of adequate pulmonary gas exchange, changes of PCO_2 are the most sensitive measure of the bellows function of the lung and chest wall. Values less than 40 mm Hg indicate alveolar hyperventilation and thus imply a state of adequate ventilatory reserve. Alveolar hyperventilation may be a response to hypoxemia, metabolic acidosis, or irritation of neural receptors in the lung. By contrast, $PaCO_2$ exceeding 40 mm Hg defines alveolar hypoventilation and correlates with severe obstruction and a generally dismal prognosis. It has often been noted that hypercapnia appears with a less severe degree of obstruction in patients with obstructive bronchitis than in those with emphysema. This is presumed to occur because of a greater V/Q mismatch in patients with bronchitis than in the patients with emphysema, where both alveolar and capillary units are lost in relatively matched units. The poor prognosis associated with hypercapnia is explained not only by its correlation with severe airflow obstruction but also by its origin in airflow obstruction. Hypercapnia in patients with COPD can also result from depression of central drive following oxygen administration, muscle fatigue associated with end-stage COPD, or the inappropriate use of sedative medications to calm the patient with dyspnea. Whereas a low PaO_2 can be treated with supplemental oxygen, a rising PCO_2 in a patient with COPD often requires intubation and mechanical ventilation.

Exercise testing

Exercise tests are being used with increasing frequency in the evaluation of patients with COPD. Compared with resting pulmonary function tests, they permit an integration of contributions from many organ systems, including the heart, lungs, muscles, blood cells, and nervous system; in many instances an improved perspective of the relationship between functional impairment and symptoms can result. For example, a patient may have progressive exertional dyspnea. Initial evaluation reveals chronic obstructive lung disease, coronary artery disease, obesity, and overall poor cardiovascular fitness. Documentation of disease does not signal which organ system contributes to the presenting symptom, dyspnea. Data from exercise testing can more precisely point to which functional impairment best correlates with the onset of symptoms. For example, a reduction of arterial oxygen saturation or a marked rise of minute ventilation suggests impairment of lung function; by contrast, the early onset of metabolic acidosis during exercise (anaerobic threshold) suggests a cardiovascular limitation. Some conditions, such as bronchospasm, can be specifically elicited during exercise and may not be detected during resting measurements. Also, some patients with COPD may develop hypoxemia with exercise yet have adequate oxygen tensions at rest. These patients might benefit from supplemental oxygen therapy, but documentation of desaturation during exercise should precede the prescription of oxygen. An excellent review of clinical exercise testing has been written by Jones and Campbell.[15]

Radiography

The major values of the chest radiograph are the exclusion of unusual diseases that have symptoms similar to those of COPD and the exclusion of disorders that commonly complicate the clinical course of a patient with COPD.

Although the overwhelming majority of patients with clinical signs of obstruction have asthma, emphysema, or bronchitis, several other causes of airway obstruction are initially suggested by the presence of an abnormal chest radiograph. Cystic fibrosis (CF) is an example. Patients with milder CF are surviving with increasing frequency into late adolescence and adulthood, presumably because of improved treatment of infections. Radiographic findings include accentuated lung markings, atelectasis, bronchiectasis, or signs of recurrent pneumonia. Although these findings are not diagnostic, they are infrequently seen in patients with bronchitis, asthma, or emphysema, and therefore they alert the clinician to the possibility of CF. Alternatively, the presence of bronchiectasis, detected by routine radiography, can also be caused by prior severe lung infection in a non-CF host, and these patients have a clinical presentation that may be difficult to distinguish from smoking-induced COPD. Further confirmation is obtainable by either linear or computerized axial tomography. Contrast bronchograms are used only when surgical resection is contemplated. Radiography is also valuable in documenting bullous disease of the lung or foreign body obstruction, the symptoms of which are wheezing and dyspnea.

Chest radiography is also invaluable for the detection of many of COPD's complications. The most common of these are infections such as pneumonia and acute infectious bronchitis. The incidence of these infections is high because of the impaired host defenses resulting from either the underlying lung pathology or, on occasion, therapy with corticosteroids. Other complications associated with COPD that can be detected radiographically include focal atelectasis from mucus plugs and spontaneous pneumothorax. Cor pulmonale may also be suspected on the basis of an enlarged right ventricle and prominent pulmonary arteries. Since

COPD patients are also at risk for lung cancer, the chest radiograph is also used for early detection of tumors. Unfortunately, the benefits of cancer screening of patients with COPD with biannual or yearly chest radiographs has not been shown to improve survival.

Several radioisotopic techniques exist with which to assess regional lung function. Those most widely used are xenon-133 (^{133}Xe) to assess regional ventilation and technetium-99m (^{99m}Tc) to assess regional perfusion. These tests are well tolerated by patients with severe lung disease but have little or no impact on the overall direction of health care. One exception is the evaluation of the lung cancer patient before surgical resection. Quantitative assessment of ventilation and perfusion in the upper and lower regions of both lungs permits a semiquantitative assessment of the lung function that will prevail after either lobectomy or pneumonectomy.

TREATMENT

The primary treatment goals include reversal of the airway obstruction and management of complications that result from chronic respiratory impairment. The medical management of each of these factors is addressed in this section.

Smooth muscle bronchodilators

Three major categories of smooth muscle bronchodilators are compared in Table 26-3. They are beta$_2$-sympathomimetics, theophylline, and anticholinergics. Although the greatest response is noted in patients with bronchial asthma, bronchial smooth muscle relaxation also benefits patients with COPD from mixed causes. In patients with predominant emphysema and limited bronchodilator reversibility, these agents are still of value but primarily because of non-bronchodilator effects.

Sympathomimetic bronchodilators such as epinephrine

and ephedrine have been available for many years and are potent bronchodilators. The newer beta-agonists are remarkable for several features: preservation of potency, prolonged duration of action, and reduced cardiac stimulation. The use of aerosol cannisters of metaproterenol or albuterol relieves bronchospasm within several minutes. Elderly patients or those with neuromotor impairment may find the technique difficult to master and may prefer a compressor-driven nebulizer, delivering a continuous flow of medication for 10 to 15 minutes. The same bronchodilators are also available for oral administration. Although they offer a longer duration of action, their use is associated with an increased incidence of systemic symptoms, such as hand tremors and general irritability. The subcutaneous route is reserved for patients with acute severe bronchospasm. Cardiac stimulation may be greater with this mode of delivery, limiting its use in the elderly or individuals with known cardiac disease. Some evidence also suggests that the aerosol route is as effective as the subcutaneous route, in terms of both onset of action and potency of bronchodilation.[21]

Theophylline remains one of the most widely used medications for the treatment of COPD, in part because of its potency and in part because few complications seem to occur with either short- or long-term use. Its rate of metabolism can be extraordinarily variable between patients, requiring some monitoring of serum levels when the agent is started or the dosage is changed. A value between 10 and 20 μg/dl is considered therapeutic. The choice between beta-agonists and theophylline for either acute or chronic COPD depends on the severity of symptoms, as well as on patient tolerance. With severe bronchospasm both agents are generally used, since their pharmacologic modes of action are distinct. Although the tremor-producing effects of beta-agonists are often more severe than those of theophylline, the latter produces more gastrointestinal irritation and may not be tolerated in patients with peptic ulcer disease. In

Table 26-3. Bronchodilator therapy of ambulatory patients with COPD*

Agent	Onset (min)	Peak	Duration (hr)	Usual dose
Sympathomimetic				
Inhaled (metaproterenol)	2-5	10-60 min	2-6	0.3 ml in 2 ml saline
Oral (metaproterenol)	10-20	15-60 min	3-4	10-20 mg q8h
Anticholinergic				
Inhaled (ipratropium)	15-30	30-180 min	3-5	36 μg (2 puffs) qid
Theophylline				
Oral (anhydrous)	—†	4-8 hr	12-24	300 mg 2 or 3 times per day

*A comparison of the time to onset of effect, time to peak effect, and typical duration of effect (in minutes or hours) of three major categories of bronchodilators (sympathomimetics, anticholinergics, or theophylline).
†Oral theophylline is not usually given as a single-dose bronchodilator, and time of onset of action is unknown.

addition to its role as a bronchodilator, theophylline has several other valuable properties, including stimulation of the central nervous system drive, improved clearance of mucus from the lung, and enhanced contractility of the diaphragm. This wide spectrum significantly adds to the value of this group of medications in the treatment of COPD.

Anticholinergics such as atropine have excellent bronchodilator properties that compare favorably with the beta-agonists in potency when administered by aerosol.[25] Although many patients using aerosolized anticholinergic agents have responses similar to those obtained with the usual sympathomimetic agents, some patients have greater bronchodilator response. The effects are particularly valuable in patients with disease of large airways, such as bronchitis. Atropine, although used successfully for the treatment of bronchospasm, has the theoretic disadvantage of excessively drying secretions and promoting mucus plugs. Although demonstrated in vitro, alteration of volume or viscosity of sputum has not been observed in the clinical setting with aerosolized administration of atropine.[25] However, in response to the concern of mucus plugging, congeners of atropine have been developed with even less mucus-drying properties. Ipratropium (Atrovent) has been available for use in Europe as a metered cannister for several years; approval by the Food and Drug Administration for its use in the United States now exists.

Alteration of bronchial mucus or its clearance

In addition to smooth muscle spasm, some aspects of COPD are related to mucus in the airways. Patients with bronchial asthma have been observed to have lung volumes that remain at 60% to 70% of predicted levels when bronchospasm has been apparently successfully treated.[17] Much of this volume restriction is probably caused by the persistence of mucus plugs. It remains unclear whether this is the result of an increased volume of mucus exceeding the capacity of the normal clearance system, impaired tracheobronchial clearance mechanisms (that is, reduced cough or mucociliary clearance), or alteration of the physiochemical properties of the mucus itself.[24] Whichever the mechanism, there is substantial evidence, from radioisotope tests, of a reduced rate of mucus clearance from the large bronchi and trachea of asymptomatic smokers as well as patients with obstructive lung diseases.[13]

These same radioisotopic techniques have also been used to show alterations of mucus clearance with various bronchodilator agents.[13] From this data it is currently believed that both beta-sympathomimetic and theophylline bronchodilators improve mucus clearance from the lung in patients with COPD. On the other hand, atropine inhibits mucus clearance to a modest degree; however, this effect is readily reversed with the simultaneous administration of a beta-agonist. Furthermore, the newer anticholinergics, such as ipratropium, do not have this unwanted effect on mucus clearance.

Corticosteroid therapy

The proper role of corticosteroid therapy has been difficult to define in patients with bronchial asthma, and its use in the treatment of patients with bronchitis and emphysema is equally difficult. When bronchial spasm or bronchial edema does not respond sufficiently to beta-sympathomimetics, theophylline, or antibiotics, corticosteroids are often remarkably effective at improving lung function. It is only because of their serious and potentially life-threatening side effects that these medications are not used routinely. The incidence of side effects found with parenteral use may be substantially reduced by the use of aerosolized corticosteroids in metered cannisters. The systemic absorption is minimal, and, at a dose of 2 puffs every 8 hours, an effect equivalent to 5 to 10 mg of prednisone daily can be achieved.

Supplemental oxygen therapy

Two important roles exist for the routine use of supplemental oxygen in patients with COPD: to reduce pulmonary hypertension with either amelioration or prevention of cor pulmonale and to improve tissue oxygen delivery. Achievement of either of these goals may contribute to a longer survival in patients with severe obstructive lung disease.

Pulmonary hypertension, defined by a mean pulmonary arterial pressure exceeding 20 or 25 mm Hg, is one of the chief factors contributing to death in patients with COPD.[6] The hypertension is the result of a combination of factors, including hypoxia, acidosis, destruction of pulmonary capillaries, and occasionally an element of pulmonary thromboembolism. By far, hypoxia is the most important factor.[12] As a result of this relationship, treatment of pulmonary hypertension is aimed primarily at raising arterial Po_2 above 60 mm Hg. In most patients with COPD this is readily obtained, requiring only 2 to 4 L/minute of supplemental oxygen. Unfortunately, the improvement of pulmonary hypertension is relatively modest; the value of oxygen may largely reside in its capacity to prevent further progression of hypertension. In the NOTT study,[18] continuous oxygen therapy for 6 months reduced pulmonary vascular resistance by 11.1%, whereas those treated with nocturnal oxygen showed a 6.5% increase.

The improvement of tissue oxygenation is the other fundamental goal of oxygen therapy. The effectiveness of this therapy, however, is difficult to evaluate. First, no precise test is currently available with which to measure total tissue oxygenation. Systemic oxygen transport (arterial oxygen content × cardiac output) and the mixed venous Po_2 provide some indication about tissue oxygenation, but both require invasive monitoring. Clinicians therefore depend on more readily available, although often imprecise, estimates of oxygen delivery. Oxygen supplementation is commonly given at a rate sufficient to raise the arterial oxygen saturation to 90%. The observation of improved exercise tolerance, increased appetite with weight gain, and improved mental status probably reflect improved oxygen delivery, but this is uncertain.

Whether by reduction of pulmonary hypertension or improvement of tissue oxygen delivery, a strong link has been found between improved survival and chronic supplemental oxygen therapy. In the NOTT study,[18] survival was twice as long in those who received continuous oxygen, as compared with those receiving only nocturnal oxygen supplementation; however, the improved survival did not correlate with the improvement of pulmonary arterial pressures in response to oxygen. When a comparison was made between patients receiving nocturnal oxygen and those receiving no supplemental oxygen, survival was again more than doubled in those receiving oxygen.[22]

CONCLUSION

The treatment of COPD is based on principles familiar to most clinicians. Until recently, much of the therapeutic effort was aimed at reducing airway resistance with a variety of bronchodilator agents. Recent pharmacologic developments have produced sympathomimetic bronchodilators with little cardiac stimulation and a prolonged duration of action. The other major bronchodilator group, theophylline, is valued not only for its capacity to relax bronchial smooth muscle but also for its potential to improve mucus clearance from the lung, promote the central drive to respiration, and improve diaphragmatic contractility. Pharmacokinetic studies of the theophyllines have led to the formulation of sustained-action agents with less gastric irritation and excellent parenteral absorption. A third bronchodilator group, the anticholinergic agents, have also seen somewhat of a revival in recent years and have properties that may make them particularly well suited for patients with COPD.

Recently methods of prolonging survival in patients with severe COPD have received greater attention. Foremost among these is the use of domiciliary oxygen as a means of improving tissue oxygenation and as a means of averting pulmonary hypertension. Studies have also been instituted to determine whether vasodilator medications are of value in the treatment of cor pulmonale, either as a complement to the role of oxygen as a vasodilator or perhaps as a less costly alternative. Finally, mechanical ventilation at home is being offered to a select group of patients with COPD and respiratory failure. The proper application of this mode of therapy will be, we believe, one of the great challenges over the next decade to clinicians treating patients with COPD.

REFERENCES

1. American Thoracic Society: Definition and classification of chronic bronchitis, asthma and pulmonary emphysema: a statement, Am Rev Respir Dis 85:762, 1962.
2. Auerbach, O, et al: Relation of smoking and age to emphysema, N Engl J Med 286:853, 1972.
3. Ayres, SM, et al: Bronchial component in chronic obstructive lung diseases, Am J Med 57:183, 1984.
4. Black, LF, and Kueppers, F: Alpha 1-antitrypsin deficiency in nonsmokers, Am Rev Respir Dis 117:317, 1978.
5. Blue, M, and Janoff, A: Possible mechanisms of emphysema in cigarette smokers, Am Rev Respir Dis 117:317, 1978.
6. Burrows, B, and Earle, RH: Course and prognosis of chronic obstructive pulmonary disease: a prospective study of 200 patients, N Engl J Med 280:397, 1969.
7. Ciba Symposium: Terminology, definitions and classification of chronic pulmonary emphysema and related conditions, Thorax 14:286, 1959.
8. Dansker, D: Gas exchange in chronic obstructive lung disease. In Montenegro, HD, editor: Chronic obstructive lung disease, New York, 1984, Churchill-Livingstone.
9. DeRenne, JP, Macklem, PT, and Roussos, C: The respiratory muscle: mechanics, control, and pathophysiology. In Murray, JF, editor: Lung disease: state of the art, New York, 1978, American Lung Association.
10. Dorhorst, AC: Respiratory insufficiency, Lancet 1:1185, 1955.
11. Faling, JL: Genetic influences in the development of emphysema in persons with normal serum proteins in emphysema, Clin Chest Med 4:377, 1983.
12. Fishman, AP: Chronic cor pulmonale, Am Rev Respir Dis 114:775, 1976.
13. Foster, WM, and Bergofsky, EH: Airway mucus membrane: effects of beta-adrenergic and anticholinergic stimulation, Am J Med 81(suppl 5A):28, 1986.
14. Foster, WM, Langenback, EG, and Bergofsky, EH: Dissociation in the mucociliary function of central and peripheral airways of asymptomatic smokers, Am Rev Respir Dis 129:633, 1985.
15. Jones, NL, and Campbell, EJM: Clinical exercise testing, ed 2, Philadelphia, 1982, WB Saunders Co.
16. Kuperman, AS, and Riker, JB: Variable effect of smoking on pulmonary function, Chest 63:655, 1973.
17. McFadden, ER, Jr, et al: Acute bronchial asthma: relations between clinical and physiologic manifestations, N Engl J Med 288:221, 1973.
18. Nocturnal Oxygen Trial Group: Continuous or nocturnal oxygen therapy in hypoxemic chronic obstructive lung disease: a clinical trial, Ann Intern Med 93:391, 1980.
19. Reid, L: Pathology of chronic bronchitis, Proc R Soc Med 49:771, 1956.
20. Reid, L: The pathology of emphysema, London, 1967, Lloyd-Luke.
21. Rossing, TH, et al: Emergency therapy of asthma: comparison of the acute effects of parenteral and inhaled sympathomimetics infused aminophylline, Am Rev Respir Dis 122:365, 1980.
22. Stuart, HC, et al: Long-term domiciliary oxygen therapy in chronic hypoxic cor pulmonale complicating chronic bronchitis and emphysema, Lancet 1:681, 1981.
23. Sutinen, S, Vaajalahti, P, and Pääkkö, P: Prevalence, severity and types of pulmonary emphysema in a population of deaths in a Finnish city, Scand J Respir Dis 59:101, 1978.
24. Wanner, A: Role of mucociliary dysfunction in bronchial asthma, Am J Med 67:477, 1979.
25. Ziment, I, and Au, JP: Anticholinergic agents in respiratory pharmacology, Clin Chest Med 7:355, 1986.

CHAPTER 27

Rehabilitation management of pulmonary/respiratory diseases

HORACIO D. PINEDA

Respiratory failure resulting from spinal cord injury, poliomyelitis, muscular dystrophy, severe scoliosis, chronic obstructive pulmonary disease (COPD), occupational diseases, and sarcoidosis is commonly encountered in the practice of rehabilitation medicine. In addition, acute respiratory complications of hospitalizations and debility such as pneumonias, pulmonary embolism, and atelectasis are frequent occurrences in inpatient practice. The physician therefore must possess a broad understanding of respiratory problems and their management.

Respiratory problems can be grouped in two general categories, restrictive and obstructive pulmonary diseases. COPD is discussed in greater clinical detail in Chapter 26. Although airway obstruction of differing degree is shared in common by patients with COPD, the pathophysiologic variations of the diseases can be significant, presenting different clinical manifestations and courses and requiring different treatments. For example, although emphysema and chronic bronchitis are both categorized as obstructive diseases, the therapeutic approaches to each are quite different. Symptoms of chronic bronchitis are excessive production of tracheobronchial secretions and hypertrophy of mucous glands. Emphysema's gradual and uniform destruction of both alveoli and terminal airways results in progressive reduction in total ventilatory function but maintains a better balance of ventilation and alveolar perfusion. Chronic bronchitis similarly results in progressive reduction in total ventilatory function caused by airway obstruction and excessive mucus secretion. Alveolar perfusion, however, is relatively preserved or impaired at a lesser extent than ventilation, resulting in severe ventilation to perfusion imbalance. Emphysema is therefore seen clinically as a relatively dry (uncongested), acyanotic, high–airway resistance disease ("pink puffer"), whereas chronic bronchitis is a congestive, cyanotic, plethoric, high–airway resistance disease ("blue bloater"). The approach to treatment differs accordingly. Although bronchodilator therapy helps both emphysema and chronic bronchitis, the patient with bronchitis needs more vigorous bronchial toilet, nebulization, and expectorant therapy than the patient with emphysema. In addition, patients with bronchitis probably need oxygen therapy much earlier than those with emphysema.

Restrictive lung diseases are conditions that result in reductions in lung volume. These diseases may be due to parenchymal, neuromuscular, or skeletal diseases. Ventilation is diminished primarily because lung expansion is restricted, respiratory muscles are weak or paralyzed, the chest wall is stiffened or its compliance is reduced. Treatment is aimed at improving ventilation by correcting the primary restricting cause. Because the airways are generally spared, bronchodilators are usually not as effective in treating these groups of diseases. Treating the specific cause, however, is very important, and antimicrobials, steroids, surgery, and mechanical ventilatory assistance are commonly employed.

Depending on the severity, both obstructive and restrictive lung diseases can lead to severe disability. Diminished lung compliance and increased airway resistance contribute to the increased work of breathing. Progression of the disease leads to a gradual reduction in effective ventilation, which can affect the blood gases. Early in the disease, attempts at compensation, such as increased rate of breathing or increased tidal volume, may succeed in maintaining acceptable blood gases, albeit at a high cost. As the disease continues, however, hypoxemia and hypercapnia may ensue. Further worsening usually results in heart failure (cor pulmonale) and finally death. The progression of the disease and the accompanying disability is often slow. Advances in technologic and pharmacologic therapy, in addition, have given added longevity to these patients. Consequently, more and more of them are apt to be referred to physicians for symptom control, endurance training, and general functional independence.

GENERAL APPROACH TO THE REHABILITATIVE TREATMENT OF PATIENTS WITH RESPIRATORY PROBLEMS

Often a referring physician has previously diagnosed the disease. However, a current and complete history and physical examination are mandatory. Current laboratory studies such as pulmonary function tests, radiographic examinations, and blood gas determinations are also essential. The physician must identify several important points about function: adequacy of ventilation, ability to clear tracheobronchial secretions adequately, physical endurance or capacity, and psychologic effect of the illness on the patient.

Adequacy of ventilation

Adequacy of ventilation can be assessed by careful observation of skin color, character of breathing (labored or comfortable), and pattern of breathing at rest, during exercise, and asleep. More precise evaluation of ventilation is reflected in the patient's blood gas levels. Hypoventilation must not be confused with hypoxemia because patients may be hypoxic even while hyperventilating (for instance, with a pulmonary embolism). Hypercapnia probably best reflects hypoventilation. This distinction is important because hypoxia is best treated by oxygen inhalation, and hypercapnia and hypoventilation by assisted ventilation.

Clearing tracheobronchial secretions

The patient's ability to eliminate tracheobronchial secretions must be evaluated carefully because failure to identify this problem can lead to serious, even catastrophic, consequences. Patients with weak or inadequate expiratory muscles or those who cannot perform a Valsalva maneuver (for instance, because of vocal cord paralysis) may not be able to generate enough expiratory force to remove secretions. This is particularly true when secretions are found in conjunction with infection. Retained secretions may predispose the patient to mucus plugging, infection, or atelectasis. The patient's ability to handle this problem can be evaluated by asking the patient to cough spontaneously or with assistance (for instance, abdominal pressure) both in the sitting and supine positions. The ability to move secretions by each method should be noted. In addition, maximum expiratory force (MEF) can also be measured. An MEF of 90 cm H_2O or higher may indicate the ability to perform a productive cough.[1] The amount, character, and consistency of the secretions must also be noted. Based on this evaluation, the therapeutic approach may involve preventive (that is, an antibiotic, decongestants, and a bronchodilator), conservative (that is, an assistive cough and postural drainage), or invasive (that is, endotracheal suctioning and bronchoscopy) management.

Physical endurance or capacity

Diminished endurance and exercise capacity are the usual consequences of COPD. Progressive respiratory failure, which reduces the patient's maximum oxygen consuming ability ($\dot{V}o_2$ max), or the adoption of a progressively sedentary way of life (usually forced on by dyspnea) contribute to a diminished exercise capacity. In many cases the patient's cardiopulmonary fitness level is much lower than can be attributed to the severity of the disease itself. Years of deconditioning probably contribute to this status. Recognizing and estimating the patient's exercise capacity are important in planning a safe and appropriate reconditioning program aimed at improving endurance and exercise capacity.

Psychologic effects

Anxiety frequently accompanies respiratory insufficiency. In many cases and with extreme degrees of anxiety, it leads to panic, which in itself can exacerbate the patient's symptoms. Dyspnea is not unlike drowning and is an extremely unpleasant sensation. Like any stress, each patient responds differently. Many handle or try to control the anxiety, but some cannot. To prevent the unpleasant feeling of shortness of breath, patients instinctively avoid conditions that bring it on, including physical activity. How well patients handle their anxiety often determines the patient's compliance with and the success of a pulmonary rehabilitation program.

ESTIMATING FUNCTIONAL CAPACITY

Quantifying the disability resulting from lung disease is useful in itself. However, defining the residual functional capacity is even more crucial.

Since restoration of the patient to his or her best potential is the goal, knowledge of the patient's remaining physical capacity is quite important to enable the physician not only to prescribe an adequate exercise program but also to identify the patient's safety limits.

Traditionally, functional disability has been equated with the degree of deterioration determined by pulmonary function tests (PFTs). The Social Security System (SSS) Disability criteria, for example, uses forced expiratory volume after 1 second (FEV_1), forced vital capacity (FVC), and maximum voluntary ventilation (MVV) to measure disability. Relying on PFT parameters alone, however, is significantly inadequate. For example, recent work correlating PFT parameters and exercise tolerance in COPD patients has shown that the best parameter (FEV_1) accounts for only 56% and 60% of the observed variation in oxygen consumption and external work respectively.[5]

Exercise testing has recently been recommended as an important measurement in evaluating disability resulting from pulmonary disease.[2,3,4] This is an important concept for the physician. Pulmonary function testing (PFT) prin-

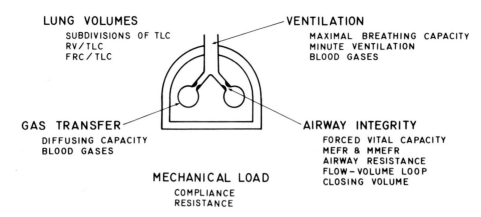

Figure 27-1. Different pulmonary function testing modalities grouped under specific subfunctions they measure. (From Haas, A, et al: Pulmonary therapy and rehabilitation, principles and practice, Baltimore, 1979, Williams & Wilkins Co.)

ciples and techniques should be familiar to the physician. Figure 27-1 diagrams the more common PFT parameters.

Pulmonary function evaluation

Pulmonary function evaluation is generally subdivided into tests for airway integrity (by measuring inspiratory and expiratory flow rates), lung volumes (total lung capacity [TLC] and subdivisions), ventilation (minute ventilation, maximum voluntary ventilation [MVV], and blood gases), lung and chest wall mechanics (compliance), and membrane parameters (diffusion capacity [DCO]). Obstructive lung disease in general shows significant air flow impairment with relatively slight volume impairment. Restrictive lung diseases, on the other hand, reduce lung volumes, membrane parameters, and lung and chest wall mechanics, while leaving air flow parameters relatively unimpaired. During pulmonary function evaluations, the patient's PFT values are compared to normal standards. The sum total of the effects of pulmonary diseases are best reflected in the patient's arterial blood gas levels. The reader is referred to Chapter 26 in which the topic of blood gases is discussed in detail.

Exercise capacity

Exercise capacity is estimated by performing a pulmonary exercise test. The determination measures not only the patient's maximum oxygen consumption ($\dot{V}O_2$ max), which serves to gauge cardiopulmonary fitness (Table 27-1), but provides other information as well. The anaerobic threshold during exercise can be identified and correlated with the patient's heart rate or with external work. Exercise-induced bronchospasm is determined whenever indicated. In addition, the traditional cardiac parameters of maximum heart rate (HR max), electrocardiographic changes (ST depression and arrhythmias), and blood pressure response can be monitored. Exercise testing is important both as a diagnostic tool and as a guide to providing an individualized, safe, appropriate exercise prescription for the purpose of improving endurance or exercise tolerance.

Table 27-1. Maximal oxygen uptake of women and men

Age (yrs)	Maximal oxygen uptake (ml/kg/min)				
	Low	Fair	Average	Good	High
Women					
20-29	<24	24-30	31-37	38-48	49+
30-39	<20	20-27	28-33	34-44	45+
40-49	<17	17-23	24-30	31-41	42+
50-59	<15	15-20	21-27	28-37	38+
60-69	<13	13-17	18-23	24-34	35+
Men					
20-29	<25	25-33	34-42	43-52	53+
30-39	<23	23-30	31-38	39-48	49+
40-49	<20	20-26	27-35	36-44	45+
50-59	<18	18-24	25-33	34-42	43+
60-69	<16	16-22	23-30	31-40	41+

Data from Preventive Medicine Center, Palo Alto, California, and from a survey of published sources. From The American Heart Association: Exercise testing and training of apparently healthy individuals: a handbook for physicians, 1972, The Association. Reproduced with permission.

To better understand exercise testing, one should consider the heart and lung as one functional unit because failure of either system reflects on the function of the other (Figure 27-2). Humans require oxygen to metabolize food and generate the energy required for performing physical work (aerobic metabolism). If energy demands exceed the person's oxygen supply, energy production can be achieved anaerobically, though inefficiently, for a limited period. Oxygen is absorbed from the air through the pulmonary alveoli and carried in the blood, primarily bound to hemoglobin inside the red blood cells. Oxygen-rich blood is distributed throughout the body by the heart, a vital organ also dependent on oxygen. Peripherally, blood releases oxy-

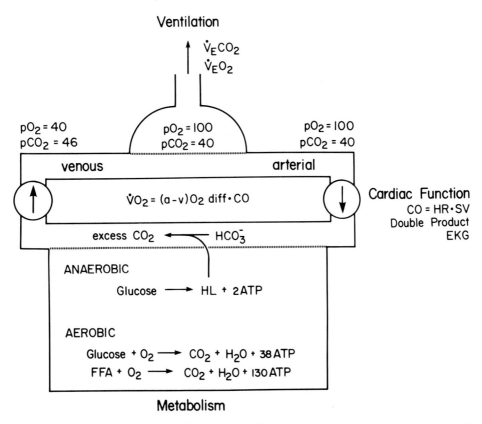

Figure 27-2. Schematic summary of important cardiopulmonary occurrences during exercise and common parameters that are frequently monitored during stress testing. At muscle level, relative efficiencies of aerobic and anaerobic metabolisms in generating high-energy phosphates, necessary for muscle contractions, are shown. See text for more detailed explanation.

gen to the tissues, which use it to metabolize food (glucose and free fatty acids) and to generate high-energy phosphates (adenosine triphosphate, or ATP) through the tricarboxylic acid cycle. If energy demand exceeds oxygen supply, generating the ATP through anaerobic metabolism can temporarily meet this demand. This inefficient means of energy generation cannot be sustained indefinitely. Production of acids (for example, lactic acid) causes changes in pH and, when buffered in the blood, can produce excessive amounts of CO_2. The anaerobic threshold, therefore, may be heralded by increased levels of lactic acid found in exercising patients. Indirectly, this may be seen in patients when increasing CO_2 production progressively stimulates ventilation, but (in spite of increased ventilation) oxygen consumption remains flat or fails to increase proportionately. An aerobic threshold therefore is indicated in a monitored patient by the intersection of the ventilatory equivalent for oxygen (VEO_2)* and the ventilatory equivalent for carbon dioxide $(VECO_2)$.† The higher the patient's maximum oxygen consumption, the higher his capacity to do physical work and

the more fit he is. By correlating $\dot{V}O_2$ max with the patient's HR response, one can regulate the exercise program by the heart rather than by measuring $\dot{V}O_2$ directly. Some laboratories use oxygen pulse $(\dot{V}O_2/HR)$ to estimate cardiac and pulmonary function as a unit. Based on the formula for $\dot{V}O_2$ being equal to arterio-venous O_2 $[(a - \bar{v})O_2]$ difference times cardiac output (CO) where

$$CO = (HR) \text{ heart rate} \times (SV) \text{ stroke volume}$$

$$\dot{V}O_2 = (a - \bar{v})O_2 \, (HR) \times (SV)$$

$$O_2 \text{ pulse} = \dot{V}O_2/HR = (a - \bar{v})O_2 \times SV$$

Although $\dot{V}O_2$ max determination is important, correlating this with the patient's actual physical performance is equally significant. Although a patient with high $\dot{V}O_2$ max is expected to perform better than one with a lower $\dot{V}O_2$ max, two people with the same $\dot{V}O_2$ max do not necessarily perform the same physical task equally well. To illustrate, suppose two patients with the same $\dot{V}O_2$ max equivalent to 3 METs were asked to run a constant speed of 3.5 mph. If both men weigh the same, but one is short and stocky, whereas the other is tall and lanky, the taller patient will most likely run for a longer period. Because of the difference in body build, the tall man's stride is longer than that of

---

*$(VEO_2) = \dot{V}e/\dot{V}O_2$.

†$(VECO_2) = \dot{V}e/\dot{V}CO_2$.

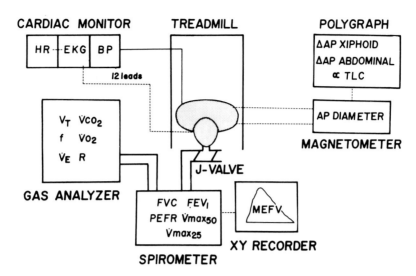

Figure 27-3. Idealized exercise testing setup in which, at any given exercise lead, pulmonary, cardiac, and chest wall parameters can be simultaneously monitored. *HR*, Heart rate; *EKG*, electrocardiogram; *BP*, blood pressure; V_T, tidal volume; $\dot{V}_E$, minute ventilation; *f*, frequency of breathing; *R*, respiratory exchange ratio; $\dot{V}CO_2$, CO_2 production; $\dot{V}O_2$, O_2 consumption; *FVC*, forced vital capacity; *PEFR*, peak expiratory flow rate; FEV_1, forced expiratory volume after 1 second; $\dot{V}MAX_{50}$, maximum expiratory flow at 50% forced vital capacity; $\dot{V}MAX_{25}$, maximum expiratory flow at 25% forced vital capacity; *MEFV*, maximum expiratory flow volume curve; *AP*, change in AP diameter.

the shorter fellow, who takes many more steps to cover the same distance. If we can quantify external work accomplished, in addition to measuring O_2 consumption, we can estimate the patient's efficiency in doing that specific task. We use the general formula

$$\text{Efficiency} = \text{Output/input} \times 100$$

where output is external work accomplished and input is the oxygen cost of the exercise. Figure 27-3 illustrates an ideal experimental exercise testing method.

Nocturnal breathing

Of special interest are the nocturnal breathing problems of severely affected respiratory patients. In severe COPD and neuromuscular and musculoskeletal respiratory impairment, hypoventilation is the ultimate result. During sleep, however, ventilation can be even more difficult. In some patients, nocturnal ventilatory assistance is needed. To identify such patients, a sleep study is usually necessary. Such a study ideally requires knowledge of the patient's ability to ventilate during sleep. To assess this, we must be able to monitor depth of sleep, ventilation, O_2 saturation, PCO_2, chest wall excursions, and air flow. One study is illustrated by Figure 27-4.

An electroencephalogram can record the depth of sleep. Air flow can be measured using thermistors placed before the patient's nostril or mouth. The frequency and depth of chest wall motion can be plotted by magnetometers or strain gauge. Simultaneous recordings of percutaneous O_2 saturation and PCO_2, air flow, and chest wall movements can

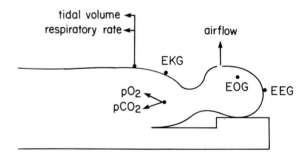

Figure 27-4. Typical sleep study setup. Depth of sleep can be monitored by electroencephalograph and electro-oculograph. Simultaneous recordings of air flow, electrocardiographic changes, chest wall motion, and percutaneous blood gas levels can show presence or absence of sleep apnea or periodic breathing pattern. In addition, character (obstructive or central) of problem, as well as its severity, can be deduced.

be done at any depth of sleep. Airway obstruction can be detected, for example, by vigorous chest wall motions with no concomitant increase in air flow recordings, coupled with a simultaneous drop in PO_2 and rise in PCO_2. Central depression may be indicated by a progressive drop in chest wall and diaphragmatic motion, air flow, and PO_2 and increasing PCO_2. Distinguishing central depression from obstructive apnea is important, since the treatments for these conditions are different. Central depression requires mechanical ventilation, stimulants, or electrical pacing, whereas obstructive apnea may be relieved by positioning, mouthpieces, or tracheostomy.

TREATMENT MODALITIES

The box at right outlines the modalities available for the management of respiratory diseases. As in any other condition, the use of one or a combination depends on indications balanced by side effects or contraindications.

Medications
Bronchodilators

Bronchodilators are the mainstays in treating COPD and are discussed in Chapter 26. This group of drugs is effective in reversing bronchoconstriction and reducing airway resistance. Indirectly, bronchodilators facilitate the elimination of tracheobronchial secretions. They are generally divided into xanthine derivatives (for example, aminophylline) and beta-sympathetic agonists (for example, isoproterenol, metaproterenol, and salbutamol). These medications come in different preparations for oral, intravenous, inhalational, or rectal delivery. More recently, the use of parasympathetic agents has been revived. Newer agents that can diminish parasympathetic tone with minimal cardiac and drying effects are being introduced.

Expectorants

Expectorants liquefy secretions to make tracheobronchial toilet easier. These drugs act either by water bonding or by molecular splitting of hydrogen and disulfide bonds. Combined with proper hydration and physical therapy modalities, the reduced viscosity of the secretion greatly enhances elimination. Glyceryl guaiacolate, potassium iodide, and terpin hydrate are the commonly used preparations.

Mucolytic agents

Mucolytic agents also reduce the viscosity of mucus by breaking down the mucopolysaccharide component. Effective in both mucoid or purulent secretions, these medications are administered as aerosols. Because they are mildly irritating to the mucosa, they can cause bronchospasm if given alone. It is therefore generally recommended that they be administered with bronchodilators. *N*-Acetyl-L-cysteine is probably the most common preparation used.

Antibiotics

Antibiotics are indicated for patients with infections of the tracheobronchial tract. Many patients with chronic pulmonary insufficiency can barely ventilate themselves adequately, despite optimal bronchodilator therapy. The presence of any infection of the respiratory tract with the resulting inflammation and increased mucus production quickly disrupts the delicate respiratory balance, causing significant discomfort if not potentially life-threatening consequences. Infections should be treated safely and ade-

quately. Culture and sensitivity studies should dictate the choice of antibiotics to administer. In general, however, patients with a high risk of pneumonia or respiratory failure are given broad-spectrum antibiotics at the earliest sign of infection.

Corticosteroids

Corticosteroids possess anti-inflammatory, antiallergic, and antistress properties. Many patients with chronic lung disease who are refractory to standard bronchodilator ther-

---

COMMON TREATMENT MODALITIES FOR RESPIRATORY DISEASES

I. Medications
   A. Bronchodilators
      1. Xanthines
      2. Beta-adrenergic
   B. Expectorants
   C. Mucolytics
   D. Steroids
   E. Antibiotics
   F. Parasympatholytics
   G. Antiallergic
II. Aerosols
   A. Humidification
   B. Nebulization
      1. Saline
      2. Bronchodilators
      3. Steroids
III. Oxygen
   A. O_2 tent
   B. Nasal O_2
   C. Ventimask O_2
   D. O_2 administered with compressors or ventilators
IV. Mechanical ventilation
   A. Positive pressure devices
      1. Pressure regulated
      2. Volume regulated
   B. Negative pressure devices
      1. Drinker respirator
      2. Chest piece respirator
   C. Miscellaneous devices
      1. Pneumobelt
      2. Rocking Bed
      3. Electrophrenic pacer
V. Physical therapy
   A. Breathing exercises
   B. Postural drainage
   C. Reconditioning
   D. Glossopharyngeal breathing
   E. Behavior modification
      1. Relaxation
      2. Hypnosis
   F. Biofeedback

apy can obtain relief only with the addition of corticosteroids to the standard regimen. Similarly, steroids may also be used in some restrictive parenchymal disease (for example, sarcoid) with surprisingly good results. Because of their potentially serious side effects, however, steroids must be used judiciously. Although some patients require long-term, low-dose maintenance therapy, steroids should be given only at the lowest dose and for the shortest course possible. Steroids come in intravenous, oral, and aerosol preparations.

Antiallergens

Disodium chromoglycate, an antiallergic agent given by aerosol, is sometimes used in patients with COPD to maintain as symptom free a state as possible. Given in conjunction with bronchodilators, this agent often reduces the need for steroids. It is indicated for maintenance therapy, not for acute bronchospastic episodes.

Oxygen therapy

Oxygen is indicated whenever hypoxemia exists or the arterial blood level is inadequate. Only a minimum amount of oxygen is given to raise the arterial oxygen tension to acceptable levels. Although 80 to 100 mm Hg is the acceptable level of Po_2 in normal persons, no hard and fast rule stipulates at what Po_2 level oxygen therapy is indicated in any particular patient or to what level Po_2 should be raised. Certainly, an ideal target is to restore Po_2 to normal levels. Since oxygen can cause toxic side effects when given at high concentrations for long periods, it is prudent to accept a slightly subnormal Po_2 level if the alternative means using very high inspired-oxygen concentrations. Oxygen can be administered by nasal cannula, mask, or tent or added to a mechanical ventilator.

Low-flow oxygen may be given to respiratory patients before and during physical work or exercise. During exercise, it delays the feeling of dyspnea and provides patients with enough stamina to perform the minimum exercise necessary to create a healthful effect. The side effects of oxygen therapy must always be kept in mind. Oxygen toxicity is characterized by a syndrome similar to acute respiratory distress syndrome (ARDS). Care should be taken in giving oxygen to infants because it can cause retrolental fibroplasia. Similarly, chronically hypercapneic patients often develop apnea when the anoxic drive is satiated by high concentrations of added oxygen.

Physical therapy
Breathing exercises

The purpose of breathing exercises is to facilitate ventilation, strengthen the respiratory muscles, minimize early airway collapse, and regulate rate and depth of breathing during physical activity. Breathing exercise techniques vary with different respiratory problems. Obstructive and restrictive lung diseases require different approaches to optimize

alveolar ventilation. In obstructive lung diseases (for instance, emphysema), the main problem is increased airway resistance and early airway collapse. Patients are taught the technique of pursed-lip breathing to slow down the respiratory rate, prolong the expiratory phase, and increase peripheral resistance to delay ostensibly terminal airway collapse. Prolonged expiration not only slows down the respiratory rate but also provides more time to release trapped air which causes hyperinflation of the chest, a condition that reduces the mechanical effectiveness of the diaphragm, restricting it from rising to its natural resting position.

Patients with restrictive pulmonary disease who suffer from reduced lung volume and decreased compliance benefit more from breathing exercises that increase inspiratory capacity. This is accomplished by a prescription of exercises to strengthen inspiratory muscles either by abdominal weights that increase resistance to diaphragmatic descent or by inspiratory resistors.

The use of incentive spirometers also encourages deep inspiration and provides visual feedback on the goal. In patients who have very weak inspiratory muscles, glossopharyngeal breathing (a method of increasing vital capacity [VC] by successively gulping air using oropharyngeal contractions) can help the patient attain high VC levels without mechanical ventilators. The increase in VC is accomplished, however, at the expense of respiratory rate.

Regulating the rate and depth of breathing can be accomplished at rest and during exercise. The most commonly employed techniques are counting, cadence (for example, 2 counts for inspiration and 4 for expiration), visual tracking of a preprogrammed pattern (biofeedback technique), or auditory tracking. Studies on the effect of music on breathing patterns show that music therapy may someday be developed into a breathing exercise modality.

Whatever technique is used, the focus is on the final goal of adequate alveolar ventilation. Reducing atelectasis, minimizing respiratory muscle fatigue, and reducing air trapping are secondary goals.

Postural drainage

Problems caused by tracheobronchial secretions result either from overproduction or impaired drainage. The consequences of retained secretions (for instance, atelectasis, pneumonia, and impaired ventilation) can be annoying at the least or fatal at the most. Excessive production of mucus is observed whenever the bronchial mucosa is inflamed or irritated from inhaled fumes or particulates, infections, or allergies. In addition to the use of expectorants, mucolytics, bronchodilators, and antibiotics, management of excessive tracheobronchial secretions also includes such physical modalities as postural drainage with vibration and percussion and assisted coughing using gravity. In postural drainage the patient assumes different positions to drain particular lung segments (Figure 27-5). Manual vibration and percussion (cupping) of the chest wall overlying the segment

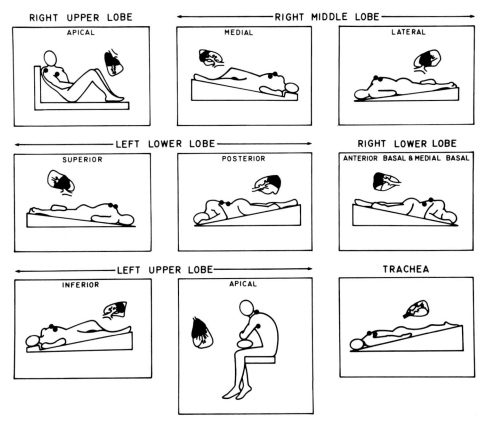

Figure 27-5. Postural drainage positions commonly employed in clearing various lung segments. (From Haas, A, et al: Pulmonary therapy and rehabilitation, principles and practice, Baltimore, 1979, Williams & Wilkins Co.)

in question, coordinated with active coughing, facilitates clearance. Auscultation identifies areas of congestion that need intensive drainage. In patients whose expiratory muscles are impaired (for instance, in quadriplegia, poliomyelitis, or muscular dystrophy), diminished capacity to generate the minimum expiratory force prevents them from producing an effective cough. In addition to hydration, expectorants, and postural drainage, these patients require assisted coughing. This technique requires an assisting person to apply a force over the patient's upper abdomen after a full inspiration. The force applied against the patient's closed glottis, which is then suddenly released, enables him or her to move the secretions effectively. Although this technique is effective, it cannot be used for patients with bleeding problems or with enlarged spleens.

Relaxation exercises

Dyspnea and the feeling of asphyxiation can cause panic among patients who have pulmonary disease. The anxiety exacerbates their problem. Sedatives were administered in the past, but the use of biofeedback seems to offer more hope for better treatment. Breath pacing using prepro-grammed visual breathing patterns coupled with electromyographic monitoring also is used. Studies in these areas are currently in progress.

Reconditioning exercises

Patients with respiratory impairment commonly experience shortness of breath on physical exertion. Consequently, they often refrain from unnecessary physical activities. However, months and years of a sedentary life-style predispose the patient to physical and cardiovascular deconditioning that results in a much lower exercise capacity than his or her lung disease alone explains. One goal of rehabilitation is to restore these individuals to as high a level of function as their medical condition allows. A reconditioning program, therefore, is designed to gradually improve general functional capacity and physical endurance through gradual, progressive, submaximal physical exercises. The use of supplementary low-flow oxygen supply is usually indicated in the following circumstances:

1. The patient's resting P_{O_2} is so low that the added oxygen demands of a reconditioning exercise program may make it unsafe (in general, a resting P_{O_2} of 55

or lower would probably require added oxygen).

2. The patient's initial endurance is so low that the minimum exercise necessary to have an effect is not met.
3. The patient is psychologically dependent on oxygen.

Although repetitive, submaximal, long-duration exercise promotes endurance, prescribing a program can become complicated, particularly when the patient's respiratory problem is severe. A program should be safe, effective, and affordable and produce long-lasting results. Although pulmonary exercise testing is an ideal starting point in developing an exercise prescription, the availability and cost consideration can become prohibitive. From a practical viewpoint, exercise testing is usually reserved for patients with severe conditions or medical complications. Mildly to moderately involved patients can be safely started after monitoring heart rate and electrocardiographic patterns during graded exercises. Treadmill or bicycle exercises are preferred modalities, although ski and rowing machines may also be used. The patient is started at a low-level, warm-up exercise lasting 3 to 5 minutes. While heart rate and subjective responses are monitored, the level of exercise is increased gradually every 3 to 5 minutes. Heart rate is generally kept at or below 75% of the predicted maximum. Whenever indicated, low-flow (2 L/min) oxygen is given by nasal cannula. PO_2 at rest and during exercise can be checked if capillary blood gas analysis equipment is available. Percutaneous PO_2 skin electrodes are also used but at times are unreliable. In most cases electrocardiographic monitoring by telemetry and observation by a trained therapist are adequate in safely accomplishing a reconditioning program. In addition to heart rate response, S-T changes, serious arrhythmias, and inappropriate blood pressure response, subjective complaints of fatigue, shortness of breath, and angina must be heeded. After reaching the desired level of exercise, the patient is maintained through a home exercise program at or slightly below the level tolerated during the monitored exercise. The patient's progress outside can be followed closely using a diary; the patient mails a record of average exercise activities back to the physician at regular intervals.

Mechanical ventilation

Mechanical ventilatory aids assist or even completely take over a patient's ventilation. The main indication for use of these devices is inadequate ventilation, indicated by a rising arterial PCO_2 level and usually accompanied by low PO_2. Hypoventilation can occur acutely or appear gradually over a period of months or years. Acute conditions such as severe lung infections, adult respiratory distress syndrome, or respiratory muscle denervation (for example, in spinal cord injury) can dramatically impair effective ventilation. In the rehabilitation setting, however, it is more common to prescribe ventilatory aids to chronic and progressively worsening conditions such as muscular dystrophy, amyotrophic lateral sclerosis, and severe obstructive lung diseases, many of which require 24-hour ventilatory assistance.

Positive and negative pressure ventilators

Mechanical ventilators can be classified as positive-pressure, negative-pressure, and miscellaneous devices. Positive-pressure ventilators pump air under pressure intermittently through the airways and into the lung at a predetermined rate, volume, or pressure setting. These machines allow passive exhalation. Ventilators may be pressure or volume regulated. Pressure-regulated machines are set with a predetermined pressure. Volume-regulated machines complete cycles preset by volume. The cycling rate may be set separately. Negative-pressure ventilators augment inhalation by creating negative pressure around the chest wall or the body as a whole. This is accomplished by encasing the patient's torso in a rigid tank with the head and neck exposed to the atmosphere. A vacuum is then generated within the tank, allowing inspiration to take place because positive atmospheric air pressure enters the chest through the air passages and into the alveoli. The ventilation rate and amount of negative pressure can be adjusted to accomplish adequate alveolar ventilation.

Although either method works if applied and used properly, positive-pressure respirators are more commonly used because they are small, portable, easier to use, clean, and relatively inexpensive. Inherent disadvantages exist, however; danger of barotrauma and infection is more evident with positive-pressure ventilators. Negative-pressure ventilators are bulky and susceptible to leaks and render the patient less accessible to nursing care. A portable chest piece negative-pressure device is inefficient and difficult to fit. These machines use electrically powered pumps and can run on house current or battery. Added oxygen may be applied to enrich the inspired air when indicated.

Pneumobelts

Several devices that are used but do not strictly fall under the previously discussed machines include pneumobelt, rocking bed, and electrophrenic pacemakers. A pneumobelt is a large canvas cuff or corset encasing a rubber bladder applied over the patient's abdomen. The bladder can be inflated by an electric air pump intermittently. When inflated, it exerts increased abdominal pressure, thus pushing the diaphragm higher than its normal resting level, and reduces functional residual capacity and dead space. When the bladder is allowed to deflate, the abdominal pressure falls and the diaphragm goes down with the descending viscerae. When timed with inspiration, this rhythm effectively augments the patient's tidal volume. Although its use is difficult to learn, the pneumobelt is effective. It can be mounted on a wheelchair and does not interfere with speech.

Rocking beds

Rocking beds are mounted on a central fulcrum, allowing them to tilt up or down by an electric motor. A patient on the bed in a head-down position facilitates exhalation by the weight of the abdominal viscerae pressing on the diaphragm. Conversely, a shift to the head-up position facilitates inspiration. The descending viscerae augment diaphragmatic contraction. The rate of tilting can be set to meet the needs of each individual patient.

Electrophrenic pacemakers

An electrophrenic pacemaker may aid breathing in patients with central hypoventilation or very high spinal cord injuries with intact diaphragmatic enervation and no serious parenchymal disease. A stimulating electrode is implanted beside the phrenic nerves. These electrodes are connected to a subcutaneously implanted radio receiver. When the pacemaker is used, an external radiopacemaker is taped on the skin overlying the receiver. The radiopacemaker electrically triggers the phrenic nerves, causing diaphragmatic contractions.

Tracheostomy

Tracheostomies are intended to ensure an accessible airway, diminish dead space, facilitate tracheobronchial suctioning, and prevent aspiration. Tracheostomy tubes are surgically placed over the anterior trachea through a skin incision. They are made of either metal or plastic material with or without an internal cannula. To ensure a tight seal around the tracheostomy tube within the trachea, a cuff is usually provided if the purpose is for mechanical ventilation or for preventing aspiration. When the cuff is inflated, no voice production is possible. To enable speech, the cuff is deflated or a fenestra (hole) is provided along the shaft of the tube to allow air to pass through the vocal cords. Tracheostomy cuffs should be low pressure and not inflated for prolonged periods. Pressure on the tracheal mucosa can cause irritation, pressure necrosis, bleeding, or even trachiectasis. A tracheostomy should be maintained only as long as the indication for it exists. Tracheostomy inner cannulas must be cleaned daily. The tracheostomy stoma must be kept clean and dry, and excessive granulation controlled by occasional cauterization. For patients whose ventilation depends on the tracheostomy tube, its patency should be checked regularly. As the patient's ventilation improves, gradual corking can be used to slowly wean the patient.

REFERENCES

1. Cook, CD, Mead, J, and Orzales, MM: Static volume: pressure characteristics of the respiratory systems during maximal expiratory efforts, J Appl Physiol 19:1016, 1964.
2. Disability evaluation under Social Security: A handbook for physicians, HEW Publication No. SSA 79-10089, Baltimore, 1979.
3. American Medical Association: Guides to the evaluation of permanent impairment, Chicago, 1971, the Association.
4. Kass, I, et al: Evaluation of impairment disability secondary to respiratory disease, Am Thorac Soc News 7:20, 1981.
5. Pineda, H, et al: Accuracy of pulmonary function tests in predicting exercise tolerance in chronic obstructive pulmonary disease, Chest 86:564, 1984.

ADDITIONAL READINGS

Astrand, PO, and Rodahl, K: Textbook of work physiology: physiological bases of exercise, New York, 1977, McGraw-Hill.

Haas, A, et al: Pulmonary therapy and rehabilitation principles and practice, Baltimore, 1979, Williams & Wilkins Co.

Wasserman, K, and Whipp, BJ: Exercise physiology in health and disease, Am Rev Respir Dis 112:219, 1975.

CHAPTER 28

Medical management of geriatric rehabilitation

MICHAEL L. FREEDMAN AND BARBARA Z. BERK

GOALS OF GERIATRIC REHABILITATION

Geriatric rehabilitation is the principle and practice of rehabilitation medicine applied to geriatric medicine. A multidisciplinary team of physical and occupational therapists, speech pathologists, nurses, psychologists, and medical social workers, nutritionists, and others operate under the leadership of a physiatrist.

The concept of geriatric rehabilitation began when physicians were faced with many elderly, immobile patients.[1] They realized that it was crucial for these patients to maximize the functional activities of daily living (ADLs), such as personal hygiene, eating, toileting, and dressing. Later, geriatric medicine came to include more acute problems and preventive medicine concepts. It was believed that exercises and activities to maintain vital systems would retard deterioration of physical and psychologic processes.[3] Especially in the elderly, usual activities must be continually performed to maintain functional capabilities.[20]

About two thirds of disabled people are over 65 years of age. The elderly's goals of rehabilitation may be different from those of younger patients, since they are more concerned with sustaining their independence by just continuing their ADLs. The following are goals of rehabilitation in the elderly:

1. Emphasis on activities of daily living (ADLs) to sustain independence
2. Understanding that improvement occurs in slow increments
3. Realization that full function often will not be regained
4. Socialization and stimulation
5. Early mobilization, since there is greater deterioration of physiologic and psychologic processes with immobility
6. Restoration of capabilities after recuperation from illness

Elderly people usually do not expect restoration to their youthful life-styles and vocations, but only to improve and maintain what function is left to them.[36] Also, they have fewer opportunities than younger people to engage in activities that help them maintain their skills, such as working or participating in stressful activities or sports. Their goal is to gain enough independence to avoid institutionalization.

Another goal of rehabilitation is to help the elderly maintain their state of health, as well as treat illnesses. This takes into consideration the preventive aspect in maintaining former capabilities and in restoration after recuperation from illness. For example, cardiac rehabilitation is useful in reconditioning the cardiovascular system in a sedentary person, as well as after recuperation from a myocardial infarction.

Rehabilitation and its results are complicated by the presence of multiple medical conditions. Geriatric patients commonly have more than one disease. A patient may have several disabilities for which the treatments are contradictory and complicated. For example, strenuous physiotherapy may aggravate existing cardiopulmonary function. The elderly have cardiac, respiratory, and hematologic disorders, and their ability to respond to increased demands for oxygen are limited. Therefore it is much more difficult for them to expend increased energy, such as that needed to walk with a prosthesis after a below-knee amputation.[42]

The prevalence of coronary heart disease and hypertension is higher in the elderly. They also have less reserve for more stressful situations. They may be called on to use their upper extremities more often in an isometric effort, which calls for a greater amount of cardiac work. The rehabilitation team must be aware of the onset of an acute myocardial infarction or the development of arrhythmias.[20]

Because of cerebrovascular compromise and decreased baroreceptor activity with a resultant diminution of reflex tachycardia, the elderly should arise slowly and carefully to avoid orthostatic hypotension.[25]

Many diseases impair cerebral oxygen delivery. Age alone is the cause for up to a 25% decrease in brain blood flow, and therefore the elderly have a decreased ability to maintain consciousness and are more susceptible to syncope. Oxygen delivery to the brain is further decreased by such conditions as anemia, chronic pulmonary disease, and heart disease. If an acute illness such as pneumonia or a coronary thrombosis is superimposed on one of these conditions, confusion or syncope may appear.[25]

AGING

Aging, a basic biologic process that occurs in almost all animal species, may be defined as a gradual decline in cell body functions ultimately leading to the death of the organism. There is a maximum life span or biologic limit to a species' longevity. In humans the life span seems to be 80 to 120 years. The range represents biologic variation among individuals. If we eradicated all disease and accidents, humans could all potentially live to about 100 years of age.

It is important to differentiate between physiologic and chronologic aging. There is a tremendous variability in how people age, and the chronologic age does not necessarily define a person's physiology. Even though changes are inevitably associated with aging, these occur at different rates in different individuals. Many physicians have seen an 85-year-old patient who looks and acts as if he is 65, and the converse. Certainly illness leads to incapacity and premature aging. People in the past were considered old at ages we now consider young because they underwent many illnesses. Since diseases are now postponed in most people until later life, more and more people are living to advanced ages (85 years and more).

Physiologic changes with aging

Aging brings on inevitable physiologic changes as outlined in the box at right. Pharmacokinetic, psychologic and sociologic changes also occur with age. There are incremental losses in the function of vital organs such as the cardiovascular and pulmonary systems.[18] Exercise tolerance and maximal oxygen uptake (VO_2 max) decrease with age. There are also declines in the maximal heart rate, stroke volume, cardiac output, and arterial-venous oxygen difference with exercise.[43] These decrements are greater after bed rest, reflecting a loss of cardiovascular fitness, and improve with physical training, even in the elderly.[14,30]

Respiratory function declines with age. This may be caused by exposure to a noxious atmosphere in addition to aging of other systems whose activities are coordinated with the lungs, such as the heart, muscles, and brain. There is a progressive marked loss of protective laryngeal reflexes.[29] The configuration of the chest wall changes, the elasticity

---

PHYSIOLOGIC CHANGES WITH AGING

1. Cardiovascular
   a. Decreased exercise tolerance
   b. Decline in VO_2 max (maximal oxygen uptake)
   c. Decreased maximum heart rate
   d. Decreased stroke volume
   e. Decreased cardiac output
   f. Decreased arterial-venous oxygen difference with exercise
   g. Decreased sensitivity of baroreceptors
2. Pulmonary
   a. Change in configuration of chest wall
   b. Decreased elasticity of lung parenchyma
   c. Dilation and breakdown of airways
   d. Pulmonary vasculature thickened and fibrotic
3. Renal
   a. Decreased renal cortical mass
   b. Decreased renal blood flow
   c. Decreased glomerular filtration rate
   d. Decreased urine-concentrating ability
   e. Decreased renal tubular secretion
4. Musculoskeletal
   a. Decreased muscle mass
   b. Increased body fat content
   c. Decreased total body water
5. Gastrointestinal
   a. Decreased gut motility
   b. Increased gastric emptying time
   c. Decreased hepatic mass and blood flow
   d. Decreased efficiency of P-450 enzymatic system

---

of the lung parenchyma decreases, the airways become dilated and break down, and the pulmonary vasculature thickens and becomes fibrotic.[21]

The changes in renal function associated with aging are well known. Renal cortical mass and blood flow decrease. There is a progressive decline in glomerular filtration rate, urine-concentrating ability, and renal tubular secretion. Because of decreased muscle mass and therefore decreased production of creatinine, the serum creatinine level usually does not rise in the face of decreased kidney efficiency.[28]

As a person ages, the number and bulk of muscle fibers decrease, leading to a diminished lean body mass. Fibrous tissue replaces some muscle fibers. Bone becomes less dense because of lack of estrogen (in women), decreased calcium intake, and abnormalities in calcium and protein metabolism. There is wear and tear on articular surfaces. Body fat increases, and body water decreases.[28]

Gastrointestinal tract changes include decreased gut motility, increased gastric emptying time, and decreased gastric acid production. A tendency toward inflammatory changes of the gastrointestinal tract with aging alters specialized cellular function and leads to changes in absorption and secretion. The number of absorbing cells may decrease, and active transport systems may be modified. Hepatic mass and hepatic blood flow are less. There is decreased efficiency of the P-450 enzymatic system.[8,28]

Changes in pharmacokinetics with aging

Changes in pharmacokinetics occur with aging.[8,13] These include how various medications are affected in the processes of absorption, metabolism, excretion, and distribution. The response of target cells to drugs is also altered. The blunted baroreceptors are less sensitive to beta-blockers, but there are increases in end organ sensitivity to some agents such as opiates and warfarin. Approximately two thirds of drug reactions are caused by agents used to treat diseases of the central nervous or cardiovascular system.[45] A few examples of changes in pharmacokinetics with aging follow:

1. Fat-soluble drugs usually have a longer duration of effect.
2. Hydrophilic drugs are more concentrated and have a more potent effect.
3. Absorptive changes may influence drug concentrations.
4. Polypharmacy may cause adverse drug interactions.
5. Decreased renal function prolongs the half-lives of certain drugs.

The rate of absorption in the elderly may be due to decreased gut motility and increased gastric emptying time. Constipation, which results from decreased motility, may prolong the effect of a drug that would otherwise have been eliminated from the body. Diminished gastric secretion with a resulting increase in gastric pH may affect the absorption of some drugs.

Metabolism of a drug determines the level of active drug and its excretion from the body. In elderly patients receiving multiple drugs, drug interactions are more frequent with resultant changes in the metabolic rate of one or all medications. Because of decreased hepatic blood flow owing in part to a decreased liver mass, some drugs are eliminated at a slower rate, including their half-lives. The cytochrome P-450 system metabolizes many drugs that act on the central nervous system. Cimetidine, an H_2 blocker frequently prescribed for elderly people, inhibits hepatic blood flow and the cytochrome P-450 system. Therefore, any psychotropic drug has a greater peak level for a longer time when it is taken with cimetidine.[11]

Most medications are excreted by the kidneys. After 70 years of age the rate of excretion of drugs is one-half to one-third that in a younger person.[28]

Changes in fat and water content in the body are reflected in the distribution of various drugs ingested. Fat-soluble drugs are stored in the increased fat depots of the body, causing a longer duration of the drug effect. Since total body water is less, hydrophilic drugs are more concentrated and therefore more potent. These effects should be considered when prescribing medications.

A lower serum albumin level in elderly patients leads to a greater free fraction of drugs that are highly protein bound, and therefore these drugs have a more potent effect.

Psychologic problems with aging

The psychologic well-being of patients and their caregivers must be appreciated. Several factors determine the progress and final results of the rehabilitation process[26]:

1. Various medications that cause or aggravate depression
2. Rigid personality traits
3. Feelings of helplessness and dependence on caregiver
4. Isolation
5. Loss of privacy
6. Loss of familiar surroundings in hospital or nursing home

The personalities of the patient and all those involved with the patient are intrinsic factors, but extrinsic factors such as stressful surroundings and medications add to this complex picture. Personality traits and motivation are key elements in the rehabilitation processes of relearning and adaptation. Personality traits include an individual's feelings and responses to stimuli. A more rigid personality may not respond to changes as readily as a more flexible one. Motivation is the attitude of mind that imparts a sense of purpose and direction and makes one want to be independent and active.[37]

An aging person may feel a general sense of loss in that youth is gone and will never return. This feeling is compounded when the older patient undergoes a sudden loss of function that probably will never fully return and has to learn to cope with this.

Being institutionalized has a major psychologic impact on rehabilitation in the elderly.[22] When hospitalized, a patient loses familiar surroundings, intimate family relationships, and most personal belongings. Privacy is minimized, relationships are superficial, and contacts are restricted. The patient becomes subservient to an orderly routine and cannot assert himself or herself. Apathy and withdrawal into a fantasy world is a common response. This may initiate a state of helplessness and depression that interferes with the rehabilitation process.[4] Institutionalization may also lead to cognitive losses that mimic a state of dementia. The physician must be alert to differentiate these states.[6] Jackson[19] examined a geriatric rehabilitation pilot project on an acute care medical unit. This program was attempting to prevent the negative effects of hospitalization on the elderly. She found that the elderly involved in the program were eventually more self-sufficient and less confused than the controls.

Situational depression usually does not warrant therapy with psychotropic medications. Drugs and physical restraints should be avoided because they only lead to more confusion, result in falls, or cause immobility.[31] Supportive care and counseling should be tried first. When confused, the elderly respond more readily to gentle encouragement. Measures for management of situational depression in a rehabilitation center include the following:

1. Careful recording and review of medications
2. Avoidance of psychotropic medications
3. Avoidance of physical restraints
4. Counseling and gentle encouragement
5. Simulated home environment
6. Stimulating environment
7. Early discharge

When admitted to a rehabilitation ward, the elderly patient must be given a great deal of attention. There should be some attempt to simulate the patient's home environment because many aged people become confused when taken away from their familiar surroundings.[4] The surroundings should be made more stimulating, and the patient should be treated as a responsible and respected individual. Optimism and enthusiasm should prevail. There should be comfortable furniture and facilities for the handicapped. Comfortable temperature levels and physical aids such as wheelchairs and eating utensils are essential. A complete list of medications taken by the individual should be recorded and reviewed, since they may initiate or aggravate the depressive state.

Early discharge should be a major goal for an elderly patient. As soon as the patient can participate maximally in the activities of daily living with or without aids, appliances, or home services (such as a visiting nurse service), arrangements should be made with the relatives or caregiver. The patient may be considered for a day hospital where individual treatment and care are rendered and where there may be recreational and social activities with special adaptations.

ROLE OF THE GERIATRICIAN

The role of the geriatrician in the rehabilitation of the elderly is twofold. First, the physician must understand the primary medical events that preceded the disability and were responsible for it. Proper management must be given so the disorder does not recur (for example, that falls are avoided) or worsen (that contractures do not follow inflammatory arthritis). Second, medical problems must be managed as they arise as a result of loss of function and immobility.[24] Some examples are decreased general conditioning and decreased cardiovascular fitness, joint stiffness and contractures, muscle wasting, decubitus ulcers,[2] urinary incontinence, constipation, aspiration from depressed gag reflexes and gastric tubes, phlebitis and pulmonary emboli, accelerated osteoporosis with or without fractures, pneumonia, and altered mental status.

MAJOR GERIATRIC PROBLEMS

The major geriatric problems, which are closely interrelated, include the five "I's": incompetence or dementia, incontinence, immobility, impaired homeostatis, and iatrogenic problems. All of these problems result from degenerative processes.

Incompetence

Various disorders cause incompetence in the aged. the most common are Alzheimer's disease, multi-infarct dementia, depression, and benign forgetfulness of senescence.

Alzheimer's disease is organic; senile plaques and neurofibrillatory tangles can be found in pathologic specimens of the brain.[41] There is a gradual progression from occasional forgetfulness to marked loss of cognition and higher intellectual functions and eventually to immobility and incontinence.

Multi-infarct dementia has a sudden onset with remissions and exacerbations. The patient usually has risk factors for cerebrovascular disease and may be emotionally labile.

In geriatric depression the patient has a history of memory difficulties but does not become severely demented. Dementia and depression usually can be differentiated by neuropsychologic testing.[10]

Benign forgetfulness of senescence, with minimal memory impairment, appears gradually with the patient complaining of cognitive deficits. This disorder can be distinguished from Alzheimer's disease in that with benign forgetfulness details of an event may be temporarily forgotten, while in dementia events are completely forgotten and never recalled again.

Reversible causes of dementia must be determined. A thorough history and physical examination, including a neurologic examination, are obtained. Laboratory data, including a complete blood count, blood urea nitrogen (BUN) and creatinine levels, liver function tests, electrolyte levels, calcium and glucose levels, thyroid function tests, vitamin B_{12} and folate levels, toxicology and drug screening, serologic tests, electrocardiography, chest radiology, and computerized tomographic scan of the brain, are used to discover hematologic, metabolic, hepatic, or renal disorders, vitamin deficiencies, drug or chemical intoxication, tertiary syphilis, congestive heart failure, arrhythmias, subdural hematomas, brain tumors, and normal pressure hydrocephalus.[39]

Reisberg and co-workers[34] at the New York University have devised a scale for cognitive decline and Alzheimer's disease. They list seven progressively worse phases seen clinically (Table 28-1).

No treatment for Alzheimer's disease has been established as effective. Early in the course of the illness, ergot alkaloids may improve mood. Recently the use of lecithin in the diet to increase the amount of acetylcholine neurotransmitter in the brain has been studied but seems to be of no value. Summers[40] recently published some encouraging results suggesting that tetrahydroaminoacridine may be useful in long-term palliative treatment of patients with Alzheimer's disease. However, this drug may prove too toxic for general use. Pharmacologic therapy may control agitation and help

Table 28-1. Global Deterioration Scale for cognitive decline

Stage of decline	Characteristics
1. None	Normal
2. Very mild	Subjective complaints of forgetfulness; poor concentration
3. Mild	Cannot function in demanding situations; denial
4. Moderate	Mild Alzheimer's disease; memory deficits; decreased ability to perform more complex tasks as handling money; defense mechanisms
5. Moderately severe	Moderate Alzheimer's disease; disoriented; cannot survive alone
6. Severe	Severe Alzheimer's disease; requires assistance with activities of daily living; incontinence; loss of will power
7. Very severe	Verbal ability and psychomotor skills eventually lost; eventual stupor and coma

Modified from Reisberg, B, et al: Am J Psychiatry 139:1136, 1982.

the patient sleep. Benzodiazepines control anxiety and have been used to manage irrational behavior. Lorazepam and alprazolam, which do not have active metabolites, are short-acting agents with greater flexibility in dosage.[11] Neuroleptics such as haloperidol (Haldol) and thioridazine (Mellaril) have been effective. A frequent side effect of haloperidol is the development of extrapyramidal symptoms, but the sedative effect is low. The usual dose of haloperidol is 0.25 to 6 mg daily. Thioridazine may cause fainting and dizziness when the patient arises and frequently produces ejaculation problems in older men. This drug is more sedating than haloperidol, but extrapyramidal symptoms are milder. The usual starting dose of thioridazine is 10 mg at bedtime, and dosages are increased to up to 300 mg a day every 2 weeks to meet the patient's needs.[11]

Many patients with dementia have a concomitant depression that worsens the symptoms of the dementia.

Incontinence

The incidence of incontinence in the institutionalized population over 65 years of age is about 50%. Recent studies have shown that this condition is often manageable in the elderly.[35,38] The five clinical classes of urinary incontinence are urge, stress, overflow, reflex, and functional.

Urge incontinence is accompanied by a strong desire to void before and during incontinence. The usual cause is detrusor (bladder muscle) hyperactivity in which the bladder escapes central nervous system inhibition and contracts repeatedly.[9]

Stress incontinence is associated with coughing and sneezing that causes a sudden increase in intra-abdominal pressure. Atrophic vaginitis or urethritis can lead to this type of incontinence by affecting the strength of the internal urethral smooth muscle sphincter and often can be relieved by estrogen cream. Also, there may be urethral hypermobility from changes in the posterior urethrovesical angle caused by weakness of the pelvic muscles.

Overflow incontinence occurs when the bladder is over-distended. The bladder may be hypotonic and not generate enough pressure to overcome urethral resistance, resulting in a large residual volume. Overflow incontinence may also be due to bladder outlet obstruction caused by an enlarged prostate or by fecal impaction. Hypotonicity may be neurogenic from a herniated disc or peripheral neuropathy.

Reflex incontinence occurs when a neurologic impairment such as a spinal cord lesion results in loss of voluntary control of urination. There is no sensation of impending urination.

With functional incontinence the patient is unable to get to the toilet in time. This may be because the patient is confused, restrained, or immobile.[12,38]

Incontinence may be acute or chronic. Medications such as diuretics, anticholinergics, sedatives, muscle relaxants, and some antihypertensives may cause acute incontinence. Other causes of acute, intermittent urinary incontinence include urinary tract infection, acute confusion, fecal impaction, polyuric states, bladder tumors or stones, and lack of estrogen in postmenopausal women.

Chronic incontinence is most often caused by detrusor hyperactivity or uninhibited bladder and is usually classified clinically as urge incontinence. It also may be caused by stimulation of the bladder by tumors or stones. Another mechanism of chronic incontinence is detrusor hyporeflexia, which leads to overflow incontinence. In this case the bladder is hypotonic and distended with a large residual volume. Detrusor hyporeflexia occurs in neurologic conditions such as diabetes mellitus, tabes dorsalis, and alcoholic neuropathy.[38] Medications such as anticholinergic drugs or muscle relaxants may precipitate this type of incontinence.

Elderly people may have more than one type of incontinence, which is classified as mixed incontinence. Established incontinence may be due to abnormalities in the detrusor or outlet (urethra).[35,38] For successful treatment of an incontinent patient, the cause should be determined. A record of daily accidents, the circumstances, and the amount of urine lost should be kept. Recent medications should be reviewed. For example, prazosin, an alpha-adrenergic blocker, can cause stress incontinence by its effect on the urethra.[17]

Laboratory tests should include a urinalysis and urine culture, if indicated. When the patient has frequent infections, an intravenous pyelogram should be done to rule out

Table 28-2. Treatment of urinary incontinence

Disorder	Therapy
Spastic bladder (detrusor instability)	Imipramine, 25-150 mg qd; oxybutynin, 5 mg tid; propantheline, 7.5-30 mg tid
Hypotonic bladder	Bethanechol, 20 mg tid; phenoxybenzamine, 10-60 mg qd; intermittent catheterization
Urethral obstruction	Relief of obstruction; sphincterotomy; phenoxybenzamine, 10-60 mg qd
Urethral insufficiency	Weight loss; pelvic exercises; pessary; surgery; estrogens; phenylpropanolamine, 25-50 mg bid; imipramine, 25-150 mg qd

an obstructive lesion. A polyuric syndrome should be ruled out if BUN, glucose, and calcium levels are normal. Urodynamic evaluation may be obtained when stress incontinence with outlet obstruction or overflow incontinence is suspected. In addition, the bladder should be catheterized for residual urine, which is present in obstructive states or with a hypotonic bladder.[35,44]

After the patient has been evaluated, treatment can begin (Table 28-2). Voiding schedules and disposable undergarment protectors can be used with great benefit. Disposable undergarments and good skin care are important for patients who do not respond to drug therapy.

Several new drugs are being administered to treat incontinence.[34,37] In detrusor instability, imipramine, 25 to 150 mg daily; oxybutynin, 5 mg two to four times daily; and propantheline, 7.5 to 30 mg three times a day, are used. In addition, alpha-adrenergic stimulants may be useful to increase urethral resistance. With the problem of detrusor hyporeflexia, bethanechol, 10 to 30 mg three times a day, and phenoxybenzamine, 10 to 60 mg daily, have been used but may cause side effects. If urethral obstruction cannot be corrected, phenoxybenzamine, 10 to 60 mg daily, may be tried. Recently prazosin, an alpha-antagonist, has been used with some success in obstructive uropathy in women.[17] To restore the integrity of the urethral mucosa, estrogen (in women)[5,27] and alpha-adrenergic agents[5] can be used.

Immobility

Immobility in the elderly is caused by various conditions. The consequences of immobility include the following:
1. Decreased general conditioning
2. Decreased cardiovascular fitness
3. Joint stiffness and contractures
4. Muscle wasting
5. Accelerated osteoporosis with or without fractures
6. Decubitus ulcers
7. Thrombophlebitis and pulmonary embolism
8. Constipation
9. Incontinence
10. Pneumonia
11. Altered mental status

Decreased mobility can be prevented or slowed. The destruction of joint cartilage in osteoarthritis and a vertebral or hip fracture secondary to osteoporosis (reduction in the quantity of bone) may lead to immobility. Osteoporosis may itself be accelerated by immobility. Degenerative arthritis may flare up with pain leading to immobility and eventual contractures. Through range-of-motion exercises, physiotherapy, and occupational therapy, the aged individual may improve.[32] Nonpharmacologic methods are tried first and involve educating the patient to modify the use of the affected joints and rest at appropriate intervals. For pain and an anti-inflammatory effect, the patient may be given analgesics including preparations of aspirin or acetaminophen with or without codeine. Anti-inflammatory drugs, such as ibuprofen, 400 to 600 mg orally four times a day, sulindac, 150 to 200 mg orally twice a day, naproxen, 250 to 375 mg orally twice a day, or piroxicam, 20 mg once a day, can be used. Intra-articular corticosteroids such as triamcinolone can also be used but no more than four times a year and at intervals of not less than 1 month.[32]

Osteoporosis, which leads to fractures, pain, and immobility with its sequelae, must be anticipated several years before menopause. It is questionable whether the use of calcium, fluoride, calcitonin, or estrogen in postmenopausal women can reverse or even alleviate the process of bone loss.

Strokes, usually from thrombotic arteriosclerotic events or embolic events caused by atrial fibrillation or peripheral thromboembolism, cause paralysis and inevitable muscle wasting. Dysarthria and dysphagia are other manifestations of a cerebrovascular event. The physiotherapist, occupational therapist, and speech therapist can combine their expertise to help the patient improve.[33] Immobility from any cause decreases general conditioning and cardiovascular fitness. Various exercises should be instituted as a protective measure. Peripheral vascular disease, usually aggravated by diabetes mellitus, may lead to amputation of one or both extremities. The patient may obtain a prosthesis and eventually learn to walk with the help of a physiotherapist.

Impaired homeostasis

Homeostasis, the ability to maintain a satisfactory internal environment despite a less than optimal external environment, requires relay of messages through the nervous or endocrine systems. Thus a close relationship must exist between a central controlling system and receptors and effectors.[22] The internal receptors are the baroreceptors, whose sensitivity is diminished with aging. This results in the development of postural hypotension and dizziness. External receptors are in the skin and help to detect temperature changes. A loss or diminution of these receptors with aging explains the poorer ability of the elderly to recognize temperature changes. Also, decreased muscle mass in the elderly leads to less shivering and therefore less heat production.[22]

A sense of one's position in space is provided by interaction between the vestibular system and multiple sensory inputs. An imbalance between the labyrinthine vestibular system and the senses results from an abnormality of either component, and in the elderly such an imbalance is often caused by medications and injury.[15]

Impaired homeostasis from imbalance of the vestibular system or loss of the sense of sight and sound may cause unsteadiness and falls. The disorder perhaps most commonly referred to the geriatrician is falling from unsteadiness. Balance requires a prompt response to changes in vestibular, visual, and proprioceptive input.[22] Improvement in vision may reduce falls.

The decrease in proprioception in the elderly is compounded by arthritis, amputation of an extremity, and cerebrovascular disease. The elderly have blunted baroreceptor reflexes and on arising may experience orthostatic hypotension because they cannot compensate with a reflex tachycardia. This may lead to falls. Older people must learn to arise slowly and carefully.[16] Various aids such as canes and walkers are helpful to assist with ambulation, and new eyeglasses and hearing aids may improve sight and hearing.

Dizziness may be constant or intermittent (see the box at right). Depression, medications, and systemic illnesses may cause constant dizziness. Intermittent dizziness usually results from visual disorders, peripheral neuropathy, and vestibular disorders. The labyrinthine vestibular dysfunction may be central or peripheral. Involvement of the vestibular portion of the brainstem (central) may be due to increased intracranial pressure, acoustic neuroma, seizures, or vascular insufficiency. Peripheral causes with involvement of the semicircular canals, saccule, utricle, and eighth nerve may be manifest as benign positional vertigo, acute labyrinthitis, Meniere's disease, and perilymphatic fistula. Cervical spondylosis may cause balance problems, and it has been shown that cervical decompression relieves vertigo. Therefore mobilizing exercises rather than a cervical collar may be indicated.[15]

The reflexes must be intact to respond to environmental changes. Many falls are associated with medical conditions as arthritis or Parkinson's disease, for instance, and these disorders may respond to a rehabilitation program.

The treatment of impaired homeostasis is usually symptomatic, managed according to its cause. Offending drugs should be eliminated if possible. Depression, systemic diseases, sensory disturbances, and vestibular dysfunction should be treated.

MANAGEMENT OF DIZZINESS

Constant dizziness

1. Treat depression, if present.
2. Discontinue psychotropic agents, ototoxic antibiotics, and cardiac adrenergic inhibitors.
3. Treat any metabolic or endocrine disorder.

Intermittent dizziness

1. Correct refractive error: prescribe eye patch for diplopia.
2. Treat peripheral neuropathy (if caused by vitamin B_{12} deficiency or diabetes mellitus). The patient may use an aluminum walker to become aware of spatial orientation transmitted by the trunk and extremities.
3. Check for labyrinthine vestibular dysfunction (involvement of vestibular portion of brainstem or semicircular canals).

Iatrogenic disease

The elderly are usually taking several medications for multiple medical conditions. These medications may complicate the rehabilitation process by interacting with one another, or their side effects may compound the effects of the immobile state and lead to such problems as urinary incontinence or constipation. The patient should be carefully assessed, and any necessary drug treatment provided or omitted. The common side effects of major drug classes are shown in Table 28-3.

Postural hypotension, which leads to falls, is one of the most serious side effects of medications in the elderly. With psychotropic drugs, small bedtime doses are given to prevent this side effect. Antihypertensive agents, which are vasodilatory, and diuretics, which in addition to salt deprivation cause a decrease in blood volume, may contribute to a fall in blood pressure in the upright position. These drugs should initially be administered in low doses, which should be increased only with caution. Blood pressure should not be lowered as rapidly and aggressively as in younger individuals.

Anticholinergic drugs are widely prescribed. They include antidepressants, psychotropics, antihistamines, and antispasmodics. These drugs can cause confusion, arrhythmias, overflow incontinence with urinary retention, and constipation and can precipitate acute narrow-angle glaucoma.

Confusion in the elderly can be caused by almost any drug. If confusion is a complaint after a new drug is started, even if the blood level of the drug is in the therapeutic range, the drug should be discontinued and the patient should be observed.

Table 28-3. Side effects of commonly used drugs

Side effect	Drugs
Confusion	Analgesics, anticholinergics, antidepressants, anticonvulsants, anti-inflammatory agents, antiparkinsonian agents, barbiturates, beta-blockers, benzodiazepines, calcium channel blockers, cimetidine, digitalis preparations, hypoglycemics, lidocaine, vincristine
Anticholinergic effect	Antidepressants, antispasmodics, antihistamines, psychotropics
Postural hypotension	Antihypertensives, psychotropics, calcium channel blockers, opiates, antiparkinsonian drugs
Cardiac effect	Digitalis preparations, beta-blockers, calcium channel blockers, antiarrhythmics, antidepressants, psychotropics
Renal effect	Aminoglycoside antibiotics, diuretics, nonsteroidal anti-inflammatory drugs
Neurologic effects	
Convulsions	Lidocaine, antidepressants
Ataxia	Anticonvulsants
Peripheral neuropathy	Vinca alkaloids, nitrofurantoin
Extrapyramidal symptoms	Phenothiazines, butyrophenones, metoclopramide, antidepressants

Table 28-4. Degenerative diseases in the elderly that lead to need for rehabilitation*

Disease	Possible problems
Stroke	Paralysis, dysarthria, dysphagia
Peripheral vascular disease	Amputation
Impaired homeostasis (vestibular, sensory)	Falls, fractures
Orthostatic hypotension (decreased baroreceptor sensitivity)	Falls, fractures
Arthritis	Immobility, contractures
Osteoporosis	Fractures, pain, immobility
Central nervous system and peripheral nervous system disorders	Incontinence, immobility
Dementia	Inability to perform activities of daily living

*The presence of multiple diseases leads to polypharmacy and therefore to adverse drug effects and interactions.

CONCLUSION

Most rehabilitation in the elderly is concerned with the management of conditions that result from degenerative diseases (Table 28-4). The physician must be aware of the particular problems of the elderly so preventive and therapeutic goals can be set.

Drugs that have negative inotropic effects include the beta-blockers, calcium channel blockers, and various antiarrhythmic agents. They can precipitate congestive heart failure in an aged patient who may already have compromised cardiac function.

Renal function, which is already probably diminished in the elderly, is compromised by aminoglycoside antibiotics, diuretics, and anti-inflammatory drugs.

More frequently in the elderly, lidocaine causes convulsions, anticonvulsants cause ataxia, vinca alkaloids and nitrofurantoin cause peripheral neuropathies, and phenothiazines and butyrophenones cause extrapyramidal symptoms. Also, tardive dyskinesia and akathisia or motor restlessness may be seen after administration of the major tranquilizers.[7] In Alzheimer's disease, haloperidol more often produces extrapyramidal side effects than thioridazine does.

Allergies and hematologic, gastrointestinal, and dermatologic side effects of drugs are seen equally at all ages. Medical personnel must be aware of the dangers of medications; often success depends on discontinuing drugs rather than adding new ones.

REFERENCES

1. Agate, J: Rehabilitation of the elderly patient—ways and means, Int Rehabil Med 7:109, 1984.
2. Anderson, KE, Jensen, O, and Kvorning, SA: Prevention of pressure sores by identifying patients at risk, Br Med J 1:1370, 1982.
3. Applegate, WB, et al: A geriatric rehabilitation and assessment unit in a community hospital, J Am Geriatr Soc 31:206, 1983.
4. Avorn, J, and Langer, E: Induced disability in nursing home patients: a controlled trial, J Am Geriatr Soc 30:379, 1982.
5. Beisland, HO, et al: Urethral spincteric insufficiency in postmenopausal females: treatment with phenylpropanolamine and estriol separately and in combination; a urodynamic and clinical evaluation, Urol Int 39:211, 1984.
6. Cohen, BS: Geriatric rehabilitation, Am Fam Physician 30:133, 1984.
7. Critchley, EMR: Drug induced neurological disease, Br Med J 1:862, 1979.
8. Crooks, J, et al: Pharmacokinetics in the elderly, Clin Pharmacokinet 1:280, 1976.
9. deGroat, WC, and Booth, AM: Autonomic systems to the urinary bladder and sexual organs. In Dyck, PJ, et al, editors: Peripheral neuropathy, ed 2, Philadelphia, 1984, WB Saunders Co.
10. Diamond, E: Testing cognitive function in the elderly, Geriatr Consult 4:21, 1985.

11. Freedman, ML: Organic brain syndrome in the elderly, Postgrad Med 74:165, 1983.
12. Gellick, MR, Serrell, NA, and Gellick, CS: Adverse consequences of hospitalization in the elderly, Soc Sci Med 16:1033, 1982.
13. Greenblatt, DJ, and Sellers, EM: Drug disposition in old age, N Engl J Med 306:1081, 1982.
14. Greenland, P: Cardiac fitness and rehabilitation in the elderly, J Am Geriatr Soc 30:607, 1982.
15. Greer, M: How serious is dizziness, Geriatrics 36:34, 1981.
16. Gribbin, B, et al: Effect of age and high blood pressure on baroreflex sensitivity in man, Circ Res 29:424, 1971.
17. Hedlund, H, and Anderssen, KE: Effects of prazosin in patients with benign prostatic obstruction, J Urol 130:275, 1983.
18. Holm, K, and Kirchhoff, KT: Perspectives on exercise and aging, Heart Lung 13:519, 1984.
19. Jackson, MF: Geriatric rehabilitation on an acute care medical unit, J Adv Nurs 9:441, 1984.
20. Jones, RH: Physiological basis of rehabilitation therapy. In Williams, TF, editor: Rehabilitation in the aging, New York, 1984, Raven Press.
21. Keltz, H: Pulmonary function and disease in the aging. In Williams, TF, editor: Rehabilitation in the aging, New York, 1984, Raven Press.
22. Kenney, RA: Physiology of aging. In Geokas, MC, editor: The aging process, Philadelphia, 1985, WB Saunders Co.
23. Konshalo, DR: Age changes in touch, vibration, temperature, kinesthesis, pain sensitivity. In Bioren, JE, and Schaie, KA, editors: Handbook of the biology of aging, New York, 1977, Van Nostrand-Reinhold.
24. Kottke, FJ, and Anderson, EM: Deterioration of the bedfast patient, Pub Health Rep 80:437, 1965.
25. Lipsitz, L: Diagnosis and management of syncope, Geriatr Consult, July/August 1985, p 26.
26. Loebel, JP, and Eisdorfer, C: Psychological and psychiatric factors in the rehabilitation of the elderly. In Williams, TF, editor: Rehabilitation in the aging, New York, 1984, Raven Press.
27. Mohr, JA, et al: Stress urinary incontinence: a simple and practical approach to diagnosis and treatment, J Am Geriatr Soc 31:476, 1983.
28. Myers-Robfogel, MW, and Bosmann, HB: Clinical pharmacology in the aged: aspects of pharmacokinetics and drug sensitivity. In Williams, TF, editor: Rehabilitation in the aging, New York, 1984, Raven Press.
29. Pontoppidan, H, and Beecher, HK: Progressive loss of protective reflexes in the airway with advance of age, JAMA 174:2209, 1960.
30. Payne, FE, and Boineau, JP: Cardiac rehabilitation, Am Fam Physician 22:152, 1980.
31. Powell, C, Edmund, L, and Fingerote, E: Freedom from restraint: consequences of reducing physical restraints in the treatment of elderly persons, Ann R Coll Phys Surg Can 16:343, 1983.
32. Quinet, RJ: Osteoarthritis: increasing mobility and reducing disability, Geriatrics 41:36, 1986.
33. Redford, JB, and Harris, JD: Rehabilitation of the elderly stroke patient, Am Fam Pract 22:153, 1980.
34. Reisberg, B, et al: The global deterioration scale for assessment of primary degenerative dementia, Am J Psychiatry 139:1136, 1982.
35. Resnick, NM, and Subbarao, VY: Management of urinary incontinence in the elderly, N Engl J Med 313:800, 1985.
36. Rusk, HA, and Lee, MH: Rehabilitation of the aging, Bull NY Acad Med 47:1383, 1971.
37. Silverstone, B: Social aspects of rehabilitation. In Williams, TF, editor: Rehabilitation in the aging, New York, 1984, Raven Press.
38. Snustad, DG, and Rosenthal, JT: Urinary incontinence in the elderly, Am Fam Physician 32:182, 1985.
39. Steel, K, and Feldman, R: Diagnosing dementia and its treatable causes, Geriatrics 34:79, 1979.
40. Summers, WK, et al: Oral tetrahydroaminoacridine in long-term treatment of senile dementia, Alzheimer type, N Engl J Med 315:1241, 1986.
41. Terry, R, and Davies, P: Dementia of the Alzheimer type, Annu Rev Neurol 3:77, 1980.
42. Van Alste, JA, et al: Exercise testing of leg amputees and the result of prosthetic training, Int Rehabil Med 7:93, 1985.
43. Wenger, NK: Cardiovascular status: changes with aging. In Williams, TF, editor: Rehabilitation in the aging, New York, 1984, Raven Press.
44. Williams, ME, and Pannill, FC: Urinary incontinence in the elderly, Ann Intern Med 97:895, 1982.
45. Williamson, J, and Chopin, JM: Adverse reactions to prescribed drugs in the elderly: a multicenter investigation, Age Ageing 9:73, 1980.

SUGGESTED READINGS

Andrews, K: Rehabilitation of conditions associated with old age, Int Rehabil Med 7:125, 1985.

Clark, GS: Functional assessment in the elderly. In Williams, TF, editor: Rehabilitation in the aging, New York, 1984, Raven Press.

CHAPTER 29

Geriatric rehabilitation management

MATHEW LEE AND MASAYOSHI ITOH

For the past few decades the phrase "geriatric rehabilitation" has been widely used by both medical professionals and the lay public. "Geriatric" is formed from words of two languages: *geras,* a Greek word meaning old, and *iatric,* an English word meaning related to medical treatment or healing. Thus geriatric rehabilitation may be defined as the restoration of the disabled older person to maximum capacity—physical and emotional. Geriatric rehabilitation may be viewed as a subspecialty of rehabilitation, like pediatric or adult rehabilitation, and does not deal with a specific disease or disability.

Improvements in medical and scientific technology and in public health have dramatically increased life expectancy in the United States. In 1900 only 4% of the U.S. population had reached 65 years of age, but by 1980 this had increased to 11%. By the year 2030, more than 50 million, or 17% of the United States population, will be in this group.[8]

The definition of the older person, the aged, or the elderly has been a controversial subject. The concept of "old" differs greatly depending on geography and culture. Even within a cultural group, the concept of "old" changes from one generation to another. The most influential factor in the concept seems to be life expectancy. Some claim that old people are those over 65 years of age, since for some time that was the federally mandated age for retirement and eligibility for Social Security benefits. However, these political and socioeconomic considerations cannot be used in the scientific definition of "old." Since the mandatory retirement age was extended to 70½ years in 1983, has the public's conception of old age changed? In general, the concept of old differs according to each individual's perception.

The elderly are referred to in various ways, such as senior citizens or golden agers. Although a relatively new tier classification of the aged seems euphemistic, from the viewpoint of social science it may be useful to classify those between ages 65 and 75 as "young old," those between 75 and 85 years as "old," and those 85 years and older as "old old."

Medical scientists recognize that terms such as old, aged, senior citizen, or any other new or old designation has no scientific basis, since a scientific term is customarily defined more specifically. The use of chronologic age as the tool for defining old age may necessitate making too many exceptions. It may be more rational to define the aged as those who belong to the top 10% or even 12% of the demographic curve of a given population. This concept depends on the life expectancy and demographic curve of that group at a specific time period; thus the "aged" may change in chronologic age, but a more realistic picture is created. For example, according to the U.S. census of 1980, individuals 65 years and older made up approximately 11% of the population, fitting the proposed definition appropriately. The aged have influenced the political, social, and economic arena in such issues as retirement age and pension planning. Another consideration in geriatrics involves the significance of biologic and physiologic changes commonly seen among those who have reached advanced age.

In Eastern cultures the elderly are respected for their contribution to society and the wisdom they have gained through experience. On the other hand, in occidental cultures, particularly urban America, the aged are frequently viewed as a social burden, an unproductive population. It is sad to see well-known comedians mimic the mannerisms and appearance of the aged with a shuffling gait and hearing impairment to evoke laughter from an audience. The elderly who appear in television advertisements often appear unintelligent rather than as role models for youth.

Many groups in our society are deprived socially and economically on the basis of sex, race, ethnicity, or religion. The aged population also falls into such a category; the

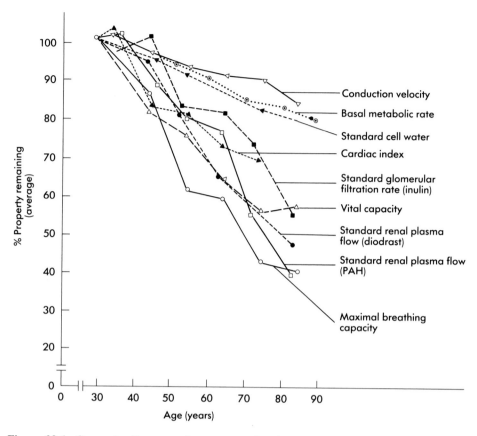

Figure 29-1. Composite diagrams of percentage of various functional capacities or properties remaining at various ages. Human cross-sectional data are derived from extensive work of Shock and co-workers.[55,56]

difference between the two groups is that the aged grew into their category whereas the others were born into theirs. The deprived status of the elderly makes geriatric rehabilitation more complex and challenging.

The early Roman saying, "Old age is a disease itself," is no longer acceptable in modern medicine. However, knowledge of the physiologic changes that occur with senescence is essential in evaluating any elderly individual. Impairment of many functions begins at about 30 years of age. Although functional decrements at the cellular level may not exceed 15%, total organic performance may depreciate by 40% to 60%. A graphic representation of physiologic decline in older persons appears in Figure 29-1.[52,55]

It should be emphasized that these declines are a gerontologic process and are not caused by the various illnesses that are highly prevalent in the elderly. When such conditions are compounded with the chronic diseases commonly found among this population, physical rehabilitation of the disabled elderly presents unique problems.

The physical restorative regimen, such as physical, occupational, or speech therapy, for the elderly disabled population is fundamentally the same as for any other age group. Because other chapters in this book describe testing and

diagnostic methods and detailed restorative techniques for a host of disabling conditions, this chapter is devoted to the unique aspects of geriatric rehabilitation.

CHARACTERISTICS OF GERIATRIC REHABILITATION

It is important to distinguish the goals of geriatric rehabilitation from the rehabilitation needs of patients in younger age groups. Although the fundamental principles are identical, there are unique distinctions in the rehabilitation of the elderly population. These features may be classified into two broad categories: conceptual and practical.

According to Rusk,[48] rehabilitation is the "ultimate restoration of a disabled person to his maximum capacity— physical, emotional and vocational." The word "restoration" means the act of bringing back or putting back into the former or original state. When Rusk's definition of rehabilitation is taken literally, the maximum achievement of the rehabilitation process is the attainment of premorbid function or ability. Although theoretically rehabilitation is most appropriate for those who have achieved physical, mental, educational, and vocational goals before becoming disabled, rehabilitation medicine is not confined to these limitations. For example, a disabled child may need to complete a formal education, including higher education or vocational training. Physically this child may not be able to regain premorbid capacity or to have normal growth, but he or she can certainly exceed the premorbid functional level educationally, vocationally, and emotionally. Adults who were manual or physical laborers may need vocational retraining so they can be gainfully employed within their physical limitations. Motivation, intellectual capability, and aptitude are prerequisites to completing the vocational rehabilitation program.

An elderly disabled person had probably retired from employment before the onset of the disability, and thus the educational and vocational aspects are not pertinent. Since an elderly disabled individual may have been functioning independently until the onset of the disability, the highest achievable goal for this person is the recovery of premorbid function.

Theoretically achievable goal

The theoretically achievable goal (TAG) is the ultimate attainment in rehabilitation that a disabled person can reach under the most ideal conditions: physical, intellectual, mental, physiologic, social, economic, and environmental. For example, even if all of the other conditions are ideal, a disabled person who lacks motivation because of a dependent personality cannot achieve the TAG. Although the TAG is greatly influenced by age, it can vary within the same age group, depending on the individual.

To illustrate TAG, a weighted score is assigned to certain essential activities or physical functions:

Activities of daily living (maximum 50 points)	Points
Independent in bowel and bladder care	10
Independent in feeding	10
Independent in grooming	10
Independent in dressing	10
Independent in communication	10

Mobility (maximum 10 points)	
Independent in ambulation	10
Independent in mobility without ambulation	5
Independent in transfer activities	5

Educational, vocational, and avocational activity (maximum 40 points)	
Regain all or most of premorbid vocational and/or avocational functions	15
Completion of formal or higher education	20
Completion of vocational training or retraining	20

The highest score (100) for a child or young adult includes independence in all activities of daily living (ADLs), independence in ambulation or mobility transfer, and completion of education and vocational training or retraining. An elderly person can score as many as 75 points, which includes independence in ADLs, ambulation or mobility, transfer, and the restoration of all or most premorbid avo-

cational functions. Figure 29-2 shows the difference in the total TAG score according to age group.

A 63-year-old patient had his right leg amputated below the knee because of diabetic gangrene of the foot. He was fitted with a patellar tendon–bearing prosthesis and continued to work as an office clerk until his retirement at 65 years of age. At the time of the below-knee amputation, his TAG was 75 points (as described previously for an elderly person) and thus his achievement was 100% of TAG. After retirement he maintained his home, doing minor repairs and gardening, went to the supermarket weekly to shop for his wife, and took occasional fishing trips. At 67 years of age, owing to occlusion of the left femoral artery, he underwent a left above-knee amputation and was fitted with an above-knee prosthesis. Since he had led a rather active retirement life, it was unlikely that he would be able to regain all or most of his avocational functions, even with a successful prosthetic rehabilitation program. Therefore the most likely TAG score is 60 points (50 points for independence in ADLs and 10 points for independence in ambulation). At present he is able to ambulate with two prostheses and two canes or a walker for a distance of approximately 30 feet. He uses a wheelchair for long-distance mobility, and his wife now goes to the market. He was totally independent in all areas of ADLs. Thus he has accomplished 100% of his TAG, totaling 60 points.

Although it is desirable that a geriatric disabled person attain 100% of TAG (75 points), obtaining 60 points is a great accomplishment. In geriatric rehabilitation, complete independence in all ADLs and in mobility is the most realistic goal. One must be careful in setting the TAG; it is necessary to take all conditions into consideration and set neither an overly optimistic nor an overly pessimistic TAG.

There are subtle differences between the response of a geriatric and nongeriatric patient to restorative processes. In a geriatric patient, aside from the fact that the functional level to be achieved is more limited, the restorative process is extremely slow. Elderly people are more prone to having physically good days and bad days.[26] Therapists may find inconsistent progress because, without any overt reason, the elderly can be full of vitality one day and feel weak, achy, and not "quite up to" the next day. It is not known whether this peculiar phenomenon is related to general physical decline in older patients as mentioned previously (Figure 29-1).

Psychologic condition

An elderly disabled individual's psychologic condition can also hinder the rehabilitation process. Depression, which in a majority of cases is situational, is a common feature of these patients. Before the disability the individual might have been depressed because of loneliness or socioeconomic hardship. With the addition of a disability, the person is no longer free to choose activities and must depend on physical assistance from others. In addition to feeling

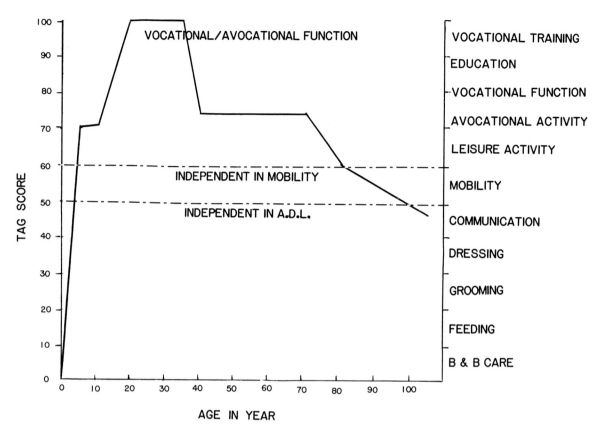

Figure 29-2. Theoretically achievable goal (TAG) score according to age. Score sharply increases in early life, reaches maximum at approximately 20 to 35 years of age, and gradually declines as age advances.

anger and frustration, the patient may experience wounds to an already diminished pride when told what, how, and when to do by young nurses and therapists who may be the same age as the patient's grandchildren.

Since the depressed patient cannot be expected to be an active participant in each and every therapeutic activity, the members of the rehabilitation team may conclude that he or she is not motivated. Motivation and rewards are so inseparable that if there is a slight ray of hope, such patients usually respond positively, becoming more active and perhaps more enthusiastic participants in the restorative process. It is therefore important for rehabilitation team members to comprehend the predicament of the aged disabled and to provide constant encouragement as well as a support system for the patients.

Before the initiation of the treatment program a thorough physical examination, with an emphasis on cardiovascular and pulmonary function, should be performed so appropriate precautionary measures may be taken during treatment, especially during exercise activities.

Physical condition

The most common cardiac disorders among the elderly are arteriosclerotic heart disease, hypertensive heart disease,

and congestive heart failure. Arrhythmias and electrocardiographic abnormalities have an increased incidence with aging.[9] Various exercise tests have been developed that provide accurate information on cardiac response to exercise but require different testing apparatuses and special technicians.* Often an exercise prescription for physical therapy notes only a cardiac precaution, which generally means checking the pulse and blood pressure before and after an exercise and, if the increase in these parameters exceeds a safe preset rate or value, altering the exercise or forbidding it completely.

These "cardiac precautions" may not be sufficient to ensure safe exercise for the elderly disabled, particularly those with abnormal electrocardiograms. A relatively inexpensive and simple method of monitoring cardiac response to exercise without additional technical assistance is telemetric electrocardiography. In contrast to exercise tests that use treadmill or ergometers in a testing room or laboratory, telemetric electrocardiograms can be taken during such actual exercise as progressive resistance, ambulation, or elevation. Telemetry can be used for the geriatric above-knee amputees: after the patient has been fitted with a pylon,

---

*References 7, 20, 37, 41, 51, 53.

the heart can be monitored with telemetric electrocardiography during ambulation exercise. Thus the feasibility of prescribing an above-knee prosthesis can be determined.

The efficiency of telemetry may be compromised by its limited range and the interference of background electronic noise. Interference can be particularly acute in an urban area where electronic traffic is heavy; however, it can be diminished and the range extended by the installation of antennae in strategic locations (such as above the ambulation area). Rather than using makeshift steps in a physical therapy gymnasium for elevation exercises, the installation of a remote antenna above the staircase of the hospital building permits monitoring of cardiac responses in a more realistic environment.

Cardiopulmonary functions decrease with age.[6,30,57] Some changes in cardiopulmonary function are the result of the physiologic alterations caused by aging, and others are related to diseases that are highly prevalent among the older population. An often overlooked factor is physical deconditioning not directly associated with gerontologic processes or age-related illnesses, but exceedingly common among the elderly population. Both diminished physiologic function and deconditioning resulting from inactivity are great hindrances to progress during rehabilitation. Many factors are involved in deconditioning. It is commonly believed that aged people have very sedentary life-styles. An elderly person who prefers the energetic pursuit of all types of physical activities may be so affected by the cultural and social pressures of younger people and peers who accept this behavioral norm that he or she chooses to conform to the stereotype.

Another common situation is overcompliance with a physician's instructions. For various reasons physicians give their elderly patients instructions to "take it easy" or "take a rest." Almost all older people can readily accept this advice, even though they may not comply with instructions concerning medication or diet. Without detailed instructions as to when and how long to rest or understanding the meaning of "take it easy," older patients become fearful of engaging in any type of physical activity and become victims of self-imposed immobilization.

Physical inactivity is common among patients with an organic mental syndrome. Depression can also drive an elderly person to excessive bed rest. When depression is compounded by a slight degree of physical discomfort (such as arthralgia or neuralgia), the incentive for physical inactivity is augmented.

When a state of physical deconditioning is detected, the various exercise tests described previously may be necessary to rule out disease processes and to establish a baseline condition. Physical reconditioning should be instituted promptly, but the intensity and progression of exercises for older patients must be gentler and slower than for younger deconditioned individuals. One of the most commonly used pieces of exercise equipment is a bicycle ergometer that can be modified for operation from a wheelchair using both upper and lower extremities.[6] A treadmill would not be suitable equipment for the elderly disabled because of possible perceptual, visual, balance, or coordination problems.

As previously noted, physical training or reconditioning should start with a suitable exercise test, measuring vital signs at least before and after exercise or monitoring them throughout the exercise period. Increment of load or resistance exercises should be more gradual than with a healthy young person. It usually takes at least 4 to 6 weeks for the elderly disabled to reach maximum functional level. If exercise training is instituted concurrently with other physical therapy modalities and occupational therapy, the total energy expenditure must be within the patient's tolerance and endurance. As the reconditioning process progresses, more physical demands can be tolerated, necessitating close communication between the therapy services and the work physiology laboratory where the reconditioning exercises are given.

Not every geriatric patient must undergo physical reconditioning training. Those who have no clinical signs or indications of cardiopulmonary complications and whose physical inactivity is due only to a current disability that will be relatively brief can proceed quickly to the restorative process.

SUSCEPTIBILITY

The word "susceptibility" is commonly used in epidemiology and immunology. It has been used in the past to refer to a lack of immunity to an infectious disease. Immunity is generally understood as the capacity of an individual, when exposed to infection, to remain free of illness or infection.[54] Susceptibility and immunity are opposite host reactions to a disease. If a specific population is highly susceptible to a certain disease or condition, that population is at high risk for the disease or condition[26]; the presence of susceptibility is equal to the absence of immunity and vice versa. Originally the concept of susceptibility and immunity was applied solely to infectious diseases or organisms; however, it is now commonly used to describe the risk of a population or individual in other instances.

Susceptibility is influenced by such factors as age, sex, nutritional status, cultural and educational background, economic condition, and naturally or artificially acquired immunity. Two examples of age-related susceptibility are greenstick fracture and Colles' fracture, both of which occur commonly in the forearm under similar circumstances. Young children are more susceptible to the former because of the high elasticity of their bones; the elderly are more susceptible to the latter because of osteoporotic bones. Persons in their teens and twenties have the highest rate of automobile accident mortality among all age groups. On the other hand, elderly pedestrians have as high an incidence of injuries as young people involved in vehicular accidents.

There appear to be certain characteristics of susceptibility to physical disabilities among the aged population. Although a decline in cardiopulmonary function does not in itself cause neuromuscular disability, it is an important factor in this type of disability. For example, arteriosclerosis can often cause stroke, possibly resulting in paralysis, and peripheral vascular insufficiency, possibly resulting in amputation of a lower extremity. Advanced cerebral arteriosclerosis may result in senility or parkinsonism. Long-standing diabetes mellitus may lead to peripheral neuropathy and amputation because of gangrene. Osteoporosis and osteoarthritis, which are common among the aged, may result in fractures and disabling chronic pain or deformities. A change in gait or diminished vision or hearing may be a causative factor in various household and pedestrian accidents.

Each of these "susceptibilities" alone may not result in disability, but instead may cause a chain of events. For a disease condition to develop, there must be simultaneous interaction of three causative factors: host, agent, and environment.[27] This is an important concept in planning geriatric rehabilitation and preventing disability.

Hip fracture

Fracture of the proximal end or neck of the femur is a common injury among elderly white women.[2,5,14,23,40] One might simply blame postmenopausal osteoporosis; however, such fractures have a lower incidence among black and Mexican-American women, which suggests some genetic differences. Almost all hip fractures are caused by a trauma, usually a fall, which may be due to a shuffling gait, diminished vision from a cataract or glaucoma, incoordination, prolonged reaction time, vertigo, or environmental factors. Vertigo may be caused by a transient cerebral ischemic attack resulting from arteriosclerosis of the cerebral arteries, hypertension, antihypertensive medication, a hypoglycemic agent, nutritional deficiency, or even dehydration. It has been reported that the frequency of falls increases in nursing homes on "laxative day."[1] When an elderly woman is receiving a nocturnal sedative, she may experience vertigo on awakening to go to the bathroom. A wet or highly waxed floor, throw rugs, electrical extension cords, or toys on the floor, poor lighting, a stepladder, or a lack of a bannister or presence of an unsafe one can make a fall likely. Worn-out house slippers, which tend to produce an unstable shuffle, are also hazardous.

The preceding environmental factors, in combination with individual "host" (patient) factors, contribute to the cause of a fall. The force of energy created by a fall is the "agent."

There are various speculations about the mechanism of a hip fracture. A direct force on the greater trochanter and torsion motion of the lower extremity, particularly at the level of the neck of the femur and with minuscule or no apparent force, are often cited mechanisms. Another theory holds that a fall is the result of a fracture rather than the fracture being the result of a fall. Although the neck of the femur can normally withstand a great amount of stress, an osteoporotic femur is especially vulnerable. A sudden muscle contraction to maintain body balance may cause a fracture. Once the fracture occurs, the length of the legs decreases and the diminished muscle tension may not be sufficiently effective to stabilize the joint, resulting in a fall. However, patients seldom claim to have had severe pain in the hip or knee immediately before a fall. This is probably because the interval between the fracture and the fall is so short that the patient may not recall the sequence of events.

The combination of hip fracture and hemiplegia is not uncommon among the elderly population. A highly significant correlation was found between the side of a previous hemiplegia and the side of a subsequent hip fracture.[15] Many investigators agree that in a majority of cases the hip fractures sustained were ipsilateral to hemiplegia.[10,22,42,45] Mulley and Esply[42] observed that such fractures often occur within 1 year of the stroke, possibly because stroke patients tend to fall to the affected side as a result of impaired locomotor function and the development of disuse osteoporosis in the hemiplegic limb as the genesis of hip fracture in hemiplegic patients.

A stroke and a fracture of the hip may occur almost simultaneously. At the onset of a stroke the individual experiences vertigo or loss of consciousness, loses control of the muscles, and consequently falls to the side of the hemiplegia. Unfortunately, the fracture is often undetected for some time. The primary care physician may be preoccupied with lifesaving measures and stabilizing the obvious stroke symptoms. The patient is often unable to communicate or may think that the pain is part of the stroke symptoms. The paralysis of the lower extremity itself makes recognition of the fracture more difficult. A poor functional recovery has been noted in cases with an interval of less than 1 week between stroke and fracture.[45]

Decubitus ulcer (see Chapter 11)

Decubitus ulcers are often seen in elderly debilitated patients.[4,38] Lesions are of great concern in such institutions as skilled nursing facilities that provide health care to predominantly elderly populations. In New York State the prevalence of decubitus ulcers in a skilled nursing facility is given high priority in the assessment of the quality of care in that facility. If the prevalence is higher than that established by statewide criteria and no special justification can be identified, a deficiency indicative of poor quality medical care is cited.

Decubitus ulcers are a debilitating, sometimes fatal, condition for which long-term treatment is required. The mechanism of development of a decubitus ulcer is a far more complex process than generally believed (Figure 29-3).

Some patients have diminished skin sensation, particularly with regard to tactility and pain sensation. Other elderly people suffer from nutritional deficiencies resulting in diminished subcutaneous fat tissue, hypoproteinemia, anemia,

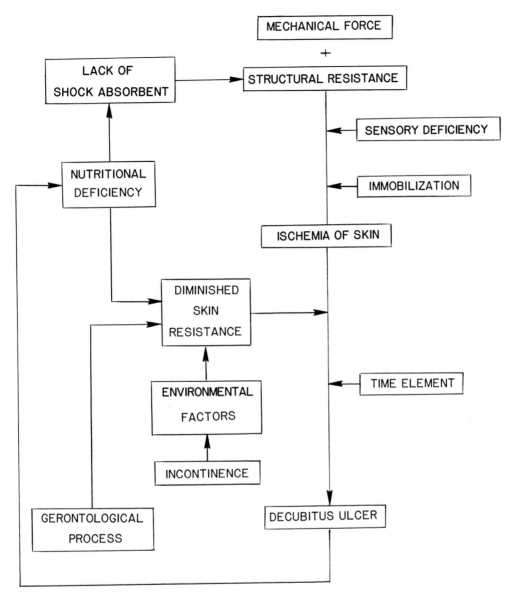

Figure 29-3. Interrelationship between various causative factors of development of decubitus ulcer. Once decubitus ulcer develops and is not treated properly, vicious cycle is formed and more ulcers develop elsewhere on skin.

ascorbic acid deficiency, and other impairments. Poor blood circulation to skin, localized endogenous oligemia resulting from peripheral vascular disease, and loss of skin elasticity and lubrication are also closely related to the aging process.

Decubitus incidence is higher among elderly persons with organic mental syndrome,[3,47] situational depression, or chronic pain, who tend to spend long periods in bed. Some individuals stay in bed in one position for hours.

The moisture, chemicals, and microorganisms resulting from prolonged exposure of the skin to urine and feces diminish its integrity. Incontinence is closely related to organic mental syndrome or depression, in the absence of any other neurologic dysfunction. Organic mental syndrome in this case is not necessarily synonymous with senility. Elderly individuals may show all the signs of acute organic mental syndrome after severe dehydration for a period as short as 48 hours. In such cases the patient's general physical condition improves rapidly after hydration, but it may take several months for the mental condition to return to the predehydration level.

Even in the absence of a major illness, a physically or mentally inactive elderly person becomes debilitated and takes on the host characteristics that conribute to decubitus ulcers.

SPECIAL CONSIDERATIONS

Although all types of disabling diseases and conditions can be found among older people, a few deserve special consideration because of their high incidence.[21]

Hemiplegia

A study in southern Alabama, which is not in the so-called stroke belt, revealed the crude incidence of stroke to be 135 per 100,000 people and the age-adjusted incidence to be 159 per 100,000 population.[17] While this study reported mortality of 24% within 3 months of a stroke, it is lower than the mortality reported in other studies from Western countries.[16,31,43] The Alabama study shows that 57% of strokes occur in persons 65 years or older. Because of their age this group of patients frequently has multiple concomitant diseases. For example, diabetes mellitus is found in 25% of stroke patients, cardiac abnormalities and hypertensive cardiovascular disease are present in well over 50% of stroke patients.[33] Many individual and social burdens resulting from strokes would be obviated by the application of multifactorial primary prevention, consisting of dietetic-hygienic measures, hypolipidemic and antihypertensive agents,[39] and rehabilitation measures, before stroke occurs.[24]

The treatment of geriatric patients with hemiplegia must be carried out in the context of their physiologic condition and social circumstances. Specific concomitant conditions, as well as varying degrees of physiologic deterioration, can be expected to complicate the effects of brain damage resulting from stroke. Aside from diabetes mellitus and hypertensive cardiac abnormalities, osteoarthritis and arteriosclerosis are common in the elderly stroke patients. Although rehabilitation procedures should be carried out, they must be clinically realistic and closely geared to social planning. Discharge to the patient's family is usually preferable but not always possible. Frequently there is no surviving spouse or any receptive children, and in some situations the patient's condition dictates institutionalization. Various levels of care facilities are available, depending on the clinical requirements. Wherever the patient lives, maintenance rehabilitation should be continued.

Hip fracture

A survey of 10,250 patients of both sexes in the municipal hospitals of New York City revealed that 5% had recent or old hip fractures and that 87% of all of the hip fractures were in people 55 years of age and over.[48] Over a recent 30-year period there was a continuous increase in the incidence of hip fracture, particularly in the oldest age group and in men.[18,28] Early open reduction and internal fixation, or insertion of a prosthesis and early ambulation, have greatly reduced mortality in patients with hip fractures. However, unless timely surgical and restorative care is provided, patients may permanently lose the ability to walk.

Postsurgical bed rest should be as brief as possible to prevent cardiopulmonary complications and the deconditioning of general physical capacities. Regardless of the surgical procedure used, and in the absence of significant contraindications, active range-of-motion exercises should be started at the earliest possible time following the operative procedure. A patient may stand, not bearing weight, in the parallel bars 48 hours after surgery, provided there are no surgical complications. Caution should be used at all times to prevent falls.

The duration of non-weight-bearing ambulation depends on the type of surgical procedure used and the postoperative radiographic findings. If an impacted subcapital fracture cannot be pinned, weight bearing should not be allowed for about 6 to 8 weeks and the patient must remain in traction until a bony union occurs.[32] When the surgical reduction or insertion of the prosthesis is satisfactorily performed, the patient should be able to start partial weight-bearing ambulation within a week after surgery. Partial weight-bearing ambulation is always a controversial subject. Unless special equipment is used, it is not possible to measure the weight bearing on the affected limb during the stance phase. A technique in which the toes barely touch the ground is a common practice in partial weight bearing. In reality such a method is the same as not bearing weight. Another common method of partial weight bearing is almost hopping during the stance phase on the fractured limb, or applying a lift to the shoe of the noninvolved side. Neither method is recommended, since the former requires considerable physical agility and the latter may cause low back pain. Unless a patient can perform a partial weight-bearing gait satisfactorily, safely, and comfortably, this phase of ambulation training should be omitted. Instead, the patient should proceed to full weight bearing on the tenth to fourteenth postoperative day.

During ambulation exercises, safety should be of the utmost concern to the rehabilitation team. Although crutch walking or ambulation with a walker is often suggested for partial weight bearing, unless the patient exhibits excellent coordination, muscle power, and balance, it is far safer for an elderly patient to ambulate on the parallel bars during this phase of training.

Recent studies have revealed that extraordinarily high pressure is exerted on the femoral head during the rise from a sitting position[19,34]; when the patient uses a cane for support, loading of the hip joint is only 5% greater than if a single crutch is used. These findings suggest that a reassessment of the current restorative care routine of a hip fracture patient is needed. Perhaps when the patient is able to ambulate safely in the parallel bars, the period of crutch walking outside the parallel bars can be shortened or eliminated and the patient can proceed to ambulation with a cane more rapidly.

When a patient complains of pain during weight bearing, a careful investigation is warranted. Although a complaint of pain on the lateral aspect of the thigh is common, such pain usually subsides without treatment unless there is a sign of infection. However, pain in the knee or the medial aspect of the thigh is usually a sign of a disorder or an abnormality on the head of the femur or acetabulum. Aseptic necrosis of the head of the femur, infection, or slippage of the nail or screw must be treated surgically.

Amputation

Prolongation of life expectancy has as its corollary an increase in the incidence of lower extremity amputation among the elderly owing to the high incidence of vascular insufficiency related to arteriosclerosis and diabetes mellitus.

Geriatric amputees are more likely to present problems in rehabilitation because of a decrease in cardiopulmonary capacity, poor neuromuscular coordination, visual impairment, weakened musculature, or the limitations in range of joint movement that impose restrictions on the intensity of preprosthetic and prosthetic training programs. The goals of prosthetic rehabilitation for geriatric amputees should be realistic. Their most common need is the restoration, to premorbid levels, of activities of daily living and recreation. This is a good example of TAG.

Even within the limited goals of geriatric prosthetic programs, most elderly amputees have more difficulty than other amputees unless the patient has excellent coordination, balance, and cardiopulmonary function and is highly motivated. A unilateral above-knee geriatric amputee is at high risk of ultimately becoming a bilateral amputee. When an above-knee prosthesis is prescribed for an elderly person, safety takes priority over function. Thus a selection of its components, weight, ease of use, and alignment of the prosthesis require special considerations (see Chapter 41).

There is a high incidence of cardiac disease among geriatric amputees, a complication that often precludes the use of a prosthesis. Therefore, to help elderly amputees become as functional and active as possible, one should not hesitate to provide a wheelchair and a prosthesis when either or both are indicated. Often the use of a wheelchair requires much less energy expenditure than that used for a prosthesis. On discharge from the hospital, the patient should receive some type of home care services to meet general health and prosthetic needs (for example, adjustment of malfitting socket resulting from stump shrinkage; repair of components if necessary).

When there has been a single amputation, preventive foot care for the remaining limb is of vital importance. The patient and family should be trained in all aspects of this activity, and the remaining limb should be examined by a health-care professional at frequent and regular intervals.

Gait patterns

Often older persons develop peculiar gait patterns that can become incapacitating. The existence of these gait anomalies has long been recognized and repeatedly studied.[12,46] A pathologic gait creates difficulty in walking and climbing stairs and can result in serious accidents. An abnormal gait, which is characterized by a decrease in motor power and unsteadiness, is often erroneously referred to as senile paraplegia.

Critchely[11] classified gait disorders according to the site of the CNS or skeletal system involvement as follows: (1) cortical, (2) subcortical, (3) spinal, and (4) muscular. Another classification was recommended earlier by Lhermitte,[35] a French investigator. The etiology of gait disorders among geriatric patients could be further defined in terms of decline in functions and conditions that mark the physiology of the older person.

Senile gait disorders are likely to escape the examiner's attention during the course of a routine clinical examination. On examination in the customary sitting or reclining position, certain older patients show little if any diminution of muscle strength. However, when the patient's gait is tested, obvious changes can be observed. When these people begin walking, they look frantically for support and take short, shuffling steps; frequently after a few such steps their knees buckle. This gait pattern was referred to by nineteenth century French clinicians as l'astasie trepidante and is sometimes called Petren's gait.[44]

If the errant gait remains uncorrected, as it frequently does, the patient gravitates to bed, with all of its attendant ill effects. Bracing is ineffective and often aggravates the problem. Treatment consists of strengthening of the muscles impaired by disuse atrophy, the liberation of joints restricted by fibrous ankylosis, and as much amelioration of the poor gait pattern as possible. Individual elements of gait, standing stance, and swing phase must be practiced separately and then fused into the best rhythmic motion possible for the patient being treated. Personal supervision and constant encouragement by the therapist are essential.

Chronic pain

Pain is a universal suffering of humans, and an enormous amount of money is spent to cure or control it. Pain is also closely identified with aging. A young person who experiences dull and ill-defined joint pain or muscle ache commonly says, "I must be getting old." Whether the higher incidence of pain among the elderly is myth or fact, it requires serious attention because pain not only is a physical discomfort and disabling, but may be followed by secondary joint contracture and other undesirable effects, as well as emotional depression.

Pain is classified into three groups: acute, chronic, and malignant.[13] Acute pain is characterized by a sudden or progressive increase in intensity (which is usually very high) for a relatively short period, rapid abatement with appropriate treatment, and a predictable prognosis. The prognosis for alleviation of acute pain is usually good. Acute pain, which is always disabling during its existence, can be caused by trauma or an acute inflammatory condition, including an infectious process.[25]

Chronic pain is an ill-defined condition. It may follow acute pain or have a slow and gradual onset over a period of time. Its intensity is usually less severe than that of acute pain but may fluctuate, even within a day. It is often described as dull, annoying, or aching. Chronic pain may subside with or without treatment but may recur without any apparent cause, in which case it is called recurrent chronic pain. The cause is not always identifiable. Even when the cause is apparent, there may be little correlation between the magnitude of the cause and the chronicity and severity of the pain. The prognosis for treatment of chronic pain is generally poor. Chronicity sometimes follows an acute pain episode. Usually, as the acute phase subsides completely, a dull aching pain persists or occurs intermittently in the same anatomic location. Some examples include posttraumatic conditions such as fracture, joint sprain, or a spinal disc disorder.

Pain is frequently associated with malignant tumor, and its intensity and location depend greatly on the organ involved. Although this type of pain often requires strong analgesics such as morphine or codeine, the goal of management is the development of a pain-free state without impairment of mental faculty.

Chronic pain is the type that most often affects the aged population. Cervical radiculopathy from osteoarthritic changes, low back pain from degenerative disc disease, and arthralgia from osteoarthritis and osteoporosis are common etiologic factors. Although the pain may not be extremely severe, its presence may decrease physical activity, cause excessive fatigue, and disturb sleep. As a result, the persistence of chronic pain can induce moderate to severe depression. One should not interpret too literally the comment "I have pain all the time and have gotten used to it" from an elderly patient. No matter how often one suffers from pain, each episode is fresh and produces great discomfort. The patient's remarks may in fact be an expression of resignation, hopelessness, and helplessness that are part of an underlying depression. The depressed emotional status and pain may force the individual into self-imposed inactivity or immobilization, thus beginning a vicious cycle.

Chronic pain should not be dismissed as a routine complaint of the elderly. The anatomic cause should be studied first, but the investigative methods should if possible be limited to noninvasive diagnostic procedures. Regrettably, clinical examinations and tests do not always reveal convincing evidence of the pain-causing condition. Tolerance to pain differs greatly from one individual to another, and psychosocial factors influence the perception of pain. Therefore, in the absence of conclusive anatomic changes, it is not appropriate to conclude that the individual is malingering or hysterical. Crue's definition of pain, "anything a patient said it is,"[13] is an appropriate and important concept in the interpretation of an elderly patient's complaints of chronic pain.

A fundamental principle in the management of chronic pain, particularly among the elderly, is the maintenance of a conservative approach. The results of surgical intervention for chronic pain in any age group are not convincing. General anesthesia, postsurgical immobilization, and prolonged postoperative physical inactivity often cause irreversible ill effects in the elderly. The surgical approach therefore should be a last choice in treatment, especially for the elderly. Often the realistic goal of chronic pain management is not to eliminate pain but to make it tolerable. Rather than addictive analgesics, mild analgesics or sedatives often prove effective and may be taken in conjunction with a physical therapy regimen.

Various physical therapy modalities such as general conditioning exercises, range-of-motion exercises, traction, heat or cryotherapy, and ultrasound treatment should be used as intensively and for as long as required. Many modalities can be self-administered, but precise instructions concerning the frequency, intensity, and methods must be provided to the patient. In some instances the patient should be referred to a psychologist or social worker for assistance with the developing coping mechanisms.

It is important for the elderly to comprehend the cause and mechanism of chronic pain and the goal of the treatment regimen. The patient must know that any treatment prescribed for chronic pain may not totally eliminate the distress and some pain is inevitable. If the treatment assists the patient in maintaining a level of activities of daily living and a healthy emotional status, a certain definitive measure of success has been achieved.

Preventive rehabilitation

The susceptibility of the aged to disability is discussed in detail earlier in the chapter. No matter how temporary it may be, the onset of a disability is a grave experience for a person of any age, resulting not only in loss of productivity but in inconvenience in all physical activities as well and necessitating dependency on another person for assistance in performing even simple tasks. When a seemingly temporal disability affects an older person, it may create secondary disabilities with serious consequences. Even if an elderly disabled person recovers completely from a disability, the restorative process is much slower than for a younger individual. Therefore the importance of prevention of disability is more acute for the elderly population than for their younger counterparts.

Disability may be classified into two categories: primary and secondary. Primary disability is the direct consequence of an illness or trauma such as hemiplegia following cerebral artery thrombosis or hemorrhage, or inability to ambulate after fracture of the neck of the femur owing to a fall. Secondary disability is absent at the onset of the primary disability but gradually develops and is as disabling as the primary type.[50] Examples of secondary disability are joint contracture, disuse atrophy of muscles, osteoporosis, and decubitus ulcer.

Primary disability

The prevention of primary disabilities involves the elderly themselves, as well as people who provide services to them. Elderly individuals should visit a physician at least annually to detect early signs of the various age-related diseases that are the potential causes of primary disability. Those who have such a disease must have regular checkups to ensure proper maintenance of the condition. For example, uncontrolled hypertension or diabetes mellitus is a potential cause of severe disability.

The primary care physician must remain vigilant in the prevention of disability. A careful history should include inquiry about any symptom the patient has noticed lately, food and fluid intake, emotional status, housing conditions, composition of the household, and other socioeconomic information including the presence or absence of a support system and the degree of adherence to any medication regimen.

The physical examination should include not only the routine items but also vision, hearing, peripheral blood circulation, skin sensation, foot hygiene, and gait. Counseling the elderly patient is as important as the early diagnosis and proper treatment of various illnesses as a means of prevention. Physicians and nurses are the most appropriate professionals to provide such counseling.

Although compliance with the prescribed medication regimen is essential in controlling the disability causing the disease, the prescription alone is not enough. A physician or nurse should explain the reason for and the purpose of a medication, as well as the possible result of noncompliance, without causing undue anxiety. The explanation must be in language the patient can easily understand.

Counseling and guidance must be as concrete and precise as possible, avoiding vague statements, generalizations, or implications. For example, a person who is currently or will be taking hypotensive drugs, sedatives, or hypoglycemic agents should be warned about the possibility of experiencing dizziness or loss of balance. However, since elderly people frequently need a more detailed explanation, it would be preferable to state that an elderly person taking such medication may experience dizziness when the body position is changed from a supine or sitting position to an upright standing position. In anticipation of the onset of dizziness, such individuals should hold onto the arm of a chair or the mattress of a bed as they stand up. When they are sufficiently balanced in an upright standing position and experience no dizziness, they should proceed to walk. When an elderly person is ascending or descending a staircase, one hand should always be on the handrail; the person should never go up or down the staircase carrying an object with both hands. An elderly person should not use a stepladder placed in the middle of a room, since a loss of balance makes a fall inevitable. These are examples of instructions that are specific enough for the elderly to remember and follow.

The patient should be instructed to eliminate hazardous conditions in the place of residence. Tidy housekeeping is the first step to the creation of safe living conditions. Adequate room lighting is frequently overlooked. For example, a visually impaired elderly person may want to go to the bathroom at night. Since the patient may have taken a sedative before retiring, it is possible that he or she may be slightly confused upon awakening. In this case a nightlight may represent a simple but efficient means of providing safe living quarters. Only conscientious, deliberate, and concerted efforts by the elderly and those who provide care or assistance to them can create such an environment.

With regard to osteoporosis and falls that cause hip fracture among elderly women, there has been a renewed interest recently in the prevention of the metabolic disturbances that give rise to osteoporosis. The main focus of these efforts is on increasing calcium intake in the form of supplemental calcium tablets or adjustments in the diet. However, merely increasing calcium intake is not sufficient to prevent osteoporosis. Therefore treatment combines diet and appropriate exercises.

Immobilization or the absence of mechanical stress to the skeletal system can cause demineralization.[29,36,58] The ill effects of physical inactivity, one of the characteristics of elderly people, lead to deconditioning, as previously mentioned. In some respects it may be more important for the elderly to lead a physically active life than for the younger population.

Since osteoporosis among women seems to begin during the menopausal years, preventive measures should be started long before the onset of the condition. Since osteoporosis is a slow, progressive condition, the effects of any preventive methods must be assessed through decades of careful follow-up studies.

A fall is a sudden unplanned displacement of an individual's center of gravity from a higher to a lower level. At its end the body usually rests on the ground or floor in a stationary position. A loss of balance does not necessarily result in a fall. Those who have good body coordination, such as professional athletes, can regain body balance without falling.

A fracture is not the inevitable result of a fall. An infant may fall dozens of times a day without any appreciable injury because of the child's low center of gravity and flexible bones. On the other hand, a fall by an elderly person may result in a fracture because the center of gravity is high and the bones of both sexes are osteoporotic in varying degrees.

The elderly woman of the 1980s was born before 1910, a time when female athletes were unheard of and physical education courses for female students were uncommon. The women of that era were expected to be relatively sedentary. Without physical education classes or athletic training, they could not easily develop good balance or physical coordination, making this age group highly susceptible to falls.

Young women of today are far more physically active in their daily lives than their elder counterparts. Many of them engage in competitive sports, leading one to speculate that as those women age there will be a decline in their susceptibility to falls. Women now in their forties and fifties should be encouraged to continue their physical activities into their golden years.

Secondary disability

The prevention of a secondary disability is a major responsibility of the rehabilitation team. Before the era of surgical reduction of hip fracture, the mortality of hip fracture patients was high because prolonged immobilization resulted in the development of venous thrombosis, hypostatic pneumonia, and decubitus ulcer. The elderly are known to have osteoporosis without such episodes, but when immobilization or prolonged bed rest is imposed, the process of demineralization is accelerated. Prolonged physical inactivity owing to immobilization or bed rest not only results in situational depression, but somehow favors the development of confusion and senility. In view of this multitude of ill effects, the duration of physical inactivity for the elderly must be absolutely minimal.

Contracture is another frequently observed secondary disability. Among the causes of contracture among primary disability victims are imbalance between the agonist and antagonist muscles, positioning, and pain. An imbalance between the agonist and antagonist muscles may be due to one being flaccid or spastic, as in the case of hemiplegia, or to loss of insertion of one of the antagonists, frequently found among above-knee amputees. Flexion contracture is more often observed than extension contracture. Since the nature of the primary disability dictates the type and location of contracture that develops, all necessary prophylactic measures such as muscle-strengthening exercise, passive rangeof-motion exercises, resting splints, proper positioning, and control of pain must be instituted at the onset of the primary disability and continued as long as necessary.

Another preventable but sometimes fatal secondary disability is decubitus ulcer. Host factors for decubiti include the following:

1. Neurosensory deficiency
   a. Central
   b. Peripheral
2. Nutritional deficiency
   a. Diminished subcutaneous fat tissue
   b. Hypoproteinemia
   c. Ascorbic acid deficiency
3. Gerontologic process
   a. Localized endogenous oligemia
   b. Loss of skin elasticity
4. Immobilization
5. Incontinence
6. Lack of health education

Among these host characteristics, nutritional deficiency should be detected as early as possible and a high-protein diet, supplemental vitamin C intake, and treatment of anemia should be provided. In general, the food intake of the elderly is far less than that of younger people. In addition, if an elderly person is suffering from an organic mental syndrome or depression or is on prolonged bed rest, the appetite may decrease further. Mild psychotropic medication and out-of-bed exercise may be helpful in restoring the desire for food.

When self-imposed immobilization or bed rest is observed, its cause should be investigated, and depending on the reason, counseling by a psychologist or social worker, psychotropic medication, or analgesics may be necessary to encourage the patient to get out of bed and resume activities.

If a clinical examination and tests indicate that the patient is in the high-risk population for developing decubiti, a decubitus precaution regimen should be established. This program, aside from the nutritional treatment mentioned previously, consists of psychologic or psychiatric intervention, control of pain, minimization of the bedfast period, special skin care (lubrication and massage of the vulnerable part of the body), and frequent change of body position in bed or a wheelchair. Skin care should be initiated while the skin area still maintains its integrity rather than after erythema or a grade I decubitus ulcer is in evidence.

Although control of host characteristics is sometimes difficult, agent and environmental factors are more readily controlled.

Agent factors include the following:

1. Mechanical force
   a. Gravitational pull
   b. Shearing force
   c. Counterforce (structural resistance)
2. Time element
   a. Duration
   b. Frequency

Mechanical force is the main agent factor. Although gravitational pull cannot be eliminated, the counterforce is controllable. The concentration of pressure on the bony prominence can be avoided by using a mattress that decreases the counterforce and lessening the amount of concentrated pressure by distributing body weight over a wider weightbearing surface. The concentration of pressure is also decreased by elimination of creases in the bedding material. Shearing force may be created when nurses crank up the head portion of the bed, transfer the patient into or out of bed, or suddenly change the patient's body position during morning or afternoon care. All these maneuvers must be performed slowly and gently. Frequent change of body position is a general measure of considerable importance.

Environmental factors include the following:

1. Humidity
2. Ventilation
3. Temperature
4. Contamination
   a. Chemical
   b. Microbiologic
5. Immobilization

Immobilization of the body in one position in bed or in a wheelchair for a long period and contamination of the skin area by urine or feces predispose the patient to decubiti. These factors can be eliminated or minimized by meticulous cleanliness and frequent change of body position. The interrelation among various causative factors that ultimately results in the development of a decubitus ulcer is shown in Figure 29-3. Once the causative factors and the mechanism of evolution of the decubitus ulcer are identified, various preventive methods can be developed.

Secondary disabilities are often more disabling than primary ones. Once they begin to develop, it takes a long period of expensive intervention to reverse the process. Thus an energetic effort must be made to prevent the development of secondary disabilities.

Although acceptance of the concept of preventive rehabilitation[27] is relatively new, it has been a daily practice of the rehabilitation team for a long time. For example, although passive exercises are often used to increase the range of joint movement, they also prevent contracture. Although progressive resistive exercises are intended primarily to increase muscle strength, such exercises also prevent disuse atrophy of the muscles.

Preventive rehabilitation should not be confined to a rehabilitation setting but must be practiced in the community. Although preventive rehabilitation in an acute rehabilitation service and a skilled nursing facility focuses on the prevention of secondary disabilities, preventive rehabilitation in the community must address the prevention of primary and secondary disabilities.

Not every disabled geriatric patient can return to the community, but some are fortunate enough to pursue as normal a life as possible within their physical capabilities in their own environment. These patients should be followed up through appropriate community home health care services, outpatient clinics, caregivers, family members, friends, and home health aides, who must be trained in various exercise programs and the use of various devices for the prevention of secondary disabilities.

The occurrence of one primary disability does not confer an immunity to the onset of another one. For example, geriatric hemiplegic patients have a tendency to fall and may incur a hip fracture. A preventive action to avoid this additional primary disability with its added poor prognosis may be attained by training such patients in falling techniques to minimize the possibility of serious trauma. As another example, geriatric patients with a unilateral below-knee amputation necessitated by peripheral vascular insufficiency or diabetes mellitus are at high risk for losing the other lower limb. In general, geriatric unilateral below-knee amputees who are properly fitted with a prosthesis can be very functional in activities of daily living. However, a bilateral amputation seriously reduces this capacity. Preventive care requires meticulous foot hygiene and regularly scheduled professional examinations to determine the need

for more aggressive treatment or for reconstructive surgery of the arterial blood supply.

Rehabilitation medicine has always focused on the geriatric population. However, the continued improvements in acute medical care and the remarkably increased longevity of humans during the past 30 years place the application of rehabilitation concepts and techniques for the elderly into a position of great prominence and priority.

REFERENCES

1. Barberi, EB: Patient falls are not patient accidents, J Gerontol Nurs 9:165, 1983.
2. Bauer, RL, et al: Risk of postmenopausal hip fracture in Mexican American women, Am J Public Health 76:1020, 1986.
3. Berecek, KH: Etilogy of decubitus ulcers, Nurs Clin North Am 10:157, 1975.
4. Bliss, MR, McLaren, R, and Exton-Smith, AN: Preventing pressure sores in hospital: controlled trial of large celled ripple mattress, Br Med J 1:394, 1967.
5. Bollet, AJ, Engh, G, and Parson, W: Epidemiology of osteoporosis: sex and race incidence of hip fracture, Arch Intern Med 116:191, 1965.
6. Boston, AG, et al: Ergometry modification for combined arm-leg use by lower extremity amputees in cardiovascular testing and training, Arch Phys Med Rehabil 68:244, 1987.
7. Bruce, RA: Principle of exercise testing. In Naughton, J, and Hellerstein, H.K, editors: Exercise testing and training in coronary heart disease, New York, 1973, Academic Press, Inc.
8. Butler, RN: Introduction. In Haynes, SG, and Feinleib, M, editors: Second Conference on the Epidemiology of Aging, Washington, DC, 1980, NIH Pub No 80-968, Dept of Health and Human Services.
9. Caird, FI, and Kennedy, RD: Epidemiology of heart disease in old age. In Caird, FI, Dall, LC, and Kennedy, RD, editors: Cardiology in old age, New York, 1976, Plenum Press.
10. Christodoulou, NA, and Dretakis, EK: Significance of muscular disturbances in the localization of fractures of the proximal femur, Clin Orthop 187:215, 1984.
11. Critchley, M: On senile disorders of gait, including the so called "senile paraplegia," Geriatrics 3:364, 1948.
12. Critchley, M: Neurologic changes in the aged, J Chron Dis 3:459, 1956.
13. Crue, BL, et al: Observations on the taxonomy problem in pain. In Crue, BL, editor: Chronic pain—further observation from City of Hope, New York, 1979, Spectrum Publications.
14. Farmer, ME, et al: Race and sex difference in hip fracture incidence, Am J Public Health 74:1374, 1984.
15. Gallagher, JC, Melton, LJ, and Riggs, BL: Examination of prevalence rates of possible risk factors in a population with a fracture of the proximal femur, Clin Orthop 153:158, 1980.
16. Garraway, WM, et al: The declining evidence of stroke, N Engl J Med 300:449, 1979.
17. Gross, CR, et al: Stroke in South Alabama: incidence and diagnostic feature—a population base study, Stroke 15:249, 1984.
18. Hedlund, R, and Lindgrew, U: Trauma type, age and gender as determinants of hip fracture, J Orthop Res 5:242, 1987.
19. Hodge, WA, et al: Contact pressures in the human hip joint measured in vivo, Proc Natl Acad Sci USA 83:2879, 1986.
20. Hodgson, JL, and Buskirk, ER: Physical fitness and age, with emphasis on cardiovascular function in the elderly, J Am Geriat Soc 25:385, 1977.
21. Holmes, EF, Lee, M, and Fleming, WL: Long-term illness and the effect of the aging process on health. In Leavell, HR, and Clark, EG, editors: Preventive medicine for the doctor in his community, ed 3, New York, 1965, McGraw-Hill Book Co.

22. Hooper, G: Internal fixation of fractures of the neck of the femur in hemiplegic patients, Injury 10:281, 1979.

23. Itoh, M, and Dasco, MM: Rehabilitation of patients with hip fracture: a clinical study of 126 cases, Postgrad Med 28:134, 1960.

24. Itoh, M, and Lee, MHM: The future role of rehabilitation medicine in community health, Med Clin North Am 53:719, 1969.

25. Itoh, M, and Lee, M: Epidemiology of pain, Bull Los Angeles Neuro Soc 44:14, 1979.

26. Itoh, M, and Lee, MHM: Rehabilitation for the aged. In Jackson, O, editor: Physical therapy of geriatric patient, New York, 1983, Churchill-Livingstone, Inc.

27. Itoh, M, and Lee, MHM: The epidemiology of disability as related to rehabilitation medicine. In Kottke, FJ, Stillwell, GK, and Lehmann, JF, editors: Handbook of physical medicine and rehabilitation, ed 3, Philadelphia, 1986, WB Saunders Co.

28. Johnell, O, et al: Age and sex patterns of hip fractures—changes in 30 years, Acta Orthop Scand 55:290, 1984.

29. Kazasian, LE, and Von Gierker, HE: Bone loss as a result of immobilization and chelation: preliminary results in *Macaca mulatta*, Clin Orthop 65:67, 1969.

30. Keltz, H: Pulmonary function and disease in the aging. In William, TF, editor: Rehabilitation in the aged, New York, 1984, Raven Press.

31. Kotila, M: Declining incidence and mortality of stroke? Stroke 15:255-259, 1984.

32. Kumar, VN, and Redford, JB: Rehabilitation of hip fractures in the elderly, Am Fam Phys 29:173, 1984.

33. Lee, MHM, and Itoh, M: Rehabilitation of the elderly stroke patient, Mediguide 1:1, 1984.

34. Lewin, R: Pressure measured in live hip joint, Science 232:1192, 1986.

35. Lhermitte, J: Etude sur la paraplegies des vieillard, Paris, 1907, Maretheux: La myosclérose rétractile des vieillards et ses syndromes acintéo-hypertoniques, Encephale 23:89, 1928.

36. Lutwak, L.: Chemical analysis of diet, urine, feces and sweat parameters related to the calcium and nitrogen balance studies during Gemini VII flight (Exp M7), Washington, DC, NASA Contractor Report, 1966, NAS9-5375.

37. Master, AM, and Oppenheimer, ER: A simple exercise tolerance test for circulatory efficiency with standard tables for normal individuals, Am J Med Sci 177:223, 1929.

38. Michocki, RJ, and Lamy, PP: The problem of pressure scores in a nursing home situation: statistic data, J Am Geriatr Soc 24:323, 1976.

39. Miettinen, TA, et al: Multifactorial primary prevention of cardiovascular disease in middle-aged men: risk factor changes, incidence and mortality, JAMA 254:2097, 1985.

40. Moldawer, M, Zimmerman, SJ, and Collins, LS: Incidence of osteoporosis in elderly whites and elderly Negroes, JAMA 194:859, 1965.

41. Montoye, HJ, Willis, PW, and Cunningham, DA: Heart rate response to submaximum exercise: relation to age and sex, J Gerontol 23:127, 1968.

42. Mulley, G, and Espley, AJ: Hip fracture after hemiplegia, Postgrad Med J 55:264, 1979.

43. Pakarinen, S: Incidence, aetiology and prognosis of primary subarachnoid hemorrhage, Acta Neurol Scand 43(suppl 29):1, 1967.

44. Petrén, K: Ueber den Zusammenhangzwischen anatomischbedingten und functionelen Ganstorung im Greisenalter, Arch Psychol 33:818; 34:444, 1900.

45. Poplingher, AR, and Pillar, T: Hip fracture in stroke patients: epidemiology and rehabilitation, Acta Orthop Scand 56:226, 1985.

46. Ross, AT: Some neurologic causes for difficulty in walking, Postgrad Med 15:40, 1954.

47. Rudd, TN: The pathogenesis of decubitus ulcers, J Am Geriat Soc 10:48, 1962.

48. Rusk, HA, and Hilleboe, HE: Rehabilitation. In Hilleboe, HE, and Larimore, GW, editors: Preventive medicine, Philadelphia, 1965, WB Saunders Co.

49. Rusk, HA, et al: Hospital patient survey, New York, 1956, Goldwater Memorial Hospital.

50. Ryder, CF, and Daitz, B: Prevention of disability. In Selle, WA, editor: Restorative medicine in geriatrics, Springfield, Ill, 1963, Charles C Thomas, Publisher.

51. Sheffield, LT, Roitman, D, and Reeves, TJ: Submaximum exercise testing, J South Carolina Med Assoc 65:18, 1969.

52. Shock, NW: Aging—some social and biological aspects, Pub No 65, Washington, DC, 1960, American Association for the Advancement of Science.

53. Skinner, JS: The cardiovascular system with aging and exercise. In Brunner, D, and Jokl, E, editors: Physical activity and aging, Baltimore, 1970, University Press, Inc.

54. Startwell, PE, and Last, JM: Epidemiology. In Last, JM, editor: Public health and preventive medicine, New York, 1980, Appleton-Century-Crofts.

55. Strehler, BL, editor: The biology of aging, Pub No 6, Washington, DC, 1960, American Institute for Biological Science.

56. Strehler, BL: Time, cells and aging, ed 2, New York, 1977, Academic Press, Inc.

57. Wegner, NK: Cardiovascular status: changes with aging. In Williams, TF, editor: Rehabilitation in the aging, New York, 1984, Raven Press.

58. Whedon, CD, Lutwak, L, and Neuman, W: Calcium and nitrogen balance: in a review of medical results of Gemini VII and related flights, J.F.K. Space Center, F. 1967, NASA SP-121.

CHAPTER 30

Pediatric rehabilitation

CYNTHIA L. SMITH

Pediatric rehabilitation is concerned primarily with the management of pediatric disorders, both congenital and acquired, in which a major characteristic is some type of functional loss—neuromuscular, musculoskeletal, or orthopedic. Thus knowledge of pediatrics is needed as well as the principles of rehabilitation medicine. The practitioner must be able to accurately assess a child's organic illness, any associated disorders and functional deficits stemming from the illness, and the impact on the child and family. All findings are related to the normal growth and development and expected behavior at the child's age level from birth to adulthood.

This chapter outlines the key aspects of the pediatric rehabilitative assessment, the hallmarks of normal growth and development, and the basic features and management of specific disorders often treated by pediatric physiatrists.

PEDIATRIC REHABILITATIVE ASSESSMENT
History

The history should be taken in a relaxed, comfortable, and objective, nonjudgmental fashion. The first aspect covered is the gestation and birth of the patient because many pediatric disorders have their roots in the prenatal or perinatal period. This should include length and character of gestation; illnesses, complication, and medications during gestation; history of prior gestations; labor and method of delivery; birth weight; and recollection of the child's neonatal behavior.

The second aspect of the history involves development, including gross motor, fine motor, language, and social milestones. Attempts should be made to differentiate slowed progress from regression of milestones. Also at this point a functional inventory should be obtained, outlining what the child is able and unable to do and what compensations have been made by the child or the family to improve function.

The third aspect of the history is the diagnostic and interventional history, that is, what diagnostic steps have already been taken and what therapeutic interventions have been or are being tried (therapies, medications, surgery, orthoses, equipment, and so forth). To pinpoint specific medical problems, the child's general health and nutritional status should be ascertained by general review of systems.

If the child is of school age, a scholastic history should be obtained, including school, grade, and performance.

Finally, a detailed family history is obtained to determine the presence of any familial pattern to the disability or illness.

Physical examination

Examination must take into account the child's developmental stage. Observations made in taking the history can give a wealth of information before the actual examination. Specifically, activity level and method of interacting with parent and the environment can be delineated.

Parents should be allowed to undress younger children and hold or be near them for most of the examination. Parents can also be instrumental in getting a young child to demonstrate gross motor skills such as creeping, crawling, or walking.

A period of interactive play between the child and examiner may give information on vision, hearing, and most cranial nerves. This "play" period permits inspection and palpation of body parts and some fine motor evaluation.

After fine and gross motor skills are tested, range of motion, tone, and reflex testing should be done. The examination culminates with procedures involving instruments, including evaluation of sensation and use of the stethoscope, blood pressure cuff, oto-ophthalmoscope, and tongue blade.

For older children, unless extreme modesty demands that they undress alone, observation of dressing skills gives some information about ability to perform activities of daily living and perceptual motor abilities.

The following specific areas of investigation should be noted:

1. Serial height, weight, and head circumference should be recorded and charted to compare with age-equivalent percentiles. Chronologic age may be corrected for gestational age in premature infants during the first year of life.
2. Notations should be made of any dysmorphic features, including epicanthal folds, low-set ears, unusual facial features, and abnormalities of fingers or toes.
3. Any asymmetries or length discrepancies of the extremities should be noted.
4. The spine should be inspected for curvature indicative of excessive kyphosis, lordosis, or scoliosis.
5. The skin may give information about possible phakomatoses, abnormal weight bearing, and even child neglect or abuse.
6. Joints should be examined for signs of inflammation, effusion, or contracture.
7. Organ examinations should include the lungs, heart, and abdomen.
8. The neuromuscular examination should outline tone, reflexes, active and passive range of motion, strength and coordination, abnormal movement patterns, and the child's motor development skills.
9. The sensory examination in young children may be limited to touch or pinprick testing. One should be cautious not to interpret reflex withdrawal as volitional response. The face should reflect a volitional response to a noxious stimulus.
10. Suspicion of a hearing or visual deficit, including strabismus, should prompt a referral to a specialist for further evaluation.

Diagnosis and plan of care

With full history and physical data in hand, a diagnostic impression and habilitative or rehabilitative plan are formulated and discussed with the parent and patient in language that each understands. An outline of further diagnostic testing is also given at this time, including any referral for full psychologic and developmental testing.

Almost uniformly, the next concern of parents is the prognosis. With neither undue pessimism nor optimism, prognostic information should be conveyed as completely as general knowledge of the disability allows. Short-term goals include preventing secondary complications such as contracture, scoliosis, and skin problems and encouraging positive developmental achievements. Long-term goals are the achievement of emotional maturity, self-reliance, and self-esteem. Both strengths and deficits of the child are addressed. Parents more easily accept the many uncertainties that accompany some disabilities if they are presented with

a complete therapeutic plan designed to help the child achieve optimal functioning.

At this critical point the partnership between the physician and parent begins. Although over the course of a child's rehabilitation the physiatrist is the major coordinator of the multidisciplinary team, he or she should also function to assist parents in achieving good parent skills, which are frequently difficult to develop with a disabled child, in learning to act as an advocate for the child, and in coping with the often unwieldy medical and educational systems. Valuable assistance for the parents can also be found in support groups and systems when indicated. Overall, the therapeutic plan should be designed to cause the least stress for the family unit, with flexibility exercised in regard to work schedules of parents, child-care schedules, home-based program options, and hospital-based needs. In this way the plan will receive optimal compliance and participation and achieve maximal results.

Normal growth and development

The ability to identify abnormalities of growth and development requires a working knowledge of their normal course. The following are growth parameters that may be considered in the evaluation of a child:

1. A newborn is expected to double in weight by 5 months of age and triple in weight by 1 year.
2. Height increases by 50% within the first year. Twice the body length at 2 years is taken as an estimate of eventual adult height.
3. Children tend to grow more over the summer months and especially during puberty.
4. Growth generally ceases 2 years after menarche in girls.

These factors have practical applications; for example, fitting new prostheses and orthoses in the fall ensures longer wear. In dealing with scoliosis, monitoring must be frequent, preferably every 3 months, during periods of rapid growth. Certain orthopedic procedures involving bone, such as triple arthrodesis, should be delayed until bony maturation has occurred.

Weight should be monitored from birth and related to gestational age. Although birth weight of 2500 g or less is considered low, determination should be made whether the child is truly small for gestational age (SGA) or actually premature and therefore appropriate for gestational age. This determination, which helps in diagnosis and prognosis, is based on obstetric history (estimation of dates) and newborn neurologic examination, usually using the Dubowitz scale for scoring.[22] SGA infants are at risk for congenital anomalies and may also have a history of congenital viral infection, usually toxoplasmosis, cytomegalovirus disease, rubella, herpes, or syphilis. Premature infants, on the other hand, are at risk for anoxic or hemorrhagic central nervous system damage.

The head circumference reflects the growth of the brain.

It should be routinely monitored until 2 years of age; in cases of abnormality, this monitoring should continue until a normal pattern is reached. Serial measurements should follow percentiles for growth similar to those on standardized charts. A "crossing" of percentile lines, either accelerated or decelerated in pattern, is cause for concern. Deceleration may signal defective brain development or even premature closure of the cranial sutures. Rapid acceleration may signal hydrocephalus or a mass lesion. All these conditions require investigation and intervention when indicated. Hydrocephalus is most often associated with tumor, spina bifida, intracranial hemorrhage, or infection. Microcephaly often follows anoxic encephalopathy.

Development refers to the acquisition and refinement of skills. It involves both the maturation of the central nervous system and the processing of experiential information. Based on the work of Gesell and Amatruda, the development of children is usually examined in the following four major categories and compared with age-matched controls[43]:

1. The gross motor area includes preambulatory, ambulatory, and higher-level physical activities.
2. Fine motor and adaptive behavior includes prehension, manipulation, and sensorimotor integration that contribute to daily living skills.
3. Language behavior includes both receptive and expressive communications.
4. Personal social behavior refers to the acquisition of societal and cultural behavioral standards.

Developmental screening tests, the most widely accepted of which is the Denver Developmental Screening Test, are used to select children who are below expected norms and require more in-depth evaluation.[26]

Delays in specific areas give clues to aid further diagnostic evaluations. Isolated delays in gross and fine motor abilities may be based on neuromuscular dysfunction, whereas language delay has been found to be the best predictor of cognitive impairment. Obviously, exceptions to these general rules exist. An example is the expressive language delay often seen with athetoid cerebral palsy or spastic cerebral palsy with associated pseudobulbar palsy from bilateral cortical damage. This delay may not reflect true cognitive function level.

Isolated language delays may also indicate a hearing impairment or early infantile autism. Recently Capute, Shapiro, and Palmer[14] devised an excellent language screening tool, the Clinical Linguistic and Auditory Milestone Scale (CLAMS), for office screening of children from birth to 36 months. This scale is standardized for both receptive and expressive milestones and correlates well with infant development scales such as the Bayley Scales, which tend to focus on visual motor abilities.[4]

In general, the newborn's behavior is governed by primitive reflex activity because the central nervous system is immature. A sequential process of maturation occurs. Motor development moves in a cephalocaudal direction as primitive infantile reflexes are suppressed and replaced by pos-

Table 30-1. Infantile reflex development

Reflex	Stimulus	Response	Time of suppression or emergence	Clinical significance
Primitive reflexes: present at birth, suppressed with maturation				
Asymmetric tonic neck	Head turning or tilting to side	Extension of extremities on the chin side, flexion on occiput side	Suppressed by 6-7 months	Obligatory abnormal at any age; persistent suspicious of CNS pathology
Symmetric tonic neck	Neck flexion	Arm flexion, leg extension	Suppressed by 6-7 months	Obligatory abnormal at any age; persistent suspicious of CNS pathology
	Neck extension	Arm extension, leg flexion		
Moro	Sudden neck extension	Arm extension abduction followed by flexion-adduction	Suppressed by 4-6 months	Abnormal if persists
Tonic labyrinthine	Head position in space, strongest at 45° angle to horizonal		Suppressed by 4-6 months	Abnormal at any age if hyperactive or if persistent
	Supine	Predominant extensor tone		
	Prone	Predominant flexor tone		

Data compiled from various sources (references 5, 8, 14, 22, 37, 39, 54, 55, 59, 64, 66, 76, and 77). From Molnar, G, and Kaminer, R: Growth and development. In Molnar, G, editor: Pediatric rehabilitation, Baltimore, 1985, Williams & Wilkins Co. *Continued.*

Table 30-1, cont'd. Infantile reflex development

Reflex	Stimulus	Response	Time of suppression or emergence	Clinical significance
Positive supporting	Tactile contact and weight bearing on sole	Leg extension for supporting partial body weight	Suppressed by 3-7 months and replaced by volitional standing	Abnormal at any age if obligatory or hyperactive; suggests spasticity of legs
Rooting	Stroking the corner of mouth, upper or lower lip	Moving tongue, mouth, and head toward site of stimulus	Suppressed by 4 months	Searching for nipple; diminished in CNS depression; obligatory persistence may be immature CNS development
Palmar grasp	Pressure or touch on palm, stretch of finger flexors	Flexion of finger	Suppressed by 5-6 months	Diminished in CNS depression; absent in lower motor neuron paralysis; persistence suggests spasticity, i.e., cerebral palsy
Plantar grasp	Pressure on sole just distal to metatarsal heads	Flexion of toes	Suppressed by 12-18 months	Absent in lower motor neuron paralysis; persists and hyperactive in spasticity, i.e., cerebral palsy
Automatic neonatal walking	Contact of sole in vertical position tilting the body forward and from side to side	Automatic alternating steps	Suppressed by 3-4 months	Variable activity in normal infants; absent in lower motor neuron paralysis of legs
Placing	Tactile contact on dorsum of foot or hand	Flexion to place leg or arm over obstacle	Suppressed before end of first year	Absent in lower motor neuron paralysis or extensor spasticity of legs

Physiologic postural responses: emerge with maturation, present throughout life, modulated by volition

Reflex	Stimulus	Response	Time of suppression or emergence	Clinical significance
Head righting	Visual and vestibular	Align face vertical mouth horizontal Prone Supine	Emerge at 2 months 3-4 months	Delayed or absent in CNS immaturity or damage or motor unit disease
Body, head righting	Tactile proprioceptive vestibular	Align body parts	Emerge from 4-6 months	Delayed or absent in CNS immaturity or damage or motor neuron disease
Protective extension or propping	Displacement of center of gravity outside of supporting surface	Extension-abduction of extremity toward side of displacement to prevent falling	Emerge between 5-12 months	Delayed or absent in CNS immaturity or damage or motor unit disease
Equilibrium or tilting	Displacement of center of gravity	Adjustment of tone and trunk posture to maintain balance	Emerge between 6-14 months	Delayed or absent in CNS immaturity or damage or motor unit disease

Table 30-2. Milestones in child development

Age	Gross motor	Fine motor adaptive	Personal-social	Speech and language	Cognitive	Emotional
Newborn	Flexor tone predominates; in prone position, turns head to side; automatic reflex walking; rounded spine when held sitting	Hands fisted; grasp reflex; state-dependent ability to fix and follow bright object	Habituation and some control of state	Cry; state-dependent quieting and head turning rattle or voice	*Sensorimotor period* (0-24 months); reflex stage	*Basic trust vs. basic mistrust* (first year); normal symbiotic phase—does not differentiate between self and mother
4 months	Head midline; head held when pulled to sit; in prone position lifts head to 90° and lifts chest slightly; turns to supine	Hands mostly open; midline hand play; crude palmar grasp	Recognizes bottle	Turns to voice and bell consistently; laughs; squeals; responsive vocalization; blows bubbles, "raspberries"	"Circular reaction"—interesting result of an action motivates its repetition	"Lap baby," developing sense of basic trust
7 months	Maintains sitting, may lean on arms; rolls to prone position; reaches with one arm in prone position; bears all weight; bounces when held erect; cervical lordosis	Intermediate grasp; transfers cube from hand to hand bangs objects	Differentiates between familiar person and stranger; holds bottle; looks for dropped object; "talks" to his mirror image	Uses single and double consonant-vowel combinations		At 5 months began to differentiate between mother and self, i.e., beginning of separation individuation; has sense of belonging to central person
10 months	Creeps on all fours; pivots in sitting; stands momentarily; cruises; slight bowleg; increased lumbar lordosis; acute lumbosacral angulation	Pincer grasp; mature thumb to index grasp; bangs two cubes held in hands	Plays peek-a-boo; finger feeds; chews with rotatory movement	Shouts for attention; imitates speech sounds; waves "bye-bye"; uses "mama" and "dada" with meaning; inhibits behavior to "no"	Can retrieve an object hidden in his view	Practicing phase of separation—individuation, practices initiating separations; "love affair with the world"
14 months	Walks alone with arms in high guard or midguard; wide base, excessive knee and hip flexion; foot contact on entire sole; slight valgus knees and feet; pelvic tilt and rotation	Piles two cubes; scribbles spontaneously; holds crayon full length in palm; casts objects	Uses spoon with overpronation and spilling; removes a garment	Uses single words; understands simple commands	Differentiates available behavior patterns for new ends, e.g., pulls rug on which toy is lying	Rapprochement phase of separation—individuation; ambivalent behavior to mother *Stage of autonomy vs. shame and doubt* (1-3 years); issue of holding on and letting go; pleasure in controlling muscles and sphincters

Data compiled from various sources (references 12, 25, 27, 30, 31, 37, 43, 47, 48, 51, 63, 67, 73, and 74). From Molnar, G, and Kaminer, R: Growth and development. In Molnar, G, editor: Pediatric rehabilitation, Baltimore, 1985, Williams & Wilkins Co.   *Continued.*

Table 30-2, cont'd. Milestones in child development

Age	Gross motor	Fine motor adaptive	Personal-social	Speech and language	Cognitive	Emotional
18 months	Arms at low guard; mature supporting base and heel strike; seats self in chair; walks backwards	Emerging hand dominance; crude release; holds crayon butt end in palm; dumps raisin from bottle spontaneously	Imitates housework; carries, hugs doll; drinks from cup neatly	Points to named body part; identifies one picture; says "no"; jargons	Capable of "insight," i.e., solving a problem by mental combinations, not physical groping	
2 years	Begins running; walks up and down stairs alone; jumps on both feet in place	Hand dominance is usual; builds eight-cube tower; aligns cubes horizontally; imitates vertical line; places pencil shaft between thumb and fingers; draws with arm and wrist action	Pulls on garment; uses spoon well; opens door turning knob; feeds doll with bottle or spoon; toilet training usually begun	Two-word phrases are common; uses verbs; refers to self by name; uses "me," "mine"; follows simple directions	*Preoperational period* (2-7 years); able to evoke object or event not present; object permanence established; comprehends symbols	
3 years	Runs well; pedals tricycle; broad jumps; walks up stairs alternating feet	Imitates three-cube bridge; copies circle; uses overhand throw with anteroposterior arm and trunk motion; catches with extended arms hugging against body	Most children toilet trained day and night; pours from pitcher; unbuttons; washes and dries hands and face; parallel play; can take turns; can be reasoned with	Three-word sentences are usual; uses future tense; asks "what," "who," "where"; follows prepositional commands, i.e., "put it under"; gives full name; may stutter in eagerness; identifies self as boy or girl; recognizes three colors	Preoperational period continues; child capable of deferred imitation, symbolic play, drawing of graphic images, mental images, verbal evocation of events	*Stage of initiative vs. guilt* (3-5 years); deals with issue of genital sexuality
4 years	Walks down stairs alternating feet; hops on one foot; plantar arches developing; sits up from supine position without rotating	Handles a pencil by finger and wrist action, like adults; copies a cross; draws froglike person with head and extremities; throws underhand; cuts with scissors	Cooperative play-sharing and interacting; imaginative make-believe play; dresses and undresses with supervision distinguishing front and back of clothing and buttoning; does simple errands outside of home	Gives connected account of recent experiences; questions "why," "when," "how"; uses past tense, adjectives, adverbs; knows opposite analogies; repeats four digits		

Table 30-2, cont'd. Milestones in child development

Age	Gross motor	Fine motor adaptive	Personal-social	Speech and language	Cognitive	Emotional
5 years	Skips; tiptoes; balances 10 seconds on each foot	Hand dominance is expected; draws man with head, body, and extremities; throws with diagonal arm and body rotation; catches with hands	Creative play; competitive team play; uses fork for stabbing food; brushes teeth; is self-sufficient in toileting; dresses without supervision except tying shoelaces	Fluent speech; misarticulations of some sounds may persist; gives name, address, age; defines concrete nouns by composition, classification, or use; follows three-part commands; has number concepts to 10		*Stage of industry vs. inferiority* (5 years to adolescence); adjusts self to inorganic laws of tool world
6 years	Rides bicycle; roller skates	Prints alphabet; letter reversals still acceptable; mature catch and throw of ball	Teacher is important authority to child; uses fork appropriately; uses knife for spreading; ties shoelaces; plays table games	Shows mastery of grammar; uses proper articulation		*Stage of industry vs. inferiority* continues
7 years	Continuing refinement of skills		Eats with fork and knife; combs hair; is responsible for grooming		*Period of concrete operational thought* (7 years to adolescence); child is capable of logical thinking	

tural responses and volitional control. Table 30-1 describes selected infantile reflexes relevant to motor behavior, as well as the physiologic postural responses that replace these reflexes.[58] The postural responses form the framework for all further motor development. Primitive reflexes are illustrated in the Primitive Reflex Profile devised by Capute and associates[15] to objectify and score normal and abnormal reflex responses. Most primitive reflexes, with the exception of plantar grasp and placing, are suppressed by 7 months of age. An obligate response or hyperactivity or persistence is considered abnormal, as is absence of a response during its expected time frame. Persistence of reflex activity indicates delayed central nervous system (CNS) maturation, whereas absence may indicate neuropathic or myopathic weakness.

Table 30-2 outlines the major milestones in child development, including both cognitive and emotional development, as well as four other descriptive areas.

CNS dysfunction in certain pediatric disabilities may lead to attention deficits, perceptual difficulties, and the inability to conceptualize, which interfere with both higher scholastic achievement and the attainment of skills of daily living. A person who is mildly retarded but educable may be expected to achieve academic skills to approximately fourth-grade level.[58] Thereafter, limited judgment and ability to abstract hamper further cognitive growth. Physically disabled children, even if they are cognitively normal, experience great difficulty in achieving the separation and self-sufficiency that characterize an adolescent's transition from dependency to adulthood. Understanding the developmental process is a prerequisite to formulating a treatment plan and supportive guidance that will be effective in assisting these disabled children to become well-adjusted adults.

PEDIATRIC REHABILITATION OF SPECIFIC DISORDER GROUPS
Spina bifida syndrome

Neural tube defects are among the most common serious congenital malformations and include anencephaly, encephalocele, and spina bifida aperta or cystica (including meningocele and myelomeningocele). The overall risk of neural tube defects is 1:1000; the risk increases by 20 to 30 times after one affected child.[32] The condition is thought to be caused by a combination of environmental factors acting on a genetic predisposition toward failure of neural tube closure around day 29 of gestation.

Anencephaly and encephalocele are associated with dismal prognoses. Anencephaly is an absence of brain formation. Anencephalic children are stillborn or die in the early neonatal period. In encephalocele a part of the brain lies outside the calvarium. Families of children with these disorders should be referred for genetic counseling because they are at increased risk for recurrence, as stated previously, or for the occurrence of spina bifida. Genetic studies show that maternal serum alpha-fetoprotein can be examined between the fourteenth and sixteenth weeks of gestation to indicate the presence of a defect.[56] If findings of these tests are positive on repeated sample, amniocentesis or ultrasonography is performed to confirm or deny the diagnosis.

Spina bifida occurs at a rate of 0.5:1000 and refers to a syndrome of multiple structural anomalies reflecting abnormal development of the neural tube and its surrounding structures before birth. Myelodysplasia is any associated malformation of the spinal cord and roots as part of the spina bifida syndrome and is seen in myelomeningocele and some cases of meningocele. Spina bifida occulta may be associated with pigmentation, hair tufts, or dermal sinuses of the sacral area, which may also overlie associated myelodysplasia. Spina bifida occulta with normal skin is usually asymptomatic and may be found in 20% of the normal population.

This section deals with the management of the spina bifida cystica conditions, including meningocele and myelomeningocele. The management of these children is usually accomplished by a multidisciplinary approach that addresses the four major areas of deficits: hydrocephalus, which is present in 90% of cases; paraplegia or paraparesis with associated sensory deficit, the degree of severity depending on the level of the lesion and the degree of cord and root disruption and dysplasia; neurogenic bowel and bladder; and spinal deformities and bone abnormalities. Since tumors and lipomas invading the spinal cord may create similar deficits and management problems, this discussion may have application in such cases also.

Evaluation

In the newborn period, correct assessment of spinal disorders demands a detailed examination. Treatment decisions may depend on its accuracy, although in the present political and medicolegal climate of the United States, most children receive early aggressive treatment.

In the immediate evaluation the physician determines whether the lesion is open or closed. If it is open, neurosurgical closure is undertaken within the first 48 hours of life to decrease the risk of infection of the CNS.[50] These infections have been linked to decreased intelligence.[52] Closed (covered) lesions may await delayed repair.

Also at the initial examination, anatomic location of the lesion is noted, although this may not accurately reflect impaired neurologic level. The presence of kyphosis, scoliosis, and other associated anomalies is observed, as are head circumference and fullness and size of the fontanelles. A baseline computerized tomographic (CT) scan of the head should be obtained.

Hydrocephalus, if present, is treated by shunting, usually via a ventriculoperitoneal route, which allows for growth and has fewer complications than the ventriculoatrial shunts of the past. Treatment of hydrocephalus gives an optimal opportunity for the development of normal intelligence. With time, revisions of the shunt may be required because of malfunction, infection, or growth.

Motor and sensory levels are also estimated from the initial examination. Motor level is determined by response to noxious stimulation above the level of the lesion. Major motor groups are observed for movements and estimation of motor power. Hip flexion alone signifies an L1 level (iliopsoas), and hip flexion and adduction denotes an L2 level. Weak quadriceps function with active but weak knee extension and flail foot without any ankle motion elicited is designated as L3 level. Strong quadriceps and active ankle dorsiflexion (tibialis anterior) signifies an L4 level. Ankle inversion is accomplished by the tibialis posterior muscle innervated by L4-5, and ankle eversion is accomplished by the peroneal muscles, which mainly receive L5-S1 innervation. Ankle plantar flexion and hip extension are achieved by S1 level musculature. In the newborn period, estimation of motor level may be somewhat difficult but is considered relatively accurate if the baby is in an awake, responsive state. Motor level correlates most closely with the prognosis for functional ambulation. Patients with lesions at a low thoracic level usually are wheelchair dependent in adulthood. Lesions at upper lumbar levels may permit ambulation with long-leg braces or a reciprocation orthosis, but these patients require wheelchairs for long distances. Problems created by lesions at a low lumbar level are usually compensated for by the use of ankle-foot orthoses in adulthood. Such lesions generally allow the patient to ambulate, although sometimes only with crutches or a cane. Patients with lesions at sacral levels may need ankle-foot orthoses or shoe modifications but are generally good walkers.[1]

Sensory level may be discerned by pinprick examination from a caudal to cephalad direction. An accurate positive response should have emotional content, such as crying, anger, or extreme surprise. Both sides of the body should be examined, one side at a time.

The bladder status is observed for dribbling or distention. An intravenous pyelogram should be obtained in the early weeks as well as blood urea nitrogen (BUN) values, creatinine levels, urinalysis, and culture testing.

Treatment

The earliest physiatric interventions in the newborn period may be explaining the various aspects of the special disorder to the parents and helping them become comfortable in the care and handling of their child. Teaching and reassurance are useful in reinforcing the care of surgical sites if not yet healed; describing signs and symptoms of infection and hydrocephalus; reassuring parents that a child may lie on a well-healed surgical site or turn his head to the side on which a shunt is placed; educating parents regarding the care of insensate skin and the precautions that must be taken against burns from water, sun-warmed car seats and strollers, and radiators, as well as the dangers of extreme cold; showing the parents how to wrap a baby's legs (to avoid the froglegged positioning of a child with a thoracic level lesion); and teaching positioning and stretching techniques to treat existing contractures and prevent further deformity.

During the first year of life, children should be examined by the multidisciplinary team every month. The hips and spine are watched closely for any developing deformities. Subluxations and dislocations are particularly common in high lumbar lesions owing to unopposed action of the hip flexors and adductors. Vertebral anomalies, such as bar vertebrae or hemivertebrae, may cause a rapid progression of scoliosis. Spine and rib radiographs should be examined closely for these commonly associated abnormalities. Also, orthopedic serial casting for attempted correction of clubfeet may be started in this period.

After the child is 6 months old, orthopedic surgical correction of severe deformities may be undertaken. Orthopedic interventions are aimed at providing proper alignment for sitting and standing. The goals of surgical intervention are to restore muscle imbalance, release contractures that have not yielded to vigorous stretching programs, especially if unilateral and leading to obliquity and secondary scoliosis, and correct any congenital or progressive bone deformity. If possible, orthopedic procedures are combined to decrease the number of hospitalizations and the periods of immobility that contribute to disuse osteoporosis. Infants with thoracic level paralysis are wrapped, with the hips and knees in extension and the feet positioned in neutral with resting splints. When they are large enough, they are placed in a hip stabilization brace with Knight spinal attachment and a ratchet joint at the hip; they are kept in 15-degree hip abduction. Foot alignment is managed with a Dennis-Brown bar and shoes. They are usually well tolerated for sleeping and help the child develop sitting skills by giving added trunk support. Infants with high lumbar level lesions require the same type of orthotic management. In addition, a program of stretching and range of motion is crucial for preventing contractures and deformity from muscle imbalance.

Iliopsoas lengthening or transfer to the greater trochanter may be performed when the child is between 9 months and 2 years of age. The surgery is followed by intensive bracing, stretching, and exercise.[53] Lesions at lower lumbar levels require close monitoring of hip joints as well as vigorous stretching at all joints to maintain range of motion.

Bladder status must also be followed closely. Frequent urinary tract infections from incomplete emptying of a flaccid bladder may occur. Either flaccid distention or detrusor-sphincter dyssynergia of a spastic bladder may lead to reflux. Any of these conditions may require intermittent catheterization at an early age. Long-term follow-up study of clean intermittent catheterization has shown that, with use of this modality, renal damage occurs in less than 3% and febrile urinary tract infections in less than 10% of patients.[41] Renal function remains stable, and improvement is noted radiologically in reflux and hydronephrosis.[40] If reflux does not improve with catheterization, vesicostomy may be performed, and if indicated ureteral reimplantation or bladder augmentation can be considered at a later date.

If an infant proves difficult to catheterize at an early age, the Credé maneuver may be used to empty a flaccid bladder, provided that full emptying is achieved and reflux is not present. (The Credé maneuver should not be done if there is reflux.) However, a clean intermittent catheterization program should begin as early as possible in such cases.

Constipation in infancy is managed with dietary manipulation (prunes, prune juice, and so on). Other aids are Malt-Supex and glycerin in liquid enema or suppository form. If constipation is avoided and a regular bowel maintainence program is established in the early years, socially acceptable bowel continence is more easily achieved before school age.

Follow-up by public health nurses and home-based early intervention programs help to reinforce care techniques and provide support to the parents during these early months.

During the preschool and childhood years, much attention is given to motor milestones and ambulation skills. Prone mobility devices or spina bifida carts may give a child early independent mobility with which to explore his environment. A parapodium or swivel walker may be introduced for children with lesions at the thoracic or high lumbar level. This allows the child to view the world from an upright perspective, stimulates better bone mineralization, improves acetabular formation and lower extremity alignment, and frees the arms for bimanual activities. Most children can learn to swivel the parapodium with the use of a rolling walker for early "ambulation." Children with active hip flexors may be fitted with a reciprocating hip extension orthosis (bilateral long-leg braces with a pelvic band and cable mechanism that, with active hip flexion on one side, aids hip extension on the other side). This permits a reciprocal four-point gait pattern and decreases the compensatory lordosis that may develop as a result of paralyzed hip extensors.

Children with lesions at the L3-4 level are braced with

long-leg orthoses to maintain good lower extremity alignment during the early years of rapid growth; they later develop adequate knee stability. Those with flail ankle resulting from an L3 lesion require solid ankle support or valgus correction T-straps for support if metal braces are used. At a later age these children may also require bone surgery for foot stabilization and mediolateral stability. In L4 lesions the foot assumes calcaneus deformity because of unopposed tibialis anterior action, and the patient requires anterior stop or limited motion ankle joints in the orthosis. Various tendon transfers may be used orthopedically in attempts to balance the feet of patients whose lesions are at the lower lumbar levels (L4-5), but most still require the support of orthoses postoperatively to maintain good correction. If deformity persists in later childhood, bone correction may be necessary.[71]

S1-2 levels generally produce foot extrinsic-intrinsic imbalance with resultant pes cavus or claw toes. Because the ambulation skills of these patients are not limited but the feet are insensate, the feet must be well supported and cushioned and closely observed to detect pressure areas or ulcerations. If shoe modifications fail to give adequate protection and relief, surgical correction should be considered.

All bracing in spina bifida children should be accompanied by explicit instructions regarding wearing schedule and skin monitoring for areas of redness. The physiatrist is the key figure in relaying this information to parents and children, as well as being responsible for the fitting and follow-up monitoring of all braces and orthoses.

During the preschool and school years, parents need reiteration of the long-term ambulation goals for their children, as outlined previously. The physiatrist must stress the importance of mobility for independence during these years, including the significance of good wheelchair mobility skills in those who will not be able to walk outside the homes. Parents should also begin to focus on developing their child's self-care and social skills, leading eventually to emancipation of the child during adolescent and adult years.

For purposes of socially acceptable urinary continence, parents can be taught the clean intermittent catheterization technique during the child's preschool years when continence is normally attained. Barring severe visual perceptual deficits, most children can learn to catheterize themselves by 7 or 8 years of age. The clean intermittent catheterization program often requires additional pharmacologic intervention to achieve good control. Anticholinergic agents such as propantheline (Pro-Banthine) and oxybutynin (Ditropan) are used to increase bladder storage capacity, and alpha-adrenergic medications such as pseudoephedrine are used to increase intraurethral tension and prevent dribbling. These agents have few side effects, and no long-term complications have been noted over many years of use.[40]

When the child reaches the expected age of bowel continence, bowel training begins with the goal of establishing a regular routine to achieve reflex emptying. Dietary ma-

nipulation, stool softeners, and digital stimulation or use of a daily glycerin suppository or enema is used to attain this goal.[79] Establishing bowel and bladder control is crucial during early childhood, since incontinence in adolescence and adulthood presents a major barrier to social and vocational goals.

Before they enter school, all children with spina bifida should undergo psychologic testing to estimate their intelligence and identify specific strengths and deficits. Most children with this disorder are of low average intelligence, but many have visual perceptual deficits, organizational and attentional difficulties, or language or academic problems in specific areas. The "cocktail party" empty chatter of many of these children has been well described,[20] and a recent study showed that many with hydrocephalus exhibited distractibility that contributed to language deficits.[35] Many spina bifida children can be "mainstreamed," but the treatment team is dependent on the educational system for any additional educational resources, adaptive physical education, school-based therapy, or psychologic support that may be needed. The physiatrist can assist parents in coordinating educational planning.

Serial psychologic evaluations may be indicated throughout the school years because deterioration in school performance may signal shunt dysfunction and increased hydrocephalus. A CT scan and neurologic intervention may also be needed.[24]

Spinal deformities, including scoliosis, kyphosis, and lordosis, may pose difficult management problems. If a deformity is present at birth, surgical correction may be attempted at the time of initial closure of the myelomeningocele. As the child grows, the deformity may develop or progress. Repeated clinical and x-ray examinations are mandatory to detect problems early and allow intervention. A high, rapidly progressing scoliosis with associated spasticity and weakness of the arms should raise suspicions of hydromyelia, which requires neurosurgical attention.[33] Bracing for spinal deformities is usually done with plastic body jackets. If these do not arrest the progression, spinal fusion may be warranted, although as much time as possible is given to allow spinal growth. However, it is better to have a short, straight spine than a longer spine shortened by severe deformity. Fusion may require an anterior approach and instrumentation owing to the absence of posterior elements at the spina bifida site. The goal of management is a vertical spine over a level pelvis.

Neuropathic fractures on the basis of paralysis, immobility, or limited weight bearing are common. The patient may not feel pain but may have only a swollen, warm limb. The immobilization for healing should be as brief as possible to avoid the cycle of immobilization-refracture-immobilization-refracture.

Attention to skin care of insensate areas must be reinforced as children become heavier and more active, giving more opportunity for poor pressure relief and repeated trauma. These children should be taught to examine their bodies from an early age. They must be aware that seemingly innocent exposures to heat or cold may result in burns or ulcerations. Decubitus care is covered elsewhere in this book, but it should be noted here that the source of skin irritation should be investigated to prevent recurrence of decubiti.

Adolescence places increased stress on a young person with spina bifida. Establishing ego identity and achieving functional independence are the developmental goals of this period. To achieve the optimal outcome, the groundwork must have been laid in childhood by parents who understand the importance of encouraging mobility, transfer, and self-help skills, as well as continence programs. Adolescents with spina bifida are still beset with concerns regarding sexual changes and functioning, educational and vocational goals, and feelings of isolation exacerbated by their multifaceted condition.

Attention to many of the areas of concern discussed previously must continue through the patient's adolescence. It is also important for the physiatrist to involve the patient in vocational counseling, recreational programs, peer support groups, and individual or family counseling as needed. The nurses who earlier taught bowel and bladder regimens often help in counseling these young adults on sexual functions and concerns. If bladder incontinence remains a problem, the discussion of incontinence prostheses by the urologist may be indicated. A detailed discussion of the psychosocial and psychosexual problems encountered by adolescents with spina bifida may be found in the recent study by Hayden.[34] The physiatrist should be actively involved in this final stage of growth and development to help the patient achieve a stable, healthy adjustment to adult life.

Cerebral palsy

Cerebral palsy is a group of clinical disorders of movement and posture resulting from a nonprogressive injury to an immature brain.[3] Because the insult involves brain damage, associated deficits are common. Nelson and Ellenberg[62] demonstrated a prevalence in 1978 of 5.2:1000 births after the Collaborative Perinatal Project analyzed the prospective follow-up of 54,000 pregnancies. The etiology of cerebral palsy varies. The injury may occur anytime during pregnancy, around the time of birth, or in the early years of life.

Prenatal causes include any source of intrauterine anoxia or decreased blood flow to the fetus, including placental insufficiency, maternal hypertension, maternal hypotension or respiratory compromise, or maternal infections, especially those associated with congenital viral infections of the newborn. Problems in the labor and birth process, including placenta previa, prolonged umbilical cord compression, or abruption of the placenta, may contribute to perinatal asphyxia. Of note, however, is a recent follow-up study in which Nelson and Ellenberg[60] reviewed Apgar scores of 49,000 infants. Of infants who survived with Apgar scores

of 3 or less at 10 minutes or later, 80% were free of major handicap at early school age. In comparison, 75% of the children from this series who developed cerebral palsy had 5-minute Apgar scores of 7 to 10. This supports the belief that a substantial proportion of cerebral palsy is due to factors other than intrapartum asphyxia.

Postnatal causes of cerebral palsy include head trauma, cerebrovascular accidents, meningitis, encephalitis, poisonings, and toxins. The pathophysiologic mechanism is usually anoxia (lack of oxygen or inability to utilize oxygen) or ischemia (lack of blood supply). These factors may combine to result in hypoxic-ischemic encephalopathy. A specific toxic effect of bilirubin, a breakdown product of red blood cells that has a preferential affinity for the basal ganglia, has been identified less frequently since Rhogam treatment of sensitized mothers and exchange transfusion of affected infants has decreased the incidence and sequelae of erythroblastosis fetalis.

Cerebral palsy can be divided into two major groups: spastic (pyramidal) and extrapyramidal. A third group of mixed types, containing elements of both major groups, also exists.

Subgroups of the spastic types are defined topographically, referring to the limbs involved: hemiplegia (involving two limbs on the same side of the body), double hemiplegia (involving all four limbs with arms more affected than legs), quadriplegia (involving all four limbs with the lower limbs slightly more affected than the arms), and diplegia (involving all four limbs with the legs markedly more affected than the arms). All of the spastic types of cerebral palsy are characterized by muscle hypertonus (clasp-knife type), extreme hyperreflexia, a tendency to develop contractures, and extensor plantar responses of affected extremities.

The extrapyramidal groups of cerebral palsy show characteristically more lead pipe–type hypertonus, milder hyperreflexia, and involuntary movement disorders, including athetosis, chorea, dystonia, or any combination of these. Ataxic cerebral palsy is uncommon. In such cases it is crucial to rule out the presence of a brain tumor or a familial neurodegenerative condition.

The physicians at the John F. Kennedy Institute advocate the addition of functional and therapeutic classifications. Their full classification listing appears in the box on p. 418.[78]

Evaluation

The diagnosis of cerebral palsy begins with a detailed history of birth weight; gestational, labor, and birth difficulties; the neonatal course; and the history of prior pregnancies. In 20% to 30% of cases, no etiologic source or event is found.[75] Delayed motor development with failure to meet milestones may be the parents' initial complaint. In addition, parents may be concerned about asymmetric limb use, abnormal movement patterns, exaggerated toe walking, or feeding difficulties.

JOHN F. KENNEDY INSTITUTE CLASSIFICATION OF CEREBRAL PALSY

Clinical

A. Spastic
 1. Hemiplegia
 2. Double hemiplegia
 3. Quadriplegia
 4. Diplegia
B. Extrapyramidal
 1. Choreoathetosis
 2. Rigidity
 3. Ataxia
 4. Tremor
C. Mixed
 1. Primary spasticity
 2. Primary extrapyramidal

Function

Class I: No practical limitations
Class II: Slight to moderate limitation
Class III: Moderate to great limitation
Class IV: No useful activity

Therapeutic

Class A: No treatment required
Class B: Extensive bracing or other apparatus; multidisciplinary team required for long-term habilitation
Class D: Long-term institutionalization required

From Vining, EPG, et al: Am J Dis Child 130:643, 1976. Copyright 1976, American Medical Association

A detailed neurologic examination between 6 months and 1 year of age usually reveals the early signs of cerebral palsy: tone abnormalities, exaggerated deep tendon reflexes, obligate or persistent primitive reflex patterns (discussed earlier in this chapter), abnormalities in posture, and delayed motor development and abnormal movement patterns, especially if other milestones have been met normally. One study found that the most reliable individual sign of high risk at the 4-month examination was excessive muscle tone in the neck extensors, arms, legs, or trunk.[23] Asymmetric hand use with early "fisting" or "cortical thumb" positioning in the second 6 months of life is an early sign of hemiparetic cerebral palsy. Late development of walking with persistence of toe walking and a high guard position of the arms may indicate the spastic diplegic form.

In extrapyramidal cerebral palsy, before the development of an overt movement disorder, early signs may be subtle. They include persistence of the primitive reflexes, tone abnormality with variability and shifts from hypotonus to hypertonus as the child is moved in space, and poor feeding and suck.[78] The involuntary movement pattern often develops in the second year of life.

Despite all of these early indicators, caution must be exercised in diagnosing cerebral palsy. In follow-up examination of a large number of children with the classic early signs of cerebral palsy, many of them had normal motor development at 7 years of age, although many had other disorders, including learning and speech difficulties.[61] Obviously, findings such as these also illustrate the inherent difficulties in evaluating the various treatment approaches. Diagnostic difficulties are certainly compounded when the child also has severe cognitive deficits.

Several maneuvers during the first-year examination may help to evaluate tone and reflex abnormalities. If the child, in being pulled to a sitting position, extends hips and knees and goes directly to stand, this is an early sign of lower extremity hypertonicity. Also, ventral suspension should allow a 2-month-old to align the head with the horizontal and a 4-month-old to bring the head above horizontal. Delay in doing so may indicate hypotonia, whereas earlier attainment may indicate excessive extensor tone and exaggeration of the primitive tonic labyrinthine reflex. Scissoring in vertical suspension indicates hypertonic hip adductors.[36] Hypotonia may be demonstrated by excessive range of motion at major joints. Taft[75] found that persistent asymmetric tonic neck and crossed extensor reflexes are diagnostically the most helpful primitive reflexes.

During the second year of life a full-blown picture of upper motor neuron CNS dysfunction evolves. Hemiparetic children may fail to develop protective reactions on the involved side. Diplegic children, who may be hypotonic during the early months, demonstrate increasing lower extremity spasticity, scissoring, extensor tone, and exaggerated positive supporting reactions. Quadriparetic children may initially show either decreased or increased tone, but the added presence of exaggerated deep tendon reflexes can often differentiate these lesions from other causes of hypotonia (neuromuscular or myopathic diseases.) A few children may remain hypotonic or atonic.

Differential diagnosis requires the exclusion of progressive CNS disorders, neuropathic disorders, myopathic diseases, dysmorphic syndromes with associated cerebral malformations, and endocrinopathies with motor delay.

Several deficits and conditions are associated with cerebral palsy. From 40% to 60% of this population falls within the mental retardation range of intelligence, with more severe mental dysfunction being associated with the quadriparetic, rigid, or atonic types.[57] Therefore cognitive testing should be done, with care taken that the tests used do not require motor skills and that expressive language problems do not falsely lower test results.

Cognitive deficit, hearing deficit, aphasia, or poor oral motor control may cause communication problems. These problems should be evaluated by experienced speech and language pathologists; if cognition allows, communication boards or electronic communication training can be used by children whose motor problems preclude understandable speech.

In addition, psychologic, speech, and hearing evaluations should be performed by professionals skilled in working with this population. Seizure disorders are common, most often in the spastic groups. Strabismus (associated in up to 75% of cases[9]), field cuts, and even cortical blindness may be concomitant visual problems. Feeding and drooling problems may result from bilateral cortical involvement (pseudobulbar palsy) or bulbar involvement. Perceptual difficulties may be present and can interfere with the acquisition of functional skills of daily living.

Treatment

Therapeutic intervention with this population usually involves a large multidisciplinary team. The pediatrician or physiatrist may coordinate the effort, which includes parents, physical therapists, occupational therapists, social workers, special educators, psychologists, orthopedists, and later, vocational counselors. The goal of intervention is maximization of the patient's ultimate functional ability. Aspects include parent education and support, environmental enrichment for the child, and medical and therapeutic treatment.

Many physiotherapeutic methodologies have been applied to the treatment of cerebral palsy. The method used most commonly is the Bobath neurodevelopmental technique, which attempts to inhibit or modify abnormal tone, posture, and reflexes in hopes of facilitating normal posture and movement patterns.[6] This approach is used in conjunction with passive range of motion and stretching of major joints to prevent contractures or deformity.

Orthotic intervention is used to put a joint at a better mechanical advantage, improve alignment, help prevent contracture, and give improved stability and posture. Lightweight plastics have made braces easier to wear and more cosmetically acceptable, as well as allowing more refined correction of reducible deformities. One disadvantage of plastic braces is the reduced adjustability to accommodate growth.

Orthopedic intervention helps prevent secondary deformity, correct existing deformity, and improve function. The most common procedures include hip adductor tenotomies, hamstring releases, and Achilles tendon lengthenings for lower extremity spasticity. Upper extremity procedures are usually aimed at reduction of wrist flexion and forearm pronation of the spastic arm. A more detailed account of orthopedic intervention in spastic conditions may be found in Chapter 38.

Upper extremity functional training emphasizes eye-hand coordination and trunk and shoulder stability. Arm movements, grasp, and fine motor dexterity training follow. Toys of various size, shape, and texture are used for the additional sensory stimulation.

A recent neurosurgical approach to the treatment of spastic cerebral palsy is selective posterior rhizotomy. This procedure involves sectioning selected posterior rootlets (subdivisions of the dorsal or sensory root) to decrease the sensory arc of the spinal reflex circuit and thereby any abnormal or exaggerated spastic motor response. Although the procedure is still relatively experimental, early results have been promising.[65]

Early intervention programs have been instrumental in treating children with cerebral palsy. Whether such an approach has a direct effect on the motor disorder remains to be proved. However, these programs do encourage the acquisition of new skills by enriching the child's experiential world and by educating parents in therapeutic, adaptational, and coping approaches. The aim is to prevent experiential deprivation and poor infant-parent interactions from compounding the child's organic deficits. Adaptations in handling and emphasis on home management help parents adjust to the difficult task of bringing up a disabled child. For school-age children, a home program of maintenance exercise should be combined with adaptive physical education and leisure activities. A carryover of functional training in the home and at school is necessary for success in these areas.

As these children become adults, assistance may be sought from the physician in making the transition from school to a vocational setting and from a dependent to an independent living situation, as the level of disability and, more important, ability allows.

Rheumatologic disorders

A physiatrist is often involved as part of a multidisciplinary team in the management of children with rheumatologic conditions. The most common of these conditions is juvenile rheumatoid arthritis (JRA). JRA is divided into three major types, depending on the onset and course: systemic onset, polyarticular onset, and pauciarticular involvement.

Systemic onset JRA is characterized by high spiking fevers (above 40.5° C) with associated irritability, listlessness, and anorexia. Physical findings may include generalized adenopathy and an evanescent salmon-colored rash. Arthralgias may be the only initial joint symptom. Arthritis may not occur until months after the onset of systemic symptoms. Splenomegaly, myocarditis, pericarditis, pleuritis, and anemia may also occur, and the white blood cell count may be elevated. Approximately 20% of JRA children have this systemic onset, possibly with recurrent systemic episodes. Polyarticular arthritis develops in most of these patients; destructive arthritis and moderate disability occur in approximately one third.

Polyarticular onset JRA affects approximately 50% of the JRA population. Four or more joints are involved. These children appear ill, with fever, anorexia, and listlessness. Rash, adenopathy, and mild organomegaly may be present. The joints most frequently involved are the knees, ankles, feet, hands, and wrists. Erythema and tenderness are sometimes present. Differential diagnoses include rheumatic fever, serum sickness, and drug reaction.[13] The presence of positive rheumatoid factor in this group denotes a greater chance of erosive arthritis and moderate residual disability.[69]

Approximately one third of JRA patients have pauciarticular involvement of one or a few joints. This group has few systemic features. The knee is the most commonly affected joint, but the hip, the ankle, elbow, or wrist may be affected. The most important and potentially dangerous manifestation is chronic iridocyclitis, which occurs in half this group. This condition requires frequent slit-lamp examinations. If it is left untreated, glaucoma, band keratopathy, and cataracts may develop, resulting in blindness.[13] Boys in the pauciarticular group should be screened for HLA-B27. Those who have positive test results should be closely monitored for the development of ankylosing spondylitis.[69]

Most children with JRA enter into remission and reach adulthood without significant disability. However, 25% have unremitting disease, leading to deformity and functional deficits. Self-care skills and the ability to walk are lost in 10%.[10] All children with rheumatologic disease require supervision and physical management in collaboration with the medical management of their disease to achieve optimal outcome.

Evaluation

History should include a full review of the child's day, including presence or absence of morning stiffness; ability to groom, bathe, and dress; walking ability; and overall endurance level. Physical examination includes inspection and palpation of all joints with range-of-motion measurements and notation of heat, swelling, or synovial thickening. The spine is examined for range of motion and evidence of scoliosis. The legs are measured for leg length discrepancies, which may develop because of inflammation in the region of the epiphyseal plate, leading to bony overgrowth.[44]

Treatment

Treatment regimens for joint disease depend on the activity of the disease. In acute stages of inflammation, resting the joint in a functionally advantageous position, applying heat, and encouraging the child to do as much for himself as possible may be all that can be done. As joint inflammation subsides, exercise is reintroduced, with care taken not to overload and reexacerbate the joint's condition. Therapy may be more aggressive during periods of remission.

The key to the rehabilitative approach in pediatric joint disease is the home-based program. In one series the physical status of 51% of the children was maintained or improved with only regular daily activities.[7] It is imperative that parents understand the clinical course of JRA so they will cooperate in the ongoing program of exercise, splinting, and therapeutic play.

Exercise programs for these children address range of motion, strength, and endurance. Range-of-motion exercise is given to increase range or prevent further loss of range.

In very severe disease, when joint fusion appears unavoidable, it is important to put the joint in the most functional position for fusing. Strengthening of surrounding muscles helps prevent joint deformity. Isometric exercises may help avoid atrophy and loss of strength in acutely painful joints. Endurance is increased by encouraging these children to resume their usual play activities as soon as acute symptoms subside. Active assisted range of motion is advanced to full active exercise and stretching as soon as possible.

Rest periods should be interspersed with activity throughout the day. During rest periods, and especially during television time, the child should lie prone with the feet extended over the edge of the couch or bed for gravity-assisted stretch of the hip and knee flexors. These children should also be taught to sleep without pillows. During acute phases a soft collar may be indicated for comfort.

Play activities, especially gross motor activities such as walking, running, and climbing, are encouraged for toddlers. Tricycle riding is also therapeutic. Upper extremity activities, including throwing balls and rolling and manipulating play dough or clay, are used to gain wrist extension and work hand joints. Drawing, model building, and weaving may be of interest to older children.

Physical education classes for schoolchildren should be adapted to avoid contact sports.[44] Swimming is one of the best activities for children with rheumatic disease. It combines the heat for relaxation with the buoyancy of the water for greater ease of movement.[2] A daily stretching program should be part of the child's routine. Cervical spine range-of-motion exercises are included if the cervical spine is involved in the child's disease. Temporomandibular joints may be exercised simply by chewing gum.[44]

Activity of daily living training for children with joint disease emphasizes joint protection. Children are taught the most energy-efficient means of performing tasks with the least stress on joints. Warm morning baths alleviate morning stiffness. Bathing aids such as grab bars, shower chairs, and shower hose attachments may be used to increase functional independence. Bath play and exercise are encouraged. Adaptive equipment such as dressing aids and built-up utensils for eating and writing is often helpful.

Splinting is an important adjunct to exercise. Resting splints are used during acute exacerbations to rest the joints in functional positions. In periods of remission they are worn during sleep for passive control. Cock-up splints for wrists and posterior shell splints for knee extension are the most commonly used. Corrective splints or dynamic splints are worn to increase range of motion. Serial splints should be bivalved to allow range of motion between periods of splinting.[70] Some patients need knee-ankle-foot orthoses for support during ambulation. Dial locks at the knees may allow passive stretch to treat knee flexion contractures. Footwear should be soft and flexible with good arch support; sneakers often suit this need. Platform adaptation of rollators or walkers may protect the wrists and the small joints of the hands when ambulatory aids are needed. Small finger splints may be used to limit flexion or extension to prevent boutonnière or swan-neck deformities, respectively.

All of the aforementioned principles apply not only to JRA but to other rheumatologic disorders as well, including ankylosing spondylitis, dermatomyositis, and scleroderma. In addition, children with ankylosing spondylitis should have emphasis placed on postural training, especially chest expansion and spine extension in combination with therapeutic heat and analgesia.[70] Children with dermatomyositis experience inflammation of skin and muscle. Pain and tenderness preclude active exercise during acute stages. Many of these children develop subcutaneous calcification that may be unresponsive to most modes of treatment. Periarticular calcification often limits joint range of motion. Physical therapeutic intervention includes range-of-motion exercise and splinting to prevent deformity. Surgery may be required. Spontaneous extrusion of calcium may produce infection-prone ulcerations. In children with scleroderma, if Raynaud's phenomenon is associated, protection from cold must be stressed. Vigorous stretching programs are incorporated, including facial exercises.[70]

With close follow-up and family involvement, the goal is to minimize the musculoskeletal deformities of children with rheumatologic conditions.

Head injury

Injuries are the leading cause of death for children after the first year of life. One study by Kraus and associates[45] found that nearly one half of deaths in U.S. children between 1 and 14 years of age in 1980 were secondary to trauma. Their study found an annual brain injury rate of 185 per 100,000 when the injury was defined as physical damage or functional impairment of cranial contents by acute mechanical energy exchange exclusive of birth trauma. The same study found falls to be the major cause (35%), with recreational activities contributing 29% and motor vehicle accidents 24%; all other causes accounted for 12%. Bicycles were involved in over 20%. In a follow-up study by Mahoney and associates[49] on the long-term outcome of children with severe head trauma and coma lasting longer than 24 hours, 38% died. The average length of coma for survivors was 15 days; 29% were normal at follow-up and 53% had mild cognitive or behavioral problems (61% of those had similar problems before the injury). Also, 9% had severe intellectual and motor problems. Children younger than 2 years of age had worse outcomes.

The patients seen by the pediatric physiatrist for rehabilitative purposes are from the more severely involved groups. The physiatrist coordinates a team of professionals whose aim is to optimize the natural recovery course and prevent secondary complications. The first goals are maintaining the patient's medical well-being, determining that all associated injuries have been managed appropriately, and monitoring for and treating secondary problems. Rehabilitation should begin in the intensive care unit, with close attention to skin care, range of motion, positioning, and resting splints to prevent contractures. When acute medical and surgical problems have stabilized and a head trauma patient is able to show some awareness of the environment, the patient should be transferred to an acute rehabilitation setting. In this early phase, close attention is given to the areas of concern discussed in the following paragraphs.

Initial management

Feeding and swallowing. If a child is not yet on a full regular diet when transferred to the rehabilitation facility, close attention must be paid to feeding and swallowing ability. A therapist competent in dysphagia treatment should evaluate the situation; in addition, videofluoroscopy may be needed before the diet can be expanded. Problems with thin liquids often signify neurogenic swallowing difficulty; difficulty with hard-to-chew solids may indicate oral motor incoordination.[18]

If physical examination reveals severe depression of the gag reflex or severe delay of the swallowing reflex, the patient should be fed by nasogastric tube until structured therapy is given and improvement can be demonstrated. With appropriate precautions and restrictions, aspiration should be avoided.

Tracheostomy use and care. Suctioning is performed to keep mucus from plugging the tube, but the patient is weaned from frequent suctioning as soon as possible. If the patient does not tolerate use of smaller tracheostomy tubes or continues to have mucus plugs, evaluation for tracheal granuloma or stenosis should be done.

Fever and urinary care. Fever is often caused by a urinary tract infection. Indwelling catheters are removed as soon as possible, but fluid intake is maintained and intermittent catheterization performed until spontaneous voiding is resumed. Urinary condom drainage in boys may be indicated until a toileting program is feasible to retrain volitional control. Girls may be managed with diapers or incontinence briefs with close attention to skin integrity.

If a urinary tract infection is not the source of fever, close examination of ears, lungs, skin, and throat is required. If there is a history of open head trauma or skull fracture, central nervous system infection must be ruled out. Only when multiple searches for a source have proved negative can fever of central origin be entertained as an etiology.

Hypertension. Transient hypertension may initially require medical intervention, but medications often can later be gradually withdrawn.

Agitation. Pain that a patient cannot express must always be considered a possible source of agitation in a patient recovering from trauma. Often an empiric trial of analgesics is indicated to rule out this possibility. Agitation is also recognized as a part of the natural progression of recovery in head trauma patients. Management of agitated behavior includes reducing external stimuli, providing a secure environment, and maintaining a set routine of daily activities to lessen the patient's confusion. If all else fails, restraints may be used to protect the patient from harming himself or others. Pharmacologic intervention may include haloperidol in low dosage.

Hypercalcemia. Long bone fractures and immobilization may contribute to hypercalcemia in these patients. Nausea and anorexia may be subtle signs. Hypercalcemia may be treated with fluids, diuretics, and calcitonin.[19]

Heterotopic ossification. Heterotopic ossification may be seen as a complication, particularly in older adolescents, and may be manifest as heat, swelling, and erythema near major joints; occasionally heterotopic ossification mimics a fracture. Bone scan may show radioactive iodine uptake before routine radiographs demonstrate the ectopic bone deposition. Medical management involves etidronate sodium. Surgical intervention may be undertaken if joint mobility is affected.

Skin care. Meticulous skin care is needed to prevent decubitus ulcers. The management of decubiti is discussed elsewhere in this text.

Visual problems. Visual problems may include strabismus, field cuts, extraocular muscle palsies, or optic nerve atrophy. Close ophthalmologic management and follow-up are indicated for any of these problems.

Nutritional management. The involvement of a dietician is often helpful. In the early phase of recovery, nutritional supplements may be needed. If hyperphagia becomes a part of the later stages of recovery, caloric restriction may be needed to avoid obesity.

Hearing loss. If hearing loss is suspected, an audiologic examination may be indicated. In an uncooperative patient, brainstem audio-evoked potentials may be helpful.[72]

Seizures. Posttraumatic seizures are common but are not seen in the majority of head-injured patients. The highest rate of seizures is seen with missile injuries, and adults are more likely to have posttraumatic seizures than are head-injured children. Children who are younger than 2 years of age are more prone to seizures than those over two.[46] About 5% of head-injured children have seizures within the first week after injury, and seizures develop in 10% to 20% over the next 4 years.[38,68]

Within the pediatric age group, phenobarbital and phenytoin are most frequently used anticonvulsants for posttraumatic seizure disorders or prophylaxis. These medications should always be withdrawn slowly, after a 1- to 3-year seizure-free period.[18]

• • •

When all associated medical conditions and complications have been recognized and treated, the child is on a clear pathway for the recovery process and rehabilitative efforts. Meticulous nursing care must be ongoing, including skin care, bowel and bladder retraining, and nutritional and feeding assessments.

Rehabilitation

Motor dysfunction in children with head injury may range from chronic decerebration to spasticity or a combination of spasticity, ataxia, and dystonia. Initial management includes vigorous range-of-motion exercises, inhibition of pathologic postures, splinting to prevent contractures, and serial casting for contracture reduction. Medications to attempt to control spasticity include diazepam and dantrolene sodium. The possible hepatotoxicity of dantrolene mandates close monitoring of liver enzyme levels. Nerve blocks or soft tissue releases, lengthening, and transfers may also be useful in managing motor problems. Ataxia may be treated with cuff weights for the patient or weighting the walker. Dystonic postures sometimes respond to trihexphenidyl, an antiparkinsonian drug. Side effects like those with atropine should be watched for and monitored. Physical therapy measures in retraining include stimulation and inhibition techniques, therapeutic exercise, transfer training, and functional and ambulation training in the usual sequences. Success in these areas depends of course on progressive cognitive recovery. Children unable to regain ambulatory status need seating and mobility aids.

Occupational therapy interventions begin with positioning, range of motion, and splinting during the coma period. As the patient enters a lighter coma, an environmental stimulation program is begun. A prefeeding assessment of facial, tongue, and jaw muscle function is initiated, as well as observation of gag, cough, and swallowing abilities. During the confused or agitated state of recovery, efforts are made to minimize stimuli and to structure and simplify the environment. Constant reorientation may be necessary. As agitation subsides, confusion and disorientation may persist. Orientation groups and an orientation journal are often helpful during this period. Simple games and crafts may be used to reeducate, strengthen, and coordinate fine motor abilities. Continued repetition of self-care tasks is emphasized to retrain the child in problem-solving and sequencing skills. As a child's behavior becomes more appropriate, more structured assessments and tasks are performed and visual perceptual retraining is begun as needed. Later phases of treatment include higher skills such as community skills, the planning of leisure time, homemaking skills, and improvement of judgment and problem-solving abilities.

Intellectual and memory deficits are common in head-injured persons and tend to be more handicapping than physical disability for this group. Some degree of cognitive impairment is common in injuries that produce posttraumatic amnesia of at least 2 weeks. In one prospective study, no cognitive sequelae were demonstrated with posttraumatic amnesia less than 24 hours in duration.[17] Overall, visuospatial and visual motor skills showed more impairment than verbal skills. Recovery was most rapid in the early months but often continued into the second year after injury. In a related study the incidence of psychiatric sequelae in head-injured children was increased in those with combined severe head injury and psychosocial adversity.[11] The risk was also influenced by the child's preaccident behavior and cognitive level. Within the broad spectrum of psychiatric problems encountered, the only pattern specific to the head-injured group was of marked socially disinhibited behavior. New psychiatric disorders showed a dose-response relationship with the degree of posttraumatic amnesia, the degree of intellectual impairment, and the presence of neurologic abnormalities.

Cognitive remediation is undertaken by psychologists within the overall rehabilitation plan for this group of children. Neuropsychologic assessments attempt to delineate specific areas of deficits. Besides general cognitive ability, areas such as memory, perception, language skills, and visuospatial and visuo-motor skills are evaluated. Memory impairment may be one of the most serious deficits because it impedes the ability to learn and integrate new concepts. Often, improving attention difficulties helps to improve memory. Problem-solving skills are also practiced within a cognitive remediation program. It has not yet been scientifically demonstrated in what way or to what degree cognitive remediation assists in the recovery of these patients.[42] However, in light of the extent to which this population continues to show a wide range of deficits, ongoing monitoring and intervention seems appropriate in the first 1 to 2 years. A study by Fuld and Fisher[28] demonstrated a need for close neuropsychologic follow-up of patients with attention to the stress of returning to school. For children demonstrating continued posttraumatic intellectual impairments, delayed return to a regular school setting may be indicated, as well as adjustment of the school program to limit stress when the child does return. The physiatrist, as coordinator of the inpatient rehabilitative care of these children, must be aware of such needs and work with parents, psychologists, and educators to ensure appropriate postinjury educational settings. Physical, occupational, and speech therapy may be coordinated through school with supplemental therapy as needed on an outpatient or at-home basis.

Five percent of survivors of severe closed head trauma exhibit a persistent vegetative state with no behavioral responses arising from the cortex. Despite having eye movements and prolonged periods of eye opening, these patients show no recognition and do not speak.[29] The physiatrist must play a supportive role for families in such case, helping to arrange either total home care or institutionalized care, recognizing the extreme emotional and financial stress involved in such situations.

CONCLUSION

It is difficult to delineate the practice of pediatric rehabilitation in one chapter. Other major categories of disability, such as neuromuscular diseases and spinal cord injury, are discussed in detail in other chapters. The cornerstone of the practice of pediatric physiatry is the ability to direct appropriate medical and therapeutic decision making based on a full account of the child as a total being. The child's natural setting of family, home, school, and community must be understood and incorporated into the total care plan. The physiatrist's goal is to achieve optimal functioning within the child's abilities and to lessen the disruption that a disease process brings to the child's life.

REFERENCES

1. Badell-Ribera, A: Myelodysplasia. In Molnar, G, editor: Pediatric rehabilitation, Baltimore, 1985, Williams & Wilkins Co.
2. Baldwin, J: Pool therapy compared with individual home exercise therapy for juvenile rheumatoid arthritic patients, Physiotherapy 58:230, 1972.
3. Bax, MCO: Terminology and classification of cerebral palsy, Dev Med Child Neurol 6:295, 1964.
4. Bayley, N: Bayley scales of infant development, New York, 1969, The Psychological Corp.
5. Bobath, K: The motor deficit of patients with cerebral palsy, Clinics in Developmental Medicine no 23, London, 1972, Spastics Society.
6. Bobath, K: A Neurophysiological basis for the treatment of cerebral palsy, Lavenham, Eng, 1980, Spastics International Medical Publications.
7. Boone, JE, Baldwin, J, and Levine, C: Juvenile rheumatoid arthritis, Pediatr Clin North Am 21:885, 1974.
8. Brazelton, TB: Behavioral competence of the newborn infant. In Avery, GB, editor: Neonatology: pathophysiology and management of the newborn, Philadelphia, 1981, JB Lippincott Co.
9. Breakey, AS: Ocular findings in cerebral palsy, Arch Ophthalmol 53:852, 1955.
10. Brewer, EJ, Giannini, EH, and Pearson, DA: Juvenile rheumatoid arthritis, Philadelphia, 1982, WB Saunders Co.
11. Brown, G, et al: A prospective study of children with head injuries. III. Psychiatric sequelae, Psychol Med 11:63, 1981.
12. Burnett, CN, and Johnson, EW: Development of gait in childhood, Dev Med Child Neurol 13:196, 1971.
13. Calabro, JJ, Katz, RM, and Maltz, BA: A critical reappraisal of juvenile rheumatoid arthritis, Clin Orthop Rel Res 74:701, 1971.
14. Capute, AJ, Shapiro, BK, and Palmer, FB: Marking the milestones of language development, Contemp Pediatr 4:4, 1987.
15. Capute, AJ, et al: Primitive reflex profile, Baltimore, 1977, University Park Press.
16. Cassady, G: The small-for-date infant. In Avery, GB, editor: Neonatology: pathophysiology and management of the newborn, Philadelphia, 1981, JB Lippincott Co.
17. Chadwick, O, et al: A prospective study of children with head injuries. II. Cognitive sequelae, Psychol Med 11:49, 1981.
18. Chamovitz, I, et al: Rehabilitative medical management. In Ylvisaker, M, editor: Head injury rehabilitation: children and adolescents, San Diego, 1985, College Hill Press.
19. Cristofaro, RL, and Brink, JD: Hypercalcemia of immobilization in neurologically injured children: a prospective study, Orthopedics 2:485, 1979.
20. Diller, L, et al: Verbal behavior in children with spina bifida. In Swineyard, C, editor: Comprehensive care of the child with spina bifida manifesta, Rehabilitation monograph, New York, 1966, New York Medical Center.
21. Donovan, WH: Physical measures in the treatment of juvenile rheumatoid arthritis, Arthritis Rheum 20:553, 1977.
22. Dubowitz, IMS, Dubowitz, V, and Goldberg, C: Clinical assessment of gestational age in the newborn infant, J Pediatr 77:1, 1970.

23. Ellenberg, JH, and Nelson, KB: Early recognition of infants at high risk for cerebral palsy: examination at age four months, Dev Med Child Neuro 23:705, 1981.

24. Epstein, F: Diagnostic and management of arrested hydrocephalus. In Cohen, MM, editor: Monographs in neural sciences, Basel, 1982, S Karger.

25. Erikson, EH: Childhood and society, New York, 1963, WW Norton.

26. Frankenburg, WK, and Dodds, JB: The Denver Developmental Screening Test, J Pediatr 71:181, 1967.

27. Freud, A: Normality and pathology in childhood: assessment of development, New York, 1965, International Universities Press.

28. Fuld, PA, and Fisher, P: Recovery of intellectual ability after closed head injury, Dev Med Child Neurol 19:495, 1977.

29. Gerring, JP: Psychiatric sequelae of severe closed head injury, Pediatr Rev 8:115, 1986.

30. Gesell, A, et al: The first five years of life, New York, 1940, Harper & Row.

31. Gesell, A, and Ilg, FL: The child from five to ten, New York, 1946, Harper & Row.

32. Golden, GS: Neural tube defects, Pediatr Rev 1:187, 1979.

33. Hall, P, et al: Scoliosis and hydrocephalus in myelocele patients, J Neurosurg 50:174, 1979.

34. Hayden, PW: Adolescents with meningomyelocele, Pediatr Rev 6:245, 1985.

35. Horn, DG, et al: Distractibility and vocabulary deficits in children with spina bifida and hydrocephalus, Dev Med Child Neurol 27:713, 1985.

36. Illingworth, RS: The diagnosic of cerebral palsy in the first year of life, Dev Med Child Neurol 8:178, 1965.

37. Illingworth, RS: The development of the infant and young child, normal and abnormal, Edinburgh, 1975, Churchill-Livingstone.

38. Jennett, B: Epilepsy after non-missile head injuries, ed 2, Chicago, 1975, William Heinemann.

39. Johnson, EW: Examination for muscle weakness in infants and small children, JAMA 168:1306, 1958.

40. Kass, EJ: Current urological management of the child with myelodysplasia, Clin Proc Children's Hospital National Medical Center 38:156, 1982.

41. Kass, EJ, et al: The significance of bacilluria in children on long-term intermittent catheterization, J Urol 126:223, 1981.

42. Kirn, TF: Cognitive rehabilitation aims to improve or replace memory functions in survivors of head injury, JAMA 257:2400, 1987.

43. Knoblock, H, and Pasamanick, B: Gesell and Amatruda's developmental diagnosis: the evaluation and management of normal and abnormal neuropsychologic development of infancy and early childhood, Hagerstown, Md, 1974, Harper & Row.

44. Koch, B: Rehabilitation of the child with joint disease. In Molnar, G, editor: Pediatric rehabilitation, Baltimore, 1985, Williams & Wilkins.

45. Kraus, JF, et al: Incidence, severity, and external causes of pediatric brain injury, Am J Dis Child 140:687, 1986.

46. Levin, HS, Benton, AL, and Grossman, RG: Neurobehavioral consequences of closed head injury, New York, 1982, Oxford University Press.

47. Lowry, GH: Growth and development in children, Chicago, 1975, Year Book Medical Publishers.

48. Mahler, ML: Thoughts about development and individuation, Psychoanal Study Child 18:307, 1963.

49. Mahoney, WJ, et al: Long-term outcome of children with severe head trauma and prolonged coma, Pediatrics 71:756, 1983.

50. Matson, DD: Neurosurgery of infancy and childhood, Springfield, Ill, 1969, Charles C Thomas Publisher.

51. McGraw, MB: Neuromuscular maturation of human infant, New York, 1963, Hafner Press.

52. McLone, DG, et al: Central nervous system infections as a limiting factor in the intelligence of children with myelomeningocele, Pediatrics 70:338, 1982.

53. Menelaus, MB: Progress in the management of the paralytic hip in myelomeningocele, Orthop Clin North Am 11:17, 1980.

54. Milani-Comparetti, A, and Gidoni, EA: Pattern analysis of motor development and its disorders, Dev Med Child Neurol 9:625, 1967.

55. Milani-Comparetti, A, and Gidoni, EA: Routine developmental examination in normal and retarded children, Dev Med Child Neurol 9:631, 1967.

56. Milunsky, A, and Alpert, E: The value of alpha-fetoprotein in the prenatal diagnosis of neural tube defects, J Pediatr 84:889, 1974.

57. Molnar, GE: Cerebral palsy. In Molnar, GE, editor: Pediatric rehabilitation, Baltimore, 1985, Williams & Wilkins.

58. Molnar, G, and Kaminer, R: Growth and development. In Molnar, G, editor: Pediatric rehabilitation, Baltimore, 1985, Williams & Wilkins.

59. Molnar, GE, and Taft, LT: Pediatric rehabilitation. I. Cerebral palsy and spinal cord injuries, Curr Probl Pediatr 7:1, 1977.

60. Nelson, KB, and Ellenberg, JH: Apgar scores as predictors of chronic neurologic disability, Pediatrics 68:36, 1981.

61. Nelson, KB, and Ellenberg, JH: Children who "outgrew" cerebral palsy, Pediatrics 69:529, 1982.

62. Nelson, KB, and Ellenberg, JH: Epidemiology of cerebral palsy. In Schoenberg, BS, editor: Advances in neurology, New York, 1978, Raven Press.

63. Okamoto, T, and Kumamoto, M: Electromyographic study of the learning process of walking in infants, Electromyography 12:149, 1972.

64. Paine, SR, et al: Evolution of postural reflexes in normal infants and in the presence of chronic brain syndromes, Neurology 14:1036, 1964.

65. Peacock, WJ, and Arens, LJ: Selective posterior rhizotomy for the relief of spasticity in cerebral palsy, South Afr Med J 62:119, 1982.

66. Peiper, A: Cerebral function in infancy and childhood, ed 3, New York, 1963, Consultants Bureau.

67. Piaget, J, Inhelder, B: The psychology of the child, New York, 1969, Basic Books.

68. Rosman, NP, and Oppenheimer, EY: Posttraumatic epilepsy, Pediatr Rev 3:221, 1982.

69. Schaller, JG: Juvenile rheumatoid arthritis, Arthritis Rheum 20:165, 1977.

70. Scull, SA, Dow, MB, and Atheya, BH: Physical and occupational therapy for children with rheumatic diseases, Pediatr Clin North Am 33:1053, 1986.

71. Sharrard, WJW: Specific orthopedic problems. In Brocklehurst, G, editor: Spina bifida for the clinician, London, 1976, Spastics International Medical Publications.

72. Starr, A, and Achor, LJ: Auditory brain stem responses in neurological disease, Arch Neurol 32:761, 1975.

73. Statham, L, and Murray, MP: Early walking pattern of normal children, Clin Orthop 78:8, 1971.

74. Sutherland, DH, et al: The development of mature gait, J Bone Joint Surg 62A:336, 1980.

75. Taft, LT: Cerebral palsy, Pediatr Rev 6:35, 1984.

76. Twitchell, TE: Attitudinal reflexes, Phys Ther 45:411, 1965.

77. Twitchell, TE: Normal motor development, Phys Ther 45:419, 1965.

78. Vining, EPG, et al: Cerebral palsy, a pediatric developmentalist's overview, Am J Dis Child 130:643, 1976.

79. White, JJ, et al: A physiologic rationale for the management of neurologic rectal incontinence in children, Pediatrics 49:888, 1972.

CHAPTER 31

Rehabilitation nursing

MARIAN T. MIGNANO

Hickey defines rehabilitation as "a dynamic process in which a disabled person is aided in achieving optimum physical, emotional, psychological, social or vocational potential in order to maintain dignity and self-respect in a life that is as independent and self-fulfilling as possible."[9] Themes central to rehabilitation are restoration to optimal functioning and optimal wellness and a return to an acceptable quality of life, albeit within an altered life-style. In the rehabilitation process the patient and family are treated as the unit of disability. As such, they require the individual and collective inputs of interdisciplinary team members if their needs are to be met effectively.

Rehabilitation nursing occupies a special niche in the fields of rehabilitation and nursing. Through an intertwining of its independent and interdependent realms of practice, rehabilitation nursing becomes a vital force in rehabilitative care for disabled persons. With its development as a specialty area of practice within nursing, rehabilitation nursing has enhanced the nursing discipline and expanded its scope. Both aspects of its unique spheres of influence warrant separate consideration.

SIGNIFICANCE OF NURSING IN REHABILITATION OF DISABLED PATIENTS

As members of a distinct discipline involved in the rehabilitation of disabled patients, rehabilitation nurses have primary responsibility for all aspects of daily patient care. The nurse uses specialized knowledge and understanding to nurture, protect, and foster the growth and development of disabled persons with complex health-care needs. Within the independent realm of practice, the nurse makes nursing decisions that anticipate and prevent the formation of secondary disability and that maintain and promote management of the primary disability. Disuse atrophy, contractures,

pressure sores, and hypostatic pneumonia are preventable occurrences that the nurse guards against by implementing protocols for positioning, body alignment, passive range-of-motion exercises, turning, skin care, pressure relief, and airway patency. Formulating nursing diagnoses that comprehensively address the patient's and family's total needs promotes the development of plans of care that are outcome oriented. Based on initial and ongoing assessments, nursing diagnoses may include alterations in health maintenance, nutritional status, bowel and bladder elimination, activity, sleep and rest, comfort, safety, sensation, perception, self-concept, role relationships, sexuality, and stress tolerance. Each diagnosis leads to a set of nursing interventions that assists the nurse to meet the needs of the patient and family and to develop their abilities to independently carry out specific aspects of care that fall within nursing's purview. Such aspects include bowel and bladder routines, skin care regimens, respiratory care programs, and activity tolerance techniques.

As a core member of the interdisciplinary rehabilitation team, the nurse collaborates and consults with physicians, psychologists, therapists, and other health professionals to achieve the best possible rehabilitation outcomes. The interdisciplinary team approach is one of the hallmarks of practice in the rehabilitation setting. Rusk, a leader in the field of rehabilitation, clearly conveyed this when he wrote,

We learned early that there had to be a total approach—to meet not just the physical needs of the disabled person but also the emotional, social, vocational, and educational needs. The goal was always to teach the client to live the best life possible, taking into consideration the disability but, infinitely more important, the abilities that were left. In other words, one had to treat the "whole person". This responsibility could never be met by a single professional approach; it required a team consisting of a physician, rehabilitation nurse, physical therapist, occupational therapist, social worker, speech pathologist, prosthetist, orthotist, psychologist, recreational therapist, nutritionist, home economist, and other specialists.*

At a basic level the interdisciplinary team approach facilitates coordination and information sharing among the disciplines, and at an advanced level it fosters complex problem solving, interdependence, and accountability as a whole.

Within their interdependent realm of practice, rehabilitation nurses have primary responsibility for daily contacts with the patient and family to ensure that the comprehensive treatment plan is carried out. The nurse takes all the skills the patient has learned in the various therapies, such as physical therapy, occupational therapy, and speech therapy, and helps the patient practice these skills during mealtime, dressing, and toileting. To accomplish this, the rehabilitation nurse must possess in-depth knowledge of the other disciplines' work and an ability to use that knowledge in clinical applications. The nurse communicates with the interdisciplinary team on an hour-to-hour basis to integrate and reinforce their work with patients and families. As a result, skills and abilities are mastered sooner rather than later. Interdependent practice is at its best when it promotes consultation among interdisciplinary team members. The interdisciplinary team is the resource the nurse uses when the usual problem-solving techniques do not achieve desired outcomes. For example, consultation with the occupational therapist on the use of assistive devices may be indicated to help a female paraplegic patient master a self–intermittent catheterization program. Conversely, the rehabilitation nurse acts as a consultant to the interdisciplinary team. An example is a consultation requested by the therapist to determine whether the patient, who has experienced decreased activity tolerance owing to side effects from medication, can withstand therapy. This process of mutual advice and consent ensures ongoing problem solving and effectively uses the distinctive expertise of individual team members within an interdependent perspective.

Interdependent practice evolves into transdisciplinary practice. This is particularly so for the rehabilitation nurse who serves as a vital link for communication flow and exchange among interdisciplinary team members on a daily basis and during regularly scheduled interdisciplinary meetings. Through constant observation and monitoring of the patient's and, by extension, the family's daily physical and emotional progress, the rehabilitation nurse becomes a first-line appraiser of the efficacy of the treatment plan. Because of its transdisciplinary approach, rehabilitation nursing is the "glue" that holds the rehabilitation process together for the patient and family. The nurse interprets the treatment

plan for and with them, identifies any new sources of concern, and brings these back to the interdisciplinary team for problem-solving purposes. Transdisciplinary practice requires that the nurse coordinate care with the discharge plan. The patient and family are encouraged to participate in transitional experiences such as self-care days, self-medication administration, independent living experiences, and therapeutic passes that help ready them for discharge. Referrals to community resources including visiting nurse associations, support groups, and outpatient clinics help guarantee that rehabilitative progress will be sustained and continued after discharge. Thus transdisciplinary rehabilitation nursing not only hastens recovery by maximizing the time spent by patients and families in the rehabilitation setting, but also promotes successful community reintegration through a coordinated discharge planning process that begins at admission and continues long after discharge.

SIGNIFICANCE OF REHABILITATION NURSING TO NURSING DISCIPLINE

While rehabilitation nursing is of primary importance to the field of rehabilitation, it is of equal importance to the field of nursing. In the mid-1970s rehabilitation nursing emerged as a formally recognized specialty area of practice. Through the succeeding years rehabilitation has become a concern of all nurses rather than just that of specialists. By learning about the specialized skills of rehabilitation nurses, nurses working in settings scattered throughout the health care spectrum have expanded their scope of practice. In acute care hospital settings, the patient is often totally dependent on the nurse for maintenance of biologic life processes. During the survival phase of an acute illness there is a need for constant preventive rehabilitative nursing care. On entering the recuperative phase the patient benefits greatly from an active rehabilitation program. In this era of prospective payment systems and shortened hospital stays, the recovery phase frequently takes place in the home care setting. Patients and families need nurses with skills in rehabilitation who can help them progress to self-sufficiency. As the U.S. population ages, many more persons are living with chronic illness and disability. Their needs are handled in ambulatory care settings where there is a growing demand for nurses versed in gerontologic and rehabilitation nursing.

The significance of rehabilitation nursing's contribution to the discipline of nursing must also be viewed from the vantage point of its own professional growth as a specialty. The Association of Rehabilitation Nurses (ARN) was founded in 1974, and its mission has been to "promote and advance professional rehabilitation nursing practice through education, advocacy, and research to enhance the quality of life for those affected by disability."[9] Major purposes of the organization include the following[9]:

1. To advance the quality of nursing service throughout the community

---

*Murray, R, and Kijek, JC, editors: Current perspectives in rehabilitation nursing, St. Louis, 1979, The CV Mosby Co.

2. To offer educational opportunities that promote an awareness of and interest in rehabilitation nursing and improve expertise on all levels
3. To facilitate exchange of ideas in rehabilitation programs

The ARN has established two important mechanisms to ensure that high-quality rehabilitation nursing service is provided to the disabled population. The first mechanism is standards development. The Standards of Rehabilitation Nursing Practice, developed in conjunction with the American Nurses' Association in 1986, identify specific competencies of rehabilitation nurses.[1] These standards serve as the framework for guiding professional practice and professional performance in all types of rehabilitation settings, and they promote accountability on the part of rehabilitation nurses to the public, the profession, and external regulatory bodies, such as the Joint Commission on Accreditation of Hospitals (JCAH) and the Commission on Accreditation of Rehabilitation Facilities (CARF). The second mechanism is the certification process. Certification within the specialty of rehabilitation nursing is a method of self-governance that rehabilitation nurses voluntarily undertake to demonstrate that they have acquired requisite knowledge and expertise in their specialty. Eligibility requirements include at least 2 years of practice in rehabilitation nursing and current registered nurse licensure. Nurses who pass the certification examination are given the title of Certified Rehabilitation Registered Nurse (CRRN), which is deemed a high honor within the rehabilitation nursing community. There are more than 1800 Certified Rehabilitation Registered Nurses nationwide, and the numbers continue to grow.

In 1976 the ARN created the Rehabilitation Nursing Institute (RNI) to act as its educational and research arm. Since its inception the RNI has developed and engaged in educational activities that disseminate information about rehabilitation nursing to nurses working in rehabilitation and nonrehabilitation settings. It has promoted nursing research primarily through awareness raising and secondarily through a proposal review and approval process for grant funding. Some examples of current research include examining how to achieve better compliance with skin care regimens in the spinal cord–injured population[4] and how to identify patients at risk of falling in a rehabilitation center.[6] Although nursing research is still in its infancy, rehabilitation nurses realize that the specialty will continue to identify and develop itself through its scientific research. The ARN also sponsors an annual educational conference and publishes a professional journal, "Rehabilitation Nursing," to keep rehabilitation nurses abreast of developments within the broad field of rehabilitation and within specialized programs throughout the country. Pursuits such as these enable rehabilitation nurses to remain on the cutting edge of using new knowledge and new ideas in their practice settings.

Growth within specialty practice signals growth for the nursing professional as a whole. Similarly, advances within the profession spur the development of specialty practice. One major contribution rehabilitation nursing has made to the discipline of nursing has already been mentioned. Rehabilitative nursing care has become an integral part of nursing's overall service to patients irrespective of setting. On the other hand, the nursing profession has contributed to the rehabilitation nursing specialty through its development of general theories of nursing. Because rehabilitation nursing is eclectic, major constructs from several nursing theories, such as Roy's adaptation model or Orem's self-care theory, have found their way into rehabilitation nurses' application of knowledge in the practice setting. Through this process of constant interchange, the climate within specialty practice and within the profession remains ripe for creative change. The result is improved practice on all levels, and the beneficiaries are patients and their families.

COMPONENTS OF CLINICAL REHABILITATION NURSING

Clinical rehabilitation nursing is a composite of its philosophy, purpose, practice, and art. Its philosophy points the way. Its purpose describes the why and wherefore of its existence. Its practice and art are the what and how of the work rehabilitation nurses do. Each component is woven into the total fabric of clinical rehabilitation nursing, and each must be considered carefully to arrive at a thorough understanding of clinical rehabilitation nursing.

Philosophic principles of rehabilitation nursing

Rehabilitation nursing is governed by a set of philosophic principles that describe values or beliefs about the nature of man and the nurse as helping agent.

Holism

The concept of holism was introduced by Smuts in 1926. He was convinced that evolutionary processes indicated "the gradual development and stratification of progressive series of wholes, stretching from the inorganic beginnings to the highest levels of spiritual creation."[8] Holism has brought the essential unity of man back into focus. It opposed mechanistic views of man as a collection of parts or Cartesian views of man's duality as mind separate from body. Rogers emphatically stated that human beings "are not disembodied entities, nor are they mechanical aggregates. They are identifiable in their totality. They behave as a totality. . . . Man is a unified whole possessing his own integrity and manifesting characteristics that are more than and different from the sum of their parts."[12]

Holistic man has long been the phenomenon central to rehabilitation nursing's concern. Each person is viewed as unique and multidimensional. For the rehabilitation nurse no two hemiplegic patients, or no two spinal cord–injured patients, are exactly alike. Patients bring the totality of their persona to the rehabilitation process, and they require an individualized plan that meets the needs of the "total person." From a holistic perspective, each event in the life process is an opportunity for growth and for developing new strengths:

Great ceramics are not made by putting clay in the sun; they come only from the white heat of the kiln. In the firing process some pieces are broken, but those that survive the heat are transformed from clay into porcelain; and so it is, it seems, with sick, suffering and crippled persons. Those who, through medical skill, opportunity, work and courage, survive their illness or overcome their handicap and take their place back in the world have a depth of spirit that you and I can hardly measure. They have not wasted their pain.*

The nurse who views illness or disability in this way has a golden opportunity to help patients transcend their disabilities by developing new abilities and arriving at new meanings.

Self-care

Orem defines self-care "as the practice of activities that individuals initiate and perform on their own behalf in maintaining life, health, and well-being."[11] Four premises underlie self-care[13]:

1. Self-care demands and self-care activities are always embedded within sociocultural settings. Although self-care activities may vary in different settings, the broad concepts remain universally applicable, and the significance of both the client's and the nurse's sociocultural context is always acknowledged.
2. Self-care responsibilities are assumed by functioning adults for themselves and for those dependent on them. Adults prefer self-care options whenever they are available.
3. Self-care abilities may vary during a lifetime, as do the demands for self-care. A child cannot meet self-care demands but is developing self-care potential; an adult is (potentially) fully able to function as a self-care agent; an old person as clinging to self-care prerogatives but becoming increasingly less able to fulfill them.
4. The greater the ability to perform self-care and meet self-care demands, the greater the level of health and life satisfaction.

Self-care activities meet the needs of the whole person. They include cognitive, social, psychologic, and physical activities, which are interrelated in every individual. By carefully evaluating the person's self-care system, the nurse designs a nursing system that may be wholly compensatory, partly compensatory, or supportive and educative in assisting that person to overcome self-care deficits. The range of potential nursing diagnoses and nursing interventions is far

---

*Rusk, HA: Foreword. In Murray, R, and Kijeck, JC, editors: Current perspectives in rehabilitation nursing, St. Louis, 1979, The CV Mosby Co.

reaching. A nurse's efforts to help disabled persons regain control over self-care activities focus on health promotion.

Optimal wellness

The World Health Organization has defined health as a "state of complete physical, mental and social well-being and not merely the absence of disease or infirmity."[7] Health and overt illness or disability are not static states; state of health is a continuum that ranges from peak wellness to death, as illustrated in Figure 31-1. Most individuals fall somewhere in the middle. Dunn coined the term "high level wellness" in 1959 to describe "an integrated method of functioning which is oriented toward maximizing the potential of which the individual is capable, within the environment where he is functioning."[9] Each person holds the responsibility for attaining his or her wellness. For a disabled person, special consideration is given to overcoming self-care deficits that hinder the achievement of a high level of wellness. Through a process of needs assessment and evaluation of outcomes, the rehabilitation nurse and the interdisciplinary team help the patient regain control of health and wellness through self-care, as diagrammed in Figure 31-2. From a holistic and self-care perspective, health can be defined as "the state of being able to initiate and perform self-care activities which sustain life processes, maintain integrated functioning, promote normal growth and development, and prevent or control disease and disability and their effects."[13] Optimal wellness is the culmination of the rehabilitation process. Rehabilitation is a lifelong, continuous process for disabled individuals, as is the attainment and maintenance of an optimal level of wellness. Whenever a disability progresses in severity, the person's optimal wellness must be redefined and new strategies for achieving control over self-care activities must be mapped out.

Purpose of rehabilitation nursing

Guided by these philosophic beliefs, clinical rehabilitation nurses seek to restore disabled individuals to maximal functioning and maximal wellness. To achieve this, rehabilitation nurses "use themselves as therapeutic tools in active partnership with the disabled or potentially disabled individual and in collaboration with other health care providers to promote health and independence."[9] They assume many different roles in their therapeutic use of self. They are caregivers, coordinators, collaborators, educators, patient advocates, and consultants. The interpersonal process that takes place between the nurse, the patient, and the family is the integrating component that brings these professional nurse roles together and renders them effective. As the patient, family, and other associates come to know the nurse and the nurse comes to know them, an in-depth relationship develops. It gathers in intensity throughout the rehabilitation process and allows the essential caring element in nursing to reach its fullest expression. The nurse generates a comforting sense that needs will be recognized

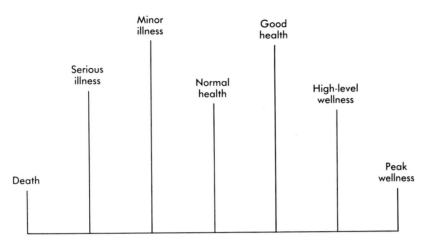

Figure 31-1. Dunn's health-illness continuum. (From Steiger, NJ, and Lipson, JG: Self-care nursing: theory and practice, Bowie, Md, 1985, Brady Communications Co, Inc.)

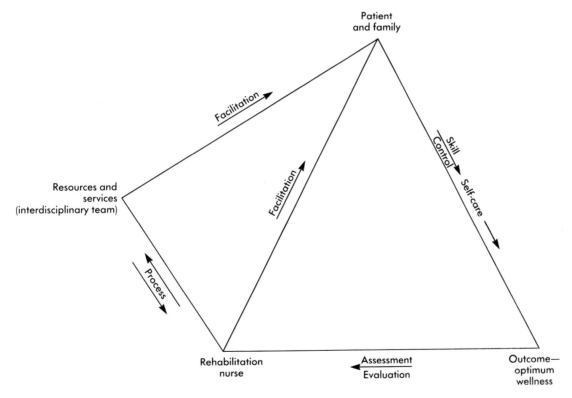

Figure 31-2. Achieving optimum wellness through the rehabilitation process. (Modified from Giese, P, and Davis, A: Rehab Nurs 6:14, 1981.)

and met on a continuing basis. Caring does not mean that the rehabilitation nurse is the sole provider of patient care. Rather, the nurse gently but persistently reinforces the contractual agreement inherent in the rehabilitation model, namely, that the patient and family must become active agents in self-care. In clinical rehabilitation nursing the caring role is barely distinguishable from the teaching role, since every encounter with the patient and family is a teaching encounter in which the nurse helps them assume responsibility for meeting self-care needs. The nurse also provides invaluable support and assistance to the patient and family as they adjust to the consequences of the disability. The patient may be apathetic, anxious, depressed, or angry, and the family may feel insecure or overwhelmed. The nurse, in collaboration with the psychologist and social worker, intervenes to help them cope with the impact of disability. The investment in time and effort is worthwhile because the patient and the family slowly come to realize that there is life after disability. Dramatic cures are rare, but the nurse conveys a sure sense that steady gains will be made and that with everyone's help the patient will return to the community in control of his or her life.

Practice of rehabilitation nursing

The practice of clinical rehabilitation nursing is predicated on the belief that every person is unique, is a member of a family cluster, and has self-care needs that must be met to attain and maintain optimal functioning and optimal wellness. Practice is the skillful use of knowledge to meet identified needs. A model of patient needs in rehabilitation includes the following:

1. Respiratory
2. Personal hygiene and grooming
3. Eating, drinking, and eliminating
4. Mobility and skin care
5. Temperature
6. Cardiovascular
7. Safety
8. Knowledge and achievement
9. Socialization

The aim of practice is to teach the patient and family all they need to know and do to attain independence in self-care. The family's role in this process cannot be overstated. They not only provide the patient with emotional support and encouragement, but often assume responsibility for meeting ongoing rehabilitation needs when severe physical or cognitive impairment exists. Through the teaching process, the nurse steadily relinquishes professional control as the patient and family learn skills and abilities until finally they know more about the patient's care than the nurse does. Specific nursing management strategies help to meet patient and family needs. The following section highlights what clinical rehabilitation nurses do in actual practice.

Nursing management strategies

Respiratory needs. Patients with chronic obstructive pulmonary disease (COPD), spinal cord injury or impairment, traumatic head injury (depending on level of consciousness), and neuromuscular disease may have difficulty breathing. Nursing management strategies are guided by the nature of the disease (obstructive versus restrictive) and the treatment plan devised by the physician. The nurse teaches techniques that promote lung inflation, such as diaphragmatic breathing, assistive cough techniques, incentive spirometry, and intermittent positive-pressure breathing (IPPB) with or without the use of bronchodilators.

Diaphragmatic breathing is a useful technique for a COPD patient who needs to increase expansion and emptying of the lungs. This technique becomes routine and automatic with regular practice and is relatively easy to perform. Assistive cough techniques, such as the one-handed abdominal thrust or the two-handed lateral thrust, are part of the daily respiratory care maintenance program for all spinal cord–impaired patients who have lesions affecting the major ventilatory muscles. If the patient has a tracheostomy or an acute respiratory infection, the nurse may carry out assistive cough as often as every 2 hours in addition to periodic suctioning. Nurses use incentive spirometry as a necessary adjunct to daily respiratory care when inspiratory volume is decreased. The patient may initially find it difficult to raise the flow rate indicator to the prescribed level but becomes proficient in deep inhalations with practice. Outcomes for the patient include prevention of atelectasis and increased vital capacity. The physician may prescribe IPPB with bronchodilators. The nurse cautions a patient to keep exhalations relaxed and passive during IPPB sessions and to cough periodically to raise pooled secretions. Since certain bronchodilators alter the heart rate, the nurse monitors the patient's pulse rate closely during each treatment for signs of intolerance.

A nursing plan of care for daily respiratory maintenance includes patient and family instruction in adequate hydration so secretions remain liquified; fluid intakes of 2000 to 3000 ml are recommended provided there are no contraindications. Frequent changes of position when in bed and a schedule for time out of bed are important to promote loosening of secretions and drainage of different segments of the lungs. The patient is instructed in signs and symptoms of respiratory changes, such as elevated temperature, increased respiratory rate, decreased performance in incentive spirometry, or change in the color of secretions. The patient is also cautioned to avoid exposure to risk factors that predispose to respiratory complications, such as smoking or exposure to persons with a respiratory infection.

Personal hygiene and grooming needs. A personal hygiene program is a requirement for all persons regardless of type of disability. A daily bath or shower with a mild soap guards against the effects of heat and moisture buildup on the skin. Shower times are scheduled to comply with the patient's preference. Energy conservation must also be considered. An elderly patient may benefit more from an evening shower so maximal energy levels are available during the day. Specific bathing aids, such as bath benches, shower and commode chairs, Rifton bath chairs for the pediatric population, or shower stretchers are selected and used depending on the patient's functional disability. The Rifton bath chair keeps a young child in a comfortable and secure position during a bath. The shower stretcher is particularly useful for a spinal cord–injured patient who is not ready to assume an upright position. Additional assistive devices, such as long-handled brushes and wash mitts, may be needed. Since the patient and family require consistent instruction and practice with items they will use in the home environment, appropriate selection is an important part of the care plan.

Occupational therapists play a key role in introducing specific techniques for meeting patients' bathing, grooming, and dressing needs. Communication between the nurse and the occupational therapist is essential to ensure that the nurse reinforces skills acquired by the patient. If a patient with a left hemiplegia is being taught one-handed technique for dressing the upper body, the patient should practice this each morning with the nurse standing by to provide cues as necessary. The same process is followed with the lower extremity dressing technique until the patient is able to function independently in the entire operation.

Eating, drinking, and elimination needs. Many patients enter the rehabilitation setting in a nutritionally weakened state. Trauma, surgery, disease, or superimposed infections can exact significant nutritional tolls on disabled patients. As metabolic demands are increased, the body's reserves of protein, fats, and vitamins is depleted. Dysphagia and self-feeding deficits may lead to further nutritional losses. Since rehabilitation necessitates tremendous outlays of energy, active participation is not possible for patients whose nutritional deficits are allowed to continue uncorrected. Returning patients to optimal nutrition levels requires the collaborative efforts of interdisciplinary team members.

The nurse, physician, and nutritionist work closely together to assess the patient's nutritional status. Actual body weight in relation to ideal body weight, real food and fluid intake, current energy requirements, and laboratory values are carefully considered before an action plan is determined. In some instances the patient is placed on a high-protein, high-calorie diet coupled with nutritional instruction. The nurse uses calorie counts, intake and output records, and interim weights to monitor the patient's daily nutritional status. If oral intake falls precipitously below basic requirements or if weight loss is unabated, a combination of oral and enteral feedings is started. Establishing a time for enteral feedings that is least disruptive to the patient's daily rehabilitation program is an important consideration. For this reason the nurse often administers enteral feedings overnight and discontinues them in the early morning. Checking for correct tube placement before initiating the feeding, monitoring stomach residuals for absorption rates, and observing for signs and symptoms of intolerance such as diarrhea, abdominal distention, flatulence, and nausea are part of the nurse's plan of care while the patient remains on enteral feedings.

Many patients with mechanical swallowing impairments require a dysphagia program to meet their special needs. In most rehabilitation settings these programs are administered jointly by the nurse, nutritionist, occupational therapist, and speech therapist. The nurse reinforces nutritional instruction with the patient and family; the rationale for avoiding water and thin liquids and for selecting foods of a certain consistency is reviewed. Thick shakes and nectars are kept on hand to maintain adequate fluid intake, and medications are crushed to facilitate swallowing. The patient is instructed to eat all meals in high-Fowler's position and to remain upright for 30 minutes after eating to prevent aspiration of food and fluid. The nurse monitors patient tolerance to pureed foods and recommends advancing the diet to mechanical soft when appropriate. The nursing care plan incorporates teaching accomplished in occupational therapy and speech therapy. With the nurse's assistance and guidance, the patient practices self-feeding techniques, with or without the use of upper limb assistive devices and tongue movement skills, during mealtimes.

Patients with spinal cord injury, multiple sclerosis, spina bifida, stroke, diabetic neuropathies, and head injury often require a detailed plan of care to meet their elimination needs. Neurologic, neuromuscular, cognitive, and perceptual impairments are taken into account before a nursing management strategy is chosen. The goal is to promote bladder and bowel elimination in a way that gives the patient as much control and independence over these vital functions as possible.

Initially the nurse may assume total responsibility for meeting a patient's bladder management needs. Intermittent catheterizations are usually carried out every 4 hours if the patient is unable to void spontaneously. To avoid overdistending the bladder, the catheterization schedule must not permit more than 600 ml of urine to accumulate at any one time. The nurse balances fluid intake and output over a 24-hour period, and the catheterization schedule is advanced to catheterization every 6 or 8 hours based on the patient's elimination patterns. Often the nurse increases daytime fluid intake and limits evening fluid intake to avoid interrupting the patient's sleep for catheterization. If spontaneous voiding does occur, the nurse checks the patient for residual urine levels. When these consistently fall below 100 ml, intermittent catheterization can be discontinued. For many patients, spontaneous voiding does not signal a return of control over urinary function but simply a return of reflex bladder activity. A male patient can learn to capitalize on this by using an external urinary collecting device such as a condom catheter attached to a leg bag to contain the flow of urine as the bladder reflexively empties. A female patient is less fortunate, since external collecting devices are less suited to the female anatomy; thus intermittent catheterizations must remain the primary method of bladder management. If the patient's physiologic control over bladder function is not impaired, a voiding schedule may help to restore continence.

Discharge planning for a patient with urinary impairment poses a distinct challenge for the nurse because of the type and extent of the problem and the suitability of the plan to the home, work, and social situation. The nurse encourages the patient and family to participate in final decisions; often they need to learn about more than one management technique. For example, an intermittent catheterization schedule may have to be interrupted by placement of an indwelling Foley catheter during a social occasion when no bathroom is available. Once a plan is selected, the nurse provides adequate time for practice sessions with the patient and family. A male patient may need to learn clean intermittent catheterization technique and how to apply and care for an external urinary collecting device. Identifying when and how to irrigate his bladder may be part of the plan. Recognizing signs and symptoms of urinary tract infection such as cloudy, foul-smelling urine and an elevated temperature is part of the learning process. Adequate hydration and a careful balance of intake and output are stressed. The patient and family should be told that over-the-counter medications such as Sudafed and cold remedies can affect a bladder management routine. The patient should preview urinary equipment supplies for clean intermittent catheterization to ensure appropriate selection for home use, such as prepackaged catheterization kits or plastic sound catheters for clean intermittent catheterization.

Bowel management routines are required for control of constipation, diarrhea, and incontinence resulting from neurogenic or cognitive and perceptual impairments. Certain basic strategies are used in all instances regardless of the problem. A key strategy is to attempt to normalize bowel function by establishing a consistent evacuation time. The patient is instructed to take advantage of the gastrocolic and duodenocolic reflexes, which generate propulsive mass movements throughout the large intestine within 30 minutes of a meal; toileting half an hour after eating promotes bowel elimination. The routine should coincide with the patient's preference, for example, each day after breakfast or after supper. Fluid intakes of 2000 to 2500 ml per day, dietary adjustments, and a daily activity program are other assistive modalities included in each patient's plan of care. Adding bulk and fiber to the diet via consumption of whole grains and fresh fruits and vegetables and administering stool softeners and mild stimulants can help to correct constipation. Diarrhea can usually be controlled with diet and antidi-

arrheal agents, but causes such as fecal impaction must be ruled out. Neurogenic bowel dysfunction may be reflexic or areflexic. A patient with the reflexic type can be helped to avoid bowel accidents primarily through the establishment of a daily habit time. Patients are taught to excite a reflex response by inserting a finger into the external rectal sphincter. If this is ineffective, it should be followed by insertion of a suppository. Assistive devices such as digital stimulators and suppository inserters are used as necessary to help the patient regain independence in bowel management. Some patients can progress to an alternate-day routine, since they learn to determine the adequacy of stool volume after daily evacuation. The patient is cautioned not to change the timing of a bowel routine, since the body takes 3 to 5 days to adjust to the change and additional problems such as constipation or fecal impaction may result. A neurogenic areflexic bowel often causes continuous oozing of stool. To prevent this, the nurse instructs the patient to avoid medications except those that add bulk so the stool remains firm. A patient with strong abdominal muscles can use them to advantage by bearing down during evacuation and then manually disimpacting the stool. A disinhibited patient who is cognitively impaired requires direction and assistance to toilet at the same time each day. Patients and families are taught to follow the specific protocol and cautioned to avoid changes in diet, fluid intake, medications, and activity. They learn that bowel accidents are exceptions to the rule and can be avoided. Instructions in preventing constipation, impaction, and diarrhea and the causes and solutions to the problems, should they arise, complete the educational program provided by the nurse.

Mobility and skin care needs. Prolonged inactivity causes profound physiologic and biochemical changes in practically all of the body's organs and systems.[7] To prevent the deleterious consequences of immobility, such as muscle atrophy, osteoporosis, phlebothrombosis, decreased ventilatory expansion and perfusion, renal lithiasis, and pressure sores, the nurse devises a preventive maintenance program that begins when the patient is admitted to the rehabilitation setting. Turning and positioning schedules, sitting tolerance routines, range-of-motion exercises, and pressure relief techniques are important components of such a program.

Turning is initially carried out as frequently as every 2 hours, and adjustments to this schedule are made gradually. If there is no visible hyperemic skin response to a 2-hour turning schedule, lying time is increased by half-hour increments to a maximum of 4 hours in any one position. Proper positioning in bed follows the principles of correct body alignment with special attention to the position of the head, neck, trunk, and extremities. Halo devices for patients with cervical injuries increase mobility without disturbing spinal alignment during position changes. As recovery progresses, patients are mobilized as soon as possible to an out-of-bed sitting routine. The nurse collaborates with the physician and the physical therapist to increase the patient's sitting tolerance while minimizing any adverse physiologic responses. For example, a spinal cord–injured patient first receives a careful trial in tilt position with monitoring for signs and symptoms of orthostatic hypotension. Tilt position is advanced slowly until the patient is able to tolerate a fully upright position. The nurse continually assesses proper positioning during out-of-bed activities. Lap boards or arm boards may provide needed support for a hemiplegic patient's affected side. Elevated leg rests may be required to decrease edema and pain in the lower extremities. In time the nurse teaches the patient to recognize abnormal posture and to make self-corrections. A range-of-motion exercise program can be set up with the physician and physical therapist to maintain joint mobility and prevent contractures. Patients with increased spasticity may require leg and hand splints. The nurse uses pressure-relieving devices to disperse pressure evenly over the body part or to protect the patient from shearing and friction injuries. Most patients with disorders of sensation and movement require a combination of two types of pressure relief devices, such as waterbeds, cushions, silica foam pads, eggcrate mattresses, sheepskins, and heel and elbow protectors. These protective aids are important adjuncts to the plan of care but are not substitutes for frequent changes of position.

Impaired mobility is intimately tied to skin breakdown. The nurse instructs the patient and family in the reasons for pressure sore formation, signs of development, stages of ulcer formation, and measures for prevention. The patient and family are taught to carry out a daily skin care maintenance program that includes skin inspection. The patient must check pressure zones along all bony prominences each day for signs of unremitting erythema. Should this occur, the patient is warned to eliminate all pressure on that site until normal skin tone returns. Regular position changes, particularly when the patient is in a wheelchair, are also necessary. The patient can be taught to do wheelchair push-ups and to slightly shift body weight every 2 hours. Discharge planning includes instruction in pressure relief devices the patient will use at home. Clothing that can cause shearing injuries should be avoided. Instructions in daily skin hygiene and adequate food and fluid intake complete the program of daily skin care maintenance.

Temperature regulation needs. Abnormal elevation or lowering of a patient's temperature is often a warning sign that an infectious process has started. During the time that the infection is not controlled by medication, the nurse strives to return the temperature to normal or near-normal levels by cooling or warming techniques. Febrile states can be managed with tepid alcohol sponge baths, antipyretic agents, and hypothermia blankets. Abnormally low temperatures require extra coverings over the patient and the administration of warm fluids; occasionally hyperthermia blankets are needed. Patients and families are instructed in recording the temperature accurately, and the patient should know his or her normal temperature. Discharge planning

requires that the nurse instruct the patient and family in early warning signs and symptoms of an infection and that a plan be made to secure medical assistance when an infection is present. Prevention is the best course, and instruction should focus on measures most applicable to the patient's disability, such as avoiding exposure to others with an active infection, careful skin hygiene and skin inspection, and adequate hydration to flush the urinary tract.

Temperature regulation is especially challenging in patients with injury at a high level of the spinal cord. These patients are poikilothermic in response to environmental extremes of heat and cold. Exploring the environment for contributory factors is an important part of the care plan when these patients are hyperthermic or hypothermic. If a patient has an elevated temperature, the nurse may administer cool fluids in ample quantities, decrease room temperature, and remove layers of clothing. Sponging with cool water or hypothermia blankets may be added if the temperature is grossly elevated. For subnormal temperatures, the nurse may give warm fluids, add extra blankets, and decrease room temperature. If these measures fail, an underlying infection has to be ruled out. Teaching the patient and family to take an accurate temperature and to develop an action plan that prevents or corrects the poikilothermic response are musts. Controlling room temperatures in the home is stressed so body temperature is maintained at normal levels. Leisure activities are explored to assist the patient to pursue these wisely without untoward effects. For example, a patient who expects to be in the warm sun for an extended period needs to increase the intake of cool fluids and keep clothing to a minimum. For watching cold weather sports such as football, the patient should dress warmly and drink hot fluids periodically throughout the game. The patient and family must be on the alert for changes in mentation, which are warning signs of alterations in body temperature. Restlessness or irritability may indicate a rise in temperature, whereas decreased alertness or drowsiness may signal a drop in temperature. The patient and family learn to check the environment for contributory factors and make necessary adjustments. Preparation for discharge includes a plan to secure medical assistance if the temperature abnormality persists despite modifications in environmental control.

Cardiovascular needs. Cardiovascular dysfunction is commonly encountered among patients treated in the rehabilitation setting. Diagnoses such as congestive heart failure, coronary artery disease, dysrhythmias, peripheral vascular disease, diabetes mellitus, stroke, and spinal cord injury require astute medical and nursing management if patients are to successfully undergo an active rehabilitation program and avoid complications such as venous stasis, fluid overload, and hypotensive or hypertensive episodes.

The control of venous stasis includes the application of thromboembolic stockings or Ace wraps, joint range-of-motion exercises, and elevation of the foot of the bed or of leg rests. The patient is carefully fitted with antiembolic stockings and instructed in proper application. Rolling them down or bunching them up locally constricts blood flow and increases stasis rather than correcting it. Antiembolic pneumatic compression devices may be prescribed and used overnight to prevent venous stasis in particularly susceptible patients. If anticoagulant therapy is ordered, it should be administered at the same time each day or spaced evenly throughout the day to keep blood levels constant. Patients should be taught to recognize signs of toxic levels, such as easy bruisability, bleeding from the gums, hematuria, or tarry stools, and to report these immediately.

Fluid overload can be averted by carefully following a regimen of prescribed medication and monitoring the patient's weight. The patient is instructed to correlate abnormal overnight weight gain, usually of 3 pounds or more, with increased fluid retention. Initially the patient may be weighed daily before breakfast and then once or twice a week as the weight becomes controlled by medication. The presence of pedal or sacral edema and symptoms of dyspnea on exertion are also carefully monitored and reported promptly to the physician. The activity schedule must promote cardiac function and decrease stress. The patient learns to pace activities within the limits of endurance. Alternating periods of rest with periods of activity provides a healthy balance.

Postural or orthostatic hypotension can occur as a sequela to prolonged bed rest, treatment with antihypertensive or antidepressant medications, or spinal cord injury. In all instances the key to minimizing the blood pressure decrease that occurs with position change is to change the patient's position slowly. A patient who has been on prolonged bed rest dangles the legs over the side of the bed first before transferring to a chair; if the patient's pulse rate and blood pressure remain stable and there is no dizziness or faintness, the nurse proceeds with the transfer. Patients receiving medications that cause orthostatic hypotension can be taught to avoid abrupt changes in position by slowly changing from a supine to a sitting position and from a sitting to a standing position. The patient's equilibration is checked by taking the blood pressure after the position change and comparing it to the patient's baseline measurement. Spinal cord–injured patients with a tendency to develop postural hypotension require slowly progressive elevation before a ninety-degree sitting position is achieved. The patient is readied by raising the head of the bed to the prescribed level at least 15 minutes before transfer to a wheelchair. Thromboembolic stockings are applied to increase venous return, and an abdominal binder is used to support the abdominal musculature. A reclining wheelchair with elevated foot pedals is selected because it maintains the patient at the proper angle and can be tipped back to help resolve orthostatic symptoms should they occur. Throughout the process there is careful monitoring of the patient's blood pressure, pulse rate, respirations, and subjective complaints as the angle of the sitting position is gradually increased to a fully upright one; explaining the rationale for slowly increasing tilt position helps to allay the patient's and family's anxieties. They are carefully instructed in signs and symptoms of a hypotensive response and the interventions that correct it.

Hypertension is most often controlled with medication or a combination of medication and diet and is monitored by frequent determinations of blood pressure and elicitation of subjective complaints. In a patient with high spinal cord injury, autonomic dysreflexia may pose a special threat and may lead to stroke if it is not brought under prompt control. Stimuli that precipitate a dysreflexic response, such as bladder distention, fecal impaction, renal calculi, and pressure sores, must be eliminated or at least minimized. The acute episode is a serious emergency in which nursing intervention is a first order of response. Although symptoms vary, most patients complain of a throbbing headache and have highly elevated blood pressures. An attempt should be made to identify the source of the noxious stimulus. Catheterizing the patient may be required to relieve bladder distention. Bladder irrigation may be indicated if there is reason to suspect that urinary flow is blocked. Fecal impactions may be present and should be quickly relieved by disimpaction. Restoration of proper positioning can alleviate pressure on decubitus ulcers. A decrease in symptoms and a return to baseline blood pressure levels indicates that the crisis is over. Because autonomic dysreflexia is a frightening occurrence, the patient and family need to acquire sufficient knowledge and skill to deal with it. They must be taught what autonomic dysreflexia is, how to prevent it, how to recognize signs and symptoms of it, and what actions alleviate it. Practice sessions with the nurse standing by to provide guidance and expert advice are useful, since the patient and family must be prepared to take calm, quick action during this emergency situation.

Safety needs. Meeting the safety needs of patients is a pressing concern for nurses caring for disabled individuals. Disorders of movement, sensation, communication, perception, and cognition are prevalent and require that the nurse maintain constant vigilance over patients to protect them from harm. Specially designed protective protocols assist with accident prevention, particularly patient falls, and promote safe management of confused or agitated patients. These strategies form part of a larger plan designed by the nurse, physician, physical therapist, occupational therapist, speech therapist, and psychologist to assist patients who have multiple impairments that compromise safety.

Patients in rehabilitation centers are vulnerable because they exhibit many of the conditions and factors associated with falling. These include disorientation, physical handicaps, urinary and bladder impairments, and increased age. These patients also have complicating factors such as poor vision, cardiac disorders, ataxia, and hypotension.[6] Active assistance with transfer activities is important in preventing patient falls. An impulsive patient needs frequent reminders to call for assistance before attempting a transfer from bed to chair. Both side rails may have to be kept up when the patient is in bed, and a protective vest restraint secured around the patient when out of bed to limit impulsive movements. Clearance by the appropriate team members is a requirement before patients are deemed safe to perform transfers unaided. Since most patients are confined to wheelchairs, proper selection is an important consideration. Antitipping devices, reversible seat belts (secured in back of the patient), and long-handled brakes are necessary safety aids for many patients. Patients and family members learn to perform wheelchair activities safely so accidents such as tipping too far backward or leaning too far forward are avoided. Clutter in patients' rooms and hallways is kept to a minimum so pathways remain unobstructed. The nurse rearranges room furniture frequently so important articles are within easy view and reach of patients. Planning for home safety is equally important. The patient needs to learn what to do in case of a fall at home when unattended. If the patient is alone for extended periods, the purchase of an electronic safety call-in system may be warranted. If this is beyond the patient's resources, a schedule of daily visits at planned times by neighbors or friends may be the best substitute.

Patients with disorders of tactile sensation require a plan that protects them against skin surface injuries that may occur after brief exposure to extremes of heat and cold. Teaching the patient to test water temperature of a bath or shower with a bath thermometer may be included in the instructional program. The patient learns to handle hot and cold fluids carefully during mealtimes. Assistive eating devices may be needed for safe consumption of food and fluids. Patients are cautioned to allow hot fluids to cool off or cold ones to warm up and to use protective bibs during eating to catch and absorb any spillage.

Cognitively impaired patients require a set routine, simple instructions, repetition, and memory aids to maintain and promote safety. Large, brightly colored appointment calendars can be posted at the patient's bedside and taken to therapy sessions to decrease confusion and forgetfulness. Smaller versions can be secured to the arm of the patient's wheelchair along with the patient's name and room location so personnel can assist in transit to and from class. For patients who exhibit periods of agitation and combativeness, measures such as decreasing sensory input, removing environmental hazards, and placing the patient in a quiet area for short intervals help to restore calm and provide for patient safety. Specific behavioral management techniques can be devised in collaboration with the psychologist. Family members are instructed in the significance of the impairment and in techniques to improve the patient's functioning. The family may need extra support if the patient may be unsafe and cannot be left alone for any prolonged period during waking hours. In such cases, the nurse develops strategies

that provide for adequate "relief" periods for family members so their own health is not compromised.

Knowledge and achievement needs. Ongoing patient and family education and recognition of gains made in meeting self-care needs are prominent aspects of daily nursing practice. At New York University Medical Center's Rusk Institute of Rehabilitation Medicine, the nurse encourages patient and family participation in two additional modalities, the Self-Medication Program and the Patient-Family Education Program, to enhance knowledge and promote decision making and effective planning and management of self-care.

The Self-Medication Program, which places the patient in control of his or her own medication administration, is not suitable for every individual. The greatest limiting factor is mental status rather than physical impairment. For those who meet the criteria, the nurse explains the program and monitors their performance after they pass a pretest administered by the pharmacist. The nurse and pharmacist share teaching responsibilities regarding purpose, dosage, and side effects of the medications prescribed. Each patient is supplied with a self-medication record, but it remains the nurse's responsibility to monitor compliance and inform the patient of changes in the medication regimen. One of the most difficult aspects for patients to master is adhering to established administration times. This becomes easier when administration times are selected to coincide with the patient's home schedule, but consistent reinforcement remains important. As the patient develops an indepth knowledge of the medication therapy, changes in dosage and frequency of administration are more easily incorporated.

The Patient-Family Education Program consists of a series of formal classes on specific topics that are presented to patients and families in a group setting. Three distinct series—stroke, spinal cord injury, and skin inspection and pressure sore prevention—have been developed. Each series includes six to 10 sessions. Teaching responsibilities are interdisciplinary; the patient education coordinator, staff nurses, pharmacist, and nutritionist share responsibility for instruction. Although the primary emphasis is on preventive management, the sessions also facilitate group interaction to enhance problem-solving skills. Peer and family support becomes evident as questions arise and discussion ensues relevant to patient and family needs. Standardized content and methods ensure that a basic amount of information is conveyed during each session. The Patient-Family Education Program has met with great success in our setting. It is an important adjunct to the informal teaching sessions that occur daily between the nurse and the patient and family, and establishes health-promoting behaviors as patients and families learn to adapt and adjust to the disability.

Socialization needs. Disability brings with it many losses, depending on the severity of the impairment. Patients may experience loss of a body part, loss of body function, role changes, and life-style changes. An initial period of grieving is expected, and patients often withdraw into themselves and away from others during this time. Once a patient starts to make gains in skill acquisition and achieves some measure of success in self-care activities, he or she begins to take fresh interest in the world. The nurse capitalizes on this by encouraging the patient and family to participate in diversional activities as a part of their daily schedule and to begin to explore community resources that will be of interest to them when the patient is discharged. Participation in activities sponsored by the therapeutic recreation department, such as cooking activities, photography workshops, and trips to special events, reinforces the patient's developing skills and abilities. By attending events outside the rehabilitation setting, the patient has the opportunity to be seen in a wheelchair and to test the responses of nondisabled individuals. The patient can start to work through feelings about being a part of a minority group of disabled persons. Brainstorming sessions are encouraged because they allow the nurse time to explore socialization plans with the patient and family. Dining out, attending social gatherings, using public transportation, joining support groups, and pursuing educational or leisure pursuits are examples of topics discussed during such sessions. Patients and family members have the opportunity to share their worst fears and to assist with planning strategies that promote healthy socialization. Whenever possible, the patient and family are urged to try out these activities throughout the patient's hospital stay. For example, a day pass on the weekend may be used to dine out in a favorite restaurant. Handling transport to and from the restaurant, checking for accessibility of bathroom facilities, and arranging for comfortable wheelchair seating are planned in advance. Outcomes of the experience are evaluated, and if there were pitfalls, the plan is reformulated and tried again on a later pass.

Art of rehabilitation nursing

Against this background of what rehabilitation nurses do in actual practice, is the added dimension of how they do it that captures the art of nursing. Defining this final component completes the description of clinical rehabilitation nursing. By its very nature, the art of nursing is subtle, ephemeral, and yet essential. Without it the tapestry is incomplete.

Art is the application of knowledge and skill to bring about desired results.[14] Weidenbach described the art of nursing as a helping process, and she stated that "the secret of the helping art, however, lies in the importance the nurse attaches to her thoughts and feelings and the deliberative use she makes of them as she observes her patient, identifies his need-for-help, ministers to his need and validates that the help she gave was helpful.[14] In time and with experience the rehabilitation nurse is able to fine-tune this helping ability and quality of caring. As described by Benner, "expert human decision makers bring a deep background understanding to the situation, so that they can grasp the whole

and attend to the most salient aspects. They do this by sharing in the meanings embedded in the situation."[2] An excerpt from her book *From Novice to Expert* clearly illustrates this point. The encounter described takes place between an experienced nurse and an elderly female patient. The patient, who has sustained a stroke, is noticeably depressed over the weakness of her right hand and has refused to go to physical therapy.

Expert Nurse: I just sat down and listened and talked to her. I did not say that I wanted her to go to physical therapy, but that was my intention. I said to her that she was showing some progress. "Think about two days ago: today you can move your fingers a little bit more. You have made progress because of the exercise. If you keep doing these exercises, I expect that you will be able to have more use of your hands." I encouraged her—pointing out the positive things because she was only zeroing in on the negative things and looking at how much she didn't have. . . . I just went through all the things that I hadn't seen the day before. After our talk she went to physical therapy.*

The expert nurse grasped the meaning behind the patient's refusal, acted on it, and succeeded in achieving a positive health outcome for this patient.

"The nurse's art brings with it a gentle power, a sense of autonomy and a commitment to facilitate health. In particular it brings a renewed awareness of the special way in which human caring is intrinsic in nursing practice."[3] Artful practice is not only a helping process; it is a healing process that brings about transformative changes. By establishing a one-to-one relationship with the patient and family, the nurse helps them meet identified needs, incorporate new knowledge, master new skills and abilities, and arrive at new meanings. The transition from disability to optimal wellness and from dependence to optimal independence is not easy, but with artful nursing as a mainstay, it reaches fruition permeated by a sense of human caring.

Through the practice of its art and emerging science, rehabilitation nursing plays a singular role in the care of disabled persons. This role will certainly become more critical and more complex in the years ahead as the ranks of the disabled increase, the health care marketplace changes, and the health care dollar shrinks. England predicted that the current labor intensiveness of the comprehensive rehabilitation team may "no longer be practical . . . and the result may be new kinds of rehabilitation professionals, perhaps including 'supertherapists' whose skills cross current disciplinary boundaries."[5] Whatever the challenges, it is certain that rehabilitation nursing will be responsive to them as it fulfills its mission to provide expert care for the disabled and potentially disabled members of society.

---

*Benner, P: From novice to expert, Menlo Park, Calif, 1984, Addison-Wesley Publishing Co, p 48.

REFERENCES

1. American Nurses' Association and Association of Rehabilitation Nurses: Standards of rehabilitation nursing practice, Kansas City, Mo, 1986, American Nurses' Association.
2. Benner, P: From novice to expert, Menlo Park, Calif, 1984, Addison-Wesley Publishing Co.
3. Connell, M-T: Feminine consciousness and the nature of nursing practice: a historical perspective. In Topics in clinical nursing, Rockville, Md, 1983, Aspen Systems Corp.
4. Dai, Y-T, and Catanzaro, M: Health beliefs and compliance with a skin care regimen, Rehab Nurs 12:13, 1987.
5. England, B, editor: Medical rehabilitation services in health care institutions, Chicago, Ill, 1986, American Hospital Publishing, Inc.
6. Grant, J, and Hamilton, S: Falls in a rehabilitation center: a retrospective and comparative analysis, Rehab Nurs 12:74, 1987.
7. Kottke, FJ, Stillwell, GR, and Lehmann, JF, editors: Krusen's handbook of physical medicine and rehabilitation, Philadelphia, 1982, WB Saunders Co.
8. Krieger, D: Foundations for holistic health nursing practices, Philadelphia, 1981, JB Lippincott Co.
9. Mumma, C, editor: Rehabilitation nursing: concepts and practice, a core curriculum, ed 2, Evanston, Ill, 1987, Rehabilitation Nursing Foundation.
10. Murray, R, and Kijek, JC, editors: Current perspectives in rehabilitation nursing, St. Louis, 1979, The CV Mosby Co.
11. Orem, D: Nursing: concepts of practice, ed 3, New York, 1985, McGraw-Hill Book Co.
12. Rogers, M: An introduction to the theoretical basis of nursing, Philadelphia, 1970, FA Davis Co.
13. Sullivan, T: Self-care model for nursing. In New directions for nursing in the '80s, Kansas City, Mo, 1980, American Nurses' Association.
14. Weidenbach, E: Clinical nursing: a helping art, New York, 1964, Springer Publishing Co, Inc.

ADDITIONAL READINGS

Anna, D, et al: Implementing Orem's conceptual framework, J Nurs Admin 8:8, 1978.

Bondy, K: Developing a research base for practice, Rehab Nurs 8:9, 1983.

Caplan, A, et al: Ethical and policy issues in rehabilitation medicine, Hastings Center Report, Special Supplement, New York, 1987, The Hastings Center.

Chaska, N, editor: The nursing profession: a time to speak, New York, 1983, McGraw-Hill Book Co.

Chinn, PL, and Jacobs, MK: Theory and nursing, a systematic approach, St. Louis, 1983, The CV Mosby Co.

Doheny, M, et al: The discipline of nursing, East Norwalk, Conn, 1987, Appleton & Lange.

Earnhardt, J, and Frye, B: Understanding autonomic dysreflexia, Rehab Nurs 9:28, 1984.

Granger, C, Seltzer, G, and Fishbein, CF: Primary care of the functionally disabled, Philadelphia, 1987, JB Lippincott Co.

Gee, Z, and Passarella, P. Nursing care of the stroke patient, Pittsburgh, 1985, AREN Publications.

Giese, P, and Davis, A: The role of the nurse clinician in a rehabilitation outpatient setting, Rehab Nurs 6:14, 1981.

Hickey, J: The clinical practice of neurological and neurosurgical nursing, Philadelphia, 1981, JB Lippincott Co.

Illis, LI, Sedgwick, EM, and Glanville, HJ, editors: Rehabilitation of the neurological patient, Boston, 1982, Blackwell Scientific Publications.

Knust, S, et al: Integration of self-care theory with rehabilitation nursing, Rehab Nurs 8:26, 1983.

Martin, N, Holt, N, and Hicks, D, editors: Comprehensive rehabilitation nursing, New York, 1981, McGraw-Hill Book Co.

Maloney, M: Professionalization of nursing, Philadelphia, 1986, JB Lippincott Co.

Matthews, P, and Carlson, C: Spinal cord injury, a guide to rehabilitation nursing (Rehabilitation Institute of Chicago procedure manual), Rockville, Md, 1987, Aspen Publishers, Inc.

Orem, D: A concept of self-care for the rehabilitation client, Rehab Nurs 10:33, 1985.

Pires, M: Rehabilitation nursing—a special role, Headlines 1:1, 1987.

Robinson, J, editor: Coping with neurological problems proficiently, a nursing skillbook, Springhouse, Penn, 1982, Intermed Communications, Inc.

Spearing, C, et al: Incentive spirometry: inspiring your patient to breathe deeply, Nursing 87 7:50, 1987.

Steiger, N, and Lipson, J: Self-care nursing: theory and practice, Bowie, Md, 1985, Brody Communications Co, Inc.

Swearingen, P: Addison-Wesley paperback photo atlas of nursing procedures, Menlo Park, Calif, 1984, Addison-Wesley Publishing Co.

Thompson, T: A self-medication program in a rehabilitation setting, Rehab Nurs 12:316, 1987.

Tortorelli, B, et al: Intermittent self-catheterization: a learning packet, Rehab Nurs 9:31, 1984.

Washburn, K: Physical medicine and rehabilitation, Garden City, NY, 1981, Medical Examination Publishing Co, Inc.

PART V

MUSCULOSKELETAL DISORDERS

CHAPTER 32

Rehabilitation of fractures in adults

JOSEPH D. ZUCKERMAN AND MARY LYNN NEWPORT

Optimal rehabilitation after fracture requires a comprehensive approach. The ultimate goal of the treatment of any fracture is to restore the injured area to its preinjury level of function. This return of function can be achieved only by close adherence to the well-known principles of fracture management and rehabilitation. Fracture care should take place within the context of the functional rehabilitation of the injured area; conversely, rehabilitation should have an important place in even the earliest phases of fracture care.

A comprehensive care plan has several important components. First is to obtain fracture healing with anatomic or near-anatomic alignment. Second is to restore full range of motion to the joints adjacent to the fracture, as well as to the nonadjacent joints in the same extremity. Third is to regain normal muscle strength in the injured areas and adjacent muscle groups. Fourth is to prevent the complications of fracture treatment, particularly those severely affecting rehabilitation, such as reflex sympathetic dystrophy. These components are not meant to be sequential; they take place concurrently throughout fracture care and rehabilitation.

This chapter discusses the important principles of fracture rehabilitation, including the pathophysiology of fractures and principles of fracture treatment. Addressed next are rehabilitation techniques commonly used to restore function after fracture. Finally the complications of fracture treatment and their impact on the rehabilitation process are discussed.

PATHOPHYSIOLOGY OF FRACTURE

A fracture involves disruption of more than just the bone itself. Periosteum, with its associated blood vessels and nerve fibers, is also disturbed. Blood vessels and lymph channels in the surrounding soft tissue are injured with resulting hemorrhage and edema. Further hemorrhage occurs from the fractured ends of bone secondary to the trauma inflicted on the intramedullary blood supply. More severe fractures with greater displacement of bone fragments generally cause greater soft tissue injury. This is significant because the severity of the soft tissue injury is important to the quality and speed of fracture healing. An appreciable amount of the blood supply to the bone enters through the periosteum and is derived from the surrounding soft tissue. The disruption of this soft tissue envelope, as occurs in open fractures with muscle injury, for instance, may compromise blood supply, which in turn may inhibit fracture healing. In addition, injuries to ligaments, tendons, and joint capsule produce periarticular scarring that may ultimately limit joint range of motion. In this situation, although the fracture has healed, the final result may be severe functional compromise of the extremity.

Microscopically, osteocytes at the fracture site are deprived of their blood supply and become necrotic. Necrosis of soft tissue also occurs if its blood supply has been compromised. An inflammatory reaction is produced with acute vasodilation and plasma exudation, which in turn produces acute tissue edema. Inflammatory cells, initially polymorphonuclear leukocytes and then macrophages, enter the fracture area. As this initial inflammatory reaction subsides, the reparative phase begins.

The sequence of events of the reparative phase of fracture healing is well known. Disruption of intramedullary and periosteal blood vessels produces a hematoma that envelops the fractured bone ends. Within the hematoma, fibrin produces a scaffolding upon which subsequent reparative processes develop. Pluripotential mesenchymal cells are brought into the hematoma by invading capillaries and granulation tissue derived primarily from the periosteum. These pluripotential cells then produce collagen, cartilage, or bone, depending on the pH, oxygen tension, and electrical potential of their microenvironment.[1] Collagen production provides a further scaffolding upon which the process of bone formation begins. Side chains on collagen react with calcium and phosphate ions to initiate the conversion of soft callus to hard callus. The mass of collagen, cartilage, and immature fiber (woven) bone encircles the fractured bone ends and leads to a gradual increase in fracture stability.

As stability increases, the remodeling phase of repair begins. Osteoclasts resorb the poorly organized bone trabeculae, and osteoblasts lay down new struts of bone along the lines of force affecting the bone. Electrical forces produced by tension and compression within the bone partially modulate the activity of the osteoclasts and osteoblasts. Remodeling generally takes place for at least 1 year after fracture but may last considerably longer.

As the bone heals, so does the surrounding soft tissue. The lymphatic system resorbs edema and the fluid phase of hematoma but not the proteins. These proteins increase the fibrosis that inevitably occurs in the wake of significant injury. The best treatment for this fibrotic reaction, which may be inconsequential in some fractures but the most debilitating feature in others, is prevention. This is accomplished by reduction and stabilization of the fracture to prevent further soft tissue injury, elevation of the affected part to minimize swelling, and mobilization of the uninjured parts of the limb. Motion not only prevents stiffness of uninvolved joints, but also facilitates the resorption of edema.

Some amount of fibrosis is inevitable after a fracture, but severe fibrosis may lead to tendon and muscle adhesions and joint capsule contraction. Tendon adhesions limit joint motion and are especially significant in the flexor tendons of the hand, which require extensive excursion and smooth gliding for finger motion. Similarly, muscle bound down by adhesions cannot contract adequately for proper joint motion and strength. Joint capsule contraction after immobilization of injury can be the most difficult soft tissue problem to rehabilitate. Capsular contraction and scarring are best prevented by active motion if the joint is not immobilized. If the joint must be immobilized, it should be in a functional position, with the periarticular soft tissues in a lengthened state to prevent shortening and contracture.

All of these factors can be exacerbated if the fracture is treated surgically. The surgical procedure itself is a form of controlled soft tissue injury. Muscle and fascia must be incised, and muscle and periosteum must be stripped from bone for proper surgical exposure. This interferes with the blood supply to the bone and increases hematoma and edema around the fracture. Use of a tourniquet during the procedure may further increase these problems. On the other hand, surgical stabilization of the fracture generally permits more aggressive measures to reduce swelling and fibrosis. With the fracture stabilized, joints can be mobilized more easily and muscles can work more extensively to decrease edema. Rigid stabilization eliminates motion at the fracture site,

which would cause more soft tissue injury. In addition, fracture fixation in the lower extremity eliminates or minimizes the necessity for treatment by traction and recumbency.

Fracture treatment

Specific treatment for fractures depends on the location of the fracture, as well as its configuration. Some bones (for example, the humerus) tolerate large degrees of angulation and rotation because deformity is accommodated by the large range of motion at the glenohumeral joint. Other bones such as the radius and ulna require precise reduction and rigid stabilization to regain pronation and supination.

As a general principle, fracture treatment requires immobilization of the joint above and below the fracture. This presupposes that the fracture is nondisplaced or minimally displaced, or that it can be reduced (aligned) and adequately immobilized by external means. The periosteum and surrounding soft tissues—the "soft tissue envelope"—add significantly to the stability of the fracture. If they are severely damaged, the fracture is more unstable. The initial displacement and comminution are important factors in determining stability. If the fracture cannot be reduced adequately or cannot be held reduced by cast immobilization, surgical reduction and internal fixation are usually necessary. Fixation can usually be accomplished by screws or pins, a screw and plate combination, or some form of intramedullary device that acts as an internal splint.

Other fractures that generally require open reduction and internal fixation (ORIF) are displaced intra-articular fractures. Joint surfaces can tolerate only minimal displacement before joint function is compromised. Optimal treatment consists of anatomic reduction of the joint surface, followed by stable fixation. This combination restores joint congruity, thereby decreasing the risk of arthritis (although damage to the articular cartilage at the time of injury can be an equally important factor in the subsequent outcome). If stable fixation of the intra-articular fracture has been accomplished, early motion of the joint can be instituted. The motion of the joint improves the nourishment of the cartilage, contributes to remodeling, and encourages repair of the articular cartilage injury with fibrocartilage.[22]

Fractures fall into four broad categories: stable fractures that require little treatment, moderately stable fractures that require some form of immobilization, unstable fractures that require more extensive immobilization of one joint above and below the fracture, and grossly unstable fractures that cannot be immobilized by casting but generally require surgical intervention for an optimal result.

Stable fractures

Stable fractures require little or no immobilization for healing, and a good functional result can be anticipated. They include, among others, nondisplaced radial head fractures, rib fractures, isolated nondisplaced ulna fractures, and impacted proximal humerus fractures (Figure 32-1). These fractures involve little soft tissue damage, are inherently stable, and have few muscular forces acting across the fracture site to cause displacement. In these instances rehabilitation begins as soon as the initial symptoms subside. Usually, progressive range-of-motion exercises can begin on the third or fourth day after injury and are followed by progressive strengthening exercises after 3 or 4 weeks.

Moderately stable fractures

Moderately stable fractures require some form of immobilization to prevent further displacement but allow significant activity of the joints surrounding the fracture. For instance, midhumerus fractures generally require only a plaster or polyethylene sleeve for the upper arm, allowing relatively free shoulder and elbow motion. Distal radius fractures (Colles' fracture) may require only a short arm

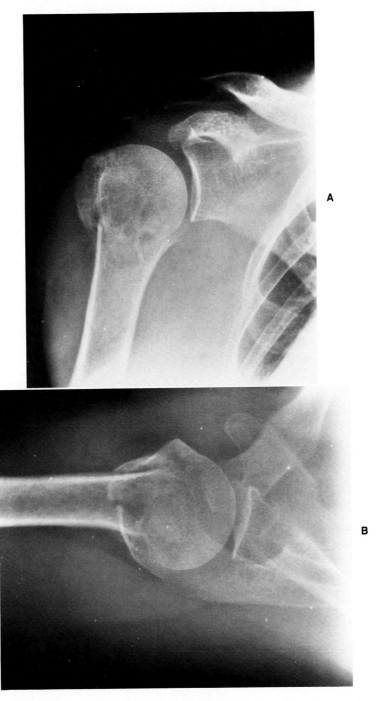

Figure 32-1. Stable fracture of proximal humerus in 69-year-old woman, showing excellent alignment on anteroposterior (**A**) and axillary (**B**) views. She was placed in sling and started on AAROM program as soon as initial discomfort diminished.

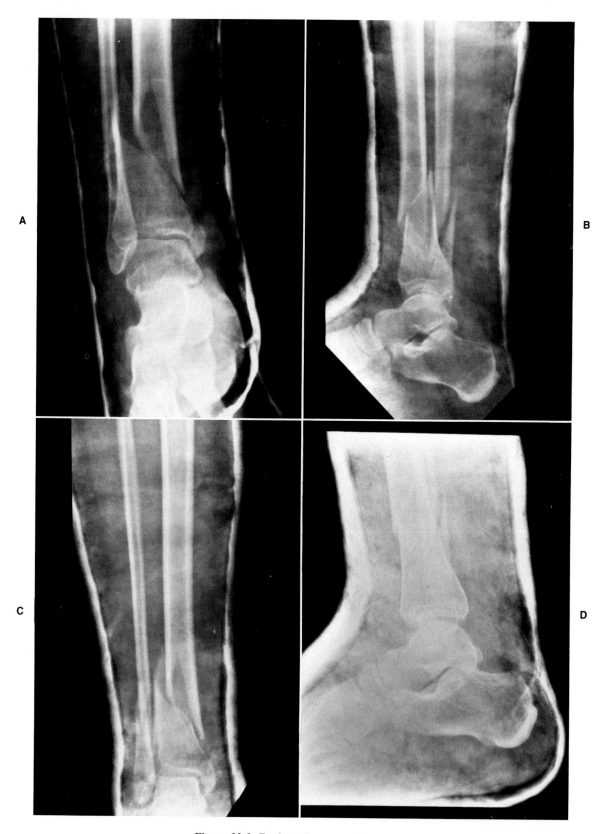

Figure 32-2. For legend see opposite page.

cast, leaving the fingers and elbow free. Metatarsal fractures may require a short leg cast, but many can be treated without immobilization (although weight bearing must still be limited). Also, fractures that have been treated surgically with ORIF sometimes require a small measure of protection postoperatively, when fixation is not absolutely rigid.

Unstable fractures

Unstable fractures may be nondisplaced or minimally displaced initially but tend to shift position if not immobilized. This category includes displaced fractures that were successfully manipulated into alignment but require immobilization to maintain the reduction (Figure 32-2). These fractures require immobilization of the affected bone to include the joints above and below the fracture. Immobilization of the proximal and distal joints decreases the angulatory and rotatory forces acting on the fracture, as well as the muscular deforming forces across the fracture.

Plaster or fiberglass casts are generally used for unstable fractures. Plaster has the advantage of being easily molded to provide secure fixation, especially in fractures that are difficult to reduce. Fiberglass has the advantage of being lightweight: approximately one-third the weight of plaster for the same strength of cast. It is not as easily molded as plaster, however, and is best used for nondisplaced fractures, after ORIF, or for fractures after 2 to 3 weeks of immobilization in a plaster cast, when better stability has been attained.

A cast-brace is a modified form of cast immobilization that can be fabricated from either plaster or fiberglass. It is unique because it has hinges that allow motion in one plane at one or two adjacent joints. The hinges can be blocked to allow a limited range of motion if desired. Cast-braces generally control rotational and angulatory forces but minimize stiffness by allowing controlled joint mobilization. Fractures that can be treated with cast-bracing include some tibia fractures and some distal femur fractures.

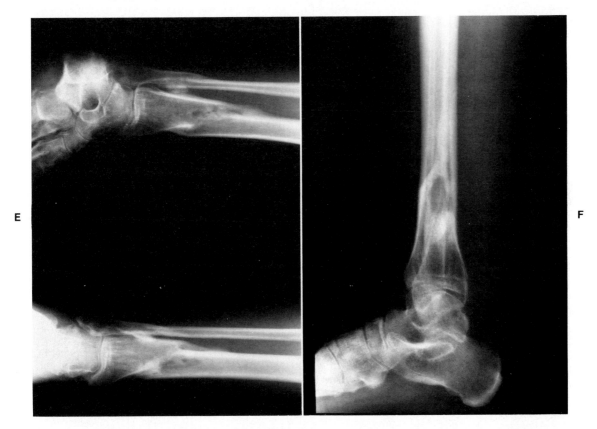

Figure 32-2. Unstable tibia and fibula fracture in 21-year-old woman, sustained when she slipped on ice. **A** and **B,** Initial radiographs showing unacceptable alignment. **C** and **D,** Closed reduction was performed under anesthesia, and better alignment was obtained. She was maintained in long leg fiberglass cast, ambulating with touch-down weight bearing with crutches. After 12 weeks, short leg cast was applied and full weight bearing was allowed. Cast was removed 6 weeks later, and rehabilitation program progressed. **E** and **F,** Radiographs obtained 6 months after injury, showing fracture healing. At that time patient was ambulating well and had near-normal range of motion in knee and ankle.

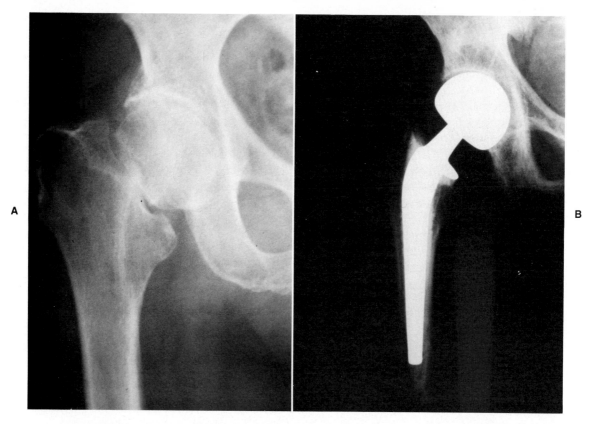

Figure 32-3. A, Displaced fracture of femoral neck in 78-year-old man, sustained after a fall. It was treated with a bipolar endoprosthesis **(B),** which allows ambulation with weight bearing as tolerated 48 hours after surgery.

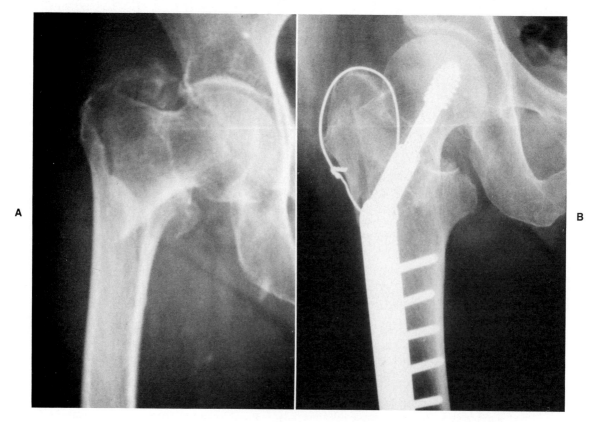

Figure 32-4. A, Comminuted intertrochanteric hip fracture in 82-year-old woman, who fell while walking. It was treated by ORIF to allow weight-bearing ambulation 2 days after surgery **(B).**

Grossly unstable fractures

Grossly unstable fractures include those in which closed reduction and casting are known to be inadequate in obtaining or maintaining adequate alignment, and those in which an attempt at closed reduction has been unsuccessful. Also included in this category are fractures that may be easily and successfully treated with traction but for which ORIF is far more attractive because of the decreased risk of malunion and avoidance of prolonged recumbency. These include most hip (Figures 32-3 and 32-4) and femur fractures (Figure 32-5). Grossly unstable fractures generally require surgical treatment for optimal results. Advantages of surgical intervention include minimization of recumbency (especially for those with lower-extremity fractures), early mobilization of adjacent joints, early return of general mobility, and, in some instances, early protected weight

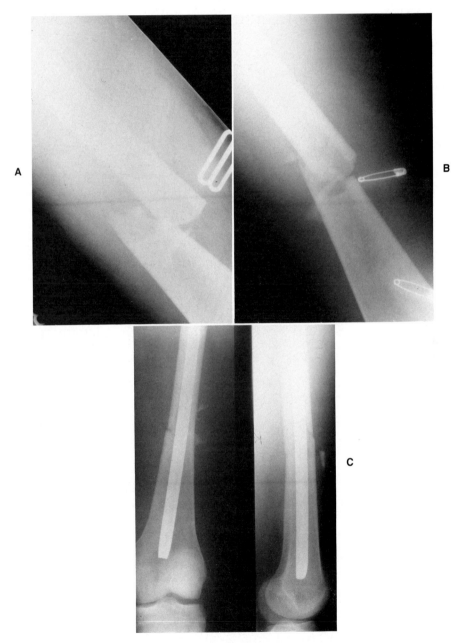

Figure 32-5. A and **B,** Closed femoral shaft fracture in 28-year-old man, sustained in motorcycle accident. **C,** Intramedullary rod was placed on night of injury. Quadriceps-setting exercises were started on second postoperative day. Crutch-walking ambulation was begun on third postoperative day. Patient was discharged 8 days after surgery, ambulating independently with crutches, with knee range of motion from 0 to 100 degrees. Patient was ambulating without assistive devices 8 weeks after fracture, with full range of motion in knee.

bearing. For intra-articular fractures early motion improves cartilage repair and limits intra-articular adhesions (Figure 32-6).

The disadvantages of ORIF include anesthetic risks, infection, and interference with the normal physiology of fracture healing and skeletal function. Most surgical fracture treatment involves use of a plate and screws for fixation. The plate is much more rigid than the bone and therefore absorbs much of the stress that would be transmitted to the

bone. This is known as stress shielding. Stress shielding causes resorption of bone under the plate and also limits the remodeling of bone at the fracture site. Bone requires stress to maintain its physiologic strength (Wolff's law) and remodel properly. In addition, internal fixation devices are generally removed after the fracture heals. This requires a second surgical procedure with the attendant risks. Removal of the fixation devices temporarily weakens the bone until the screw holes fill in with new bone and the stress-shielded

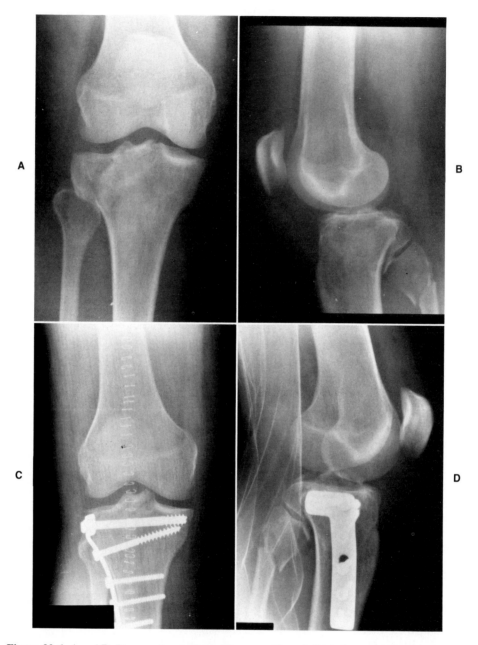

Figure 32-6. A and **B,** Depressed comminuted fracture of lateral tibial plateau in 51-year-old man, sustained when struck by car. **C** and **D,** Patient underwent ORIF with bone grafting to restore joint surface congruity. Continuous passive motion exercises were started 3 days after surgery. Hinged cast brace was used for immobilization, and patient was kept on program of non-weight-bearing ambulation for 3 months.

areas undergo physiologic remodeling. Despite these disadvantages, ORIF remains an important treatment of unstable fractures.

Intramedullary devices are also useful in the treatment of unstable long bone (femur, tibia, humerus) fractures (Figure 32-5). The principle of intramedullary fixation is to provide an internal splint for the bone while allowing the bone to absorb its normal stresses. This allows bone healing and remodeling to occur in a more normal fashion and bone strength to increase more rapidly to preinjury levels. Removal of the intramedullary device can be performed with minimal compromise of bone strength. Intramedullary devices are considered to be load sharing, whereas plates and screws are load-bearing devices.

The role of traction is usually limited to short-term use immediately before the operation or for long-term use in fractures that are so comminuted that ORIF is not indicated or cannot provide adequate fixation, for example, comminuted acetabular fractures in elderly patients. Traction treatment brings an increased risk of the problems of recumbency—cardiopulmonary compromise, thrombophlebitis, urinary retention—as well as fracture malunion. In addition, while traction may require immobilization of the involved extremity, it is important to maintain proper function of the uninvolved extremities and limit the effects of "deconditioning."

REHABILITATION AFTER FRACTURE

The specific rehabilitation program used for upper and lower extremity fractures depends on the fracture type and location, the treatment employed, and the preferences of the treating orthopedic surgeon. The limitations of this chapter make it unrealistic to discuss a rehabilitation program for each specific fracture. Instead, we first discuss the principles of fracture rehabilitation that are applicable to all fractures regardless of location or mode of treatment. Then we discuss the different components of fracture rehabilitation, including useful local modalities, gait-training techniques, range-of-motion exercises, and muscle strengthening. Included in these discussions are specific examples of fractures, their treatment, and the timing of the prescribed rehabilitation program.

Principles of fracture rehabilitation

Although fracture patterns, location, and treatment vary greatly, there are a few important principles that have broad applicability.

First, all joints that do not require immobilization should be mobilized early to maintain function. For example, a patient with a distal radius fracture treated with a short arm cast should start range-of-motion exercises of the shoulder, elbow, and interphalangeal joints as soon as possible to prevent stiffness. This principle is extended to the uninvolved extremities as well.

Second, gait training should be instituted as soon after injury as possible. This helps to prevent the problems of recumbency, particularly in the elderly population. For lower extremity fractures, assistive devices (walker, crutches, cane) are usually necessary for variable amounts of time after fracture.

Third, mobilization of the injured areas should begin when adequate fracture stability exists. This should be performed in a atraumatic manner to avoid additional soft tissue injury.

Fourth, local modalities should be used for pain control and reduction of muscle spasm. These simple measures are preferred over medications because their effects are local and not systemic. (An example of this is the drowsiness often experienced with the use of oral analgesics.)

Fifth, muscle strengthening of the involved areas should begin as fracture stability allows. Isometric exercises are most often used initially, with progression to isotonic strengthening when joint range of motion has been regained and fracture healing and stability allow resistive exercises.

Local therapeutic measures

The use of local modalities can be an important adjunct in both early and late treatment and in rehabilitation of fractures. Various modalities may be useful at different stages of treatment. In the acute phase of injury, which is characterized by swelling and hemorrhage, local cooling measures may be helpful.[14] These measures cause vasoconstriction, which reduces swelling and bleeding. Cold has an analgesic effect as well—either directly, through an effect on the sensory nerve endings and pain fibers, or indirectly, by the relief of associated muscle spasm. It is usually applied in the form of ice or gel packs, with care taken to avoid direct application to skin surfaces. These measures are beneficial in reducing pain and swelling in the first 48 to 72 hours following fracture. Cold can also be used to reduce postoperative swelling in fractures treated surgically. Studies have shown a reduced need both for cast splitting and for analgesics when ice is used postoperatively.[23]

In the rehabilitation stages after fracture, local cooling measures can also be effective as an analgesic. This is particularly true during the mobilization of previously immobilized or surgically treated joints. Periarticular musculature often develops spasms that can be relieved by cold application. Cold also reduces local inflammation from the trauma of mobilization. Moreover, pain relief is obtained by the effect of the cooling measures as a counterirritant, which has been shown to increase the pain threshold.[21]

Therapeutic heat applications are primarily useful in the later stages of fracture treatment, after the acute injury phase has passed and mobilization has begun. Heat causes a number of physiologic responses that are important in fracture rehabilitation.[14] These include the abilities to increase extensibility of collagen, to decrease joint stiffness, to produce pain relief, and to relieve muscle spasm. We prefer to use heat before and during joint mobilization, applying it to the joint and periarticular muscles. The choice of heating modality depends on equipment availability and on whether superficial or deep heat is desired. We most often use hot packs because they are simple, inexpensive, and easily available and because a patient can be instructed in their use at home. Conversion modalities (ultrasound, short waves, diathermy) produce a deep-heating effect that has the advantage of a greater depth of penetration but can be used only in the hospital or office setting. Therapeutic heat is contraindicated in areas of diminished sensation and for confused patients. In addition, it should not be used in areas of compromised vascularity, since the temperature elevation increases metabolic demands without an adequate increase in blood flow. We do not use therapeutic heat in diabetic patients following lower extremity fractures because of compromised vascularity and diminished sensation resulting from diabetic neuropathy.

Transcutaneous electrical nerve stimulation can be an effective method of controlling pain during the rehabilitation process.[18,25] It can be applied to the painful extremity during the rehabilitation program, which should allow a greater participation in the exercises and a faster recovery of function. It can be safely used by most patients, who have the option of adjusting both the amplitude of the stimulation and the location of the electrodes in response to the severity and location of the pain. The device is usually employed for short sequences of impulses at a frequency of three to five per second. The intensity of the impulses is usually three to five times the pain perception threshold.[16]

Gait training after fractures

Gait training is a very important part of the rehabilitation process after fractures. The ability to walk with assistive devices greatly enhances functional recovery. Weight bearing by one or both lower extremities stimulates recovery of bone mass and muscle function. It also adds to the patient's psychologic well-being by providing the sense of a return of independence.

The methods of gait training used following fracture depend on a number of factors, including location of the fracture (upper versus lower extremity), type of fracture treatment, need for restricted weight bearing (non weight bearing, partial weight bearing, full weight bearing), type of immobilization (long leg cast versus hinged cast brace), and patient characteristics (age, prefracture ambulatory status, associated medical problems). The best way to approach this area of rehabilitation is to discuss the different clinical situations one encounters.

Upper extremity fractures cannot be neglected as an indication for gait training. Younger patients and most older patients with upper extremity fractures generally recover ambulatory ability without difficulty. However, gait training may be necessary in selected patients. This is especially true in older patients who have preexisting balance problems and must rely on one or both upper extremities for support. It is not uncommon for an elderly patient with a proximal humerus fracture that is treated with a shoulder immobilizer to use a cane for ambulation until regaining use of both upper extremities.

Lower extremity fractures are by far the primary indication for gait training after fracture. The ease with which gait training proceeds depends on weight bearing and the type of immobilization used. Non-weight-bearing, partial weight-bearing, or full weight-bearing (that is, weight bearing as tolerated) gait training is generally ordered. Non-weight-bearing training is usually prescribed for intra-articular fractures, whether treated surgically or nonsurgically, because weight bearing carries a high risk of displacement of articular surfaces with resulting joint incongruity. For example, a patient with a displaced tibial plateau fracture treated surgically with excellent restoration of the articular surface is usually prescribed early range-of-motion exercises but remains on a non-weight-bearing program for 3 months following the fracture (Figure 32-6). A non-weight-bearing program is also recommended for unstable fractures that were reduced and immobilized, since weight bearing may cause fracture displacement and loss of reduction (Figure 32-2). A non-weight-bearing gait requires the use of assistive devices, usually including crutches or walkers. Walkers are used by older patients because they provide more support and require less balance than crutches. This brings up an important point about the non-weight-bearing gait of elderly patients. One often sees this type of gait training ordered for elderly patients following surgical treatment of hip fractures or following other lower extremity fractures; it is mentioned only to make strong recommendations against it. A non-weight-bearing status is essentially impossible for older patients to maintain after lower extremity trauma. This is true whether the fracture is treated surgically or nonsurgically and whether immobilization is used or not. In fact, it represents a situation that puts the patient at risk for falling and sustaining additional injury. Treatment of lower extremity fractures in elderly patients should be planned to allow weight bearing whenever possible. Touch-down weight bearing, in which the foot is placed on the floor as a means of balance, is strongly preferable to a non-weight-bearing gait in patients for whom weight bearing must be restricted.

Partial weight bearing is used most commonly in patients who require protected weight bearing because of the nature of their fracture, but for whom limited weight bearing is desired for balance, to stimulate fracture healing, and to maintain bone mass in the injured extremity. Partial weight bearing also often includes progressive weight bearing as the healing progresses. For example, a closed tibia-fibula fracture treated with closed reduction in a long leg cast may be kept on toe touch-down weight bearing for the first 4 to 6 weeks (Figure 32-2). If the radiograph shows evidence of callus formation, partial weight bearing is begun in an effort to stimulate healing. It is started at a point when fracture displacement is no longer a significant risk. The patient can then progress to full weight bearing as tolerated.

It is important to be very specific when requesting partial weight-bearing gait training. Otherwise, the therapist does not know whether "partial weight bearing" means 5% or 95% of body weight. The treating physician must develop an overall treatment plan that specifies the extent of partial weight bearing and must communicate this to the therapist.

We often use orders for partial weight bearing in a patient after intramedullary nailing for a transverse midshaft femur fracture (Figure 32-5). The intramedullary nail is a load-sharing device in which some weight bearing is desirable to provide impaction at the fracture site. We allow weight bearing of up to 25% of body weight as the postoperative discomfort subsides and quadriceps function returns. We generally increase this to 50% at 2 to 3 weeks postoperatively as soft tissue healing progresses. Progression to full weight bearing is allowed at about 6 weeks, when fracture callus is evident on the radiograph.

Full weight bearing or weight bearing as tolerated is used initially in stable fracture patterns in which there is little or no risk of displacement. This usually follows a brief period of limited weight bearing while swelling and discomfort subside. A nondisplaced medial malleolus fracture without injury to the lateral aspect of the ankle is a stable fracture that is usually treated in a short leg walking cast. In this situation full weight bearing is allowed as soon as the post-injury discomfort subsides. Full weight-bearing gait training is most often used in the later stages of rehabilitation of unstable fractures, as healing progresses and stability is achieved. This may be when a fracture callus is radiographically evident, or may be somewhat arbitrary when fractures have been treated with open reduction internal fixation. Rigid fixation of fractures promotes healing by primary osteosynthesis (absence of external callus). Weight bearing is allowed in this situation based on the anticipated healing rates for the bones involved. When ankle fractures, which occur primarily in metaphyseal (cancellous) bone, are treated by internal fixation, 6 weeks is generally required for healing. At this point, weight bearing can be increased. This is in contrast to tibial shaft fractures (disphyseal or cortical bone) treated by rigid plate fixation; they require a much longer time before sufficient healing occurs to allow progressive weight bearing.

Range of motion

An essential component of the rehabilitation of fractures is maintenance of range of motion of the affected joints. Permanent joint stiffness following fracture can be a devastating functional disability. The best treatment for post-fracture joint stiffness is prevention. Any fracture treatment protocol must include a plan for joint mobilization to obtain the best functional outcome. Loss of joint motion following fracture occurs either because of the fracture location (intra-articular or periarticular) or as a result of the required immobilization.

The first step in joint mobilization following fractures is to maintain full range of motion of all uninvolved joints. This includes the joints of the uninvolved extremities. For example, a patient placed in a spica cast for a pelvic fracture should be started on a program for upper extremity range-of-motion exercises (as well as strengthening, since the upper extremities are responsible for bed mobility). Another example is a patient in a short arm cast for a distal radius (Colles') fracture. In this situation it is essential to provide an active range-of-motion program for the ipsilateral shoulder and elbow, as well as the metacarpophalangeal and interphalangeal joints, since these joints are prone to joint stiffness even though they are not included in the cast.

The nature and timing of the mobilization of injured areas depend on the fracture location and the method of treatment. Fractures that involve joint surfaces usually require open reduction and internal fixation to restore joint congruity and allow early range of motion. Fractures adjacent to joints (metaphyseal) or in the diaphyseal portion of long bones also have an effect on adjacent joint function because of the associated soft tissue injury. For example, a displaced tibia fracture with significant contusion of the posterior compartment's muscles causes scarring and possible restriction of ankle and toe plantar flexion (Figure 32-2). Extended immobilization prevents early stretching of these injured areas, which may lead to additional scar formation. This in turn makes eventual mobilization more difficult. However, if the same tibia fracture is treated with open reduction and rigid internal fixation, only short-term immobilization is necessary. This allows joint mobilization to begin earlier, with more prompt return of adjacent joint motion. This is not in and of itself a reason to treat tibia fractures surgically, but it is a factor to be considered in planning treatment.

Four types of range-of-motion exercises are commonly used: passive, active assisted, active, and resistive. Each type is useful in different clinical situations.

Passive range-of-motion (PROM) exercises are useful in the early postfracture period, when associated muscle injury prevents active range of motion or when muscle contraction for joint motion is undesirable. The primary goal of PROM exercises is to prevent contractures and formation of adhesions. It implies that there is no active participation by the periarticular musculature—that is, no muscle action occurs. This may or may not be true clinically. In the early postinjury phase passive motion may be limited by the protective contraction of the antagonist muscle groups secondary to pain and splinting. This usually subsides with time and can be minimized by initiating PROM exercises through a limited arc. To be certain that no damage is being caused, this arc must be painless or minimally painful.

PROM exercises provide a number of benefits, including preservation of gliding motion of tendons, preservation of muscle fiber lengths, and decreased intraarticular and periarticular scar formation. In addition, PROM has been shown to enhance nourishment of articular cartilage and to assist in the resorption of hemarthroses.[20] In the late 1970s clinical use of continuous passive motion (CPM) machines began, the idea of which was based on experimental data showing that CPM promoted repair of articular cartilage injury with hyaline-like cartilage rather than fibrocartilage.[22] CPM machines were initially available for the knee but are currently available for most major joints of the body: the ankle, shoulder, elbow, and wrist. They have been very useful in the rehabilitation of intra-articular fractures that have been stabilized surgically. For example, 3 days after open reduction, internal fixation, and bone grafting of a depressed tibial plateau fracture (Figure 32-6), the CPM machine can be used to initiate motion. Passive motion is desired in this situation to minimize joint loading and prevent displacement of fragments. It enables range-of-motion exercises to begin in the early postoperative period, thereby improving the eventual return of function.

Active assisted range-of-motion (AAROM) exercises are the first step in muscle reeducation. The exercises are accomplished by active muscle contraction by the patient with the assistance of the therapist or the patients themselves. This allows active muscle function and at the same time prevents excessive strain on the periarticular musculature. AAROM is useful in the early phases of rehabilitation after stable fractures that do not require immobilization have occurred or after removal of immobilization devices in the early phases of joint mobilization. It is also useful early in the period following surgical stabilization of fractures. For example, after a stable proximal humerus fracture, early AAROM can be instituted (Figure 32-1). The patient begins with forward elevation performed in a supine position. The supine position minimizes the effects of gravity and the weight of the arm. Often the uninjured upper extremity is used to "assist" the injured extremity through the range of motion when the patient's own musculature cannot function independently. The therapist can also perform the same assistive function. The benefit of having the patient assist is that therapy can be continued between sessions with the therapist.

Another example of the need for AAROM is knee extension following surgical stabilization of a patella fracture. It is often difficult to achieve the final 30 degrees of full extension following this injury and surgery. In AAROM the quadriceps initiates knee extension, and at the point when further extension is not possible actively, the therapist (or the patient's other limb) assists extension to overcome gravity, thereby completing the arc. As muscle function improves and is indeed reeducated, the assistive component decreases and the motion becomes completely active.

Active range-of-motion (AROM) exercises are performed entirely by the patient, who voluntarily contracts and relaxes the muscles that control a specific motion. It is the next step in the progression from AAROM. Once muscular control has been established, the patient continues to move the involved joints through the largest possible range of motion. This not only preserves joint function but also increases strength. AAROM exercises make it possible to regain at least antigravity muscle strength (grade 3 out of 5). Once this is accomplished, the rehabilitation program takes one of two different directions.

When a normal or near-normal range of motion exists, additional muscle-strengthening exercises are indicated. These take the form of resistive range-of-motion (RROM) exercises. These exercises are performed against resistance that may be provided by the therapist or by mechanical devices (weights, pulleys, springs, rubber tubing). RROM exercises are usually not initiated until fracture healing has occurred. For example, following ORIF of a humeral shaft fracture, AROM and AAROM exercise of the elbow may be initiated. However, resistive exercises significantly increase the stress at the fracture site, which may excessively stress the fraction fixation. In the worst case fixation may become lost, requiring additional surgery, or position may shift, requiring immobilization and discontinuation of early range-of-motion exercises. Therefore resistive exercises should be considered the final phase of muscle rehabilitation, reserved for the time when fracture healing is adequate to withstand the additional stresses.

When AROM exercises have restored only a partial range of motion, stretching exercises are often used. Stretching consists of gentle forced motion, usually applied by the therapist or the patient with or without mechanical aids. The therapeutic use of stretching is to restore the normal joint range of motion in areas where limitation of this range is caused by loss of soft tissue elasticity—that is, the presence of soft tissue contracture. Stretching must be performed carefully to prevent the possibility of additional injury. It generally causes a feeling of discomfort for the patient, but it should never evoke acute pain. Any discomfort should subside 15 to 20 minutes after the exercises are completed. Excessively forceful stretching will cause additional muscle injury, which begins the cycle of hemorrhage-inflammation-fibrosis-contracture, thereby reducing further the range of motion. Stretching is best performed gently over an extended period. The muscle to be stretched must be maximally relaxed to produce the desired effect. As with resistive exercises, stretching should not be performed until fracture healing is adequate to withstand the additional stress. Stretching is most effective when performed by the therapist, who also instructs the patient in self-stretching exercises so they can be repeated between visits with the therapist. It is important for anyone performing stretching exercises to respect the biologic tissues involved so as to prevent further injury and complications.

Stretching can be very helpful in many situations involving fracture rehabilitation. For example, following rehabilitation after extended immobilization in a long leg cast for a tibia and fibula fracture, a patient may have a knee range of motion from 10 to 120 degrees and normal muscle strength. Gentle stretching should achieve full extension and improve flexion. Another method of stretching is to use overhead pulleys following proximal humerus fractures. After fracture healing, patients often have significant restriction of forward elevation of the involved shoulder. The overhead pulley allows the uninjured extremity to stretch the affected shoulder gently and regain range of motion. This can be performed at home as well as under a therapist's supervision. The patient must be informed about all the necessary precautions to prevent any additional injury.

Strengthening

Muscle strengthening is an important component of fracture rehabilitation. Return to normal strength is essential to complete the rehabilitation process. Methods of muscle strengthening generally involve three types of exercise techniques. Isometric exercises are those in which muscle tension increases without a change in the muscle fiber length—that is, no movement is produced. This is particularly useful for immobilized limbs. Isotonic exercises produce a change in muscle fiber length as muscle tension increases; movement is produced. This type of exercise is useful when joint range of motion has been regained. Isokinetic exercises rely on machines that can apply variable resistance throughout the range of motion of the limb. This is believed to represent a more effective technique in muscle strengthening. It is most useful in the final stages of fracture rehabilitation before return to unrestricted, strenuous (athletic) activity.

Strengthening is often considered the final stage of fracture rehabilitation; however, ideally it begins early in the rehabilitation process. For example, quadriceps-setting and straight leg–raising exercises (isometric contraction) should be performed when a long leg cast is immobilizing a tibia and fibula fracture. These exercises can be performed in the cast and help to limit the amount of quadriceps atrophy present at the time of cast removal.

As noted previously, AAROM and AROM exercises strengthen the muscles being used. These are isotonic exercises, in which the resistance is the weight of the limb and antigravity strength can be developed. When appropriate, weights can be used to provide resistive exercises. This further increases muscle strength. However, resistive exercises for strengthening should not be used until fracture healing or stability is sufficient to withstand the increased stress.

In designing a muscle-strengthening program it is important to differentiate between exercises designed for power and those designed for endurance. Exercises for power are strengthening exercises that should precede any endurance type of exercise. Weak, atrophied muscles must be restored to near-normal strength before endurance exercises are started. Endurance exercises are designed to increase tolerance. Unlike power exercises, which rely on a few repetitions with maximal active effort, endurance exercises are based on many repetitions performed at a submaximal effort. The combination of isometric, isotonic, and isokinetic strengthening exercises provides the necessary elements for recovery of muscle function following fracture.

COMPLICATIONS OF FRACTURES

Complications of fractures involve those specific to the involved bone, such as malunion and nonunion, as well as more wide-ranging physiologic disturbances. Nearly all complications can be minimized by vigorous treatment and meticulous attention to detail. The elderly are most prone to all complications for a variety of reasons. First, aging—with its physiologic changes and general limitation of activities—can produce osteoporosis of varying degrees. Osteoporotic bone is more likely to fracture, heals with less strength, and holds internal fixation devices poorly. This results in a higher incidence of malunion and device failure. Second, impaired eyesight, balance mechanisms, and muscle strength, as well as cardiac disturbances and neurologic deficits, increase the risk of falling. Almost all fractures in the elderly are a result of low-energy injuries such as falling, the most common being fractures of the hip and wrist. The same factors that contribute to the risk of fracture also make rehabilitation more difficult. Third, impaired vascular status can contribute to poor skin healing, infection, and deep venous thrombosis, and impaired cardiopulmonary reserves can lead to atelectasis, pneumonia, and increased anesthetic risks.

Younger patients are at risk for these same systemic complications. However, in this age group they are more often the result of multiple trauma. The most important contributing factor to the development of systemic complications in the young or elderly is recumbency. Recumbency may be a necessity (when the patient is in traction) or may be incidental (when the older patient, perhaps not so cooperative or poorly motivated, is not properly mobilized). Many problems can be associated with recumbency, the most common being atelectasis and pneumonia. The simple act of moving from supine in bed to upright in a chair is enough to improve pulmonary ventilation and perfusion and thereby limit pulmonary complications. Genitourinary stasis and gastrointestinal hypomotility are also minimized by activity. All of these complications are readily addressed by early fracture stabilization[3] or by some form of mobile traction device that allows the patient out of bed while continuing the traction on the lower extremity.[16]

Early mobilization also diminishes the risk of deep venous thrombosis and pulmonary embolus, which is greatest in the elderly.[24] Motion and muscle action diminish venous stasis and prevent subsequent thrombus formation. These are also minimized by use of compressive stockings, intermittent pumping devices, and antithrombotic medications, such as aspirin or dextran.[7-11] Warfarin (Coumadin) is perhaps the most effective of these medications but is difficult to monitor properly and, along with heparin, is associated with an increased risk of bleeding complications.

These systemic complications are of paramount importance because they are the most frequent cause of death in the elderly after a major fracture.[24] In the younger population pulmonary embolus and pneumonia are also of major importance, but a more significant threat arises from fat embolism after long bone fractures and adult respiratory distress syndrome (ARDS)—the sequelae of vigorous resuscitative efforts after severe multiple-system trauma.

Complications specific to fractures themselves are not uncommon and can cause significant problems in subsequent rehabilitation. Fracture malunion and nonunion are minimized by proper immobilization and use of ORIF with bone grafting when necessary. Stress increases the rate and quality of fracture healing and is produced by muscle forces in the upper and lower extremity and by weight bearing in the lower extremity. Weight bearing can occur, of course, only when the fracture pattern and treatment allow it.

Malunion of long bones is better tolerated in certain bones, such as the humerus, than in others. In general, however, malunion leads to unequal distribution of forces across nearby joints and can result in arthritis. Nonunion can be secondary to soft tissue interposed between the fracture ends, significant soft tissue stripping with decreased blood supply to the bone, or inadequate reduction and immobilization. It is associated with prolonged periods of immobilization, often occurs in the face of infection, and can require multiple surgical procedures. All of these lead to progressive muscle atrophy, disuse osteoporosis, and joint capsule and ligament contracture, which in turn can create substantial problems in rehabilitation once the fracture has healed.

Infection is seldom a complication of closed fractures treated in a closed manner but is a significant risk with open fractures. There is also a small risk of infection when closed fractures are treated surgically. Infection can cause a significant degree of additional swelling (and resultant fibrosis), as well as destruction of adjacent soft tissues and bone. The risk of infection is minimized in open fractures by immediate, thorough debridement of vitalized soft tissues and appropriate antibiotic therapy. The fracture itself is then treated by casting or ORIF. Infection associated with ORIF for closed fractures is minimized by meticulous surgical technique, with gentle handling of soft tissues and prophylactic perioperative antibiotics.

Stiffness can be a major obstacle to the successful treatment of fractures and can ultimately be the major cause of disability. It can occur remote from the fracture, in joints that were immobilized and in joints that were not immobilized yet were not moved by the patient. In joints not immobilized, stiffness is best and most easily prevented by encouraging range of motion in all uninvolved parts several times a day and encouraging normal use of the uninjured extremity. Stiffness of joints near a fracture can occur in

one of two ways. Intra-articular fractures are associated with intracapsular hemorrhage, which then leads to intra-articular fibrosis; contracture of joint capsule and ligaments can occur if the joint is not immobilized in a position that maximally stretches these structures. Stiffness can therefore be minimized by immobilization in the proper position or, in the case of fractures treated by ORIF, by early motion.

Reflex sympathetic dystrophy (RSD) can be a relatively common complication following orthopedic injury. Historically it has been referred to as causalgia, Sudeck's atrophy, reflex dystrophy, posttraumatic dystrophy, and shoulder-hand syndrome. The different names reflect differing presentations and manifestations. The exact cause of the condition is not clearly understood, but most authors agree that an abnormal sympathetic reflex is present. The major symptom is pain out of proportion to the objective findings. The most common physical finding is generalized edema, often accompanied by stiffness and skin discoloration.

The earliest stage of this disease occurs within the first 3 months after injury. It is characterized by increasing pain, usually constant in nature and often described as a burning sensation. The pain is exacerbated by light touch, temperature changes, passive or active motion, and emotional changes. Swelling increases during this period, rather than decreasing as one might expect. The swelling is soft and pitting and responds somewhat to elevation. The limb is warm and erythematous and shows evidence of hyperhidrosis. Early stiffness exists, as does osteoporosis, which may be evident radiographically as early as 3 to 4 weeks after injury.

The second stage of RSD begins at about 4 months and lasts up to 12 months after injury. Pain reaches a peak during this period, persists, and is especially exacerbated by motion. Swelling becomes more brawny and is less affected by elevation. Redness diminishes, and eventually the limb becomes cool and pale or cyanotic. Hyperhidrosis diminishes. Stiffness becomes progressively worse, and there may be evidence of early periarticular thickening or fibrosis.

The late stage may last several months or even years. Pain may or may not dissipate during this phase. Swelling abates, leaving only the periarticular fibrosis. Stiffness is generally pronounced, and there is little hope of regaining functional motion at this junction. The skin is pale, dry, cool, and glossy.

The etiology of RSD has been difficult to ascertain because no laboratory model is suitable. Lankford[13] thinks that three conditions must be present for RSD to develop: a persistent painful stimulus, either traumatic or acquired; a diathesis for the disease (personality may play a role or the patient may have a tendency for increased sympathetic activity—hyperhidrosis, cold hands or feet, and so on); and an abnormal sympathetic reflex. Livingston hypothesized that chronic irritation of a peripheral sensory nerve secondary to trauma and soft tissue injury increases afferent sensory input, which results in an abnormal state of activity in the internuncial neuronal pool.[15] This then creates a large intracord burst of activity and subsequently produces continuous stimulation of sympathetic efferent fibers. The defect therefore is in the neuronal central processing system.

Melzack and Wall offered further credence to this hypothesis.[19] Their gate control theory of pain proposed that an inhibiting fine-control mechanism of specialized cells exists within the substantia gelatinosa of the dorsal horn. These form a functional unit within the spinal cord, which is capable of modulating input from small (C) and large (A) fibers. They suggested that selective stimulation of small (pain) fibers suppresses the substantia gelatinosa and "opens the gate," whereas stimulation of the large fibers inhibits the substantia gelatinosa and "closes the gate." This may explain why deep friction massage, which stimulates the large (A) fibers, is beneficial to RSD.[6]

The diagnosis of RSD is made on the basis of primary signs, which include pain, swelling, stiffness, and discoloration. Secondary signs, present in the majority of patients, include osteoporosis, temperature changes, trophic changes, vasomotor instability, and palmar fibromatosis. Differential diagnosis may be difficult, especially in the early stages of the disease. Tenosynovitis, disuse atrophy, senile osteoporosis, peripheral neuritis, and peripheral vascular disease should all be considered.

Early recognition is of paramount importance and often greatly simplifies treatment. If early RSD is suspected, judicious physical therapy and medications (analgesics, tranquilizers, anti-inflammatory agents) may alleviate most or all symptoms. AROM acts in a fashion similar to deep friction massage in stimulating the large (A) fibers and closing the gate to the small (C) unmyelinated pain fibers.

Once RSD has been established and early conservative measures have proved unsuccessful, the treatment of choice is a sympathetic blockade to interrupt the abnormal sympathetic reflex. The most effective and reliable modality is a stellate ganglion (upper extremity) or lumbar sympathetic (lower extremity) block, with a local anesthetic agent such as lidocaine or bupivacaine. If used early in the course of disease, one block may be sufficient. In general, however, more than one is required, usually to a maximum of four or five. An effective block warms and dries the skin and produces return of a more normal coloration, a marked decrease in pain, and, in the case of a stellate ganglion block, a Horner's syndrome. Careful range-of-motion exercises are begun immediately after the block to make full use of the period when pain is diminished. Peripheral nerve blocks can also be performed. These block sympathetic, sensory, and motor function. The effects of peripheral blocks do not last as long as those of sympathetic blocks, but peripheral blocks can be performed more often because they produce less local reaction.

Chemical sympatholytic agents can also be effective in obtaining sympathetic blockade. Guanethidine seems to be the most effective of these agents.[17] This drug is used in the same manner as intravenous regional anesthesia with the Bier block method. Guanethidine serves as a false transmitter because it is taken up by the sympathetic nerve endings, displacing norepinephrine. Sympathetic blockade in this manner can last up to 3 or 4 days. Reserpine used in a similar fashion has had less reliable results.[2] The complications of these two medications are generally of little consequence but can include prolonged orthostatic hypotension, dizziness, somnolence, nausea, and vomiting. Neither has yet been approved by the Food and Drug Administration for other than experimental intravenous use.

Oral corticosteroids, usually in the form of prednisone, can have a significant benefit in improving symptoms,[4,12] although they probably should be used only as an adjunct to sympathetic blockade.[13] Steroids most likely decrease inflammation of the primary disorder and stabilize the capillary basement membrane. Reduction of vascular permeability limits plasma exudation, swelling, and resultant fibrosis.

Sympathectomy is the treatment of last resort. It should be used only if previous attempts at sympathetic blockade have been at least temporarily or partially successful.

The mainstay of treatment for RSD regardless of modality is judicious physical therapy. Forced motion and aggressive attempts can increase the pain and worsen the condition. Gentle range-of-motion exercises and massage not only decrease stiffness but may help in the treatment of RSD itself.

REFERENCES

1. Bassett, CAL: Current concepts of bone formation, J Bone Joint Surg 44A:1217, 1962.
2. Benzon, HT, Chomka, CM, and Brunner, EA: Treatment of reflex sympathetic dystrophy with regional intravenous reserpine, Anesth Analg 59:500, 1980.
3. Border, JR, et al: Trauma and delayed sepsis. In Burke, JF, and Hildick-Smith, GY, editors: The infection-prone hospital patient, Boston, 1976, Little, Brown & Co.
4. Christensen, K, Jensen, EM, and Noer, I: The reflex dystrophy syndrome response to treatment with systemic corticosteroids, Acta Chir Scand 148:653, 1982.
5. Evarts, CM, and Feil, EJ: Prevention of thromboembolic disease after elective surgery of the hip, J Bone Joint Surg 53A:1271, 1971.
6. Frazer, FW: Persistent post-sympathetic pain treated by connective tissue massage, Physiotherapy 6:211, 1978.
7. Harris, WH, et al: Comparison of warfarin, low-molecular-weight dextran, aspirin, and subcutaneous heparin in prevention of venous thromboembolism following total hip replacement, J Bone Joint Surg 56A:1552, 1974.
8. Harris, WH, et al: Aspirin prophylaxis in venous thromboembolism after total hip replacement, N Engl J Med 297:1246, 1977.
9. Harris, WH, et al: High- and low-dose aspirin prophylaxis against venous thromboembolic disease in total hip replacement, J Bone Joint Surg 64A:63, 1982.
10. Harris, WH, et al: Prophylaxis of deep-vein thrombosis after total hip replacement: dextran and external pneumatic compression compared with 1.2 and 0.3 gram of aspirin daily, J Bone Joint Surg 67A:57, 1985.
11. Hartman, JT, et al: Cyclic sequential compression to the lower limb in prevention of deep venous thrombosis, J Bone Joint Surg 64A:1059, 1982.

12. Kozin, F, et al: The reflex sympathetic dystrophy syndrome. I. Clinical studies: evidence of bilaterality and of periarticular accentuation, Am J Med 60:332, 1976.

13. Lankford, LL: Reflex sympathetic dystrophy. In Omer, GE, Jr, and Spinner, M, editors: Management of peripheral nerve problems, Philadelphia, 1980, WB Saunders Co.

14. Lehman, JF, and DeLatour, BJ: Diathermy and superficial heat and cold therapy. In Kottke, FJ, Stillwell, GK, and Lehman, JF, editors: Krusen's Handbook of physical medicine and rehabilitation, Philadelphia, 1982, WB Saunders Co.

15. Livingston, WK: Pain mechanisms: a physiologic interpretation of causalgia and its related states, New York, 1943, Macmillan Co.

16. Mays, J, and Neufeld, AJ: Skeletal traction methods, Clin Orthop 102:141, 1975.

17. McKain, CW, Urban, BJ, and Goldner, JL: The effects of intravenous regional guanethidine and reserpine: a controlled study, J Bone Joint Surg 65A:642, 1983.

18. Melzack, R: Prolonged relief of pain by brief intense transcutaneous somatic stimulation, Pain 1:357, 1975.

19. Melzack, R, and Wall, PD: Pain mechanisms: a new theory, Science 150:971, 1965.

20. O'Driscoll, SW, Kumar, A, and Salter, RB: The effect of continuous passive motion on the clearance of hemarthrosis from a synovial joint: an experimental investigation in the rabbit [abstract] Proc, Orthop Res Soc 8:32, 1983.

21. Ottoson, D: The effects of temperature on the isolated muscle spindle, J Physiol 180:636, 1965.

22. Salter, RB, et al: The biological effects of continuous passive motion on the healing of full thickness defects in articular cartilage: an experimental investigation in the rabbit, J Bone Joint Surg 62A:1232, 1980.

23. Schanbel, HJ: The local use of ice after orthopedic procedures, Am J Surg 72:711, 1946.

24. Sikorski, JM, and Hampson, WG: The natural history and aetiology of deep vein thrombosis after total hip replacement, J Bone Joint Surg 63B:171, 1981.

25. Thorsteinsson, G, et al: Transcutaneous electrical stimulation: a double-blind trial of its efficacy for pain, Arch Phys Med Rehabil 58:8, 1977.

CHAPTER 33

Arthroplasty rehabilitation

THEODORE WAUGH

HISTORICAL REVIEW
Lower extremity

It is commonly believed that the modern history of arthroplasty began in 1891 with the implantation of an ivory ball and socket joint as an experimental procedure in Berlin.[6] The techniques employed during the first part of the twentieth century were developed to free painful and ankylosed joints by reshaping the articular surfaces and interposing a wide variety of materials, both organic and inorganic, such as ivory, Bakelite, chromized pig's bladder, skin, and fascia lata. Following years of experimentation with such materials as glass and Pyrex, Smith-Peterson first used cobalt-chromium-molybdenum molds for arthroplasty of the hip. In the early 1950s Austin Moore developed a hip replacement device fixed by an intramedullary stem that was longer and more anatomic than those used in other femoral head replacement devices of the time. Surgeons recognized that both the mold arthroplasty and femoral head replacement had limitations and that frequently pain relief was inadequate. Since the problem of arthritis was common to both the acetabular and femoral surfaces, it seemed these should both be addressed. Also, firm fixation was needed because stem looseness was frequently painful.

In 1951, at the SICOT meeting in Copenhagen, Kiaer and Jansen presented their work on the use of polymethylmethacrylate as a grouting agent in hip surgery. In 1953, at the Hospital for Joint Diseases in New York, Haboush performed a small series of procedures using this material but with failure because of infection. Charnley and Smith must be credited with recognizing the real value of methylmethacrylate as a fixing agent and with the development of total hip replacement using this material. McKee, Watson-Farrar, and Ring developed hip replacement devices that depended on metal-to-metal contact, but Muller and

Weber also devised prostheses closely resembling that of Charnley with a metal femoral component articulating with polyethylene acetabular device, both fixed by methylmethacrylate. The devices used today have generally been developed from these earlier types.

Better "cementing" techniques and improved mechanical fixation have developed, and sintered and fiber-metal surfaces appear to encourage bone and fibrous ingrowth into the devices. The acetabular sockets are now metal backed, which provides a supportive surface for the polyethylene. These can be threaded or have a sintered or fiber-metal layer of the same material applied as a coating. The femoral hip protheses have been refined with respect to shape and contour. Stainless steel is now rarely used, having been replaced by cobalt-chromium-molybdenum (vitallium) and titanium alloys that have better physical characteristics. Although many surgeons cement femoral protheses, others rely on surface fins to stabilize the devices in cancellous bone or on biologic ingrowth into sintered or fiber-metal surfaces.

Knee replacement developed similarly. Fascial arthroplasties were replaced by condylar replacements, which were not generally successful until the introduction of a prosthesis developed by Gunston while he was working with Charnley.[7]

Over the next several years a plethora of devices were developed in the United States and elsewhere. These designs gradually began to duplicate the articular surface of the distal femur more accurately and provide articulation for the patella. If ball-and-socket joints were simple to design for the hip, the polycentric hinge characteristic of the knee associated with terminal rotation, or screwing home, made design difficult. Fixation of femoral resurfacing devices is usually easily accomplished by methylmethacrylate, but cemented tibial resurfacing devices frequently loosened. If the tibial component was to have a substantial stem that could provide fixation or transfer weight-bearing forces to the stronger periphery of the tibia, it was impossible to retain the cruciate ligaments. Today a few designs continue to retain the cruciate ligaments, but knee arthroplasty is technically easier if the cruciate ligaments are excised. Similar methods of fixation have been explored in the knee and hip, but there appears to be less urgency in this regard because the results of total knee replacement using methylmethacrylate as a fixing agent have become increasingly satisfactory and predictable. Cruciate retention dictates biologic ingrowth as fixation, but while immobilization of the sintered or fiber-metal surface to bone is desirable to achieve ingrowth, it may be counterproductive in attempting to retain motion.[15] The early knee devices did not address the patellofemoral joint, but today this joint is commonly included in the total knee replacement. There is some evidence that in the absence of patellar disease it may not be necessary to replace the patella.

Ankle replacement developed along with replacement of the knee, but it never gained the popularity of either hip or knee replacement because ankle arthrodesis is such an excellent reconstructive alternative. A major problem with ankle replacement has been the high failure rate from loosening with methylmethacrylate fixation. With the use of sintering, however, loosening as a complication has been largely obviated. Thus the procedure can now be recommended with greater confidence in the special circumstances where it may be the procedure of choice.

Arthroplasty of the toes was for many years a resection procedure and generally worked well. Swanson developed a Silastic insert that can be used to replace the proximal articular surface of the proximal digit of the hallux. This acts as a spacer and prevents the shortening associated with all resection arthroplasties.[10]

Upper extremity

In both the lower and upper extremities the objective of arthroplasty is to provide a painless range of motion, but stability is of greater importance in the lower extremity because of one-legged support during the gait cycle. In the upper extremity a certain measure of instability can be accepted and more importance is attached to the range of motion. In general the same implant materials are used in both, but silicone rubber is used more frequently in the upper extremity.

Total shoulder replacement has been brought to an advanced stage of development through the work of Neer and others. Neer's oldest device is a hemiarthroplasty developed for comminuted fractures of the humeral head. More recently, paralleling the developments in treatment of the lower extremity, resurfacing of the humeral head and glenoid have been increasingly used. Shoulder devices have been classified according to the degree of constraint imposed by the linkage of the humeral and glenoid components. Thus in the Neer prosthesis the humeral head and glenoid cavity are resurfaced but are not connected, in contrast to the Post and Gestina types where the humeral and glenoid components are fixed to each other as well as to the bone. The situation is somewhat similar to that in the hip, since the humeral components use the intramedullary canal of the humerus for fixation. Unfortunately, because of the anatomic constraints of the glenoid cavity, it is much more difficult to achieve fixation of the glenoid device than the acetabulum. Methylmethacrylate fixation has been used, but there would seem to be considerable advantage to biologically fixed glenoid components.

Hinge replacements of the elbow have been used since the 1950s, but they presented serious problems with loosening. Use of methylmethacrylate made it possible to achieve better fixation of the medullary stems into the humerus and ulna, but absorption at the bone-implant interface has been a significant problem. Hinge devices have given way to surface replacement of the humerus and ulnar fossa, although such replacements demand intact ligamentous support. Fractures of the radial head have been satisfactorily treated by radial head resection; however, Swanson introduced a Silastic stemmed replacement of the radial head that functioned as an articular spacer. In circumstances where a loss of spacing increased elbow instability, this device has been valuable.

The treatment of arthritis of the wrist is somewhat controversial. Many hand surgeons use proximal row carpectomy, whereas others insert implants. If stability is more important than motion, wrist arthrodesis may be the procedure of choice, as in the ankle. Like the radial head, the distal ulna may be resected, as by the Darrach procedure, but Swanson has advocated replacement of the distal ulna by a prosthesis, particularly when resection arthroplasty has failed or distal dorsal instability is marked.

Individual bones of the carpus can be successfully replaced by silicone prostheses. These include the scaphoid and lunate bones with comminuted avascular necrosis or pseudarthrosis. The prostheses are not applicable for generalized arthritis of the carpus or gross instability with loss of ligamentous support.

Arthroplasty of the metacarpophalangeal joints may be necessary for hand function. In the past, this was largely accomplished by resection arthroplasty, but recently there have been attempts to use silicone implants and various articulated joint replacements. Fixation has been improved in some devices by methylmethacrylate and biologic ingrowth.

Because the purpose of metacarpophalangeal and occasionally interphalangeal joint arthroplasty of the hand is to provide painless motion, the patient must realize that such procedures cannot restore the ability to perform heavy work. Staging is important for success; tendon repair and synovectomy must be performed before reconstruction and tendon imbalances or bone and joint malalignment must be corrected.

• • •

Arthrodesis of joints imposes little demand on the patient. Arthroplasty, to be successful, necessitates cooperation between the patient and surgeon and recognition of the role of rehabilitation in achieving an excellent result. Often the results of arthroplasty of the hand, wrist, elbow, shoulder, and knee depend more on the postoperative rehabilitation than on the surgery itself. Successful arthroplasty demands that the patient actively participate in achieving the final result. Physical and occupational therapy play a tremendous role in the outcome.

LOWER EXTREMITY
Hip

In total hip replacement several variables during the course of surgery dictate postoperative rehabilitation. Surgical approaches to the hip joint can generally be divided into anterior and posterior approaches, with several variations of each. In an anterior approach the capsule lies under the tensor fascia lata muscle. Therefore this muscle must either be detached distally or separated from the gluteus medius along a fairly well-demarcated line with the tensor muscle then retracted distally. Generally part of the anterior gluteal musculature must be detached from the anterior surface of the trochanter if osteotomy of this bone is not to be performed. The anterior capsule is excised, and if necessary the posterior capsule is detached from the acetabulum. Many surgeons believe that the anterior approach allows the most accurate positioning of the prosthetic acetabulum, with good visualization even in the most difficult procedures.[1] However, in some situations, such as revision surgery, the presence of a large amount of scar tissue, or an obese patient, it may not provide adequate exposure. Under these circumstances osteotomy of the trochanter must be performed. At closure the trochanter is reattached, usually with wire or screws. Adjustment of the length of the abductor muscles, sometimes to their physiologic length, is possible. If osteotomy of the trochanter is not performed but the gluteus medius is particularly detached, this muscle and the tensor fascia should be reattached. Anterior surgery is associated with temporary weakening of the internal rotators of the hip, and at least 6 weeks is necessary for the insertion of these muscles to heal.

The posterior approaches split the gluteal musculature and necessitate cutting the insertion of the short external rotators. Most surgeons can perform a posterior approach more rapidly than the anterior, but the incidence of postoperative dislocation is higher.

In total hip replacement it is important that the postoperative joint be stable in the usual positions the patient assumes. With the anterior approach the position of maximal instability is in adduction and external rotation. Stability is improved by correct positioning of the prosthetic components and maintenance of proper neck length. With the patient fully anesthetized, the prosthetic hip should be reducible with modest difficulty but still be stable. A prosthesis with an overly long femoral neck can lengthen the extremity, and an overly short neck can increase the chance of dislocation.

The method of fixation dictates the postoperative therapeutic regimen. Methylmethacrylate is most secure at the time of polymerization, which is 90% accomplished within 10 minutes, although additional polymerization occurs over the next few days. Therefore stability of the prosthesis is at its maximum early in the rehabilitation process. When biologic fixation is being attempted, ingrowth occurs within 5 weeks if apposition between bone and device is satisfactory; however, it is customary to allow an additional week for security. Whether this period should be one of no weight bearing or partial weight bearing is unclear and may depend on the mechanical fixation of the device within the acetabulum and femur. Many elderly patients in whom I have inserted sintered hip devices have borne weight fully on the extremity without ill effects after leaving the hospital 10 to 14 days following surgery. It may be that more weight bearing is desirable with well-fixed prostheses.

Cemented prosthetic components with intact trochanter

When the prosthesis is cemented and the trochanter is intact, therapy begins on the first postoperative day with anterior tibial and quadriceps setting exercises. The lower extremity is positioned in mild abduction and neutral rotation, preventing external rotation. To avert thrombophlebitis, the patients routinely receive anticoagulants and wear supportive stockings. On the second day dangling at the bedside and sitting in a high hip chair are permitted. Active quadriceps exercises are added. On the third day the patient is out of bed learning to ambulate using a walker with the foot gently positioned on the floor and about 25 pounds of weight bearing. On the fifth day, if the patient's stability permits, Lofstrand crutches are introduced. The exercise program the patient will carry out at home is started in the hospital by the therapist (see box on p. 460). Weight bearing can be increased to 50 pounds. On the seventh postoperative day the patient begins instruction in ascending and descending stairs, and on the eighth day the patient practices entering and exiting a bathtub or shower and the front and back seats of a mock-up automobile.

When stable and afebrile with wound healing well advanced, the patient may be discharged and followed up in the office. The box on p. 461 lists instructions the patient should receive at discharge. At home the patient should continue the exercises, but if his or her ability to do so is

---

TOTAL HIP REPLACEMENT HOME EXERCISE PROGRAM

Perform the following exercises two times a day. Each exercise is to be done 10 to 15 times. Avoid pain or fatigue.

Position: Perform the following exercises lying on your back. While performing exercises, count out loud so as not to hold your breath.

1. Isometric exercises:
   a. Gluteal sets: Tighten your buttocks, hold for a count of 3, and release.
   b. Abduction: Tighten the muscles that spread your legs. STOP!! Remember, *do not* allow your legs to move. Hold for a count of 3, and release.
   c. Quadriceps set: Tighten your thighs, pressing the back of your knees into the bedsheet. Hold for a count of 3, and then release.
   d. Ankle isotonics: With your legs straight, raise your ankle for a count of 3 and release, then turn ankle down for a count of 3.
2. Hip and knee flexion: Slide your heel up the sheet, toward the head of the bed, bringing your knee toward your chest. Hold for a count of 3, then slide your heel back down the sheet to starting position.
3. Modified straight leg raise: Slide your heel up the sheet, toward the head of the bed. Raise your leg toward your head. Hold for a count of 3, and slowly lower your leg without bending the knee.
4. Abduction: Slide operated leg out to side from other leg, keeping your knees and toes pointing straight up toward the ceiling. Do not lift your leg off the bed. Return to starting position.

Position: Perform the following exercises in the sitting position. Sit in a straight back chair with thighs supported.

5. Knee range of motion: Sitting with feet flat on the floor, straighten your leg. Hold for a count of 3, then slowly lower. Straighten your leg halfway. Hold for a count of 3, then slowly lower.
6. Postural exercises:
   a. Neck rolls: Gently turn your head in a circular direction, first circling to the right and then to the left.
   b. Shoulder rolls: Gently stretch shoulder blades: up, back, down, and forward.

Position: Perform the following exercise standing alongside a countertop.

7. Mark time in place: March in place. Do not bring knees higher than hip level.

---

*These abduction exercises may be modified if trochanteric osteotomy was carried out at surgery.

questionable, provision should be made for scheduled home physical therapy. Three to 4 weeks postoperatively the patient may be seen in the office, the wound examined, and weight bearing gradually increased to full, with crutches. Generally the patient should continue to position the limb in abduction and neutral rotation and to use an elevated toilet seat until 6 weeks, when the capsule can be assumed to be healed. At 6 weeks a crutch on the postoperative side may be abandoned and a cane substituted for the contralateral crutch in 2 more weeks. Ambulation within the limits of discomfort, as well as abduction and internal rotation exercises, should be encouraged. By 2½ to 3 months after surgery, most patients are free of the cane, except perhaps for long walks, and the strength of the abductor musculature should be evaluated by the Trendelenburg test. If the abductor muscles are weak and the patient limps, or if abductor strength has returned to a good level but the patient limps from habit, additional therapy is desirable to correct any deficiencies. For most patients, active and passive range of motion returns to normal. When it does not, corrective stretching exercises may be indicated. Loss of previously present motion in the hip may indicate the development of hypertrophic bone; radiographs help to detect this. Patients can resume milder sports such as golf and doubles tennis at 6 months postoperatively if radiographs are satisfactory and physical examination indicates near-normal muscle strength. The limits placed on a patient depend on the surgeon's interpretation of the stability of the fixation and the radiographic appearance of the prosthetic components.

Hip replacement with ingrowth fixation and the trochanter intact

In a patient with ingrowth fixation and an intact trochanter, rehabilitation is the same as that for cemented fixation until the fourth postoperative day when the foot can be placed flat on the floor with very light weight bearing (about 15 pounds). This appears to be preferable to toe touching, which is difficult for older patients to learn and probably places greater stress on the hip joint from muscular tension. Weight bearing is not increased until ingrowth has occurred.

At 6 weeks postoperatively the patient returns for radiographic examination, which generally indicates close apposition of the prosthesis to the overlying bone. In some areas there may be fuzzy radiolucency suggesting bone ingrowth. The raised toilet seat and abduction pillow are discontinued, and the patient is advised to begin partial weight bearing with crutches (30 pounds of foot pressure, which can be determined using a set of bathroom scales). In the seventh week, weight bearing is increased to 50 to 60 pounds using crutches or a walker, and in the eighth week weight

---

DO'S AND DON'TS FOLLOWING TOTAL HIP REPLACEMENT

1. Keep a pillow between legs while in bed.
2. Sleep on either side with a pillow between legs.
3. When home, put one or two firm pillows on any low chair to build up the height. Continue to use your raised toilet seat.
4. Do not cross legs.
5. Do not pivot on operated leg.
6. Do not put on your own shoe, sock, or stocking, without the use of your long-handled shoehorn or stocking assist.
7. While sitting or standing, do not bend over to pick up any object from off the floor. Use reacher provided.
8. When ascending stairs, lead with your good leg. When descending stairs, lead with your crutches and the operated leg.

---

bearing is increased to 75 pounds, or half body weight. By the ninth week the patient discards the crutch on the operated side and at the end of the week returns for radiographic evaluation. If results continue to be satisfactory, the patient substitutes a cane for the contralateral crutch when walking around the home. By the tenth week the crutch is discontinued and the patient is advised to establish a regular schedule of increased walking distance, using the cane for support on long walks only. Reexamination is important to verify correction of the muscle atrophy normally associated with arthritis and reconstructive surgery. By the eleventh week there should be decreasing dependence on the cane and strong emphasis on walking normally with avoidance of limp.

I encourage walking as much as possible, but no matter how well the patient feels and how satisfactory the radiographs appear, I do not permit a return to sports such as golf, doubles tennis, and skiing until 6 months. Before resuming this type of activity, the patient should be reevaluated to ensure that muscles have recovered enough to permit mild athletics.

Total hip replacement with trochanteric osteotomy and either methylmethacrylate or biologic fixation

When there has been total hip replacement with osteotomy of the trochanter and with methylmethacrylate or biologic fixation, rehabilitation is identical to the ingrowth program except that at 6 weeks the radiographic evaluation includes the healing of the trochanteric osteotomy. The films show whether sufficient healing has occurred to permit the resumption of weight bearing. If the radiographs do not show this to be sufficient, the patient should continue light weight bearing, although the abduction pillow and elevated toilet seat can be discontinued. If radiographs confirm satisfactory healing 8 to 9 weeks after surgery, partial weight bearing

can be started, progressing to half body weight with crutches over the ensuing 2 to 3 weeks. At 10 to 12 weeks the crutch on the operated side can be discontinued, and 1 or 2 weeks later a cane can be substituted on the opposite side. The patient must be followed carefully to verify satisfactory increase in abduction strength and the elimination of abduction limp. Whether such a patient can participate in recreational sports depends on the return on muscle strength and range of motion. Under no circumstance should this be permitted earlier than 6 months after surgery, and generally 1 year should elapse.

Patients with posterior surgical approaches are generally treated much the same as those with anterior approaches, but in view of the tendency to instability in flexion, greater care must be taken with sitting in the early period. In revision surgery and in primary procedures performed for congenital dislocation or subluxation of the hip, where extensive bone grafting is required, the postoperative regimen is dictated by both the radiologic evidence of bone healing and the appreciation of the significant time interval required for vascularization of large bone grafts. In some cases it may be several months before a patient with a homologous graft can be safely permitted to progress beyond partial weight bearing. Because of the nature of such procedures, outlining a rehabilitation plan is fruitless. The regimen must be individualized by the surgeon.

Knee

The early results of total knee replacement arthroplasty were acceptable from the point of view of pain relief, but motion was only slightly improved. Unfortunately, the early designs often loosened and failed, and a common misconception arose that knee replacement was far less successful than hip replacement. Today, with improved component designs, knee replacement produces not only complete pain relief but also improved motion and lasting firm fixation, free from loosening and prosthetic settling. Arising from a chair requires 93 degrees of flexion, and ascending and descending stairs requires 83 degrees.[8] The use of passive motion machines early in the postoperative period has not only decreased the incidence of thrombophlebitis but also increased the early range of motion.

Knee replacement is usually performed through a medial parapatellar approach. This necessitates sectioning the quadriceps expansion medially, extending proximally into the quadriceps tendon and distally medial to the insertion of the patellar tendon. The insertion of the femoral prosthesis requires approximately 120 degrees of flexion, but unfortunately this amount is rarely retained. Depending on the particular prosthetic design, patellar replacement may make the patella more prominent and put added tension on the repair. However, disruption of the incision is rare and need not be an important consideration in postoperative rehabilitation. The major determinant of rehabilitation is the method of fixation. Biologic fixation appears to have discrete

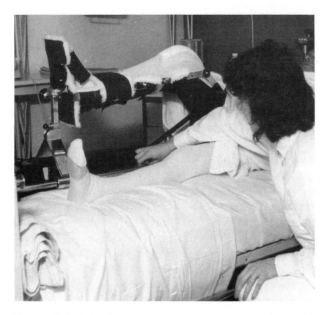

Figure 33-1. After knee surgery, patients are started in passive motion machine as soon as wound drains are removed. Flexion is increased daily to tolerance with full extension. Four hours of treatment daily is given in divided sessions.

advantages in the hip and ankle, but there is little evidence that this technique offers an improvement in total knee arthroplasty.

After surgery most patients are immediately immobilized in a bulky Jones pressure dressing with an overlying splint, which is retained for at least 24 hours. Quadriceps and anterior tibial setting exercises are instituted on the first postoperative day, but the start of movement depends on the removal of any wound suction catheters. Once catheters are removed, passive motion can begin. This can be readily accomplished by a passive motion machine, in which the flexion and extension stops can be set (Figure 33-1).[2] On the second postoperative day the patient can sit in a bedside chair and continues the passive motion regimen with gradually increasing flexion. Active quadriceps motion and ambulation with a walker are begun on the third day, with the amount of weight bearing dependent on the type of fixation. If the prosthetic components are fixed with methylmethacrylate, weight bearing is allowed to tolerance, whereas with biologic fixation only resting the foot on the floor or toe touching is permitted. Exercises are continued and increased during the 10 to 12 days of hospitalization. Most patients can flex the knee to 90 degrees or beyond before discharge. Manipulation under anesthesia is rarely indicated or desirable.

Before discharge of a patient with a device that depends on biologic ingrowth for fixation, lateral radiographs are taken in flexion and extension to verify the absence of rocking of the tibial component. If none is found, the patient is advised to continue active motion during the 6 weeks re-

quired for biologic ingrowth and is warned of the disastrous effect that weight bearing might have on the end result. If movement of the prosthesis is shown, the patient should be placed in a long leg cast in extension until 6 weeks after surgery. By the time the cast is removed, the knee is relatively stiff and even with manipulation will probably not gain the 105 degrees of flexion desired.[5] Newer sintered tibial components have employed screws and keels to provide additional fixation of the tibial component.

Patients with methylmethacrylate fixation are encouraged to use crutches for the first 6 weeks after surgery and to continue a daily program of active and passive exercises for the knee (see box opposite). If the exercises are performed religiously, the quadriceps will regain strength and the motion gained at surgery will be retained. The patient must be instructed carefully in what is required and the importance of these exercises. Most elderly patients profit from frequent visits by a physiotherapist to ensure that the program is being followed on a regular basis.

At 6 weeks postoperatively, patients with biologic fixation are examined radiologically to visualize the prosthesis-bone interface. The patient must be carefully positioned so this critical area can be seen. If ingrowth appears to be proceeding well, the patient is started on a gradually increasing weight-bearing program identical with that used for hip replacement patients. For those who have had methylmethacrylate-fixed devices inserted, walking aids are gradually reduced, first by one crutch and then by substitution of a cane for the other crutch. The bone is gradually strengthened by avoiding undue stress on the interface in the early phases of healing. With time the bone reorganizes and becomes stronger in keeping with the altered biomechanics of the new joint replacement. A cane should be used until muscle strength has returned to a good level and the limb is stable.

Ankle

Total ankle replacement is far less commonly performed than knee or hip replacement. Arthritis of the ankle joint usually follows trauma such as a fracture of the plafond, widening of the mortice secondary to unreduced fractures of the fibula, instability caused by tearing of the lateral ligament complex, and rheumatoid arthritis.[3] Because of the ankle's excellent design, it is largely immune to osteoarthritis. Ankle arthrodesis, if properly performed with placement of the fused joint in neutral to 5 degrees of plantar flexion, results in little disability. Therefore ankle arthroplasty is indicated only in special circumstances when there is bilateral ankle involvement, the subtalar joint is fused, or the patient is elderly. The procedure is effective in removing pain, but failures have occurred from loosening and settling of the tibial component. Fortunately, this serious drawback has been largely obviated by the use of sintered tibial and talar components. The procedure is normally carried out through an anterior approach. Skin healing is critical because of the superficial position of the ankle joint.[13,14]

TOTAL KNEE REPLACEMENT HOME EXERCISE PROGRAM

Perform the following exercises two times a day. Each exercise is to be done 10 to 15 times.* Avoid pain and fatigue.

Position: Perform the following exercises lying on your back. While performing exercises, count out loud so as not to hold your breath.

1. Isometric exercises:
   a. Gluteal sets: Tighten your buttocks, hold for a count of 3, and then release.
   b. Quadriceps sets: Tighten your thighs, pressing the back of your knees into the bedsheet. Hold for a count of 3, and then release.
   c. Modified quadriceps sets: Place a firm towel roll under your ankle. Press the back of your knee down into the bed. At the same time, begin to stretch your toes up toward your nose. Hold for a count of 3, and then release.
   d. Ankle isotonics: With your legs straight, raise your ankle up for a count of 3 and release, then turn ankle down for a count of 3 and release.
2. Hip and knee flexion: Slide your heel up the sheet toward the head of the bed, bringing your knee toward your chest. Hold for a count of 3, then slide heel back down the sheet to starting position.
3. Straight leg raise:
   a. First exercise: With your leg straight, repeat the quadriceps set exercise. At the same time turn your ankle up and raise leg toward your head. When it is raised as far as possible, without bending the knee, hold for a count of 3 and slowly lower your leg to the starting position.
   b. Second exercise: Slide your heel up the sheet, toward the head of the bed. Raise your leg toward your head. Hold for a count of 3, and slowly lower your leg without bending the knee.
4. Terminal extension: Place a firm pillow roll under your knee. Press your knee down into the pillow roll as you raise your foot toward your head. Hold for a count of 3, and then slowly return foot to the bed.

Position: Perform the following exercises in the sitting position. Sit in a straight back chair with thighs supported.

5. Knee stretch:
   a. First exercise: Sitting with knees bent and feet flat on the floor, place the good leg over the operated leg. Begin to push the operated leg back further with the assist of the good leg. Hold this position for a count of 3, then release.
   b. Second exercise: Place a 3-pound weight around your ankle. Sitting with feet flat on the floor, straighten your leg. Hold for a count of 3, then slowly lower. Straighten your leg halfway. Hold for a count of 3, then slowly lower.

*Start with five repetitions and increase by one repetition each day. Do not exceed 15 repetitions.

Separation of the skin edges and necrosis are all too common but may in part be due to inadequate care and handling of the skin or to undermining of the skin edges. Because of loosening, many surgeons have stopped cementing ankle components and have changed the postoperative routine accordingly. To ensure good ingrowth, patients are placed in a short leg plaster cast immediately after surgery. Because the results of total ankle replacement are to some extent correlated with dorsiflexion, the postoperative cast must maintain the position achieved at surgery. As the prosthetic components are inserted in maximum plantar flexion, dorsiflexion tends to compress the sintered surfaces against the bone of the tibia and talus, setting the stage for maximal potential ingrowth.

Six weeks after surgery the cast is removed and radiographs are taken. As in the case of the knee, the ankle must be positioned properly to ensure that the x-ray beam is parallel with the surface of the device. If the interface is shown to be satisfactory, the patient is started on progressive weight bearing similar to the regimen used in the hip and the knee. After the cast is removed, a close-fitting ankle corset can be worn for the next 6 weeks. The corset seems to reduce swelling of the distal calf and foot and provides external support during calf muscle rehabilitation. Patients are taught flexion and extension of the ankle and permitted to exercise the subtalar joint. Despite the removal of pain and the redevelopment of strength in the calf muscles, the tendency to walking with the leg in external rotation can be difficult to correct. Usually by persistence in forcing the patient to walk more slowly and correctly, a normal gait can be regained after arthroplasty.

Foot

Anthroplasty of the foot is generally confined to the metatarsophalangeal and interphalangeal joints. Arthroplasty of the first metatarsophalangeal joint is the most commonly performed procedure. Excision of the proximal portion of the proximal phalanx and exostectomy of the head of the first metatarsal have been carried out for many years for the treatment of hallux valgus. In the past, it was unusual to use a transfixation pin across the joint, but this adjunct has become increasingly popular because it holds position and permits fibrous tissue ingrowth by separating the proximal phalanx from the metatarsal head. Swanson has developed a Silastic spacer for the base of the proximal phalanx to provide more stability with retention of anatomic length.

Similar procedures are performed on the other metatarsophalangeal joints, often for disabling rheumatoid arthritis. The decision of whether to use a transfixing pin or wire depends on the degree of stability that exists when the arthroplasty is performed. Excisional arthroplasties tend to produce significant instability of the metatarsophalangeal joint; to avoid postoperative dislocation of the joint, insertion of a Kirschner wire may be a good routine.

Arthroplasty of the interphalangeal joint of the hallux or the proximal or distal interphalangeal joints of the other digits is less commonly performed, but similar principles apply and internal fixation is used for stability and maintenance of correction. With pins in place patients are permitted to walk in a postoperative wooden-sole shoe. A pad can be inserted to elevate the metatarsals if the metatarsophalangeal joints are fixed in neutral position; with arthroplasty and internal fixation of the interphalangeal joints this is generally unnecessary. The wires are retained in position for approximately 4 weeks, and when they are removed, the patients are permitted progressive ambulation as tolerated. A resumption of normal activities occurs over the next few weeks and is generally painless.

UPPER EXTREMITY
Shoulder

Replacement of the humeral head for treatment of fractures began in 1951. Over the years this procedure has given good results in patients with a normal glenoid cavity and good shoulder musculature. During the early 1970s attempts were made to design fixed-fulcrum prostheses that would eliminate the need for an intact rotator cuff. Unfortunately, this design was associated with a high failure rate, and consequently a return was made to the original hemiarthroplasty, modifying the top and edges so the prosthesis could be articulated with a polyethylene glenoid surface.[9] Other designs are used, such as the Swanson bipolar with the humeral and glenoid components joined, an overhanging glenoid component designed by MacNab and English, and some very constrained types, such as the Post and Gestina, in which the humeral and glenoid components are fixed to the bone and also to one another. My experience has been largely with the Neer prosthesis, and for that reason his rehabilitation program is outlined here. Severe arthritis of the shoulder is much less common than similar disease in the knee and hip. Primary osteoarthritis is relatively infrequent, but secondary degenerative arthritis is associated with

a number of arthritides resulting in articular damage, such as metabolic disorders, old septic arthritis, trauma to the articular surface from severe cuff tears, and chronic dislocation or fractures involving the articular surface. Some of the more common secondary causes are the infractional diseases such as sickle cell anemia, Gaucher's disease, and lupus treated with steroids. One of the most important causes of severe arthritis of the shoulder is rheumatoid arthritis. Neer has found it valuable to classify rheumatoid disease of the shoulder into three grades of severity (low, intermediate, and severe) with three types of involvement (dry, wet, and resorbative). These differentiations are valuable in surgical prognostication with respect to the intactness of the cuff and quality of the bone available for shoulder reconstruction.

Several approaches to total shoulder replacement may be used, but the long deltopectoral approach is considered best because it improves the potential for rehabilitation.[9] Other approaches require detachment of the anterior or middle part of the deltoid and result in weakening. With the long deltopectoral approach the deltoid is retracted laterally with abduction of the arm and the subscapularis tendon is divided medial to the bicipital groove. The long head of the biceps is retained, and any rotator cuff tears present are repaired. The glenoid fossa must be carefully prepared because relatively little material is available for fixation. The subchondral bone is preserved. Fixation is generally accomplished with polymethylmethacrylate, although sintered devices have been used. Erosion of the glenoid fossa, as occurs in rheumatoid arthritis, may necessitate bone grafting to ensure correct orientation of the device stem. Because of the anatomy and function of the shoulder, little stability is provided by either the glenoid fossa or the surrounding ligaments. The surrounding muscles play the critical role in stability, so great care must be taken in closure to ensure that contracted muscle tendon units are lengthened and cuff defects are mobilized and repaired without tension. Occasionally, additional procedures, such as an acromioclavicular arthroplasty or deltoidplasty, are needed for a sound satisfactory result.

Postoperatively the extremity is usually immobilized in a sling and swath. With large shoulder cuff repairs an abduction brace may be helpful, and a light spica cast is useful for patients with marked instability.

The rehabilitation program is of great importance in achieving an excellent result. Because variations exist in stability, muscle intactness, and degree of repair carried out, rehabilitation goals must be individualized. Neer described three exercise phases: (1) local heat and passive or assisted motion, (2) active exercises, and (3) muscle-stretching and resistive strengthening exercises. Phase 1 begins on the sixth postoperative day and phase 2 is added on the eleventh day. Neer recommended mild heat and analgesies before the exercise routines. Patients in phase 3, such as those with nonfunctioning deltoid and rotator cuff muscles, have an exercise program prescribed that is aimed at retaining stability and achieving external rotation and elevation but still permits the activities of daily living.

Total shoulder replacement is a procedure that requires specialized training to perform. Many surgical variables must be taken into account if an excellent result is to be obtained. In general the indications are similar to those of arthroplasty elsewhere: pain and the inability to perform, or great difficulty with, the activities of daily living, resulting in a significant reduction in the quality of life. While generally associated with an improvement in motion, this is not usually considered a reason for performing total shoulder replacement.

Elbow

The elbow consists of two joints, the ulnohumeral and the radiocapitellar. The function of the former is flexion and extension, and the latter is associated with rotation of the forearm.

The ulnohumeral joint has a wide range of motion, which is important in daily living. Therefore arthrodesis of this joint in 90 degrees of flexion, the desired position for unilateral fusion of the elbow, significantly impairs function. Also, it is one of the most difficult arthrodeses to achieve, and none of the many procedures available is associated with a high fusion rate. As a result, arthroplasty is an attractive alternative. It is unlikely to be successful if the muscles monitoring the joint are weak or inadequate or if the ankylosis is extra-articular. As in all arthroplasties, infection is generally considered a contraindication. For anatomic reasons, whatever type of arthroplasty is intended, the elbow is approached posteriorly by detaching the triceps at the aponeurosis proximally or through a midline splitting of the aponeurosis, triceps muscle, and periosteum, with exposure gained through medial and lateral retraction. In the past, it was customary to free the ulnohumeral joint and cover the end of the humerus with some interposed material such as fascia lata or freeze-dried dura mater, and to treat the radio-capitellar joint by covering the radial head with the same interposing material or excising the head. Because the motion of the ulnohumeral joint is essentially flexion and extension, uniaxial hinges with stems were used in the 1960s. Unfortunately, these generally loosened but were tried again with the advent of polymethylmethacrylate fixation.

Arthroplasty of the radiocapitellar joint alone can be performed by excision of the radial head with fairly good success. If preserving the spacing of the joint is necessary, insertion of a Silastic radial head implant may be desirable. More recently, various unconstrained surface replacements have been developed for the ulna and humerus, such as that of Ewald and others. These show definite improvement over the older techniques.[4] After interpositional arthroplasty the elbow is immobilized in 90 degrees of flexion for approximately 2 weeks. The cast is then splinted, or a posterior

molded splint made, to begin active exercises of the head. By 3 weeks postoperatively protected active motion of the elbow is started, but recovery of function is generally delayed because of the necessity of redeveloping strength in the active elbow flexors and extensors. During the early stage it is desirable to protect the elbow from varus-valgus instability. The protocol for total elbow replacement is outlined in the box on p. 466.

Wrist

The classical solution to functionally limiting arthritis of the wrist is arthrodesis, placing the joint in the position of function at about 15 degrees of extension. Most surgical techniques, and there are a wide variety, include the use of a bone graft from the radius to either the proximal carpal bones or the base of the third metacarpal. When motion must be retained, proximal carpal row excision as an arthroplasty has been used. Articular implants for the wrist have been devised by Voltz, Swanson, and others. The results of these replacements and proximal row carpectomy have not been altogether satisfactory, causing many surgeons to suggest that arthrodesis is preferable, especially for patients who must perform fairly heavy work. Voltz recommends that candidates for wrist arthroplasty be carefully studied to evaluate motor function, particularly the wrist extensors, since many patients with arthritis lose volitional control. Electromyography is helpful in evaluating the activity level of muscles. A biofeedback program may be desirable to regain active control. Postoperatively, the wrist must be splinted until volitional control is regained.[12]

The fingers can be exercised regularly, and isometric exercises of the forearm arm muscles started. Following cast removal in 3 to 4 weeks, active flexion and extension and radial and ulnar deviation exercises are started, as well as pronation and supination of the forearm. Steady progress in achievement of an active range of motion is to be expected over the next 2 months, but if motion appears somewhat inadequate, passive stretching of the joint may be started. Arthroplasty of the radial-ulnar joint is usually accomplished by the Darrach resection of the distal ulna. Swanson advocated a Silastic replacement of the ulnar head dorsal subluxation and the failure of ulnar head resection, as well as for the usual indications. The postoperative regimen is similar to the preceding except that the forearm is placed in a cast in supination for a few weeks before removal and the start of an exercise program.

Many surgeons recommend the use of a rolled-up piece of fascia or tendon as a spacer for the scaphoid and lunate bones, but Swanson advocated the use of silicone, particularly for pseudarthrosis, avascular necrosis, or localized degenerative changes.[10] He advised postoperative plaster cast immobilization, which in the case of the scaphoid bone is a long arm-thumb spica cast. For the lunate bone a short arm cast with the wrist in slight extension suffices. Because of immediate postoperative swelling the cast be either split

EWALD'S TOTAL ELBOW REPLACEMENT PROTOCOL

These guidelines are subject to change relative to the precise surgical procedure performed and the patient's progress.

Preoperative physical therapy

1. Preoperative evaluation with careful attention to shoulder motion on operative side
2. Preoperative pulmonary therapy instruction (deep breathing and coughing)
3. Instruction in postoperative exercise regime
4. Instruction in transfers using nonoperative extremity for assistance when necessary or feasible

Preoperative occupational therapy

1. Assessment of upper extremity range of motion and ability to perform activities of daily living, including bathing, toileting, dressing, and grooming
2. Hand status recorded to determine whether range of motion and strength deficits at the elbow have resulted in decreased functional abilities of the hand; ulnar nerve distribution checked for sensation and strength
3. Assessment of home situation and discharge situation
4. Patient instruction; explanation of postsurgical activities of daily living techniques and precautions

Day of surgery

1. Postoperative pulmonary therapy as necessary
2. Elbow in commercial posterior splint, usually at close to 60-degree flexion; check positioning
3. Hand maintained in elevated position with pillows

Postoperative day 1

1. Pulmonary therapy
2. Gentle hand and wrist active exercise on operated extremity; check for ulnar nerve deficit
3. Correct positioning as necessary

Day 2

1. Chest, hand, and wrist exercises as on postoperative day 1
2. Patient ambulation with elbow in splint and supported by sling when upright or sitting in chair
3. Gentle assisted shoulder flexion on operative side, giving careful manual support protection above and below elbow joint and preventing medial and lateral stress on joint

Days 3 to 6

1. Pulmonary therapy continued as necessary; ambulation as tolerated by patient
2. Active, assisted, range-of-motion (ROM) exercises to elbow, including progressive flexion, extension, supination, and pronation, when approved by surgeon; all exercises performed with elbow at side; placement of prosthesis is to be protected for 6 weeks for capsular healing; all exercises must be done *only* with upper *arm* in *adducted position*
3. Elbow replaced in splint following exercise and kept in sling for upright activities

Day 7

1. Splint adjusted to maximum extension for night use only, when approved by surgeon
2. ROM exercises as before; independent sessions encouraged

Days 8 to 10

1. Hand to mouth exercise, keeping upper arm adducted and using some forward flexion of shoulder
2. Use of splint and sling during day discontinued if appropriate
3. Assessment of patient's ability to put on and take off elbow sling; sling adapted as necessary
4. Ulnar nerve function documented
5. Feeding ability evaluated and encouraged to reinforce hand-mouth exercise.

Physical therapy day 11 to discharge

1. ROM and all permitted activities with elbow held in adducted position for 6 weeks postoperatively; no resistive exercises or activities added to program
2. Instruction in appropriate use of sling as determined
3. Final evaluation

Occupational therapy day 11 to discharge

1. Instruction in sagittal plane activities of daily living, including dressing, bathing, grooming, feeding, and toileting; identification of dominant extremity and instruction in appropriate precautions
2. Evaluation for instruction in use of adapted equipment as necessary
3. Final evaluation

Activities to avoid

1. No lifting, except spoon, fork, or knife, maximum weight 1 pound
2. No carrying handbag on operated side
3. No abduction or internal or external rotation of shoulder
4. No jarring or pounding motions
5. No pushing motions against resistance
6. No tennis, golf, or throwing sports *under any circumstances*

initially or applied a few days after surgery. After 6 to 8 weeks the plaster is removed and active exercises are begun, but radiographs of the wrist must be taken to ensure that the implant does not become subluxated or dislocated.

Swanson also recommended the use of a Silastic implant for the trapezium or in resection arthroplasty of the basilar joint of the thumb. Certainly the motion generated at the base of the thumb is a desirable feature as long as stability is not lost. Apparently the key is meticulous capsule ligament reconstruction to prevent instability, as is also the case with spacer implants for the scaphoid and lunate bones.

Hand

Metacarpophalangeal joint motion is extremely important in hand function, and a variety of techniques have been used to restore motion in these joints. However, with any arthroplasty of the hand the timing in relation to other necessary procedures is of critical importance. Thus, in rheumatoid arthritis, ulnar drift must be corrected and tendon procedures performed before arthroplasty; otherwise the latter is doomed to fail. The classical arthroplasties of Fowler and Vainio are essentially resection procedures but use the resection to obtain tension release of the soft tissues. Because of the inherent instability and limitation of flexion, many surgeons such as Flatt, Niebauer, and Swanson used joint prostheses to increase motion and limit instability.[10] Postoperatively the hand is placed in a compression dressing and elevated. Later, Kirschner stabilizing wires are removed and motion is instituted. Dynamic splints play an important role in improving flexion and reducing the risk of recurrent ulnar drift.

There is less indication for arthroplasty of the proximal interphalangeal (PIP) joints. Carroll performed a resection of the distal one fourth of the proximal phalanx followed by 6 weeks of traction on the middle phalanx by a Kirschner wire. Swanson used a Silastic implant for reconstruction of a stiff PIP joint, a swan-neck or boutonnière deformity. He advised starting exercises within 3 to 5 days after surgery if no tendon function has been performed.[11] Because of the tendency of the distal interphalangeal (DIP) joint to move rather than the PIP, it may be necessary to immobilize the DIP joint with a splint or a Kirschner wire. If the arthroplasty was performed for a swan-neck deformity, it should be immobilized in 10 to 20 degrees of flexion. If the procedure was for a boutonnière deformity, the PIP joint should be maintained in extension. Active flexion and extension exercises can be started in 10 days or so.

Arthroplasty of the DIP joint is least often performed. Swanson has a double-hinged implant that can be used for resection arthroplasty of these joints, which are much more commonly treated with arthrodesis. Postoperatively the DIP and PIP joints are splinted in full extension, after which the DIP joint is immobilized for an additional 4-week period and motion is permitted in the PIP joint. Active flexion and extension exercises follow.[11]

REFERENCES

1. Charnley, J: Total hip replacement by low friction arthroplasty, Clin Orthop 72:7, 1970.
2. Coutts, RD, et al: The effect of continuous passive motion on total knee rehabilitation, presented at AAOS Fifteenth Annual Meeting, Anaheim, Calif, March 15, 1983.
3. Evanski, PM, and Waugh, TR: Management of arthritis of the ankle, Clin Orthop Rel Res No. 122, January-February 1977.
4. Ewald, FC: Personal communication, January 14, 1987.
5. Fox, JL, and Poss, R: The role of manipulation following total knee replacement, J Bone Joint Surg 63A:357, 1981.
6. Gluck, T: Referat uber die Durach das moderne Chirurgische Experiment, Arch Klin Chir 41:186, 1891.
7. Gunston, FH: Polycentric knee arthroplasty, J Bone Joint Surg 53B:272, 1971.
8. Kettlekamp, DB: Knee mechanics related to surgery in arthritis, AAOS Instructional Course, Washington, DC, 1972.
9. Neer, CS, Watson, KC, and Stanton, FJ: Recent experience in total shoulder replacement, J Bone Joint Surg 64A:319, 1982.
10. Swanson, AB: Flexible implant resection arthroplasty in the hand and extremities, St Louis, 1973, The CV Mosby Co.
11. Swanson, AB, Swanson, G de G, and Leonard, J: Post-operative rehabilitation program in flexible implant arthroplasty of the digits. In Hunter, JM, et al, editors: Rehabilitation of the hand, St Louis, 1978, The CV Mosby Co.
12. Voltz, RG: Personal communication, January 5, 1987.
13. Waugh, TR: Total knee arthroplasty in 1984, Clin Orthop 192:40, 1985.
14. Waugh, TR, Evanski, PM, and McMaster, WC: Irvine ankle arthroplasty: design, operative technique and preliminary results, J Bone Joint Surg 58A:729, 1976.
15. Waugh, TR, Evanski, PM, and McMaster, WC: Irvine ankle arthroplasty: prosthetic design and surgical technique, Clin Orthop Rel Res 114:180, 1976.

CHAPTER 34

Surgical management of scoliosis

GORDON L. ENGLER

INDICATIONS FOR SURGERY

When it appears that conservative measures will no longer maintain or correct a significantly developed case of scoliosis, a thorough examination of the patient and the radiographs often lead the physician to recommend surgery. Although it is usually a last resort, it may actually be a more conservative route for the scoliosis patients who would endure long years of conservative management only to require surgery at a later date.

To assist the physician in decision making, there are several indications for surgery.

Magnitude of curve

In general, curves of 20 degrees or less may be carefully watched for progression during adolescent growth. However, when a curve is progressive or exceeds 20 degrees, some form of treatment is usually necessary to prevent further progression. A brace has been the standard treatment for many years. Recently, however, electronic devices that stimulate muscle contraction at night have been used with some success.

When a curve exceeds 40 or 45 degrees, a brace or other conservative measures are usually inadequate to prevent further progression, and surgical correction becomes necessary. There are, however, gray zones. A curve of 38 degrees with other problems may require surgery, whereas a stable curve of 42 degrees in an adult male might never require surgery. These are unusual exceptions to the basic rules.

Pain

Pain is a rare symptom in a healthy child with idiopathic scoliosis. If present, it should alert the physician to determine whether it has some neurologic basis. In an adult, however, pain may be a sequela of an adolescent idiopathic

curve. Usually this occurs in curves of greater than 40 degrees and is often caused by arthritic changes.

Progression

Significant progression of scoliosis to a magnitude greater than 40 degrees despite active treatment with the brace is usually an indication for surgery. These curves are unusual but do occur during adolescent growth. On rare occasions curves might progress in an adult to 40 degrees or more and require surgical correction.

Rotation

The degree of rotation of the thoracic rib cage does not always correlate with the magnitude of the curve. Some curves of 40 degrees may have very little rotation of the thoracic rib cage, whereas curves of 25 degrees may have significant rotation, with a large right thoracic rib prominence. When this rotational deformation becomes severe, surgical correction may be required to prevent further deformity. The brace is often more effective in preventing and correcting the rib prominence by exerting a direct force on the rib angle. The electronic muscle stimulator type of conservative treatment cannot accomplish this goal.

Flexibility

A patient's flexibility is a two-edged sword. Although a relatively inflexible curve prevents correction by brace, the same rigidity prevents progression once the brace treatment has been completed.[13] Often a very flexible child is well corrected with the brace but still requires surgical treatment because the curve progresses after the brace has been removed.

Balance

One large structural curve can often create a marked imbalance of the truncal alignment. If this becomes manifest, it is often cosmetically necessary to correct the spine with surgery rather than prescribe brace treatment for a period of time. One of the early manifestations of the brace program is the development of a secondary curve, which allows the largest structural change to be split into two smaller curves and provides the child with a more cosmetically appealing balanced spinal alignment.

Age of patient

It is usually recommended that surgery not be performed on a child with an immature skeleton—that is, whose growth has not yet begun. Nevertheless, this old attitude of waiting until growth has stopped often deprives the patient of appropriate surgery at a period when optimal correction can be obtained. One cannot wait too long, or this ability will be lost and adequate correction will be impossible. If progression exceeds 45 or 50 degrees despite brace treatment, surgery is usually indicated even if the child has not completed full growth. In general, 50% of growth should be attained by the time of surgery.

Wedging of the intervertebral disc

The invertebral disc is often wedge shaped, thus preventing correction with conservative measures such as a brace. In these cases surgery is often required because of the curve's rapid progression and deformity. When the wedging of the intervertebral bodies themselves is seen, brace treatment is often more effective because of the adaptational growth of the bony elements of the spine in the brace.

Lateral spondylolisthesis

In an adult, large lumbar curves often result in lateral slippage of the vertebral body on its subjacent segment. This may lead to nerve impingement and often pain. This becomes in the adult patient an indication for surgery to correct and stabilize both the scoliosis and the lateral vertebral displacement.

Pulmonary deficit

Curves of greater than 60 degrees in the thoracic region usually result in some degree of pulmonary deficit in the adult patient.[14,15] To prevent this from developing, surgery is often recommended in a child whose curve may progress to that magnitude or in the adult when the pulmonary deficit becomes manifest.

Thoracic lordosis

Usually the normal spine has a certain kyphosis in the thoracic region. A moderately round back is an acceptable posture. In some people, for unknown reasons, the spine is absolutely straight or "caves in" at that level. When this is combined with scoliosis, it makes brace treatment difficult because pressure from the brace pad further accentuates this narrow anteroposterior dimension of the thoracic cage.[14]

This results in a markedly narrow dimension of the chest and causes pulmonary problems. When thoracic lordosis is seen, surgery is often recommended earlier, and brace treatment is often contraindicated. It is therefore not unusual to see a 30- or 35-degree scoliosis curve requiring surgery when a marked degree of thoracic lordosis or hypokyphosis is present.

Gray zone

In the face of many of the problems already mentioned, it is often necessary to watch and wait to determine whether surgery is necessary. Surgery can always be performed, and unless significant progression of the curve demands immediate surgery, it is often wiser to wait 6 months to ensure that the surgical procedure is absolutely necessary.

In summary, it can be seen that the curve magnitude (related to the bone age and cosmetic appearance of the patient) often play a significant role in deciding about surgical intervention. In general, it can be assumed that a curve of greater than 50 degrees will worsen slowly over the years after the completion of growth. A curve of greater than 45 degrees in a growing child may increase even if bracing is continued. Thoracic lordosis may increase and cause further pulmonary deficiency.

In the lumbar area a curve of more than 40 degrees may worsen with time. This may lead to further cosmetic deformity because of an unbalanced truncal alignment. The lateral spondylolisthesis may cause pain in the adult, although it is rare in the adolescent.

PREOPERATIVE EVALUATION

Once the decision for surgery has been made, radiographs are required to evaluate the entire spine. Usually, standing anteroposterior and lateral radiographs make it possible to determine the nature of the curve, assess the thoracic lordosis, and rule out the presence of spondylolisthesis. Lateral bending or traction radiographs may assist the surgeon in deciding the placement of the spinal instrumentation. Furthermore, if the curve is not flexible, the surgeon may consider a two-stage procedure with anterior release of the spine followed by traction and subsequent posterior fusion with instrumentation.[2,17]

Pulmonary function tests are often obtained before surgery to determine the capacity of the patient's lungs and evaluate appropriate safety measures for anesthesia during the surgical procedure. In patients with neuromuscular disease, there have been occasions in which pulmonary function worsens after traction has been applied to the spine. In such a case correction of the spine must be either abandoned or performed carefully to prevent a serious pulmonary problem arising as a direct result of the surgery. In general, if the P_{CO_2} is elevated or the vital capacity is less than 25% of the predicted value, postoperative ventilatory support will probably be required.

Because of the nature of the surgery, blood transfusions may be required. The use of autologous blood in recent years has given a great measure of safety to the patient and prevented the possible hazard of blood transfusions: 5 weeks before surgery, the patient's blood can be banked and then transfused back at the time of the surgery.

The selection of the fusion level is an extremely important aspect of scoliosis surgery. In general, when performing an anterior spinal fusion for scoliosis, the surgeon must fuse all the vertebrae, with widening of the disc space on the curve convexity. In the posterior spinal fusion with instrumentation, the surgeon must include all the rotated vertebrae in the fusion mass. One must avoid fusion to L4 or below in double structural scoliosis curves. Some difficulty arises in the determination of the length of the fusion if the lumbar curve appears very flexible and is corrected on traction or side bending. Instrumentation and fusion to the stable vertebra is the basic requirement for the procedure.

Anesthetic considerations include induced hypotension. Nitroprusside, trimethaphan, or nitroglycerin can reduce the mean blood pressure to 50 or 60 mm Hg, thereby reducing blood loss during the surgical procedure. There have been discussions regarding the hazard of this technique. Some authors believe that, with reduced perfusion in a spinal vessel that has undergone elongation and attenuation, diminution of blood flow to the cord may result in neurologic deficit.[6]

Spinal cord monitoring, by either the wake-up test or the evoked-potential spinal cord monitor,[9] allows safe correction of severe spinal deformity. Some alterations in anesthetic agents might be required depending on the type of monitoring carried out. In general, halothane and ethrane must be avoided to allow for somatosensory evoked potentials, and muscle relaxants must be avoided during the surgery to allow for the wake-up test.

A spinal frame often assists in the reduction of blood loss by reducing abdominal pressure on the patient and therefore lessening venous engorgement in the spinal area (for example, the Batson plexus).

SPINAL INSTRUMENTATION
Posterior spine

Although several different methods of spinal instrumentation are currently employed to correct spinal deformity, the single most important aspect of all spinal surgery involves the attainment of a spinal fusion. These techniques require meticulous and exact dissection, careful spinal decortication of all posterior elements available for the fusion, and autologous bone grafting of all the instrumented levels.

Any spinal instrumentation eventually fails and breaks because of cyclic loading if a solid bony fusion is not obtained. If, for some special case, a fusion is not to be achieved, the spinal instrumentation must be protected by external immobilization for a period of time and then re-

moved before removal of the external immobilization device (for instance, the brace). Furthermore, it has been shown that instrumented spinal segments that are not fused undergo cartilage changes at the facets of mobile spinal segment.

The Harrington instrumentation rods were developed in the 1950s by Dr. Paul Harrington.[3,7,8,12] His original work involved spinal instrumentation of scoliosis in polio patients. In his first cases he used the instruments without creating a spinal fusion. He realized early on that spinal fusion is necessary for long-term spinal stabilization and maintenance of correction. The ¼-inch distraction rod may or may not be used in combination with the ⅛-inch compression assembly on the convex side of the curve. Usually the compression rod is used only in cases of significant kyphosis in association with the scoliosis. It also, at times, increases the stability of the instrument construct, improves the kyphosis, and, when used in the lumbar spine, preserves some of the lumbar lordosis. The compression rod should not be used in patients with thoracic lordosis or curves over 85 degrees.

In general, curve correction of 45% to 55% can be accomplished with the Harrington distraction instrumentation. Moderate rotational correction can be anticipated. A postoperative cast or brace is required for approximately 6 months from the date of surgery for adequate healing of the spinal fusion.

In the 1970s Luque developed the posterior Luque spinal instrumentation (also known as segmental spinal instrumentation, or SSI).[1] The technique involves the implantation of two ¼-inch or ³⁄₁₆-inch L-shaped rods along each side of the spine. The spine is affixed to the rods at each level by 16- or 18-gauge wires passed beneath the laminae. By prebending the rods to cause correction but allow for residual uncorrectable curves, the spine can be approximated to the rods and affixed by the segmental spinal wires. The wires are passed beneath the lamina before the final application of the instrumentation. The rods are further contoured to preserve the sagittal curve. Eventually the rods are wired together to improve the mechanical construction.

Although for some patients postoperative casts or bracing is avoided, there has been no universal acceptance of this idea. A simple postoperative brace is often used. The primary use of Luque instrumentation has been neuromuscular scoliosis where some neurologic deficiency already exists.

Some of the disadvantages of Luque instrumentation include a higher intraoperative blood loss and a higher risk of iatrogenic neurologic injury, especially paresthesia. Inadvertent injury to the dura or nerve root by the passage of the sublaminar wires has caused many surgeons to abandon this technique in idiopathic scoliotic patients. Furthermore, the device is extremely difficult to remove, since the relatively stiff 16- or 18-gauge wires often cause injury to the dura or neural tissues when pulled from the sublaminar space. Some evidence has recently been presented that shows the adverse effect of long-term sublaminar wiring.[10]

Sublaminar wires have been used with Harrington rods by many surgeons in recent years. Being affixed to the spine at each end with the Harrington hooks gives the Harrington rod some advantages over the Luque rods, which are simply laid along the side of the spine and affixed by the wires. Contouring of the Harrington distraction rod can be accomplished with the square-ended distraction system. The supplemental sublaminar 16-gauge wires are used to affix the apical vertebrae and thus accomplish a transverse load on the spinal deformity while still stabilizing the end vertebrae by the Harrington hooks. This technique has been useful in the correction of thoracic lordosis. A brace may not be necessary after the operation.

Further development of the segmental spinal stabilization technique was developed by Drummond in the 1980s. His Wisconsin system of instrumentation involves contoured square-ended Harrington distraction rods on one side of the spine and a contoured C-shaped ³/₁₆-inch Luque rod on the convex side of the spine. Segmental 18-gauge wires are passed through the base of the spinous processes bilaterally with small Drummond "buttons." This fixation of the segments of the spine to the rods on both sides of the spine affords good correction and stabilization. The double wires and buttons on each spinous process do not include the end vertebrae, which are stabilized by the usual Harrington hooks. At the superior and inferior end of the Harrington distraction rod, this cross-linkage of rods through the base of the spinal process affords the good fixation. Often a brace or cast can be avoided in the postoperative situation.

The most recent advancement in spinal instrumentation comes from a development in France in the 1980s by Cotrel and Dubousset. The Cotrel-Dubousset spinal instrumentation (CD device) attempts to correct scoliosis by conversion of the thoracic lordosis.[4] By a system of implants, vertebral derotation is accomplished. Although some distractive forces are applied, it is the vertebral derotation that causes a correction in the sagittal plane of the scoliosis. Since this technique is rather new, its long-term results have not yet been determined.

The CD device involves the use of 7 mm rods with a roughened surface, open and closed pedicular and laminar hooks, pedicular screws, and a transverse linkage rod system. The technique involves the determination of the hook placement in preoperative radiograph. Pedicular hooks are placed in the thoracic area, and a contoured rod is placed on the concave side of the thoracic spine. A second rod is then placed on the convex side of the curve. Initial distraction and compression are applied to the spine. With special instruments a derotation of the spine is then carried out with preservation of the sagittal alignment. All screws and hooks are tightened. Usually a brace or cast is not used in the postoperative period.

The advantages of the CD device include the preservation of the sagittal curve and the rotational correction, which is often approximately 40% in the thoracic and 20% in the lumbar spine.

Its drawbacks include its greater technical difficulty, involving a high degree of "fiddling" with a great number of hooks and screws. Rigid, large curves (such as in adult scoliosis) are difficult to derotate or correct. The implant is quite massive and has a high profile, often limiting its use for thin children. Finally, it is an expensive system of metal, often costing in excess of $1000 for a single implant device system.

Anterior spine

To achieve access to the anterior spine, an approach is usually carried out along the lateral aspect of the thoracic or lumbar region. Usually the approach is accomplished at the level of the upper vertebra to be fused. If the curve to be fused is above T10, a formal thoracotomy is required. For curves from T11 through L1, a thoracotomy in combination with a retroperitoneal transdiaphragmatic approach must be carried out. If the anterior fusion is limited to L1 through L5, a retroperitoneal approach is made below the diaphragm.

Developed in Australia in the 1960s by Dwyer, one early form of anterior spinal instrumentation involved vertebral screws, vertebral staples, and a titanium cable passed between the screw heads on the convex side of the curve.[16] The technique involved an anterior approach to the spine with total disc removal between the vertebral segments to be fused. Rib or iliac graft blocks are placed anteriorly to prevent production of kyphosis when the vertebral bodies are brought together. Instrumentation at all levels with widened discs is accomplished on the convexity. Some correction of rotation may be accomplished by posterior placement of the screw head at the apex of the deformity. The cable is inserted through the screws and crimped sequentially after tension is achieved.

The Dwyer instrumentation provides excellent correction for thoracolumbar curves with only a 20% rotational correction. Its greatest advantage, however, involves the fact one can fuse fewer levels than those required with the posterior instrumentation and fusion.

A disadvantage of the Dwyer system is the production of a local kyphosis at the level of the instrumentation. The Dwyer system's use in the thoracic spine is prohibited because further production of kyphosis in this region is undesirable. A postoperative cast or brace is usually required.

Developed in Germany in the 1970s by Zielke, the Zielke-VDS anterior instrumentation gained popularity because of its abilities to derotate and to achieve correction in the sagittal plane of the scoliosis.[11] The technique required is similar to that of the Dwyer device, but it uses vertebral screws, half staples, and a ⅛-inch threaded rod with nuts rather than a titanium cable. This rigid rod prevents the production of kyphosis as is often seen with the Dwyer device. The correction is excellent, usually 60% to 90% correction of scoliosis and 40% correction of rotational deformation.

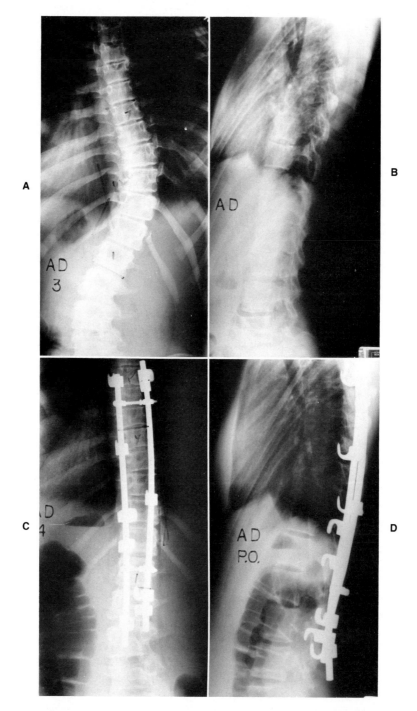

Figure 34-1. Patient A.D. **A,** Preoperative anteroposterior radiograph demonstrating right thoracic adolescent idiopathic scoliosis. **B,** Preoperative lateral radiograph demonstrating marked thoracic lordosis. **C,** Postoperative anteroposterior radiograph demonstrating spine fusion with Cotrel-Dubousset instrumentation. **D,** Postoperative lateral radiograph demonstrating correction of thoracic lordosis with Cotrel-Dubousset instrumentation. Note increased anteroposterior chest dimension as compared to preoperative view.

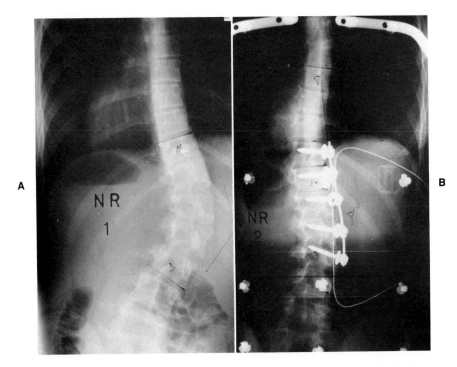

Figure 34-2. Patient M.R. **A,** Preoperative anteroposterior radiograph demonstrating adolescent idiopathic right thoracolumbar scoliosis. **B,** Postoperative anteroposterior radiograph showing anterior spine fusion with Zielke (ventral-derotation-spondylodesis) instrumentation (brace visualized).

Complications

Among the immediate postoperative complications of spinal instrumentation, a neurologic injury to the patient during the procedure is the most serious. If the spine undergoes distraction beyond the capability of the vascular supply to accommodate for the new position, an ischemic episode results and leads to neurologic deficiency. This usually involves the entire transverse section of the cord, and paraplegia is the outcome. If it is recognized early, within 4 hours, immediate removal of the spinal instrumentation must be carried out. This has resulted in recovery in a great percentage of cases. Systemic steroids may be administered in this early phase.

To prevent this neurologic injury during the course of surgery, some form of spinal cord monitoring should be carried out,[9] either the wake-up test or monitoring of the somatosensory evoked potential.

A postoperative infection requires irrigation drainage and the institution of antibiotic therapy. Prophylactic antibiotics often are used before and during the surgery. These antibiotics are then delivered postoperatively for several days in an attempt to prevent the occurrence of a postoperative infection. Once irrigation drainage has been instituted, the implants are often left in place while the drainage devices are closed over the wound. In those cases antibiotic therapy is usually continued for several weeks.

Although rare, malnutrition may occur during the two-stage (anteroposterior) procedure in cases of neuromuscular or paralytic scoliosis with prolonged intravenous infusion. Hyperalimentation is sometimes required.

In cases of posterior spinal fusion the occurrence of a pneumothorax is quite unusual but nevertheless must be considered if blood gas abnormalities are seen. A postoperative chest radiograph is required, and a pneumothorax, if present and 10% to 20% or greater, must be treated with a chest tube.

Dural tears caused by direct instrument intrusion must be closed. Management of this complication often requires neurosurgical consultation during surgery.

To prevent incorrect placement of the fusion level, preoperative radiographs must be reviewed and an intraoperative radiograph taken so the preoperative situation can be duplicated at the time of surgery.

Abnormal sagittal alignment of the lumbar spine (for instance, flat back) must be avoided. Vigorous distraction of the lower vertebra (such as L5) of a lumbar scoliosis results in the lower spine pitching forward. To avoid this, one should contour the lumbar rod at the time of the instrument insertion. Furthermore, rod malrotation can be avoided by using square-ended rods with square-holed lower hooks. Great care must be taken when contouring the rods to accommodate for both thoracic kyphosis and maintenance of lumbar lordosis.

The late complications of spinal instrumentation include a pseudarthrosis.[3,5,7] In adolescents its incidence is probably 1% or less. This incidence increases in the adult to approximately 15% to 20% in the 30- to 40-year age group. Pain is usually present after 6 months as an early indication of a pseudarthrosis. Eventually cyclic loading on the rod may cause the instrument to fail (fatigue fracture), and rod breakage may become evident on the radiograph. If the pain persists and curve progression is noted after the occurrence of pseudarthrosis is identified, it must be repaired by removal of the broken instrumentation and possible reapplication of new instrumentation. Rod or wire breakage is usually the result of a pseudarthrosis and can be painful if allowed to persist untreated. Removal of the Luque sublaminar wires may be hazardous.

Back pain has been implicated as a late result of elongated spinal fusions. One report states that 70% of adults with long spinal fusions to L4, L5, or both experience some back pain, whereas only 38% of patients fused to L1-L3 as the distal segment experience the same type of back pain.

If flat back syndrome (loss of lumbar lordosis) occurs, extension osteotomy of the lower end of the fusion or at the midlumbar spine might be required to correct the abnormal posture. If the fusion level is too short superiorly, kyphosis above the instrumentation may result. Superior extension of the fusion above the end of the previous fusion site is required.

POSTOPERATIVE MANAGEMENT

Most techniques, as already stated, involve use of some form of postoperative immobilization. This can be either a full-body cast or a body brace. The brace is worn on a full-time basis but may be removed for a stand-up shower once each day. The decision for a cast or removable brace is made by the individual surgeon.[18] It depends on the technique used and the cooperation of the patient.

During the cast or brace immobilization it is important to maintain the patient's pulmonary function. Some breathing-enhancement device is often used. An incentive spirometer apparatus is beneficial during postoperative immobilization.

Exercises may be performed to maintain tone of both the upper and lower extremities. Isometric and gentle range-of-motion exercises with the extremities can be carried out without jeopardizing the spinal fusion, which is protected by the cast or brace.

Activities of daily living may be performed. Rest periods require recumbency, but this may be diminished as the postoperative period progresses. In the initial postoperative period the patient usually rests in a semirecumbent position on a couch or reclining chair. Four weeks after the operation, patients are usually able to return to school on a limited basis, provided that they are permitted a rest period in the middle of the day. This program should continue for the remaining period of immobilization.

Sports are to be avoided during the postoperative healing process but may be resumed on a limited basis once the spinal fusion has fully healed. In general, calisthenic and noncontact sports may be resumed, but gymnastics (which use an apparatus), contact sports, and trampoline play are to be avoided. More hectic sports, such as downhill skiing, can be resumed if the patient was proficient in that sport before the surgery. It is not recommended if they were unpracticed before the surgery.

OTHER FORMS OF SCOLIOSIS

Although 75% of those scoliosis cases seen in the office are idiopathic, the other 25% can be divided into three major groups. Congenital scoliosis makes up 10%, the paralytic scoliosis another 10%, and the neuromuscular and associated diseases make up the final 5%. In this last group, neurofibromatosis and Marfan's disease are but two of many varieties of illnesses associated with scoliosis. Each individual disease process—and the development and progression of the scoliosis in the patient—dictate what methods and techniques must be used to correct the spine surgically. Certainly, as in the idiopathic group, the attainment of a solid spinal fusion is the one single factor for the surgeon to accomplish. It is to this end that all methods of surgical stabilization with instrumentation are directed.

Once the spine has been fused, it is hoped that the level of daily activities will improve. That is, a bedridden patient may become a wheelchair patient, and the wheelchair patient may become a partial ambulator. If this is not possible, some benefit might at least be realized in a new ease of care, improvement in or less progression of pulmonary deficiency, and comfort of the already handicapped patient. It is to this end that all methods of rehabilitative devices and therapy are directed.

REFERENCES

1. Allen, BL, Jr, and Ferguson, RL: L-rod instrumentation for scoliosis in cerebral palsy, J Pediatr Orthop 2:87, 1982.
2. Bjerkreim, L, Carlsen, B, and Korsell, E: Preoperative Cotrel traction in idiopathic scoliosis, Acta Orthop Scand 53:901, 1982.
3. Cochran, T, Irstam, L, and Nachemson, A: Long-term anatomic and functional changes in patients with adolescent idiopathic scoliosis treated by Harrington rod fusion, Spine 8:576, 1983.
4. Cotrel, Y, and Dubousset, J: A new technic for segmental spinal osteosynthesis using the posterior approach, Rev Chir Orthop 70:489, 1984.
5. Cummine, JL, et al: Reconstructive surgery in the adult for failed scoliosis fusion, J Bone Joint Surg 61:1151, 1979.
6. Cunningham, JN, Jr, Laschinger, JC, and Spencer, FC: Monitoring of somatosensory evoked potentials during surgical procedures on the thoracoabdominal aorta. IV. Clinical observations and results, J Thorac Cardiovasc Surg 94:275, 1987.
7. Curtis, RS, et al: Results of Harrington instrumentation in the treatment for severe scoliosis, Clin Orthop 144:128, 1979.
8. Duhaime, M, et al: Treatment of idiopathic scoliosis by the Harrington technique: experience from the Ste-Justine Hospital, Montreal, Chir Pediatr 23:17, 1982.
9. Engler, GL, et al: Somatosensory evoked potentials during Harrington instrumentation for scoliosis, J Bone Joint Surg 60:528, 1978.

10. Geremia, GK, et al: Complications of sublaminar wiring, Surg Neurol 23:629, 1985.

11. Griss, P, and Jentschura, G: Early results of operative treatment of scoliosis using the anterior derotation spondylodesis technique (VDS-Zielke) [author's translation], Z Orthop 119:115, 1981.

12. Hall, JE, Herndon, WA, and Levine, CR: Surgical treatment of congenital scoliosis with or without Harrington instrumentation, J Bone Joint Surg 63A:608, 1981.

13. Halsall, AP, et al: An experimental evaluation of spinal flexibility with respect to scoliosis surgery, Spine 8:482, 1983.

14. Holden, WE, Carr, WA, and Beals, RK: Position dependence of pulmonary function in a patient with lordoscoliosis, Eur J Respir Dis 68:146, 1986.

15. Kumano, K, and Tsuyama, N: Pulmonary function before and after surgical correction of scoliosis, J Bone Joint Surg 64:242, 1982.

16. Michel, CR, Onimus, M, and Kohler, R: The Dwyer operation in the surgical treatment of scoliosis, Rev Cir Orthop 63:237, 1977.

17. Nachemson, A, and Nordwall, A: Effectiveness of preoperative Cotrel traction for correction of idiopathic scoliosis, J Bone Joint Surg 59:504, 1977.

18. Tolo, V, and Gillespie, R: The use of shortened periods of rigid postoperative immobilization in the surgical treatment of idiopathic scoliosis, J Bone Joint Surg 63A:1137, 1981.

ADDITIONAL READINGS

Benson, DR, and Newman, DC: The spine and surgical treatment in osteogenesis imperfecta, Clin Orthop 159:147, 1981.

Carr, WA, et al: Treatment of idiopathic scoliosis in the Milwaukee brace, J Bone Joint Surg 62:599, 1980.

Daruwalla, JS, and Tan, WC: Spirometric pulmonary function tests before and after surgical correction of idiopathic scoliosis in adolescents, Ann Acad Med Singapore 14:475, 1985.

Dutroit, M, et al: Surgical treatment of scoliosis of 100 degrees and greater in children and adolescents (neurological and myopathic scoliosis excluded): apropos of a series of 66 cases, Rev Chir Orthop 71:549, 1985.

Fabian, IA: Dominant coping behaviors of one adolescent female hospitalized for surgical correction of scoliosis, Matern Child Nurs J 14:9, 1985.

Ferguson, RL, and Allen, BL, Jr: Staged correction of neuromuscular scoliosis, J Pediatr Orthop 3:555, 1983.

Fisk, JR, Winter, RB, and Moe, JH: The lumbosacral curve in idiopathic scoliosis: its significance and management, J Bone Joint Surg 62:39, 1980.

Kahanovitz, N, Brown, JC, and Bonnett, CA: The operative treatment of congenital scoliosis: a report of 23 patients, Clin Orthop 143:174, 1979.

Kostuik, JP: Recent advances in the treatment of painful adult scoliosis, Clin Orthop 147:238, 1980.

Kostuik, JP, Errico, TJ, and Gleason, TF: Techniques of internal fixation for degenerative conditions of the lumbar spine, Clin Orthop 203:219, 1986.

Kostuik, JP, and Hall, BB: Spinal fusions to the sacrum in adults with scoliosis, Spine 8:489, 1983.

Kumano, K, et al: Energy expenditure during exercise on a treadmill before and after surgical correction of spinal deformities, Nippon Seikeigeka Gakkai Zasshi 60:439, 1986.

Lascombes, P, et al: Comparative study of the Armstrong and Harrington technics in the treatment of idiopathic scolioses, Chir Pediatr 27:69, 1986.

Leong, JC, et al: Surgical treatment of scoliosis following poliomyelitis: a review of one hundred and ten cases, J Bone Joint Surg 63A:726, 1981.

Lindh, M: Energy expenditure during walking in patients with scoliosis: the effect of surgical correction, Spine 3:122, 1978.

Mayer, PJ, et al: Post-poliomyelitis paralytic scoliosis: a review of curve patterns and results of surgical treatments in 118 consecutive patients, Spine 6:573, 1981.

Mazur, J, et al: Efficacy of surgical management for scoliosis in myelomeningocele: correction of deformity and alteration of functional status, J Pediatr Orthop 6:568, 1986.

Nykoliation, JW, et al: An algorithm for the management of scoliosis, J Manipulative Physiol Ther 9:1, 1986.

Riseborough, EJ: Irradiation-induced kyphosis, Clin Orthop 128:101, 1977.

Shevchenko, SD: Complications, errors and hazards of the surgical correction of the spine and thorax in severe forms of scoliosis, Ortop Travmatol Protez 3:63, 1985.

Slabaugh, PB, et al: Lumbosacral hemivertebrae: a review of twenty-four patients, with excision in eight, Spine 5:234, 1980.

Stanitski, CL, et al: Surgical correction of spinal deformity in cerebral palsy, Spine 7:563, 1982.

Stoll, J, and Bunch, WH: Segmental spinal instrumentation for congenital scoliosis: a report of two cases, Spine 8:43, 1983.

Swank, S, et al: Surgical treatment of adult scoliosis: a review of two hundred and twenty-two cases, J Bone Joint Surg 63A:268, 1981.

Tolo, VT, and Gillespie, R: The characteristics of juvenile idiopathic scoliosis and results of its treatment, J Bone Joint Surg 60B:181, 1978.

Viviani, GR, et al: Biomechanical analysis and simulation of scoliosis and surgical correction, Clin Orthop 208:40, 1986.

Youngman, PM, and Edgar, MA: Posterior spinal fusion and instrumentation in the treatment of adolescent idiopathic scoliosis, Ann R Coll Surg Engl 67:313, 1985.

Zagra, A, Lamartina, C, and Zerbi, A: The Risser plaster corset as the only method of correction in the surgical treatment of scoliosis: a study of 150 cases, Ital J Orthop Traumatol 11:67, 1985.

CHAPTER 35

Medical management of scoliosis

JACOB J. GRAHAM

Appropriate and effective management of scoliosis cannot be undertaken without definition of terms, methods of clinical and radiographic diagnosis, and above all, knowledge of the natural history of this disease. Epidemiologic studies have helped to clarify the magnitude of the problem and the curves to treat.

DEFINITIONS

Scoliosis is a lateral curvature of the spine, usually with rotational elements. It may be nonstructural or structural. A structural curve is not completely correctable on lateral bend, whereas a nonstructural one is (Figure 35-1). An example of a nonstructural curve is one caused by inequality of leg length. An irritative scoliosis is an antalgic curve, that is, one that develops in response to pain. Until the pain is relieved, it too is not completely corrected on lateral bend in the direction of the pain. Idiopathic scoliosis (sometimes referred to as genetic scoliosis) constitutes the largest subdivision of the structural curvature group (about 80%). Idiopathic scoliosis can be divided by age into the infantile type (birth to 3 years), the juvenile type (3 to 10 years), the adolescent type (10 years to maturity), and the adult type (maturity to old age). A curve is described by its location in the spine and by the direction of its convexity, for example, right thoracic scoliosis. It is quantified by measurement of the supplementary angle formed by the intersection of perpendiculars dropped from the end vertebrae (Cobb method),[14] the end vertebrae being those maximally tilted into the concavity of the curve (Figure 35-2). A curve or curves are compensated if a plumb line dropped from the occiput or from the spinous process of C7 falls through the natal cleft.

Curves of the spine in planes other than lateral are kyphosis and lordosis. Kyphosis is a sagittal plane curvature of the spine with its apex directed posteriorly. Lordosis is

a sagittal plane curvature of the spine with its apex directed anteriorly (Figure 35-3). Kyphosis and lordosis are normal spinal curvatures necessary for balance and function of the spine. An abnormal kyphosis may be either a hyperkyphosis (round back) or a hypokyphosis (flat back). An abnormal lordosis is similarly defined; its excess or hyperlordosis is a swayback deformity, and its deficiency is a flat back. Kyphosis and lordosis may coexist with scoliosis. Kyphoscoliosis has been used to describe an advanced kyphotic deformity of thoracic or thoracolumbar curves. In reality, the deformity is attributable to the rib hump that develops as a result of spinal rotation, which throws the spine into a lordotic position. Dickson[16] called lordosis the significant deformity in idiopathic scoliosis, believing it to be the precipitating pathologic factor in the development of a curve.

Scoliosis other than idiopathic is defined by the presence of associated disease conditions (such as neuromuscular scoliosis), which does not mean that the condition necessarily has an etiologic relationship to curve development, or by the presence on radiograph of such manifest skeletal abnormalities as hemivertebra (congenital scoliosis). In congenital scoliosis the bony abnormalities may be considered to have caused the curve.

The classification in the box on p. 479 is adapted from the official classification of the Scoliosis Research Society.

PATHOGENESIS AND ETIOLOGY

The etiology of idiopathic scoliosis is unknown. It is probably multifactorial. The genetic pathway has been regarded as a sex-linked (X chromosome) autosomal recessive with incomplete penetrance and variable expressivity.[51] Disorders of muscle, connective tissue growth, and neurologic function have all been suspected as causative factors. Results of studies to date are either conflicting or inconclusive. For example, Nordwall and Willner[36] and Burwell, Dan-

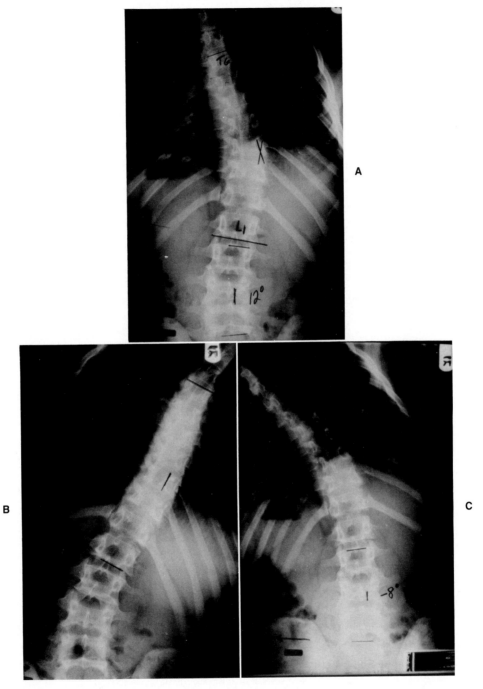

Figure 35-1. A, Idiopathic structural right thoracic curve of 35 degrees with functional left lumbar component of 12 degrees. **B,** On right lateral bend, thoracic curve is 10 degrees, indicating by its failure to correct completely that it is structural curve. **C,** On left lateral bend, left lumbar curve is overcorrected to −8 degrees, confirming that it is functional curve.

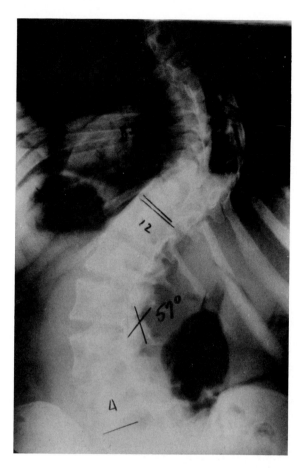

Figure 35-2. This curve is described as right thoracic left lumbar curve (S curve), which identifies its location in spine and directions of its convexities. It is quantified by Cobb method of measurement.

gerfeld, and Vernon[13] reported scoliotic patients, especially female, to have a greater than normal stature, but Veldhuizen and co-workers[46] could not substantiate this. Dickson,[17] as noted, believed that uneven vertebral growth (increase in the anterior height of the apical vertebra) was the precipitating cause of the thoracic lordosis, which in turn initiates scoliosis because the lordotic position can be assumed only by rotation. The frequent association of neurologic disorders with scoliosis points toward the neurologic pathway as the etiologic route. Disorders of the posterior column pathway have been implicated by demonstration of alterations in vibratory response and in proprioception in patients with idiopathic scoliosis.[5,50,52] As interesting as these studies may be, they still do not provide a practical guide for management, and effective clinical control of the disorder remains pragmatic.

NATURAL HISTORY
Epidemiology

Epidemiologic studies, principally school screenings, have shown a wide variation in the prevalence of sco-

liosis.[11,18,40] An average of 4% to 5% of North American schoolchildren between 12 and 14 years of age have scoliosis when this is defined as a visible rotational deformity on forward bend and a measurable curve of 5 degrees or more on a standing radiograph.[33] However, if one defines scoliosis as curves with an angular value of 10 degrees or greater, an average of 2% have scoliosis.[3,25,29] Weinstein[47] has shown that, when age 16 is the endpoint, 2% to 3% have curves of 10 degrees or greater. The prevalence (proportion of the population affected at a particular time) drops to 0.3% to 0.5% with curves greater than 20 degrees, to 0.1% to 0.3% with curves greater than 30 degrees, and to less than 0.1% with curves greater than 40 degrees. Generally, about three per thousand (0.3%) require some form of active treatment.[33] There is an equal sex incidence with small curves of 10 degrees or less, but a female preponderance for large curves, reaching a female prevalence of 10:1 for curves greater than 30 degrees.

Natural history in untreated adults

Past studies, particularly from homogeneous populations in Sweden, painted a dismal picture indicating increased morbidity and mortality, decreased work ability, and poor psychosocial adjustment in adults with untreated scoliosis. Other studies from Iowa by Ponseti, Friedman, and Weinstein[47-49] have shown that 40% to 60% of patients complained of backache, a figure comparable to that in the general population. Lumbar and thoracolumbar curves, particularly if associated with lateral vertebral shift, cause slightly more pain. Simmons[22] and Kostuik[23] have pointed out that the quality of pain is worse in scoliotic adults than in the normal population.

Curve progression

Determining the prognosis at first visit is generally not possible.[26-28,37] Curves can progress, remain the same, or (rarely) resolve. Curve progression is probably best defined as a sustained increase of 5 degrees or more. Curve progression is not necessarily synonomous with a progressive curve requiring treatment. A progressive curve is generally one that in childhood, before the end of spinal vertebral growth, is 30 degrees or more. Progression in childhood and adolescence is most likely to occur during periods of rapid growth. There are two such critical periods of growth velocity: from birth to 2 years and the postpubertal period. The juvenile group, which constitutes 12% to 16% of scoliosis, is a period of relatively slow growth, generally permitting observation without treatment or part-time brace-wearing. However, this factor is counterbalanced by the fact that the onset is early with great remaining growth time. Infantile scoliosis is rare, and in about 90% it resolves by 2 years of age (generally the right thoracic curves). Left thoracic curves, S curves, and those with a rib-vertebra (RV) angle greater than 20 degrees or in phase II (see "Radiographic Evaluation") are most at risk of progression.

CLASSIFICATION OF SCOLIOSIS

Structural scoliosis

I. Idiopathic
   A. Infantile (0-3 years)
      1. Resolving
      2. Progressive
   B. Juvenile (3-10 years)
   C. Adolescent (10 years to maturity)
   D. Adult (maturity to old age)
II. Neuromuscular
   A. Neuropathic
      1. Upper motor neuron
         a. Cerebral palsy
         b. Spinocerebellar degeneration
            i. Friedreich's disease
            ii. Charcot-Marie-Tooth disease
            iii. Roussy-Levy disease
         c. Syringomyelia
         d. Spinal cord tumor
         e. Spinal cord trauma
         f. Other
      2. Lower motor neuron
         a. Poliomyelitis
         b. Other viral myelitidies
         c. Traumatic
         d. Spinal muscular atrophy
             i. Werdnig-Hoffman
            ii. Kugelberg-Welander
         e. Myelomeningocoele (paralytic)
      3. Dysautonomia (Riley-Day)
      4. Other
   B. Myopathic
      1. Arthrogryposis
      2. Muscular dystrophy
         a. Duchenne (pseudohypertrophic)
         b. Limb-girdle
         c. Facioscapulohumeral
      3. Fiber-type disproportion
      4. Congenital hypotonia
      5. Myotonia dystrophica
      6. Other
III. Congenital
   A. Failure of formation
      1. Wedge vertebra
      2. Hemivertebra
   B. Failure of segmentation
      1. Unilateral (unsegmented bar)
      2. Bilateral
   C. Mixed
IV. Neurofibromatosis

V. Mesenchymal disorders
   A. Marfan's
   B. Ehlers-Danlos
   C. Others
VI. Rheumatoid disease
VII. Trauma
   A. Fracture
   B. Surgical
      1. Postlaminectomy
      2. Postthoracoplasty
   C. Irradiation
VIII. Extraspinal contractures
   A. Post-empyema
   B. Post-burns
IX. Osteochondrodystrophies
   A. Diastrophic dwarfism
   B. Mucopolysaccharidoses (for example, Morquio's syndrome)
   C. Spondyloepiphyseal dysplasia
   D. Multiple epiphyseal dysplasia
   E. Other
X. Infection of bone
   A. Acute
   B. Chronic
XI. Metabolic disorders
   A. Rickets
   B. Osteogenesis imperfecta
   C. Homocystinuria
   D. Others
XII. Related to lumbosacral joint
   A. Spondylolysis and spondylolisthesis
   B. Congenital anomalies of lumbosacral region
XIII. Tumors
   A. Vertebral column
      1. Osteoid osteoma
      2. Histiocytosis X
      3. Other
   B. Spinal cord

Nonstructural scoliosis

I. Postural scoliosis
II. Hysterical scoliosis
III. Nerve root irritation
   A. Herniation of nucleus pulposus
   B. Tumors
IV. Inflammatory (for example, appendicitis)
V. Related to leg length discrepancy
VI. Related to contractures about the hip

From Moe, J, et al: Scoliosis and other spinal deformities, Philadelphia, 1978, WB Saunders Co.

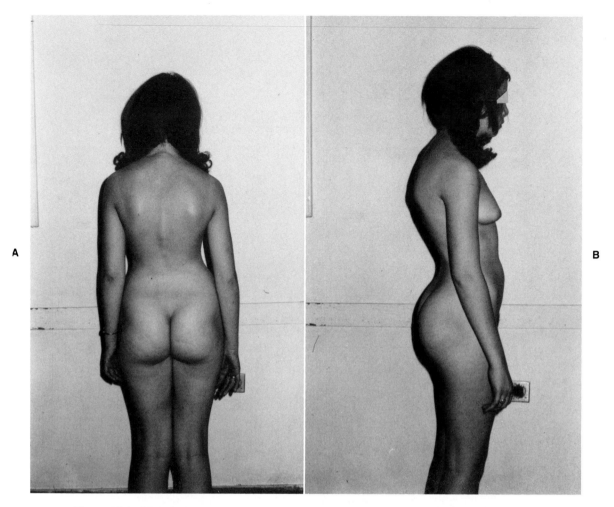

Figure 35-3. Clinical appearance (**A,** posterior and, **B,** lateral profile view) of adolescent girl with thoracic hyperkyphosis resulting from thoracic vertebral epiphysistis (Scheuermann's disease). There is associated minimal scoliosis (often seen) and compensatory lumbar hyperlordosis.

Most idiopathic adolescent scoliosis progresses to some degree during the growth period, but the change may not be significant. An estimated 5% to 24% of curves progress during adolescence.[28] The variation in this figure relates to the size of the curve and to the patient's gender. Early age at onset, truncal shift, absence of menses, recent rapid growth spurt, and family history of scoliosis are all factors suggesting guarded prognosis. Curve pattern should also be considered; probably lumbar curves are least likely, and double curve patterns most likely, to progress.

Accurate measurement of a curve is critical in determining curve progression. There can be a variation of 3 to 5 degrees in value of angular measurement depending on such factors as interobservor error and variation in the incidence of the x-ray beam to the plane of the film. Curve progression can be said to occur when an increase of 5 degrees or more is maintained on consecutive examinations. Lack of continuity of increase distinguishes curve progression from the progressive curve.

Risk of curve progression in maturity

Weinstein and Ponsetti[47,48] showed that curves greater than 30 degrees can progress and that the magnitude of the increase generally is significantly greater when an angle of 50 degrees is reached. They identified radiographic progression factors: for thoracic curves a Cobb angle of greater than 50 degrees, apical vertebral rotation greater than 30%, and a Mehta angle greater than 30 degrees; in lumbar curves a Cobb angle of greater than 30 degrees, apical vertebral rotation greater than 30%; curve direction, translatory shifts, and relation of L5 to the intercrestal line; for thoracolumbar curves a Cobb angle greater than 30 degrees, apical vertebral rotation greater than 30%, and translatory shifts; and for combined curves a Cobb angle greater than 50 degrees.

Pulmonary function

Pulmonary function is affected only by the thoracic curves. Measurable deficit of pulmonary function has been demonstrated even in mild and moderate scoliosis.[31] How-

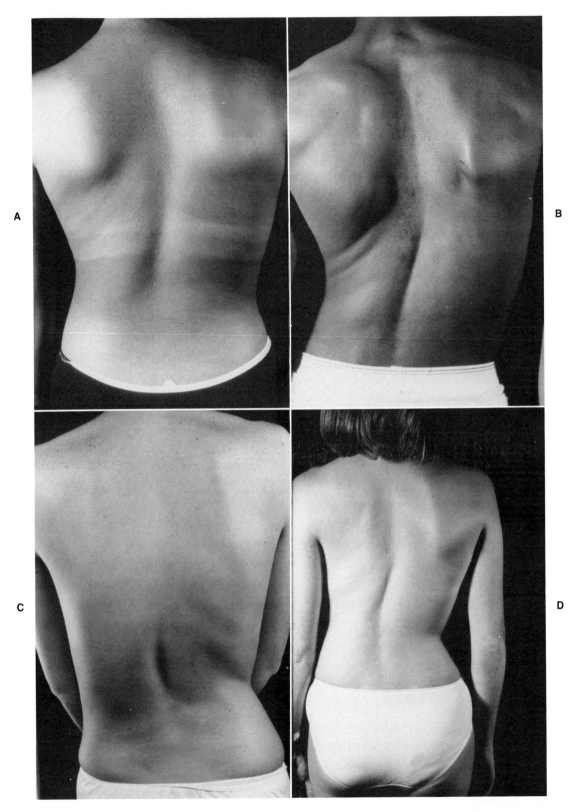

Figure 35-4. A, Typical thoracic curve. **B,** Thoracolumbar curve. **C,** Lumbar curve. **D,** Double S curve (thoracic and lumbar).

ever, the amount of decrease is easily tolerated. As the curve approaches 100 degrees there is a significant reduction in vital capacity, Po_2, and FEV_1, all because of restrictive lung disease with alveolar hypoventilation and consequent arteriovenous shunting. Cor pulmonale has occurred in these severe cases.

DIAGNOSIS

The diagnosis of idiopathic scoliosis is based on the history and clinical and radiographic examination. The usual history is detection of deformity during a period of rapid growth. Symptoms are rare in children and adolescents. As mentioned, there is often a family history of scoliosis. A history of associated diseases may point to other types of scoliosis. A complicated delivery may raise suspicion of cerebral palsy and hence neuromuscular scoliosis. Drug ingestion in pregnancy can raise suspicion of congenital osseous defects (congenital scoliosis).

Physical examination

Characteristic findings on physical examination are torso asymmetries such as scapular asymmetry (prominence or winging on one scapula); waistline asymmetry (prominent hip owing to unequal definition of iliac crests, often mistaken as a short extremity with a prominent hip); unequal shoulder height; or presence of a truncal list or decompensation measured as the distance a plumb line dropped from either the occiput or C7 falls to one side of the natal cleft (Figure 35-4). The forward bend test described by Adams[2] is the most reliable means of detecting early rotation (Figure 35-5). This is done with the patient bending forward at the waist with the arms hanging forward, hands and arms opposed, and knees straight. The test is best viewed from the rear but should also be viewed from the front to detect high curves and from the side to appreciate alterations in the normal thoracic kyphosis. Bunnell[12] has described the use of an inclinometer, similar to a spirit level on sailboats, to measure the angle of trunk inclination (ATI) (Figure 35-6). An ATI of 5 degrees is significant. The use of flexible rules to create profile maps of the truncal regions was described as early as 1901 by Schulthess,[30] and the Shriner flexible rule was recently introduced.[39]

Attention should be paid to the character of the kyphos on forward bend. If it is smooth and gradual, even though larger than normal, it can be consistent with a postural round back. If it is exaggerated and angular, one must be suspicious of a bony disorder, usually thoracic vertebral epiphysitis, which may be associated with a mild degree of scoliosis.

Radiographic evaluation

The basic radiographic examination should be a single anteroposterior view of the erect spine. Although a 14 × 36 inch film includes the entire spine, it entails more radiation,

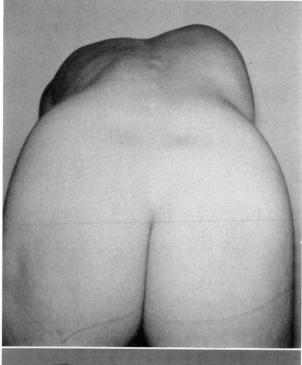

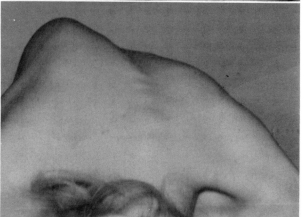

Figure 35-5. Forward bend test of Adams when viewed, **A,** from rear and, **B,** front, which in this case is particularly revealing of high curve.

and a 14 × 17 inch film from the iliac crests up is sufficient for most patients of average height. Nash[35] has shown that if a posteroanterior rather than an anteroposterior view is used, there is less breast irradiation and the quality of the radiograph is adequate for scoliosis evaluation and measurement. Radiographs reveal four characteristic curve patterns: thoracic, thoracolumbar, lumbar, and thoracic and lumbar (S curve) (Figure 35-7). Thoracic curves have their apex between T8 and T11; 90% are convex to the right with an upper end vertebra at T5-6 and a lower end vertebra at T11-12. Thoracolumbar curves have their apex at T11-12 and the lower at L1-2. Lumbar curves are usually convex

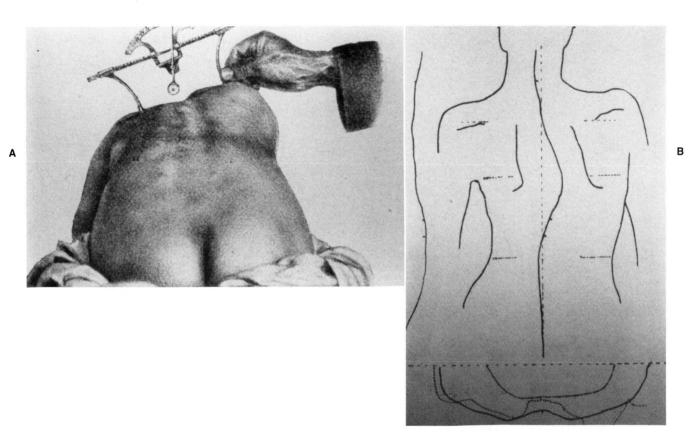

Figure 35-6. A, Inclinometer and, **B,** profile map drawings made from flexible rule, both designed and used by Schulthess in 1901, years before modern inclinometer of Bunnell and Shriner flexible rule.

to the left (70%) and have their apex at L1-2; the upper end vertebra is T11-12 and the lower is L3-4. S curves are usually (90%) to the right in the thoracic area and to the left in the lumbar area and usually extend from T5-6 to T10 in the thoracic area and from T11-12 to L4 in the lumbar area. Other curve patterns, which are much less common, include cervicothoracic (apex at C7-T1), double thoracic, and thoracic thoracolumbar.[47] Sometimes there are small triple or quadruple curve patterns, which tend to be inherently stable. A left thoracolumbar curve is quite common in minimal curves early in onset. Abnormalities such as hemivertebra indicate congenital scoliosis.

Structural idiopathic scoliosis can be diagnosed on a single radiograph without dynamic lateral bend studies. The radiograph shows one or more of the following structural changes: vertebral wedging, wedging of the disc spaces, vertebral rotation beyond the norm, a curve that crosses the midline, returns, and crosses again, and lateral vertebral shift (translatory shift) (Figure 35-8). The last is a lateral translation of a vertebra in relation to the vertebra below it reflecting early segmental instability. In this lateral spondylolisthesis, one vertebra slides laterally on its inferior vertebra, usually in the lower lumbar spine.

Curve measurement is important. The Cobb method of measurement[14] has been adopted by the Scoliosis Research

Society (Figure 35-9). The end vertebrae of the curve are selected, an end vertebra being defined as one that tilts maximally into the concavity of the curve. A parallel line is drawn on the end-plate or pedicle shadows of these vertebrae, and the supplementary angle formed by the intersection of perpendiculars drawn from these lines is the Cobb angle.

Radiographic signs of spinal maturity should be noted. The most commonly used is the Risser sign,[38] which is the appearance and subsequent completion of ossification of the iliac apophyses. This is quantified from 1 to 5 and measures the march medially of the ossific center toward the sacroiliac joint and its eventual fusion with the crest by 18 to 21 years of age. The Risser sign, also called capping, usually appears in girls about the time of the first menses. Risser noted that in as much as one third of the population, the ossific center does not reach the sacroiliac joint but stops short of it about one third of the way across the iliac crest (Figure 35-10). Concurrent with the appearance of the iliac apophysis is the apophysis for the head of the rib, usually best seen in the lower ribs. The vertebral ring apophyses also start to appear about this time, and their eventual fusion with the vertebral body is the final arbiter of the end of spinal vertebral growth.

Measurement of the amount of vertebral rotation on radiograph is best done using Nash and Moe's technique (Figure 35-11).[34] Four grades of rotation are defined reflecting

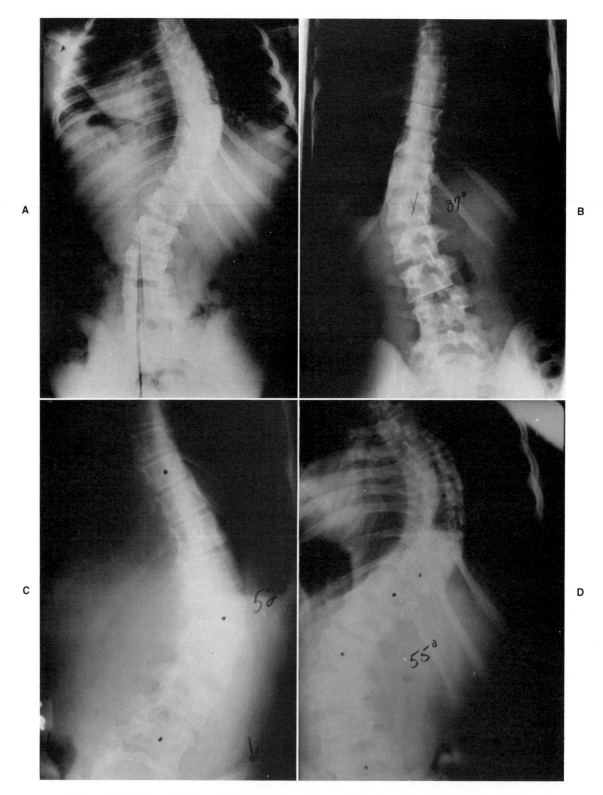

Figure 35-7. Characteristic radiographic curve patterns of, **A,** thoracic, **B,** thoracolumbar, **C,** lumbar, and, **D,** thoracic and lumbar (S curve).

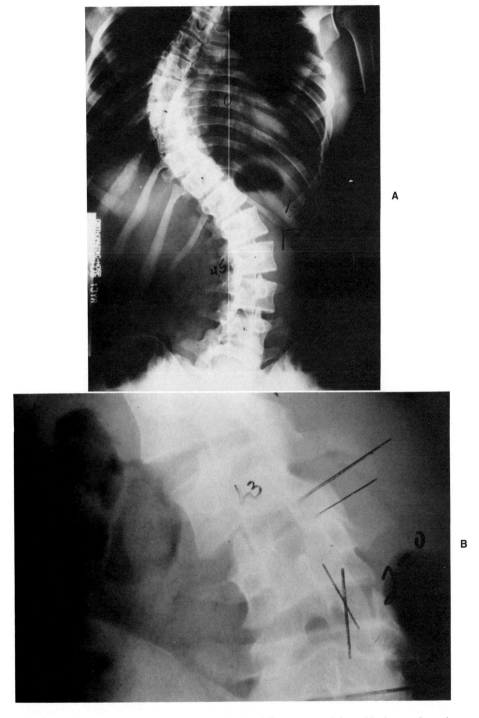

Figure 35-8. A, Single radiograph showing vertebral and disc space wedging with abnormal rotation and curve crossing midline to and fro. **B,** Cone radiograph focused on lateral vertebral (translatory) shift, also known as lateral spondylolisthesis.

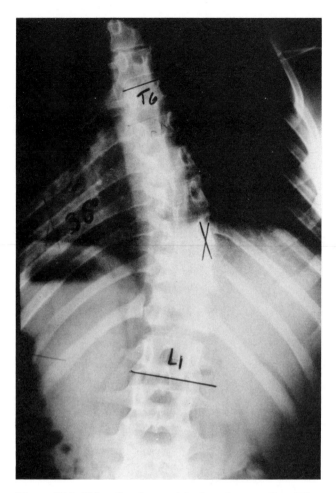

Figure 35-9. Thirty-five degree right thoracic curve from T6 to L1. Thirty-five degree angular value was measured using Cobb method. Parallel lines were drawn through end plates (or pedicles) of end vertebrae, perpendiculars were erected from these, and supplementary angle formed by their intersection was angular value of curve.

the degree of migration of the convex pedicle shadow away from the edge of the vertebral body and toward its center. Symmetric pedicle shadows are zero rotation. Grade I rotation occurs when the pedicle shadow moves away from the side of the vertebral body, progressing to grade II when the shadow is in the middle of the relevant half of the vertebral body, to grade III when it is in the center of the body, and to grade IV when it is beyond the center.

Mehta's angle,[32] or rib-vertebral angle difference, was first described by Mehta as a prognostic aid in infantile idiopathic scoliosis (Figure 35-12). The apical vertebra is selected, and lines are drawn through the adjacent ribs on each side bisecting the head and neck. The angle they make with a perpendicular erected from a line drawn parallel with the inferior end plate of the vertebral body is measured. If the difference between the angles on the two sides is greater than 20 degrees, there is an 80% chance that the scoliosis

will be progressive rather than resolving. Mehta also noted two phases of the curvature. Phase I was the separation of the rib head from the vertebral body on the convex side at the apex; phase II described their overlapping, regarded as a poor prognostic sign.

School screening

School screening, which has been mandated in many states, has unearthed a number of minor curves, largely because of the sensitivity of the tests used. When screening was first implemented, a large number of previously severe cases were discovered and successfully treated by orthopedic surgery with improved technologies of orthoses and spinal instrumentation. The number of treatable cases has decreased, and the incidence of patients currently requiring treatment appears to range between 0.3% and 0.6%. There is danger of high overreferral with school screening if, for example, a Cobb angle of 5 degrees and an ATI of 5 degrees are used as criteria. The effectiveness (particularly cost effectiveness) of school screening has not been universally accepted. The British Scoliosis Research Society, using the Bunnell ATI index of 7.5 degrees and a Cobb angle of 20 degrees or greater, is still studying the problem and has not yet reached any final conclusions.

MANAGEMENT
Indications for treatment

As more cases have been studied and more knowledge gleaned about the life history of persons with scoliosis, no consensus has developed on when and how to treat the disorder in early stages. Certain factors have been identified as placing the curve at risk for progression, particularly in girls before skeletal maturity. They are double curve patterns, young age, absence of menses (68% chance of progression before menarche, as compared with 33% after), absence of or low Risser sign, larger curve magnitude at initial detection, and sex (females at risk at a ratio of 10:1).[47]

In light of the preceding factors, avoidance of overtreatment is best obtained by observing the minimal curve initially at 4-month intervals in a premenarchal child. Photographic recording at the first visit is of inestimable value in determining the presence or absence of progression at later dates and minimizing the number of radiographs needed. Moiré topography has also been used as a nonradiation method of monitoring curve progress[1]; this is a noninvasive stereophotogrametric method used to produce a three-dimensional shape of the trunk by casting contour lines on the photograph. It has not gained general acceptance, largely because of cumbersomeness and expense of the equipment, which make it ill suited for the average office facility. Sahlstrand,[42] in analyzing its use, believed that it had many pitfalls and that there was no correlation between moiré asymmetry and the Cobb angle. Despite this, he felt

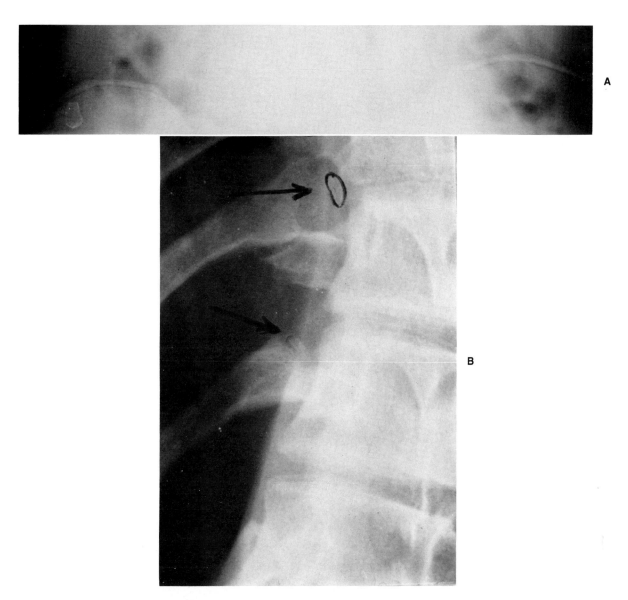

Figure 35-10. Radiographic signs of spinal maturity. **A,** Risser capping sign (stage 4). There are five stages: (1) when apophysis first appears; (2) when it is halfway across; (3) when it is three quarters of the way over; (4) when iliac apophysis has reached its most medial excursion; (5) when apophysis fuses with iliac crest (which may occur as late as 18 to 21 years of age). **B,** Appearance of rib apophysis.

that it had some value in following cases as a complement to physical examination.

In the absence of progression, intervals between visits to the physician can be progressively lengthened. Standing height and leg lengths should be serially recorded to give growth parameters. A flowsheet for recording this information is helpful.

In a skeletally immature child with a curve of less than 20 degrees, treatment should be implemented when there is progression of 10 degrees. In measuring on a radiograph there can be a 3- to 5-degree error, so 10 degrees is a safe parameter. A child with lesser progression, however, is a candidate for treatment if the curve is 20 to 30 degrees, and if the curve is 30 degrees or greater, one should not wait for progression but should prescribe bracing. A persistent truncal shift with a curve less than 20 degrees can also be taken as an indication for bracing in a skeletally immature child. An algorithm can be easily constructed as a guideline.

Bracing

Goals of treatment in bracing are primarily prevention of progression and secondarily improvement in deformity. Un-

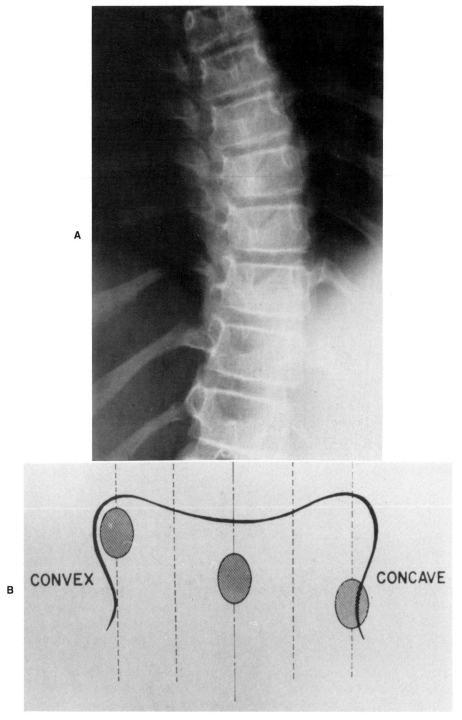

Figure 35-11. A, Radiographic cone view illustrating grade I rotation of apical vertebra. Apical vertebra is usually the one with maximum rotation and therefore the one selected for measurement. **B,** Diagrammatic representation of vertebral body and quadrants it is divided into for purposes of measuring degree of displacement and therefore grade of rotation of pedicles (after Nash and Moe).

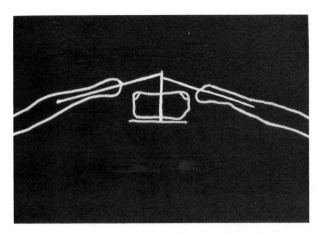

Figure 35-12. Technique of measuring rib-vertebra (RV) angle of Mehta.

fortunately, the latter objective is rarely attained in the long run. Enthusiasm about initial improvement with the brace has been replaced by sobering reality with the gradual return to the pretreatment angular value after the brace is discontinued.

Bracing of various forms has been used since antiquity, but it was not until the late 1940s that Blount and Schmidt introduced the Milwaukee brace with first a chin piece and then a throat mold for the treatment of scoliosis (Figure 35-13). Although it was meant originally for postoperative immobilization, it was adapted for nonoperative treatment on a rigorous basis of 23-hour-a-day brace wear. Its use was coupled with an exercise program both in and out of the brace and was promoted with evangelical enthusiasm, even being hailed as helping improve character. Subsequent studies began to show that little if any permanent improvement was effected. Furthermore, in many of the patients treated there was no documentation of curve progression before treatment, raising the question as to whether these curves would have continued to worsen. Despite this, clinical improvement was apparent, particularly in the thoracic curves with rib hump; this improvement was due to the flattening of the hump by plastic deformation of the ribs by the pressure pad, without correlation with decrease in the angular value of the curve. With increasing recognition of the lack of permanence, coupled with the rigors of a regimen that often made the treatment worse than the disease, various forms of underarm brace (thoracolumbar spinal orthosis, or TLSO) began to appear even on a part-time basis (Figure 35-14).

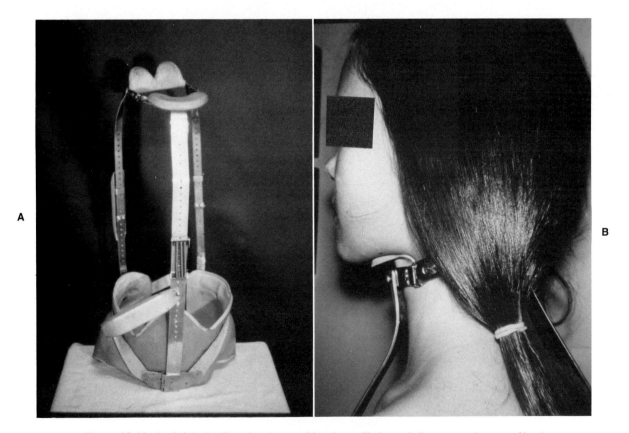

Figure 35-13. A, Original Milwaukee brace with submandibular pad. Pressure pads were affixed at various points to uprights. **B,** Subsequent throatpiece designed to eliminate mandibular pressure. (Courtesy Dr. Walter Blount.)

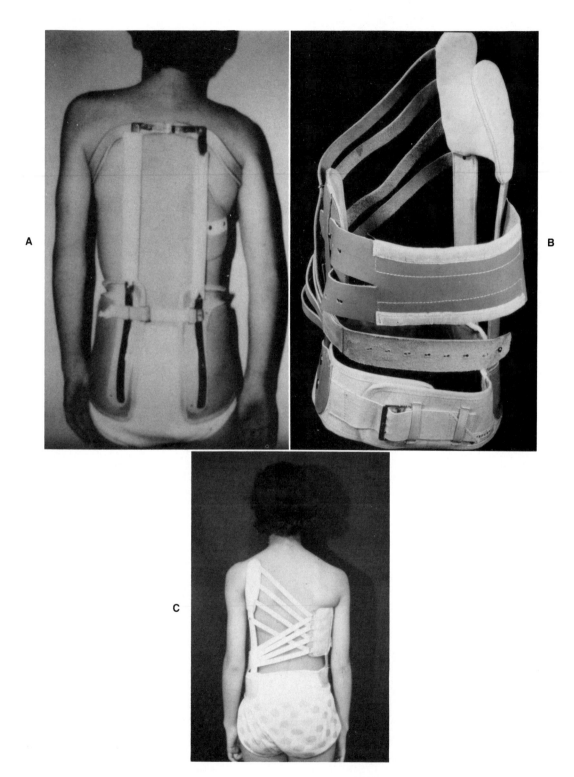

Figure 35-14. Examples of underarm orthoses. **A,** Topless Milwaukee brace with thoracic pad. **B,** Quadrilateral brace employing three-point pressure principle as seen on patient. **C,** Where the three points of pressure are upper and lower ends of quadrilateral frame and pressure pad.

Progression is probably halted in 85% to 90% of the cases. There is great variation in response to brace treatment. If the brace is effective, a prompt reduction in curvature within the first 6 months can be expected with slow return to the original angular value as the brace is discontinued. The type of brace used and the daily amount of brace wearing remain questions of individual judgment. Bracing is generally continued until the end of spinal vertebral growth, at which time gradual weaning from the brace is effected. Bracing is aborted in the face of continued progression of sufficient degree to warrant surgery. This angular value can vary, but Weinstein and colleagues[48] have shown that curves in excess of 30 degrees can progress in maturity. When a curve reaches the 45- to 50-degree range, there is greater risk of progression. Since bracing is most successful in curves less than 40 degrees, and since 20 degrees appears to be the average starting point for implementing bracing, it becomes apparent that there is a narrow spectrum for brace treatment. Only a prospective study of bracing will give a definitive evaluation of its worth. A combined institution study by the Scoliosis Research Society is under way.

Exercises

Much has been written about the use of exercise in treating scoliosis. Such exercises as the creeping and crawling exercises of Klapp[24] have been described as useful to selectively bend against the different apices of the curves and effect active correction. Blount[6] discussed the need for exercise in conjunction with brace treatment. He emphasized active extension to move the apical body prominence away from the pressure pad of the brace. Dworkin and co-workers[19] used a biofeedback method from Rockefeller University employing circumferential strings attached to a beeping computer. The computer sensed variation in string length and, by beeping, encouraged the patient to bend actively against the apex of the curve, which encouraged corrective exercises and facilitated correction. This was reported with optimism but with insufficient results to justify conclusions.

There is no documented evidence to indicate that exercises are effective in treating a curve. However, they are important in two ways. First, they can effect postural improvement by helping correct associated round back and swayback deformities and, by teaching patients to maintain their scapulae in a more symmetric relationship to each other in the frontal plane, mask the underlying rib deformities. Second, they can help maintain spinal flexibility and muscle tone and thus guard against aching discomfort from muscle and ligament fatigue. Such fatigue can occur with the imbalance of spinal mechanics that results from even a mild curve, secondary to abnormal ligamentous and muscle tension. Symmetric extension exercises of the paraspinal and scapulothoracic muscles help the patient keep the scapulae more equally in the frontal plane and help level the shoulders, resulting in better-looking posture. The asymmetric lateral bend and Williams exercises can be quite effective in relieving symptoms of fatigue.

Electrospinal stimulation

Electrospinal stimulation of spinal musculature must still be regarded as an experimental method of treatment. It was reported initially by Axelgaard[4] as having an 84% success rate, but this has dropped to only a 26.8% success rate in further studies by Sullivan and co-workers.[45] Davis and associates[14a] demonstrated that electrospinal stimulation probably has the best results when used to treat flexible curves of 25 to 35 degrees with normal or increased kyphosis, an ATI of 12.5 degrees or less, and a Risser grade of 2 or less. Rowe[41] demonstrated poor compliance with the Scolitron because of skin problems and equipment failure and indicated greater satisfaction with the brace. On the other hand, Houghton[21] in England, using secret pressure cells that liberated a dye when a brace was worn, demonstrated poor compliance with the brace.

Indications for surgery in adults

Pain is the main indication for surgery in an adult with scoliosis. One must be satisfied that the frequency and intensity of pain are sufficient to alter life-style and justify surgical intervention. Therefore, before resorting to surgery, emphasis should be placed on using physical therapy, exercises, and spinal supports to treat pain. Psychosociaal factors are of great importance, and psychologic profiling can be invaluable before surgery. Careful documentation of disability, which comes only with long acquaintance with the patient, must be made. Surgery in an adult is accompanied by much greater morbidity than in an adolescent. A report presented to the Scoliosis Research Society in 1986 by Sponseller and co-workers[44a] noted 20 complications, including eight reoperations in 46 adult patients treated surgically between 1972 and 1982. When questioned by an independent investigator, not the surgeon, the patients stated that they had no significant change in the subjective assessment of their pain. However, 75% believed that they had a decrease in their peak pain level, but 16% had an increase. In 58% there was a reduction in their general pain level, while 18% had an increase. Sixty-one percent felt that they had increased function, while 35% said that they had decreased function.

NEUROMUSCULAR SCOLIOSIS

Neuromuscular scoliosis differs from idiopathic scoliosis in that loss of neural and muscular control dictates the deformity and that potential for curve progression may be present after skeletal maturity even in a smaller curve. With an upper motor neuron lesion (such as cerebral palsy) and resultant spasticity, or with a lower motor neuron lesion (such as spinal muscular atrophy or poliomyelitis) and resultant flaccidity, the final common pathway affected is skeletal muscle. In muscular dystrophy the neural system is unaffected and the skeletal muscle is directly involved. The loss of muscular or neural control, or both, produces spinal deformity in a high percentage of cases. The frequent association of sensory and autonomic dysfunction with altered mental capacity makes management especially difficult. Increasing spinal deformity in a patient with loss of neural and muscle control can quickly reduce the level of independence, robbing the patient of walking or even sitting ability. Since many of the neuromuscular lesions are present at birth or shortly afterward, deformity can start early in life and be relentless and progressive. Constant vigilance is necessary. Checkups should be twice yearly; radiographs should be taken as a baseline at the start of treatment and at least annually thereafter.

Early bracing is necessary rather than waiting until a significant deformity is established. Brown and Swank[10] advocated support as soon as a measurable consistent spinal deformity of 20 degrees is present. However, one should not hesitate to treat lesser curves, particularly when they are associated with truncal overhang. Bracing provides spinal support and helps maintain alignment in the flaccid collapsing curve; it can retard but not prevent curve progression. If there are associated sensory deficits with potential for pressure sores, the brace must be carefully supervised. However, it is not contraindicated. In a spastic patient with a rigid curve, bracing is more difficult and less likely to succeed unless the curve is mild.

Bracing until maximum truncal height is obtained is desirable, but it is essential to abandon bracing and proceed with surgery at the first indication that the brace is failing and the curve is progressing significantly.

For the wheelchair patient, specialized seating systems can provide spinal support and with molded inserts can provide sitting balance when pelvic obliquity exists. Such supports and spinal braces (for example, TLSO) provide freedom of upper extremity use. Without them, the hands are often used to support the spine while the patient is seated, depriving the patient of their much needed use for other necessary functions. Thoracic cutouts in the plastic jackets must be generous to avoid reducing chest expansion in a flaccid patient.

CONGENITAL SCOLIOSIS

Management of congenital scoliosis depends on whether there is potential for asymmetric vertebral growth and accompanying progressive scoliosis. Thus proper classification with attention to the accurate anatomy of the defect is essential. A bilateral failure of segmentation does not produce deformity, but a unilateral one does because of its inhibition of growth on the concave side with continued unopposed growth on the opposite (convex) side. A balanced congenital scoliosis requires no treatment other than general exercises. A congenital curve with unequal growth

requires surgery, no matter how early the age. It cannot be helped by a brace. Braces have been thought to have some value in prevention of progression in compensatory curves associated with congenital scoliosis, but this is extremely limited.

SCOLIOSIS WITH MYELOMENINGOCELE

Scoliosis with myelomeningocele can represent a mixture between the congenital and the paralytic deformities. The neurologic lesion associated with myelomeningocele can lead to the development of a paralytic curve, initially of the flexible collapsing type and subsequently, with curve progression, of more rigidity and deformity. The spina bifida may be only one osseous manifestation of multiple skeletal deformities such as unilateral failure of segmentation and with it asymmetric growth, rigidity, and relentless progression. The more proximal the neurologic lesion, the greater the incidence of spinal deformity (100% of T12 paraplegia, 5% when the lesion is at S1, according to Moe and associates[33]).

Development of paralytic curves is usually gradual before 10 years of age but increases in rate of progression at the time of the adolescent growth spurt. The curves are often a long C type extending into the sacrum or pelvis, which together can be considered the lowest vertebra of the curve, with resultant pelvic obliquity. When severe enough and fixed, they interfere with sitting balance and defy orthotic correction.

The congenital curves behave as do other congenital curves, present at birth and with early rigidity and early progression if the potential for asymmetric growth exists. Curves can be a mixture of congenital and paralytic with features of both.

Orthotic treatment is feasible in treating the paralytic component and has two goals: to retard curve progression and try to obtain maximum torso length until fusion, generally after age 10, and to maintain trunk balance so as to facilitate sitting and avoid loss of function associated with progressive spine deformity. The timing of bracing is the same as for other paralytic curves.

ABNORMAL KYPHOSIS AND ABNORMAL LORDOSIS

Sagittal plane curvatures evolve from the straight infantile spine as antigravity curves that develop to maintain balance and erect posture. The thoracic kyphos also provides accommodation for cardiac and pulmonary organs. The cervical lordosis, thoracic kyphosis, and lumbar lordosis give an elongation potential to the spine, making it a flexible structure with undulating length that is of use in ambulation, running, and other physical activities.

The excesses of sagittal plane curvature, particularly hyperkyphosis or round back and hyperlordosis or swayback, have been vexing treatment problems to physicians, patients, and particularly parents (Figure 35-15). Much has been learned about these disorders during the past 20 years. Normal values have been stated to be 20 to 40 degrees for thoracic kyphosis, 40 to 60 degrees for lumbar lordosis, and 50 degrees for cervical lordosis (Moe and co-workers[33]). Methods of measurement of the curves are the same as used for measuring the scoliotic curve. A wide range of clinical disorders can accompany kyphosis, ranging from the cosmetic with mild symptoms of ligament and muscle fatigue to severe deformity with back pain, cardiopulmonary compromise, and even rarely paraplegia.

Excesses of sagittal plane curvatures are either functional or structural. Functional curvatures such as postural round back result from weakened anterior and posterior spinal ligamentous and muscle supporting structures. Weakened spinal extensor muscles, for example, result in decreased tension on the convexity with increasing kyphosis. Weakened abdominal muscles lead to loss of compression force with increased lordosis.

Structural sagittal curvature is best exemplified by thoracic vertebral epiphysitis. Often bearing the name of Scheuermann,[43] who defined its radiographic changes, it is

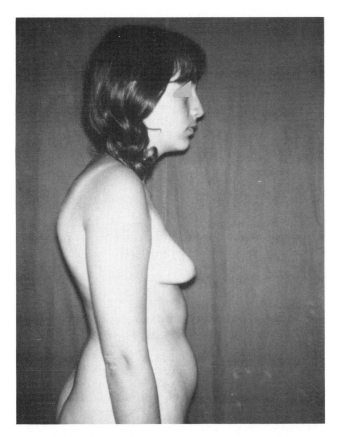

Figure 35-15. Patient with Scheuermann's disease exhibiting abnormal sagittal plane curvatures, hyperkyphosis from abnormal thoracic vertebral formation, and hyperlordosis secondary to hyperkyphosis.

the main clinical condition in this category. It is characterized by failure of the anterior vertebral column owing to disorganization of the end-plate disc structures with Schmorl's nodes and resultant wedging of the thoracic vertebrae. Sorenson[44] further refined its definition as three or more apical adjacent vertebrae with wedging of 5 degrees or more, as well as structural disorganization of the end-plate disc complex. Some wedging of the midthoracic vertebrae can be seen normally, but not exceeding 5 degrees, just as posterior wedging of the fifth lumbar vertebra may be noticed as a normal manifestation of lumbar lordosis.

Postural round back and swayback, being nonstructural, are usually flexible and can best be treated by exercises to strengthen the weakened structures and stretch any that have become contracted through unequal opposing muscle pull. Bracing is rarely necessary, but in severe cases where curves approach 70 degrees it can be helpful, even on a part-time basis of night wearing. Bracing can also be used if deformity persists despite diligent attempts at exercise. However, bracing is no substitute for exercises and must be done in conjunction with them. Without motivation to exercise, treatment will fail. The parents' understanding and cooperation are essential.

Tight hamstrings often accompany round back and swayback and have been implicated as etiologic factors by causing posterior pelvic rotation with compensatory increases in lumbar lordosis and thoracic kyphosis. That one curve reacts to the other is illustrated by the dramatic decrease of a postural thoracic round back with effective pelvic tilt and decrease of lumbar lordosis. Hamstring stretches are an integral part of the exercise program, which generally includes symmetric extension exercises of the paraspinal and scapulothoracic muscles, abdominal muscle exercises, pelvic tilt, and Williams flexion exercises.

Thoracic vertebral epiphysitis should be treated. Otherwise, deformity, psychologic handicap, pain, degenerative arthritis, and rarely cardiopulmonary compromise and paraplegia can be the sequelae.

Orthotic devices to carry out and maintain correction consisted initially of extension casts, often applied in sections, to first flex the lumbar spine and decrease the lordosis and then extend the thoracic spine to decrease the kyphosis. The casts were supplanted by the Milwaukee brace, with good results, including correction of vertebral wedging and kyphos, being reported within 1 year. Unlike scoliosis brace wearing, the brace need not be continued until vertebral skeletal maturation or, for that matter, on a full-time basis. After an initial period of full-time brace wearing, part-time bracing is permissible. However, follow-up studies have shown loss of correction of as much as 60%.[15] Underarm bracing has also been used when the highest apical vertebra is T8. Its effectiveness, particularly in controlling the forward thrust of the cervical spine, remains questionable. Electrospinal stimulation has been used; the final outcome is yet to be determined.

When structural kyphosis approaches 65 to 70 degrees, the likelihood of effective brace treatment is remote and surgery should be considered.

REFERENCES

1. Adair, IV, van Wyck, MC, and Armstrong, CWD: Moire topography in scoliosis screening, Clin Orthop 129:165, 1978.
2. Adams, F: Lectures on the pathology and treatment of lateral and other forms of curvature of the spine, London, 1865, John Churchill & Sons.
3. Asher, M, Greene, P, and Orrick, J: A six year report: spinal deformity screening in Kansas school children, J Kans Med Soc 81:568, 1980.
4. Axelgard, J, Nordwall, A, and Brown, JO: Correction of spinal curvatures by transcutaneous electrical muscle stimulation, Spine 8:465, 1983.
5. Barrack, RL, et al: Proprioception in idiopathic scoliosis, Spine 9:681, 1984.
6. Blount, WP, and Moe, JH: The Milwaukee brace, Baltimore, 1973, Williams & Wilkins Co.
7. Bradford, DS, et al: Scheuermann's kyphosis and roundback deformity: results of Milwaukee brace treatment, J Bone Joint Surg 56A:749, 1974.
8. Brooks, HL, et al: Scoliosis: a prospective epidemiological survey, J Bone Joint Surg 57A:968, 1975.
9. Reference deleted in proofs.
10. Brown, JC, and Swank, S: Paralytic spine deformity. In Bradford, D, and Hensinger, R, editors: The pediatric spine, New York, 1985, Thieme Inc.
11. Bunnell, WP: A study of the natural history of idiopathic scoliosis, Paper presented at 17th Annual Meeting of the Scoliosis Research Society, Denver, Sept 1982.
12. Bunnell, WP: The angle of trunk rotation: an objective criterion for spinal screening, Orthop Trans 7:429, 1983.
13. Burwell, RG, Dangerfield, PH, and Vernon, CL: Anthropometry and scoliosis. In Zorab, PA, editor: Scoliosis: Proceedings of the Fifth Symposium held at the Cardiothoracic Institute, Brompton Hospital, London, September, 1976, New York, 1977, Academic Press, Inc.
14. Cobb, JR: Outline for the study of scoliosis, AAOS Instructional Course Lectures 5:261, 1948.
14a. Davis, RD, et al: Efficacy of electrical surface stimulation versus bracing in the treatment of idiopathic scoliosis—a comparative study. Paper presented at 21st Annual Meeting of Scoliosis Research Society, Hamilton, Bermuda, Sept 1986.
15. DeMauroy, JC, and Stagnara, P: Résultats à long terme du traitement orthopédique: réunion du groupe d'étude de la Scoliose Aix en Provence 1:60, 1978.
16. Dickson, RA, et al: School screening for scoliosis: cohort study of clinical course, Br Med J 73:265, 1980.
17. Dickson, RA, et al: The pathogenesis of idiopathic scoliosis: biplanar spinal asymmetry, J Bone Joint Surg 66B:8, 1984.
18. Drummond, D: The natural history of spine deformity. In Bradford, D, and Hensinger, R, editors: The pediatric spine, New York, 1985, Thieme Inc.
19. Dworkin, B, et al: Behavioral method for the treatment of idiopathic scoliosis, Proc Natl Acad Sci USA 82:2493, 1988.
20. Reference deleted in proofs.
21. Houghton, G, et al: Monitoring true brace compliance, Paper presented at 21st Annual Meeting of Scoliosis Research Society, September, 1986.
22. Jackson, RP, Simmons, EH, and Stripins, D: Incidence and severity of back pain in adult idiopathic scoliosis, Spine 8:749, 1983.
23. Kostuik, JP, and Bentiroglio, J: The incidence of low-back pain in adult scoliosis, Spine 6:268, 1981.
24. LeGrande-Lambling, Y: Therapeutic exercises. In Licht, S, editor: Exercises for scoliosis, New Haven, Conn. 1958, Waverly Press.
25. Lonstein, JE: Screening for spinal deformities in Minnesota schools, Clin Orthop 126:33, 1972.
26. Lonstein, JE: Prognostication in idiopathic scoliosis, Orthop Trans 5:22, 1981.
27. Lonstein, JE, Carlson, JM: Prognostication in idiopathic scoliosis, Orthop Trans 5:11, 1980.
28. Lonstein, JE, and Carlson, J: The prediction of curve progression in untreated idiopathic scoliosis during growth, J Bone Joint Surg 66A:1061, 1984.
29. Lonstein, JE, et al: Voluntary school screening for scoliosis in Minnesota, J Bone Joint Surg 64A:481, 1982.
30. Luning, A, and Schulthess, W: Atlas und Grundriss der orthopadischen Chirugie, Munchen, 1901, Verlag von dF.
31. Mankin, H, Graham, J, and Schack, J: Cardiopulmonary function in mild and moderate idiopathic scoliosis, J Bone Joint Surg 46A:52, 1964.
32. Mehta, MH: The rib vertebral angle in the early diagnosis between resolving and progressive infantile scoliosis, J Bone Joint Surg 54B:230, 1972.
33. Moe, J, et al: Scoliosis and other spinal deformities, Philadelphia, 1978, WB Saunders Co.
34. Nash, CL, and Moe, JH: A study of vertebral rotation, J Bone Joint Surg 61A:371, 1979.
35. Nash, CL: Risks of exposure to X-rays in patients undergoing long-term treatment for scoliosis, J Bone Joint Surg 61A:370, 1979.
36. Nordwall, A, and Willner, S: A study of skeletal age and height in girls with idiopathic scoliosis, Clin Orthop 110:6, 1975.
37. Ponseti, IV, and Friedman, B: Prognosis in idiopathic scoliosis, J Bone Joint Surg 32A:381, 1950.
38. Risser, JC: The iliac apophysis: an invaluable sign in the management of scoliosis, Clin Orthop 11:111, 1958.
39. Rogala, E, and Drummond, DS: The Shriner's flexicurve assessment of scoliotic hump deformities, J Bone Joint Surg 61B:245, 1979.
40. Rogala, EJ, Drummond, DS, and Gurr, J: Scoliosis: incidence and natural history—a prospective epidemiological study, J Bone Joint Surg 60A:173, 1978.
41. Rowe, DE: Comparison of patient acceptance of scolitron and brace treatment of idiopathic scoliosis, Paper presented at 21st Annual Meeting of Scoliosis Research Society, Hamilton, Bermuda, Sept 1986.
42. Sahlstrand, T: The clinical value of moire topography in the management of scoliosis, Spine 2:409, 1986.
43. Scheuermann, H: Kyphosis dorsalis juvenilis, Orthop Chir 41:305, 1921.
44. Sorenson, KN: Scheuermann's juvenile kyphosis, Copenhagen, 1964, Munksgaard.
44a. Sponseller, PD, et al: Long-term follow-up of adult scoliosis treated surgically, Paper presented at 21st Annual Meeting of Scoliosis Research Society, Hamilton, Bermuda, Sept 1986.
45. Sullivan, JA, et al: Further evaluation of the scolitron treatment of idiopathic adolescent scoliosis, Spine 11:903, 1986.
46. Veldhuizen, AF, Baas, P, and Webb, PJ: Observations on the growth of the adolescent spine, J Bone Joint Surg 68B:724, 1986.
47. Weinstein, SL: Adolescent idiopathic scoliosis: prevalence, natural history, treatment, indications, Monograph sponsored by SRS and AAOS Committee on the Spine, 1985.
48. Weinstein, SL, and Ponseti, IV: Curve progression in idiopathic scoliosis: long term follow-up, J Bone Joint Surg 65A:447, 1983.
49. Weinstein, SL, Zavala, DC, and Ponseti, IV: Idiopathic scoliosis: Long-term follow-up and prognosis in untreated patients, J Bone Joint Surg 63A:702, 1981.
50. Wyatt, MP, et al: Vibratory response in idiopathic scoliosis, J Bone Joint Surg 68B:714, 1986.
51. Wynne-Davies, R: Familial scoliosis: a family survey, J Bone Joint Surg 50B:24, 1968.
52. Yamada, F, et al: Etiology of idiopathic scoliosis, Clin Orthop 184:50, 1984.

CHAPTER 36

Orthopedic management of children with cerebral palsy

NICHOLAS A. TZIMAS

The most frequent musculoskeletal disorders encountered by the pediatric orthopedist in a rehabilitation center are cerebral palsy, spina bifida, and to a lesser degree, congenital limb deficiencies and neuromuscular disorders. Musculoskeletal injuries and infections, bone tumors, bone dysplasias and metabolic conditions, and such regional disorders as congenital hip dislocations, Legg-Perthes disease, and knee and foot deformities such as clubfoot are not often seen in a rehabilitation center and are therefore excluded from this discussion. Spine and hand disorders are discussed in Chapters 28, 32, 33, 35, and 36. The definition, etiology, and clinical manifestations of cerebral palsy and drug and physical therapy modalities in its management are discussed in Chapter 30.

It is estimated that 15% to 20% of children with cerebral palsy are candidates for surgical treatment. The major goals of treatment are prevention of deformity, correction of deformity that is already established, and improvement of the overall function and attainment of the highest possible degree of habilitation and rehabilitation.

GENERAL ASPECTS OF ORTHOPEDIC CARE

Braces and splints are important adjuncts in the management of a child with cerebral palsy. They are used for support and positioning. A splint can be used preoperatively to place a joint in the position to be surgically attained, thus indicating the postoperative result. Braces are also used to control the involuntary movements in athetosis that impede ambulation.

About 95% of surgery is performed on spastic children. Surgical indications in athetosis are limited to the mixed forms (spastic-athetotic) and to severely athetotic patients with painful hip dislocations. Certain patients with rigidity can occasionally benefit from surgery, which often facilitates nursing care. Surgery is not used in cerebral palsy patients to control tremor or ataxia.

When surgery is indicated, it should be performed early (Figures 36-1 and 36-2). In operations on the soft tissues at more than one joint level, surgery should be carried out in a proximodistal direction (hip to ankle) by an experienced surgeon who has a thorough understanding of joint deformity pathomechanics and joint interdependence.

Surgery should not be performed on very young children who have had neither preparatory physical therapy nor the time to learn basic motor skills. Premature surgery may be counterproductive and effectively reduce a child's functional potential.

Since spasticity affects muscles spanning more than one joint, surgery at a single joint level does not improve the overall function. On the contrary, it may have adverse effects on neighboring joints whose muscles have not been operated on, since joints act interdependently. For example, lengthening of the triceps surae tendon at the ankle in a spastic paraplegic child without simultaneous lengthening of the knee flexors (hamstrings) gradually increases the knee flexion deformity, the triceps having been weakened by the lengthening operation. In domino fashion the increased knee flexion causes flexion deformity at the hip and calcaneus at the ankle. The triceps surae, restricted in range, is weakened further, as are the hip extensors. The patellar tendon of the quadriceps muscle, in the constantly flexed position, becomes longer and the patella rides high. In such a case, rehabilitation is protracted, even after the eventual lengthening of the knee flexors and use of long leg braces. One-stage, multiple-joint operations have additional benefits: there is one hospitalization, one exposure to anesthesia, one stage of rehabilitation, and decreased expenses. The child does not have to be prepared psychologically time and again.

The operations, in upper and lower extremities, are performed with the child in the supine position and in a proximodistal direction (hip to ankle). It is difficult to perform

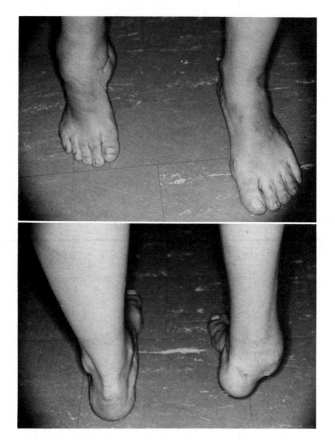

Figure 36-1. Late deformities of right foot of 24-year-old untreated patient with spastic hemiplegia.

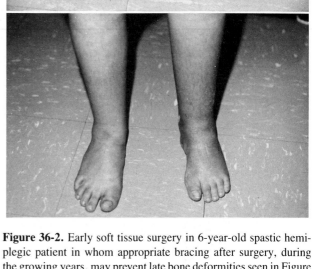

Figure 36-2. Early soft tissue surgery in 6-year-old spastic hemiplegic patient in whom appropriate bracing after surgery, during the growing years, may prevent late bone deformities seen in Figure 36-1.

lengthening, for example, of the hamstring muscles, when the hip adductors are tight and do not permit leg abduction.

TYPES OF SURGICAL PROCEDURES IN CEREBRAL PALSY

It is not practical to present all the surgical procedures that have been described or that are used to treat patients with cerebral palsy. This presentation covers experiences in the New York University Medical Center. Surgery in cerebral palsy is directed mainly to the soft tissues—muscles, tendons, and occasionally, fascia. An attempt is made to lengthen and thereby temporarily weaken the contracted prevalent muscles (mostly flexors) so their antagonists can be strengthened by therapy and integrated functionally with the agonists. Bone operations are reserved for long-standing deformities, for cases in which soft tissue procedures are inadequate for deformity correction (Figure 36-3), and for hip dislocations and rotary leg deformities. Operations on nerves (neurectomies) are rarely performed, except when ambulation is not expected and neurectomy (for example, sectioning the obturator nerve) will facilitate nursing care.

In order of decreasing frequency, the following surgical procedures are most commonly used:

I. Muscle and tendon
  A. Division
  B. Excision
  C. Lengthening
  D. Transfer
  E. Shortening

II Bone
  A. Arthrodesis operations
    1. Foot—triple arthrodesis (after 12 years of age)
    2. Subtalar joint—rarely performed, children 4 to 9 years of age
    3. Wrist—fusion; rarely performed
  B. Osteotomies
    1. Femoral intertrochanteric, varus derotation osteotomy
    2. Pelvic—Chiari
    3. Tibial and fibular derotation osteotomy (rarely)

III. Nerve—anterior obturator or total obturator neurectomy (rarely)

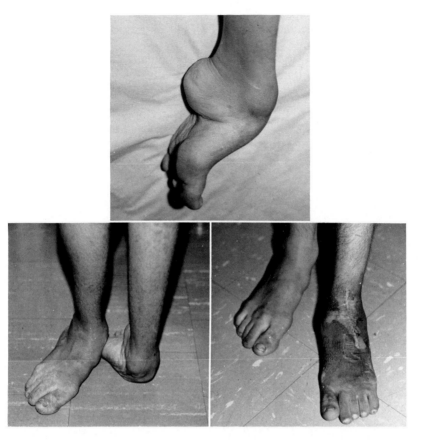

Figure 36-3. Severe equinovarus deformity of left foot in spastic hemiplegic patient treated late with soft tissue and bone operations in order to obtain plantigrade foot.

Muscle and tendon operations
Division

The most frequently performed operation on the muscle or tendon is division, or release, from its points of attachment, proximally or distally. In the upper extremity, for example, division of the distal attachment of the pronator teres to the radius increases forearm supination and elbow extension. In the lower extremity, complete division of the tendon of the adductor longus and partial of the tendinous origin of the adductor gracilis and, on occasion, of the adductor brevis muscles allows increase and abduction and decreases hip flexion and internal rotation of the leg. In time the divided muscles reattach by fibrous tissue to the previous points of attachment, but they remain in general weaker than before—a desirable condition. With weaker adductors the therapist is able to strengthen the hip abductor and extensor muscles (gluteals).

Extensive adductor muscle division, especially when combined with tenontectomies of the medial hamstrings (which act also as internal rotators of the leg), will result in severe hip weakness and external rotation deformity of the leg to the point that ambulation becomes very difficult or impossible. This is further compounded when, in addition, an imbalance exists or is created in the adductor-abductor muscle groups of the same limb or on the other side. The pelvis, on the side of the stronger adductors, rises and tilts in the opposite direction. It may also tilt forward or rotate in a certain direction, depending on the action of the unbalanced muscle forces around the hip. The leg of the adducted side becomes shorter. The hip of the same side may dislocate and cause additional leg shortening. Changes in the position of the pelvis bring adaptive changes to the superimposed spine and secondary spinal deformities (Figure 36-4). It is therefore evident that only judicious adductor tendon and muscle division can prevent these complications. Many surgeons advocate transfer of all or some of the three adductors (longus, gracilis, and brevis) to the ischial tuberosity. I believe that muscle division is much preferable to transfer because it not only reduces muscle pull but also maintains the muscles in their normal habitat and with the same line of muscle action.

Tendon excision

Partial tenontectomy is carried out on the tendons of the gracilis and semitendinosus muscles at the knee. Both are long, multiarticular muscles and more difficult to control in cerebral palsy patients. By virtue of their distal attachment, in relation to the knee joint's axis of rotation, they have a

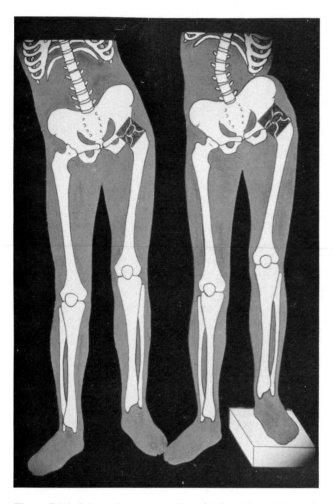

Figure 36-4. Schematic representation of deformities to hips, pelvis, spine, and lower extremities resulting from unbalanced muscle forces in hips. The stronger left hip adductor muscles caused dislocation of left hip, tilting of pelvis, shortening of left lower extremity, and lumbar lordosis. Similar deformities may occur with stronger abductor muscles in opposite (right) hip.

greater rotary effect (torque: muscle force times perpendicular distance from axis of rotation) and consequently deform the knee in flexion more than the other knee flexors, namely the semimembranosus and biceps femoris muscles, which have attachments very close to the knee joint and a lesser bending moment.

A piece of tendon, about 2 inches in length, is excised from each of the tendons of the gracilis and semitendinosus muscles, above their points of attachment to the tibia (pes anserinus). They are thus converted to simpler monarticular muscles, which act mainly as hip extensors. Hip extension is almost always a weak function in cerebral palsy.

Proximal division of the hamstrings at the point of origin in the region of the ischial tuberosity, as advocated by some authors, is not recommended because weakening of the extension produces hip flexion deformity. The continued action distally of the hamstrings and gracilis still causes knee

flexion deformity in spite of some temporary weakness of the hamstrings from their proximal release.

To reduce tightness in the semimembranosus muscle, its distal aponeurotic envelope is divided sharply over about two thirds of its circumference (without injuring muscle fibers) before becoming the tendon of insertion. If there is any residual knee flexion deformity after the gracilis and medial hamstrings have been lengthened, attention is turned to the tendon of the biceps femoris, which is divided within the muscle fibers of its short head. If there is tightness of the iliotibial band unilaterally, the iliotibial band and the lateral intermuscular septum are also divided through the same small lateral incision.

Simple tenontectomy of the hamstring muscles at the knee is preferable to their transfer, either anteriorly to the quadriceps or patellar tendon or posteriorly to the lower femur. After simple tenontectomy the cut proximal ends of the tendons stick to the surrounding tissues or, at times, following the lead of their tendon sheaths, reunite by a fibrous band with their distal ends, forming a weaker connection than the previous one. With the reduction in flexion power the quadriceps length adjusts and its function improves. Transfer of the hamstrings anteriorly not only reduces the ability of the knee to flex but also increases disproportionately the extensor power in the knee. This may create an extension contracture with a high-riding patella and, at times, genu recurvatum.

Similarly, transfer of some of the hamstring muscle to the lower femur posteriorly (Eggers' procedure[4]) creates an extension contracture of the knee with recurvatum and limits the forward and backward excursion of the leg in walking; the effect is greater if all the hamstring muscle is transferred. The leg is literally tied to the pelvis posteriorly by the transferred hamstrings to the lower femur. This transfer prevents forward excursion, while anteriorly the shortened quadriceps (through its pelvic attachment of the rectus femoris) prevents its backward excursion. Other factors, such as tightness of the tendon of the triceps surae, may further aggravate the knee deformity into excessive genu recurvatum. Secondary pelvic and trunk adjustments to the altered position of the joints in the lower extremities in the form of anterior pelvic tilt and excessive lumbar lordosis may make ambulation impossible.

Tendon lengthening

The most frequently performed and probably the oldest orthopedic operation[3] is the lengthening of the triceps surae tendon (tendo Achillis). It is performed for equinus foot deformity, for equinovalgus in spastic paraplegia, or for equinovarus in spastic hemiplegia. The equinovarus deformity in spastic hemiplegia is due not only to the contracture of the triceps surae muscle but also to shortening of the posterior tibial muscle.

In spastic paraplegics the role of the posterior tibial muscle is secondary, and the presenting equinovalgus foot de-

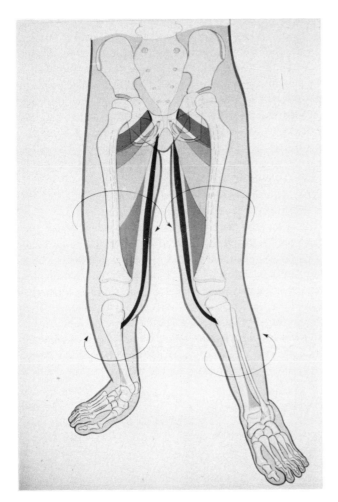

Figure 36-5. Adductor muscles in the spastic paraplegic patient produce flexion, adduction, and internal rotation deformities in hips and compensatory flexion, abduction (valgus) deformities in knee, external rotation of leg, and valgus deformity of foot associated with hallux valgus.

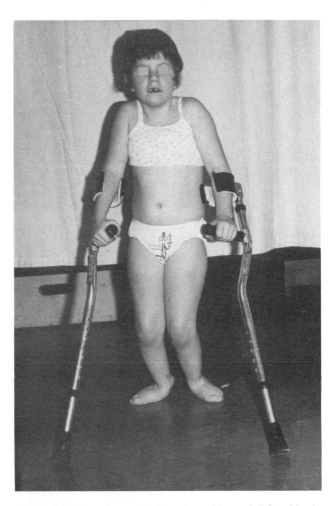

Figure 36-6. Spastic paraplegic patient with usual deformities in hips and knees and rocker bottom deformities of feet.

formity follows a different chain of events. The hip adductors adduct, flex, and internally rotate the thigh. The adduction of the hip causes abduction (valgus) of the knee, external rotation of the leg, and valgus of the foot. The tissues in the sole of the foot are displaced laterally, and secondary toe deformities (for example, hallux valgus) appear (Figure 36-5). There are several additional factors involved in the development of equinovalgus: the displaced weight-bearing line, medially, to the area of the body support by the foot; the ligamentous relaxation present in some patients; and the tightness of the triceps surae tendon, which does not permit the foot to dorsiflex at the ankle joint but at the subtalar joint; at this joint dorsiflexion occurs together with foot pronation. All of these favor development of the equinovalgus or, at times, rocker bottom foot deformity in the spastic paraplegic (Figure 36-6). Lengthening of the triceps surae tendon, followed by positioning of the foot in appropriate shoes or braces, may be all that is necessary to

correct the foot deformity in a growing child at an early stage.

There are a variety of lengthening operations of the contracted triceps surae. We prefer to lengthen the common tendon (not the gastrocnemius aponeurosis, as would be the case in pure gastrocnemius contracture[1]) by a Z-plasty operation.

The subcutaneous, partial, multilevel tenotomy performed by some surgeons is a blind procedure, leading at times to calcaneus foot deformity when the entire triceps surae tendon is inadvertently divided. Moreover, it is not feasible to obtain the necessary amount of tendon lengthening by such a closed method.

The next most frequent tendon lengthening is that of the posterior tibial tendon. It is performed through a small medial incision in the lower third of the leg at the level of the musculotendinous junction and within enveloping muscle fibers. Its proximal and distal parts are thus kept in proximity by muscle fibers after division.

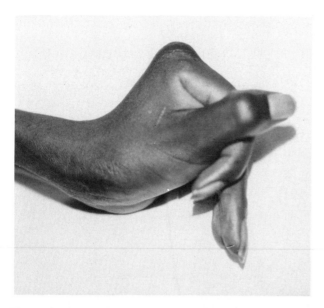

Figure 36-7. Poor result from an ill-advised transfer of extensor carpi ulnaris tendon to dorsum of wrist in a dystonic hemiplegic patient; result is severe extension of wrist, flexion of fingers at metacarpophalangeal joint level, and a totally useless hand.

Tendon transfer

Tendon transfers are not usually successful in cerebral palsy. They should not be performed in athetotic patients, in whom the results are uniformly poor. The tendon transfer we perform most frequently is the transfer of the flexor carpi ulnaris, either around the ulnar border of the forearm or through the interosseous membrane to the attachment of the extensor carpi radialis brevis. This procedure corrects or minimizes flexion adduction deformity of the wrist and enhances finger function. With proper patient selection, it has given acceptable functional results[7]; however, in inappropriate cases (for example, dystonic patients), the results of such a transfer are decidedly poor (Figure 36-7).

In a less frequently used operation the posterior tibial tendon is transferred to the dorsum of the foot (second cuneiform) subcutaneously or, preferably, through the interosseous membrane. The transfer of the posterior tibial tendon is mostly done in equinovarus foot deformity in spastic hemiplegic patients, in whom lengthening of the triceps surae and, at times, of the posterior tibial tendon does not correct the varus deformity with forefoot adduction. It is preferable, however, to perform the tendon transfer after foot stabilization (triple arthrodesis) at the age of 12

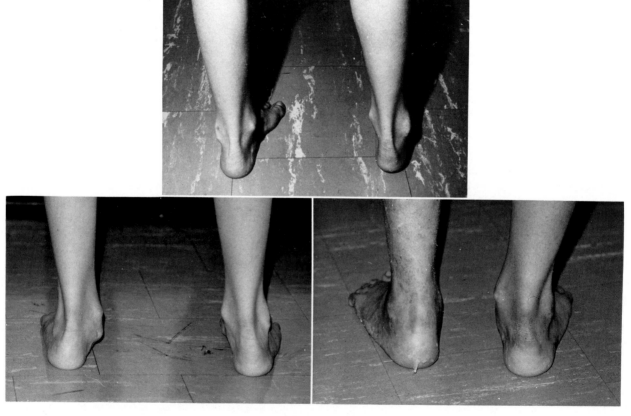

Figure 36-8. Valgus deformity of left foot secondary to transfer of posterior tibial tendon to dorsum of foot, necessitating triple arthrodesis for its correction.

years or later. In some patients the transfer of the posterior tibial tendon to the dorsum may unbalance the foot and create valgus foot deformity with abduction of the forefoot (Figure 36-8).

The posterior tibial transfer should not be done simultaneously with heel cord lengthening, since strong pulling by the anterior tibial may draw the foot into dorsiflexion (in the face of a weakened triceps surae muscle), and a calcaneus foot deformity will ensue. In any case the posterior tibial tendon transfer always reduces functional capacity of the foot. The foot may remain rigid in a position of 90 degrees, unable to dorsiflex because of the tightness of the triceps surae tendon and unable to plantar flex because of tightness imposed by the transferred posterior tibial tendon to the dorsum of the foot.

Other tendon transfers around the foot are not advised. We do not transfer the anterior tibial to the dorsolateral aspect of the foot because it causes valgus deformity of the foot with dropping of the first metatarsal owing to unbalanced action of the peroneus longus, the natural antagonist of the anterior tibial muscle. On the other hand, transfer or tenotomy of the peroneus longus produces a varus deformity of the foot, elevation of the first metatarsal and dorsal bunion, with the head of the first metatarsal protruding dorsally and the great toe in flexion (hallux equinus) (Figure 36-9).

Tendon shortening

Tendon shortening is not performed, except for shortening of the tendons of the radial extensors of the wrist during transfer of the flexor carpi ulnaris to the extensor carpi radialis brevis. In the lower extremity this procedure is

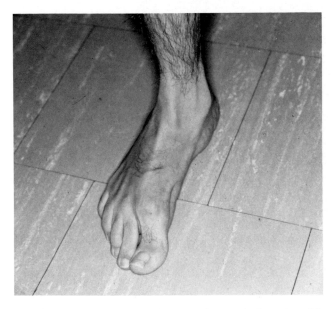

Figure 36-9. Hallux equinus in a spastic paraplegic patient following release of peroneus longus tendon.

sometimes tried when the tendon of the triceps surae was previously overlengthened. The shortening attempts to correct the calcaneus foot deformity. This is a difficult problem to solve, especially when lengthening of the triceps surae tendon has been of long standing. Correction of the calcaneus foot may never be obtained, even after triple arthrodesis, transfer of the anterior tibial tendon to the os calcis, tenotomy of the peroneus longus, and so on.

Bone surgery
Arthrodeses

Arthrodeses, or joint fusion operations, have been especially useful in feet with equinovarus deformity (spastic hemiplegia) or equinovalgus (spastic paraplegia). The subtalar, talonavicular, and calcaneocuboid joints are fused after the removal of appropriate bone wedges to correct the deformities (triple arthrodesis). The best results are obtained in the correction of the equinovarus foot deformity (Figure 36-10). Triple arthrodesis is performed after the age of 12 years, when there is sufficient bone maturity in the foot. Earlier, and between the ages of 4 and 9 years, the subtalar joint is fused extra-articularly (Grice procedure). This procedure, however, has been overused. It should not be performed without simultaneous lengthening of the tight triceps surae. Failure to do so produces a rocker bottom foot deformity, since the compensatory dorsiflexion of the foot, with pronation at the level of the subtalar joint, is lost by the fusion. In addition, patients with relaxed joint ligaments do not fare well, since with recurrence of the equinus the foot may assume the varus position through the ankle and remaining foot joints.

In the upper extremity, fusion of the wrist is rarely performed in older patients who have had long-standing wrist deformity and who do not appreciably benefit from splinting, physical therapy, and tendon transfer of the flexor carpi ulnaris.

Osteotomies

The most common type of osteotomy involves the femur at the intertrochanteric level. It is done to correct coxa valga and anteverta, which are frequently associated with the most severe cases of cerebral palsy and with hip dislocation (Figure 36-11).

Pelvic osteotomies (Chiari type,[2] Figure 36-12) are occasionally used to deepen a deficient acetabulum that results in hip dislocation. The results of the surgery in obtaining satisfactory hip joint function are rather poor.

In the rare rotary problem in the lower extremity that is caused by tibial torsion (mostly internal), a derotation tibial and fibular osteotomy is indicated for its correction.

Dislocation of the hip

Hip dislocation in cerebral palsy is caused by the strong action of the hip adductor and flexor muscles, the absence of abductor muscle function, and the lack of weight bearing.

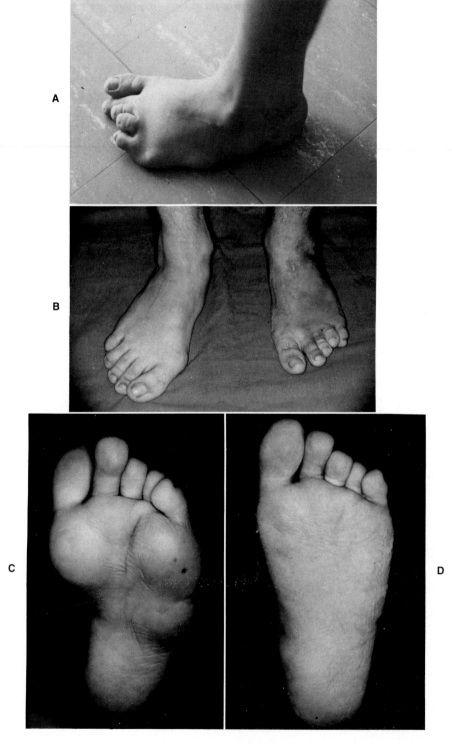

Figure 36-10. Equinovarus left foot deformity in spastic hemiplegic patient. Before (**A**) and after (**B**) correction with triple arthrodesis. Plantar aspect of same foot before surgery (**C**) and after surgery (**D**).

To prevent or correct hip dislocation, the first priority is to weaken the adductor-flexor muscle group, strengthen the abductor group, and enhance standing and weight bearing. Our experience has been limited regarding iliopsoas tenotomies to reduce hip flexion and adduction or iliopsoas tendon transfers to the greater trochanter that attempt to create an abductor gradient to prevent the dislocation. Iliopsoas transfer has been done primarily in children with spina bifida.

We have also tried to reduce hip flexor activity by tenotomy of the rectus femoris tendon and partial release of the origin of the tensor fasciae latae and sartorius.

If after a period of adductor lengthening and weight bearing the hips are still subluxated from coxa valga and anteverta, a subtrochanteric valgus derotation osteotomy is indicated to position the femoral heads into the acetabula.

Finally, when the acetabular cavity is too small to accommodate the femoral head, a pelvic osteotomy above the acetabulum, with displacement of the lower part of the pelvis containing the acetabulum medially (Chiari), improves the position of the femoral head and increases hip stability.

Nerve operations

Peripheral neurectomies, such as of branches of the posterior tibial nerve to the soleus muscle or of the medial nerve in the muscles of the forearm (pronator teres), have not been used in our practice. In very severe spasticity or rigidity, anterior or total obturator neurectomy may be necessary to facilitate groin hygiene and nursing care. More recently, posterior rhizotomy has been used to relieve spasticity, and the results have been encouraging. Earlier in the century, Foerster[6] successfully reduced spasticity by dividing posterior nerve roots in the lumbar and cervical regions. Fasano[5] recently refined the technique and reported his results with selective stimulation of the rootlets comprising the posterior root and division of the ones associated with an abnormal muscular response.

POSTOPERATIVE CARE AND REHABILITATION

Except for some cases of bone surgery in which a specific period of time (6 to 12 weeks) is necessary for healing, patients are quickly mobilized postoperatively and placed on an intensive program of physical therapy and gait training, usually 1 week after the operation. They are

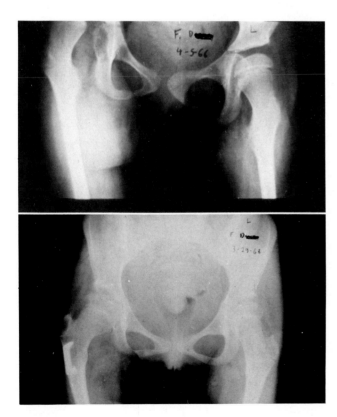

Figure 36-11. Dislocation of right hip in spastic quadriplegic patient corrected with a varus derotation femoral intertrochanteric osteotomy.

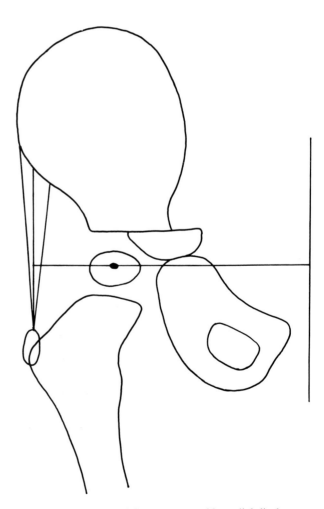

Figure 36-12. Chiari pelvic osteotomy with medial displacement of lower part of inominate bone for correcting shallow and deficient acetabulum.

encouraged to bear weight with short leg casts that are applied following lengthening of the triceps surae tendon and kept on for 5 weeks. In the past, the leg casts were kept on for longer periods of time and the postoperative rehabilitation was delayed until the casts were removed. Such prolonged immobilization encourages diffuse fibrosis and atrophy of the already weakened muscles and reduces functional recovery.

Following cast removal, long leg braces are frequently used over a period of time to protect weak muscles, prevent secondary joint deformities, and to aid the patient in acquiring a sound gait pattern. The braces particularly control the ankle and, to a lesser degree, the other joints.

The failure to obtain good results from surgery is multifaceted. In addition to such factors as the severity and the extent of involvement, the child's mental and emotional status and motivation, the absence of previous competent physical therapy, parental cooperation, and social conditions, the following situations are conducive to poor results:

1. Failure to assess properly the entire chain of deformities, not only the presenting one
2. Undercorrection or overcorrection of the deformity. It is better to undercorrect than to overcorrect, since overcorrection may produce an irreversible deformity. The undercorrection may necessitate only additional surgery.
3. Failure to maintain the correction of a deformity by prolonged use of splints and braces and expert physical therapy
4. Failure to recognize the fact that the child is growing and the effects of growth on the recurrence of the deformity

SUMMARY

We have presented a review and rationale for the surgical management of children with cerebral palsy. Early diagnosis is the key to better management. Spasticity can be diagnosed in the first 6 months of life. Athetosis is usually diagnosed later when the involuntary movements have appeared (third or fourth year). A history of perinatal problems, delay in psychomotor development, and persistence of abnormal reflexes, beyond a certain age, particularly if symmetric, are important determinants in diagnosis and prognosis. A dedicated rehabilitation program, balanced by appropriately timed early surgery—especially of soft tissues—constitutes the sine qua non of successful management and maximal functional results.

REFERENCES

1. Baker, LD: A rational approach to the surgical need of the cerebral palsy patient, J Bone Joint Surg 38A:313, 1956.
2. Chiari, K: Medial displacement osteotomy of the pelvis, Clin Orthop 98:55, 1974.
3. Delpech, MJ: Tenotomie du tendon d'Achille, Chirurgie Clinique de Montpellier, ou observations et reflections tirées des travaux de chirurgie clinique de cette École, Paris, 1823, Gabon.
4. Eggers, GWN: Transplantation of hamstring tendons to femoral condyles in order to improve hip extension and to decrease knee flexion in cerebral spastic paralysis, J Bone Joint Surg 38A:827, 1952.
5. Fasano, VA, et al: Surgical treatment of spasticity in cerebral palsy, Child's Brain 4:289, 1978.
6. Foerster, O: On the indications and results of the excision of posterior spinal nerve roots in men, Surg Gynecol Obstet 16:463, 1913.
7. Green WT, Banks, HD: Flexor carpi ulnaris transplant and its use in cerebral palsy, J Bone Joint Surg 44A:1343, 1962.

CHAPTER 37

Rehabilitation of athletic injuries

JEFFREY MINKOFF AND ORRIN SHERMAN

RUSK INSTITUTE AND THE INTRODUCTION OF THE CYBEX

The Rusk Institute has gained fame as a center for rehabilitation. Although it is particularly known for its work with various paralytic disorders, its less widely proclaimed influence in the field of sports medicine should not go unnoticed. In fact, the most celebrated rehabilitative apparatus currently used in sports medicine was largely introduced to the medical literature by the physicians and workers at Rusk. In the late 1960s the works of Hislop and Perrine,[12] Moffroid, Whipple, and Hofkosh[16] and Thistle and co-workers[24] brought to light the benefits of a new form of exercise known as *isokinetics*. Although isokinetic modes, or those that provide resistive training at a constant velocity, were used in laboratory research as early as the 1920s,[14] commercially available forms were not readily available until the 1970s, when the Cybex isokinetic machinery was introduced to the public.

SPORTS MEDICINE

Sports medicine has been a burgeoning specialty for several decades. It gained impetus in the 1950s when television expanded the numbers of spectators. The Kennedy physical fitness campaign elevated sports consciousness to a new and higher level. Eventually the glorification of the superstars and their astronomic earnings throughout the 1970s added measurably to the burdens and tensions of the sports physician. Orthopedic surgeons have spearheaded the sports medicine movement with the help of cardiophysiologists, trainers, therapists, and other specialists.

Unfortunately, sports orthopedists have been on occasion the subject of peer derision. Allegations against them have ranged from "glory mongering" to an inability to practice real medicine. For the most part these attitudes are a product of misinformation about a specialty in which there has been an admitted commercialism and a wholesaling of "shake and bake" sports injury modalities by self-proclaimed experts. Others know it is no simple task to make an on-the-field, split-second decision with momentous implications, or to perform a screening examination for a multimillion dollar contract, or even to deal with athletes who refuse to abstain from sports in the face of severe injury, disability, or degenerative disease. Sports orthopedists distinguish themselves from their colleagues by permitting an athlete of any level the most expedient return to activity with optimal allowable function by considering the patient's goals and the risks and consequences of continued participation or treatment.

Among the principal vehicles by which these goals are accomplished are muscle-conditioning systems. For many athletes, muscle education may obviate a surgical procedure. Moreover, surgery for an athletic injury cannot be successful without subsequent muscle reeducation. Physical therapy for muscle reeducation is a ubiquitous and vital feature in all treatment of athletic injury. The muscle training must impart a specificity: a shot-putter's arm cannot be rehabilitated in the same way as the arm of a baseball pitcher, nor can a fencer's leading leg be managed in the same way as the leg of a place kicker. The limb segment action modes are different for each of these activities with respect to work, power (work rate), and the angular accelerations and decelerations of each involved articulation.

TRAUMATIC AND ATRAUMATIC INJURIES

Before a discussion of individual sports injuries, it is worthwhile to explore some factors more basic to the reader's knowledge. There are reasons why injuries or afflictions occur in certain individuals. Obviously, a contact sport such as football, rugby, or ice hockey creates more numerous and serious injuries than noncontact sports. The individual's style of play is a critical factor; some athletes are injury prone. Moreover, the player's position may make injury more likely—for instance, the hockey player who always skates to his off wing, the defensive back stopping hefty runners in full flight, and the kickoff returner.

It has been postulated that somatotype is important in susceptibility to injury, and more particularly that loose-jointed individuals are more prone to ligamentous injuries or sprains.[17] This has not been substantiated by subsequent researchers,[13] but it is known that hyperelastic disorders such as Ehlers-Danlos and Down syndromes lead to increased frequencies of patellar and other subluxations. Some activities are properly performed only with excessive laxity: ballet and gymnastics, for example. In these activities inadequate joint laxity may lead to injuries.

Training camps and screenings are held for athletes even though they are young and in generally good health. The purpose is to detect aberrances in their flexibility and power, as well as to detect medical abnormalities. For example, an affliction common to runners and skaters is the groin pull. Contrary to common belief, such strains are a consequence not so much of muscle tightness as of a weakness that allows the muscle to be damaged by tensile forces. The weaknesses of the adductor groups that are determined during screenings in camp are usually harbingers of muscle or tendon strains soon to follow. Players with chronic afflictions, such as tibiofemoral or patellofemoral instabilities, insidiously lose strength in the involved extremity if constant strengthening is not performed throughout the year. A failure to maintain strength predisposes to injury.

Some afflictions are traumatic in origin and leave little doubt as to their cause. However, there exists a whole spectrum of "sports tumors" that appear only after an athletic trauma has triggered symptoms. The evaluation of any medical problem must include an earnest history, a thorough physical examination, and the ordering of any auxiliary tests appropriate to the problem. The standard review of differential categories must never be abandoned; developmental, anatomic, vascular, metabolic, traumatic, neoplastic, and neurologic categories of diagnosis must be considered. A black athlete may have leg pain caused by sickle cell infarction. An athlete looking sluggish may be on drugs, have a cardiomyopathy, or be anemic.

An athlete with a nontraumatic onset of symptoms is even more suspect of having an insidious, underlying, nonathletic disorder, especially if the symptoms are unilateral and progressive. Onsets solely attributable to athletic injury but without overt trauma are most often a consequence of a relative structural insufficiency, such as a subluxating patella or excessive rotatory laxity of the tibiofemoral articulation. They may also be a consequence of a relative overuse best known as the overuse syndrome. For example, a pitcher throwing hundreds of pitches per day over a period of years

damages the glenoid labrum, rotator cuff, olecranon fossa, and medial capsule of the elbow. Ascertaining the particular cause for a group of symptoms is the only means by which a prophylactic program can be developed to anticipate and thwart their occurrence.

SHOULDER INJURIES

The shoulder has more degrees of freedom in its motion than any of the other major joints of the body. The layperson is usually surprised to learn that the glenohumeral joint is not truly a ball and socket and that the glenoid is the lateral extremity of the scapula. Whereas the femoral head is so well contained within the acetabulum that its stability is ensured by the bony configuration of the hip joint alone, the humeral head is apposed to, but not contained within, the glenoid. The glenohumeral joint is therefore an inherently unstable joint, relying exclusively on its capsular and muscular investments for stability. The frequency of glenohumeral dislocation attests to its unstable character.

Acute injuries

The most frequent nonosseous acute sports injuries to the shoulder region are glenohumeral subluxations or dislocations, acromioclavicular separations, and less often, acute ruptures of the rotator cuff. First-time glenohumeral subluxations or dislocations in athletics typically occur in those under 30 years of age, most often as a result of a fall or a leverage injury, such as might be sustained by arm tackling in football. The extremity is usually immobilized in a cross-chest position for several weeks to reduce pain and to permit collagenous contracture of the offended capsule. No matter what degree of immobilization is administered, however, the recurrence rate is extremely high: 80% to 90%.[11,21]

The humeral head is usually displaced anteriorly. Surgical repair or reconstruction is rarely considered after a single occurrence. Since prevention of recurrence is virtually impossible, the principal reason for any immobilization should be to curtail symptoms. Postinjury symptoms are rarely substantial for more than 48 hours, when reduction has been either spontaneous or at least early. I begin early motion and resistance exercises. This helps to avert unnecessary, early recurrences caused simply by poor glenohumeral muscle control during the performance of simple activities of daily living. Slowly performed, low-resistance low-repetition exercises are begun in forward flexion, abduction, horizontal abduction and adduction, and even internal and external rotation in varying degrees of abduction. External rotation is performed especially slowly, and the arcs of each direction of exercise are governed by tolerance and comfort. Frequently the patient is fitted with a dislocation harness that check-reins excessive abduction and external rotation of the humerus (Figure 37-1). This permits relatively safe participation in most sports, as long as the affected arm is not used for throwing. Before any participation, re-

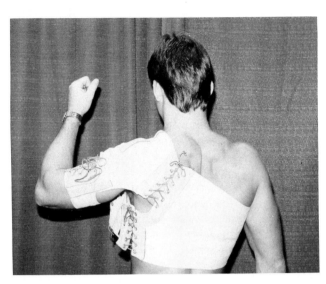

Figure 37-1. Shoulder dislocation harness. Restriction of shoulder motion can be adjusted with laces. (Courtesy Bruce Bennett.)

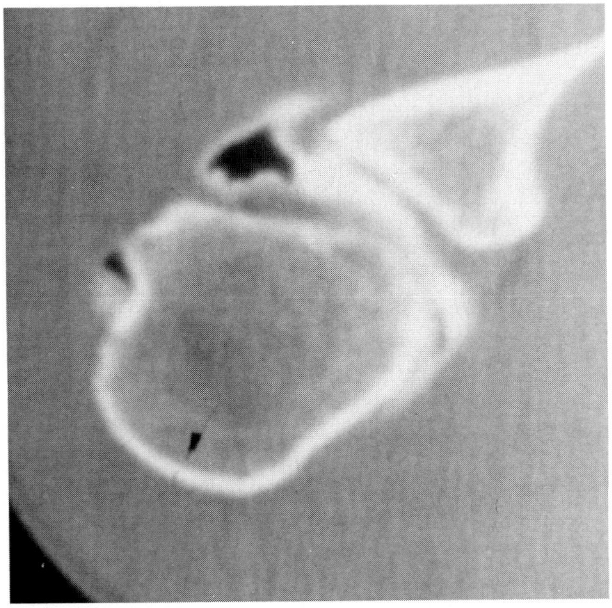

Figure 37-2. Computerized tomographic arthrogram of shoulder. Anterior is to right; glenoid is at upper right and humeral head at lower left. *Solid arrows,* Anterior capsule stripped from scapular neck; *hollow arrow,* distorted anterior labrum.

habilitation progresses by increasing the loads, repetitions, velocities, and arcs of each exercise direction—ultimately with a combination of machines capable of variable-resistance isotonics and isokinetics.

At the time of the acute episode the treating physician must be alert to the possible presence of tuberosity fractures and axillary nerve or brachial plexus traction injuries, none of which are rare sequelae of the injury. Obviously, plain radiographs and a neurovascular examination are necessary adjuncts to the evaluation. In some instances an acute shoulder injury has been sustained with the patient unaware of a glenohumeral separation—the patient may experience only severe pain. Glenohumeral subluxation or dislocation should be suspected in such patients. For professional athletes, who need an immediate prognosis and determination of ability to return to play, computerized tomographic (CT) arthrography of the shoulder is warranted. This study can demonstrate the capsular and labral abnormalities of an instability that is suspected but not corroborated by the history and physical examination (Figure 37-2).

The acromioclavicular separation, or "shoulder separation," is usually caused by a fall or impact on the point of the shoulder. The force of the impact determines the quantitative disruption of those structures resistant to the dislocation of the distal end of the clavicle from the acromion: the acromioclavicular joint capsule and ligaments, the coracoclavicular ligaments (conoid and trapezoid ligaments), and the trapezius and deltoid muscles. In the most severe forms each of these structures has been disrupted, allowing

a superior and subcutaneous dislocation of the clavicle equivalent to type V of Rockwood's classification.[20]

Acromioclavicular joint separations (ACJSs) are common in football quarterbacks and especially in professional ice hockey players. There is barely a veteran hockey player in the locker room without at least one elevated clavicle. Since the clavicle is the only strut connection between the axial and appendicular portions of the skeleton, its role in stabilizing the shoulder girdle has been a stimulus for aggressive treatment. A few decades ago it was common to operate on an ACJS and to transfix the joint with pins, screws, or sutures. The degree of separation has a bearing on future symptoms. The natural history of the disorder is well described in the work of Cox.[4]

Surgery for less than the most dramatic ACJS carries a morbidity that probably outweighs its potential benefits. Prolonged immobilization followed by prolonged rehabilitation virtually precludes the return of a throwing athlete during the season in which the injury was sustained. The joint, although reduced, might become painfully arthritic or even develop osteolysis. Infections are devastating. Pins have been reported to migrate through the spinal cord, mediastinum, and lungs. Of particular significance in a throwing athlete, the cicatricial response to surgery may cause a loss of shoulder motion, which may be more devastating than a loss of stability for some athletes. To avert these sequelae some workers have resorted to complex riggings by which the clavicle is forced downward while the flexed elbow is forced upward. In the past, the most popular of these immobilizers was the Kenny Howard strap. Maintaining whatever reduction had to be achieved required prolonged immobilization (4 to 6 weeks) and constant and severe pressure by the harness. The consequences were often an incomplete reduction, protracted recovery, and pressure sores over the superior margin of the clavicle.

This small historical background might make it less surprising that currently most elite sports physicians rarely resort to surgery[5] or to elaborate strappings. Instead the symptoms are permitted to abate with use of such supportive measures as slings, ice, and anti-inflammatory medications, and then the shoulder is initiated into a program of resistive exercises.

Frequently it is possible to begin the exercises within 24 hours of the injury. In 13 years with a professional hockey team, the senior author (J.M.) performed only one operation on a player for an ACJS and only a single additional procedure in a private practice confined exclusively to sports injuries. In only one case was a secondary arthroplasty necessary to relieve a painful restriction of motion resulting from nonoperative treatment. The ability to intervene later

with an arthroplasty is one reason for avoiding primary surgical treatment. The major reasons, however, are the very limited disabilities ordinarily caused by the injury and the expeditious return to athletics afforded by muscle rehabilitation as a singular treatment.

Within minutes of an ACJS the athlete is often capable of abduction, since the middle portion of the deltoid is largely uninvolved. The anterior tissue disruptions inhibit forward flexion ability and especially horizontal abduction, each because of a combination of pain and weakness. Reasonable restoration of these functions, allowing a return to contact sports, ordinarily takes 3 to 5 weeks for an ACJS of an intermediate or severe grade. It is often easiest to begin the rehabilitation process with water exercises. In a pool the arm is buoyant, circumferentially braced by the hydrostatic pressure, and strengthened by movements against the column of water being displaced. As out-of-water symptoms dissipate, antigravity exercises are performed with free weights and then machines. Horizontal abduction is typically the last arc of pain and weakness to overcome, and when this has been accomplished, the player may return to athletics. In contact sports a return may be permitted sooner when the shoulder is protected against impact injury by special shoulder pads (Figure 37-3). Although protection is important, the most essential feature for a return to participation is the strength-controlled motion. This satisfies the almost half century old wisdom of Nicholl,[18] who maintained that a limb with range but no power is in its extreme form a flail limb.

KNEE INJURIES
Decision to operate or rehabilitate

The knee is the most frequently afflicted joint in athletics. The most debilitating knee problems are experienced as a consequence of major ligament disruptions, especially those involving the cruciate ligaments. Although the community of sports orthopedists collectively recommends immediate, or at least early, repair or reconstruction of these ligaments, there is a place for conservative management. Proponents of early surgical intervention indicate that only surgery is capable of restoring athletic function to the unstable knee while helping to avert the progressive degenerative consequences of frictional shear between the bearing surfaces of the tibia and femur. Unfortunately, surgery does not always lead to stability; success rates are between 70% and 90% for different series. Ensuing joint stiffness as a complication may be a worse experience than the instability for which the surgery was attempted. Infection, patellar pain, and other complications may also diminish the success of surgery. The benefits of surgery as an inhibitor of arthritic progression have been expounded but never clearly proved.

An estimated 20% to 30% of persons with unstable knees can acceptably negotiate a reasonable activity schedule with temperance, therapy, and bracing in the absence of sur-

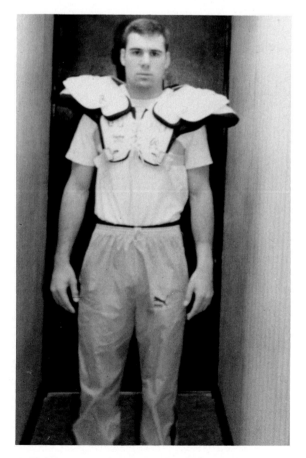

Figure 37-3. Protective pads for acromioclavicular joint injuries. This football type of shoulder pad is cantilevered to move with arm and is lined with cushioning material.

gery.[19] The activity level, specific sport, and compliance of an individual are paramount issues. A professional athlete's career may be terminated by unsuccessful surgery. A basketball player, who needs to jump and to decelerate rapidly, has virtually no chance to resume a career after cruciate rupture, whether treated by surgery or by nonsurgical management.

It is probably safe to say that successful surgery is the best choice for an athlete with a disability attributable to a ruptured cruciate ligament. Since an unconstrained instability ultimately leads to progressive degenerative changes, there is a concurrence of opinion that early surgery may help to prevent such changes. Of course, opinion and approbation do not necessarily conform with the truth.

Since surgery of any quality results in an imperfect knee, it is sometimes best to permit a patient to experience life with the afflicted knee in order to determine its level of function before any consideration of surgery. This is more often appropriate for an older, less competitive athlete than for a zealous youthful athlete.

Time may influence a decision for or against early surgery. Another obviously critical issue in decision making relates to the nature and severity of the instability and its associated pathology. Nevertheless, an objective quantification of these elements does not quantify the perceived disability. Owing to great variations in individual structure, proprioceptive ability, activity demands, and cerebral influences, individuals with the same severe grade of instability may express a gradient of perceived disability ranging from an awareness of some problem to marked trepidation about even a minor misstep.

Classifications of instabilities are complex and beyond the scope of this chapter. Furthermore, the number of disorders associated with anterolateral rotatory instability (ALRI) and anteromedial rotatory instability (AMRI), for example, is high and precludes a discussion of more than a general approach to instability (Table 37-1).

Diagnosis of disorders

It is important to establish as specific a diagnosis as possible before assuming the responsibility of making a recommendation about surgery. Although a gross instability is usually readily recognized, it may be masked by pain and voluntary guarding, a hemarthrosis too large to allow knee

Table 37-1. Pathologic conditions associated with ALRI and AMRI in 30 patients

	Number	Percentage
Torn anterior cruciate ligament	28	100
Nonfunctional anterior cruciate ligament	2	
Median meniscocapsular ligament–musculotendinous unit complex	30	100
Lateral meniscocapsular ligament–musculotendinous unit complex	30	100
Torn lateral meniscus	23	77
Torn medial meniscus	21	70
Acute subluxation of patella	5	17
Laterally hypermobile patella	4	13
Partial tears of posterior cruciate ligament	5	17
Torn plica	2	7
Acute peroneal nerve compression	2	7
Chondral fractures		
Lateral tibial plateau	1	3
Lateral femoral condyle	1	3
Fractures		
Avulsion of tibia with lateral capsular sign	3	10
Fractured xiphoid process of patella	1	3
Degenerative changes		
Chondromalacia of patella	1	3

From Terry, GC, and Hughston, JC: Orthop Clin North Am 16:33, 1985.

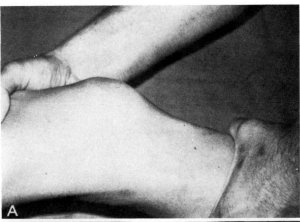
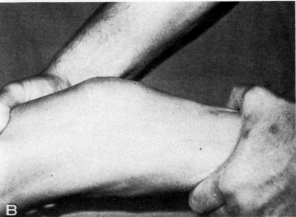

Figure 37-4. Lachman test demonstrating anterior cruciate ligament injury. **A,** Tibia reduced. **B,** Tibia subluxated anteriorly. (From Torg, JS, Conrad, W, and Kalen, V: Am J Sports Med 4:84, 1976.)

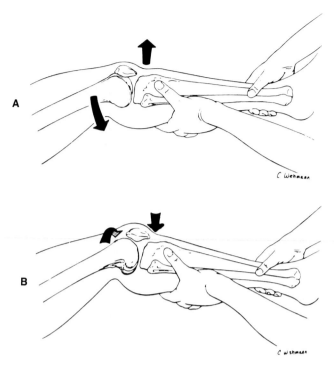

Figure 37-5. Flexion-rotation-drawer test for anterior cruciate ligament injury with tibia subluxated **(A)** and reduced **(B).** (Courtesy Dr. F.R. Noyes. From Crenshaw, AH, editor: Campbell's operative orthopaedics, ed 7, St. Louis, 1987, The CV Mosby Co.)

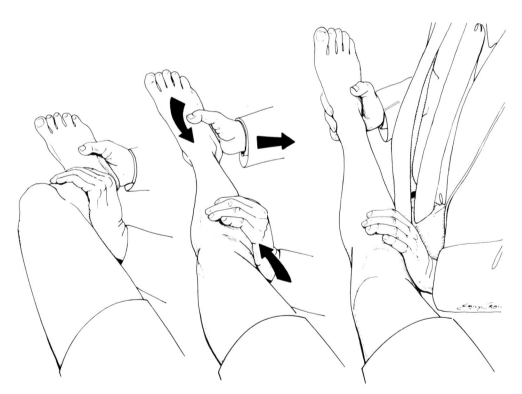

Figure 37-6. Pivot shift test for anterior cruciate ligament injury. *Left,* Tibia reduced. *Middle,* Anterior tibia displacement. *Right,* Completion of maneuver. (Courtesy Dr. J.C. Hughston. From Crenshaw, AH, editor: Campbell's operative orthopaedics, ed 7, St. Louis, 1987, The CV Mosby Co.)

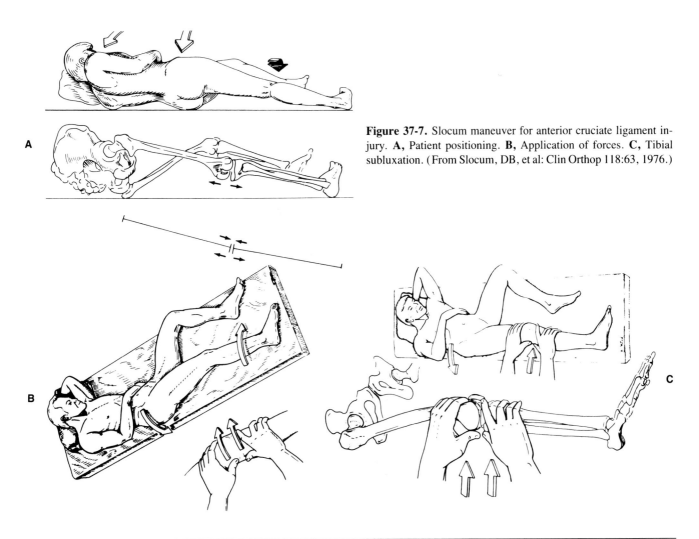

Figure 37-7. Slocum maneuver for anterior cruciate ligament injury. **A,** Patient positioning. **B,** Application of forces. **C,** Tibial subluxation. (From Slocum, DB, et al: Clin Orthop 118:63, 1976.)

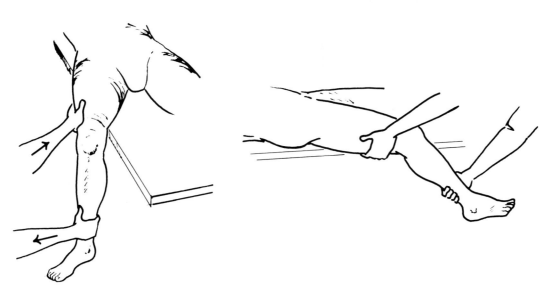

Figure 37-8. Abduction stress test for medial instability. (From Hughston, JC, et al: J Bone Joint Surg 58A:159, 1976.)

motion, or other factors. Few torn ligaments are truly reparable, but those that are should be approached with early surgery. A fractured joint surface should not be neglected, nor should a meniscus, which may be reattached or repaired most effectively by early surgery.

Options available for diagnostic specificity include the following:

1. History. A loud pop generally signifies a ruptured cruciate ligament but may also represent an acute patellar dislocation, torn meniscus, or osteochondral fracture; a definite separation between the tibia and femur leaves little doubt about the presence of a ruptured ligament.

2. Physical examination. A number of commonly employed physical maneuvers are helpful in delineating the format of instability. These are portrayed in Figures 37-4 through 37-12.

3. Radiographs. A plain radiograph is used to look for ligament and capsular avulsions (Figure 37-13). An arthrogram is used for meniscal lesions (Figure 37-14). CT arthrography is used for posterior cruciate ligament and masses (Figure 37-15).

4. Magnetic resonance imaging (MRI). MRI clearly demonstrates lesions of the menisci, posterior cruciate ligament, anterior cruciate ligament (to a degree), and extracapsular soft tissues (Figure 37-16).

5. Examination under anesthesia. Anesthesia eliminates all guarding influences to allow a more accurate examination.

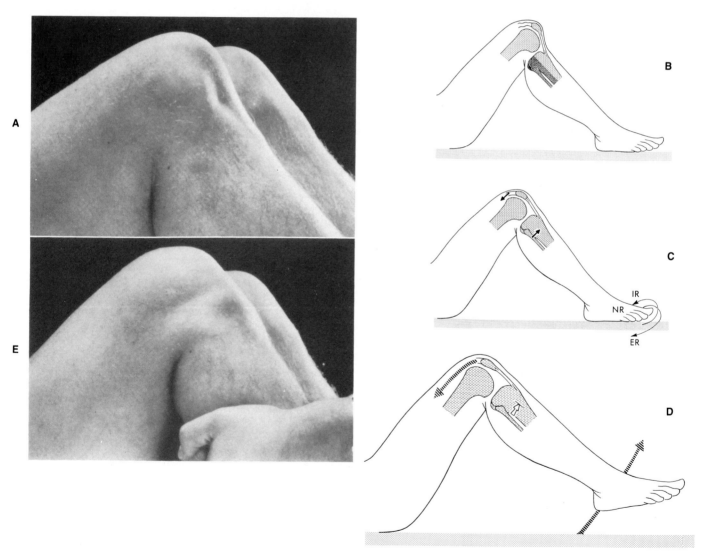

Figure 37-9. Posterior drawer test for posterior cruciate ligament injury. **A** and **B,** Posterior tibial subluxation. **C,** Tibial rotational influence. **D,** Quadriceps contraction and tibial reduction. **E,** Manual reduction. (From Muller, W: The knee: form, function, and ligamentous reconstruction, New York, 1983, Springer-Verlag.)

6. Ligament testers. These devices have been available for several years. The most commonly used is the KT-1000 (Figure 37-17), which allows an objective determination of anteroposterior instability.[22] More sophisticated units, such as the Genucom, allow a measurement of rotatory and translational instability. The simple testers, such as the KT-1000, can be used on an awake or anesthetized patient.

7. Arthroscopy. Arthroscopy is an extreme and invasive diagnostic technique. Although it clearly documents lesions of the cruciate ligaments, menisci, and articular surfaces, it fails to demonstrate many abnormalities of the capsule and extracapsular structures. Large quantities of irrigating fluid may extravasate through capsular rents. The resulting tissue edema may adversely affect any subsequent open surgery. Arthroscopically assisted cruciate ligament reconstructions have become popular, so it seems almost foolish to perform a diagnostic arthroscopy as a mere prelude to a subsequent reconstructive arthroscopy, even though there is a minimal risk with arthroscopy.

Choosing a diagnostic approach is rarely difficult for an orthopedic surgeon; most often the diagnostic avenues are used for research documentation and for proof to the patient that a given disorder exists. Patients with major instabilities usually require reconstruction and should probably proceed directly to arthroscopically assisted reconstructive procedures. Patients refusing surgery regardless of disability or

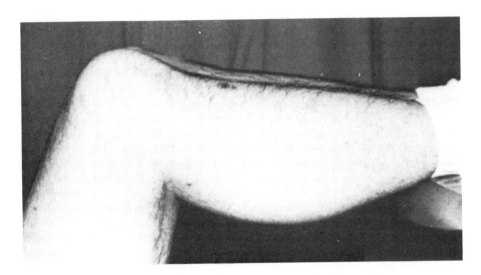

Figure 37-10. Posterior sag sign (Godfrey's sign) for posterior cruciate ligament injury. (From Godfrey, JD: Curr Pract Orthop Surg 5:56, 1973.)

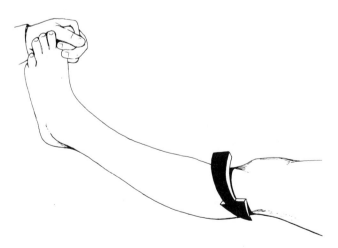

Figure 37-11. External recurvatum test for posterolateral instability. (Courtesy Dr. J.C. Hughston. From Crenshaw, AH, editor: Campbell's operative orthopaedics, ed 7, St. Louis, 1987, The CV Mosby Co.)

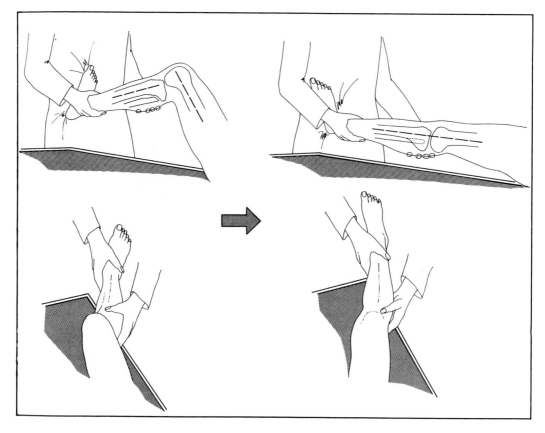

Figure 37-12. Reverse pivot shift test for posterior cruciate ligament injury. *Left,* Posterior tibial subluxation. *Right,* Reduced position. (From Jakob, RP, Hassler, H, and Staeubli, HU: Acta Orthop Scand 52[suppl 191]:1, 1981.)

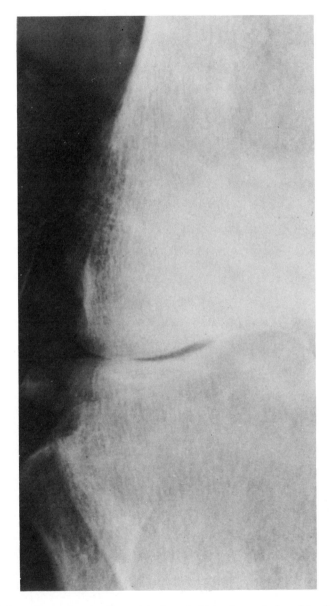

Figure 37-13. Lateral capsular sign (bony detachment of lateral capsule from lateral tibial plateau), highly suggestive of anterior cruciate ligament injury. (From Insall, JN, editor: Surgery of the knee, New York, 1984, Churchill-Livingstone. By permission of Churchill-Livingstone.)

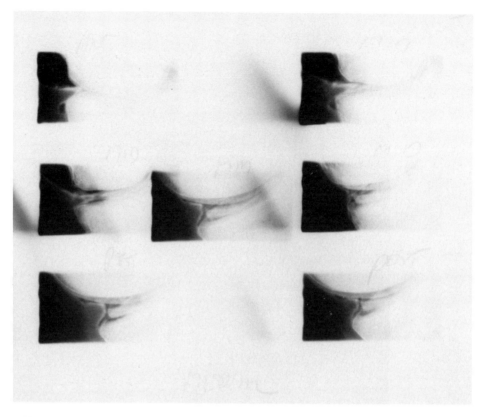

Figure 37-14. Arthrogram demonstrating vertical tear in posterior horn of medial meniscus.

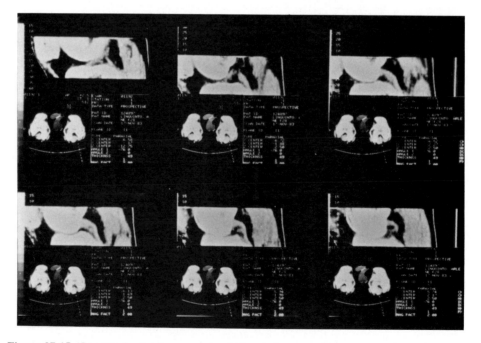

Figure 37-15. Computed arthrotomogram (sagittal cut) demonstrating torn posterior cruciate ligament.

disorder need not pursue a complement of diagnostic tests. Arthroscopically assisted reconstructions are major operations. Patients deserve to know in advance of their surgery whether to anticipate a simple arthroscopy or an additional reconstructive operation that will result in a multiweek disability. Only diagnostic deliberation in advance of a procedure can reasonably anticipate the length of postsurgical disability.

Rehabilitation of knee after injury

When a nonoperative approach to an instability has been elected by the patient and surgeon, the options for treatment are limited. They include activity modulation, strength rehabilitation, and bracing. Clearly, the less decelerating activities are less likely to produce "giving-way" episodes than are jumping, cutting, and rapid-rotating activities (such as basketball, soccer, and fencing). Braces must have rigid multipoint fixation to be effective, and "being effective" means reducing, not necessarily eliminating, the perception of instability. Many such braces are manufactured throughout the world. Examples of braces employed in the United States appear in Figure 37-18.

Rehabilitation is vital, but the axioms born of experience must be abided for an understanding of its role. The multiple

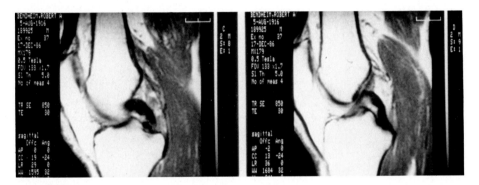

Figure 37-16. Magnetic resonance image (sagittal cut) showing anterior and posterior cruciate ligaments.

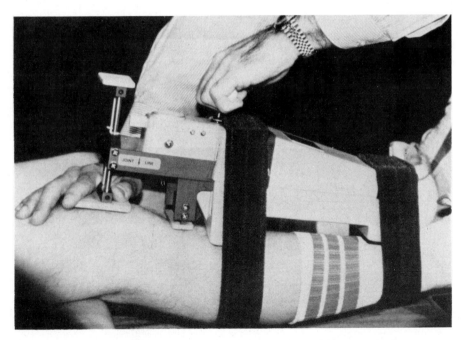

Figure 37-17. KT-1000 knee ligament arthrometer. (From Sherman, OH, Markolf, KL, and Ferkel, RD: Clin Orthop 215:156, 1987.)

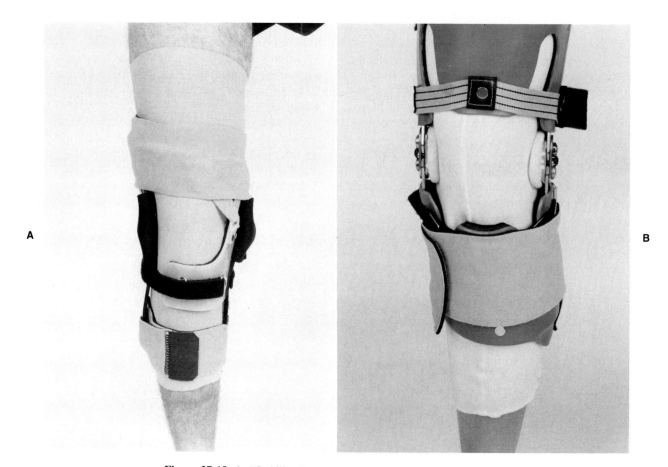

Figure 37-18. A, "Stabilizer" brace. **B,** Total knee control (TKC) brace.

forms of strengthening increase the stability of the joint, but only to a degree. Even when strengthening has little effect in controlling instability, it must be continued if only to maintain a locomotor force and to inhibit atrophic dysfunction, which occurs spontaneously in unstable knees that are not trained. Many stimuli and injury forces occur much more rapidly than a muscle's contractile response. In such instances the muscle-strengthening programs are ineffectual as a prophylaxis against injury. Still, the aftermath disability must be curtailed more substantially in a strength-maintained knee than in a strength-delinquent knee.

There is no unified accord among experts concerning an ideal program for rehabilitation. Whether it is better to train isokinetically or isotonically, concentrically or eccentrically, at high or low speed, or to concentrate on a particular muscle group such as the quadriceps or hamstrings is in dispute. There is no pat answer.

The resistive loads needed to restore a knee with cruciate damage to athletic function may disrupt any remaining ligament fibers. Nevertheless, this risk must be assumed by a patient who refuses surgery and attempts a return to athletics. In such instances the level of initiation of a program of rehabilitation must be predicated on a level of tolerance. After acute injuries, rest, ice, compression, and elevation

(RICE program) are typically instituted. Next, strengthening is begun. However, pain intolerance to loading the knee through a range of motion may limit the program to submaximal isometrics, modalities, hydrotherapy, continuous passive motion, and electrostimulation. When pain and swelling have resolved sufficiently, loading through various arcs of motion may be started with free weights or available accommodative variable resistance machinery of the isotonic and isokinetic types.

Modern or machine rehabilitation is a culmination of more than 50 years of accrued knowledge. Almost 40 years after Blix described the length-tension curve of a muscle, Steinhaus[23] promulgated the overload theory, which forms the basis for progressive strengthening. It is currently called progressive resistance exercise. DeLorme wrote that the best way to gain strength is a progression of heavy resistance with a low-repetition pattern.[6]

Clarke[3] recognized that a muscle's maximal efficiency occurred in the middle of the arc of motion, a concept basic to the design of the isotonic variable-resistance machinery (such as the Universal or Nautilus machines). Machine inventors have so far been relatively unsuccessful in capitalizing on the report[7] that an ability to lift weight has no bearing on the ability to perform rapid movement. The best

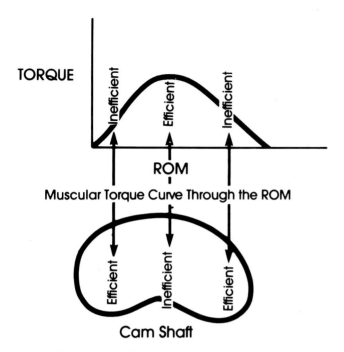

Figure 37-19. Relationship of muscular torque curve and cam that provides isotonic variable resistance. (From Davies, GJ: A compendium of isokinetics in clinical usage and rehabilitation techniques, ed 2, LaCrosse, Wisc, 1985, S&S Publishers.)

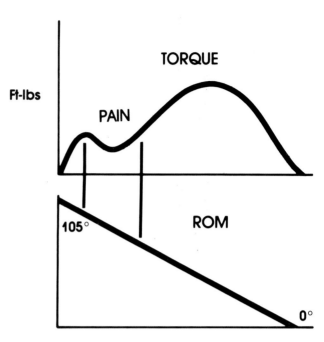

Figure 37-20. Isokinetic accommodation to pain. As pain occurs, force on dynamometer decreases and stylus drops to accommodate to force change. (From Davies, GJ: A compendium of isokinetics in clinical usage and rehabilitation techniques, ed 2, LaCrosse, Wisc, 1985, S&S Publishers.)

of machines can drive a joint at only several hundred degrees per second, far below its physiologic activity velocity. In 1958 Hellebrandt and Houtz[9] reported that the rate of work (power) is more important than the work quantity for function. Whether working toward strength, power, or endurance, the operative word is Steinhaus' "overload." The cam principle used by Nautilus to allow muscles to be efficient in more than just the middle of the arc is an embodiment of the striving for overload (Figure 37-19). However, muscle reeducation programs are always an arbitration between the desire to institute progressive resistance and the subject's tolerance of pain, swelling, and injury. The postinjury knee is no exception to this arbitration. In 1967 Hislop and Perrine[12] described the benefits of a new system of exercise machinery. This isokinetic system not only allowed for muscle efficiency but also permitted an accommodation to pain (Figure 37-20). Many types of machine have debuted over the last two decades, some emphasizing isotonic exercise forms and others, isometric forms. Within each category there appeared a spectrum of emphasis between concentric and eccentric modalities. Of particular importance to the training of the cruciate-deficient, unstable knee are the machines with antishear devices that inhibit anterior translation of the tibia relative to the femur (Figure 37-21). The availability of any given machine to an individual, the individual's tolerance to a given machine, and in some instances a needed specificity of training offered by a given machine are all determinants of the overload program to be performed.

The basic mechanisms of exercise types offered by single, alternate-leg, and reciprocal-leg training available by some machines, as well as a summary of comprehensive loading machines and machines that demonstrate and record workloads or performance, are cited in Tables 37-2 and 37-3.

Rehabilitation of postreconstruction cruciate ligament–deficient knee

Rehabilitation of the postreconstruction, cruciate ligament–deficient knee is a particularly sensitive and controversial subject. This is especially the case in the overwhelming majority of patients, in whose knees a tissue substitute (autograft or allograft) has been used to replace the absent ligament. The graft is insidiously reworked by the process of vascularization and creeping substitution, with long periods of structural weakness and limited tensile resistance. Protection from weight bearing, avoidance of active extension, and other load-avoidance measures must be practiced for reasonably long periods (without allowing undue wasting of the extremity) lest the graft or its fixation be disrupted.

Discussion

The current thinking with regard to reconstructed and unreconstructed cruciate ligament–deficient knees is outlined on pp. 521 and 522:

Table 37-2. Attributes of some popular machines

	Cybex	Biodex	Kin Com	Lido	Hydrafitness	Ariel	Kaiser	Universal	Nautilus	Eagle	Weight stacks
Basic mechanism											
Electronic	X	X	X								
Hydraulic				X	X	X					
Compressed air							X[1]				
Weight stacks								X	X	X	
Exercise type											
Isokinetic (constant speed)	X	X[2,3]	X[2-4]			X[2]					
Isometric (constant length)	X[5]	X[5]	X[5]		X[5]						
Isotonic (constant tension; variable speed in arc)					X		X	X	X	X	
Compressive loading[6]								X	X	X	
Leg press					X		X				X
Antishear mechanisms	X	X		X							
Workload setting	X[7,8]	X[7]	X[7]	X[7]	X[7]						X[9]
Recording ability											
Hip	X	X	X	X	X	X					
Knee	X	X	X	X	X	X					
Ankle	X	X									

[1]Cam II.
[2]Eccentrics.
[3]Passive mode.
[4]Less impact than Cybex.
[5]Each machine has locking mechanism.
[6]No knee-extension machines.
[7]Can restrict workload to certain level by watching indicator.
[8]Cybex-Fitron.
[9]Can monitor quantity of weight used (no dials).

Table 37-3. Leg patterns of common isotonic and isokinetic machines

	Does only one leg	Does one or both legs	Alternating legs	Concentric exercise	Eccentric exercise
Isokinetic					
Cybex	X			X	
Biodex	X			X	X
Kin Com	X			X	X
Lido	X			X	
Ariel	X			X	X
Isotonic					
Eagle		X		X	X
Hydrafitness			X	X	
Nautilus		X		X	X
Universal		X		X	X
Kaiser*		X	X	X	X

Modified from Slocum, DB, et al: Clin Orthop 118:63, 1976.
*Kaiser is reciprocal: concentric and eccentric.

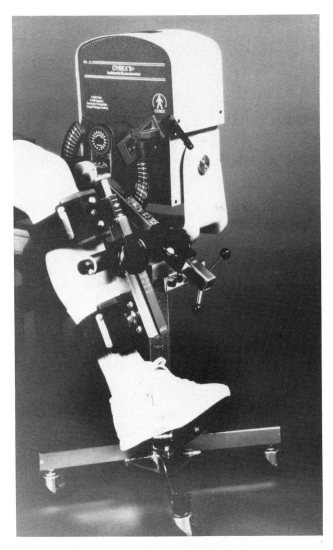

Figure 37-21. Johnson antishear device attached to isokinetic dynamometer. It is bar that rests on front of shin.

I. Historical considerations
  A. The anterior cruciate ligament is important in preventing disability and instability.
  B. Rotation plays a major role in instability.
II. Natural history of progression
  A. Unstable knees undergo progressive deterioration.
  B. A certain percentage of patients have acceptable results with activity reduction, bracing, and rehabilitation.
III. Hamstrings and cruciate ligament
  A. Biomechanical considerations suggest that hamstrings are a restraining element. Neither the origin of this theory nor proof of its truth has been shown.
  B. There is no relative deficit of hamstrings to quadriceps strength ratios with chronic anterior instability.
IV. Collagen and strain
  A. Tendon and ligament collagen have the crimping pattern of their fibers affected by the graft materials used and their tensioning when inserted.
  B. Collagen failure occurs through breaks in cross-bonding links, which do not form to any substantial degree until several months into the healing process.
  C. Collagen aligns and gathers strength in the direction of applied force.
  D. Some tension favors healing.
V. Biomechanical properties
  A. A number of biomechanical tests are performed to determine the characteristics of the collagen tissue. The results of these tests are a function of multiple variables, making it impossible to deduce in vivo characteristics for any given case.
  B. All tests have been based on "starting graft strength," which may be of limited importance.
  C. Fixation is a more critical concern than collagen strength during the initial weeks after a repair or reconstruction.
  D. It seems apparent that a noncycled or a single-test loading failure provides inaccurate information.
  E. A slow loading failure may be more pertinent to the early rehabilitation phase than a rapid loading failure thought to cause most cruciate ruptures in sports activities.
  F. Quantitated loads to failure in the laboratory are nonconvertible to practical usage in rehabilitation.
  G. One in vivo study suggests safe forces for several activities.[10]
  H. Exercising with the knee extended more than 35 to 40 degrees is dangerous, according to several authors.[1,10]
  I. From the important work of Arms and co-workers,[1] the following may be deduced.
    1. Passive motion may be safe in both flexion and extension throughout a full arc of motion.
    2. The least strain for passive motion occurs at 35 degrees.
    3. Varus and internal rotational stress should be considered dangerous.
    4. Eccentric exercise may be dangerous at angles more extended than 60 degrees.
    5. Isometric exercises in the extended range

(less than 45 degrees) are potentially dangerous.

VI. Joint compression and rotation
  A. Sufficient compression loading in extension appears to increase joint stability.
  B. Internal rotation increases the tensile force to the ligament.

VII. Bicycling
  A. Several authors indicate that low-load bicycling is a relatively safe early activity.[10,15]
  B. Full-revolution cycling requires 100 degrees of flexion.

VIII. Exercise versus ligament strength
  A. High-frequency endurance training increases the strength of ligamentous tissue.
  B. Such endurance training has preoperative and late postoperative implications.

IX. Immobility and atrophy
  A. Immobility decreases tensile strength of ligaments, interferes with cartilage nutrition, and promotes joint stiffness and muscle wasting; it should be avoided.
  B. Postreconstruction strength of the anterior cruciate ligament may take 6 months or more to reach 50% of its full level.

X. Electrostimulation
  A. Electrostimulation's benefits to strengthening are controversial.
  B. It may be effective in pain reduction during the restoration of muscle use and range of motion.

XI. Passive motion
  A. Passive motion is important in overcoming atrophic effects.
  B. Intermittent or interval-continuous passive motion is most commonly used with no known optimal pattern.
  C. Passive motion's stress can strengthen ligaments or avulse fixations.

XII. Neurophysiology
  A. Injury or surgery alters neuroproprioceptive perception, motor unit responsiveness, and electromechanical delay, each of which can be improved with training.
  B. Golgi-like organs are present in the cruciate ligaments of humans.
  C. Training of the unaffected extremity may produce beneficial cross-over effects.

XIII. Strength rehabilitation
  A. Strength rehabilitation is vital and is often restricted by the patient's fear of damage.
  B. Isometrics are often used early.
  C. Dynamic exercises are instituted later on.
  D. Progressive strengthening over time is based on the overload principle.

E. Forces produced on the anterior cruciate ligament are unknown for most exercise forms.
  F. Antishear devices may be helpful.
  G. Co-contraction of the hamstrings with the quadriceps muscle does not appear to inhibit the forces produced by the quadriceps.
  H. Data recordings help to follow progress.
  I. High-speed agility exercises are needed in addition to strengthening exercises.

Whether reconstructed or not, the knee will never be normal. If strength is not continuously maintained, it spontaneously dissipates as does knee locomotor ability. Prophylactic bracing and activity counseling are vital adjuncts to the treatment regimen.

Another frequently hard to treat knee problem of athletes is the abnormal patella. A host of terminologies have been used to describe afflictions relating to this sesamoid bone: chondromalacia, patellar subluxation, patellar tendinitis, and patellar maltracking, to name a few. The fact is that all of these diagnoses are intimately related and are almost invariably caused by some aberrance of patellar glide, incongruence with the femoral groove, or relative laxity. The resistant and ubiquitous character of patellofemoral disorders is not confined to white populations. They are the most common problems seen by sports orthopedists in the People's Republic of China, where about one quarter of the world's population transports itself by foot and by bicycle.

The complexities of patellar tracking are attributable to an infinite variety of structural combinations. The patella may be too small or too large for the femoral groove, or the acclivity of the respective facets of each structure may lack sufficient depth or may demonstrate poor congruence. This may be true for all arcs or only limited arcs of motion. The patella may be relatively too high or too low. The rotational alignment between the femur and tibia may create tethers and whips in motion glide. The Q angle is a commonly used index of difficulty and represents the linear or angular lines of pull of the rectus–patella–patellar tendon mechanism. It is generally held that this angle should not exceed 20 degrees.

However, this traditional angle is based on a static measurement in the passively extended knee only. It is equally, if not more, important to determine what we consider the "potential Q angles," or those angles that are measurable at varying degrees of flexion and tibial rotation (Figure 37-22). In this fashion arcs of motion prone to producing particular stress to the patellar mechanism may be ascertained—that is, the resultant vectors produced by the quadriceps and patella may be grossly perceived.

Although the "chondromalacic" patellofemoral disorders are unfortunately lumped into a group, their individual characteristics are as varied as fingerprints. For this reason, rehabilitation and surgery for these disorders are not predictably successful.

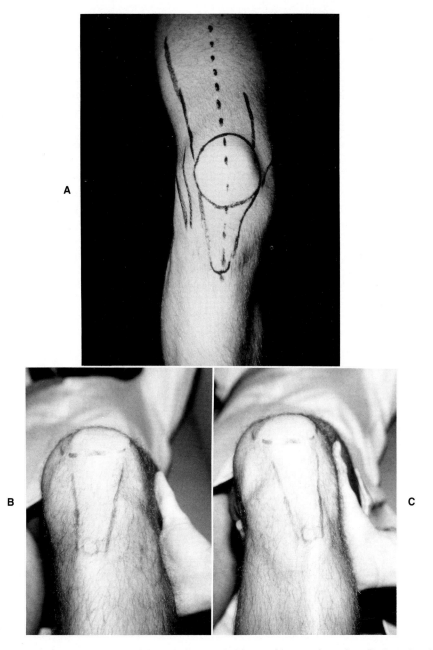

Figure 37-22. A, Measurement of Q angle in extended knee with neutral rotation. **B,** Q angle with knee in flexion and tibial internal rotation. **C,** Q angle with knee in flexion and tibial external rotation.

When the knee is extended from a flexed position, the patella usually rises out of the femoral groove at about 40 degrees less than full extension. This produces a biomechanical inflection and frequently a point at which there is a hitch or jerk or cessation of patellar glide. Again, it is difficult to predict in advance of training whether a patient will best tolerate free weights, concentrics, eccentrics, only limited arcs, or something else. Strengthening is nevertheless a critical treatment designed to impart a greater control over the movement aberrances of the patella (to increase stability and reduce retinacular and tendon pain).

A quantity of dogma has arisen with respect to rehabilitation of patellofemoral disorders. For example, full-arc knee-extension exercises and avoidance of low-speed Cybex training have been repeatedly denounced by authors of rehabilitation programs. Although it is often true that these formats produce pain about the patella, no arc or format of strengthening should be forsaken at the outset unless ex-

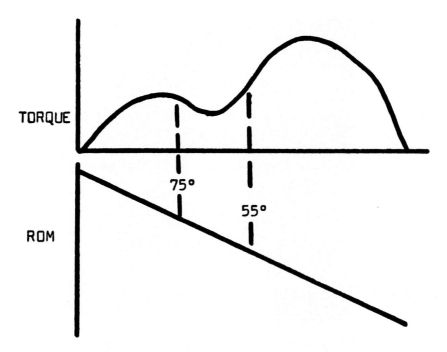

Figure 37-23. Isokinetic torque curve deformation objectively documented at specific points in range of motion. (From Davies, GJ: A compendium of isokinetics in clinical usage and rehabilitation techniques, ed 2, LaCrosse, Wisc, 1985, S&S Publishers.)

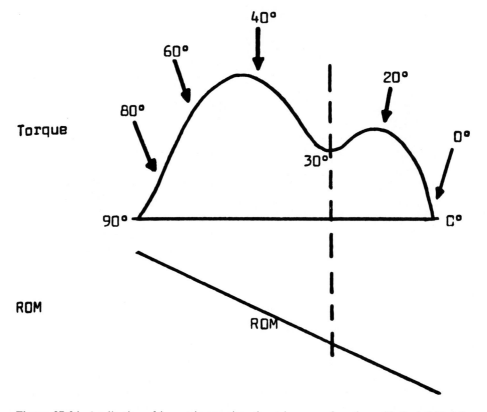

Figure 37-24. Application of isometric exercises through range of motion with "painful" deformation. Isometrics were applied every 20 degrees throughout range of motion. (From Davies, GJ: A compendium of isokinetics in clinical usage and rehabilitation techniques, ed 2, LaCrosse, Wisc, 1985, S&S Publishers.)

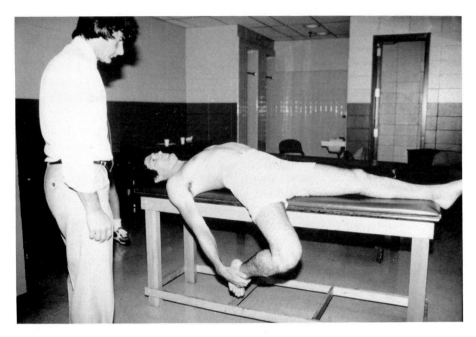

Figure 37-25. Demonstration of correct technique for quadriceps stretching.

periential trial has proven it to be painful for a given subject.

For most of these problems the format of rehabilitation predominantly evolves on a trial-and-error basis. Clues to its initiation are sometimes deduced from historical data. For example, a patient whose pain occurs primarily with stair descent and not at all with stair ascent may be presumed to have a glide disorder confined largely to the more extended range of the knee (the only range used in descent). A patient with a sense of painful slipping of the patella on a variety of movements will most likely require a patellar brace to perform resistive exercise without pain. By serial and pointed questions in the initial examination, troublesome arcs and other provocative vectors may be excluded from the initial therapy. Variable and accommodating resistance machinery has permitted the resolution of many more of these problems than was once possible with the simple isotonic exercises afforded by free weights. Recording machines, such as the Cybex, may demonstrate arcs to be avoided in programs (Figure 37-23), and the multiple-angle isometric testing system may be helpful in starting up a program without a need to force the knee through a painful range of motion (Figure 37-24).

In many instances quadriceps stretching is as important as strengthening (Figure 37-25). A contracted quadriceps inhibits vertical glide of the patella and accentuates tension at the insertions of the rectus muscle, patellar tendon, and retinacula onto the patella. Intractable pain, present for months, is sometimes relieved after a single such stretch performed in the office.

When therapy and bracing fail—regardless of the numbers of changes in arcs, loads, speeds, machine types, and repetition patterns—surgery may have to be considered. When successful, such surgery often reduces but rarely eliminates all symptoms attributable to the disorder. The size of the patella, the groove and facet depths, the tilts, rotations, and other bony factors are not alterable by surgery. Only the glide influences exerted by the muscles and retinacula are alterable by incision, reorientation, or both.

ELBOW INJURIES

The most common athletic injuries or afflictions about the elbow are "tennis elbow" and posterior compartment impingement. Tennis elbow, or lateral epicondylitis (more commonly than medial epicondylitis), may appear precipitously or insidiously. The term implies a frequent association with the game of tennis but by no means an exclusive one. It is an extra-articular disorder, posing no medical danger to those who choose to ignore the symptoms. Instead it produces disability primarily as a result of the pain it inflicts on its bearer.

The common tendon of the extensor muscles of the wrist attaches to the humerus at the anterolateral aspect of the lateral epicondyle. The area of insertion is inordinately small, creating a great stress concentration for the bulk of inserting fibers. Presumably these fibers are readily avulsed or otherwise damaged by repetitive impact loading such as that created by tennis. Pathologic studies[8] and our own observations during surgery have failed to find a grossly apparent pathologic lesion. The tenderness that results from the elusive pathologic entity tennis elbow is consistently elicited over tne anterior aspect of the epicondyle and sometimes along the extensor muscle mass. The diagnostic sine qua non is the creation of pain in the aforementioned locations by the simple application of resistance to the dorsiflexing wrist. A very acute case of this is exemplified by the patient who claims that lifting a cup of coffee is extremely painful.

Tennis elbow is one condition for which surgical success in most series exceeds 90%. However, if left unabused, the elbow will usually experience a progressive reduction in inflammation. The injection of cortisone or its analogs is a common practice that frequently produces apparent success in less severe cases. The word "apparent" is used because, although the inflammatory pain may be curtailed, the underlying disorder or pathomechanics still exist. Furthermore, the adverse affects of steroids on tendons is well documented in the literature. Orally administered anti-inflammatory agents may be similarly effective on a temporary basis.

It is more realistic and practical to avoid stopgap treatments and to make an attempt to identify the source of the problem. As is typical of disorders derived from repetitious activity, the inciting possibilities are multiple. The most obvious are overuse and excessive frequency and intensity of play, especially when the technique is inefficient and stressful. Moderation and instruction on correct use are the obvious, although infrequently observed, antidotes.

Tennis elbow is uncommon in people under the age of 30 years. The reasons for this are not entirely clear, but it is reasonable to assume that it takes that long to degenerate a quantity of the targeted tissues and to develop some weakness or contracture of the overused extremity. Virtually without exception, individuals with tennis elbow demonstrate weakness of the ipsilateral shoulder girdle in multiple directions. There is often an associated contracture of the dorsiflexor muscles manifested by a reduction in palmar flexion at the wrist while the elbow is extended. The weak

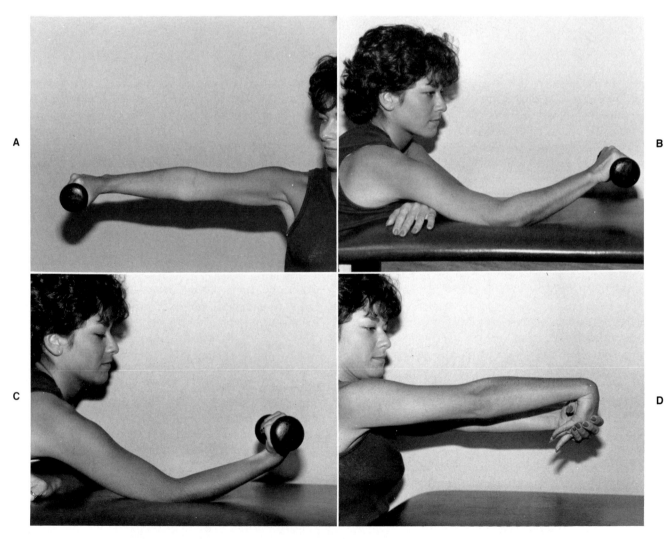

Figure 37-26. Tennis elbow exercises. **A,** Strengthening shoulder girdle. **B,** Strengthening wrist dorsiflexors. **C,** Strengthening pronator-supinator groups. **D,** Stretching of wrist extensors.

shoulder muscles—the pronator-supinator groups, the dorsiflexors of the wrist, and the intrinsic muscles of the hand—must be strengthened to make the extremity resistant to the actions that ordinarily provoke symptoms. Similarly, stretching the wrist extensors is important in preventing tensile avulsion effects, in much the same way that one must stretch the adductors to help overcome adductor strain (groin pull) in the hip (Figure 37-26).

Tennis elbow bands or circumferential forearm braces (Figure 37-27), such as the Froimson band, are placed about the extensor mass just distal to the elbow joint. These braces often help to reduce or control pain by several mechanisms. They diffuse the concentration of stress at the small insertion site on the epicondyle. They support the attenuated muscle group and, by virtue of compression, inhibit the transmission of sudden jerking forces to the inflamed epicondylar region. The efficacy of such bracing may be pretested in the office by wrapping the proximal forearm with an elastic bandage and exerting resistance to the dorsiflexing wrist. Failure to inhibit the epicondylar pain signifies a low probability that a brace would reduce pain. Other bracing systems for relief of tennis elbow have been designed to limit wrist motion, thereby reducing the distal excursions of the extensor mass.

Abstinence or moderation of play reduces existing inflammation. Orally administered or injected anti-inflammatory agents can often reduce the perception of an existing pathologic condition without altering it. Bracing may help control symptoms but does not alter the condition. Strengthening and stretching exercises provide no immediate solution, but they are necessary for the ultimate function and protection of the extremity in subsequent usage.

A brief discussion of posterior compartment impingements of the elbow is needed. In essence, they are most often characterized by posterior elbow pain in association with repetitive movements that require an extension thrust at the elbow (to full or even incomplete extension). Activities that might precipitate such symptoms are baseball pitching, fencing, and javelin throwing. Olecranon-humeral instability, osteoarthritis, or loose bodies may be responsible for inflammatory pain emanating from extension and thrust activities. When instability is partially responsible, strengthening and bracing may be needed to control the motion more effectively. When evidence exists of loose bodies or arthritic spurs, arthroscopic or open surgical debridement is often needed to reduce impinging spurs, synovium, or bodies. In all cases it is often helpful to employ an elbow brace that blocks the terminal extension arc and thereby the pain (Figure 37-28). Activity moderation, anti-inflammatory pharmaceutical agents, and therapeutic modalities are additional adjuncts to treatment.

ANKLE INJURIES

Ankle sprains are among the most common of sports injuries. Most commonly the foot folds beneath the ankle in plantar flexion and inversion. The most often torn of the three groups of lateral ankle ligaments is the anterior talofibular ligament. Many loose-jointed individuals are subject to recurrent sprains with a minimal aftermath or disability;

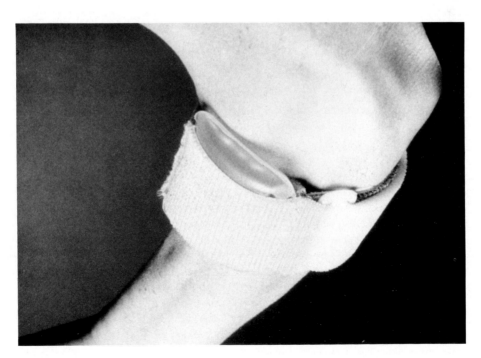

Figure 37-27. Circumferential forearm brace used in treatment of tennis elbow.

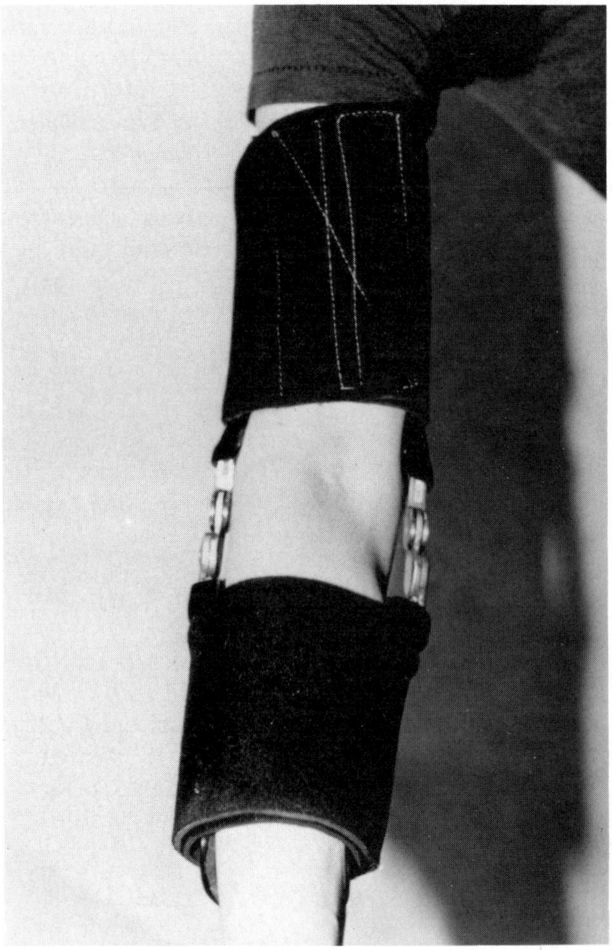

Figure 37-28. Elbow extension block brace.

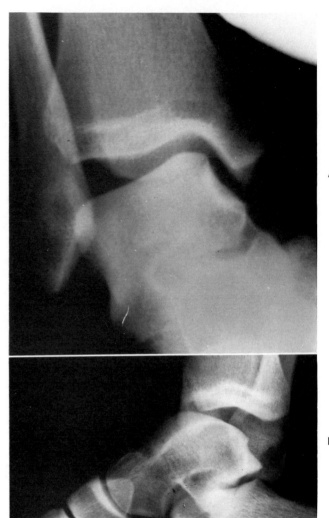

Figure 37-29. A, Anteroposterior stress radiograph of ankle demonstrating lateral tibiotalar distraction. **B,** Lateral stress radiograph of ankle demonstrating anterior drawer of talus relative to tibia. (From Crenshaw, AH, editor: Campbell's operative orthopaedics, ed 7, St. Louis, 1987, The CV Mosby Co.)

however, most people develop immediate swelling about the lateral aspect of the ankle and a variable period of disability and pain lasting from 3 to 6 weeks on the average. When more than a single ligament complex is disrupted, a significant and chronic instability may result with the appearance of lateral tibiotalar distraction as well as an anterior drawer of the foot relative to the ankle (Figure 37-29).

Most sprains are treated with ice, elevation, and partial or total relief of weight bearing until the acute symptoms have dissipated. Compression and stabilization by means of Ace bandages, paste boot wraps, or even casts may be more practical in some cases. After the acute phase (7 to 14 days

on the average), the ankle is mobilized with a motion program, strengthened with progressive resistance exercises, and introduced to a progression of weight bearing as tolerated.

In medical centers with treatment policies inclined toward early surgical repair of major sprains, early double-contrast arthrography is performed in an attempt to ascertain the quantitative disruption of the capsular structures (Figure 37-30). Most authors promulgating this approach to sprains hail from the South.[2] Cox estimated that approximately 20% of Annapolis midshipmen manifest symptoms of chronic ankle instability that might have been thwarted by timely surgery.

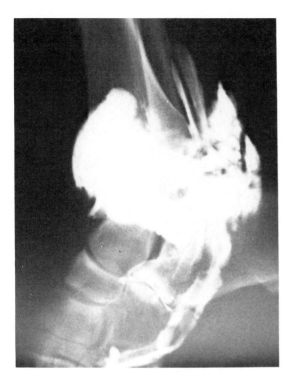

Figure 37-30. Arthrogram of ankle with dye extravasation laterally representing disruption of capsuloligamentous structures. (Courtesy Dr. HM Black, Jr. From Crenshaw, AH, editor: Campbell's operative orthopaedics, ed 7, St. Louis, 1987, The CV Mosby Co.)

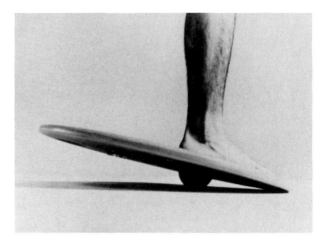

Figure 37-31. BAPS board used to develop proprioceptive-kinesthetic skills after ankle injuries.

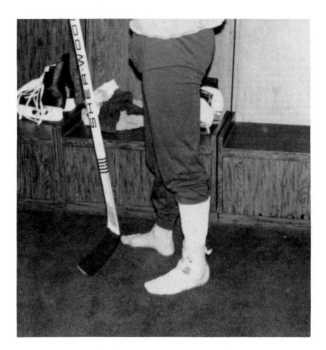

Figure 37-32. Rigid ankle brace.

Still, most individuals can exist adequately with some quantity of instability, particularly when strengthening and bracing are added to the treatment regimen. In my exclusively sports-oriented practice, not a single operation to correct an intolerable ankle instability has been strictly necessary during the last 3 years.

The physician presented with an acute "ankle sprain" must respect a differential of potentially serious problems often associated with sprainlike symptoms. The following diagnoses must be sought: peroneal tendon subluxation or retinacular rupture, tibiofibular diastasis, osteochondral fracture of the talus or tibia, tibiotalar impingement, os trigonum fractures, tarsal coalition, and stress or other fractures of the talus or fibula.

Having established the presence of an isolated sprain by whatever radiographs, scans, or arthrograms are indicated to rule out the differential diagnoses, the physician must proceed with treatment. In the wake of the florid symptoms after a primary sprain—and omnipresent in those with recurrent sprains—are two consistent necessities. The first is to strengthen the evertor muscles, which resist inversion movement. This must be accomplished with a variety of modes, speeds, and arcs for maximal effectiveness. Strengthening is necessary but inadequate as a preparation for sports movements. In this regard, balance boards and proprioceptive-kinesthetic devices designed for the ankles are important (Figure 37-31). Stretching may be needed to recapture any losses in the range of motion. Ankle braces are needed for sports, especially those requiring jumping, when there is a demonstrable residual instability. Many varieties of brace are available, and selection must be based on comfort and the degree of rigidity needed to control the joint (Figure 37-32). Surgery to correct instabilities is usually successful—and usually unnecessary. The principal risk of surgery is the potential for a stiff ankle, which inhibits the capability for agile lateral movements.

REFERENCES

1. Arms, SW, et al: The biomechanics of anterior cruciate ligament rehabilitation and reconstruction, Am J Sports Med 12:8, 1984.
2. Brand, RL, Collins, M, and Templeton, T: Surgical repair of ruptured lateral ankle ligaments, Am J Sports Med 9:40, 1981.
3. Clarke, H, et al: Relationship between body positions and the application of muscle power to movements of the joints, Arch Phys Med 31:81, 1950.
4. Cox, JS: The fate of the acromioclavicular joint in athletic injuries, Am J Sports Med 5:258, 1977.
5. Cox, JS: Acromioclavicular joint injuries in athletes. In Petrone, FA, editor: AAOS symposium on upper extremity injuries in athletes, St. Louis, 1986, The CV Mosby Co.
6. DeLorme, TL: Restoration of muscle power by heavy-resistance exercises, J Bone Joint Surg 27:645, 1945.
7. DeLorme, TL, Ferris, B, and Gallagher, J: Effect of progressive resistance exercise on muscle contraction time, Arch Phys Med 33:86, 1952.
8. Goldie, I: Epicondylitis lateralis humeri (epicondyalgia or tennis elbow): a pathological study, Acta Chir Scand (suppl) p. 339, 1966.
9. Hellebrandt, FA, and Houtz, SJ: Methods of muscle training: the influence of pacing, Phys Ther Rev 38:319, 1958.
10. Henning, CE, Lynch, MA, and Glick, KR: An in vivo strain gauge study of elongation of the anterior cruciate ligament, Am J Sports Med 13:22, 1985.
11. Henry, JH, and Genung, JA: Natural history of the glenohumeral dislocation—revisited, Am J Sports Med 10:135, 1982.
12. Hislop, HJ, and Perrine, JJ: The isokinetic concept of exercise, Phys Ther 47:114, 1967.
13. Jackson, DW, et al: Injury predication in the young athlete: preliminary report, Am J Sports Med 6:6, 1927.
14. Levin, A, and Wyman, J: The viscous elastic properties of muscle, Proc R Soc Lond [Biol], p 218, 1927.
15. McLeod, WD, and Blackburn, TA: Biomechanics of knee rehabilitation with cycling, Am J Sports Med 8:175, 1980.
16. Moffroid, MT, Whipple, R, and Hofkosh, J: A study of isokinetic exercise, Phys Ther 49:735, 1969.
17. Nicholas, JA: Injuries to knee ligaments: relationship to looseness and tightness in football players, JAMA 212:2236, 1970.
18. Nicoll, EA: Principles of exercise therapy, Br Med J, p 747, 1943.
19. Noyes, FR, et al: The symptomatic anterior cruciate ligament, J Bone Joint Surg 65A:163, 1983.
20. Rockwood, CA: Injuries to the acromioclavicular joint: fractures in adults, ed 2, Philadelphia, 1984, JB Lippincott Co.
21. Rowe, CR: Prognosis in dislocations of the shoulder, J Bone Joint Surg 38:957, 1956.
22. Sherman, OH, Markolf, KL, and Ferkel, RD: Measurements of anterior laxity in normal and anterior cruciate-absent knees with two instrumented test devices, Clin Orthop 215:156, 1987.
23. Steinhaus, A: Chronic effects of exercise, Physiol Rev 13:103, 1933.
24. Thistle, HG, et al: Isokinetic contraction: a new concept of resistive exercise, Arch Phys Med Rehabil, p 279, 1967.

CHAPTER 38

Spasticity and spastic deformities

RALPH LUSSKIN AND BRUCE B. GRYNBAUM

The majority of patients treated in rehabilitation centers have diseases or trauma involving the brain or the spinal cord. After the initial flaccidity, most of these patients develop muscle spasticity. The increased involuntary muscle tone is frequently a major barrier to rehabilitation. Spasticity develops in patients with stroke, head injuries, spinal cord trauma, cerebral palsy, and degenerative-autoimmune diseases such as multiple sclerosis.

Spasticity is a difficult problem to treat. Drugs that reduce spasticity, such as diazepam, baclofen, and sodium danzolene, frequently produce somnolence, lack of coordination, and occasionally weakness. In addition, the degree of relief is often limited.[58] Chronic spasticity then progressively limits motion as the joints crossed by the spastic muscles develop functional and fixed contractures, leading to further problems and also limiting the patient's already reduced volitional control over the spastic limbs.

The number of upper motor neuron lesions that produce spasticity rises as the population ages because stroke is an important cause of prolonged disability. Spinal cord injuries from falls and motor vehicle accidents tend to affect the young, usually males, and lead to many years of disability. Gunshot wounds also contribute to disability in this group, as do head injuries and coma from intracerebral bleeding and from anoxia. Since the young are often involved, prolonged disability often results. Demyelinating disorders such as multiple sclerosis are another large group of spastic disorders. Residual cerebral palsy is seen in adults, who have lifelong problems of spasticity and spastic deformity.

Currently, the United States has an estimated 400,000 victims of stroke, 75,000 patients with multiple sclerosis, 400,000 cases of cerebral palsy, and 500,000 adults with parkinsonism.

Complicating the management of these patients are several impediments to maximum rehabilitation: neurologic and intellectual deficits, psychologic problems, unrealistic expectations, and progression of deformity. Global neurologic and intellectual impairment occurs in stroke and head injury. Serious balance abnormalities and deficits in sensory perception—auditory, visual, tactile, and proprioceptive—may exist. All these factors interfere with the patients' ability to respond to therapy and to use volitional motor function that is available.

It is well known that the young spastic person has psychologic problems. Beyond the reactive depression of the disabled may well be a personality disorder that led to the behavior precipitating the injury. Such acts as driving at high speed while under the influence of alcohol, narcotics, and other sedatives; refusing to wear seat belts; riding a motorcycle without a helmet; criminal behavior leading to a spinal gunshot wound; and drug overdose leading to coma are results of psychologic factors that persist following the injury and that continue to impede rational therapy. Any individual may have a frank psychosis or an obvious borderline personality. The same personality pattern affecting the patient may affect the family, contributing to poor patient compliance and inappropriate family support.

Elderly patients with recent-onset spasticity often suffer from profound psychologic reactions. These reactions must be faced and treated if the maximum potential for rehabilitation is to be achieved.

Unrealistic goals set by the patient or the therapist are wasteful of therapeutic resources and may impede appropriate treatment. Years may be lost in hopeless efforts to ambulate when education and vocational training would have been more appropriate.

Progression of deformity may necessitate revision of

therapy. Spastic disorders lead to joint contractures, as the limb tends to remain in the position dictated by the reflex pattern that is present. These contractures consist of a re-modeling of joint capsule and ligaments, as well as a per-manent shortening of the spastic muscle. The spastic muscle insertion develops a further mechanical advantage over its antagonist and becomes even more deforming. It should be appreciated that in the absence of intra-articular pathology such as fracture, sepsis, or arthritis, the joint contracture may be less severe than the inflexibility of the deformity might indicate. Muscle fibrosis in a shortened position may be the major determinant of the contracture, permitting ef-fective surgical release with little risk. Even capsular con-tractures can be present without intra-articular fibrosis in long-standing disease and can be released by modern sur-gical techniques.

Other factors can contribute to more disability than may be necessary. The patient or therapist may prolong a treat-ment program beyond its effective duration. For instance, if a program of stretching is not effective in 12 to 16 weeks, another 16 weeks of therapy will probably not be more effective. A brace that cannot be tolerated when applied or that becomes intolerable is probably going to fail even if it is reapplied daily for many months. If global balance de-ficiencies, volitional paralysis, or severe deformities block an ambulation training program, it will probably be unsuc-cessful no matter what efforts are expended unless specific inhibitors of progress can be eliminated.

In the remainder of the chapter we identify those problems that can be treated positively to achieve realistic goals and describe the rehabilitative, orthotic, and surgical techniques that can be applied sequentially or concurrently to achieve maximum functional recovery of the spastic adult.

NEUROLOGIC BASIS OF SPASTIC DISEASE
Definitions

Spasticity is a disorder of neuromuscular function char-acterized by an involuntary contraction of muscle groups in response to excitation of the central nervous system. It is manifest as an exaggerated stretch reflex, which at first tends to subside with continued isotonic force application. The tendon jerks are hyperactive. Sensory stimulation and psy-chologic excitation reinforce the spastic state. Volitional motor activity that stretches the spastic groups induces more spasticity and resistance to motion.

Spastic states are induced by neurologic injuries or dis-eases that impair the control of the extrapyramidal motor system, which determines the threshold of activity of the motor neurons in the anterior horn of the gray matter of the spinal cord. Cortical, thalamic, pontine, and spinal extra-pyramidal centers generate patterns of motor activity that require intricate balance to achieve proper motor control. As these centers are released from superior control, the spastic state intensifies and in time leads to progressive

deformity, which further degrades voluntary movement. The lower the level of central nervous system injury, the more profound the spasticity, for the lesions tend to be more complete, inducing more voluntary deficit, and bilateral, accompanied by a more profound sensory deficit. Thus stroke-induced spasticity is usually less profound than that caused by spinal cord injury. Demyelinating disease such as multiple sclerosis produces episodically increasing spas-ticity and paralysis.

Muscle spindles are sensory organs that are distributed throughout the voluntary muscles (striated) and that contin-uously monitor the tension and rate of change of tension of these muscles. They are the source of much information to the central nervous system and have an important role in coordinated motor activity and in generating muscle tonus (response to stretch). They are supplied by a complex set of afferent and efferent nerve fibers. The afferent fibers carry information about tension and rates of change of tension in three types of motor fibers located in the spindles (intra-fusal): the nuclear bag 1 (NB1), nuclear bag 2 (NB2), and nuclear chain (NC) fibers. These muscle fibers are inner-vated, in turn, by three types of nerve endings: trail endings and P1 and P2 plate endings. The afferent endings are of two types: primary and secondary. Each spindle has at least one primary ending, usually in the equatorial region. Sec-ondary endings are not always present and are rather dif-fusely distributed along the fiber.[26]

The motor supply, which modifies the response of the muscle spindles to stretch, is derived from two sources. First is the gamma efferent system, exclusively directed to the spindles. Second is an alpha motor system derived from alpha motor neurons that concomitantly produce motor ac-tivity in the main muscle fibers (extrafusal fibers), as well as in the muscle spindle fibers (intrafusal).

Recent electrophysiologic studies have separated the ef-ferent (fusimotor) fibers into static and dynamic groups, thus creating the basis for the complex responses of the muscle spindles to various patterns of motor activity. (For a com-plete review see Mathews.[26])

Some have postulated that a major determinant of the spastic state is the heightened response of muscle spindles from increased gamma (fusimotor) activity. Studies on alert and cooperative subjects have generated data that casts doubt on this hypothesis, however, and that indicates the alpha motor neuron is made hyperactive directly after damage to the pathways of the extrapyramidal motor system without the operation of the muscle spindle system.[4]

Tendon organs are sensory endings, located within ten-dons, that provide central nervous system (CNS) input via 1-b afferent nerve fibers. Formerly they were thought to be only inhibitory to the stretch reflex because of their high threshold. It is now understood that they provide continuous information to the CNS about the tension in the tendon and thus must play a continuous role in the control of muscle activity. This role has not been studied in spasticity, and the fate of the information they generate is not known.

Rigidity is a disorder of neuromuscular function characterized by an increase in muscle tension that is present continuously in all muscle groups but tends to be more prominent in the flexors of the trunk and limbs. In rigidity there is an even, steady resistance to passive movement, which has been likened to bending a lead pipe. Perhaps the term "plastic resistance" would be appropriate. In contrast to spasticity, no sudden release of resistance occurs during passive stretch. The tendon jerks are not hyperactive, and there is no clonus.

Rigidity is seen in many extrapyramidal diseases such as parkinsonism, Wilson's disease, striatonigral degeneration, certain drug intoxications, progressive supranuclear palsy, and calcinosis of the basal ganglia.

Degenerative changes or malfunction of the basal ganglia causes rigidity. Although a "cog-wheel" effect may be noted, the rigidity is not affected by the speed of passive stretch as in spasticity. Repetitive stretching of the trunk and extremities will decrease rigidity for some time and is of real value in the daily management of the parkinsonian patient.

Spinal cord tracts exert major effects on spasticity. Descending spinal cord tracts influence motor function in two ways: they directly command motor neurons, and they facilitate or inhibit spinal reflex pathways.[5] Facilitation of the spinal stretch reflex occurs as a result of vestibulospinal and reticulospinal descending influences.[43,49] The facilitative downflow is held in check by equally powerful inhibitory projections. The lower extrapyramidal motor centers are inhibited by higher centers, and the reticular formation of the caudal medulla is itself capable of inhibiting spinal reflexes. This bulboreticular center receives input from higher centers, including the cerebellum and cerebral cortex.[27] Patients with incomplete spinal cord injury often have greater spasticity than those with complete lesions owing to the relative sparing of descending facilitative fibers.

Brain determinants of volitional function and spasticity

The cerebral cortex, from which the corticospinal tracts descend, is influenced by the thalamus, which receives information from all the sensory systems as well as the basal ganglia and cerebellum. Muscle groups of the contralateral face, arm, trunk, and leg are represented in the primary motor cortex (Brodmann's area 4), those of the face being at the lower end and those of the leg in the paracentral lobule on the medial surface of the cerebral hemisphere. Stimulation of this primary motor cortex produces isolated movements.

The premotor area of the cerebral cortex (area 6) is also electrically excitable to produce movements, but more intense stimuli are required. Stimulation of the caudad area 6a produces responses that are similar to those elicited from area 4. These movements are abolished if area 4 is removed.

The outflow is by the corticospinal tract. Stimulation of the more superior portion of areas 6a and 6b elicits more general movement patterns, as well as bilateral tonic contractions of the muscles in the trunk and legs.

Experiments in monkeys and chimpanzees have shown that lesions confined to the precentral motor cortex resulted in long-standing flaccid paralysis accompanied by hypotonia and depressed reflexes. When the lesion in the same animals was then extended posteriorly to include area 6, the flaccid paralysis became spastic. Other experiments have demonstrated that lesions confined to area 6 resulted in spasticity without significant paralysis.[8,14]

PATTERNS OF DISEASE: THE "LIFE CYCLE" OF SPECIFIC DISORDERS
Spastic cerebral palsy in adults

Spastic cerebral palsy can be classified according to the limbs involved as hemiparesis, diparesis, or quadriparesis. In each situation progressive deformities may develop that further interfere with ambulation and hand function. This is especially true in children in whom muscle imbalance can affect the development of the growing skeleton and lead to hip dislocation.

In spastic hemiparesis gastroc-soleus and foot invertor tension leads to fixed equinus or equinovarus deformities. Prominent features of the hemiparetic gait are unequal stride length, stance phase starting with toe contact, absence of the foot-flat position, and ineffective toe clearance. Abnormal arm posture and contractures of spastic forearm pronators and of the elbow and wrist flexors can occur. The hand may develop thumb-in-palm, finger flexion, or hyperextension deformities. These deformities seriously inhibit function as the patient grows and attempts to work.

Spastic diplegia is characterized by a scissor gait. The legs are extended or slightly bent at the knees and may be adducted strongly at the hips. In quadriparesis the legs are usually more affected than the arms. Deformities as seen in hemiplegia and diplegia or paresis occur.

Stroke

Stroke is a disorder characterized by the sudden onset of one-sided weakness or paralysis, usually as a result of a cerebrovascular disorder. The vascular event is usually a thrombosis or localized hemorrhage. An embolus or subarachnoid hemorrhage may also be the cause. The disorder presents itself as a flaccid paralysis and sensory deficit. Speech is often affected if the dominant hemisphere is involved. Coma may be present. The acute phase may last up to 3 weeks and is followed by a recovery phase characterized by hypertonicity that may last 6 to 12 months. The disorder then reaches a more or less permanent plateau.

During the recovery phase, mixed deficits involving volitional motor loss (paralysis), spasticity, and sensory deficits (epicritic and protopathic) become more defined. Anosognosia (denial of self-image with rejection of the hemiplegic side) may be the most profound sensory loss.[44] The spastic component often prolongs and heightens the functional deficit and tends to increase with time.

Brunnstrom[3] has classified motor recovery from adult-onset hemiplegia into six phases. Initial flaccidity is followed by increasing spasticity and then by the development of movement synergies. This is followed by a decline in spasticity and the return of isolated movement. These stages are not discrete but consist of a continuous progression with the gradual appearance of new, overlapping stages.

When profound paralysis of the lower extremity and trunk is present in the early stages of the disorder, the strong presumption is that paralysis will preclude the recovery of functional ambulation. Gait training may be impossible. Nevertheless, when residual effective volitional function exists, residual spasticity remains as the most common disabling factor in gait. In most stroke patients, spasticity interfering with gait produces plantar flexion hyperactivity. Often this can be overcome with an adequate orthosis.

Spasticity of the hemiplegic arm may result in adduction deformity of the shoulder with loss of range of motion. Paralysis of the shoulder often produces inferior subluxation of the shoulder joint with pain and occasionally traction on the brachial plexus. Spasticity of the biceps or brachialis produces a flexed elbow; flexor spasticity deforms the wrist and fingers. The nails may be forced into the skin of the palm. Spasticity in the flexor-pronator group produces the hyperpronation deformity.

Head injury

During the acute stage of a closed head injury, especially while patients are in coma or semicoma, severe spasticity may occur. Unless patients are exercised frequently through the full range of motion of the limbs, severe joint contractures may develop. Formation of heterotopic bone in the para-articular tissues often accompanies these contractures. This bone does not involve primarily the joint capsule or the muscles but lies in the planes between them. Prevention of this bone formation following surgery to the paraplegic joint has been demonstrated with the use of disodium etidronate[50]; however, when the drug is stopped, bone forms in the para-articular tissues. In addition, some weakening of the skeleton occurs after prolonged use of this drug, as bone accretion is blocked while normal bone resorption takes place. The drug is useful in delaying and sometimes reducing or preventing heterotopic bone after head injury and should be considered in treating a comatose patient. If alkaline phosphatase levels become elevated and there is radiographic evidence of heterotopic ossification around the joints, local radiotherapy may also be effective in reducing bone formation and the resulting ankylosis. Late sarcoma formation should be prevented if the dose of x-ray therapy is kept below 1500 rem.

Indomethacin may also be of use in preventing heterotrophic bone, but it increases gastric acidity.

Spinal cord injury

Spasticity is one of the severe complications of interrupted spinal cord motor pathways. External trauma is the most frequent cause of this disorder. Tumor and infection create a state of extreme spinal cord vulnerability to additional trauma such as that encountered in spinal cord surgery. Vascular lesions are also common, since the blood supply of the cord is vulnerable. Spinal cord infarction and paraplegia may result from injuries to the aorta, aneurysms of the aorta, angiography, correction of spinal deformities, and surgery that affects the blood supply emerging from a spinal artery that sends a branch to the spinal cord.

Patients with incomplete lesions usually have more severe spasticity than patients with total transections. Spasticity frequently interferes with the rehabilitation program and limits the patient's ability for self-care. As previously stated, oral antispasticity drugs often fail to give adequate relief, even in high doses, and have side effects that further limit their usefulness.

Multiple sclerosis

Multiple sclerosis, a central nervous system disorder, may result in considerable spasticity and lead to severe contractures. Dantrolene sodium is of some help in the management of spasticity, but weakness and drowsiness may interfere. Case review in a chronic disease hospital shows more contractures and resulting decubiti in this disease than in any other single neurologic disease. Since intellectual function may be relatively spared, the problems created by spasticity and joint contractures are most difficult for the patient and family. As soon as the joint cannot be properly put through range of motion, consideration should be given to surgical methods to relieve spasticity (see Figures 38-6 and 38-7). Our rapidly increasing knowledge of immunology may offer treatment to prevent the progression of this disorder.

Parkinsonism

Rigidity in parkinsonism may lead to progressive deformities that interfere with ambulation. A toe flexion attitude within the shoe causes tip callosities and pain. Equinus and equinovarus lead to lateral plantar callosities and progressive instability of the subtalar-ankle complex. The line of weight-bearing force tends to be directed lateral to the foot in stance phase, leading to excess foot inversion on stance. This inversion causes limb buckling. Knee flexion, when present during stance, markedly increases the energy demands of ambulation.

Volitional control may be relatively unaffected. Rigidity predominates. When deformity is added, especially deformity that cannot be controlled by gentle stretching and bracing, the patient may lose the ability to ambulate, and nursing demands are increased.

TREATMENT OF SPASTICITY
Assessment for realistic goals

Assessing for realistic goals is the first step in any rehabilitation program. One must consider the cause and extent of the disorder. The prognosis for the eventual residual disability must include an assessment of the patient's potential to cooperate with the treatment program. Psychologic and intellectual evaluation is important in setting goals. The physician must understand the life cycle of the disease to determine what problems the patient will encounter 1, 2, or 10 years in the future. Issues to be considered include the effect of the spastic state on future ambulation, nursing demands, and sitting potential.

Practical evaluation of the possible effects of relief of spasticity can be obtained by motor point injections in the spastic muscles using electrical stimulation for guidance and local anesthetic for blockade. Information thus obtained can demonstrate increase in function and range of motion of the affected joints. It may be able to show if the deformity is dynamic or static and thus show what surgical approach may be useful. Dynamic deformities are corrected when the spastic muscles are blocked, whereas static (fixed) deformities persist (see Figures 38-1 and 38-3).

In some circumstances the blocks change the scissors gait of a spastic diplegic to a state of abduction overactivity, with a resultant excessively wide base. The degree of adductor release and obturator neurectomy can then be modified to better balance motor activity. In spinal injury patients, relief of spasticity in a single muscle or muscle group may at times decrease the spasticity of the entire limb.

Communication with patient and family

When spasticity can be determined to be a significant impediment to rehabilitation or when it can be seen as a potential cause of future functional impairment or can lead to such complications as contracture and sepsis, the patient and the family should be informed. One may then attempt to evaluate the potential for using local measures to reduce spasticity. If surgical measures appear potentially useful, the goals and risks of such therapy should be discussed with all concerned. Physical and occupational therapists and nurses assisting in the care of the patient should be brought into the discussion of the potential for assistance by these surgical methods. They too must understand the limitations of conservative treatments in the face of unrelenting spasticity and progressive deformity. They can play a valuable and effective role in communication with the patient.

Since the deficit in volitional control (paralysis or paresis) remains even if spasticity is reduced, the goals of treatment should be clarified for all concerned. Patients and their families can be informed that the release of spasticity of the upper extremity, especially in hemiplegia, may improve the ease of nursing care and may prevent deformities without improving the function of the arm and hand. As a rule,

increased activity decreases spasticity. Patients whose function, especially ambulation, has improved as a result of a procedure may further decrease spasticity by increased activity.

Effective rehabilitation techniques

Patient mobilization to chair, wheelchair, standing, and walking is the progression of goals in the management of spastic disorders. Each step in the process may reveal the potential for further improvement or demonstrate a plateau beyond which the patient cannot progress. Methods that reduce the spastic state may permit increased activities. Decreased spasm of hip and knee flexors may enable the patient to use a wheelchair more effectively. To this end such modalities as local heat applications and ice massage may offer some relief. Large vibrators may relieve spasticity during the application, but unfortunately there is no carryover after the application is terminated.

Active exercises are always beneficial. If the patient can and will use a nonplegic arm to assist in such activities as shoulder abduction, this activity should also promote improved function and reduce contractures.

Properly applied passive stretching one or more times a day decreases spasticity for a period of time and helps preserve the range of motion. Too forceful, rapid, or vigorous passive motion may produce local trauma. Such trauma has been thought to lead to increased heterotopic calcification and bone formation. This has not been proved, however. The major complication of passive stretching is fracture of the severely porotic bone that follows prolonged disuse and lack of weight bearing. Pain resulting from local tissue trauma heightens spasticity and leads to reduced motion. Spastic muscles must be stretched slowly and carefully. As long as a joint can be moved through its full range without an abnormal rotation being produced and without pain, stretching may improve function and prevent contracture. Once the joint cannot be fully extended passively, further stretching may not help and may hinder the recovery pattern. Another result of overenergetic stretching can be subluxation of joints. Hemarthrosis as a result of capsular tearing is accompanied by pain, by more spasticity, by lost range of motion, and ultimately by fixed contractures.

Other measures such as motor point injections, motor nerve phenolization, neurectomy, and surgical release of tendon and muscles can be employed to regain muscle balance and achieve a physiologic joint position. This can permit use of residual volitional function and can control certain progressive deformities. The technical details of these surgical techniques are important if the operations are to be successful.

Bracing in spasticity

Orthotic devices, originally designed for lower motor neuron (LMN) palsies, can be successfully applied in spastic states. Certain modifications of the LMN device are necessary to allow for the problem of the heightened response to stretch in spasticity.

Orthoses may be characterized as static (stabilizing) or dynamic (functional).

Static orthoses

The static orthosis blocks joint motion. The joint (ankle, knee, elbow, wrist, or thumb) is held in an appropriate position that permits proximal limb motion to control the distal part. Correctable flexible deformities can be stabilized in a neutral position while fixed deformities are held. Additional deformation imposed by gravitational load or unbalanced motor activity is prevented. The static orthosis can be used to reduce pain in arthritis; to control spastic deformities of the foot, ankle, and knee; and to improve volitional control of distal parts when proximal control is present. The immobilization of the device reduces feedback to the CNS from muscle spindles and tendon receptors in the affected muscle groups.

Dynamic orthoses

The dynamic, flexible orthosis uses energy stored during one phase of action to return the distal portion of a limb to the neutral position during another phase of action. The movement permitted makes the device more comfortable and lends fluidity to the action desired. The energy storage device is most often a spring or flexible plastic component. Although metal bar braces with spring assists were previously used to control paralyses and flexible deformities, there has been a major shift in technology to plastic orthoses.

The dynamic brace has major drawbacks in spasticity.[44] First, the spring device stretches spastic muscles. Stretching can create a spastic response in the limb segment encompassed by the brace and also proximally as spasm spreads to adjacent spinal segments. Second, in the presence of fixed deformities, adjusting brace axes to the distorted joint axis is very difficult. This malalignment leads to further stress on the joints—with pain added to an already complex problem.[21]

Corrective braces and casts

Corrective braces and casts are devices that correct joint deformities. Although they can be used in special circumstances, they are really surgical tools. Specially designed plaster casts, changed as the deformity changes or is corrected, can also be used to improve early fixed (nonflexible) deformities. Tone-reducing casts have been shown to reduce static and dynamic spasticity in children.[35]

Sensory deficits create major risks in the use of corrective braces and casts. They can lead to pressure ulceration, with deep and chronic infection, and to vascular compromise with the potential for limb ischemia. Peripheral nerve problems may also follow the use of corrective devices in spasticity.

One should therefore not attempt to force fixed deformities into orthoses that do not accommodate these deformities. Unfortunately, the attempt to control fixed deformities with nonaccommodating orthoses is still encountered. This error often leads to delay in appropriate corrective surgery and to unduly prolonged functional impairment.

The use of custom-made, rigid, static plastic orthoses for stabilizing the spastic limb has been an important advance in spasticity control. The tendency to attempt to brace the deformed limb in a "correct" position is much reduced when these devices are available.

Orthotic devices rarely achieve hip and shoulder control. Many attempts to support the subluxating shoulder in stroke have been of little benefit. A sling is best. Hip braces to control adduction or subluxation have not proved effective in children and are not indicated in adults.

Nerve-stimulating orthoses

Special orthoses that attempt to stimulate motor activity electrically have been tested experimentally. The direct electrical stimulation of the peroneal nerve to overcome footdrop or spastic equinus using a heel contact control has led to nerve degeneration and has not found wide acceptance.

With this experience influencing the choice of orthoses the following devices have demonstrated effectiveness.

Lower extremity orthoses

Double-bar braces attached to a shoe. The plantar stop at the ankle controls equinus, whereas the medial and lateral bars control varus (inversion) and valgus (eversion) of the foot. Varus and valgus control straps are not highly effective if the deformity is pronounced and do not correct fixed deformities. The shoe often becomes deformed.

This brace is rather heavy. Spring ankle assists may create problems in spastic states. Upper bands should be wide to distribute proximal forces and avoid placing pressure on the peroneal nerve. The heel height must be adjusted to accommodate fixed equinus or to eliminate clonus produced by the plantar-grade position in severe spasticity.

If the heel rises out of the shoe because of fixed or dynamic equinus, the calf should be weakened by neurectomy or tendon lengthening (see "Corrective Surgery in Spasticity"). These procedures can be performed under local anesthesia, and the patient can be mobilized quickly—often using the previously poorly conforming brace as a postoperative orthosis once the deforming force is corrected. If the ankle can be brought into dorsiflexion, a short leg orthosis can be used to prevent genu recurvatum (hyperextension) when this is a problem. Slight plantar flexion of the foot in a static orthosis can be used to extend the knee during stance when there is a mild dynamic flexion attitude of the knee.[44]

Plastic ankle-foot orthosis with rigid ankle. The plastic AFO with rigid ankle can be quite useful when there is proximal volitional control. Spasticity is often reduced when this device renders the gastroc-soleus nonfunctional, although knee extension stretches the gastrocnemius and may increase spasm. Deformities are accommodated. A soft heel and roll-over bar set just in front of the heel can simulate ankle function during stance phase. The opposite heel must be raised to balance the limbs if there is unilateral disease (hemiplegia). A rather normal-looking shoe can be worn.

Plastic ankle-foot orthosis with flexible ankle (posterior leaf plastic orthosis). Rigidity of the device can be varied. A stock brace is rarely satisfactory, since they are designed for LMN palsy. Flexibility (a spring) in the ankle may heighten spasticity. Inversion cannot be controlled. The heel rises out of the shoe if spasticity is significant and if the orthosis foot piece is set at a right angle to the shank.

Double-bar long leg brace with knee lock. The double-bar long leg brace with a knee lock (KAFO) usually requires a knee strap or pad and should have a high upper thigh band for better distribution of forces. This may be useful when there is hip control and when arm function permits use of an assistive device—walker, crutch, or cane. The patient must have balance to ambulate. The brace is heavy, which may help to stabilize the limb in stance and reduce over-swing. It should not be locked straight if there is a fixed-flexion deformity of the knee. If the limb cannot be straightened, the hamstrings can be released, lengthened, and loosely transposed anteriorly to balance the forces at the knee. The surgery may permit the use of a simpler orthosis.

Plastic knee-ankle-foot orthosis with metal hinges and knee lock. The plastic KAFO with metal hinge and knee lock is much lighter and more comfortable than the bar braces. They must be applied with the same caution concerning fixed deformities as bar braces.

Knee cages (plastic knee orthosis). Knee cages have limited application in spasticity. The patient must be thin and the tendency to flexion relatively mild.

Upper extremity orthoses

Rigid plastic hand-wrist splints. The major goal in the spastic upper extremity is preventing deformity caused by spasticity of the finger flexors. If this condition is not treated, fingernails may grow into the palm. Wide use of plastic palmar splints has almost eliminated such severe complications. A lightweight plastic splint holding the fingers in partial flexion and the thumb in abduction prevents contractures. The abduction of the thumb tends to decrease finger flexor spasticity in the majority of hemiplegic hands. Positioning the wrist in about 30 degrees of dorsiflexion maintains the length of the flexor tendons. Frequently the spasticity of the hand can be greatly reduced by placing the hand behind the back with the shoulder in internal rotation. At times this maneuver may permit application of a splint to the hand and wrist.

Foam hand splints. Recently plastic foam splints have been made available that place the fingers in abduction and extension. Heavy plastic prefabricated splints have limited use. Plastic prefabricated splints placing the thumb in full

opposition have a place in the positioning of a flaccid hand.

Opponens splints. Dynamic splints are of little use in treating the spastic hand. All straps should be marked to prevent the patient, staff, or family from applying them too snugly and producing swelling of the hand.

Patients with spastic upper extremity may develop marked hyperpronation of the forearm. This is usually caused by spasm and contracture of the flexor carpi radialis and can be released by surgery.

Elbow control orthoses. Rigid orthoses and inflatable splints and elbow immobilizers help prevent elbow flexion contractures. Dynamic splints may increase the degree of spasticity. Marked spasticity of the elbow flexors is a definite indication for phenol blocks or surgical release. These procedures may help relieve spasticity in the distal part of the extremity.

Shoulder splints. Subluxation of the shoulder caused by traction of the weight of the extremity is frequently seen in flaccid hemiplegics. This complication is not seen in spastic patients. If tightness of spastic pectorals develops, an airplane-type splint may be attached to wheelchair. A sling may be required to support the arm.

Corrective (serial) casts and dial lock orthoses

Corrective casts and dial lock orthoses may be of use in certain individuals. Sensory deficits make these techniques somewhat dangerous. Extra padding and careful plaster technique are important. The essential application principle is that the cast or orthosis does not force the correction; it merely takes up slack. Translational movements of the cast on the limb gradually permit more correction. After a few days the slack is again taken up by a new cast or adjustment (wedging), and thus the limb gradually straightens. This technique is useful for recent deformities only. It should not be used after 4 months from onset.

The dial lock orthosis is used in a similar way to take up slack in a joint and bring the deformity (usually knee flexion) into the corrected position. Pain or afferent stimulation of the spinal cord may accentuate spasticity. Prolonged pressure may produce pressure ulceration.

CORRECTIVE SURGERY IN SPASTICITY

Surgical intervention in spastic states has a long history, especially in cerebral palsy.[33] Many procedures are useful if applied at the right time in the right patient.[7] The goals of therapy must be clear. Overly optimistic expectations should be avoided. Nevertheless, prolonged delay in surgery does not improve results.

The underlying disorder and the clinical presentation determine the needs for therapy. In many instances relatively simple release operations can help hemiplegia caused by stroke or head injury.[23,24] Long-standing paraplegia or quadriplegia from spinal cord injury or multiple sclerosis presents a much more profound problem. Here surgical procedures that correct deformity may avoid major bone and joint resections and reconstructive plastic operations at a later date. The goal is to permit the supine and prone positions for pressure relief, to permit limb abduction for nursing care, and to aid functional improvement using residual, less impaired lower and upper extremity muscles.

Surgery for spasticity of the upper extremity

Upper extremity surgery in spastic states has had less success than in the leg. Conceptual and sensory deficits along with loss of voluntary function may preclude successful functional activities after release surgery.[33] Nevertheless, certain procedures can be useful when severe spasticity is present. These include *motor neurectomy* (musculocutaneous nerve, median nerve to pronator teres), *tendon lengthenings* (biceps, wrist and finger flexors), and *tenotomy* of the pectoralis major, subscapularis, and latissimus dorsi for severe internal rotation of the shoulder. Occasionally tendon transfers are useful when there is volitional function.[23,33]

Nerve blocks with local anesthetic are useful in evaluating patients before definitive procedures begin. Phenol blockade of the upper extremity nerves after localization with electrical stimulation and anesthetic injections can be effective.[17] Some attempts at prolonged relief of spasticity with phenol blocks of motor points or specific motor nerves have not proved completely reliable. Undesirable effects may accompany these injections, including spread of motor deficits and the onset of pain when a mixed peripheral nerve has been injected (see p. 542.) Alcohol injections of motor points may also be useful in the presence of severe spasticity and paralysis but are more often used in the leg.[44]

Shoulder pain is often produced by frozen shoulder syndrome, which develops secondary to spastic contractures of the subscapularis and pectoralis major muscles. Release of the subscapularis and pectoralis major has permitted mobilization of the shoulder and relief of the painful contracture.[2]

Flexion of the elbow

Severe elbow flexion can be treated by open phenol block of the musculocutaneous nerve or neurectomy of the musculocutaneous nerve.[11,24] Tenotomy or lengthening of the biceps and brachialis may also be useful.[41] Although capsular contractures producing fixed flexion may be present, residual deformity is often due to local spasticity that is not completely relieved (Figure 38-1).

Flexion deformities of wrist and fingers

Wrist and finger deformities are disabling when residual volitional function is blocked and when the severe flexed position makes cleaning and washing difficult. The *flexor slide operation*, which releases the flexor pronator origin, has been used in this disorder,[15] but Treanor[52] proposed more selective tendon lengthenings. Although release of spasticity

can be helpful, improved function is usually limited.[23] *Fractional flexor muscle-tendon lengthening* is limited to half the distance required to extend the finger from the point of restriction of voluntary extension to full extension.[38] Thumb and finger flexors may be lengthened as required.

One must distinguish between the functioning arm and hand that is impaired by a specific deficit or contracture and the nonfunctioning limb that is a cosmetic or hygiene problem. In the functioning limb a careful evaluation of sensory deficit and paralytic and spastic components of the disorder must be undertaken when planning surgery. Nerve blocks of the median, ulnar, and musculocutaneous nerves with local anesthetic can be used to quantify fixed and dynamic components of deformity. Proprioception and two-point discrimination sensation of less than 10 mm should be present if an attempt to restore function by tendon transfer is to be undertaken.[54]

In recent years reconstructive surgery of the upper limb that attempts to restore motor balance in hemiplegia has become more sophisticated, and results have subsequently improved.[41] Pinzur[42] groups the functional deficits as follows: elbow flexor spasticity, isolated spasticity of the wrist flexors, spasticity of the combined wrist and finger flexors with overpowered extensors, and spasticity of combined wrist and finger flexion with absent extensors. Surgery is performed under regional or general anesthesia. Elbow flexion spasticity is managed by step-cut lengthening of the biceps tendon and release of the lacertus fibrosis. Isolated wrist flexor spasticity with voluntary control of all motor groups is treated by *wrist fusion* and *lengthening of the flexor carpi ulnaris and radialis*. Combined wrist-finger flexor spasticity with overpowered extensors, including thumb-in-palm, is treated by lengthening the wrist flexors along with the flexor sublimis and profundus to the fingers. With absent wrist extensors a *tenodesis* of the wrist extensors or transfer of the flexor carpi ulnaris to the extensor carpi ulnaris is used. Results seem better than those achieved by flexor pronator origin release.

In cerebral palsy the spastic thumb-in-palm may be treated by a tendon transfer of the extensor pollicis longus, since there is often enough discrete voluntary control to permit a functional balance of the thumb.[25] This technique may be applicable in some young adults when spasticity is secondary to head injury.

Another procedure useful in children and adults with isolated thumb-in-palm deformity when there is a functioning hand is the flexor pollicis longus abductor transfer in which the flexor pollicis longus is transferred to the radial side of the thumb.[48]

Quadriplegia

Reconstructive procedures in quadriplegia may be useful but carry risks. Moberg[29] proposed a program of surgical rehabilitation in quadriplegia that eliminated previous overcomplicated reconstructions. Spasticity can interfere

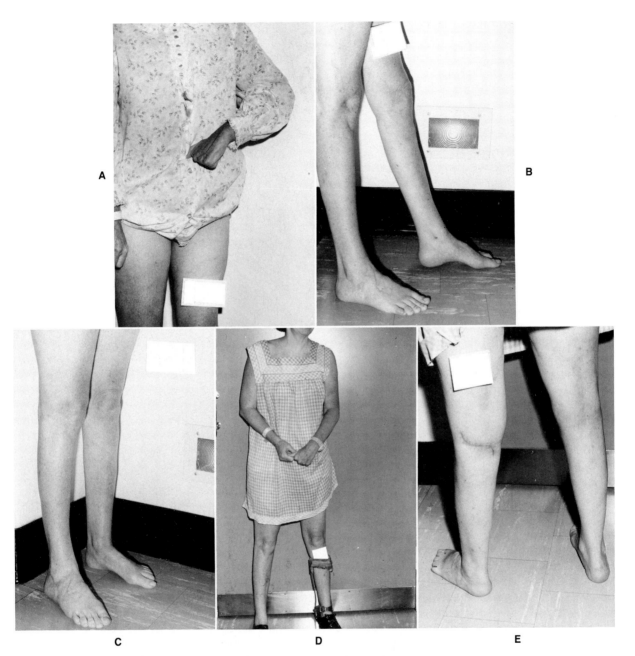

Figure 38-1. Spastic hemiplegia of 12 years' duration treated by musculocutaneous neurectomy for severe elbow flexion spasm. Spastic equinus evaluated by posterior tibial nerve block and then treated by neurectomy of posterior tibial motor branches to gastrocnemius. **A,** Left arm before surgery. **B,** Left foot and leg showing equinus deformity. **C,** Patient standing after posterior tibial nerve block. **D,** Patient standing in double-bar ankle-foot orthosis after left musculocutaneous neurectomy and posterior tibial neurectomy. **E,** Posterior view of left leg following neurectomy of motor branches of posterior tibial nerve to gastrocnemius.

with successful surgical efforts, as can inadequate assessment of the muscles to be rerouted.[13]

Certain patients benefit from a brachioradialis transfer to give wrist extension, tenodesis of the flexor pollicis longus, and arthodesis of the joint of the thumb. This transfer creates key grip without stiffening the fingers. Deltoid to biceps transfer has not given significant elbow power. Deltoid to triceps transfer has been used to improve elbow extension in tetraplegia.[6] Spasticity in the arm makes such reconstructions of questionable value.

Surgery for lower extremity spasticity

The elimination of deformity and reduction of spasticity that can result from judicious surgery in the feet and legs can be most gratifying. Increased experience has produced better-defined criteria for surgical interventions and their timing. The results of such procedures are fairly predictable, and complications have been reduced. Naturally differences exist between etiology groups. Hemiplegia from stroke or head injury usually affects the foot to a greater extent than the knee and hip. Paraplegia may produce spastic deformity in the foot, but the knee and hip deformities are more important in the nonambulator. Head injury can produce diffuse spasticity and contractures, often with para-articular ossification. Multiple sclerosis and spinal cord injury lead to severe deformities and sensory deficits. Hip dislocations and sepsis, major pressure ulceration, and pelvic osteomyelitis are frequent complications. As in many disorders, prevention of fixed deformity is better than surgery that attempts to treat the more severe complications of paralysis and sensory loss.

Next we review the specific problems encountered and the program for appropriate intervention, leaving the salvage operations for last. Many of these operations can be performed under local anesthesia, especially when isolated deformities in the foot are treated. When some sensation is present and proximal operations—hip and knee—are performed, general anesthesia may be required. In planning for surgery one should coordinate the rehabilitation plan with the surgical plan to ensure the patient's earliest possible mobilization. Intensive postoperative ventilatory support is necessary. Psychologic assistance is often required to ensure patient cooperation. Goals should be realistic. Careful preoperative functional studies are needed to evaluate exactly what needs to be done and what should not be done.

Of some importance is the usefulness of residual spastic hip and knee extension in some patients with paraplegia. This spasticity can be helpful in transfer. Reduction of spasticity may lead to reduced function—at least temporarily. This caution should be balanced by recognizing the problem of specific contractures, which become progressively disabling and ultimately contribute to ulceration and joint sepsis. Deformities that may be corrected early by tendon releases eventually require bone and joint resection if untreated. Early multiservice assessment is required once

deformities are no longer manageable by simple stretching programs or controllable by static orthoses.

Toe flexion

Toe flexion deformities are encountered in spasticity and rigidity. They are usually apparent after correction of an equinus deformity.[19] These flexed toes make donning of a shoe difficult and lead to painful toe tip callosities. The

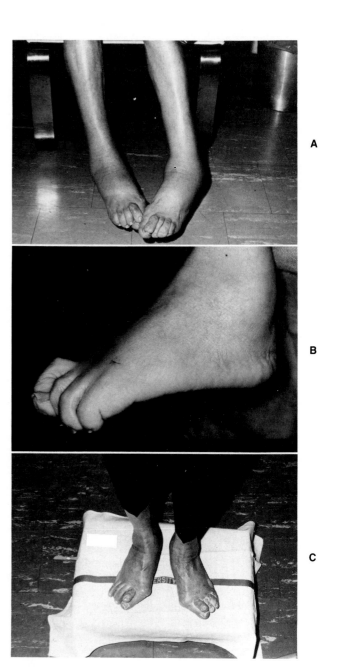

Figure 38-2. Toe flexion deformities and residual cock-up of second toe following extensor digitorum tenotomies. **A,** Claw toes in marginally ambulatory patient. **B,** Left foot with flexion deformities of toes following extensor tenotomy. **C,** Patient standing after subsequent release of long flexors of toes.

treatment is by flexor digitorum longus tenotomy performed distally at the level of the proximal phalanges or proximally at the ankle. If toe flexion is noted when equinus is being corrected, this tendon should be released. If a cast is to be applied after tendo Achillis lengthening, the flexor digitorum longus can be lengthened at the ankle at the same time (Figure 38-2).

Clawing of the toes

Clawing of the toes consists of hyperextension of the metacarpophalangeal joints and flexion of the interphalangeal joint. It leads to plantar metatarsal callosities as weight is transferred to the metatarsal heads. Phalangectomy is simple but may lead to residual clawing; fusion of the proximal interphalangeal joints combined with extensor digitorum longus and brevis tenotomy should solve the problem. Clawing of the great toe (cock-up deformity) can often be managed by lengthening of the extensor hallucis longus tendon.

Spastic equinus

Spastic equinus is encountered in hemiplegia from stroke, after head injury, and in spinal cord disease. Careful evaluation of the gait pattern should lead to an appropriate plan. The equinus and varus may be due to an overactive gastroc-soleus group alone, or there may be concurrent overactivity of the tibialis anterior, especially in swing phase.[18] If tibialis anterior overactivity is present, it should be documented because balance of the foot can be achieved only by combined posterior (gastroc-soleus and tibialis posterior) and anterior (tibialis anterior) muscle surgery. The tibialis anterior should be transferred to balance the foot in swing phase. In other patients, abnormal activity of the tibialis posterior is found throughout the gait cycle, and this muscle must be lengthened.

The evaluation of spastic equinus has been largely clinical. The position of the foot during stance and swing phase is noted. The presence of dynamic (functional) deformity is evaluated by slow and rapid manual attempts to correct the position of the foot with the knee extended and then with the knee flexed to reduce the effect of gastrocnemius stimulation. Residual deformation after slow manual correction and during quiet stance would be a static (fixed) deformity. The ability to invert and evert the foot is noted. Residual inversion (varus) spasticity with the foot in equinus is due to tibialis posterior contracture or spasticity when tested with the patient sitting. If the foot goes into varus during swing phase, the tibialis anterior is the usual deforming muscle, although the extensor hallucis longus may play a role. At times, the tibialis posterior may be overactive during swing phase.

Attempts have been made to evaluate more precisely the spastic equinus deformity. Measuring the torque required to move the ankle joint at a specific velocity may accurately assess the amount of spasticity.[34] Electromyographic (EMG)

analysis of equinovarus following stroke can yield valuable data as to the muscle firing pattern during swing and stance phase.[39] Most stroke patients demonstrate premature firing of gastrocnemius and soleus—often during swing phase. The anterior tibial, posterior tibial, and flexor hallucis longus muscles can be shown to have different patterns of activity in different subjects.

The gait cycle of hemiplegics has been studied using an ultrasound gait monitor combined with EMG and electrogoniometric recordings.[45] This method evaluates the percentages of the cycle spent in swing, stance, and double support phases. The distances between the ankles are measured by an ultrasound monitor. Three groups of ambulating hemiplegics are thus identified, depending on the slope and duration of the data generated. The cause of the gait abnormality may be identified by the EMG pattern, and the effect of equinus on the proximal joint position can be demonstrated. With more severe degrees of equinus, the patient cannot bring the uninvolved limb ahead of the spastic limb, extension of the ipsilateral knee is accentuated, and hip flexion is increased.

Dynamic EMG recording in a sophisticated gait analysis laboratory can confirm a direct observation and add to the evaluation process but is not usually available.

An inexpensive but perhaps useful tool is videotaping the patient during ambulation to permit better presurgical evaluation and postsurgical analysis.

The most important point in the evaluation of spasticity following stroke is that functional recovery may continue for as long as 9 months but that most of the recovery is seen by 3 months.[16] Certainly the presence of progressive deformity should be apparent at 6 months following onset.[55] Motor, cognitive, sensory, and balance problems should be evaluated serially to give a pattern of recovery and to isolate motor factors whose early correction might improve function and prevent severe deformities.

Equinus produced by gastroc-soleus overactivity usually produces some varus of the foot, but in many instances the foot rotates into eversion at the subtalar joint under stance phase body weight loading. This eversion leads to concomitant dorsiflexion and abduction at the subtalar joint, producing a position of valgus. This is not spastic flatfoot but is a rotational response to the equinus and loading of the foot.

A certain amount of spastic equinus can be accommodated by raising the heel of the shoe. This elevation reduces afferent stimulation from the muscle and tendons and improves spastic gait patterns. If poor balance or coronal plane deformity (varus or valgus) at the subtalar joint or severe clonus from calf (especially gastrocnemius) stretching exists, this solution is not satisfactory.

Phenol nerve block of the posterior tibial nerve has been successful in many patients in reducing spastic equinus.[40] Used early in the disorder, the block can sometimes prevent fixed equinus. Paresthesias develop in about one fourth of the patients. Weakness may be difficult to control if significant functional control of the calf exists.

Nerve blocks and phenol injections for evaluating and treating spasticity

Motor nerve blocks with short- and long-acting agents can be quickly useful in the evaluation of patients and in some instances can relieve spasticity for some time, thus permitting more effective physical therapy. These blocks can also stimulate the effects of more definitive procedures such as phenolization or neurectomy and so help the patient and family evaluate the chances of improvement after such surgery.

The posterior tibial nerve and obturator nerves are easily blocked in spastic equinus and in hip adduction deformities. Petrillo and co-workers[40] use a technique of electrical stimulation to localize the injecting needle to the region of the posterior tibial nerve 7 cm distal to the popliteal crease. The nerve is more superficial at the popliteal crease just below the deep fascia and can be located there without penetrating to bone, as described by Petrillo. As previously stated, the results of phenolization of peripheral nerves are not as predictable as after open neurectomy, but the procedure is relatively simple and usually innocuous (Figure 38-3).[17]

Phenol blocks of motor points are performed under control of electrical stimulation of the motor points. This localization is followed by local anesthetic and dilute phenol injections.

Achilles tendon lengthening

Some patients are not ambulators, but their fixed equinus deformity is so severe as to make wearing a shoe very difficult. Even wheelchair use is significantly hampered in these circumstances.

In severe spasticity in multiple sclerosis or quadriplegia, tenotomy of the Achilles tendon under local or no anesthesia corrects most equinus deformities. Minimal or no splinting over bulky soft dressings is used postoperatively.

When ambulation function is required, the tendo Achillis is lengthened (Figure 38-4). In the adult the operation can often be performed under local anesthesia, permitting adjustment of the amount of lengthening required to correct imbalance, and the amount of tension controlled to prevent overweakening, gait degradation, and calcaneus deformity. A tourniquet is not required. An attempt to gauge the amount of lengthening can be based on the amount of deformity and the patient's functional requirements. This operation has been described in cerebral palsy patients[9] but has permitted only 71% to rise to toes when walking. In this series a tourniquet was used, and the patients were under general anesthesia—two factors that make a functional evaluation during surgery difficult.

A simple Achilles tendon lengthening that has been used in many stroke patients is the *Hoke triple-hemisection tenotomy*.[55] This tenotomy can be performed under local anesthesia and consists of three hemisections of the tendon through small incisions. This permits a passive dorsiflexion force applied to the ankle to lengthen the tendon appropri-

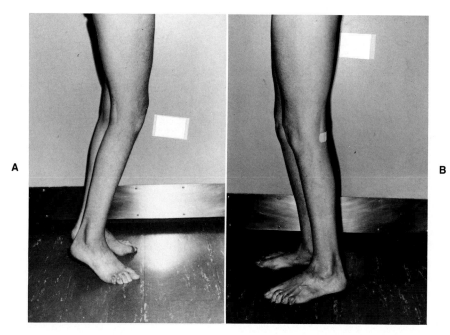

Figure 38-3. Posterior tibial nerve block used to evaluate spastic equinus. **A,** Patient standing showing bilateral equinus. **B,** Standing 5 minutes after injection of each posterior tibial nerve in popliteal region with 5 ml 1% lidocaine.

ately. A short leg cast is then applied for 6 weeks. Over-lengthening of the tendon should be avoided.

Toe "curling," or flexion deformity, is distinguished from claw toe deformity and should be managed by *tenotomy of the toe flexors* at the toes if the deformity is isolated,[19] or released in the foot[55] or at the ankle.[23]

Control of inversion, when it accompanies equinus, is based on the phase and origin of the deformity. Extension synergy—hip extension, knee extension, plantar flexion, and heel inversion during swing phase—may be treated by Achilles tendon lengthening (TAL) combined with length-ening of the toe flexors and tibialis posterior (TPL), often under local anesthesia.[23,30]

A more extensive procedure to balance the foot combines TAL, TPL, multiple toe flexor tenotomies, and the *split transfer of the tibialis anterior tendon* (SPLATT).[30,51] The

operation is used when the foot strongly inverts during swing phase. It has been quite successful in adult head trauma patients and is often combined with flexor hallucis transfer.[18]

Isolated SPLATT transfers may balance the foot nicely if spasticity is mild. Transposition of the tibialis posterior tendon to the dorsum of the foot is usually performed in LMN palsy but has been used in some cases of spasticity.[53]

For many older patients simple procedures suffice. In younger patients the reconstructive operations can be useful.

Interestingly, fixed equinus deformities usually respond to tendon division or lengthening. More extensive joint re-leases are seldom needed in spasticity. However, it is pos-sible to correct deformities associated with capsular con-tracture by combined tendon, tendon sheath, and capsular release if the neural and vascular supply to the foot is mo-bilized.[22]

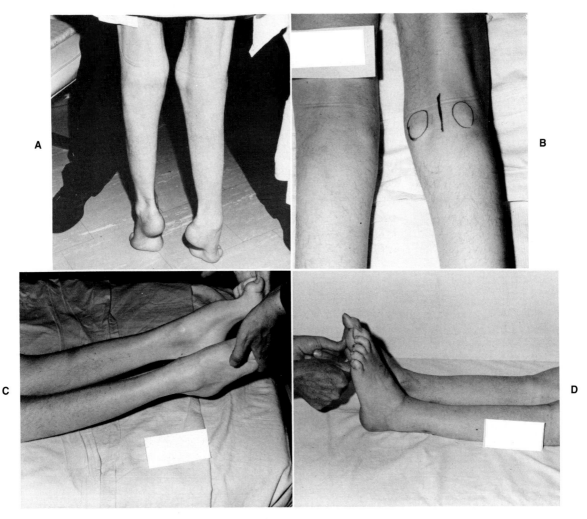

Figure 38-4. Spastic diplegia treated by tendo Achillis lengthening under local anesthesia. **A,** Patient standing with support. Severe equinus is present bilaterally. **B,** Landmarks for posterior tibial nerve block. Femoral condyles and tibial nerve are outlined. Nerve lies in middle of popliteal fossa just beneath deep fascia. **C,** Status following posterior tibial nerve block. There is little improvement in deformity. **D,** Tendo Achillis lengthenings produce plantigrade feet.   *Continued.*

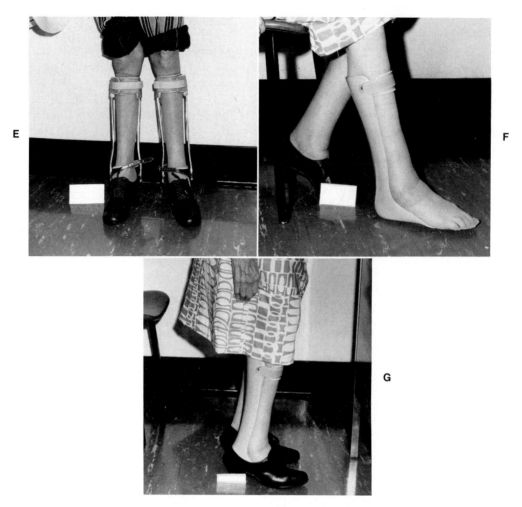

Figure 38-4, cont'd. E, Standing in double-bar ankle-foot orthosis (AFO) with lateral straps to control residual varus. **F,** Plastic AFO in use after tendo Achillis lengthening. **G,** Standing in shoe with plastic AFO following surgery.

Based on gait and EMG analysis, Pinzur[42] balances the foot and ankle 1 year following stroke using the Hoke tendo Achillis lengthening, a complete transposition of the tibialis anterior tendon to the middorsum of the foot, section of the toe flexors, and selective section of the tibialis posterior and flexor hallucis longus. Subjective and objective improvement in gait with less extension of the knee and less flexion of the hip has been demonstrated. Orthotic requirements are reduced or eliminated.

Following surgery for spastic equinus, the duration of immobilization is determined by the complexity of the surgery and the expected outcome. Simple tenotomy requires only a stabilizing orthosis to prevent recurrence or flaccid footdrop. When the Achilles tendon is lengthened by Z-plasty and when there has been a tendon transposition such as a SPLATT, 6 weeks of casting is the usual postoperative regimen. The patient can often be permitted weight bearing soon after surgery while the tendons heal. The foot and leg

are then braced for several months to permit the tendon repair to mature and the patient to return to active ambulation.

Ankle clonus may be corrected by TAL, but considerable calf strength is lost. Motor branch neurectomy to denervate the gastrocnemius remains a useful procedure. Although 3% phenol injections of the motor branches give temporary improvement, neurectomy is probably better. The motor nerve often regenerates in children with spasticity but not in adult patients.

Selective motor neurectomy under magnification has been used with good results for multiple deformities of the foot.[47]

In some instances of stroke, weakness about the ankle requires attention. This weakness may be due to gastrocsoleus or tibialis anterior paralysis. The problem is best managed by a static orthosis if spasticity exists.[55] Spring dorsiflexor assists can be used only if spasticity is not a problem.[28]

Spastic knee flexion deformity

Spastic knee flexion deformities range from mild flexion during stance phase, associated with generalized limb spasm, to severe progressive flexion at rest. Complicating hip flexion contractures may exist. Pressure ulceration about the knee may penetrate the joint, causing septic arthritis. When severe, knee flexion is a major deforming factor in lower limb spasticity and almost defies correction.

A common therapeutic error consists of allowing too long a period of passive stretching treatments while the deformity progresses; another is the attempt to control uncontrollable knee flexion with a straight orthosis.

The two surgical approaches for dynamic knee flexion deformities are *hamstring neurectomy* and *hamstring tenotomy and transposition*. Hamstring neurectomy is usually reserved for nonambulatory patients with excessive knee flexion (Figure 38-5). Hamstring tenotomy and transposition may be used on ambulatory and nonambulatory patients. In contrast to the anterior transposition of the hamstrings, sometimes performed in LMN palsy of the quadriceps, the operation in spasticity is a negative transfer and is designed to control the tendency of the divided muscles and tendons to reattach to their original insertions and thus to recover spasticity as the tendon scar contracts (Figure 38-6).

The hamstring tenotomy and transposition is an extensive operation and is often performed in conjunction with proximal releases to control hip deformity. Certain technical steps are important. The incisions on either side of the knee and distal thigh should be long and located anteriorly near or over the axis of the knee joint. This location reduces the scar's tendency to contract and produce more knee flexion. The peroneal nerve should be protected and the popliteal vessels not overstretched. The biceps femoris, sartorius, semitendinosus, and semimembranosus tendons are sutured to the quadriceps with no tension on the muscles to avoid enhancing spasticity and disrupting the suture lines. Suction catheter drainage is used postoperatively. No cast is needed and none should be applied, but a knee immobilizer splint can be applied over soft bandages (Figure 38-7).

Considerable temporary worsening of the patient's bladder and bowel control and of residual volitional function may follow this operation, especially if concomitant hip surgery is performed. The patient's requirements for nursing, rehabilitation, and ventilatory care are often increased for several weeks. With proper preoperative evaluation, the results are worthwhile. The earlier the knee flexion deformity is treated surgically, the easier the recovery and the better the results. Residual flexion often stretches out if the patient spends time in the prone position.

Severe knee flexion deformities require *distal femoral resection*. If this is performed carefully, the vascular supply of the leg is not injured. The femur is transected just above the condyle, and a subperiosteal dissection is performed with a combined cutting and coagulating electrocautery. The knee

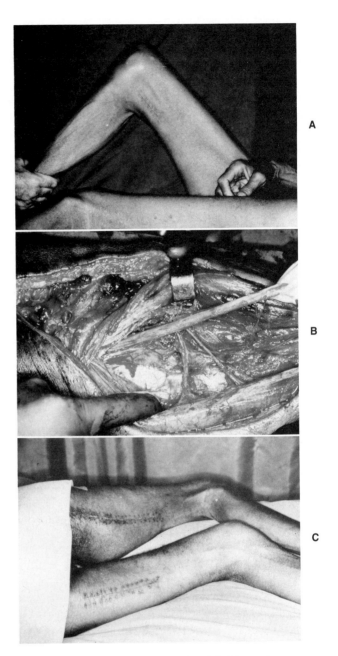

Figure 38-5. Hamstring neurectomy after failed hamstring tenotomy. **A,** Maximum knee extension after limited hamstring tenotomy. **B,** Sciatic nerve exposed by posterior thigh approach. Motor branches were identified and then resected. **C,** Posterior thighs and knees after bilateral hamstring neurectomy.

joint capsule is divided and the distal femur removed. Protective splints can be applied over very bulky soft sheet wadding dressings. When septic arthritis of the knee occurs because of pressure necrosis, this resection is the only procedure (other than amputation) that can, at times, solve the problem.

Some have attempted *soft tissue releases of severe fixed contractures of the knee*. This release leaves a large skin

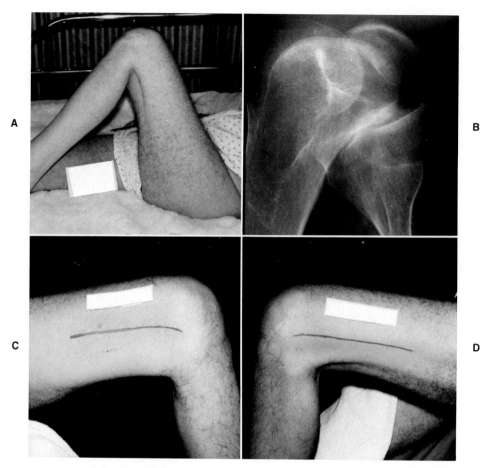

Figure 38-6. Left spastic hemiplegia owing to multiple sclerosis complicated by arthritis of hip in 38-year-old man. **A,** Preoperative status showing maximum knee extension. **B,** Preoperative radiograph of knee showing position of limb at rest. **C,** Medial view showing incision marked anterior to hamstring tendons. This prevents posterior skin and scar contracture following surgery. **D,** Lateral view showing incision marked. Note length of incision and its position anterior to biceps femoris.

defect that can be closed by a gastrocnemius flap turned back to the popliteal space and covered by split-thickness graft.[31] Circulatory and neural deficits may result from stretch of shortened vessels and nerves.

Extension deformity of the knee

Excessive extension of the knee or "stiff-legged gait," is sometimes seen. The muscle action pattern seen on EMG is variable. When the rectus femoris and vastus intermedius muscles produce the deformity, they can be released.[55] The operation is performed 4 cm above the patella; the vastus medialis and lateralis must not be divided or knee instability will result. Immediate ambulation is permitted.

Spastic deformities of the hip

Spastic deformities of the hip usually develop in non-ambulatory patients. At first they are annoying because they interfere with washing the perineum. Then they prevent the prone position, leading to sacral ulceration or trochanteric

pressure sores. At some point this problem becomes serious because septic spastic dislocation of the hip can result in penetrating ulcer into the hip joint. Osteomyelitis of the femur is bad enough, but osteomyelitis of the iliac bone at the hip is truly a grave disorder. Hip flexion contracture promotes, and is often seen in conjunction with, ischial pressure ulceration and osteomyelitis of the ischium and sacrum.

The late complications can be prevented by early muscle releases and neurectomies. This surgery can be combined with hamstring tenotomy and transposition during a single operative session—much as in the modern surgical approach to cerebral palsy.[32]

Adduction deformity is corrected by *adductor tenomyotomy* and *obturator neurectomy*. The adductor longus tendon is divided at the pubis and the adductor brevis muscular origin is divided if the muscle is contracted, as it usually is. The anterior and posterior branches of the obturator nerve are then divided and 1 cm segments excised. The obturator

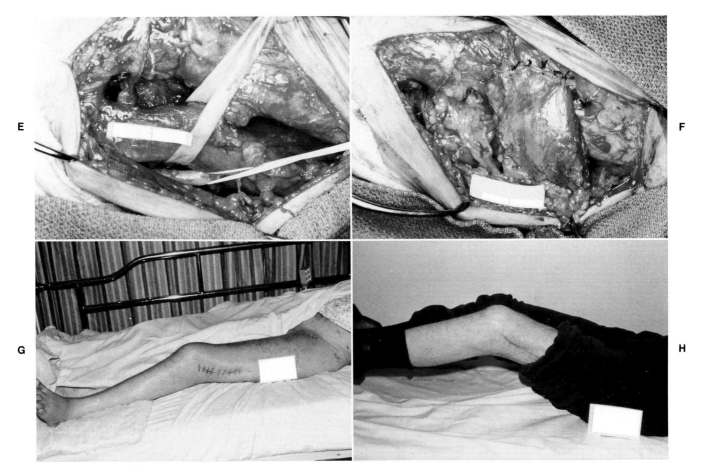

Figure 38-6, cont'd. E, Operative photograph showing biceps femoris and peroneal nerve exposed before tenomyotomy and transposition into quadriceps. **F,** Biceps femoris sutured to quadriceps without tension. **G,** Postoperative status after concomitant obturator neurectomy and iliopsoas tenomyotomy. **H,** Final status 3 months after surgery.

vessels should be identified and protected or cauterized. In the presence of mild fixed adduction, only the anterior division of the obturator nerve need be divided. In severe adduction the pectineus should be denervated as well (Figures 38-6 and 38-7).

Occasionally this operation creates an abduction attitude when severe hip abductor spasm is unmasked. A secondary *release of the hip abductors* can then be performed, often under local anesthesia.

Hip flexion is best managed by *iliopsoas tenomyotomy* at the pelvic brim. The incision is made just at the lower edge of the inquinal ligament (Poupart's), and the femoral vessels and nerve are lifted to give access to the iliacus muscle and psoas tendon.

Severe hip flexion (over 90 degrees), contracture, and dislocation are treated by *proximal femoral resection*. This salvage procedure may solve a severe, life-threatening problem. The resection should include the entire proximal third of the femur. Spasticity is relieved because muscles that are

permitted to shorten 30% no longer possess functional contractibility (Figure 38-8).

In adults these operations for proximal limb contractures should not be followed by prolonged bed rest or attempts to straighten the limbs with skeletal traction. Bilateral operations are often necessary. Adequate ventilatory support and enthusiastic nursing and physical therapy assistance are required during the postoperative recovery phase.

Heterotopic bone formation

Para-articular bone formation (myositis ossificans paralytica) is often seen after head injury, in paraplegia, and occasionally following stroke.[57] Severe burns also produce this problem. The cause has never been established. Theories include local trauma, overstretching of muscles, and venous stasis. Joint trauma and fractures are risk factors for this disorder. Overstretching has been ruled out as a causative factor.

The bone formation is between the muscles and is usually

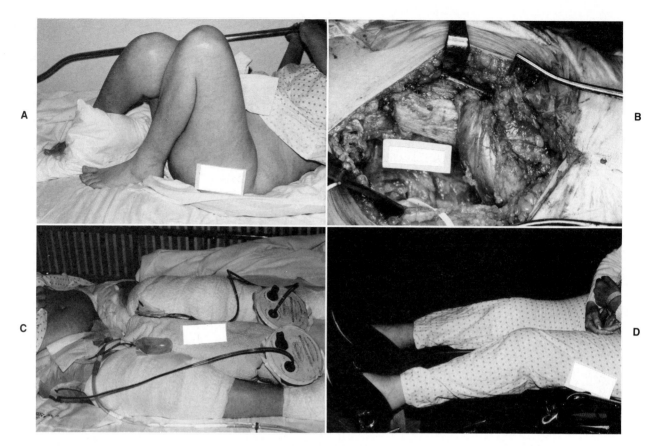

Figure 38-7. Severe lower extremity contractures in 48-year-old woman with multiple sclerosis treated by bilateral hamstring tenomyotomy and transposition and concurrent obturator neurectomy and iliopsoas tenomyotomy. **A,** Preoperative status. Sitting is impossible. Nursing care is very difficult. **B,** Operative photograph showing biceps femoris released and transposed. Peroneal nerve is visible and controlled by silicone tape. **C,** Postoperative status after bilateral medial and lateral hamstring releases and transposition, adductor tenotomy, obturator neurectomy, and iliopsoas tenomyotomy. Soft dressings are on knees and feet. Note lack of casts or splints. Suction catheters are in wounds to remove hematoma. Catheter is in bladder. Position of legs is much improved. **D,** Patient seated comfortably in chair 3 weeks after surgery.

extracapsular. It may start as a local inflammatory reaction with swelling, redness, and heat. The hip is most often involved in head injury and paraplegia. Knees, elbow, and shoulder may be involved. At first the radiograph is negative. Later soft calcific shadows appear about the joint and go on to organized bone ridges, protuberances, or complete bone bridges. Alkaline phosphatase levels rise, and bone scans are positive. Of greater importance and difficulty is the need to evaluate the end of the ossification process, a stage that unfortunately is usually difficult to determine. Although radiographic maturation may indicate the end of the active disorder and alkaline phosphatase levels may fall, surgical resection of major bone bridges or even femoral resection can be followed by reankylosis.

Treatment during the acute phase consists of passive exercises and the use of antiossification agents such as diphosphonates. These slow down the process, but bone for-

mation may well take place after the medication is stopped. In the interim the remainder of the skeleton is losing mineral as a result of disuse and the diphosphonates.

Radiotherapy can be effective but is followed by late sarcoma formation in some patients. Lower doses of radiation that are still effective may reduce the problem of late neoplasia. Nonsteroid anti-inflammatory agents are being used to block bone formation after joint surgery and injury, but hard data are lacking. These drugs have a tendency to induce peptic ulcer, which is already a problem after head injury. Antacid therapy should be used to reduce this problem.

The major positive determinant in the surgical treatment of heterotopic ossification is recovery of active motor power. If the patient can move the joint after surgery, there is more chance that motion regained will be motion retained. Bone projections that block one part of the joint's arc of motion

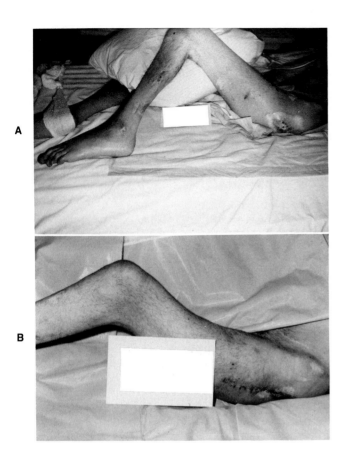

A

B

Figure 38-8. Proximal femoral resection for fixed hip deformities. **A,** Severe contractures of legs and ulceration of hip region secondary to spastic paraplegia. **B,** Status following proximal femoral resection. If hip joint is not septic, wound can be closed with reasonable chance of primary healing. When severe decubiti and septic dislocation of hip have developed, wounds must be left open to heal by secondary intention.

can be successfully removed after 18 months to 2 years. When ankylosis is complete, the extent and locations of the bone formation give some indication of prognosis. Posterior ossification about the hip and anterior bridges at the elbow are less likely to be resected successfully than anterior hip or posterior elbow bridges.[10] Interestingly, the joint itself is seldom destroyed by the prolonged immobilization of bony ankyloses, at least not in the 1 to 2 years that usually elapse between onset and surgery. This is also true in prolonged ischemic contractures.

Central nervous system surgery for spasticity

Several spinal cord procedures have been used to modify or control spasticity and other disorders of motor overactivity, such as dystonia. Walty and co-workers[56] have used *spinal cord stimulation* for spasticity in cerebral palsy and after stroke or head injury. Multilead electrodes were applied to the dorsal aspect of the spinal cord at the C4 level via laminectomy; various combinations of stimulus pattern and

frequency were studied to obtain the best response for each patient. Unilateral posttraumatic spasticity was helped, but long-term results are not available. This type of treatment is invasive and potentially hazardous but may lead to better understanding of the pathophysiology of spasticity.

When there is some voluntary function, all surgery directed at the spinal cord is apt to be associated with instances of reduced function. Since Fasano developed *selective posterior rhizotomy,* numerous surgeons have performed it, often in multiple sclerosis patients.[1,12,20] Sensory fasicles that produce muscle contractions when stimulated are divided. This operation is designed to reduce spasticity without producing a major sensory deficit. Since fascicles in the posterior roots are mixed, loss of skin sensation must occur. The surgery is extensive and tedious and not supported by animal study findings. Nevertheless, this type of therapy is now under active investigation and may well offer improved results once the techniques have been carefully developed and evaluated.

Various spinal cord incision procedures have been proposed to reduce intractable spasticity. *Lumbar myelotomy,* the longitudinal incision of the lower spinal cord in the frontal plane, seems to reduce the severe flexor spasticity seen in some cases of multiple sclerosis and spinal cord disease.[1,36] These procedures are used mainly for lower limb spasticity. The cord is incised in the sagittal and frontal planes to interrupt the reflex paths between anterior and posterior horns while attempting to avoid corticospinal tract injury. Only a few cases are reported in each series, but some results appear excellent. Interestingly, when the leg spasticity was eliminated by L1-S1 myelotomy, function in the arms improved.

Total destruction of spinal cord function has resulted from *alcohol or phenol intraspinal injections.* These procedures are somewhat difficult to control, and bladder function may deteriorate.

Embolization of the artery of Adamkiewicz to the lower thoracic and lumbar cord segments has been performed in intractable spasticity.[46] This reduced femoral and obturator nerve spasticity in paraplegia but not in quadriplegia. Unfortunately, this procedure leads to unpredictable neurologic effects because the anatomic distribution of the subject artery is variable.

Penn and Kroin[37] have injected the spinal reflex blocking agent baclofen directly into the intrathecal space via an implanted continuous infusion pump. This technology may offer prolonged relief of spasticity without the side effects of systemic administration of the drug. Preliminary results have been encouraging.

SUMMARY

Spastic paralysis presents many patterns, depending on the location and severity of the underlying disease. Cognitive and sensory deficits accompany it making rehabilitation more difficult. Nevertheless, the preservation of function and the reduction of spasticity (when necessary) have been the goals of physicians, orthopedists, and neurosurgeons. Aided by dedicated nurses, physical therapists, and orthotists, medical efforts can improve the outlook for many patients. The early application of effective surgical techniques can lead to better limb use when the specific goals are understood and when proper planning has defined the surgical plan.

For the last hundred years much attention has been directed at the intellectual training, functional exercising, and surgical correction of children with spasticity; the study of adults with spastic disorders is more recent. The increased number of adults with spasticity and their increased survival rate has presented rehabilitation specialists and orthopedic surgeons with a challenge and an opportunity. The lessons learned from treating cerebral palsy can be applied to many adults when the multiple deficits and particular vulnerabilities of individual patients are evaluated properly. Similarly, the lessons learned from treating adult stroke can be applied to children—especially information about the necessity for early and effective treatment and the requirement for careful evaluation to avoid prolonging less successful programs.

ACKNOWLEDGMENT

Douglas Barlow assisted in the preparation of material for this chapter. Funding was provided by New York University School of Medicine. Elizabeth Lusskin provided word processing and editorial assistance in manuscript preparation.

REFERENCES

1. Benedetti, A, and Colombo, F: Spinal surgery for spasticity (46 cases), Neurochirurgia 24:195, 1981.
2. Broun, RM, et al: Surgical treatment of the painful shoulder contracture in the stroke patient, J Bone Joint Surg 53A:1307, 1971.
3. Brunnstrom, S: Movement therapy in hemiplegia, New York, 1970, Harper & Row.
4. Burke, D: A reassessment of the muscle spindle contribution to muscle tone in normal and spastic man. In Feldman, RG, Young, RR, and Knoells, WP, editors. Spasticity: disordered motor control, Chicago, 1980, Year Book Medical Publishers.
5. Clemente, CD: Neurophysiologic mechanisms and neuroanatomic substrates related to spasticity, Neurology 28:40, 1978.
6. Debenedetti, M: Restoration of elbow extension power in the tetraplegic patient using the Mobery technique, J Hand Surg 4:86, 1979.
7. Dunkerley, DR: The role of surgery in rehabilitation, Int Rehab Med 7:39, 1985.
8. Fulton, JF, and Kennart, MA: A study of flaccid and spastic paralysis produced by lesions of the cerebral cortex in primates, Res Publ Assoc Nerv Ment Dis 13:158, 1934.
9. Gaines, RW, and Ford, TB: A systematic approach to the amount of Achilles tendon lengthening in cerebral palsy, J Pediatr Orthop 4:448, 1984.
10. Gartland, DE: Head injuries in adults. In Nickel, V, editor: Orthopedic rehabilitation, New York, 1982, Churchill-Livingstone.
11. Gartland, DE, Thompson, R, and Waters, RL: Musculocutaneous neurotomy for spastic elbow flexion in non-functional upper limb extremities in adults, J Bone Joint Surg 62A:108, 1980.
12. Heimburger, RF, Slominski, A, and Griswold, P: Posterior cervical rhizotomy for reducing spasticity in cerebral palsy, J Neurosurg 39:30, 1973.
13. Henty, VR, Brown, M, and Keoshian, LA: Upper limb reconstruction in quadriplegia: functional assessment and proposed treatment modifications, J Hand Surg 8:119, 1983.
14. Hines, M: The "motor" cortex, Bull Johns Hopkins Hosp 60:313, 1937.
15. Inglis, AC, and Cooper, W: Release of the flexor-pronator origin for flexion deformities of the hand and wrist in spastic paralysis, J Bone Joint Surg 48:847, 1966.
16. Jordan, C, and Walter, RL: Stroke. In Nickel, V, editor: Orthopedic rehabilitation; New York, 1982, Churchill-Livingstone.
17. Khalili, AA, and Betts, HB: Peripheral nerve block with phenol in the management of spasticity, JAMA 200:1155, 1967.
18. Keenan, MA, et al: Surgical correction of spastic equinovarus deformity in the adult head trauma patient, Foot Ankle 5:35, 1984.
19. Keenan, MA, et al: Intrinsic toe flexor deformity following correction of spastic equinovarus deformity in adults, Foot Ankle 7:333, 1987.
20. Laitinen, LV, Nilsson, SN and Fugl-Meyer, AR: Selective posterior rhizotomy for treatment of spasticity, J Neurosurg 58:895, 1983.
21. Lusskin, R: The influence of errors in bracing upon deformities of the lower extremity, Arch Phys Med Rehab 47:520, 1966.
22. Lusskin, R: Peripheral neuropathies affecting the foot: traumatic, ischemic and compressive disorders. In Jahss, M, editor: Disorders of the foot, Philadelphia, 1982, WB Saunders Co.
23. Lusskin, R, Grynbaum, BB, and Dhir, RS: Rehabilitation surgery in adult spastic hemiplegia, Clin Orthop 63:132, 1969.
24. Lusskin, R, Grynbaum, BB, and Dhir, RS: Peripheral surgery after stroke, Geriatrics 26:65, 1971.
25. Manske, PR: Redirection of extensor pollicis longus in the treatment of spastic thumb-in-palm deformity, J Hand Surg 10A:553, 1985.
26. Mathews, PBC: Muscle spindles: their messengers and their fusimotor supply. In Brooks, UB, editor: Handbook of physiology, vol 11, Bethesda, Md, 1981, American Physiological Society.
27. McColloch, WS, Graf, C, and Magoun, HW: A cortico-bulbo-reticular pathway from area 4-S, J Neurophysiol 11:501, 1948.
28. McCollough, N: Orthotic management in adult hemiplegia, Clin Orthop 131:38, 1978.
29. Moberg, E: Surgical treatment for absent single hand grip and elbow extension in quadriplegia, J Bone Joint Surg 57A:196, 1975.
30. Mooney, V, Perry, J, and Nickel, V: Surgical and nonsurgical orthopaedic care of stroke, J Bone Joint Surg 49A:989, 1967.
31. Moscana, AR, Keret, D, and Reis, ND: The gastrocnemius muscle flap in the correction of severe flexion contracture of the knee, Arch Orthop Traumatic Surg 200:139, 1982.
32. Norlin, R, and Tkaczuk, H: One session surgery for correction of lower extremity deformities in children with cerebral palsy, J Pediatr Orthop 5:208, 1985.
33. Ono, K, et al: Reconstructive surgery of the limb in the braindamaged adult, Med J Osaka Univ 20:245, 1970.
34. Otis, JC, et al: Biomechanical measurement of spastic plantarflexors, Dev Med Child Neurol 25:60, 1983.
35. Otis, JC, Root, L, and Kroll, MA: Measurement of plantar flexor spasticity during treatment with tone-reducing casts, J Pediatr Orthop 5:682, 1985.
36. Padovani, R, et al: The treatment of spasticity by means of dorsal longitudinal myelotomy and lozenge shaped grisotomy, Spine 7:103, 1982.
37. Penn, RD, and Kroin, JS: Long-term intrathecal baclofen infusion for treatment of spasticity, J Neurosurg 66:181, 1987.
38. Perry, J, and Walters, RL: Orthopaedic evaluation and treatment of the stroke patient. Instructional course lectures, Am Acad Orthop Surg 24:51, 1975.
39. Perry, J, Waters, RL, and Pervin, T: Electromyographic analysis of equinovarus following stroke, Clin Orthop 131:47, 1978.

40. Petrillo, RP, Chu, DS, and Davis, SW: Phenol block of the tibial nerve in the hemiplegic patient, Orthopedics 3:871, 1980.
41. Pinzur, MS: Surgery to achieve dynamic motor balance in adult acquired spastic hemiplegia, a preliminary report, J Hand Surg 10A:547, 1985.
42. Pinzur, MS, et al: Adult onset hemiplegia: changes in gait after muscle balancing procedures to correct the equinus deformity, J Bone Joint Surg 68A:1249, 1986.
43. Rhines, R, and Magoun, HW: Brain stem facilitation of cortical motor response, J Neurophysiol 9:219, 1946.
44. Roper, BA: Rehabilitation after a stroke, J Bone Joint Surg 64B:156, 1982.
45. Sherman, R, et al: Multiple factor gait analysis in acquired hemiplegia, Orthop Trans 9:370, 1985.
46. Shibasaki, K, Nakai, S, and Higuchi, M: Percutaneous embolization of major spinal cord artery as a treatment of intractable spasticity, Paraplegia 20:158, 1982.
47. Sindou, M, et al: Traitement du pied spastique par la neurotomic selective du nerf tibial; rusultats sur un serie de 31 cas, Neurochirurgie 31:189, 1985.
48. Smith, RJ: Flexor pollicus longus abductor plasty for spastic thumb-in-palm deformity, J Hand Surg 7:327, 1982.
49. Sprague, JM, et al: Reticulospinal influences on stretch reflexes, J Neurophysiol 11:501, 1948.
50. Stover, SL, Niemann, KMW, and Miller, JM, III: Disodium etidronate in the prevention of postoperative recurrence of heterotopic ossification in spinal-cord injury patients, J Bone Joint Surg 58A:683, 1976.
51. Tracy, WH: Operative treatment of the plantar-flexed inverted foot in adult hemiplegia, J Bone Joint Sug 58A:1142, 1976.
52. Treanor, WJ, and Riefenstein, GH: Potential reversibility of the hemiplegic posture; results of reconstructive surgical proceedings, Am J Cardiol 7:370, 1961.
53. Vanderwerf, GJIM, and Tonino, AJ: Transposition of the posterior tibial tendon in spastic equinovarus, Arch Orthop Trauma Surg 103:128, 1984.
54. Walters, RL: Upper extremity surgery in stroke patients, Clin Orthop 131:30, 1978.
55. Walters, RL, Perry, J, and Garland, D: Surgical correction of gait abnormalities following stroke, Clin Orthop 131:54, 1978.
56. Walty, JM, Reynolds, LO, and Riklan, M: Multilead spinal cord stimulation for control of motor disorders; seminar on spinal cord stimulation, New York, 1980, Appl Neurophysiol 44:244, 1981.
57. Wharton, GW, and Morgan, TH: Ankylosis in the paralyzed patient, J Bone Joint Surg 52A:105, 1970.
58. Young, RR, and Delwaide, PJ: Spasticity, N Engl J Med 304:28, 1981.

CHAPTER 39

Conditions affecting the cervical spine

HOWARD G. THISTLE

This chapter concerns the diagnosis and management of common conditions affecting the cervical spine. Many cervical problems do not produce symptoms in the neck but rather symptoms in the shoulder, arm, head, chest, or even the lower extremities. Therefore, pain in the shoulder does not necessarily mean the cause is "intrinsic," since it may have its origin distant to the joint itself.[89] Compression of a cervical root may, for example, produce minimal neck symptoms but reflect severe pain and paresthesias to the muscles and appropriate dermatome supplied by that root. If this involves the shoulder girdle, there may be marked local spasm with restriction of shoulder motion, thus mimicking primary shoulder pathology. Conversely, pain may be referred to the neck from other sites, for example, from angina. Concomitant pain may often occur in neck and shoulder and be causally related,[45] and the patient may have a mixed picture of symptoms. Therefore, without careful history taking and proper examination, the physician may be misled. The perfection of computerized tomography (with or without contrast) and introduction of magnetic resonance imaging has enabled better visualization of the cervical spine and therefore a more precise diagnosis. However, the patient's symptoms and signs must be correlated with the radiologic findings and with the pathologic changes responsible for the symptoms.[8] It is therefore essential to develop a systematic approach to the problem for proper diagnosis, for prescribing appropriate definitive therapy, and for effective results.[93]

The patient's symptoms may be acute and severe with minimal radiographic abnormality, or patients with gross radiologic changes may have no symptoms at all. Pain originating in the neck, shoulder, arm, hand, or head frequently results from irritation of cervical roots in the region of the intervertebral foramen, encroachment of the vascular supply in the vertebral canal, or invasion of the spinal cord.[12] This usually results from encroachment on space or impairment of movement and presents as pain, muscle spasm, limitation of motion, muscle weakness or wasting, or paresthesias—all or any in combination.

Since many patients with cervical spine disorders have shoulder and arm pain, it is helpful to understand the possible sites of origin. The modified classification of Craig and Witt[21] is helpful in this regard (see box).

ANATOMIC AND PATHOLOGIC CONSIDERATIONS

The basic anatomy of the cervical spine and its surrounding structures has been well described in standard anatomy texts. The reader should refer to these sources for this information; however, several points regarding the functional anatomy and related pathology should be noted here.

Motion

Motions from the second through the seventh cervical vertebrae consist of forward flexion, extension, rotation, and lateral flexion. Normally motion is in a gradual intersegmented flow pattern and is greatest in the upper part of the cervical spine.[27] At the interspace between the first and second cervical vertebrae, movement can occur independently. At both the atlantooccipital and atlantoaxial joints, there is normally 15 degrees of flexion and extension, and 45 degrees of rotation is possible to either side, with the odontoid process as the pivotal point.[40] As stated by Jackson,[46] the plane of the articular surfaces prevents lateral bending without some degree of rotation and rotation without some degree of lateral bending. Maximum flexion and extension occur in the region of C4 to C6, and this portion has the most wear and tear.[12] Any undue laxity of the joint structures allows subluxations of the joint or an abnormal range of motion between the articular surfaces.

CLASSIFICATION OF CONDITIONS PRODUCING PAIN IN THE SHOULDER AND ARM

I. Local
   A. Cuff injuries
   B. Bursitis
   C. Arthritis
   D. Fractures
   E. Tumors
   F. Immobilization
II. Vertebral column
   A. Fractures
   B. Arthritis
   C. Protruded disc
   D. Spondylitis
   E. Spondylosis
III. Spinal cord
   A. Syringomyelia
   B. Poliomyelitis
   C. Herpes zoster
   D. Tumors
IV. Brachial plexus
   A. Trauma
   B. Mechanical
      1. Cervical rib
      2. Scalene syndrome
      3. Costoclavicular syndrome
V. Peripheral nerves
   A. Trauma
   B. Tumors
   C. Neuritis
   D. Carpal tunnel syndrome
VI. Thorax
   A. Cardiac
   B. Diaphragm
   C. Sternal lesions
VII. Abdomen
   A. Gallbladder
   B. Diaphragm
VIII. Peripheral vascular
   A. Periarteritis nodosa
   B. Raynaud's disease
   C. Phlebitis
   D. Aneurysm

From Thistle, HG: Med Clin North Am 53:512, 1969.

Joints

There are three joints between each two adjacent vertebrae—the posterior or apophyseal joints, the secondary fibrocartilaginous joint (or the joint that is made by the fibrocartilaginous disc), and the adjacent surfaces of the vertebral bodies.[45] In addition, between the second and third and each subsequent vertebrae, there are two small lateral joints between the vertebral bodies. These joints are referred to as the Luschka joints, uncovertebral joints (Jackson[45]

refers to them as the lateral interbody joints). In 1858, Luschka[63] described true synovial joints situated at the posterolateral aspect of the second to seventh cervical vertebral bodies. Trolard[96] later called these articulations uncovertebrales in 1892. However, in 1960, Orofino and co-workers,[79] in studying coronal sections of the cervical spine in the fetus from the third to seventh cervical vertebrae, failed to demonstrate the presence of synovium in the region of the uncinate processes. They therefore must be considered pseudoarthroses. Orofino further stated that the changes seen in radiographs and attributed to degenerative arthritis or protruded intervertebral discs are caused by reactive osteogenesis. Hadley[37] described this new bone formation as a response to the repeated minor stresses of aging that result in collapse of the intervertebral disc. Jackson[45] suggested that the process may be hastened by external trauma.

These joints are of clinical importance for several reasons. They insulate the intervertebral discs at the posterolateral margins of the vertebral bodies and prevent the extrusion of disc material. Also, they are subject to injury, especially from lateral or oblique forces. They help to form the anterior walls of the intervertebral canals and in the presence of disease may irritate or compress the cervical roots and their accompanying vascular and sympathetic structures. Nathan,[74] in studying a series of 400 vertebral columns for the presence of osteophytes, found the incidence of osteophytes to be greater on the posterior aspect than on the anterior aspect of the cervical vertebral bodies. Morton[73] stated that nerve symptoms are more frequently caused by Luschka joint exostoses than by osteophytes arising from the apophyseal joints. Friedenberg and colleagues[31] observed that osteophytes developing from the "joints of Luschka" of the cervical spine may impinge on the vertebral arteries and their accompanying plexuses as they pass through the foramina in the transverse processes. This was also confirmed by Sheehan and co-workers,[86] who studied vertebral-basilar artery insufficiency from cervical spondylosis in 46 patients with recurrent symptoms.

The posterior articulations, "facets," are true joints, lined with synovium and lubricated by synovial fluid within the joint capsule. They are termed apophyseal joints.[12] They are capable of degenerative changes, referred to as osteoarthritis joint changes, and production of osteophytes.

Cervical discs

Nerve root compression from disc herniation in the cervical area is infrequent.[12] Unlike the lumbar area, in the cervical area disc material is rarely extruded posterolaterally or posteriorly.[45] If extruded posteriorly, it causes compression of the spinal cord rather than nerve roots. Such protrusions are limited by a number of factors: none of the nerve root fibers pass over the intervertebral disc; the nerves exit from the vertebral canal at the lateral extremes of the canal; the Luschka joints separate the nerve from the disc anulus; the anulus is thicker posteriorly and is reinforced by the two layers of the posterior longitudinal ligament; and the shape of the disc tends to keep the nucleus in the wider anterior portion. According to Jackson,[45] posterior extrusions might occur if there is undue relaxation, weakness, or an actual tear in the posterior longitudinal ligament and anulus. Most extrusions occur anteriorly or anterolaterally. When extrusions occur, they may be composed of "soft" or "hard" disc material[8]—the former mostly nuclear material and the latter mostly anular tissue—or osteophytes may form at the periosteal ligamentous attachment with calcification of the extruded disc material.[31]

Nerves

After leaving the cervical spinal cord, the dorsal sensory and ventral motor roots combine to enter the intervertebral foramen. After emerging from the foramen, the mixed nerve divides in posterior and anterior rami.

The first cervical nerve emerges between the occiput and atlas, necessitating that the other seven exit *above* the corresponding vertebrae, except for the eighth nerve, which emerges between C7 and T1. The first two cervical nerves do not pass through intervertebral foramen and, after leaving the spinal canal, travel mostly through muscle.[12] They are primarily sensory and supply the posterior and lateral portions of the scalp. They are joined by branches of C3 in forming the greater and lesser occipital nerves. The remaining nerves exit through intervertebral foramen and normally occupy only one fifth to one fourth of the cervical foraminal diameter.[8] The remainder of the space is filled with soft tissues, which may be subject to inflammation and its related sequelae. The position and angulation as the nerve passes through the foramen vary greatly, and the nerve is protected by its covering. Arachnoid and dural sleeves enclose the roots as they enter the foramen; each sleeve is separated by its interradicular septum. Once outside the foramen, the arachnoid and dura blend with the nerve sheath where the arachnoid layer ends. Here the root is covered by a periradicular sheath, which later becomes the epineural sheath of the brachial plexus. The periradicular sheath, through its bony attachments, prevents avulsion of the root from the spinal cord during a traction injury. Often there are intercommunicating fibers between two or three nerve roots, making localization of nerve root irritation difficult.[45] At the foraminal level the dorsal sensory and ventral motor components of the cervical nerve roots are often clearly demarcated and are both subject to compromise.[32] The dorsal sensory nerve roots are larger than the motor nerve roots and are located mostly in the upper portion of the foramen rostral and posterior, whereas the motor nerve roots are ventral and caudal to the sensory nerve roots and located in the lower half of the foramen.[92]

The autonomic nervous system is divided into sympathetic and parasympathetic systems. In the cervical region, Laurelle[54] found that sympathetic cell bodies are present in the cervical portion of the spinal cord at the base of the anterior horns from C4 through C8. These preganglionic sympathetic fibers leave the spinal cord with the somatic motor nerve fibers in the ventral roots of C5 through T1. Symptoms attributed to the sympathetic nervous system have been relieved by surgical decompression of the nerve root within the intervertebral foramen. Neuwirth[75] contrasts symptoms and signs related to somatic sensory and motor nerve fibers that are confined to their own areas of distribution with those of cervicosympathetic origin that have a wide topography of clinical manifestations. The sympathetic nerve trunk in the cervical area is composed of superior, middle, and inferior ganglia connected by intervening cords. The efferent branches proceed to the viscera of the neck and chest, and the afferent branches form the vertebral nerve. The vertebral nerve plexus surrounds the vertebral arteries, at least from C4 to C8, and follows the arteries through the arterial foramen of the cervical transverse process. This nerve can be mechanically irritated as it follows the vertebral artery along its course. The parasympathetic system is connected with the central nervous system in the cervical area through the oculomotor, facial, glossopharyngeal, and vagus nerves and through the cranial nerve roots of the spinal accessory nerve.[59]

Muscles and ligaments

The muscles and ligaments bear the brunt of the stresses related to movements, positional changes, and various degrees of trauma.[12] The ligaments, although lax enough to permit a great range of motion, are sufficiently resilient to control motion. Extending downward from the occipital condyles and attaching to the odontoid are the alar ligaments, which limit skull and atlas rotation on the axis. The accessory atlantoaxial ligament similarly limits rotation in this area. The transverse ligament holds the atlas to the odontoid process as it moves around it. If the odontoid is fractured, this ligament will prevent posterior dislocation of the odontoid but not anterior dislocation unless other ligaments are intact.[45] From C2 to C7 the anterior and posterior longitudinal ligaments reinforce the disc anulus and capsular ligaments and limit transverse vertebral gliding motion, as well as flexion and extension. The ligamentum flavum reinforces the apophyseal joints.

Perry and Nickel[81] divided the neck muscles into two major functional groups: the capital movers, which flex and extend the head, and cervical muscles, which flex the cervical spine. In addition, the splenius capitis and cervicis act as rotators.

Other muscles that contribute to motion are the sternocleidomastoid, scalenus, upper trapezius, and levator scapulae. In evaluating function of the cervical spine, spasm or paralysis of these muscles must be considered.

DIAGNOSIS
History

Often from a careful history alone one can postulate a diagnosis that can be confirmed by examination.[93] Inquiry must be made into past history, especially as related to trauma; into all characteristics of the pain, particularly with regard to onset, precipitating factors, relationship to movements of the neck or arm, coughing or sneezing, and patterns of radiation; into measures or maneuvers affording relief or aggravation; and into associated symptoms such as paresthesias, limitation of motion, and weakness.

Examination

For proper examination some clothing must be removed; examination through clothing enhances the danger of misdiagnosis.

Posture

The patient's general posture is observed for deviations from its normal curvatures, such as exaggerated lordosis, kyphosis, or scoliosis; for tilt of the head to one side; and for winging of the scapula. Loss of cervical lordosis or lateral tilt of the head may lead one to detect muscle spasm, scoliosis to unilateral muscle weakness, or degenerative cervical changes with a compensatory cervical curvature. Sagging shoulder girdles may indicate muscular weakness or faulty posture with consequent constant overstretching of shoulder musculature or the cervical plexus. Winging of a scapula may identify weakness of the trapezius or serratus anterior muscle; elevation of a shoulder may indicate upper trapezius spasm.

Motion of the cervical spine

It is important to observe and record ranges of motion in the cervical spine, not only as an aid in diagnosis but also as a baseline for measuring progress in treatment. Limitations of motion may be manifest in the presence of muscle spasm (for example, of the trapezius, sternocleidomastoid, or paraspinal muscles) as well as in osteoarthritis or cervical spondylosis. Abnormally excessive motion, such as that secondary to ligamentous tear, is usually not demonstrable clinically because of associated protective muscle spasm but may be evident on radiographs taken with the neck in stress positions or by cineradiography.

Palpation of the posterior spinous processes

The posterior cervical spinous processes may be palpated with the spine in a slightly flexed position. Radiation of pain into the shoulder girdle or arm resulting from forward pressure of the examiner's thumb on a posterior spinous process is suggestive of abnormal motion at that level with associated nerve root irritation.

Palpation of muscles

The muscles of the neck, shoulder girdle, and arm should be palpated for evidence of focal spasm and tenderness, so-called trigger points. Palpation of these, if extremely sensitive, may reproduce referral of pain to other areas. Frequent sites of trigger points are in the upper trapezius muscle, rhomboids, infraspinatus muscle, deltoid origin and

insertion, and in the long head of the biceps in the bicipital groove.

Palpation of the cervical plexus and scalene muscles

The cervical roots and plexus can be palpated in the supraclavicular fossa, as they emerge from between the scalene muscles, and also high in the axilla. Palpation of the roots and plexus that produces pain radiating down the arm is strong evidence for radiculitis. The scalene muscles are also palpated for evidence of spasm or local tenderness.

Head and shoulder compression tests

The examination should always include the application of pressure on the top of the patient's head with the neck in a rotated and laterally flexed position—Spurling's maneuver.[88] Pain in the shoulder or arm elicited by this maneuver indicates nerve root irritation. If pain is confined to the neck, injury or disorder of the cervical joints may be present. Referred pain produced by downward pressure of the shoulder with the head rotated to the opposite side[45] similarly suggests a radicular origin.

Inspection and palpation of the subacromial bursa and rotator cuff

Presence of local heat, swelling, and pain on palpation over the subacromial bursa are characteristics of acute bursitis. Chronic or acute injury to the rotator cuff may be suspected if there is pain on palpation of the cuff—commencing anteriorly and progressing posteriorly, palpating the tendonous insertions of the subscapularis, supraspinatous, infraspinatous, and teres minor, respectively.

Codman's jog and wince test

When downward pressure is applied on the patient's abducted arm, a sudden release of pressure produces a rebound upward impingement of the humeral greater tuberosity against the acromion process. If pain is produced in the shoulder by this maneuver (Codman's jog and wince test),[16] it is strongly suggestive of an inflamed bursa or a rotator cuff syndrome.

Range of motion of the shoulder girdle

All ranges of motion should be measured and recorded accurately. These motions normally take place at the sternoclavicular, acromioclavicular, scapulothoracic, and the glenohumeral joints, producing a smoothly integrated motion referred to as scapulohumeral rhythm.[44]

Motions at the glenohumeral joint consist of flexion, extension, internal and external rotation, adduction, abduction, and circumduction. With abduction and flexion of the glenohumeral joint, motion also occurs between the scapula and thorax and at the sternoclavicular and acromioclavicular joints. Motions of the scapula include elevation, depression, protraction, retraction, and rotation in upward and downward planes. The presence of pain with various shoulder motions must be noted and localized. Muscle spasm or injury to tendons or ligaments may be painful when the tendons or ligaments are stretched.

Palpation and test for bicipital tendonitis

To palpate the head of the biceps tendon in the bicipital groove, the humerus must be externally rotated to expose the tendon. Pain on rolling the tendon in the groove is suggestive of a bicipital tendonitis. Yergason's sign, elicited by flexing the elbow and having the patient forcefully supinate the foramen against resistance, is positive for bicipital tendonitis if the patient experiences pain in the region of the bicipital groove.

Maneuvers for neurovascular compression syndromes

Various maneuvers have been described to identify compression of the axillary vessels or brachial plexus owing to tightness or spasm of the scalene muscles or to cervical ribs. Although these maneuvers are helpful, they are not infallible,[61] and results must be interpreted in context with other clinical signs and symptoms. For example, the diagnosis of claviculocostal syndrome would be suspect if one manually obliterated the radial pulse and then reduplicated the symptoms by having the patient bring the shoulders back and down, with additional passive pressure from the examiner.[12] However, this maneuver may obliterate the radial pulse in many patients who present no symptoms, thus being of no significance. By contrast, in a study of 20 cases of clinically documented thoracic outlet syndrome, Glassberg[34] found the thoracic outlet stress test to be positive in 16 cases (80%). To perform this test, both arms are hyperabducted with the elbows flexed at 90 degrees; the hands are opened and closed for up to 3 minutes. It is significant that a supraclavicular bruit was heard in one third of the patients during the test and supraclavicular tenderness was present in 12.

Examination should include muscles supplied by cranial nerves, as well as careful grading and recording of strength in the muscles of the shoulder girdle and arm. Upper and lower extremity reflexes and sensory modalities should also be tested and noted. In the event of compression of a nerve root by a protruded cervical disc or a foraminal osteophyte, one would expect weakness in muscles supplied by that root, with possible loss of an appropriate tendon reflex and a segmental sensory deficit. If there is cervical cord compression, lower extremity reflexes may be hyperactive with plantar extensor responses.

Laboratory tests, electromyography, and radiographs

Where needed, appropriate laboratory tests, electrodiagnostic procedures, and radiographs may aid in establishing a diagnosis. Electromyography, especially, is extremely helpful in revealing early denervation and in differentiating a neuropathy from a myopathy. Nerve damage, however, may not show abnormal findings for up to 3 weeks. Nerve conduction studies can be similarly invaluable in the differentiation from, as well as the localization of, peripheral nerve entrapments; for example, they can be of great importance in differentiating between carpal tunnel syndrome and radicular cervical root pain when the sensory deficit in the hand and the rest of the extremity is equivocal or when pain is referred proximally into the forearm and shoulder from a median nerve compressed in the carpal tunnel.[82] Sensory evoked potentials may be helpful when there is a question of cervical myelopathy.

Appropriate radiographs of the cervical spine are often helpful diagnostically and should include, in addition to the standard anteroposterior and lateral views, oblique views to demonstrate a possible foraminal disorder. In cases of cervical trauma, views of the odontoid process should also be obtained. In instances of acute trauma or of recurring episodes of neurologic symptoms, stress films in flexion and extension or cineradiography may be helpful in identifying a site of instability or of abnormal motion. Roentgenograms of the shoulder to demonstrate the possible presence of calcium deposits, local osteoporosis, osteoarthritis, or other pathologic findings should be obtained in both internal and external rotation for greatest visualization.

In a recent prospective study in evaluating cervical radiculopathy, Modic and associates[71] compared the findings at surgery with those of surface coil magnetic resonance imaging (SCMR), metrizamide myelography (MM), and computerized tomography with metrizamide (CTM). They found that all three were equal for identifying disease level. CTM was most specific for identifying the type of disease and was most advantageous in contrasting bone from soft tissue without contrast material. MM provided the best images of the entire cervical spine, except where there was a block, but this method must be weighed against the need for hospitalization and its invasiveness. SCMR provided a variable alternative to the MM and, when combined with computerized tomography, provided the best examination of the cervical region.

CONSERVATIVE TREATMENT OPTIONS

The aims of conservative treatment are to relieve pain, reduce inflammation, relax muscle spasm, protect the injured part to allow healing, rebuild muscle power, and restore normal ranges of motion and function in activities of daily living.[93]

Medications
Analgesics

Since cervical spine disease may be chronic and recurrent, use of narcotics should be avoided whenever possible. Acetominophen, acetylsalicylic acid, and associated compounds can be given on a regular basis, as tolerated, and 600 mg of acetylsalicylic acid can be given as needed for pain (600 to 1500 mg four times a day as required for an anti-inflammatory effect with maintenance of a blood level of 20 to 30 mg/dl). Gastric irritation may be reduced by using buffered or enteric coated preparations.

Anti-inflammatory agents

Corticosteroids have potent anti-inflammatory activity; however, benefits must be weighed against undesirable effects, and prolonged excessive doses should be avoided. They may be given orally or by local injection. The route of administration and dosage often depend on the experience of the practitioner.

The nonsteroidal anti-inflammatory drugs (NSAIDS) have anti-inflammatory and analgesic effects. They act by inhibiting the cyclo-oxygenase pathway of arachidonic acid breakdown. Their clinical affects are variable, since each patient may respond differently. Therefore it may be necessary to try a number of different drugs before finding an effective one. The half-life of each medication may help determine the dosage; those with a short half-life (for example, ibuprofen) are given three to four times daily; those with longer half-lives, only once daily (for example, piroxicam). These medications have potentially serious side effects and contraindications and must be carefully monitored.

Muscle relaxants

Commonly prescribed muscle relaxants have been studied for their effectiveness in reducing muscle spasm in a variety of musculoskeletal disorders. The effectiveness of carisoprodol,[3] cyclobenzaprine,[11] diazepam,[39] and methocarbamol[35] have been reported singly and in combination and found to have varying effectiveness. The choice of muscle relaxant and effectiveness may also depend on the experiences of physician and patient.

Sedatives, tranquilizers, and antidepressants

Acute cervical injuries may result in extreme anxiety and depression so that the use of psychotropic medication may be helpful. Imipramine, a tricyclic antidepressant, was found in one study to be more effective than placebo in controlling chronic low back pain.[2] However, since cervical spine problems may become chronic, the use of sedatives and tranquilizers must be carefully monitored.

Anesthetics

Injection of trigger point areas of local muscle spasm with procaine is frequently effective in relieving local pain and muscle spasm[20] and increasing mobility. These trigger points often correlate with acupuncture points for pain.[68] Ethyl chloride or fluoride spray may be similarly effective.

Physical modalities
Heat

The rationale for using local heat in relieving muscle spasm and reducing inflammation has been well established.

Moist hot packs, such as Hydrocollator packs applied for 20 to 30 minutes, induce muscle relaxation reflexly by heating the skin. Short-wave diathermy applied for 20 minutes to the cervical spine or shoulder provides somewhat deeper heating. It is capable of heating musculature itself, as well as skin and subcutaneous tissues, and thus may have a direct effect on the spindle mechanism, in addition to muscle relaxation triggered reflexively through excitation of exteroceptors of the skin.[69] However, this advantage must be weighed against the expense involved. Ultrasound is also effective in heating deeper ligamentous and joint structures. Its dosage ranges from 0.8 to 1.5 watts/cm² for periods of 5 to 10 minutes. In combination with electrical stimulation, it may also be effective in relieving trigger points and providing an alternating contraction and relaxation of muscle.

Cold

The application of cold may be more effective than heat in reducing muscle spasm and associated pain. Cold applied to the skin reduces local circulation, the local metabolic rate, and the rate of conduction of impulses by peripheral nerves.[93] Edema resulting from trauma is decreased by cold application.[57] It can be applied in the form of cold packs for 15 to 20 minutes. Massaging of muscles with ice is another effective, safe, and inexpensive way to employ cold in the management of neuromuscular problems.[97]

Massage

Massage is useful in relaxing muscle spasm and improving blood flow. Too often, however, it is ordered as a substitute for more specific treatment. Since it is time consuming for a therapist and patients become fond of it quickly, it should be ordered only when specifically needed and then only for a limited time.[93]

Exercise

For conditions of the cervical spine and shoulder, a variety of types of exercises are useful. Local muscle spasm, for example, in the trapezius, often responds to maximum contraction against resistance followed by relaxation. For limited ranges of motion and tight painful muscles at the shoulder, pendulum exercises are indicated. These must be done with the arm hanging loosely and the scapular muscles relaxed. As motion increases, they are executed with a weight in the hand, progressing to wall climbing with the fingers, and later to the use of a shoulder wheel. Passive motion is to be avoided, since the production of additional pain leads only to further muscle spasm with a decrease in motion. When there are postural problems, postural exercises should be prescribed. If there is muscle weakness, resistance exercises are indicated, either with manual resistance by the therapist or by using weights or exercise equipment such as isokinetic or variable-resistance equipment. Lower extremity weaknesses and gait disturbances may be helped by using reciprocal exercise equipment such as a stationary bicycle.

Loss of function in the arm or hand may require occupational therapy. Restorative exercises for weakness and visual compensatory training for sensory deficits are important. Training in activities of daily living skills, including homemaking and the use of self-help devices, may restore a patient's independence.

Cervical traction

Traction may be applied in a constant or intermittent form and in the vertical or horizontal position. The technique of traction used and the position of the patient depend on the equipment available and the acuteness of the condition. Constant traction produces some degree of immobilization of the cervical spine and helps to relieve muscle spasm and pain. Correctly applied, it straightens the cervical spine and enlarges the intervertebral foramina to relieve compressive or irritative forces on the roots.[45]

In some instances intermittent traction is more effective in overcoming paracervical muscle spasm. It can be applied manually or with a motorized intermittent traction machine (Figure 39-1, *A*). It has been my experience, however, that in acute conditions intermittent traction may increase symptoms. This type of traction can be adjusted to the weight, period of traction, and period of relaxation desired. Traction and relaxation timing is in seconds and usually arbitrarily selected according to clinical experience. During the traction phase the paracervical muscles tend to resist the forces of pull by contracting, whereas during the nontraction phase, they relax as the forces are reduced to zero. The result is a massagelike effect leading to reduced muscle spasm and more effective subsequent traction. Because of its relaxation phase, intermittent traction permits the application of greater weights with less discomfort. The application of a Hydrocollator cervical pack before or during either form of traction augments muscle relaxation. Judovich[52] recommended injection of the scalenus muscle with procaine immediately before the use of intermittent traction.

There is no uniform agreement as to the amount of weight or traction time to produce distraction of vertebrae.[52,55] As a rule, the greater the force, the shorter the traction time used. Colachis and Strohm[17] found that a tractive force of 30 pounds for a duration of only 7 seconds can separate the

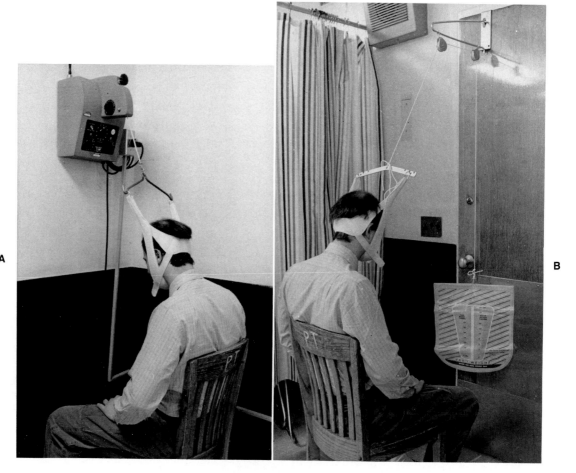

Figure 39-1. A, Intermittent motorized traction. **B,** Home traction unit.

cervical vertebrae posteriorly. The amount of separation increased with flexion of the cervical spine. Vertical traction with 5 to 10 pounds, as is often used, is inadequate because it does little more than support the head. For vertical traction, Jackson[45] advocated beginning with 15 to 20 pounds and gradually increasing to 35 to 50 pounds in more muscular individuals. Colachis and Strohm[18] evaluated traction effects on the cervical spines of 10 normal medical students, using 30 and 50 pounds of tractive force for 7, 30, and 60 seconds. They found that the amount of intervertebral separation was not influenced by the duration of the tractive force. I have found 15 to 30 minutes of vertical traction applied daily or a minimum of three times weekly to provide satisfactory results and good patient tolerance in most cases.

There is fairly uniform agreement about the position of the neck during traction.[12,17,45] Crue[22] studied 20 patients who experienced little or no relief from cervical traction in the supine position. However, with the neck flexed 20 to 30 degrees, 19 of the 20 patients had moderate to complete relief. Slight flexion opens the posterior articulations, widens the intervertebral foramina, disengages the facet surfaces, and elongates the posterior muscular tissues and ligaments.[12] Therefore, to produce the desired effect on the posterior, vertebral structures, the forces must be applied to the occiput and not to the mandible. The patient sits *facing* the unit at a distance of 1 to 2 feet, so that the angle of pull is approximately 25 to 30 degrees to the vertical. Pressure on the mandible can be avoided and the desired angle of pull augmented by using an adjustable halter. Patients who experience pain in the temporomandibular joint or teeth are

improperly positioned and the forces improperly directed.

Horizontal traction is most commonly used for hospitalized patients with acute conditions. It has the advantage of permitting prolonged traction with the patient in a more relaxed position, but since the traction time is longer, weight tolerance is less. Constant traction with hospitalization gave best results (78% good results with 13 treatments) in a comparison study of traction methods by Caldwell and Krusen.[13] However, it requires considerable expense and the use of scarce hospital beds. With this method, patients are usually started with 5 pounds for 1 to 2 hours three times daily and slowly increased as tolerated to 8 to 10 pounds for most of the day and night, with rest periods at mealtime. Since in most instances the desired objective is the same as with vertical traction, it is important that the angle of pull, usually one of slight flexion, be properly adjusted and maintained. Too commonly, patients in horizontal traction experience bitter discomfort and frequently an increase in symptoms because the traction is applied at an improper angle, forcing the neck into extension and transmitting most of the force to the mandible. Other causes of discomfort are poorly fitting head halters and excessive traction weight. To correctly attain traction forces at the occiput and to relieve forces on the mandible, the pulley should be elevated so the line of pull is directed upward and backward at an angle of approximately 45 degrees to the horizontal (Figure 39-2).

Once vertical traction has been found helpful, it may be useful to teach the patient how to apply it at home on a maintenance basis. This is obviously not possible with motorized intermittent traction and is difficult with horizontal

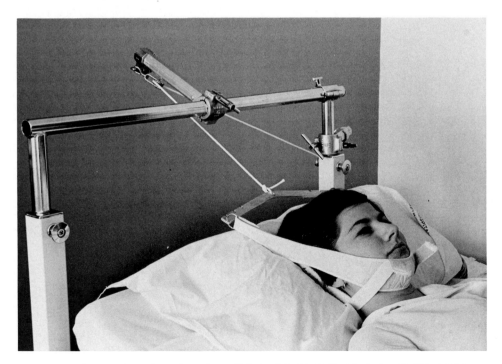

Figure 39-2. Horizontal traction. (From Thistle, HG: Med Clin North Am 53:520, 1969.)

traction. A simple home unit such as that in Figure 38-1, *B*, attaches to a door and is used with a waterbag or weights.

Orthotic devices

Cervical collars and braces. Cervical collars and braces are used to maintain varying degrees of immobilization of the cervical spine to reduce mechanical stress on its joints and ligaments.[93] They are used to treat neck disorders of traumatic and nontraumatic etiology.[38] Inflammatory reactions tend more rapidly to subside, strained or torn ligaments to heal, and painful muscle spasms to relax. Johnson and colleagues,[50] categorized conventional cervical supports into four groups: collars, extending from the head to the upper part of the thorax and made of a variety of materials; poster braces that control the head through padded mandib-

ular and occipital supports; the cervical thoracic brace, similar to the poster brace, but with rigid metal connections between the front and back components and extending farther distally over the trunk; or skeletal fixation using a halo.

The type of collar used depends largely on the degree of immobilization required. If it is used mainly as a reminder to the patient not to move the neck in extreme ranges of motion, a soft foam collar suffices. For greater immobilization, a firm foam, plastic, molded leather, or felt wraparound collar may be used, with or without the addition of a chin piece or occipital plate. To achieve maximum immobilization, a four-poster or cervicothoracic brace or halo with molded plaster or fiberglass jacket is necessary.

Immobilization of the cervical spine with a proper collar or brace is essential in a variety of acute and chronic con-

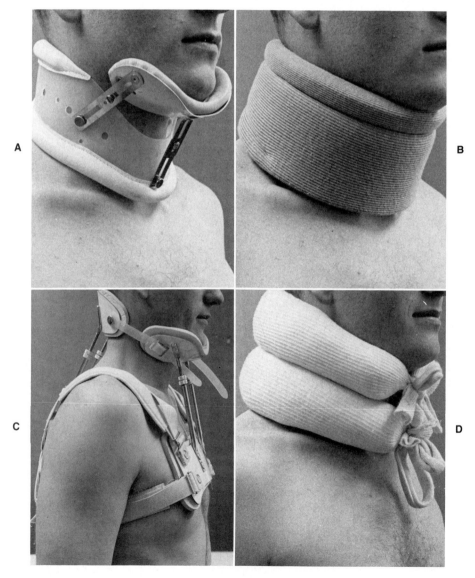

Figure 39-3. Cervical collars. **A,** Plastic foam padded collar with chin piece. **B,** Serpentine firm foam collar. **C,** Four-poster collar. **D,** Cervical ruffs for sleeping.

ditions. For most conditions it is desirable to support the neck in neutral position with the chin tucked in. The neck should be immobilized in hyperextension in spine injuries only when there is definite disruption of the posterior ligaments.[45] Positioning of the neck in hyperextension compresses the apophyseal joints, reduces the foraminal space, stretches the anterior longitudinal ligaments, and shortens the posterior ligamentous and capsular structures. Pain reduction is often a guide to correct positioning. Motions to be limited are usually extension and extremes of rotation. A collar therefore should provide adequate support under the occiput to prevent extension and, where limited rotation is desired, a chin piece is added (Figure 39-3, *A*). Fortunately, most commercially available collars are now designed to hold the head in neutral or the slightly flexed position, although some patients are still fitted with collars that limit flexion while providing little occipital support. A "serpentine" firm foam collar (Figure 39-3, *B*), factory made in a variety of widths and lengths, holds the head in a neutral position. Writing a prescription for a "standard" collar is to be thoroughly discouraged,[12] since no two necks have the same size, shape, curvature, or carrying angle.

Although collars should be made for each patient, this option is often precluded by expense and time constraints. Following fitting, the physician should check for positioning, degree of immobilization, and comfort. Improper fitting is frequently the cause of discomfort. The edges of the collar should be padded sufficiently to prevent pressure discomfort, and certain anatomic landmarks should be observed. Posteriorly its superior aspect should fit under the occiput below the superior nuchal line; if it rests against the occipital protuberance, pressure discomfort develops. The inferior border should rest on the trapezii without pressing on the lower cervical or upper thoracic spinous processes. Anteriorly the superior edge should be shaped to prevent pressure on the mandibular angles and, if a chin-piece is used, pressure should be widely distributed and not focused just on the mental protuberance. Inferiorly the collar should be cut out over the clavicles to permit pressure to be borne on the manubrium; patients should be advised to expect some initial discomfort and possible skin irritation.

Simple cervical ruffs (Figure 39-3, *D*) provide effective partial immobilization of the neck and limitation of extension. These are made of cotton surgical padding placed inside a 1-inch stockinette, leaving 6 to 8 inches in front for ties. They can be cheaply and quickly made and are comfortable. Two ruffs are usually adequate; their width may be varied by adding layers of cotton inside the stockinette. They effectively limit neck motion during sleep and are usually well tolerated, in contrast to plastic and metal collars, which do not lend themselves to comfort in bed.

When more rigid immobilization is required, a poster, cervicothoracic brace, or halo fixation must be used (Figure 39-3, *C*). Johnson and associates[50] studied the limitation of flexion-extension measured between the occiput and the first

thoracic vertebra, comparing five of the most commonly used collars and braces. The cervicothoracic brace was the most effective of the conventional orthoses studied, allowing 13% of normal flexion-extension, followed in order of decreasing effectiveness by the four-poster brace, 21%; the SOMI brace, 28%; the Philadelphia collar, 29%; and the soft collar, 74%. The halo with plastic body vest was most effective, allowing only 4% of normal flexion-extension of the whole cervical spine, as well as 4% of normal lateral bending, which was by far the best lateral immobilizer. The cervicothoracic brace ranked highest in allowing only 18% of normal rotation, whereas the halo with plastic body vest allowed only 1%. The best conventional braces in this study restricted only 45% of flexion-extension at the atlantoaxial joint; the halo restricted 75%. The conventional braces therefore were more effective in the middle and lower portions of the cervical spine. Similar studies by Fisher and associates,[29] in comparing four different conventional cervical orthoses, found that the four-poster and sternal occipital mandibular immobilization (SOMI) were most effective in restricting extension and flexion, respectively. The polyethylene and Plastizote orthoses were significantly less effective in restricting motion. Fisher also evaluated the effect of the SOMI orthosis in restricting sagittal cervical spine motion. He measured the resting chin and occipital pressures when the four-poster and SOMI orthoses were fitted in the usual manner by an orthotist and found them to be approximately 105 mm Hg. This pressure far exceeds the maximum capillary pressure of the human skin. When pressure sensors were used to fit the SOMI brace loosely at approximately 25 mm Hg, there was no significant difference in the mobility of the entire cervical spine or at any intervertebral level. Therefore, for patient comfort, it is recommended that the orthotist fit such an orthosis more loosely.

Slings. Slings are helpful in providing support and rest for an acutely painful shoulder.[93] Many types are used, from the familiar, simple, Red Cross cloth sling to the more complicated, sohpisticated ones with leather cuffs. When a sling is used, it is important to remember that the extremity must be removed from it at least once daily for gentle active exercise to preserve ranges of motion.

COMMON CLINICAL PROBLEMS
Cervical spondylosis

Cervical spondylosis is a term commonly used to describe degenerative intervertebral disc disease and vertebral body osteophyte formation, with compression of the nerve roots, spinal cord, or both. This is the concept suggested by Brain,[8] who distinguished between nuclear herniations and anular protrusions. Logue,[60] however, stated that spondylosis refers to a hard transverse ridge of fibrocartilage, bone, and fibrous tissue. Payne and Spillane,[80] noted that nuclear material may herniate through a torn anulus and become a calcified part of the ridge. Acute herniations are excluded from the definition,[85] as are osteoarthritic changes in the synovial apoph-yseal joints,[31] the latter providing no correlation with disc degeneration. In reviewing cervical spondylosis, Bradshaw[6] stated that it consisted of a circumferential osteophytosis of the vertebral rims and uncovertebral areas with or without subluxation. Although spondylosis usually occurs at several levels, changes at a single level occur in 20% of cases.[99] It is estimated that on the basis of plain radiographs of the cervical spine, 50% of people over age 50 and 75% over the age of 65 suffer from the disease.[47]

The cause of intervertebral disc degeneration is unknown, but among those suggested are congenital abnormalities,[14] aging,[12] metabolic abnormalities,[78] trauma,[8] wear and tear of normal spinal movements,[8] and interference with diffusion of nutrients from the vertebral marrow to the intervertebral disc, with resultant fibrillary change, dehydration, and fissuring of disc material.[25] The etiology of cervical spondylotic myelopathy is likewise debatable. Various theories advanced include narrowed sagittal cervical canal diameters, subluxation, compression, age, and cord ischemia.[76]

Studies have shown that the lower cervical nerve roots, particularly the posterior roots, are most severely affected by cervical spondylosis.[5] The posterior roots are larger, and compression or irritation leads to pain referred along dermatomes, accompanied by dysesthesias, weakness, and reflex changes. Irritation of the ventral nerve root creates pain along the myotome innervated by nerve roots at that level. If both ventral and dorsal roots are involved, both myotomal and dermatomal pain may occur (Figure 39-4). Common

spondylotic involvement of C6, C7, and C8 can therefore explain the "cervical angina syndrome" described by Booth and Rothman,[5] when precordial myotomal pain is present. Leban and associates[56] studied 18 women with persistent breast pain and found them to have a clear preponderance of left C7 root syndromes. Clinically, there was asymetric weakness in the myotome distribution of the ipsilateral C7 root, electromyographic abnormality of the C7 root myotome distribution, and radiologic evidence of C6-C7 interspace narrowing.

In addition to compressing the spinal cord and nerve roots, cervical spondylosis may lead to compression of the vertebral artery by osteophytes. This has been described by Sheehan and co-workers[86] as "spondylotic vertebral artery compression." Johnson and Wolf[51] described cervical radiculopathy in patients with previously asymptomatic cervical spondylosis produced by use of bifocal spectacles with consequent cervical hyperextension.

Signs and symptoms

Sandler,[85] in reviewing 19 cases of cervical myelopathy treated surgically, confirmed observations of others' previously reported clinical findings.[6-9] The significant features are sex difference (ratio of men to women, 4:1), variability in mode of onset (some patients with a preponderance of myelopathy, others with mainly radiculopathy), long duration of symptoms before seeking medical advice (a few months to several years), and an average age at onset of 55 years. In a study of 72 patients, only about one third complained of neck stiffness and pain.[6] Symptoms were intermittent or persistent pain in the upper limbs with or without radiation to the forearm and fingers and sometimes "burning" (often made worse by coughing, straining, and movements of the neck, usually rotation and lateral flexion to the contralateral side); sciatica; numbness and tingling involving one or more digits; sensory disturbances of the thighs, calves, or feet; weakness or clumsiness of the hands; stiffness of the legs with or without spasms; difficulty walking; and disorders of sphincter control (hesitancy or precipitancy of micturition or, more rarely, incontinence of both urine and feces).

Examination reveals a variety of findings referable to cranial nerves, motor and sensory systems, and tendon reflexes. Painless limitation of neck motion is common. When neck motion is painful, it is usually associated with cervical radiculopathy. Cranial nerve findings include nystagmus and Horner's syndrome. Muscle wasting in the upper extremities with fasciculations, marked spasticity, weakness, and gait disturbance in the lower extremities are observed with motor system involvement. Sensory deficits may be diffuse or localized and involve the upper and lower extremities, singly or together. A sensory level may or may not be present. One or all modalities may be involved. There may be a dissociation between vibration and position or pain and temperature sensation.[90] Patients with myelopathy, with or with-

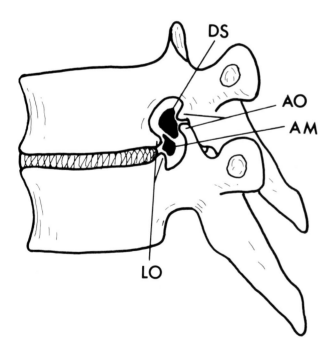

Figure 39-4. Cervical root compression (exaggerated for illustration). *DS,* Dorsal sensory root; *AM,* anterior (ventral) root; *LO,* Luschka joint osteophytes; *AO,* apophyseal joint osteophytes.

out radiculopathy, always exhibited extensor plantar responses and exaggerated knee and ankle jerks, and 50% of patients had no abdominal responses.[6] Furthermore, upper limb reflexes are usually not helpful in localizing the lesion to the cervical spine, since they may be normal, hyperactive or hypoactive, or absent completely.

Diagnosis

The diagnosis is made by careful history and physical examination in conjunction with investigative procedures. Plain radiographs of the cervical spine may be sufficient, (Figures 39-5 and 39-6) but the use of computerized tomography in combination with metrizamide myelography or magnetic resonance imaging better visualizes the cervical spine and related structures and better localizes the lesion.[72] Electrodiagnostic studies may validate root impairment and aid in localizing the root level.[12]

Treatment

A conservative versus surgical approach to the treatment of cervical spondylosis continues to be controversial, since there is no definitive treatment.[85] Medical treatment may consist of medication, bed rest, heat and massage, a variety of pain-relieving techniques, immobilization in a cervical collar, cervical traction, or manipulation.

Bradshaw[6] found that patients with a generalized cervical spondylosis and treated with polythene cervical collars respond poorly as judged by their walking, whereas those with focal spondylosis may do well. Those with radicular pain did better with a collar and usually had complete relief within weeks; sensory symptoms and signs tended not to respond. Clarke and Robinson[15] found that at least half the patients treated with collars were helped. Barnes and Saunders[4] found that results were variable and may have been related to patient compliance. Brain[10] suggested that a period of neck traction is often beneficial before wearing a collar. Cyriax[23] stated that 90% of patients with neck or radicular pain obtained relief after manipulation of the neck. Liversedge and colleagues[58] considered traction to be helpful only in the treatment of root pain. Honet and Puri[43] in a retrospective study of 82 patients with cervical radiculitis from a variety of causes, found 80% of the patients had good to excellent results when treated conservatively (medication, decreased activities, heat, firm cervical collar, and cervical traction). Of 59 patients contacted 1 to 2 years later, 71% continued to have good to excellent results. They

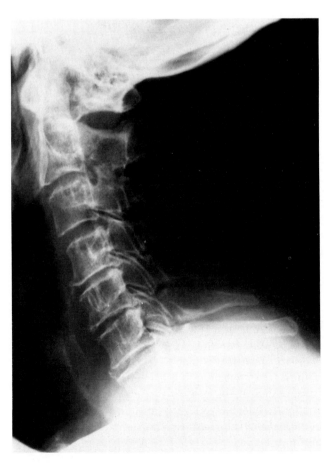

Figure 39-5. Cervical spondylosis with disc degeneration and Luschka joint osteophytes.

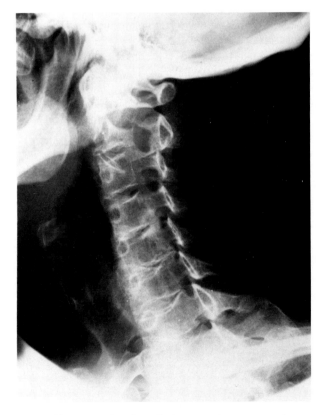

Figure 39-6. Anterior foraminal encroachment secondary to Luschka joint osteophytes.

concluded that a trial of conservative treatment is indicated; only if there is no improvement should surgery be considered. Barnes and Saunders[4] studied a number of etiologic variables in an attempt to find useful factors in predicting long-term prognosis in cervical myelopathy in 45 patients treated conservatively. They found that those who retain substantial range of movement seem more likely to deteriorate.

Indications for surgical intervention include failure of conservative treatment, rapid progression of symptoms and neurologic deficits, focal (single-level) spondylosis, and age under 50.[85] Advanced age and a short duration of preoperative symptoms have been associated with poor results.[1]

Advocates of different surgical procedures have claimed variable results.[26,33,91] The literature on cervical spondylotic myelopathy discusses the relative merits of decompressive laminectomy versus anterior surgical approaches. Gregorius and associates[36] in a study of 55 patients who underwent surgery for cervical spondylotic myelopathy and radiculopathy, found improved postoperative change in disability following anterior interbody fusion and a worsening in disability after laminectomy. Long-term follow-up in patients with myelopathy showed results varying from progressive worsening after operation, maintenance of improvement for a mean of 85 months, to deterioration after 8 to 12 years. Preoperative sphincter disturbance and lower extremity weakness was associated with a worsened postoperative disability.

Nurick[77] reviewed reports of laminectomy and found that after surgery 56% of patients were improved, 25% remained the same, and 19% were worse. Nonoperative treatment affforded almost the same results. He advocated the anterior approach for disc or osteophyte protrusion at one or two levels, whereas laminectomy would be the procedure of choice for a narrow canal with multiple protrusions. Jeffreys[48] concurred, but stated that protrusions of 4 mm required anterior decompression. It would therefore seem that both approaches have their place. Whether to perform a fusion following anterior decompression is likewise controversial and depends on the experience of the surgeon.

Patients with muscle weakness and wasting or gait disturbances should undergo restorative physical and occupational therapy whether conservative or surgical treatment is rendered. Where specific treatment has failed, maximum function should be maintained through self-help devices, equipment, and home modification.

Rheumatoid cervical myelopathy presents a clinical picture similar to that of cervical spondylotic myelopathy. Marks and Sharp,[65] in a retrospective study of 31 patients with rheumatoid cervical myelopathy, found that multiple neurologic deficits were eventually present in all patients. Paresthesias, numbness, or both were the most common presenting features and were often misdiagnosed as a peripheral neuropathy. Whether these patients underwent electrodiagnostic investigation or not is unclear. Two thirds of

the patients had a dissociation between loss of position and vibration sensation. Although atlantoaxial displacement was most common, multiple subaxial luxations were present. Occipitocervical fusion provided more frequent and prolonged neurologic improvement, although surgery was decided on the basis of general medical condition and minimal neurologic disability.

Cervical angina

The cervical angina syndrome secondary to cervical spondylosis is commonly confused with classical coronary ischemia. It most likely results from compression or irritation of the ventral nerve root, creating pain along the myotome innervated by the motor nerves of that level.[5] Spondylosis at C6 and C7 levels with C7 nerve root compromise is the suggested mechanism.[56] Precordial pain may or may not be associated with radicular dermatomal pain. The pain may be relieved by nitroglycerin[67] and is usually exacerbated by cervical spine positioning rather than exertion. Although true cardiac angina must be excluded by the usual methods, if cervical angina is suspected the diagnosis can usually be confirmed by careful history, examination, radiology, and electromyography. Treatment with a cervical collar and traction usually provides relief of symptoms.

Spondylotic vertebral artery compression

Symptoms of vertebral-basilar artery insufficiency may be produced by spondylotic vertebral artery compression.[86] This syndrome is characterized by "drop attacks" (usually precipitated by rotation or cervical spine extension), ataxia, dizziness, vertigo, blurred vision, and headache. The findings on examination are those of vertebral artery compression (cerebellar signs, cranial nerve weakness, hemisensory loss) with or without evidence of associated nerve root compression.

The diagnosis is usually made by reproducing the symptoms with rotation or hyperextension of the neck, cervical spondylosis on radiographs, and evidence on arteriography of vertebral artery compression or displacement by osteophytes. Treatment consists of immobilization of the cervical spine with a collar, thus preventing mechanical compromise of the artery. Anticoagulants have also produced good results.[86] Surgical intervention may be necessary.

Cervical disc herniation

The incidence of disc herniation in the cervical spine is much less than in the lumbar region for reasons already outlined (see "Anatomic and Pathologic Considerations"). Acute posterolateral "soft disc" protrusion with nerve root compression is relatively uncommon and is usually related to sudden physical stress for which the neck muscles are unprepared. Posterior protrusions usually cause pressure on the spinal cord. More commonly, disc degeneration causes thickening of the capsular ligaments and osteophyte formation at the margins of the lateral interbody joint.[46] This gives the appearance of a bulging disc ventral to the nerve root and is a much more chronic process. Degeneration begins in the anulus, with fragmentation associated with nuclear softening.[12] As degeneration progresses, nuclear material may protrude through the anulus, causing bulging or rupture of the posterior longitudinal ligament—the so-called hard disc. This process may result from several factors, including recent or past trauma.

The symptoms and signs depend largely on the site of the herniation. Posterolateral protrusion with unilateral nerve root compression may cause radicular pain and paresthesias with or without neck pain. Symptoms are usually aggravated by neck extension and coughing or sneezing. Spurling's sign is usually positive. Odom and co-workers[78] reviewed 175 cases of unilateral ruptured soft discs with nerve root compression that were verified by operation. Seventy percent were located at the sixth cervical interspace and 24% at the seventh interspace. Lunsford and associates[62] reported similar findings. Although compression of the sixth nerve root more frequently produced hypalgesia of the thumb and the seventh hypalgesia of the second finger, it was not uncommon to find hypalgesia in more than one finger with either root involved. A posterior or central herniation with cord compression usually is manifest as lower extremity weakness but few complaints of pain. There may also be weakness and numbness associated with atrophy in the upper extremities, depending on the duration of the disease. The diagnosis requires careful history, examination, and radiography, including computerized tomography with or without myelography. Conservative management usually includes medication, rest, and a cervical collar. When a posterolateral herniation is suspected, bed rest with continuous halter traction is the treatment of choice. If symptoms or neurologic findings do not improve, surgical intervention may be required. A 6-week period is suggested as a reasonable trial.[62] Where there is spinal cord compression, surgery may be the treatment of choice to prevent further damage to the cord.

As with cervical spondylosis, anterior versus posterior surgical procedures for herniated cervical disc remain controversial. The anterior approach has gained popularity, with from 70% to 92% improvements reported.[19,62,66] Results are the same with anterior discectomy alone or discectomy with fusion.[62,66] Many variables, including selection of patients,[77] make comparison of studies difficult. Lunsford and co-workers[62] found that with time 38% of patients reported recurrence of one or more symptoms. Deterioration rarely required further surgery. Conservative treatment was necessary in 35% of soft disc cases and 60% of hard disc cases within 1 to 6 years after surgery was performed.

Soft tissue injuries of the neck

Soft tissue injuries have been variously described as cervical sprain, "whiplash," cervical syndrome, and extension or acceleration injury. Jackson[46] stated that approximately 90% of all cervical nerve root irritation is the result, directly or indirectly, of sprain injuries of the ligamentous and capsular structures of the cervical spine. Sixty percent of these injuries cause some immediate symptoms, and the other 40% produce symptoms days, weeks, or months later. Vehicular collisions account for most of those injuries seen in clinical practice,[41] although falls, strenuous sports, sudden forces directed against the arms, and blows to the head and chin are also responsible.[46] Davis[24] described the term "whiplash" in 1945 in referring to a forced motion of the head and neck in one direction with the body suddenly moving in the opposite direction. If the forward motion of the body within a car suddenly stops, the head continues forward, but if the body and the car are suddenly propelled forward, as in rear-end collisions, the head is whipped backward.[30] In comparing rear-end collisions with front-end and side collisions, rear-end collisions generally result in the most disability.[42,64] There is built-in restraint to hyperflexion as the chin strikes the chest and restraint to lateral flexion as the head strikes the shoulder. However, the head is stopped in hyperextension only when it strikes the upper dorsal spine; movement exceeds the range permitted by anatomic structures. Front-end collisions injure mostly the posterior structures with tearing of posterior muscles and ligaments.[98]

The cervical syndrome, or whiplash, injury can be divided into three major phases: postconcussion, sympathetic shock, and myoradicular.[84] In the postconcussion phase the patient may have a variety of symptoms related to concussion (directly or by contrecoup effect) or from cerebral circulatory disturbances, and symptoms may be similar to those of patients with closed head injuries. Headache, visual and auditory disturbances, memory lapses, concentration difficulties, nervousness, and hyperirritability have been described. Torres and Shapiro[95] compared electroencephalograms from 45 patients who suffered whiplash injuries with those from 45 patients with closed head injuries. Electrical abnormalities of moderate or marked degree were found in 46% of the whiplash cases and in 44% of the head injury group. The number and distribution of focal abnormalities were similar in the two groups.

The sympathetic shock phase may be due to intraforaminal or extravertebral irritation of the cervical sympathetic nervous system.[12] Symptoms include postural dizziness, blurring of vision, and loss of ability to focus. Vasomotor disturbances may result in excessive perspiration, tachycardia, and tremors in the extremities.[28]

The myoradicular phase, as described by Rubin,[84] varies in severity according to the varying degrees of injury to the soft tissue structures. Early symptoms may be due to compression of the nerve roots within their bony canals as the joints are subluxated or to swelling and hemorrhage of capsular ligaments or injury of the vascular and sympathetic structures.[45] Rear-end collisions may result in stretching or tearing of the anterior longitudinal ligament. The disc may be avulsed from the cartilaginous plates of the vertebral bodies,[64] and anterior vertebral muscles may be torn. Posterior forces may injure the apophyseal joints.

These injuries result in a variety of musculoskeletal symptoms, of which pain, muscle spasm, and limited motion are paramount. Pain may be local or radicular, including the head, shoulders, scapulae, or arms. Spasm is frequently noted in the upper and middle trapezius and rhomboids but with nerve root involvement may be myotomal in distribution. These muscles are painful to palpation. There may be pain on swallowing because of prevertebral swelling. Attempts to move the head may create extreme pain, especially when painful muscles are stretched or the head is moved in the direction of the forces causing the injury, thereby stretching damaged tissues. There may be neurologic abnormalities in the upper extremities with nerve root compression including motor, sensory, and reflex changes.

The diagnosis of soft tissue injuries of the cervical spine is based on the history, including the exact mechanism of injury, and is supported by careful examination. The presence of painful neck and shoulder-girdle muscle spasm with painful limitation of neck and shoulder motion is common within hours of the injury. The presence of muscle weakness and sensory or reflex changes is indicative of nerve root compression with associated swelling. Cervical spine radiographs must be taken to rule out fracture or dislocation. Reversal of the normal lordotic curve is common secondary to spasm.

The most effective treatment is prevention. Public educational prevention efforts should be vigorously directed toward preventing automobile and sports injuries. Seat belts and air bags are controversial as a means of preventing neck injuries,[45] and head rests are poorly designed. Appropriate rule changes in certain sports and diving education have helped reduce serious neck injuries; because of their inherent dangers, trampolines may have no place in recreational, educational, or competitive gymnastics.[94]

Following an acute cervical spine injury, the cervical spine should be immobilized. The degree of immobilization depends on the severity of the injury. Usually a firm foam cervical collar such as the "serpentine" kind is satisfactory. The position of immobilization should be with the neck straight and the chin tucked in; collars or braces that hold the neck in hyperextension are completely wrong in principle unless there is disruption of the posterior ligaments.[45] Above all, the position should be one of comfort. Immobilization may be required for 3 to 8 weeks until tissues are healed and symptoms subside. It should be discontinued slowly and for increasing intervals as the patient gradually restores normal motion through careful exercise.

Within the first 24 hours the use of cold may be more beneficial than heat. Most patients, however, find moist heat to be comforting. Massage may also be helpful. Analgesics, muscle relaxants, and anti-inflammatory medication are useful separately or in combination. Cervical traction may be indicated, especially when there has been nerve root compression. However, care must be taken to ensure that the traction forces are directed properly. If traction aggravates symptoms, it should be discontinued.

In a review of the literature, Hohl[42] found a number of factors that favored a poor prognosis. These were identified as symptoms or findings of arm numbness or pain, a sharp cervical curve reversal, limitation of motion at one intervertebral level, wearing a collar for more than 12 weeks, and needing home traction or restarting physical therapy more than once.

Cervical osteoarthritis

Osteoarthritic changes may be found in apophyseal joints in the cervical spine. The exact etiology and mechanism of these changes are unclear. Cailliet[12] suggested that as approximation of the anterior portion of the functional unit occurs (that is, degeneration and narrowing of the intervertebral disc), reapproachment of the posterior articulation occurs with a loss of congruity of joint surfaces and compression of the cartilaginous articular surfaces. This ultimately leads to osteophyte formation, which may subsequently encroach on the intervertebral foramen. In addition, since these are true synovial joints, they are subject to inflammation with associated swelling. This may be a local process or related to a systemic disease affecting joints. Symptoms may not present for years and may be progressive or may present suddenly with minor trauma. The patient may notice only neck stiffness with local discomfort and restriction of movement, or there may be associated radicular symptoms, which when present usually prompts the patient to seek medical advice.

Radiographs may demonstrate the hallmarks of osteoarthritic changes in the apophyseal joint with or without associated osteophytes projecting into the posterior aspect of the intervertebral foramen. There may be concomitant anterior foraminal osteophytes from the Luschka joints with associated intervertebral disc space narrowing. Treatment usually includes rest, heat, analgesics and nonsteroidal anti-inflammatory medication, and a firm foam cervical collar. The head should be held in a position of maximum comfort. Traction may be of use, especially if there is a radicular component.

DIFFERENTIAL DIAGNOSIS

Fibrositis may present a confusing picture of pain and local tenderness and may be primary or secondary to an associated disease.[87] Diagnosis of primary fibrositis is based on the presence of large numbers of tender points, skinfold tenderness, and reactive hyperemia. There may be associated non-REM sleep disturbance.[72] Spasmodic torticollis, a painful and often disabling condition consisting of involuntary neck muscle contraction and thought to be associated with basal ganglia disturbances, is often confused with cervical spine pathology. However, the diagnosis can usually be based on careful history and observation of the involuntary muscle spasm. Thoracic outlet syndromes often produce pain, paresthesias, or weakness in the upper extremity. The most accurate test in diagnosis is the 3-minute elevated arm test,[34,83] which evaluates the three types of outlet syndrome—neurologic, venous, and arterial. The scapulocostal syndrome, consisting of pain and local tenderness at the site of insertion of the levator scapulae muscles to the scapula, is usually caused by poor posture and occupational fatigue.[70] Diagnosis is made by postural evaluation, site of pain and tenderness, and the absence of neurologic symptoms and signs. Shoulder-hand syndrome, or so-called reflex sympathetic dystrophy syndrome, the cause of which is controversial, consists of painful limitation of the shoulder with an associated swollen, painful, dystrophic-appearing hand. The diagnosis is usually made on a clinical and radiologic (osteoporosis) basis.[53] Carpal tunnel syndrome, resulting from pressure on the median nerve in the carpal tunnel, may be mistaken for cervical root compression. However, the distribution of pain and paresthesias associated with a positive Phalen's sign,[82] weakness of muscles in the hand supplied by the median nerve, and a median nerve conduction velocity of greater than 5 msec[49] at the wrist are all distinguishing characteristics. A large percentage of patients with carpal tunnel syndrome have an associated problem in the cervical spine. A variety of shoulder disorders may be confused with pathology in the cervical spine, especially since they may be associated with the cervical syndrome.[45] Careful history and physical examination, as previously outlined, usually direct the physician to the correct cause of the patient's symptoms.

A number of medical conditions involving the thorax and abdomen may cause referral of pain to the neck, shoulder, or arm.[21] Again, the diagnosis of these disorders depends on medical history and examination, although the tendency for patients to relate symptoms to a recent or past injury may always be misleading.

SUMMARY

The symptoms related to cervical spine pathology may be extremely protean and misleading. The physician must understand the underlying mechanisms of symptoms and possible sites of origin. A meaningful diagnosis can be established only after careful history taking and adequate examination. Investigative procedures should be used as adjuncts in making the diagnosis. Treatment is usually conservative and consists of medication, physical therapy, and orthotic devices. The success or failure of treatment often depends on individual attention to each patient. Surgical intervention may be indicated when conservative measures fail. The surgical approach may vary according to site, degree of pathology, and the surgeon's preference. Following surgery, many patients continue to require rehabilitation measures.

REFERENCES

1. Adams, CBJ, and Logue, V: Studies in cervical spondylotic myelopathy. III. Some functional effects of operations for cervical spondylotic myelopathy, Brain 94:587, 1971.
2. Alcoff, J, et al.: Controlled trial of imipramine for chronic low back pain, J Fam Pract 14:841, 1982.
3. Baratta, RR: A double-blind comparative study of carisoprodol, proxyphene and placebo in the management of low back syndrome, Curr Ther Res 20:233, 1976.
4. Barnes, MP, and Saunders, M: The effect of cervical mobility on the natural history of cervical spondylotic myelopathy, J Neurol Neurosurg Psychiatry 47:17, 1984.
5. Booth, RE, and Rothman RH: Cervical angina, Spine 1:28, 1976.
6. Bradshaw, P: Some aspects of cervical spondylosis, Q J Med 26:177, 1957.
7. Braham, J and Hertzberger, EE: Cervical spondylosis and compression of the spinal cord, JAMA 161:1560, 1956.
8. Brain, R: Spondylosis—the known and unknown, Lancet, p 687, Apr 3, 1954.
9. Brain, R: Discussion on cervical spondylosis, Proc R Soc Med 49:197, 1956.
10. Brain, WR: Cervical spondylosis, Lancet 2:718, 1952.
11. Brown, BR, and Womble, J: Cyclobenzaprine in intractable pain syndromes with muscle spasm, JAMA 240:1151, 1978.
12. Cailliet, R: Neck and arm pain, Philadelphia, 1981, FA Davis Co.
13. Caldwell, JW, and Krusen, EM: Effectiveness of cervical traction in treatment of neck problems: evaluation of various methods, Arch Phys Med Rehabil 43:214, 1962.
14. Clark, E, and Little, JH: Cervical myelopathy. A contribution to its pathogenesis, Neurology 5:861, 1955.
15. Clarke, E, and Robinson, PK: Cervical myelopathy; a complication of cervical spondylosis, Brain 79:483, 1956.
16. Codman, EA: The shoulder, Boston, 1934, Thomas Todd Co.
17. Colachis, SC, and Strohm, BR: A study of tractive forces and angle of pull on vertebral interspaces in the cervical spine, Arch Phys Med Rehabil, p 820, Dec 1965.
18. Colachis, SC, and Strohm, BR: Cervical traction: relationship of traction time to varied tractive force with constant angle of pull, Arch Phys Med Rehabil, p 815, Dec 1965.
19. Connolly, ES, Seymour, RJ, and Adams, JE: Clinical evaluation of anterior cervical fusion for degenerative cervical disc disease, J Neurosurg 23:431, 1965.
20. Cooper, AL: Trigger-point injection: its place in physical medicine, Arch Phys Med Rehabil 42:704, 1961.
21. Craig, WM, and Witt, JA: Cervical disc, shoulder-arm-hand syndrome, Postgrad Med 17:267, 1955.
22. Crue, BJ: Importance of flexion in cervical traction for radiculitis, USAF Med J 8:374, 1957.
23. Cyriax, J: Spinal disk lesions: an assessment after 21 years, Br Med J 1:140, 1955.
24. Davis, AG: Injuries of the cervical spine, JAMA 127:149, 1945.
25. Epstein, JA, and Davidoff, LM: Chronic hypertrophic spondylosis of the cervical spine with compression of the spinal cord and nerve roots, Surg Gynecol Obst 93:27, 1951.
26. Fager, CA: Results of adequate posterior decompression in the relief of spondylotic cervical myelopathy, J Neurosurg 38:684, 1973.
27. Fielding, JW: Normal and selected abnormal motion of the cervical spine from the second cervical vertebra to the seventh cervical vertebra based on cineroentgenography, J Bone Joint Surg 46A:1779, 1964.
28. Fields, A: The autonomic nervous system in whiplash injuries, Int Rec Med 169:8, 1960.
29. Fisher, SV, et al: Cervical orthoses effect on cervical spine motion: roentgenographic and gonometric method of study, Arch Phys Med Rehabil 58:109, 1977.
30. Frankel, CJ: Medical-legal aspects of injuries to the neck, JAMA 169:96, 1959.

31. Friedenberg, ZB, et al: Degenerative changes in the cervical spine, J Bone Joint Surg 41A:61, 1959.

32. Frykholm, R: Lower cervical roots and their investments, Acta Chir Scand 101:457, 1951.

33. Galera, R: Anterior disc excision with interbody fusion in cervical spondylotic myelopathy and rhizopathy, J Neurosurg 28:305, 1968.

34. Glassberg, M: The thoracic outlet syndrome: an assessment of 20 cases with regard to new clinical and electromyographic findings, Angiology 32:180, 1981.

35. Gready, DM: Parafon Forte versus Robaxisal in skeletal muscle disorders; a double-blind study, Curr Ther Res 20:666, 1976.

36. Gregorius, FK, Estrin, T, and Crandall, PH: Cervical spondylotic radiculopathy and myelopathy; a long term follow-up study, Arch Neurol 33:618, 1976.

37. Hadley, LA: The covertebral articulations and cervical foramen encroachment, J Bone Joint Surg 39A:910, 1957.

38. Hartman, JT, Palumbo, F, and Hill, BJ: Cineradiography of braced normal cervical spine; comparative study of five commonly used cervical orthoses, Clin Orthop 109:97, 1975.

39. Hingorani, K: Diazepam in backache: a double-blind controlled trial, Ann Phys Med 8:303, 1966.

40. Hohl, M: Normal motions in the upper portion of the cervical spine, J Bone Joint Surg 46A:1777, 1964.

41. Hohl, M: Soft tissue injuries of the neck, Clin Orthop Rel Res, No. 109, p 42; June 1975.

42. Hohl, M: Soft tissue injuries of the neck in automobile accidents—factors influencing prognosis, J Bone Joint Surg 56A:1675, 1974.

43. Honet, JC, and Puri, K: Cervical radiculitis: treatment and results in 82 patients, Arch Phys Med Rehabil 57:12, 1976.

44. Inman, VT, Saunders, JBDeC, and Abbot, LC: Observations on the function of the shoulder joint, J Bone Joint Surg 26:1, 1944.

45. Jackson, R: The cervical syndrome, Springfield, Ill, 1978, Charles C Thomas Publisher.

46. Jackson, R: Syndrome of cervical root compression. In McCarty, DJ, Jr, editor: Arthritis and allied conditions, ed 10, Philadelphia, 1985, Lea & Febiger.

47. Jeffreys, RV: The surgical treatment of cervical myelopathy due to spondylosis and disc degeneration, J Neurol Neurosurg Psychiatry 49:353, 1986.

48. Jeffreys, RV: The surgical treatment of cervical spondylotic myelopathy, Acta Neurochir 47:293, 1979.

49. Johnson, EW, Wells, RM, and Duran, RJ: Diagnosis of carpal tunnel syndrome, Arch Phys Med Rehabil 43:414, 1962.

50. Johnson, RM, et al: Cervical orthoses, J Bone Joint Surg 59A:332, 1977.

51. Johnson, EW, and Wolf, CV: Bifocal spectacles in the etiology of cervical radiculopathy, Arch Phys Med Rehabil, p 201, May 1972.

52. Judovich, B: Herniated cervical disc: a new form of traction therapy, Am J Surg 84:646, 1952.

53. Kosin, F: Painful shoulder and the reflex sympathetic dystrophy syndrome, ed 10, Philadelphia, 1985, Lea & Febiger. (Edited by D.J. McCarty, Jr.)

54. Laurelle, LL: Les bases anatomiques du systemes autonomes cortical et bulbo-spinalis, Rev Neurol 72:349, 1940.

55. Lawson, GA, and Godfrey, CM: A report on studies of spinal traction, Med Serv J Canada 14:762, 1958.

56. Leban, MM, Meerschaert, JR, and Taylor, RS: Breast pain: a symptom of cervical radiculopathy, Arch Phys Med Rehabil 60:315, 1979.

57. Lehman, JF, and de Lateur, BJ: Cryotherapy. In Legman, JF, editor: Therapeutic heat and cold, ed 3, Baltimore, 1982, Williams & Wilkins Co.

58. Liversedge, LA, Hutchinson, EC, and Lyons, JB: Cervical spondylosis simulating motor-neurone disease, Lancet 2:652, 1953.

59. Lockhart RD, et al: Anatomy of the human body, Philadelphia, 1959, JB Lippincott.

60. Logue, V: Cervical spondylosis: modern trends in diseases of the vertebral column, London, 1959, Butterworths.

61. Lord, JW, and Rosati, LM: Neurovascular compression syndromes of the upper extremity, Clin Symp 12:139, 1960.

62. Lunsford, LD, et al: Anterior surgery for cervical disc disease; treatment of lateral cervical disc herniation in 253 cases, J Neurosurg 53:1, 1980.

63. Luschka, Von H: Die Halbergclenke des Menschienchen Korpes, 1858.

64. Macnab, I: Acceleration injuries of the cervical spine, J Bone Joint Surg 46A:1797, 1964.

65. Marks, JS, and Sharp, J: Rheumatoid cervical myelopathy, Q J Med (New Series L) 199:307, 1981.

66. Martins, AN: Anterior cervical discectomy with and without interbody bone graft, J Neurosurg 44:290, 1976.

67. Master, A: The spectrum of anginal and non-cardiac chest pain, JAMA 187:894, 1964.

68. Melzack, R, Stillwell, DM, and Fox, EJ: Trigger points and acupuncture points for pain: correlations and implications, Pain 3:3, 1977.

69. Mense, S: Effects of temperature on the discharges of muscle spindles and tendon organs, Pflügers Arch 374:159, 1978.

70. Michele, AA, et al: Scapulocostal syndrome (fatigue-postural paradox), NY State J Med 50:1353, 1950.

71. Modic, MT, et al: Cervical radiculopathy: prospective evaluation of surface coil MR imaging, CT with metrizamide and metrizamide myelography, Neuroradiology 161:753, 1986.

72. Moldofsky, H, et al: Musculoskeletal symptoms of non-REM sleep disturbance in patients with "fibrositis syndrome" and healthy subjects, Psychosom Med 37:341, 1975.

73. Morton, DE: Anatomical study of human spinal column, with emphasis on degenerative changes in the cervical region, Yale J Biol Med 23:126, 1950.

74. Nathan, H: Osteophytes of the vertebral column; anatomical study of their development according to age, race and sex with considerations as to their etiology and significance, J Bone Joint Surg 44A:243, 1962.

75. Neuwirth, E: Current concepts of the cervical portion of the sympathetic nervous system, Lancet, p 337, 1960.

76. Nurick, S: The pathogenesis of the spinal cord disorder associated with cervical spondylosis, Brain 95:87, 1972.

77. Nurick, S: Cervical spondylosis and the spinal cord, Br J Hosp Med 13:668, 1975.

78. Odom, GL, Finney, W, and Woodhall, B: Cervical disc lesions, JAMA 166:23, 1958.

79. Orofino, C, Sherman, MS, and Schechter, D: Luschka joint-A degenerative phenomenon, J Bone Joint Surg 42A:853, 1960.

80. Payne, EE, and Spillane, JD: The cervical spine; an anatomico-pathological study of 70 specimens (using a special technique) with particular reference to the problem of cervical spondylosis, Brain 80:571, 1957.

81. Perry, J, and Nickel, VL: Total cervical spine fusion for neck paralysis, J Bone Joint Surg 41A:37, 1959.

82. Phalen, GS: The carpal-tunnel syndrome, J Bone Joint Surg 48A:211, 1966.

83. Roos, DB: New concepts of thoracic outlet syndrome that explains etiology, symptoms, diagnosis and treatment, Vasc Surg 13:313, 1979.

84. Rubin, D: Head, neck and arm symptoms subsequent to neck injuries: physical therapeutic considerations, Arch Phys Med Rehabil 40:387, 1959.

85. Sandler, B: Cervical spondylosis as a cause of spinal cord pathology, Arch Phys Med Rehabil, p 650, Sept 1961.

86. Sheehan, S, Bauer, RB, and Meyer, JS: Vertebral artery compression in cervical spondylosis, Neurology (Minneap) 10:968, 1960.

87. Smythe, HA: Nonarticular rheumatism and the fibrositis syndrome. In McCarty, DJ, Jr, editor: arthritis and allied conditions, ed 10, Philadelphia, 1985, Lea & Febiger.

88. Spurling, RG, and Scoville, WB: Lateral rupture of the cervical intervertebral discs, Surg Gynecol Obstet 78:350, 1944.
89. Steinbrocker, O, Neustadt, D, and Bosch, SJ: Painful shoulder syndromes: their diagnosis and treatment, Med Clin North Am 39:563, 1955.
90. Stern, EW, and Rand, RW: Spinal cord dysfunction from cervical intervertebral disk disease, Neurology 4:883, 1954.
91. Stoops, WL, and King, RB: Neurological complications of cervical spondylosis: their response to laminectomy and foraminotomy, J Neurosurg 19:986, 1962.
92. Teng, P: Spondylosis of the cervical spine with compression of the spinal cord and nerve roots, J Bone Joint Surg 42A:392, 1960.
93. Thistle, HG: Neckkand shoulder pain: evaluation and conservative management, Med Clin North Am 53:511, 1969.
94. Torg, JS: Epidemiology, pathomechanics and prevention of athletic injuries to the cervical spine, Med Sci Sports Exer 17:295, 1985.
95. Torres, F, and Shapiro, SK: Electroencephalograms in whiplash injury, Arch Neurol 5:28, 1961.
96. Trolard, A: Quelques articulations de la colonne vertebrale, Int Monatsschr Anat Physiol 10:3, 1893.
97. Waylonis, GW: The physiologic effects of ice massage, Arch Phys Med Rehabil 48:37, 1967.
98. Whitley, JE, and Forsyth, HF: The classification of cervical spine injuries, Am J Roentgenol 83:633, 1960.
99. Wilkenson, M: The morbid anatomy of cervical spondylosis and myelopathy, Brain 83:589, 1960.

CHAPTER 40 | Disorders of the lumbosacral spine

EDWARD S. RACHLIN

EPIDEMIOLOGY

Disorders of the lumbosacral spine are responsible for one of society's most serious socioeconomic and health problems. The magnitude of the problem is clearly demonstrated by data assembled in the United States, Great Britain, and Scandinavia. Statistics in England indicate that each year more than 2% of the population consults a physician because of low back pain. Among working people in the United States, disorders of the spine are the most frequent cause of disability in patients under the age of 45.[10,11] Swedish surveys indicate that back problems are responsible for between 9% and 19.5% of all sickness absence days.

Statistics to suggest occupational risk factors have been collected by Frymyer.[8] In a retrospective three-part study of 3920 patients, certain occupational risks were suggested. Muscle sprains occur most often in occupations involved with lifting, bending, twisting, and vibrational exposure. Three occupations having the highest risk for low back pain are truck driving, material handling, and nursing and nurses' aides. Sedentary occupations and heavy work occupations can give rise to back pain. Occupations requiring prolonged sitting were associated with problems involving the lumbar disc, whereas occupations of heavy work that required lifting and bending were associated with muscular sprains.

The maximum frequency of low back pain symptoms appears to occur between the ages of 35 and 55 years of age. Surveys in Sweden have indicated that 50% to 80% of adults at some time in their lives suffer from back pain. Employees with back problems absent from work for more than 6 months have only a 50% chance of returning to their employment and only 25% after 1 year. A greater incidence of back pain was noted with increased numbers of pregnancies in women. Anxiety, depression, and stressful life situations were more prevalent in patients with back pain.

The cause of back pain is usually explained on the basis of pathology involving the intervertebral disc, bone, joints, and ligaments of the spine. Some authors emphasize that most often the cause of low back pain is not identified. Kraus,[14] based on his evaluation of 3000 patients seen at a multidisciplinary back clinic at Columbia Presbyterian Hospital, demonstrated that more than 83% of back pain is of muscular origin. He distinguished four types of muscle pathology: muscle spasm, muscle tension, muscle deficiency, and trigger points in muscle. Muscle pathology may be the sole source of pain but most often is one factor in a disease complex. Mechanical factors alone may account for 20% of the patients with back pain. Even in those cases, muscle pathology usually plays a role. Tension myositis of psychogenic origin is the cause of the majority of common pain syndromes of the back and neck, according to Sarno.[20]

Low back pain must be viewed as a symptom of a disease complex rather than a localized mechanical problem or psychiatric problem. A diagnosis of back pain must take into account all contributing causes—psychologic, environmental, occupational, endocrinologic, mechanical derangement—and their effects on muscle pathology. In most cases of back pain there is an overlapping of pathologic states giving rise to symptoms. All aspects of the etiology must be treated if we are to succeed in rehabilitating the patient.

HISTORY AND PHYSICAL EXAMINATION

Therapeutic results depend on an accurate diagnosis and total assessment of all factors related to the occurrence of back pain. The necessity for a thorough history and physical examination cannot be overemphasized.

History taking

The physician who treats back pain must be not only knowledgeable in spinal disease, but also interested in the

---

**IMPORTANT AND OFTEN MISSED CAUSES
OF BACK PAIN**

I. Vasculogenic
   A. Abdominal aortic aneurysm
   B. Peripheral vascular disease
II. Neurogenic
   A. Nerve root tumors
      1. Neurofibroma
      2. Neurilemmomata
   B. Spinal cord tumors
   C. Diabetic neuropathy
III. Spondylogenic
   A. Multiple myeloma
   B. Secondary malignancy
   C. Osteoid osteoma
   D. Pathologic fracture (osteoporosis)
   E. Vertebral osteomyelitis
   F. Ankylosing spondylitis

From Kirkaldy-Willis, WH: Managing low back pain, ed 2, New York, 1988, Churchill-Livingstone.

patient as a person. A proper history takes time and should not be rushed. All factors contributing to back pain must be investigated. A history of trauma accompanying the complaints of back pain may not be sufficient to explain the occurrence of symptoms, the patient's progress, or the chronicity of symptoms. An attack of back pain may be precipitated by emotional or sociologic problems, tension, business strain, physical activities, work, or athletic activities to which the patient is unaccustomed. Endocrine problems such as thyroid disease or lack of estrogen may contribute to the development or prolongation of muscle pain. A complete medical and surgical history is obtained to help rule out nonspinal and often missed causes of back pain (see boxed material). A more focal history related to back pain is then taken that emphasizes the following categories:

I. Current complaints—history of the nature of onset, previous episodes, treatments, and responses to treatments
   A. Characteristics of lumbosacral pain
      1. Discogenic pain—diffuse ache, morning stiffness, low-grade pain (acute or chronic). Unusual severe pain with muscle spasm following laminectomy or chemonucleolysis may indicate disc space infection
      2. Osteoarthritic pain. Osteoarthritis of the small joints of the back can cause referred pain along sclerotogenous routes. Referred pain may be experienced in the buttocks and lower extremity, simulating a herniated disc. Trigger points may also cause referred pain often attributed to disc herniation. Morning stiffness improves

with ambulation and improvement increases with prolonged walking.
      3. Mechanical insufficiency. Pain of instability may be aggravated with forward bending or extension. This is usually aggravated with activity and relieved with rest and back immobilization.
      4. Nerve root impingement. Radicular pain may be felt only in the calf. Pain may be accompanied by paresthesia, numbness, and motor weakness following nerve root patterns. Spinal stenosis can cause pseudointermittent claudication in the lower extremities. Patients with vascular claudication will notice relief of pain when they stop walking. Symptoms occur after walking a specific distance. Pain is not completely relieved in those patients with pseudointermittent claudication after walking stops. Pain is also relieved with spine flexion. Vascular claudication does not respond to changes in back posture.
      5. Night pain. Night pain should alert the physician to the possible presence of tumor or infection. Arthritis or disc problems may also wake the patient. Upper lumbar pain may occur with rheumatoid spondylitis.
      6. Metastatic disease. Persistent pain with or without pathologic fracture not relieved with rest.
      7. Psychogenic or psychosomatic pain. Suspect a psychologic component when there are bizarre descriptions of pain and sensory complaints with a nonorganic pattern, history of psychosomatic disorders, or complaints of disability that appear out of proportion to injuries. A pain drawing may be helpful.
II. Past history of trauma or back pain. Residuals of trauma or back surgery may be a persistent cause of repeated episodes of back pain. This may be due to untreated muscle pathology, which is often present before surgery and a frequent occurrence after surgery. Following acute care, the patients should be given a follow-up rehabilitation program to eliminate the cause of their back pain and prevent attacks in the future.
III. Tension. Determine if the patient is leading a stressful life. Does he enjoy his work? Are there marriage problems? Does he work under pressure? Does he have problems with his stomach, such as duodenal ulcer, colitis, or a nervous stomach?
IV. History of postural attitudes at work. Inquire as to how his work is performed. Does work require repetitive movements? How are they performed? Does the patient remain in one position for a long time with muscle held rigidly? Hunching of shoulders and tight-

ness of the shoulders may cause pain in drivers and typists. Frequent causes of neck pain include reading in bed and watching television. This is particularly true if bifocal eyeglasses are used. The patient must be instructed in new habits of posture if a permanent relief of symptoms is to be achieved. What kind of chair or bed does the patient use? Soft chairs or bed may cause back pain symptoms. The bed should be firm. The mattress should be without springs and made of hair, firm latex, or kapok and placed on a board.

V. Physical activity and athletic history. Does the patient's work provide much exercise? In taking an athletic history details concerning the nature of the athletic activity is necessary. Tennis requires a knowledge of how often and on what surface the patient plays and whether the game is singles or doubles. A knowledge of techniques unique to a specific sport may be necessary in treating certain athletic injuries. Back pain in a tennis player may be due to the arching of the back in performing a twist serve. In this case treatment must be extended to correcting serving technique. Joggers are questioned concerning running shoes, orthotics, running surface, distance, and time. Does pain occur after hobbies such as gardening? Is pain related to housework activities such as making beds or vacuuming? Back pain during or after pregnancy may be caused by weak abdominal muscles.

VI. Endocrine imbalance. Hypothyroidism and estrogen deficiency may be a cause of muscle pain and multiple trigger points. Inquire as to dryness of skin, nails breaking, and hair falling out. Does the patient fatigue easily? Is there a need for much sleep? Does the patient have a weight problem. In estrogen deficiency, is the patient menopausal? Is menopause associated with hot flashes or nervousness? Has the patient ever taken estrogen?

VII. Emotional stability. Is the patient nervous? Is the patient in psychotherapy?

VIII. Routine inquiries. Allergy history, especially allergy to procaine or xylocaine. Is the patient on medications? Is the patient on anticoagulants? Is there pain in other parts of the body, other joints, or muscles? Multiple areas of pain may indicate a systemic disease.

IX. Dental bite problems. Grinding and clenching of the teeth may play a role in neck and upper back pain. This can be related to mechanical disturbances involving the teeth and temporomandibular (TMJ) region and demonstrate existing tension.

X. Neurologic symptoms. Does the patient have symptoms of muscular weakness, sensory loss, bladder or bowel irregularities?

Physical examination of the patient
General examination

Physical examination of the patient begins when the patient enters the office and during the taking of the patient's history. Does the patient walk in with a limp or dropfoot gait? Does the patient list to one side? This may be due to a disc lesion but is more often found to be caused by acute back muscle spasm due to muscle strain. Does the patient show signs of tension by hiking the shoulder during the interview and not relaxing the upper extremities? A general physical examination with appropriate laboratory testing is important in diagnosing the presence of systemic disease, which may be a cause of back pain. These conditions include thyroid disease and other endocrine disorders, estrogen deficiency, rheumatic diseases, and diseases influenced by stress, including cardiovascular and gastrointestinal disorders. To properly examine the patient for back problems, the patient must disrobe leaving only the undergarments on. It is not possible to thoroughly evaluate body structure and movements with the patient partially clothed or wearing the conventional examination gown. Structural measurements of skeletal abnormalities such as scoliosis, lack of chest expansion, leg length measurements, and knee and foot deformities such as pronation are determined.

Neurologic examination

The neurologic examination is performed for evidence of nerve root pressure or disc or neurologic disease. Testing is done for upper and lower motor neuron lesions. Examination includes testing for reflex loss, pathologic reflexes, sensory loss, and localized muscle weakness. Tests to stretch the sciatic nerve include straight leg raising and the Lasègue test. Testing for sacroiliac joint and hip joint pathology should be included.

Muscle examination

An examination for back pain without a thorough evaluation for muscle pathology is incomplete. Pain patterns caused by trigger points may be similar to those seen with nerve root irritation. In both instances the pain may radiate and be relieved by lying down. Palpation of muscle may reveal muscle spasm, which must be relieved before the examiner can palpate specific sensitive trigger point areas; these may sometimes be identified as knots in the muscle. This finding must be differentiated from the tenderness typical of fibrositis. In fibrositis, tenderness of the subcutis is found by rolling and squeezing the skin.

Look for signs of muscle tension. Does the patient let go or tighten up when asked to perform certain motions? Reflexes that are difficult to obtain without distraction may be a sign of tension.

Muscle deficiency of key postural muscles is determined by performing the Kraus-Weber tests.[14] These should not be performed if the patient is in acute pain. Muscle deficiency is evaluated as to muscle strength, length, elasticity, flexibility of muscle, and holding power.

Nonorganic findings

Examination of the lumbosacral spine should include investigation of nonorganic physical signs. Waddell and co-workers,[23] have described and standardized nonorganic signs of physical pathology, which can be used to identify patients who require more detailed psychologic evaluation. They have developed five types of physical signs:

1. Tenderness. Nonorganic tenderness may be superficial or nonanatomic. Superficially, the skin is tender to a light pinch over a wide area of lumbar skin that does not correspond to the distribution of a posterior primary ramus. Tenderness is abnormally diffuse and may spread and extend to the thoracic spine, pelvis, sacrum, and cervical area.
2. Simulation tests and axial loading. Low back pain is reported when the examiner applies pressure on the skull in performing vertical loading. This is done with the patient standing.
3. Rotation. The shoulders and pelvis are passively rotated in the same plane. A report of low back pain is positive. This is to be distinguished from actual root irritation, which may give rise to leg pain.
4. Distraction tests. Movements that can be carried out when the patient is being observed but not during the formal examination may have a nonorganic component. Straight leg raising is also a useful distraction test. Discrepancies in straight leg raising when the patient is lying down compared to when the patient is sitting up on the examination table extending the leg are indicative of a nonorganic finding.
5. Regional disturbances. Findings that are not substantiated by neuroanatomic patterns such as weakness of many muscles of the extremity or giving way of muscles when being tested for strength suggest nonorganic findings. Sensory disturbances of a stocking or glove type that do not respond to nerve root patterns may be nonorganic findings in the absence of disturbances that suggest multiple root involvement from spinal stenosis or repeated spinal surgery.
6. Overreaction. Overreaction consists of inappropriate verbilization, evidence of muscle tension and tremors, collapsing during the examination, and unusual facial expressions.

The finding of three or more of the five types of nonorganic physical findings is clinically significant. An isolated positive sign may be ignored. Overreaction is the single most important nonorganic physical sign. Nonorganic signs may help identify the prognosis for conservative treatment and surgery and may indicate the presence of psychosocial factors that contribute to patient rehabilitation. Compensation factors reduce the success rate of any form of treat-

ment for back pain and sciatica by approximately one third.

The physical may also require rectal and gynecologic examinations.

Laboratory workup

The type of laboratory workup indicated depends on physical findings. Routine radiographs should always include the pelvis to visualize both hips in addition to the lumbosacral spine. Further studies such as computerized tomographic (CT) scans, nuclear magnetic imaging, myelography, and electrical diagnostic studies may be indicated. Consultation may include neurologic, rheumatologic, orthopedic, and rarely, vascular consultation when arterial disease such as Leriche's syndrome is suspected as a cause of buttock and leg pain. Appropriate laboratory studies to rule out systemic disease is indicated. Bone scans may be necessary to differentiate fracture, metastatic tumor, or inflammatory process. A cystometrogram may be required if one suspects the presence of a neurogenic bladder. Epidural venography and discography have been used to confirm foraminal entrapment syndromes.

Additional consultations

Psychologic consultation should include a psychosocial evaluation.

During the history and physical examination the following nonmuscular skeletal conditions should be considered as possible causes of low back pain:

1. Gastrointestinal disorders such as peptic ulcers, pancreatitis, genitourinary pathology, kidney stones, pyelonephritis, and gastrointestinal and gynecologic neoplasms
2. Prostatitis, herpes zoster, polymyositis, polymyalgia rheumatica, and lymphoma

Malignant tumors may metastasize to bone from thyroid, breast, bronchus, kidney, or prostate.

CONGENITAL ANOMALIES

The clinical significance of congenital defects[17] is still uncertain. The incidence of congenital defects has been estimated as 0.5% to 27% in patients with backache, compared with 2% to 7% in controls.

Transitional lumbosacral vertebra

Sacralization of the transverse process of the fifth lumbar vertebra may occur unilaterally or bilaterally. A sacralized lumbar vertebra is described as sacralization. Lumbarization refers to a lumbarized sacral vertebra. The transverse process may become long and unusually broad, resembling the flat bone structure of the sacrum. It is therefore referred to as a transitional vertebra, having characteristics of both the lumbar and sacral areas. A pseudarthrosis may form at the connection of the transverse process and sacrum. This abnormality may be symptomatic. Clinically, symptoms appear as pain after 18 years of age. Pain is experienced on the side of the pseudarthrosis. Bilateral sacralization is usually asymptomatic. Pseudarthrosis is the cause of pain, which is usually not expected if the L5 transverse process is fused to the sacrum. It may be precipitated by trauma. Radiation of pain may occur in the absence of motor, sensory, or reflex exchanges. Pain is usually aggravated with activity and relieved with rest or lumbosacral support. Lateral flexion and palpation of the low back produces pain, and tenderness may be present over the sacroiliac joint on the side of the pseudarthrosis.

Wiltse[26] notes that sacralization of L5 or lumbarization of S1 probably has no effect on the incidence of low back pain. Farfan's studies on mechanical failure of intervertebral joints noted by Wiltse indicate that the presence of lumbarization or sacralization increases the incidence of rupture of the anulus fibrosis by causing abnormal positional stresses.[7]

Facet tropism

Facet joints of the same vertebral level oriented in different planes are not themselves a source of pain but contribute to disc herniation. Facet tropism increases rotary motion, which predisposes to disc prolapse. Herniation was noted to occur on the side of the more obliquely oriented facet.

Sacrohorizontal angle

Some texts refer to the sacrohorizontal angle as the lumbosacral angle or Ferguson's angle. It is formed by a line parallel to the superior border of S1 and the horizontal plane. The sacrohorizontal angle is associated with low back pain only if it is greater than 70 degrees. Radiographs should be taken in the standing position for evaluation. An increase in the sacrohorizontal angle increases lordosis and shearing stresses. These forces are greatest at the L5-S1 interspace. The increased sacrohorizontal angle has often been suggested as an explanation of pain in spondylolisthesis.

Congenital or dysplastic spondylolisthesis

Congenital or dysplastic spondylolisthesis is due to abnormalities in the arch of L5 and of the upper sacrum. The L5 vertebra slips forward on the sacrum below. The pars interarticularis may be intact in this type of spondylolisthesis. The pars, however, is often weakened and has a predisposition for fracture or separation. The treatment of dysplastic spondylolisthesis and spondylolysis depends on the symptoms. Nachemson[15] has described spondylolysis without spondylolisthesis as a "questionable cause of back symptoms." Radiologic evidence of spondylolisthesis and spondylolysis is found in 5% of the population. According to Wiltse,[25] the presence of spondylolysis and spondylolisthesis increases the incidence of disc degeneration. According to Porter and Hibbert,[18] disc symptoms are infre-

quent in patients with spondylolisthesis from sagittal widening of the central canal as the lamina is left behind in the process of forward displacement.

Differences in leg length

Pain caused by leg length discrepancy depends on whether the discrepancy is congenital or suddenly acquired. In cases of fractures a leg length difference of 1.3 cm may increase the incidence of low back pain.[17] In cases of congenital or gradually developing shortening, back pain is associated with differences greater than 4 cm. If the patient has back pain with shortening of 2.5 cm, a small lift under the heel of the short leg is indicated. One should not compensate for the entire difference in cases that are congenital or have developed gradually.

HERNIATED DISC

Over 90% of disc herniations occur in the region of the L4-L5, L5-S1 intervertebral disc spaces. They may occur at any age but most frequently are found in patients between 30 and 50 years of age.

Pathology

Herniation of the nucleus pulposus may represent one stage in the progression of disc degeneration and the subsequent changes indicative of lumbar spondylosis. This complex has been referred to as a lumbar disc syndrome. Trauma is considered to be a precipitating rather than a causative factor in disc herniations. Early signs of degeneration can be seen in the second decade of life. Herniation that occurs before the process of disc degeneration can occur in adolescence due to embryologic abnormalities (residuals of the notochord or abnormalities of the cartilage end-plate). The disc herniation causes indentations in the cartilage end-plate (Schmorl's nodes).

Biochemical and biomechanical changes caused by the aging process affect the efficiency of the disc and alter the normal anatomy. As aging progresses, hydration of the disc decreases from 88% water content in the first 10 years of life to 60% in patients in their seventies. The cellular content of the nucleus decreases in relation to the fibrous component. There is progressive decrease in chondroitin sulfate and an increase in keratin sulfate.

Narrowing of the disc space follows the process of degeneration, causing the intersegmental ligament to become lax. Ligamentous laxity with subsequent evidence of instability has been considered a cause of back pain. More recent studies have demonstrated a wide variation of mobility in the lumbar spine. Lateral views in flexion and extension of the lumbosacral spine to determine mobility reveal that an average of 3 to 6 mm of anterior displacement at the L4-L5 interspace occurs in asymptomatic individuals and that 1.5 to 3 mm displacement occurs at the L5-S1 interspace. The instability noted on radiographs and its relationship to

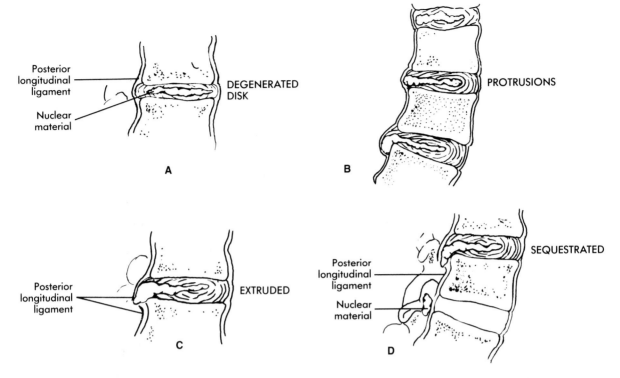

Figure 40-1. Various stages of disc degenerations and herniation. **A,** Disc degeneration. As nucleus loses water, disc space narrows and anulus bulges circumferentially. **B,** Disc protrusion. Note that posterior longitudinal ligament remains intact. **C,** Extruded disc. In extruded disc, posterior longitudinal ligament is ruptured. **D,** Sequestrated disc. Fragment has left the point of extrusion and has lodged somewhere a short distance away. Some believe that for fragment to be sequestrated, pathway between sequestrated fragment and opening in the posterior longitudinal ligament and anulus must have sealed off. (From American Academy of Orthopaedic Surgeons: Orthopaedic knowledge update I, Chicago, 1984, The Academy.)

back pain require careful investigation to determine significance for the individual patient. Radiologic findings of instability or degenerative changes must not be assumed to cause the patient's symptoms. Patients with advanced degenerative changes may have no symptoms. Radiographic changes may be coincidental in patients experiencing back pain. Disc degeneration causes bulging of the anulus fibrosis. This follows dehydration of the nucleus and is part of the aging process. Report of bulging of the anulus in CT scans should not be confused with disc herniation. With further degeneration, disc protrusion occurs with an intact posterior ligament. With a tear in the posterior ligament, the nucleus can press through, giving rise to an extruded disc. Sequestration occurs when the disc fragment has separated from its attachment and has moved away from the affected disc (Figure 40-1).

Symptoms

Most patients with a disc herniation relate a prior history of recurrent episodes of back pain. Back pain may precede disc herniation by many years. Prolonged sitting and stand-

ing can aggravate pain. Lifting may precipitate an episode of pain. Occupations that include simultaneous bending and twisting place the patient at high risk.

With progressive disc protrusion and herniation, sciatic pain with radicular pain is noted. It is not uncommon for the initial back pain to subside with the occurrence of pain down the leg. Sometimes pain is noted only in the calf. Pain in the back subsides once the nucleus pushes laterally and tension on the posterior longitudinal ligament is removed. Increase in intraspinal pressure caused by coughing, sneezing, or bearing down during bowel movements increases the pain.

Motor symptoms of muscular weakness and sensory deficits depend on the nerve root involved. L5 and S1 nerve roots are most frequently affected. Patients with lesions involving the L4 nerve root may have quadriceps atrophy and knee pain. Pain patterns follow dermatomal innervations (Figure 40-2).

Disc herniation may cause bladder and bowel dysfunction. Bladder disturbances include urinary retention, frequency, and episodes of incontinence. Neurologic and uro-

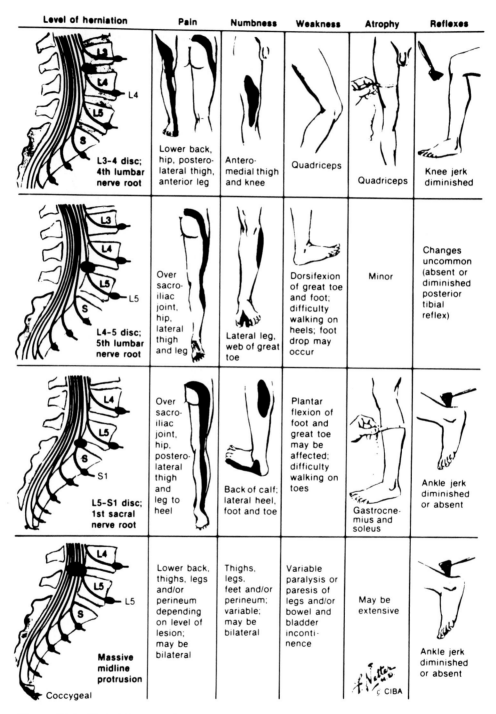

Level of herniation	Pain	Numbness	Weakness	Atrophy	Reflexes
L3-4 disc; 4th lumbar nerve root	Lower back, hip, postero-lateral thigh, anterior leg	Antero-medial thigh and knee	Quadriceps	Quadriceps	Knee jerk diminished
L4-5 disc; 5th lumbar nerve root	Over sacro-iliac joint, hip, lateral thigh and leg	Lateral leg, web of great toe	Dorsifexion of great toe and foot; difficulty walking on heels; foot drop may occur	Minor	Changes uncommon (absent or diminished posterior tibial reflex)
L5-S1 disc; 1st sacral nerve root	Over sacro-iliac joint, hip, postero-lateral thigh and leg to heel	Back of calf; lateral heel, foot and toe	Plantar flexion of foot and great toe may be affected; difficulty walking on toes	Gastrocne-mius and soleus	Ankle jerk diminished or absent
Massive midline protrusion Coccygeal	Lower back, thighs, legs and/or perineum depending on level of lesion; may be bilateral	Thighs, legs, feet and/or perineum; variable; may be bilateral	Variable paralysis or paresis of legs and/or bowel and bladder incontinence	May be extensive	Ankle jerk diminished or absent

Figure 40-2. Clinical features of herniated nucleus pulposus. (Copyright 1980 Ciba Pharmaceutical Company. Division of CIBA-GEIGY Corporation. Reprinted with permission from Keim, HA, and Kirkaldy-Willis, WH: Low Back Pain Clin Symposium 32:6, 1980. Illustrated by Frank H. Netter, MD.)

logic evaluation, including cystoscopy and urodynamic studies, is indicated in the presence of urinary bladder symptoms.

Referred pain may be due to other causes, which must be differentiated from nerve root compression. Radiating pain may result from irritation or stretching of ligaments or irritation of the periosteum or joint capsule. Trigger points in muscle may cause referred pain that simulates a herniated disc. Failure to recognize other causes of referred pain has led to frequent incorrect diagnoses of herniated disc.

Physical findings

In the acute stages the patient stands with hip and knee flexed on the affected side. Observation of the back reveals

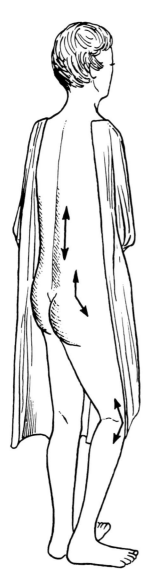

Figure 40-3. Flattening of normal lumbar lordosis in association with severe paraspinal muscle spasm. (From Finneson, BE: Low back pain, ed 2, Philadelphia, 1980, JB Lippincott Co.)

loss of the normal lordotic curve in the lumbar region (Figure 40-3). Limitation in range of motion and tenderness in the lower back with paravertebral muscle spasm is present. Sciatic scoliosis is due to nerve root pressure and may occur with tenderness along the sciatic nerve (Figure 40-4). Straight leg raising may produce pain; however, pain with straight leg raising is not specific for herniated disc. Such pain may be caused by muscle pathology. Neurologic deficits, including motor weakness, sensory deficit, and reflex changes, depend on the level of the nerve root involvement.

A cauda equina syndrome may result from a massive midline disc herniation. Symptoms of cauda equina syndrome may be acute or may progress gradually. Symptoms include back pain, pain in the back of the thighs, and perianal pain. Urinary difficulties include frequency and incontinence; bowel complaints may be present, in addition to complaints of impotence. Numbness is diffuse, extending from the buttocks to the feet, and is usually bilateral (Figure 40-5). Loss of anal reflex and perianal hypesthesia is characteristic. Although a cauda equina syndrome occurs rarely (0.2% of disc herniations), the physician must constantly be aware of this possibility, since prompt surgical decompression may play a role in decreasing permanent neurologic residuals.

Diagnostic studies

A medical laboratory workup for back pain should include a complete blood count, sedimentation rate, latex fixation, SMA-12 to include fasting blood sugar and uric acid levels, alkaline phosphatase, HLA-B27, and acid phosphatase, when appropriate for the possibility of prostatic carcinoma. A urinalysis is routinely ordered.

Radiologic studies of the lumbosacral spine should include anterior, posterior, lateral, and oblique views and with a view of the pelvis to visualize both hips. Symptoms attributed to the lower back may in fact be due to the presence of an osteoarthritic hip.

Computerized tomography (CT scan) permits noninvasive differentiation of tissue densities and may distinguish between muscle, bone, fat, nucleus pulposus, and nerve roots. In addition to the diagnosis of herniated disc, it has enabled the physician to more accurately diagnose the presence of spinal stenosis and lateral stenosis. It may be combined with a metrizamide myelogram.

Lumbar myelography is now performed using metrizamide, a water-soluble tri-ionate contrast medium. The water-soluble dye is less irritating than previous oil media, which markedly decreases the incidence of arachnoiditis.

Nuclear magnetic resonance imaging is excellent for visualizing the brain and spinal cord. It is helpful not only in diagnosing disc herniation, stenosis, and tumors but also in demonstrating demyelinization in the brain and spinal cord.

Radiologic techniques that are used less frequently to diagnose disc herniation include discography and epidural venography. Conventional tomograms may be useful for the

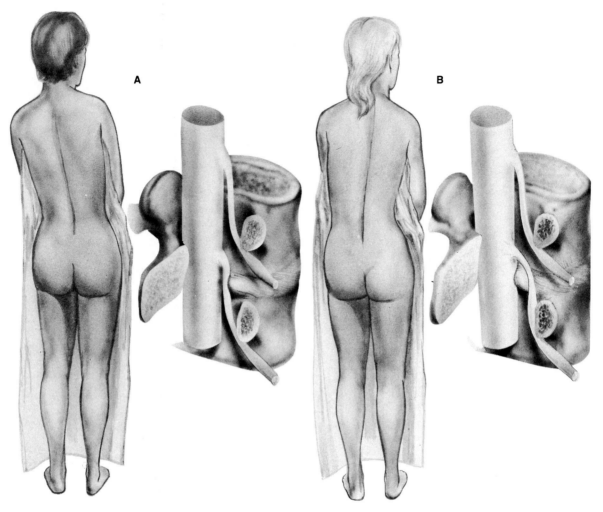

Figure 40-4. A, Herniation of disc lateral to nerve root. This usually produces a sciatic list away from side of irritated nerve root. **B,** Herniation of disc medial to nerve root and in axillary position. This usually produces sciatic list toward side of irritated nerve root. (From Rothman, RH, and Simeone, AF: The spine, ed 2, vols I and II, Philadelphia, 1982, WB Saunders Co.)

diagnosis of tumors, infection and fractures and to evaluate healing.

Electromyography and nerve conduction studies are helpful in diagnosing peripheral neuropathy caused by systemic disorders (such as diabetes), and in defining nerve root compressions.

Treatment

A patient with a herniated disc should be reassured that there is an 80% chance of recovering with conservative treatment and thus avoiding surgery. Since intradiscal pressure is lowest when the patient is lying down, bed rest is important in treating disc herniation. Intradiscal pressure or load on the disc in the third lumbar disc is 25 kg when the patient is supine, 100 kg standing, and 150 kg sitting. A period of 2 weeks' bed rest with bathroom privileges should be considered a minimum trial of bed rest. During this time,

anti-inflammatory drugs, analgesics, and muscle relaxants can be prescribed. A short course of oral steroid medication has been helpful in resistant cases of radiculopathy.

Pelvic traction may be of value, although there is no evidence that traction causes any appreciable change in the intervertebral disc. Some patients note symptomatic improvement. It is also helpful to keep patients on a program of bed rest.

Manipulation for reducing herniated disc has been advocated by Cyriax.[5] Kirkaldy-Willis[12] found that manipulation was of value in patients suffering from dysfunction owing to a posterior joint disorder or sacroiliac syndrome.

Physical therapy, including short-wave diathermy, sinewave electronic stimulation, heat or ice application, or massage, may help relieve symptoms.

Epidural steroid blocks are of value in radiculopathy; however, results are usually temporary.[24]

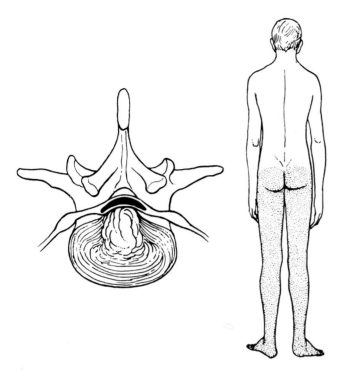

Figure 40-5. Cauda equina syndrome. (From Finneson, BE: Low back pain, ed 2, Philadelphia, 1980, JB Lippincott Co.)

After pain subsides, appropriate exercises for the lower back should be instituted. All exercise programs should include relaxation, limbering, and stretching. Exercise programs should begin with warm-up and end with a cool-down period. They should be demonstrated to the patient and, if possible, supervised for a period of time so the exercises are carried out properly. In patients with weak abdominal musculature, a lumbosacral support decreases the intradiscal pressure and is of value in early ambulation.

Surgical treatment

Surgical treatment is considered only after an adequate trial of conservative therapy. In the absence of progressive neurologic deficits, a trial of 4 to 6 weeks of conservative therapy is indicated. Indications for surgery include progressive muscle weakness, bladder or bowel difficulties, and development of cauda equina syndrome. If sciatic pain is persistent and incapacitating and is accompanied by evidence of disc herniation, surgery may also be indicated. Operating on the basis of pain alone usually gives poor surgical results. Even after disc excision, recurrent disc herniation can occur 1 week, months, or 1 year after surgery (Figure 40-6).

Surgical procedures include laminectomy with disc excision (Figure 40-7), microdiscectomy, chemonucleolysis, percutaneous discectomy, and spinal fusion. Spinal fusion may be indicated in cases of instability, after a second laminectomy, and in cases of spondylolisthesis. The most common spinal fusion performed is posterior lateral spinal fusion

(Figure 40-8). In selected cases, anterior lumbar body fusion or posterior intervertebral body lumbar fusion has been performed. These procedures are usually considered after a failed posterolateral fusion.

Psychologic factors that play a role in the patient's symptoms may be demonstrated by a pain drawing or a Minnesota Multiphasic Personality Inventory (MMPI). The MMPI is a questionnaire of 550 items designed to obtain a psychologic profile to aid in the diagnosis of neuroses and psychoses. If there is any doubt about the psychologic factors involved, it is wise for the surgeon to obtain a preoperative psychologic evaluation. Patients with poor results are often referred for psychologic evaluation and treatment only *after* surgery has been performed.

Patient education is of vital importance in conservative and surgical management. The patient must play an active role and share in the responsibility for getting well. It is not enough to get the patient over the initial attack of back pain. The patient must understand why the problem developed and how to prevent it. The physician or therapist must take the time to instruct the patient in back care. Back schools are playing an increasing role in the management of patients. Zacrisson-Forsell established the Swedish Back School in 1970. Emphasis in the Swedish program is on body mechanics based on ergonomic education. Canadian Back Education Units were established in 1974. A psychologic component was added to the training program with the aim of changing patients' attitudes toward low back pain.[9]

White founded the California Back School in San Francisco in 1976 with a more individualistic approach and emphasis on proper ergonomic techniques.

In a review of 6418 participants, the Canadian Back Education Units (CBEU) found that significant improvement occurred in patients who experienced back pain for 6 months or less. The complete CBEU consists of five classes, four weekly lectures, and a fifth review class 6 months later. Table 40-1 outlines the CBEU program.[9] The topics dis-

Table 40-1. CBEU program outline

Lecture	Lecturer	Data collection
Lecture 1	Orthopedic surgeon	Questionnaire 1 Multiple choice test 1
Lecture 2	Physiotherapist	
Lecture 3	Psychiatrist	Multiple choice test 2
Lecture 4	Psychologist or physiotherapist	
Review lecture	Physiotherapist	Questionnaire 2 Multiple choice test 3

From Hall, H, and Icetow, JA: Clin Orthop Rel Res 179:10, 1983.

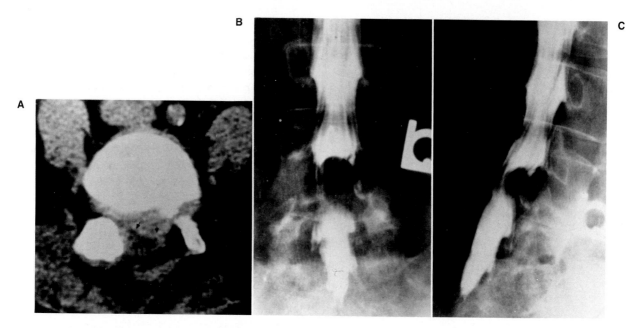

Figure 40-6. Recurrent herniated nucleus pulposus. Patient had back and leg pain 1 year after discectomy. **A,** Axial computerized tomographic scan demonstrates large extradural mass *(arrows)* extending posteriorly from disc space and compressing thecal sac. **B** and **C,** Metrizamide myelogram confirms this finding, and at surgery a large recurrent herniated nucleus pulposus was removed. (From Genant, KH: Spinal update 1984, San Francisco, 1983, Radiology Research and Education Foundation.)

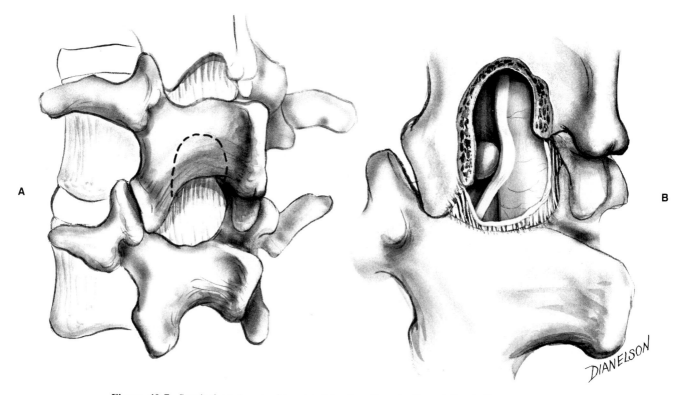

Figure 40-7. Surgical treatment of herniated lumbar disc. **A,** Dotted line indicates bone to be resected. **B,** Resection of inferior portion of lamina and removal of underlying ligamentum flavum reveals protruding disc compressing nerve root. (From Ruge, D, and Wiltse, LL: Spinal disorders, diagnosis and treatment, Philadelphia, 1977, Lea & Febiger.)

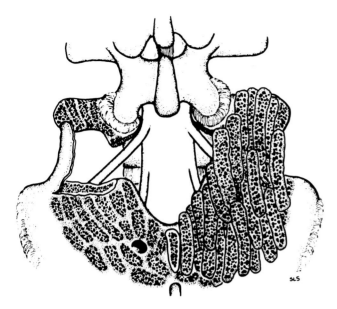

Figure 40-8. Posterolateral fusion. *(Left),* Damaging posterior joint and sacroiliac joint should be avoided during decortication. *(Right),* Bone graft should not be placed on exposed nerves. (From Kirkaldy-Willis, WH: Managing low back pain, ed 2, New York, 1988, Churchill-Livingstone. By permission of Churchill-Livingstone.)

cussed include anatomy, pathophysiology of the spine, body mechanics, psychiatric aspects of chronic pain, and the relation of emotions to muscle tension. The last lecture is devoted to low back exercises, including the teaching of relaxation techniques practiced under supervision.

One important aspect of the back school is the self-confidence it instills in patients so they can take an active role in getting well and staying well.

Preoperative and postoperative care of spinal surgery

Surgery involving the lumbosacral region is usually elective. Postoperative results improve greatly if the patients come to surgery in the best possible condition. Reconditioning of the patient should begin before surgery. Medical problems, especially overweight and endocrine imbalance (for example, thyroid, estrogen deficiency), should be taken care of preoperatively. Evaluation for muscle disorders is part of the preoperative workup. Muscle evaluation includes testing for strength, flexibility, and trigger points. Preoperative muscle tests also give information about the type of exercises the patient will later need. Conditioning of the patient before surgery decreases the length of convalescence and improves operative results. Relaxation techniques should be a part of all preoperative and postoperative exercise programs. Psychologic factors should be evaluated and treated before surgery.

Postoperative exercises are begun as soon as possible. Wearing a plaster body jacket or brace should not prevent the patient from doing appropriate exercises that will not interfere with the surgical procedure. Patients who return to work before normal strength and flexibility are achieved often become symptomatic. They experience recurrent pain, develop trigger points, and are then considered surgical failures. A surgical procedure that is technically well performed should not be allowed to fail because of poor preoperative and postoperative rehabilitation. The purpose of surgery is to increase the patient's function and permit a return to the patient's usual work. At the end of treatment the patient should be able to perform a full exercise program and be aware of how to prevent problems.

The following exercise program devised by Kraus incorporates the basic requirements for preoperative and postoperative rehabilitation.[21] It uniquely encompasses all factors that must be included for successful results. Emphasis is placed equally on relaxation, limbering, and stretching to promote flexibility and muscle strengthening of key postural muscles. In Chapter 44, Kraus discusses in detail the proper approach to treating muscle pain, including muscular deficiency, and the evaluation of trigger points before prescribing the exercise program.

Disorders of key postural muscles are best evaluated using the Kraus-Weber Minimum Muscular Fitness Test. An individualized program based on the results of the K-W Minimum Muscular Fitness Test can then be prescribed. A description of the K-W Minimum Muscular Fitness Test is included in Chapter 44 with a thorough discussion of the proper execution of the exercise program. The K-W Minimum Muscular Fitness Test can be performed preoperatively and postoperatively when the patient is not in acute pain.

The exercise program, a full series of exercises for preoperative and postoperative rehabilitation, should be performed on a gradual basis in sequence (Figure 40-9). As described in Chapter 44, exercises should start with relaxation techniques and progress gradually with limited repetitions. A partial or full program should be achieved preoperatively and postoperatively whenever possible.

I would not consider a back rehabilitation program complete until all efforts are made to enable the patient to complete the full exercise program.

Intervertebral disc space infection

It is especially important that a physician treating patients after spinal surgery be aware of the symptoms of intervertebral disc space infection. In children, disc space infection may be due to hematogenous spread. Adult disc space infections occur following spinal surgery. Vertebral osteomyelitis often involves the disc space and connecting vertebra. *Staphylococcus aureus* is the most frequently found organism.

Symptoms and signs

Pain is more severe than would be expected postoperatively and is present at rest and during the night. There is

Text continued on p. 586.

Exercise 1

Position yourself comfortably on the floor with both knees bent. Close your eyes. Take a deep breath and exhale slowly. Slide one leg out and slide it back. Slide the other leg out and slide it back. Take another deep breath. Tighten both fists, then let go. Repeat once more. When you do this exercise at the end of your exercise session, make sure that you include the alternating movement.

Take a deep breath—exhale slowly. Now shrug and breathe up. Exhale as you let go of the shrug.

Turn your head all the way to the left, then return it to the normal front and center position, and let go. Turn your head all the way to the right as far as you can, return to normal position, and let go. If you have a stiff neck, also do this exercise in a sitting position. Repeat three times.

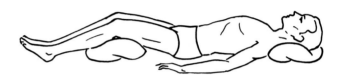

Exercise 2

Flex your knees and slowly draw your right knee up as close to your chest as you can comfortably. Return your foot to the floor, slide the leg out, and slide back. Now bring the other leg up to the chest. Return the foot to the floor, slide the leg out, and slide it back.

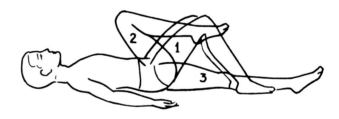

Exercise 3

Lie on your left side with your head resting comfortably on arm. Keep both knees flexed and hips slightly flexed. Slide your right knee as close to your head as is comfortably possible, then slowly extend the leg until it is completely straight. The leg is dead weight. Do the exercise three times, then turn to your right side and do the exercises with your left leg. Remember the top leg is dead weight.

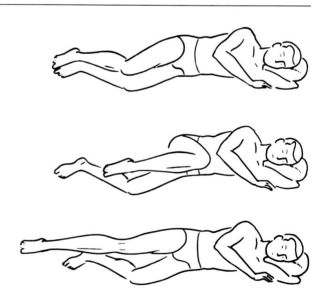

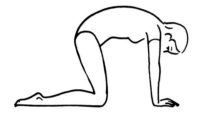

Exercise 4. Double Knee Flex

Lie on your back with both knees flexed. Pull both knees up to your chest. Then lower your legs gradually to the floor in the flexed position. Do not raise hips off the floor.

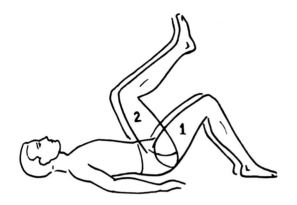

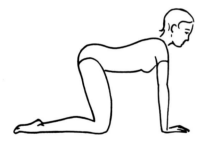

Exercise 5. Cat Back

Assume a kneeling position, resting on your hands and knees. Arch your back like a cat and drop your head at the same time. Then reverse the arch by bringing up your head and forming a U with your spine.

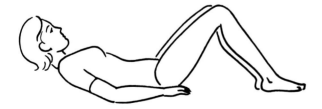

Exercise 6. Head Up, Supine

Lie on the floor, with knees flexed, hands loose by your sides. Raise your head and shoulders off the floor, bring them down slowly, and let go. Remember that fingertips should touch the top of the knee.

Figure 40-9. Exercise program devised by Kraus for preoperative and postoperative back rehabilitation. (From Ruskin, AP: Current therapy in physiatry, physical medicine, and rehabilitation, Philadelphia, 1984, WB Saunders Co.)

Continued.

Exercise 7. Bend Sitting

Sit on a chair, feet apart on the floor. Let your neck droop, then drop your shoulders and arms and bend down between your knees as far as you can. Return to an upright position, straighten up, and let go. Do not force your downward bend.

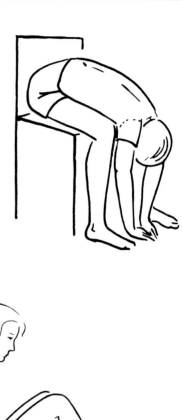

Exercise 8. Sit-up, Knees Flexed

Lie on your back with your hands clasped behind your head, knees flexed. Tuck your feet under a heavy object that will not topple over (a chest of drawers, bed, or heavy chair). Sit up, then lower yourself slowly to a lying position. You should sit up gradually, starting by raising your head, then your shoulders, and then your chest and lower end of the spine. Do not sit up by holding your trunk stiff and jerking your weight up. If you cannot do this exercise with your hands behind your neck, try to do it with your hands at your sides. Later, cross them over your stomach, and still later, when you are stronger, bring your crossed arms up to your chest and, finally, behind your neck and head. If you are unable to do this exercise at all, continue with the earlier exercises until you have gained enough strength to manage this one. Before the exercise, take a deep breath and exhale as you curl to a sitting position.

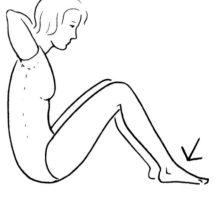

Exercise 9. Bend-Sitting Rotation

Sit on a chair; bend forward as far as possible, dropping your head and shoulders. Bend down to the left, then gradually straighten up and rest. Do the exercise again, bending to the right.

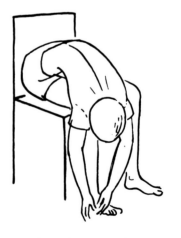

Figure 40-9, cont'd. Exercise program devised by Kraus for preoperative and postoperative back rehabilitation. (From Ruskin, AP: Current therapy in physiatry, physical medicine, and rehabilitation, Philadelphia, 1984, WB Saunders Co.)

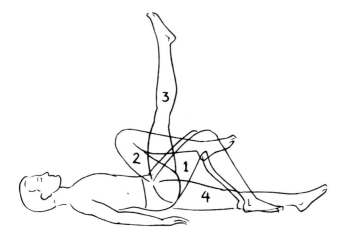

Exercise 10. Hamstring Stretch

Lie on your back, both knees flexed, arms at sides. Bring one knee up as close as possible to your face and extend the leg, pointing the toes toward the ceiling. Keep the knee locked. Lower the straight leg to the floor. Slide the leg back to a bent position. Do the same for the other leg. Bring the other leg to the shoulder. As you extend the leg, cup the heel. Lock the knee, lower the straight leg to floor, and slide the leg back to a bent position. Do the same for the other leg.

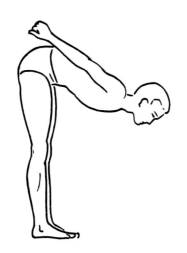

Exercise 11. Hamstring Stretch

Stand up, and with feet together, clasp your hands behind your back, keeping your back and neck straight. Bend forward from the hips. Gradually lower your trunk and go down as far as you can, raising your head until you feel stretching in the back of your legs.

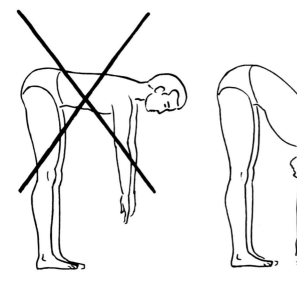

Exercise 12. Floor Touch

This is the peak exercise given in all programs. Stand and keep the feet together. First relax by inhaling and exhaling deeply. Drop your neck gradually and let the trunk "hang" loosely from the hips. Drop the shoulders and then the back gradually. Let gravity help you. Do this two or three times. When you are completely relaxed, "hanging from the hips," try to reach down as far as is easily possible. Relax again, straighten up, then repeat. Now reverse the order of exercises, going from 12 to 1.

a progressive increase in pain and muscle spasm. Marked limitation in the range of motion and tenderness in the region of the disc space is noted. Symptoms may occur 5 to 10 days and as late as 2 months following surgery. Fever usually is not present. Neurologic findings do not differ from the preoperative status.

Radiologic findings

Progressive narrowing and fusion of the disc space with bony proliferation is seen.

Laboratory studies

The sedimentation rate is usually elevated. A needle aspiration of the intervertebral disc space or biopsy under x-ray control may provide evidence of the invading organism. A bone scan is positive for infection.

Treatment

Rest and intravenous antibiotics are the treatments of choice. Ideally, one should identify the causative organism. Intervertebral disc space infection is treated conservatively unless a paravertebral abscess develops, which may require surgical drainage.

Arachnoiditis

The arachnoid is a fibrous elastic membrane that envelops the spinal cord. Inflammation of the arachnoid may be caused by infection, trauma, allergic reactions, reactions to myelographic dyes, and the trauma of spinal surgery itself.

Patients complain of back and leg pain. Symptoms are aggravated with movement. Characteristically, there is limited lumbosacral flexion, straight leg raising is positive, and paravertebral muscle spasms are present. Examination of the spinal fluid produces negative findings—normal protein levels and cell counts. A myelogram may demonstrate typical findings of arachnoiditis and confirm the diagnosis.

Both conservative and surgical treatments are often disappointing. Epidural injections of steroid offer some relief, which unfortunately is temporary.[24]

Microscopic lysis of adhesions has been performed. Cailliet[3] stated that spinal forceful flexion under anesthesia has been of value.

Patients with arachnoiditis often are referred to pain clinics for the control of chronic pain. All modalities for chronic pain have been used, including transcutaneous electrical nerve stimulation (TENS), posterior spinal column stimulation, antidepressant drugs if indicated, behavior modifi-

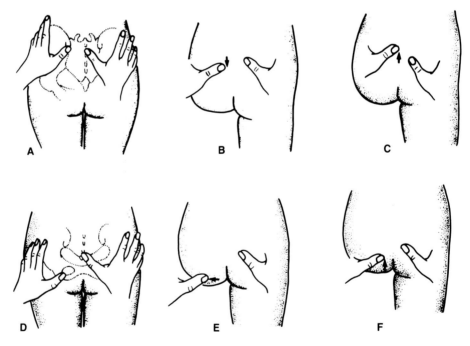

Figure 40-10. Tests to demonstrate left sacroiliac fixation. Tests for upper part of joint (**A** to **C**) and for lower part (**D** to **E**). **A,** Examiner places left thumb on posterior superior iliac spine and right thumb over one of sacral spinous processes. **B,** When movement is normal, examiner's left thumb moves downward as the patient raises left leg. **C,** When joint is fixed, examiner's left thumb moves upward as patient raises left leg. **D,** Examiner places left thumb over ischial tuberosity and right thumb over apex of sacrum. **E,** When movement is normal, examiner's left thumb moves laterally as patient raises left leg. **F,** When joint is fixed, examiner's left thumb moves slightly upward as patient raises left leg. (From Kirkaldy-Willis, WH: Managing low back pain, ed 2, New York, 1988, Churchill-Livingstone. By permission of Churchill-Livingstone.)

cation, and control of medication to prevent drug dependency.

SACROILIAC JOINT SYNDROME

In the early 1900s sacroiliac joint disorder was a fashionable explanation of low back pain. After the discovery of disc herniation, little attention was given to sacroiliac disorders, and there was a tendency to overdiagnose disc herniation. Kirkaldy-Willis[12] noted that sacroiliac joint syndrome is a commonly seen type of dysfunction, the exact cause of which is unknown.

Symptoms

Pain may be acute, chronic, or recurrent in the area of the sacroiliac joint; buttock pain is commonly referred to the posterior aspect of the thigh, leg, and groin. Symptoms are similar to those seen with L4-L5, L5-S1 posterior joint involvement.

Physical examination

Examination reveals local tenderness in the region of the sacroiliac joint and sacrosciatic notch. Differences in mobility of the joint may be detected on physical examination (Figure 40-10).

There is controversy over whether motion is present under ordinary circumstances. According to Kirkaldy-Willis some motion (3 to 5 degrees) may be present in the sacroiliac joint until late middle age, after which movement is reduced. Kirkaldy-Willis[12] believes that manipulation can benefit certain sacroiliac problems.

Cyriax[4,5] believes that movement can occur at the sacroiliac joint but it is limited to 0.25 mm. He stated that displacements of the sacrum on the ilium do not occur and that there is in fact little that can go wrong with the sacroiliac joint. He does not manipulate the sacroiliac joint.[4,5]

Injection into the sacroiliac joint with lidocaine and steroid under radiologic control can be diagnostic and therapeutic.

Treatment

Treatment may include anti-inflammatory drugs, analgesics, and physical modalities, including heat, ice, ultrasound, and diathermy. The use of a sacroiliac support may be indicated. There is no universal agreement that *manipulation* of the sacroiliac joint is indicated. Persistent pain that does not respond to conservative therapy may require fusion of the sacroiliac joint; however, surgery is rarely necessary.

It is unusual to see any evidence of sacroiliac pathology on a radiograph unless there is disruption of the sacroiliac joint accompanied by fracture of the pelvis or with the inflammatory changes and subsequent fusion of the sacroiliac joints seen in ankylosing spondylitis.

COCCYDYNIA

Coccydynia most frequently follows a traumatic event such as contusion or fracture of the coccyx or sprain of the sacroiliac joint. It may be caused by congenital deformities, infection, or arthritis of the sacrococcygeal joint.

Symptoms

The term "coccydynia" refers to pain in the area of the coccyx that extends beyond the normal expected healing time. Posttraumatic coccydynia is found more often in women. The pain is aggravated with sitting. Patients usually come for consultation carrying a cushion or foam rubber ring to sit on. Rectal pain and problems with defecation may occur. Symptoms can occur after childbirth, injuries involving the lumbosacral area, or spinal surgery (laminectomies and spinal fusions).

Physical findings

Tenderness on external palpation is usually present. A rectal examination enables the examiner to evaluate the coccyx and surrounding musculature. Palpation of the coccyx itself may detect abnormal motion or tenderness that reproduces the patient's symptoms. The examining finger may feel spasm of the pericoccygeal musculature. Spasm may be the only cause of persistent complaints, and there may be no disorder of the coccyx bone.

Patients with chronic coccygeal pain should be evaluated by a proctologist. A urologic examination may sometimes be necessary. Frequently, there is a functional overlay that requires psychologic evaluation.

Treatment

Conservative treatment should be exhausted before surgery is considered. Some patients feel more comfortable in a soft chair, and others feel worse. Most require a cushion to sit on and obtain relief from a sacroiliac support. Muscle relaxant and analgesics can be prescribed. Massage and electrogalvanic stimulation for three 1-hour treatments over a period of 10 days often relieve symptoms. If movement of the sacrococcygeal joint is painful, injection of lidocaine and steroid may be helpful. Patients are instructed in isometric gluteal exercises. Most respond well to conservative therapy. I routinely refer patients with coccydynia to a proctologist for evaluation as well as for proctologic treatment. Treatment consists of massage of the paracoccygeal muscles, electrogalvanic stimulation, and appropriate muscle relaxants or tranquilizers. Even if definite coccyx pain is present and symptoms are disabling, surgery should probably not be considered because the overall results of coccygectomy have been poor.

If the patient has a verifiable coccyx abnormality without psychologic overlay and has not responded to adequate conservative therapy performed by a proctologist experienced in treating coccydynia, the results of surgery can be very satisfactory. Nevertheless coccygectomy is rarely necessary.

PIRIFORMIS SYNDROME

The piriformis muscle may be injured by local trauma or twisting of the leg. All or part of the sciatic nerve may pass under or through the piriformis muscle. Figure 40-11 demonstrates the close relationship of the piriformis muscle to the sciatic nerve.

Symptoms

Buttock and sciatic pain caused by a disorder of piriformis muscle must be differentiated from a herniated disc. Pain may radiate as far as the ankle and toes. Symptoms of sciatic nerve entrapment, although rare, may occur. Trigger points in the piriformis muscle may cause a typical pattern of sciatic pain radiation. Tenderness of the piriformis is present. The muscle is best palpated with the patient lying on the unaffected side; the affected hip is flexed with the thigh adducted and the knee in flexion. The muscle may be painful on rectal or vaginal examination. Straight leg raising may evoke symptoms. Pain may be elicited with abduction and external rotation of the leg. Findings of the neurologic examination are usually negative, as is a radiograph of the lumbosacral spine.

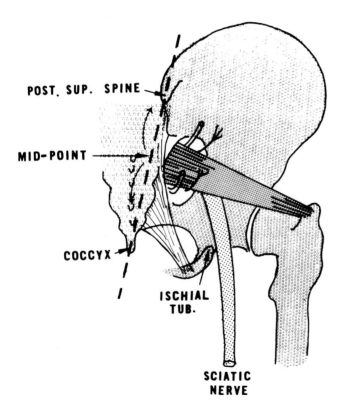

Figure 40-11. Piriformis muscle. Anatomic relationship of sciatic nerve to piriformis muscle. (From Cailliet, R: Low back pain syndrome, Philadelphia, 1981, FA Davis Co.)

Treatment

Symptoms usually respond to local injection of lidocaine, which may be combined with a steroid. If a trigger point is found, needling of the trigger point with lidocaine and appropriate follow-up care is indicated.[14]

TRAUMA
Lumbosacral sprain and strain (facet syndrome)

A lumbosacral sprain or strain includes muscle tears as well as sprain of the apophyseal joints (facet syndrome). Symptoms may be caused by bending or twisting motions. Patients with a facet syndrome characteristically complain of pain with hyperextension. First-time acute back injuries have a good prognosis. Ninety percent are relieved of pain in 6 weeks, and 95% in 3 months, regardless of treatment used.[16]

In cases of lumbosacral sprain, bed rest may be indicated for 2 to 3 days in the acute phase, but if patients can tolerate it, they should be kept ambulatory. Prolonged bed rest is indicated only in the treatment of herniated disc because it encourages rapid physical deconditioning. Psychologically, it is best for the patient to remain ambulatory and return to work as soon as possible. Patients who continue to experience low back pain usually have an inadequately treated muscle disorder. The four causes of muscle pain (spasm, tension, trigger points, muscle deficiency) must be investigated and treated accordingly. The following outline describes a regimen for the management of muscle pain[19]:

  I. Avoid bed rest.

  II. Keep ambulatory, if possible.

  III. Treat spasm and pain with ice massage, heat, ethyl chloride spray, tetanizing current for 10 minutes, relaxation and limbering exercises, gentle stretching.

  IV. Evaluate.

    A. Tension
      1. Tranquilizers, if necessary
      2. Biofeedback
      3. Psychologic evaluation

    B. Muscle deficiency
      1. Kraus-Weber muscle test
      2. Individual exercise
      3. Program to relax, limber, stretch, and strengthen muscles

    C. Trigger points—treat trigger points before starting exercise program; needle with lidocaine or saline

    D. Multiple trigger points and diffuse muscle tenderness
      1. Obtain endocrine workup
      2. Hypothyroidism
      3. Estrogen deficiency

  V. Prevent recurrences.

    A. Medical evaluation
      1. Endocrine disturbances
      2. Obesity

B. Psychologic recurrences
  1. Neurosis
  2. Anxiety
  3. Tension states
C. Exercise program and postural changes
  1. Change of work habits
  2. Specific exercise program with appropriate warm-up and cool-down periods
  3. Weight control

Sprung back

Sprung back is due to injury to intraspinous or supraspinous ligaments; it may result from lifting improperly or bending forward with the knees extended. Tenderness is noted over the posterior ligaments. Pain may be relieved by local injection of lidocaine, with or without steroid. Lumbosacral support may be necessary in the acute phase. As with all back pain, the patient must be instructed in postural lifting techniques.

Fractures

One must distinguish between three groups of spinal fractures:
  1. Fracture of the spinous and transverse processes
  2. Fracture of the vertebral bodies
  3. Fracture of the articular facets of the neural arch

Fractures of the transverse process

Fractures of the transverse process result from sudden contraction of the quadratus lumborum muscle against resistance. An avulsion fracture with tearing of muscle and fascia occurs with symptoms of an avulsion sprain injury. One or more transverse processes may be avulsed. Injury to the soft tissues (muscle aponeurosis, hemorrhage) is the most important aspect of this injury.

Treatment is symptomatic. The emphasis is on preventing adhesions. The patient may initially require a short period of bed rest but should be ambulatory as soon as possible. A lumbosacral support is indicated for several weeks after which a back exercise program should begin. Exercises are progressive and emphasize relaxation, limbering, stretching, and strengthening of muscle. Exercises should always have warm-up and cool-down periods.

Fracture of the spinous process

Fractures of the spinous processes are treated as avulsion fractures. Normal activities should resume as soon as possible, and the patient should be reassured about the benign nature of the fracture.

Fracture of the vertebral bodies

Fractures of the lumbar region most often result from flexion-compression injuries in the region of the upper two lumbar vertebral bodies and the twelfth dorsal vertebral body. Fractures limited to the lower lumbar vertebral bodies usually do not present as fracture dislocation and usually do not have neurologic involvement. Careful neurologic examination must be performed for all spine fractures. Wedge compression fractures may result from trauma or osteoporosis or tumor. Early stages of pathologic fractures causing pain and spasm may not be visible on radiographs. Early microfractures may progress to a major vertebral body collapse. In these cases a bone scan should be performed to determine if another fracture is present. A bone scan should also be performed when there is doubt concerning the differential diagnosis of a recent or old compression fracture. Serial radiographs are helpful in demonstrating the healing of recent fractures. It is not unusual for this diagnostic problem to occur when a patient with a compression fracture caused by osteoporosis sustains an injury to the back. Radiographs may indicate only that there is a compression fracture of uncertain duration. Such patients require bone scans and follow-up radiographs to determine if indeed there is a recent compression fracture.

In cases of suspected infection or tumor, a needle biopsy under CT scan guidance or open biopsy may be necessary for diagnosis. A bone scan including technetium and gallium scans may also be needed. A gallium scan helps identify the presence of infection.

Patients with compression fractures of the lower lumbar vertebral bodies that are stable and offer no danger of neurologic involvement should ambulate as soon as comfort permits. A lumbosacral support or Knight spinal brace may be used for initial pain relief, and a program of hyperextension exercises should be given as soon as symptoms permit. Stable minor fractures may require no immobilization. It is important to keep elderly patients active and use as little immobilization as necessary to prevent further osteoporosis and vertebral body collapse. In severe cases of osteoporosis and multiple compression fractures, medical evaluation and studies for possible malignancy, osteoporosis, and osteomalacia should be performed. Iliac bone biopsy, osteoporosis scanning, and appropriate laboratory work are indicated. Calcium, phosphorus, alkaline phosphatase, and special studies such as vitamin D and parathormone assay may be necessary. Based on the cause of the disorder, drugs in various combinations such as calcium, vitamin D, sodium fluoride, calcitonin, estrogen, and progesterone are being used in research studies to determine their effect on remodeling of osteoporotic bone.

Fracture dislocation with instability and spinal cord injury occurs in the thoracic lumbar junction where rotary forces are greatest. The lumbar vertebrae, L3-L4, L4-L5, are more resistant to rotation and displacement because of the configuration of the lumbar facet joints in the sagittal plane, in addition to the surrounding supporting ligaments and musculature.

Fractures of the neural arch

Stress fractures of the neural arch may involve the pedicle, pars, or lamina. Abel[1] has reported cases of stress fractures involving a laminar fracture in a jogger, bilateral pedicle fractures in a ballet dancer, and lamina and isthmus fracture in a child.

Symptoms are usually insidious and difficult to explain when radiographs are normal. Radiologic visualization may be difficult; vertebral arch views, multidirectional tomography, and CT scan may be required. If a stress fracture is considered, a bone scan should be ordered. Treatment is symptomatic—the patient should avoid activities that cause symptoms. A back support may be prescribed in the acute phase. Back exercises should begin after a period of healing and subsidence of symptoms.

LUMBAR SPONDYLOSIS

Spondylosis consists of degenerative changes involving the intervertebral disc and its adjacent structures. Hereditary factors predispose to premature disc degeneration. Patients as young as 20 years of age may have significant degenerative changes, whereas some patients in their seventies have radiographs of the lumbosacral region that are unusually free of any degenerative changes and have no symptoms of lumbar spondylosis. The degenerative process is related to aging. The presence of degenerative changes, however, need not be symptomatic. The frequency of lumbar spondylosis is not related to sex or occupation. The significance of the radiologic findings of chronic degenerative disc disease should be adequately explained to the patient. Many patients are unnecessarily made anxious by the diagnosis. Often the patient's symptoms are not related to the radiologic findings. In these cases degenerative findings are coinci-

dental. An explanation of the significance of the degenerative findings in each case is necessary.

Pathology

Chronic pathologic changes begin with dehydration of the nucleus pulposus. The height of the intervertebral disc spaces decreases, anulus fibrosis bulges, and osteophytes and spurs form. These pathologic changes can result in nerve root and canal cord impingement, giving rise to neurologic signs and symptoms. Pathologic changes are found earliest at the L4-L5 and L5-S1 intervertebral disc spaces. The posterior facet joints are synovial joints and undergo the same pathologic changes seen in other synovial joints in the body. Articular cartilage undergoes degenerative change with osteochondral fractures, thickening of the joint capsule with secondary synovitis, and the development of adhesions. Arthritic changes give rise to the symptoms of pain and joint stiffness. A summary of the pathologic progression from disc degeneration to spinal stenosis is detailed in Figure 40-12.

Symptoms

Pain is the major complaint of patients with lumbar spondylosis. Backache may precede sciatica, depending on the major disc degeneration and nerve root involvement. Back pain that radiates to the lower extremities may also occur with facet joint irritation. Leg pain is usually unilateral—less frequently bilateral. Activities such as lifting and falling may contribute to the development of symptoms. Pain is intensified by coughing or sneezing. Patients may have re-

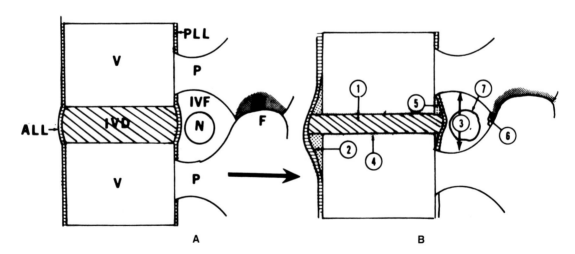

Figure 40-12. Sequence of degeneration: spondylosis. **A,** Normal functional unit: *V,* vertebral body; *IVD,* intervertebral disc; *ALL,* anterior longitudinal ligament; *PLL,* posterior longitudinal ligament; *P,* pedicle; *N,* nerve; *IVF,* intervertebral foramen; *F,* facet; *C,* cartilage. **B,** Disc *(1)* degenerates; longitudinal ligament *(2)* slackens and pulls away from vertebral body; foramen *(3)* narrows; cartilaginous end-plates *(4)* show sclerotic changes; posterior spurs or osteophytes *(5)* begin to form; degenerating cartilaginous changes *(6)* occur in facets; foraminal stenosis appears *(7)* leading to nerve root compression. (From Cailliet, R: Low back pain syndrome, Philadelphia, 1981, FA Davis Co.)

current episodes of symptoms and periods of being totally asymptomatic. Paresthesia, motor weakness, numbness, and bladder dysfunction may occur.

Physical findings

Physical findings vary with the extent of degenerative changes and the specific anatomic structures involved. The patient may have a limp and stand with the hip and knee on the affected side in flexion. Range of motion of the lumbosacral spine is limited in all directions. Extension is usually painful and more restricted than flexion. Straight leg raising may elicit symptoms when the L4-S1 disc area is involved. Neurologic findings depend on specific nerve root involvement. Atrophy, muscle weakness, and diminished or absent reflexes follow specific anatomic nerve root patterns. Neurologic findings do not necessarily indicate the level of intervertebral disc involved but are specific for the nerve root affected. An absent ankle reflex from S1 nerve root compression may be due to a lesion involving the L4-L5 or L5-S1 disc. This differentiation must be made by myelogram or CT scan. Sensory changes of numbness or paresthesia follow nerve root dermatome distribution. Sensory findings are highly subjective and unreliable as an indicator of spinal neurologic levels of involvement. Patients with back problems almost always have a muscle disorder contributing to their symptoms.

Radiologic findings

Radiologic studies help establish a diagnosis and rule out other causes of back or leg pain. A radiograph of the pelvis that includes the hips should be part of the lumbosacral radiologic examination. It is not unusual for patients with degenerative arthritic changes of the spine to have advanced arthritis of the hip, which is the main cause of their complaints. CT scan and nuclear magnetic resonance imaging demonstrate foraminal narrowing and lumbar canal narrowing. A myelogram helps visualize spinal cord and root pathology. The development of the CT scan has helped greatly in diagnosing spinal stenosis and lateral canal stenosis. As with all studies, findings must be correlated with the patient's symptoms and physical signs to determine diagnosis and treatment. One should treat the patient and not the radiographs.

Treatment

An initial brief period of bed rest may be indicated. Prolonged bed rest is detrimental and to be avoided. The patient should use a firm bed, preferably with a bed board. Anti-inflammatory drugs, analgesics, and muscle relaxants are prescribed. A lumbosacral support is used if necessary. Examination is made for muscle disorder (muscle spasm, tension, muscle weakness, and trigger points), which is treated accordingly.

Physical modalities, including massage and electrical stimulation, are prescribed according to the symptoms. In-

jection of apophyseal joints with local anesthetic has been used for diagnostic purposes.[6] Steroid injections into the synovial facet joints are infrequently performed.

Indications for surgery include persistent pain that has not responded to conservative therapy, progressive or sudden motor weakness, or bladder dysfunction. Surgery for lumbar spondylosis may require excision of the herniated disc in addition to foraminotomy, removal of osteoarthritic spurs, and decompression depending on the problem. Instability may require spinal fusion. Spinal fusion, however, is rarely indicated for patients past 60 years of age (Figure 40-13).

SPINAL STENOSIS

Spinal stenosis is a narrowing of the central portion of the spinal canal, giving rise to central stenosis, or a narrowing of the lateral part of the nerve canal, giving rise to lateral stenosis with lateral nerve entrapment. Central and lateral stenosis may occur separately or in combination and may involve one or more levels. Spinal stenosis of the lumbar canal may be primary (congenital) or secondary (acquired). Congenital narrowing of the lumbar canal rarely causes difficulties until adult life. Degenerative changes lead to further narrowing of available space with cauda equina symptoms. Causes of narrowing of the lumbar canal may be degenerative disc disease with progressive spondylosis, spondylolisthesis, extradural tumors, and bony proliferation resulting from spinal fusion. The greatest central canal narrowing occurs at the L3-L4 and L4-L5 region.

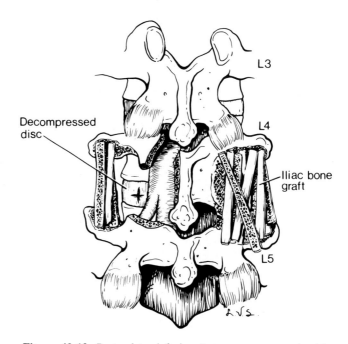

Figure 40-13. Posterolateral fusion (transverse processes) with bone graft from iliac crest. Laminectomy and decompression with posterolateral fusion. (From Morris, JM: Spine Update 1984.)

Symptoms of central spinal stenosis

Symptoms characteristic of spinal stenosis resemble the lower extremity pain of vascular occlusive disease. Symptoms usually begin with back pain progressing to classical neurogenic claudication, which must be differentiated from the intermittent claudication of vascular occlusive disease. Patients with spinal stenosis experience leg pain when walking and standing. Sensory changes and muscle weakness may also be present. Symptoms of narrowing of the lumbar canal may be caused by intermittent ischemia of the cauda equina syndrome or be posturally induced. Posturally induced pain may result from lordosis and is relieved by changing posture. The pain of ischemic neurogenic intermittent claudication, or "pseudoclaudication," is relieved by sitting down and flexing forward; in contrast, vascular claudication is relieved when walking is stopped. Pain of neurogenic onset continues after the provocative activity stops and is more sciatic in distribution. With neurogenic claudication, neurologic deficits may be present at rest or may appear after the patient exercises. Symptoms are aggravated with hyperextension.

Symptoms of lateral spinal stenosis

Two types of lateral entrapment are encountered.[11] Dynamic recurrent entrapment in the early stages of the degenerative process progresses to fixed permanent entrapment at a later stage. Lateral entrapment may accompany central stenosis or a herniated disc, giving rise to all the symptoms associated with those conditions.

Isolated lateral entrapment may cause sciatic-type pain evoked by straight leg raising. Neurologic findings are often normal. In lateral stenosis, myelogram findings are usually normal or sometimes suggest "cutting off of the nerve root sheath." Central stenosis and lateral spinal stenosis is best diagnosed by CT scan (Figure 40-14). Electromyography may provide additional evidence of nerve root involvement.

Treatment

Treatment depends on the severity of symptoms. A trial of conservative therapy is indicated unless there is progressive neurologic muscle weakness or symptoms of a neurogenic bladder. Conservative treatment includes rest, lumbosacral support, exercises or decrease postural lordosis, and treatment of muscle disorder. Vocational rehabilitation may be necessary.

Surgical treatment of stenosis requires decompression (Figure 40-15). In central stenosis an adequate amount of lamina is removed to relieve pressure on the cauda equina. If a herniated disc is present, the disc is excised. A lateral canal or lateral recess runs from the medial edge of the superior process to the foramen. Lumbar spinal lateral entrapment is sometimes referred to as superior facet syndrome. The canal is enlarged by removing the medial and anterior portions of the superior articular process. If segmental instability is present, a single- or two-level posterolateral fusion is performed.

Postoperative care is essentially the same as for disc removal. The patient is out of bed the next day and discharged in 7 to 10 days.

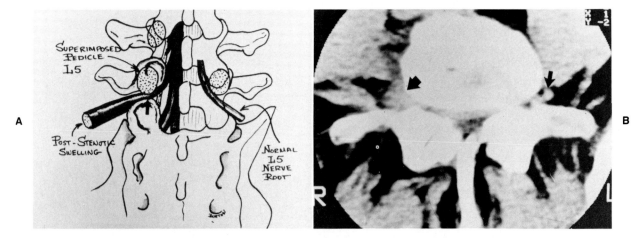

Figure 40-14. A, Bony lateral spinal stenosis at L5-S1 from hypertrophic overgrowth of superior articular process of S1 and cephalic subluxation with impingement of nerve root and marked postimpingement swelling. **B,** Axial image at L5-S1 showing severe central spinal stenosis and severe bony lateral spinal stenosis at L5-S1 on right. Although both intervertebral nerve root canals appear narrowed, patient had right-sided sciatica; severe swelling of right L5 nerve root *(large arrow)* compared with left nerve root *(small arrow)* confirm significant nerve root impingement that is present. (From Heathoff, K, and Ray, DC: Spine Update 1984.)

Kirkaldy-Willis[13] reported marked improvement is 62% of patients operated on for lateral stenosis and slight improvement in 21%. Seventeen percent were unimproved, and 66% returned to their previous occupations. He also observed that lumbar spinal stenosis was a more common cause of back and leg pain than disc herniation.

Failure to recognize lateral canal stenosis may explain some of the poor results of disc surgery. Before the use of the CT scan the diagnosis of lateral stenosis was primarily a clinical one, with the help of a myelogram, which did not always confirm the diagnosis. CT scan may be combined with a metrizamide myelogram. Symptoms do not necessarily correspond to the degree of spinal compression noted on CT scan or myelogram. CT scan, myelogram, and nuclear magnetic resonance imaging must be interpreted in light of the clinical examination.

The diagnosis of "low back syndrome" may represent various stages of lumbar spondylosis. Symptoms may be acute or chronic and result from minor or major stresses placed on the lumbosacral spine. The physician should attempt to make a more anatomic diagnosis based on specific structural pathology whenever possible.

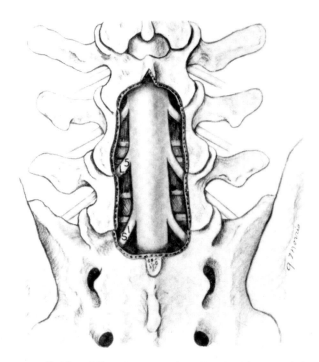

Figure 40-15. Midline decompression. We do this type of decompression most frequently. Pars and most of facets are saved. Medial portion of superior articular process is nipped off as it swings medially posterior to spinal nerve. Stability is preserved. Removing spinous processes seems to produce no clinically noticeable adverse effect. L5 spinal nerve is the one most frequently compressed in lateral canal. (From Wiltse, LL: Clin Orthop Rel Res 129:22, 1977.)

SPONDYLOLYSIS AND SPONDYLISTHESIS
Spondylolysis

Spondylolysis is a defect in the neural arch (pars interarticularis). It may occur without spondylolisthesis. It is rarely seen in patients younger than 5 years of age. It is unlikely that spondylolysis is a congenital defect in view of the fact that recent knowledge has confirmed the presence of only one ossification center in the pars instead of the dual ossification center that was thought to be present. The ratio of male to female is two to one. The incidence of spondylolysis and spondylolisthesis increases until the age of 20. There is a hereditary predisposition for spondylolysis and spondylolisthesis that occurs in 27% to 69% of members of some families, compared to 4% to 8% in the general population.

Congenital deformities such as sacral spina bifida, lack of development of the proximal sacrum, and superior sacral facet can cause a lack of posterior support, which increases the forces in the pars interarticularis and results in a stress fracture.

Wiltse[20] suggested that spondylolysis represents a "stress or fatigue fracture of the pars interarticularis." Shear stresses are highest in the pars interarticularis when the spine is extended. This defect is often found in athletes who engage in activities requiring hyperextension, such as gymnasts, weight lifters, and college football linemen.

Porter[18] compared symptoms of 131 patients with lysis of the pars interarticularis and 2229 patients without lysis during their initial referral to a back pain clinic. Symptoms associated with disc prolapse were significantly fewer in those patients with lysis of the pars.

In contrast, the most common symptom in patients with lytic defects was pain in the back or referred pain to the posterior aspect of the thighs. In Porter's study the canal diameter was measured by ultrasound.[18] In patients with spondylolisthesis, sagittal widening of the canal was noted. Widening of the canal may explain the rarity of herniated disc symptoms in spondylolisthesis, even when a disc prolapse is present.

Semon and Spengler[22] reviewed the records of 506 college-age football players over an 8-year period. There is no significant difference in time lost from games or practice sessions between patients with spondylolysis and those with normal radiologic findings. They concluded that lumbar spondylolysis is of minimal clinical significance over a short (4-year) period. With the exception of certain occupations, athletic activities that increase the risk of hyperextension injuries, and pregnancy, a patient with lysis is no more likely to develop back pain than the rest of the population. A child who is found to have spondylolysis or spondylolisthesis but is asymptomatic should not be restricted in any way. Full participation in sports is permitted. Parents should be informed of the condition and advised that reevaluation is indicated if the child is symptomatic.

CLASSIFICATION OF SPONDYLOLISTHESIS

1. Dysplastic (congenital). Congenital abnormalities of the upper sacrum or the arch of L5 permit the olisthesis to occur.
2. Isthmic. The lesion is in the pars interarticularis. Three types can be recognized:
   a. Lytic—fatigue fracture of the pars
   b. Elongated but intact pars
   c. Acute fracture of the pars (not to be confused with "traumatic," see no. 4)
3. Degenerative. This type is due to long-standing intersegmental instability.
4. Posttraumatic. This type is due to fractures in areas of the bony hook other than the pars. (Fracture-dislocation is not considered in this type of spondylolisthesis, but the differentiation may not always be clear.)
5. Pathologic. There is generalized or localized bone disease.

From American Academy of Orthopaedic Surgeons: Orthopaedic knowledge update. I, Chicago, 1984, The Academy.

Spondylolisthesis

Spondylolisthesis is a slipping forward of one vertebra on the vertebra below. Spondylolisthesis and spondylolysis occur most often at the L5-S1 level. The etiology of spondylolisthesis is classified into five types described in the box at left.

Dysplastic spondylolisthesis

Dysplastic or congenital spondylolisthesis is characterized by an inadequate superior process of the sacrum and hypoplasia of the upper sacrum, permitting the fifth lumbar vertebra and spine to move forward on the sacrum. If the pars interarticularis remains intact, a slippage of greater than 25% to 35% would cause cauda equina paralysis. Usually the pars elongates or comes apart. Dysplastic spondylolisthesis is often accompanied by congenital deformities such as spina bifida occulta. Symptoms can occur during childhood and early adolescence.

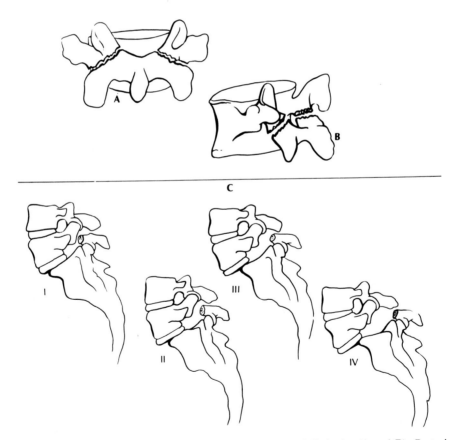

Figure 40-16. Spondylolysis may occur with or without spondylolisthesis. (**A** and **B**), Posterior and oblique views of lumbar vertebra that demonstrate congenital defect in pars interarticularis that constitutes spondylolysis. If this bony defect results in separation and anterior displacement of vertebral body, this dislocation is referred to as spondylolisthesis. **C,** Increasingly severe stages of anterior dislocation, referred to as spondylolisthesis of grades I to IV. (From Wilkinson, HA: The failed back syndrome: etiology and therapy, Philadelphia, 1983, Harper & Row.)

Isthmic spondylolisthesis

The basic lesion in isthmic spondylolisthesis is in the pars interarticularis. Three types of lesion are identified. A lytic lesion in the pars or elongation may be found. The lytic lesion is seldom seen below the age of 5. It is considered a fatigue fracture. Elongation of the pars is said to be due to microfractures. The third type of lesion, caused by an acute fracture, is rare.

Degenerative spondylolisthesis

Deformity of facet joints from osteoarthritic changes involving the intervertebral joints and facet joints disrupts facet joint integrity, which causes subsequent spondylolisthesis. This is usually seen over the age of 50 years. It is six times more common at the L4-L5 interspace. It is found more frequently when there is sacralization of the L5 vertebra.

Posttraumatic spondylolisthesis

Posttraumatic spondylolisthesis may result from fractures that involve the articular processes.

Pathologic spondylolisthesis

Pathologic spondylolisthesis may be caused by bone disease such as Paget's disease. Forward slipping of the vertebral bodies is graded according to degree. Four grades of forward displacement are distinguished: grades I, II, III, and IV. Grade I corresponds to 25% of forward displacement. The top of the sacrum is divided into four quarters in measuring the degree of spondylolisthesis, as seen in Figure 40-16.

Isthmic spondylolisthesis
Clinical findings

Spondylolysis or spondylolisthesis may cause low back pain in children; however, pain is relatively uncommon. Pain may be noted in the posterior thighs. Children may seek medical attention because of postural deformities or an abnormal gait caused by hamstring tightness. Straight leg raising may be markedly limited. The pelvis is tilted back with flattening of the normal lumbar lordosis. Flexion of the hips and knees is noted (Figure 40-17). In cases of more severe slipping, usually grade III, palpation of the lumbar region reveals palpable step-off or depression over the fifth lumbar process. The patient may demonstrate a sciatic scoliosis owing to nerve root tension. Pain in young athletes who hyperextend the back should alert the physician to the diagnosis of spondylolysis. Progression of spondylolisthesis may occur during the adolescent growth spurt. It is not common for progression to occur in adults. However, there are exceptions. Spondylolisthesis is known to progress following a surgical procedure.

Diagnosis

Diagnosis of spondylolysis and spondylolisthesis may be made on routine radiographs. A lytic defect in the pars interarticularis is most easily visible on oblique views. If radiographs are negative and pain persists, films should be repeated after several weeks just as when searching for a stress fracture. A technetium bone scan should be ordered; this may demonstrate the defect before it is visible radiologically. A tomogram may also be of value. A myelogram is performed only if symptoms persist or a neurologic deficit is present (for example, bladder or bowel difficulties, progressive motor weakness).

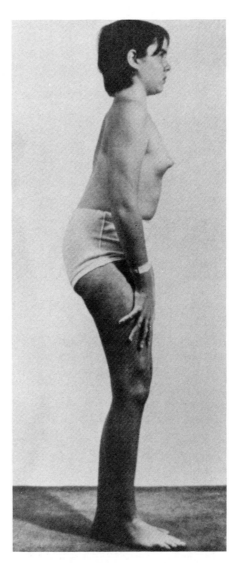

Figure 40-17. Teenager with severe hamstring tightness, typical posture, flexion of hips and knees, pelvis tilted backward, and flattening of normal lumbar lordosis. (From Rothman, RH, and Simeone, AF: The spine, ed 2, vols I and II, Philadelphia, 1982, WB Saunders Co.)

Treatment

Spondylolysis

It is common for spondylolysis to be symptomatic in adolescence. The physician should rule out disc herniation or neurologic causes of back pain such as a spinal tumor. Pain usually responds to conservative therapy. Depending on the severity of symptoms, the patient may require bed rest, plaster of Paris immobilization, or a brace followed by back and abdominal muscle exercises. Activities that produce symptoms should be avoided. Children who are asymptomatic are not restricted.

Spondylolisthesis

Children with asymptomatic spondylolisthesis should be carefully observed. Only with slips greater than 25% does Wiltse[20] recommend avoiding contact sports and activities or occupations that stress the lower back.

In grade III and IV slips, the patients may require surgery

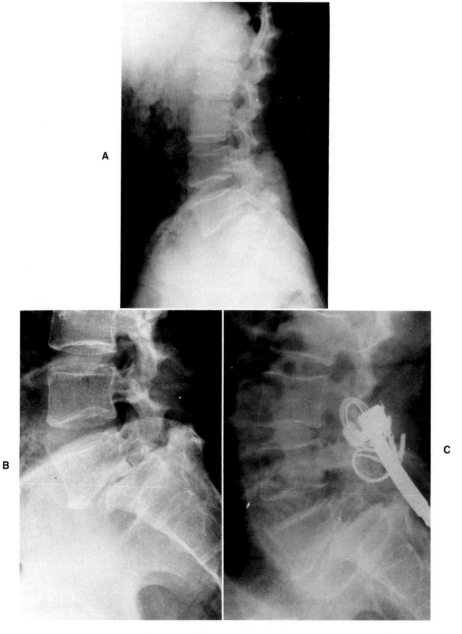

Figure 40-18. A, Radiograph taken in 1959, demonstrating defect in pars interarticularis. **B,** Progressive spondylolisthesis since 1959, with increase in back and leg pain. **C,** Spine fusion L4 to S1 with Harrington rod fixation illustrating progressive spondylolisthesis with persistent symptoms.

if they fail to respond to conservative therapy. Progression of spondylolisthesis can occur.

The treatment of adult patients with spondylolisthesis offers different challenges from those in a growing child. There is little concern for the progression of the deformity in types I and II. The exception to this is seen in Figure 40-18. Radiographs of a 60-year-old symptomatic man demonstrates progression of spondylolisthesis preoperatively, with further slipping following spine fusion. In the presence of a pars defect, however, the chances of backache increases by 25%. Conservative therapy includes lumbosacral immobilization by corset or brace, trial of bed rest if necessary, evaluation, and treatment of the muscle disorder. If surgery is necessary, those patients who experience back pain alone will improve greatly following a spinal fusion. A posterolateral fusion is the most common type of fusion performed. A one- or two-level fusion may be necessary. The facet joints are considered to be a source of pain and are included in the fusion. Reduction of the deformity is attempted only in slips greater than 50%. Most patients can be fused without attempting reduction of the deformity. Patients with radicular pain in addition to back pain require decompression in addition to a spinal fusion. Decompression as described by Gills[20] includes removing a loose neural arch and fibrocartilaginous mass at the defect site. Decompression of the L5-S1 nerve root is accomplished by the Gill procedure; in addition, the herniated nucleus pulposus found in one third of the cases is excised. The Gill procedure without fusion has been successful in treating radiculopathy in adults when the danger of further slipping is minimal. Spondylolisthesis in an adult usually does not progress unless surgery has been performed. If symptoms persist following a spinal fusion or pseudarthrosis develops following a posterolateral fusion, an alternative fusion such as the anterior approach for anterior interbody fusion or posterolumbar interbody fusion should be considered to achieve stability.

Degenerative spondylolisthesis

There is no pars defect in degenerative spondylolisthesis. The entire vertebra is slipped forward. The most frequent site is between L4 and L5. Degenerative changes and incongruity in the facet joints cause malalignment. Rotation of facets, as well as forward displacement of facets, is noted. Degenerative spondylolisthesis usually occurs after 40 years of age and is four times as common in women. Symptoms of back pain may be accompanied by radiculopathy or neurogenic claudication. Symptoms are treated conservatively (Figure 40-19). Anti-inflammatory drugs, immobilization, and physical modalities such as diathermy and ultrasound may be necessary. Muscle disorders, when present, should be corrected.

Surgery may be considered if progressive neurologic deficits are present. The surgical approach includes canal and root decompression similar to treating degenerative disc disease and spinal stenosis. A posterolateral fusion is recommended if instability is present. Autogenous bone graft is used and is usually taken from the posterior iliac crest. During a decompression procedure, care is taken to save the pars articulating processes to avoid postoperative olisthesis. If a neurologic deficit exists, a myelogram should be performed before surgery to determine whether disc excision is indicated.

The patient should be ambulatory as soon as possible after surgery. Every effort should be made to place the patient on an exercise program when healing permits to avoid further deconditioning.

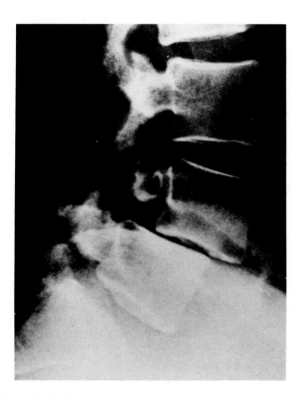

Figure 40-19. Lateral radiograph of lumbar spine of woman 45 years of age showing spondylolytic spondylolisthesis, grade I, at L5-S1 with normal intervertebral disc, and grade 2 at L4-5 with disc resorption at that level. Patient required only conservative treatment for low back pain. (From Crock, VH: Practice of spinal surgery, New York, 1983, Springer-Verlag.)

ANKYLOSING SPONDYLITIS

Ankylosing spondylitis is a systemic inflammatory disease. It is considered a separate entity from rheumatoid arthritis. Symptoms occur most frequently in young adults. It is now known to occur equally in both sexes. Low back pain and stiffness are usually the first symptoms. Pain may be present in the thoracic region. Limited spinal motion is accompanied by limited chest expansion (less than 2.5 cm). Extra-articular structures such as the eyes and heart may be involved. Iritis and aortitis are part of the symptom complex.

Characteristically, patients develop a progressive kyphosis, with ankylosis of the cervical, thoracic, and lumbosacral spine, and the hips. Associated diseases includes Reiter's disease, psoriasis, spondylitis, and inflammatory bowel disease (Crohn's disease, ulcerative colitis). Rheumatoid factor is absent. The sedimentation rate is raised in 80% of patients. HLA-B27 antigen occurs in 80%. The presence of HLA-B27 varies with different populations—8% in whites and 4% in American blacks.

Neurologic symptoms are usually absent unless a traumatic incident causes fracture and dislocation. Cauda equina syndrome can occur in the lumbar spine as a result of fracture dislocation.

Radiologic findings are characterized by bilateral sacroiliitis. Fusion of the sacroiliac joints, calcification of the anterior spinal ligament with the formation of the "bamboo spine" or "trolley track" configuration, and ankylosis of the apophyseal joints, as well as costovertebral joints are also found.

Hip radiographs may reveal bilateral hip arthritic changes or hip fusions (Figure 40-20). A bone scan detects changes in the sacroiliac joint before radiologic changes.

The major goals in treatment include prevention and correction of deformity and pain relief. Rest to avoid fatigue is an important part of management. However, the patient should also remain active, so a balance between rest and activity must be achieved. The patient's occupation should enable him or her to change positions throughout the day and not be fixed in one posture. Sports such as swimming should be encouraged. The patient must be made conscious of his or her posture and instructed in postural exercises to avoid deformity. Exercises should emphasize spinal extension and chest expansion. Examination of the hips and knees and the cervical and lumbosacral region should be performed routinely. Hip and knee flexion contractures may develop without the patient's awareness. The patient may require repeated episodes of therapy requiring stretching of the hips. Braces are used only if necessary. The patient should be observed at regular intervals and measurements taken to determine if the deformity is progressing; if it is, more aggressive therapy should be instituted.

Nonsteroidal anti-inflammatory drugs such as aspirin and indomethacin remain the drugs of choice. Steroids are rarely

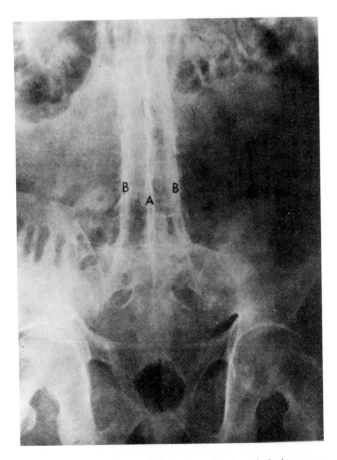

Figure 40-20. "Trolley track" configuration in ankylosing spondylitis. Parallel vertical white lines reflect ossification of interspinous ligaments (**A**) and capsules of apophyseal joints, as well as strands of connective tissue extending between these joints (**B**). Sacroiliac joints are fused. (From Rothman, RH, and Simeone, AF: The spine, ed 2, vol 2, Philadelphia, 1982, WB Saunders Co.)

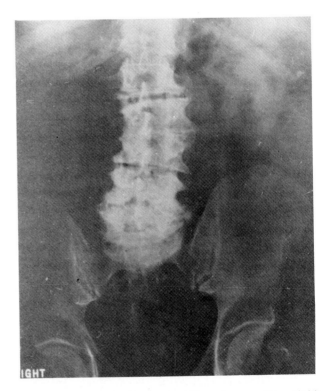

Figure 40-21. Patient with neurosyphilis and neuropathic arthritis (Charcot joint). Advance compression and sclerosis of vertebral bodies and disc degeneration are present with moderate osteophytosis. (From Rothman, RH, and Simeone, HF: The spine, ed 2, vol 2, Philadelphia, 1982, WB Saunders Co.)

used. Surgical procedures may be indicated for disabling pain or ankylosis. Ankylosis of the lumbar spine, cervical region, and hips may prevent the patient from being able to carry out the necessary activities of daily living.

Osteotomy of the lumbar spine may be performed in severe flexion deformities to improve posture and respiratory and gastrointestinal function. Hip flexion deformity should be corrected before spinal osteotomy. Patients may require recurrent intensive periods of physical therapy to relieve developing hip flexion contractures.

Ankylosing spondylitis involving the hips has been successfully treated with total hip replacements. Calcification of soft tissue following total hip replacement may occur. Irradiation has been used postoperatively to prevent calcification and ankylosis.

CHARCOT SPINE

Neuropathic arthropathy resulting from impaired pain and proprioceptive sensation can occur in the lumbar spine. It is usually a result of tabes dorsalis, diabetes, or paraplegia. Although pain may be the presenting complaint, pain severity is characteristically less than one would expect from the destructive changes apparent radiologically. Advanced signs of neuropathic arthropathy include severe osteoarthritic changes with intra-articular fractures, loose bodies, massive osteophytes, and synovial joint effusion. There is progression to marked deformity and instability. Patients may develop signs of nerve root compression with muscle weakness. Radiologic findings may resemble advanced Paget's disease, advanced lumbar spondylosis, or ankylosing spondylolitis with pseudarthrosis (Figure 40-21).

Treatment is conservative. Surgery is to be avoided because of the patient's poor healing response.

REFERENCES

1. Abel, MS: Jogger's fracture and other stress fractures of the lumbosacral spine, Skel Radiol 13:221, 1985.
2. Andersson, GBJ: Epidemiologic aspects on low-back pain in industry, Spine 653, 1981.
3. Cailliet, R: Low back pain syndrome, Philadelphia, 1981, FA Davis Co.
4. Cyriax, J: Textbook of orthopaedic medicine, vol II, Baltimore, 1971, Williams & Wilkins Co.
5. Cyriax, J, and Cyriax, P: Illustrated manual of orthopedic medicine, Wellington, Eng, 1983, Butterworths.
6. Fairbank, JDT, et al: Apophyseal injection of local anesthetic as a diagnostic aid in primary low-back pain syndromes, Spine 6:598, 1981.
7. Farfan, HF, and Kirkaldy-Willis, WH: The present status of spinal fusion in the treatment of lumbar intervertebral joint disorders, Clin Orthop Rel Res 158:198, 1981.
8. Frymoyer, JW, et al: Epidemiologic studies of low-back pain, Spine 5:419, 1981.
9. Hall, H, and Icetow, JA: Back school—an overview with specific reference to the Canadian Back Education Units, Clin Orthop Rel Res 179:10, 1983.
10. Kelsey, J: Proceedings of the First International Conference on Injuries in the Work Place: epidemiology of injuries, New York, 1984, Hospital for Joint Diseases Orthopaedic Institute.
11. Kelsey, JL, and White, AA: Epidemiology and impact of low back pain, Spine 5:133, 1980.
12. Kirkaldy-Willis, WH: Managing low back pain, New York, 1983, Churchill-Livingstone.
13. Kirkaldy-Willis, WH, et al: Lumbar spinal nerve lateral entrapment, Clin Orthop Rel Res 169:171, 1982.
14. Kraus, H: Clinical treatment of back and neck pain, New York, 1970, McGraw-Hill Book Co.
15. Nachemson, AL: The lumbar spine: an orthopaedic challenge, Spine 1:59, 1976.
16. O'Donoghue, CE: Treatment of back pain, Physiotherapy 70:7, 1984.
17. Orthopedic knowledge update. 1. Chicago, 1984, American Academy of Orthopedic Surgeons.
18. Porter, RW, and Hibbert, CS: Symptoms associated with lysis of the pars interarticularis, Spine 9:755, 1984.
19. Rachlin, ES: Musculofascial pain syndromes, Med Times J Family Med, January, 1984.
20. Ruge-Wiltse: Spondylosis. In Spinal disease, New York, Lea & Febiger.
21. Ruskin, AP: Current therapy in physiatry, physical medicine, and rehabilitation, Philadelphia, 1984, WB Saunders Co.
22. Semon, RL, and Spengler, D: Significance of lumbar spondylolysis in college football players, Spine 6:172, 1981.
23. Waddell, G, et al: Nonorganic physical signs in low-back pain, Spine 5:117, 1980.
24. White, AH, Derby, R, and Synne, G: Epidural injections for the diagnosis and treatment of low-back pain, Spine 5:78, 1980.
25. Wiltse, LL: The effect of the common anomalies of the lumbar spine upon disc degeneration and low back pain, Orthop Clin North Am 2:569, 1971.
26. Wiltse, LL: Surgery of internal disc disease of the lumbar spine, Clin Orthop Rel Res 129:22, 1977.

ADDITIONAL READINGS

Bernick, S, and Cailliet, R: Vertebral end-plate changes with aging of human vertebrae, Spine 7:97, 1982.

Brill, MM, and Whiffen, John R: Application of 24-hour burst TENS in back school, Phys Ther 65:1355, 1985.

Bromley, JW, and Gomez, JG: Lumbar intervertebral discolysis with collagenase, Spine 8:322, 1983.

Brown, M: Diagnosis of pain syndrome of the spine, Orthop Clin North Am 6:233, 1975.

Cairns, D, Mooney, V, and Crane, P: Spinal pain rehabilitation: inpatient and outpatient treatment results and development of predictors for outcome, Spinal Pain Rehabil 9:91, 1984.

Carabelli, RA: Waistbelt lumbosacral support suggestion from the field, Phys Ther 66:231, 1986.

Carron, H, DeGood, DE, and Tait, R: A comparison of low back pain patients in the United States and New Zealand; psychosocial and economic factors affecting severity of disability, Pain 21:77, 1985.

Crock, VH: Practice of spinal surgery, New York, 1983, Springer-Verlag Wien.

Cyron, BM, and Totton, WC: Articular tropism and stability of the lumbar spine, J Spine 5:168, 1980.

Deyo, AR, Diehl, AK, and Rosenthal, M: How many days of bed rest for acute low back pain? N Engl J Med 315:1064, 1986.

D'Ambrosia, RD: Musculoskeletal disorders, ed 2, Philadelphia, 1986, JB Lippincott Co.

Di Fabio, RP: Clinical assessment of manipulation and mobilization of the lumbar spine, a critical review of the literature, Phys Ther 66:51, 1986.

DonTigney, RL: Function and pathomechanics of the sacroiliac joint, a review, Phys Ther 65:35, 1985.

During, J, et al: Toward standards for posture, postural characteristic of the lower back system in normal and pathologic conditions, Spine 10:83, 1985.

Duthie, RB, and Bentley, G: Mercer's orthopedic surgery, ed 8, Baltimore, 1983, University Park Press.

Eisenstein, S: Spondylolysis, a skeletal investigation of two population groups, J Bone Joint Surg 60B:488, 1978.

Finnison, BE: Low back pain, ed 2, Philadelphia, 1980, JB Lippincott Co.

Frederickson, BE, et al: The natural history of spondylolysis and spondylolisthesis, J Bone Joint Surg 66A:701, 1984.

Genant, KH: Spinal update 1984, San Francisco, 1983, Radiology Research and Education Foundation.

Goald, JH: Microlumbar discectomy: follow-up of 477 patients, J Microsurg, vol 95, 1980.

Gross, RH: Leg length discrepancy: how much is too much? Orthopedics 307, 1978.

Hayne, CR: Back schools and total back-care programmes—a review, Physiotherapy 70:14, 1984.

Heathoff, K, and Ray, CD: Principles of the computed tomographic assessment of lateral spinal stenosis, Spine Update, p 207, 1984.

Jacoby, RK, Newell, RLM, and Hickling, P: Ankylosing spondylitis and trauma: the medicolegal implications, a comparative study of patients with non-specific back pain, Ann Rheum Dis 44:307, 1985.

Keefe, F, and Hill, RW: An objective approach to quantifying pain behavior and gait patterns in low back pain patients, Pain 21:153, 1985.

Krishnan, KRR, France, RD, and Houpt, JL: Chronic low back pain and depression, Psychosomatics 26:299, 1985.

Liang, M, and Komaroff, AL: Roentgenograms in primary care patients with acute low back pain, Arch Intern Med 142:1108, 1982.

Mall, JC, and Kaiser, JA: Critical evaluation of computed tomography versus myelography in assessing low back pain, Spine Update 1984, p. 97.

Martin, PR: Physiotherapy exercises for low back pain: process and clinical outcome, Int Rehabil Med 8:34, 1986.

Mellin, G, Jarvikoski, A, and Verkasalo, M: Treatment of patient with chronic low back pain: comparison between rehabilitation centre and outpatient care, Scand J Rehabil Med 16:77, 1984.

Mellin, G: Physical therapy for chronic low back pain: correlations between spinal mobility and treatment outcome, Scand J Rehabil Med 17:163, 1985.

Mendelson, G: Compensation, pain complaints, and psychological disturbance, Pain 20:169, 1984.

Moffett, JAK, et al: A controlled prospective study to evaluate the effectiveness of a back school in the relief of chronic low back pain, Spine 11:120, 1986.

Morris, JM: Surgical management of lumbar disc disease, Spine Update 1984, p. 118.

Newman, RI, Seres, JL, and Miller, EB: Liquid crystal thermography in the evaluation of chronic back pain: a comparative study, Pain 20:293, 1984.

Ottenbacher, K, and DiFabio, RP: Efficacy of spinal manipulation/mobilization therapy, a meta-analysis, Spine 10:833, 1985.

Pearcy, M, and Shepherd, J: Is there instability in spondylolisthesis? Spine 10:175, 1985.

Pope, MH, et al: The relation between biomechanical psychological factors in patients with low-back pain, Spine 5:173, 1980.

Posner, I, et al: A biomechanical analysis of the clinical stability of the lumbar and lumbosacral spine, Spine 7:374, 1982.

Rachlin, ES, and Kraus, H: Management of back pain, Intern Med Spec, vol 8, March 1987.

Rothman, RH, and Simeone, AF: The spine, ed 2, vols 1 and 2, Philadelphia, 1982, WB Saunders Co.

Ruge, D, and Wiltse, LL: Spinal disorders diagnosis and treatment, Philadelphia, 1977, Lea & Febiger.

Rusk, HA: Rehabilitation medicine, ed 4, St. Louis, 1977, The CV Mosby Co.

Sandstrom, J: Clinical and social factors in rehabilitation of patients with chronic low back pain, Scand J Rehabil Med 18:35, 1986.

Sandstrom, J, Anderson, GBJ, and Wallerstedt, S: The role of alcohol abuse in working disability in patients with low back pain, Scand J Rehabil Med 16:147, 1984.

Sandstrom, J, and Esbjornsson, E: Return to work after rehabilitation; the significance of the patient's own prediction, Scand J Rehabil Med 18:29, 1986.

Sikorski, JM: A rationalized approach to physiotherapy for low back pain, Spine 10:571, 1985.

Splithoff, CA: Lumbosacral junction, roetgenographic comparison of patients with and without backaches, JAMA 152:1610, 1983.

Wigh, RE, and Anthony, JF: Transitional lumbosacral discs, Spine 6:168, 1981.

Wilfling, FJ, Klonoff, H, and Kokan, P: Psychological, demographic and orthopaedic factors associated with prediction of outcome of spinal fusion, Clin Orthop Rel Res 90:153, 1973.

Wilkinson, HA: The failed back syndrome etiology and therapy, Philadelphia, 1983, Harper & Row.

CHAPTER 41

Rehabilitation of the amputee

LAWRENCE W. FRIEDMANN

The exact incidence of amputation is unknown. In the United States about 43,000 new major amputations a year occur. Most of these are due to vascular disease, so 90% involve the legs. In most recent Western series, approximately 5% were partial foot and ankle amputations, 50% below the knee amputations, 35% above the knee, and 7% to 10% at the hip. In the Orient, amputation for vascular disease is uncommon; trauma is the most common cause. In upper limb amputations, trauma is the predominant cause in adults, whereas congenital limb reduction defects are most frequent in children.

ETIOLOGY

Limb absence or loss may occur from many causes, including congenital absence, limb reduction deformity, reduplication with surgical removal of interfering parts, thermal or electrical burns, crush, vascular occlusion or injury, infection, tumors, traumatic loss, and neurogenic resorption.

The most frequent indication for amputation of the lower limb is gangrene resulting from occlusive arterial disease. The inciting cause may be relatively minor trauma occurring in a limb in a precarious state or may result from the use of heat.

In the upper limb the most common cause of amputation is trauma. The injury is most commonly due to misuse of power tools. Congenital absence or deformities of limbs, malignant tumors, infections, and trophic changes are relatively rare causes of amputation, overall.

PREOPERATIVE CARE

Preoperative evaluation and consultation by a physician with special skills and knowledge of amputations and their sequelae, such as a physiatrist, is desirable. Before surgery, the patient should be told of the functional implications of amputation and prosthetic use, including phantom sensation. The patient may be shown the prosthetic replacement if he or she requests it, but it should not be routine. The surgeon and physiatrist should allay the patient's unrealistic fears but at the same time discuss what to realistically expect after surgery and rehabilitation, taking into account the patient's general physical status, intelligence, athletic ability, and premorbid way of life and the level of amputation.

Having the patient see amputees with similar problems during their training is helpful. This can be done by ordering preoperative and postoperative physical therapy in the gymnasium while other amputees are receiving treatment. Being "accidentally" left to wait before and after treatment allows the patient to see other amputees at various stages of learning and facilitates development of a realistic frame of reference for the patient's own care and prognosis. Calling in an amputee from the outside to demonstrate is more artificial and less helpful.

In cases where amputation is not an emergency, physical and psychologic preparation of the patient and family is important. The potential amputee should be told the following in the sequence given:

1. The physicians are doing their best to save the limb. The natural course of the disease may cause loss of the body part. If it cannot be saved, every effort will be made to leave as long a stump as is consistent with good healing and the best attainable function with a prosthesis.
2. The patient's general health and care of the other limbs is vital. Walking is often possible with one leg amputated but is extremely difficult with both legs amputated above the knees. For an indefinite period, medical supervision will be required for the care of the residual limb, the protection of the other limbs, man-

601

agement of the other complications of the systemic arterial disease and any concurrent diseases, and modifications of the artificial limb.

3. The range of motion and strength of the stump and the sound limbs need to be maintained. Strengthening of the upper limbs is important for the use of crutches or a walker. Breathing and trunk exercises are required before and after surgery.

PRINCIPLES OF LEVEL SELECTION AND SURGICAL TECHNIQUE

Although surgery is but one brief episode in the life of a patient, its importance cannot be overestimated. When carried out properly, it is part of the overall integrated rehabilitation of the patient. Errors in surgery have implications far beyond the immediate period of surgery and wound healing. A poorly performed amputation markedly limits the patient's function for the rest of his or her life.

The selection of surgical level for the amputation is probably one of the most important single decisions that must be made for the amputee. The disease dictates most decisions. In malignancies, if local resection is inadvisable, ablation above the proximal joint is advised. In other cases the viability of the remaining tissues determines the most distal possible level. Functional considerations, especially in the legs, may then determine whether to ablate more proximally. Surgical judgment based on a knowledge of the patient, prosthetic availability, and other factors is the key.

With regard to the forefoot, it may be possible to remove only the necrotic tissue with successful healing. When distal metatarsal and toe amputations are contemplated, the physician should save only bone that can be provided healthy, full-thickness skin coverage. Split-thickness and insensate grafts are a poor choice for the foot because persistent pressures from footwear usually cause skin breakdown.

If only the toes and possibly the metatarsal joints must be resected, a shoe filler is needed to prevent the foot from sliding forward in the shoe. A steel shank in the sole of the shoe provides a more normal push-off and prevents unsightly curling of the front of the shoe. The steel shank should extend to the ball of the shoe, and its distal termination should be wide and flexible. A rigid leather sole is necessary. If more proximal removal is performed, a prosthesis is needed.

The most difficult choice is often between an above-knee and a below-knee amputation, since use of the prosthesis after the latter is much easier and more likely to meet with success in an older patient. With modern amputation methods, between 75% and 90% of below-knee amputations in patients with vascular disease will heal. If the foot cannot be saved because of irreversible damage, the presence of a popliteal pulse virtually guarantees healing below the knee. Even in patients who have no popliteal pulse, the value of retaining the knee is such that amputation just below the knee

is wise even in questionable cases. Skin vascularity is the crucial factor in limb survival, and evaluation methods are being upgraded. Sometimes the 10% risk of having to revise a failed, ultrashort, below-knee amputation must be accepted to try to give the patient an optimal future life-style.

A below-knee amputation should ideally be performed at the junction of the middle and upper thirds of the tibia, usually between 8 and 18 cm below the tibial plateau. A stump as short as 5 cm below the tibial plateau can be fitted with a below-knee prosthesis, but since the shank of a prosthesis is kept extended at heel strike primarily by pressure at the distal end of the tibia, a stump of this length with its short lever arm is inefficient in extending the femur on the prosthesis after heel strike, and this results in distal tibial pressure and occasionally skin breakdown. Such a short stump is difficult to keep in the socket, especially in an obese patient, and special adaptations such as polycentric knee joints or supracondylar suspension sockets may be required. Knee disarticulation is seldom performed but through the knee is a much better ablation level than above the knee, since it permits full weight bearing distally, needs no ischial seat socket, is much less traumatic for frail patients, and results in a better gait.

Above-knee amputation should be performed in such a way that available prosthetic devices can be used. Patients with amputation at this level cannot tolerate distal weight bearing. An amputation ten cm above the knee joint is desirable. A longer amputation such as the Gritti-Stokes procedure requires that the prosthetic thigh be longer than the unamputated side because almost 7 cm is needed for the internal knee joint mechanism. Furthermore, it does not tolerate weight bearing. Since the higher the amputation, the greater the loss of socket control, the stump should be no shorter than 10 cm below the crotch.

The vascular surgeon chooses the amputation level in the operating room. The surgeon observes whether and how well the skin bleeds. Even when the underlying muscles are not viable, an amputation heals provided the muscles are "shelled-out," leaving bone, subcutaneous fascia, and skin. The muscles atrophy with time anyway, are of modest benefit except for early cushioning, and demand a supply of blood that is better used to nourish the skin. A stump comprised of bone, fascia, and skin retains proprioception and is helpful in controlling the prosthesis during ambulation. If the muscular tissues enclose the bone or adhere to it, control is enhanced. The neuroma of the transected nerve must be buried deeply in the muscles; if tender, it may prevent the use of an artificial leg.

An experienced member of the amputation team should perform skin closure, since the skin is the crucial interface between the musculoskeletal structures and the prosthetic socket. Skin adherent to bone tends to tear at the edge, which can usually be prevented by tight fascial closure at a different level from that of skin closure. After healing, gentle stroking and friction massage help to mobilize a minor degree of adherence. Skin adherent to the underlying bone may require reamputation or, at the very least, prosthetic modifications.

The level of amputation for the lower limb may be classified on an anatomic or functional (prosthetic) basis. Some important technical information is summarized in the following paragraphs.

The patient uses a leg prosthesis like a stilt, balancing the full superincumbent body weight over the prosthesis with each step. The body weight is applied to a relatively small surface area, which predisposes to skin irritation and breakdown if the stump is not fashioned as a functional end-organ for use in a human-machine interface. The prosthesis must be fabricated to spread the weight where it is tolerated.

Toe amputation and transmetatarsal amputation are self-explanatory except for the terms "partial" and "complete," which are needed for intelligent limb fitting. The named amputations are many, but the major ones in the foot are the Lisfranc tarsometatarsal amputation and the Chopart tarsotarsal amputation. Both are usually condemned as leading inevitably to foot deformity with disability. However, each is useful in selected circumstances. The Chopart procedure is especially useful in children and adults in whom traumatic ablation has left enough normal plantar skin for coverage of the entire stump.

True ankle disarticulation is performed mainly as an open amputation drainage procedure in adults. The Syme amputation is not an ankle disarticulation. The supra-articular cut in the Syme procedure should not be perpendicular to the long axis of the tibia but parallel to the ground when the patient stands so as to provide a flat surface for weight bearing. Rounding the bones is a surgical error, although the sharp edges of the bone should be rasped slightly. Removal between the ankle joint and the junction of the lower and middle thirds of the tibia is called a long below-knee amputation. (The healing rate after amputation at this level in vascular disease is reduced.) Removal between that point and the junction of the upper and middle thirds of the tibia is called a standard below-knee amputation. Above that is a short below-knee amputation. An ultrashort below-knee amputation is just below the tibial tubercle. The healing rate improves with a short stump length. A knee disarticulation most closely preserves the patient's anatomy. There are various surgical modifications; the true knee disarticulation is best.

An ablation in the lowest one quarter of the femur is called a supracondylar amputation. It results in poor function with prostheses, since internal knee units cannot be used without leaving the thigh section of the artificial limb longer than the remaining side. The long above-knee amputation gives a length between 55% and 75% of a normal femur. It is an excellent functional length. Between 35% and 55% of the femoral length is a medium above-knee amputation. From the groin to 35% of the length of the femur is a short above-knee amputation. Above this point the procedure is

functionally a hip disarticulation amputation even when part of the femur remains. The hip disarticulation amputation preserves the ischial tuberosity and pelvis. The patient can bear weight through the ischial tuberosity but has no active bony lever to move a prosthesis. Amputation through the pelvis is defined as hemipelvectomy or hindquarter ablation. The hindquarter amputee must bear weight on the soft tissues and chest cage.

The surgical levels of greatest utility are the transmetatarsal, the Syme, and the standard below-knee amputation. With these procedures the vascular supply is relatively good provided the surgical level is well chosen. The next best level is the ultrashort below-knee amputation. These patients, with a 3 to 7 cm bony stump from the tibial plateau, require removal of the fibula and all of the muscles originating below the knee. They often need hamstring section for accurate prosthetic fitting. The patients bear weight on the patellar tendon and both tibial flares. They require specially constructed artificial limbs but have far better function than patients with above-knee amputation.

In the past, knee disarticulation was rightfully denigrated because the artificial limbs were so cumbersome. With newer knee designs an excellent prosthesis can now be made. The patient has full weight bearing through the knee and excellent prosthesis control. Using a long anterior flap under the femoral condyles requires that the anterior skin be very long. If the long flap has an adequate blood supply, a very short below-knee amputation can usually be performed. Where the blood supply is mediocre, it is advisable to use shorter equal medial and lateral flaps with a suture line between the femoral condyles. The scar does not interfere with weight bearing.

The higher the amputation level, the more energy expended for ambulation. A below-knee amputee walking on level ground uses between 10% and 40% more energy than a nonamputee walking the same distance. An above-knee amputee under the same conditions uses between 60% and 100% more energy. Thus a bilateral below-knee amputee uses less energy for walking than a unilateral above-knee amputee.

The sensory implications of lower limb amputation level are frequently ignored. An amputee loses the sensory input from the skin, joints, tendons, and muscles, in addition to proprioception and kinesthesis. The spinal cord and brain, receiving different sensory inputs on the two sides of the body, become confused. If the muscles are not reattached over the bone end in the normal length-tension relationship, the information given to the central nervous system is diminished and erroneous. This further interferes with the central excitatory state and thus with motor control.

The removal of a joint greatly decreases the sensory information provided to the patient. When the surgeon amputates above the knee, the patient does not know where the prosthetic foot is. A patient with even an ultrashort below-knee stump always knows that the prosthetic foot is directly below the stump in a straight line from the tibial fragment to the floor. Such a patient can walk in the dark without fear of stumbling, in contrast to an above-knee amputee.

The care of a diabetic patient with infection and gangrene is quite different from that of patients with other vascular and nonvascular diseases. Wide local excision of all infected and necrotic tissue, with the wound initially left open, is usually the most conservative approach. The wound frequently heals by secondary intention with a lower amputation, and the patient requires only minimal rehabilitation.

With regard to upper limb amputation, the technical aspects are somewhat different from those of lower limb procedures. Prostheses lack sensory feedback, and although this is of some importance in the lower limb, especially in patients who have diminished sensation in the remaining leg owing to neuropathy, it is obviously far more important in the arm amputee, since the patient needs to feel what is being grasped and manipulated for best function. If feeling is absent, the patient must use visual control at all times. The loss of sensation in an upper limb is probably the major limiting factor in the effective use of artificial arms.

A blind person cannot use an upper extremity prosthesis. If the patient is blind or may become so and the arm amputation is a long below-elbow amputation or wrist disarticulation, a Krukenberg surgical procedure should be done, resulting in a "lobster claw" hand. Although this is not cosmetically acceptable to some patients, it is the only functional stump if the person desires two-handed function. Some sighted persons who feel a need for sensate two-handed work may elect a Krukenberg stump. The procedure uses the pronators and supinators for approximating the radius to the ulna. The interosseous septum is divided, and the muscles are left in a position that allows fast, fairly forcible pinch between the residual radius and ulna. Skin with sensation is placed at the distal interosseous area so that sensate pinch is preserved. Such a stump may be covered by a cosmetic glove for social occasions. Functional prostheses can be adapted for use with the Krukenberg stump.

PROSTHETIC TEAM

The rehabilitation of the amputee may be used as a model for the concept and practice of medical rehabilitation, since it demands the coordinated efforts of many professionals in teamwork. Although the rehabilitation team for the care of amputees includes many of the workers found on other teams, it varies sufficiently to justify a separate description.

The prosthetic team includes the patient and family, employer, surgeon, physical and occupational therapists, social workers, psychologist, physiatrist, rehabilitation counselor, prosthetist, nurse, and many others. As with any team, there must be a captain, and I believe that person should be the physician. The co-captain of the team is the patient, who would be the best captain of the team if he or she had enough knowledge. At each stage of the treatment, some other member of the team usually takes precedence in functional terms, but the captain has the ultimate authority and responsibility.

Although amputations are performed by surgeons, the follow-up treatment is usually by a physiatrist, who is better suited to be the captain of the team after surgery is complete. In the amputee clinic there should be two physicians: a physiatrist and a surgeon (either orthopedic or vascular) who is well informed and experienced in amputation problems. Most amputations in the United States are performed by general surgeons with little experience in the aftercare of amputees. The only surgeons with more experience are the orthopedic surgeons, but they perform relatively few amputations in most hospitals, since most amputations are for peripheral vascular disease. The physiatrist should consult with all members of the team including the amputee, especially in difficult cases. The prescription should represent the combined judgment of this group, but in case of doubt the physiatrist should make the final decision. Effective medical care cannot be delivered by a committee.

To be an effective member of the team, the prosthetist should advise the physicians on the advantages and disadvantages of the possible prosthetic solutions for each patient. A good prosthetist can be of great help in suggesting unusual and new approaches to difficult problems. The prosthetist takes the measurements, makes the prosthesis, and evaluates it for proper fit and appropriateness.

The physical therapists perform the preprosthetic stump conditioning, range-of-motion, and general conditioning exercises. The occupational therapists teach self-care activities, prevocational and vocational skills, and other functional skills. In some instances the occupational therapy section fabricates temporary limbs. The therapists encourage good hygienic and prosthetic habits and teach the patient how to preserve the condition of the skin.

Therapists advise on any training problems they encounter and report the amputee's reaction to all phases of the program. Since the therapists see the patient much more frequently than do physicians, they become more friendly with the patient and frequently gain useful information about attitude and progress. Therapists train the amputee to use the prosthesis in all aspects of self-care and recreation.

PSYCHOLOGIC REACTIONS TO AMPUTATION

The treatment of the patient's behavioral reactions by the psychology department in conjunction with the rest of the team is one of the most important aspects of care. Because of the massive assault on the patient's body image and self-image and way of life caused by the surgical event, the patient's entire psychic defense mechanism is under stress. He or she is at this time most vulnerable but also amenable to psychic change. Previous patterns of defense may be most easily breached and modified. This stage can "make or break" the amputee. The patient may become self-pitying, self-denigrating, and withdrawn and generally a rehabilitation failure even if a surgical success. Conversely, the amputee may be brought to the point where despite the new problem he or she forges ahead to make a new life. Pity is probably the most destructive attitude in the relationship between professional personnel and the amputee. The psychologic relationship between the patient and the therapist is a sensitive one that requires careful balancing.

Psychosocial factors are important both in amputation and in fitting a prosthesis. Amputation was used as punishment in ancient times and continues to be used in Islamic countries. The concept of amputation as punishment for sin persists even in Western culture. A feeling of guilt and shame often accompanies an amputation, whether congenital or acquired.

Although stages of psychologic "mourning" for a lost body part have been described, they are not universal. The timing, depth, and sequence of the emotional reactions vary from individual to individual.

An artificial limb hides the fact of amputation from the world and thus hides the "sin" that "caused" the amputation. It also disguises the functional loss and acts as a replacement for the loss of a "loved" part of the body.

The disfigurement of the individual and the damage to the patient's body image and to self-image contribute to the development of introversion, feelings of inferiority, and self-imposed social isolation. The understanding of the psychosocial factors is important in the prescription of a prosthesis, since a prosthesis serves psychologic and social, as well as functional, needs. Even a lower limb prosthesis serves cosmetic functions. Some patients who are permanently incapable of walking and in a wheelchair nevertheless insist on and psychologically need a cosmetic lower limb prosthesis. Patients are looked on more adversely if they have an obvious physical deformity than if they do not. Artificial limb provision is also vocationally important, since it is easier for a patient with an artificial leg to get a job than for a person using crutches alone. Thus the prosthesis changes a person's income, social status, and attitude toward life.

Anger and frustration are extremely common. They may interfere with a patient's acceptance of therapy and a prosthesis. The anger is self-directed first and later is turned toward the people and situation that contributed to the limb loss and toward the medical staff. If staff members personalize the anger, they may inhibit the rehabilitation process.

Amputees who have lost a limb through trauma have had a sudden emotional shock without preparation. Those who have the slow anxiety and premonitory mourning with chronic occlusive arterial disease or malignancy adjust in a somewhat different way and appear to take amputation better. They fear loss of their second limb from the arterial disease that took the first. All amputees live in dread of injury to the contralateral limb.

A patient's worry about the effects of the limitation of function on self and family, although expressed commonly, is possibly the least important of the psychologic reactions to amputation. Reality testing is the best treatment.

Except in extreme cases the psychologic reactions to amputation are best handled by the physiatrist, the surgeon, and, when properly trained, the therapists who work with the patient. Among the psychologic defense mechanisms commonly used by amputees are withdrawal, obliteration, compensation, and substitution, depending to some extent on their preamputation personality.

Withdrawal with depressive features is the most common reaction in patients. They become hermits, their sleep patterns are disturbed, they cry easily, and they look pitiful. This is particularly true among older, psychologically insecure, or less well-educated amputees.

Obliteration, the refusal to recognize the disability, occurs often in highly educated people who come from secure backgrounds and have only mild cosmetic defects. The refusal to recognize the disability can be a good adjustment unless the disability is severe.

Compensation for the amputation can be a useful mechanism in those with moderate functional loss, since these patients become competitive and aggressive and may become fanatics about the use of their devices. They proselytize other limbless persons. For most this is an advantage, but for some who cannot excel in sports, for example, their depression and self-abnegation may increase. Another form of psychologic compensation is the fatalistic type in which the patient overaccepts the disability and does nothing to improve function. In the paranoid type of compensation the patient projects his or her own physical and emotional inadequacies onto various situations and other people, often to the patient's detriment.

Substitution is the psychologic mechanism most physicians hope for in dealing with an amputee. The patient who realizes that a change in life-style is necessary to deal with the new situation is acting in a mature and rational fashion. The patient's basic life goals need not always be changed, but the methods by which he or she attempts to meet goals will require review, since the means available to obtain them may be altered. Patients who choose substitution as a psychologic mechanism are often young, intelligent, and fairly severely handicapped. They realize that to attain their goals in life they must change their modes of behavior.

Psychologic adjustment to a prosthesis requires the patient to realize that the prosthesis is a tool for performing certain activities. The efficacy of a tool depends on its appropriateness for the job to be done and the skill with which it is used. The rehabilitation team must ensure that the job the patient seeks to perform can be done with the tools available. If the patient does not have them, either the job must be changed or new devices must be obtained and the amputee trained to use them. In rehabilitation the patient does the work; the team gives advice and guidance. The acceptance of advice depends on interpersonal relations, and that is why the therapist's advice may be taken over the physiatrist's. Patients usually have far more contact with the therapists and like and trust them more.

At least as important as giving encouragement is giving the amputee the truth. The patient must be told that prostheses have deficiencies in their present state of development. Prostheses have an unstable attachment to the skeletal system that makes them feel heavier than the limb they are replacing, even though they are usually considerably lighter. In addition, there is a false joint between the skeletal system and the artificial limb, leading to socket instability and a "bell clapper" motion. The instability may cause skin irritation, which is aggravated by the excessive perspiration in the socket. The socket decreases the body's ability to cool itself, with resultant increase in sweating, skin maceration leading to skin breakdown, infection, and pain. The friction of the harness is also irritating. Gait with a prosthesis is abnormal at best, and cosmesis is never as good as we would like.

For some amputees, particularly those with guilt feelings, the artificial limb conceals the amputation. For them appearance both at rest and in motion is of great importance, and any deviation from the normal that reveals the amputation upsets them. Other amputees find the inability to perform certain acts far more threatening than the appearance of having had an amputation, and for them cosmesis is of secondary importance. Patients with poorly resolved castration fears in childhood react more severely than others to amputation. All patients have psychologic reactions to the loss of a limb in the sense that they have lost a precious part of themselves. This may lead to depression and self-pity, although they may not be a difficult problem in some patients. Few patients need psychiatric intervention.

Another psychologic distortion produced by amputation is the incompleteness of body image. Patients feel that a part of them is gone not only physically, but also emotionally. Many feel uncomfortable unless the symmetry of the four limbs is restored. This is one value of any prosthesis, although it may be otherwise totally nonfunctional. Many patients feel themselves only half a person after the loss of both legs, even though they are functionally independent in a wheelchair. The provision of artificial legs, even if only cosmetic, may be important for them. Still other people regard a prosthesis as a tool, and this led in the past to the development of many separate tools to be attached to the wrist unit of an upper limb prosthesis. Most patients look on a prosthesis in combinations of the ways mentioned.

Phantom sensation, the feeling that the part is still there, is a normal occurrence after amputation of a limb. The physiatrist must mention the phenomenon of phantom sensation to the amputee before surgery, since some of them awake from anesthesia with the feeling that surgery was not performed. Occasionally a patient finds it difficult to reconcile the phantom sensation with the absent limb, and on rare occasions this has resulted in doubts of sanity and suicide.

POSTOPERATIVE CARE

Care of the stump immediately after an amputation is the surgeon's responsibility. The main objective is to ensure rapid wound healing with minimal scarring and adhesion of the skin to the underlying bone.

The usual method is to place a soft dressing on the wound over the drain and allow the incision to heal. An elastic bandage may be used over the dressing.

A method now diminishing in popularity is the rigid total contact dressing with a prosthesis attached immediately. The principle of the rigid dressing used alone is excellent. The socket prevents edema and helps the stump to heal. It is especially useful as an immediate prosthesis for children, for upper limb loss, or for traumatic amputees. For elderly amputees with vascular disease, however, immediate ambulation can cause serious damage except under the most meticulous supervision. An amputee team must be available 24 hours a day, 7 days a week.

A less dangerous and more easily applied dressing is the Unna semirigid dressing. It is more easily changed and is associated with fewer instances of wound breakdown. When the stringent requirements for the rigid dressing cannot be met, the Unna semirigid dressing is an excellent alternative.

Another postoperative care method is the "controlled environment treatment" developed by Redhead, in which a machine supplies air to the wound that is cleansed of bacteria with controlled humidity and temperature. This provides a perfect environment for primary wound healing. The technique is experimental but when available may become the method of choice for stump healing.

Less desirable is an inflated transparent plastic bag placed over the stump so the skin can be easily observed and postoperative edema kept at a minimum. The problems with the plastic bag are that it causes skin maceration, and in the above-knee amputee it keeps the thighs abducted and flexed, fostering the already great tendency to hip flexion and abduction contracture. A variation is use of a temporary prosthesis with an airbag inside it.

Among the factors determining the size of the stump are its muscle mass, its fluid content, and the amount of subcutaneous fat. Disuse leads to muscle atrophy, which occurs more quickly if the muscles are not reattached. The fat disappears most rapidly with pressure. Shrinkage is necessary to reduce the stump volume for the most efficient use of the permanent prosthesis. Surgeons apply shrinking devices to the postoperative stump, in some instances as early as the first day.

Stumps may be shrunken somewhat with elastic bandages. If spaces occur between the turns of an elastic bandage, window edema is common. The spaces occur because the bandage slips as the patient turns in bed or in the wheelchair. If used, bandages must be reapplied carefully at least four times a day.

I prefer elastic stump shrinking socks so proximal compression is less than distal compression, which prevents proximal tourniquet effects. The socks should be worn whenever the patient does not wear the artificial limb. A garter belt prevents them from rolling down and constricting the vessels.

If the compression provided by a stump shrinker is inadequate, a smaller size can be used, a five-ply wool stump sock can be worn under the shrinker, or elastic bandages can be applied over the shrinker. The stump shrinker prevents many of the problems found when elastic bandages are used alone. One may use two different stump shrinkers: a Bessco stump shrinker next to the skin and a Truform stump shrinker over it. A Daw sheath underneath prevents tension on the wound margin and makes the shrinkers easier to don. The Bessco sock is smooth and has more distal pressure than proximal. The Truform sock gives much more compression, but it has a pad at the distal end that usually slips down, allowing some distal induration. Using them together results in greater compression and prevents distal induration.

Shrinkage should continue until the prosthesis is worn regularly. The best method of shrinking and shaping a stump is use of an artificial limb itself. If possible, a temporary articulated prosthesis should be worn routinely after the wound is healed. The full weight of the patient's body is placed in the socket with each step. This is far more pressure on the stump than can be applied by any elastic material. It is the pressure that causes the subcutaneous fat to vanish. The limb also assists in general conditioning and permits the start of training for walking. A plaster of paris or adjustable socket is of great value, for as the stump shrinks, it can be cheaply adjusted or a smaller socket can be substituted for it. When the permanent prosthesis is made, fewer socket adjustments are needed, since most of the shrinkage has taken place. The early use of a permanent leg is inadvisable because rapid shrinkage is common, requiring multiple modifications and replacement of the entire limb in a short period of time. It is better both medically and economically to use a temporary provisional prosthesis. The socket is attached to leased components that the patient eventually returns to the prosthetist.

As the stump shrinks, adjustments are made to the socket and the alignment. The patient is discharged from the hospital and walks with the temporary limb for at least 3 months until the stump is almost its final size. The time required depends on the patient's weight and activity level. The patient usually is able to wear the permanent prosthesis for 1½ to 2 years before replacement is required.

The provisional limb also conditions the stump and the patient's cardiorespiratory and musculoskeletal systems, in addition to allowing accurate evaluation of the patient's potential as a prosthesis user, rather than solely a wearer. It permits use of various prosthetic components to determine which should be included in the permanent prosthesis.

Postoperative conditioning

The deconditioning of the patient and the residual limb must be prevented or, if it occurs, reversed. This deconditioning is physical, mental, emotional, social, economic, and vocational.

The training of the patient is done by a physical therapist for the lower limb and an occupational therapist for the upper. Physical therapy is concerned with stump conditioning, range-of-motion and conditioning exercises, and strengthening for the entire body. The physical therapist also teaches good standing, walking, climbing, and transfer techniques. The occupational therapist works on functional activities involving endurance, activities of daily living, and prosthesis use with both controls and use training. Both observe the condition of the patient's skin as it responds to the stresses imposed on it. The stump and the remaining leg are gently massaged with lanolin to keep it in good physiologic condition and to toughen it. The patient is taught to care for his or her own limbs.

The therapists are also a vital part of the psychologic rehabilitation of the amputee. The therapist performs a prosthetic evaluation and reports any problems to the clinic team. The therapist trains the amputee in the donning and doffing of the prosthesis and in use of the limb in self-care, ambulation, recreation, and the patient's job.

The therapist is the prime source of information to the team regarding the type of permanent prosthesis the patient should have. Aside from the length and condition of the residual limb, many other factors influence the choice of prosthesis components. The therapist reports the patient's responses to various components and alignment changes so the optimum final prescription can be given. Since the emotional responses are crucial, the therapist's reports help everyone.

A patient with serious cardiorespiratory disease may be incapable of tolerating an artificial limb. Hemiplegia on either side may require additional stability built into the leg.

The effective use of an artificial limb depends on the patient's neuromuscular coordination. This can be estimated by asking the patient about his or her previous agility, but the best test is a trial. A patient who cannot learn to walk well with a walker without an artificial leg often has great difficulty in using an artificial leg. It is better to overprescribe temporary artificial limbs and to use the limb for its predictive value. Patients and families are reluctant to trust a physician's experience alone when a limb is not prescribed. A failure with a provisional limb makes nonprescription more palatable. Early ambulation maintains coordination.

To prevent contractures, the stump must be moved through its full range of motion at least four times daily. The prone position discourages knee and hip flexion contractures. Active assistive exercises and active exercises against resistance are important for strengthening muscles. Endurance is enhanced by use of the temporary limb. Facilitation exercises are excellent, especially for correction of contractures, but expensive in therapists' time. The use of the provisional limb inhibits contracture formation.

High amputations may interfere with personal hygiene. A hemipelvectomy patient may have difficulty sitting on the toilet seat. Bilateral amputees need to learn transfer techniques into and out of a wheelchair and bed and onto the toilet.

Unilateral amputees can balance on one leg and walk with crutches or can use a prosthesis. The more proximal the amputation, the more difficult ambulation is, especially on rough, uneven terrain. Irregular pavement is just as difficult for walking as rocky ground. The use of a cane or crutches is important on uneven surfaces.

Unilateral hip disarticulation and hemipelvectomy patients often abandon their prostheses because crutch ambulation is faster and easier. They use their prostheses on social occasions, primarily for cosmesis. Approximately 85% of young men with this level of amputation abandon their prostheses. Fifty percent of women retain the prostheses, primarily for cosmetic reasons.

Bilateral amputees walk much more poorly than unilateral amputees because most of the functional adjustments to prosthetic use are made by the remaining limb. Where there is no remaining limb to compensate, the second prosthesis must serve. Bilateral above-knee amputees frequently do not walk, especially if they are elderly or need to walk on uneven terrain. The energy costs are great, and they prefer to use a wheelchair.

Vascular disease is systemic. The vessels of the other leg and the coronary, cerebral, and ophthalmic arteries are all involved. Each complicates rehabilitation.

Treatment should be part of a continuum in the natural history of the disease, vascular or otherwise, from prevention to cure or compensation for loss. Amputation is not a failure of medical or surgical knowledge and skill. It is an inevitable phase in the history of the illness.

The weeks following surgery are the most important in the care of the amputee. During this time the patient does or does not develop the proper attitude for successful use of the prosthesis and return to society. It is the period during which the physician must reevaluate the patient's physical, emotional, vocational, intellectual, and social strengths and weaknesses, since these determine whether a prosthesis should be prescribed and if so what type.

Temporary prostheses

If there has been an active rehabilitation program from the start, a prosthesis can be fitted as soon as the wound is healed. It is unnecessary to wait until the stump has shrunk completely or flexion contractures have been overcome, since the use of a temporary articulated prosthesis avoids or reverses many of the problems of the new amputee. Patients should be instructed in prosthetic concepts before the operation, or as soon thereafter as possible, since the more they understand about what the device can provide and what is expected of them, the better they will cooperate and the more successful will be the result. If delayed wound healing expected to last more than 4 weeks is a problem, I prescribe a bypass prosthesis so training may progress and the person may go home walking while the wound is healing. The bypass does not replace the provisional limb.

Certain conditions apart from the stump affect the use of a prosthesis. For example, a patient with serious cardiorespiratory disease may not be a candidate for any prosthesis, inasmuch as the effort in using it may jeopardize the patient's survival. Provision of a wheelchair, walker, or crutches may be safer. Stress testing is needed, and a trial with an ultralight provisional limb may be performed carefully.

Hemiplegia on either side may prevent a patient from using an artificial leg or arm. The scar of a radical mastectomy on the side opposite the arm amputation may dictate a special harness for an artificial arm or contraindicate its use. The condition of the stump must be evaluated repeatedly in the postoperative period, for it may need to be strengthened, bandaged, shaped, and toughened to receive the prosthesis. The forces acting on the stump and the device are determined by the available muscle power, gravitational forces, and inertia. There is always some motion between a socket and the underlying skin, muscle, and bone. Work is force exerted over a distance. The work output of a prosthesis is equal to the work the patient puts into it (work input), minus frictional and other mechanical losses. Thus, for a prosthesis to be effective, both the muscular force the stump can impart to it and the distance through which the part can move (range of motion) are important.

The effective use of an artificial limb depends greatly on the patient's neuromuscular coordination (athletic ability). An amputee who has always been agile, learned to dance easily, and excelled in sports and in handicrafts has little difficulty in learning to use an artificial limb. Conversely, a patient who has always been considered clumsy may find learning to use an artificial appliance difficult. A patient who cannot learn to walk well with a walker without an artificial leg will probably not be able to walk well with an artificial leg. However, since success is sometimes possible, I tend to err on the side of overprescribing provisional artificial limbs. This gives the patient a chance to prove to himself or herself, the family, and me whether or not the limb is feasible. At the same time, my concern for safety has led me to prescribe many devices that improve stability, such as thigh corsets, knee friction locks, and pelvic bands.

For an amputee over 55 years of age, I also prescribe a wheelchair for convenience and energy conservation.

If a patient is not yet a candidate for even a provisional prosthesis because of medical complications, but needs to be out of bed, a pylon prosthesis may be prescribed. It helps the patient stand, which improves cardiorespiratory reserve, prevents decubitus ulcers, and simply motivates the patient. Because a pylon prosthesis has no joints, it may result in poor gait patterns and thus must be discouraged for use in gait training after 10 days unless it will be used permanently.

Use of an immediate temporary articulated prosthesis is inadvisable for patients with vascular disease but should be applied in a patient with limb amputation for malignancy or trauma and in children. It reduces pain and edema and gives the patient some idea of how the prosthesis works and what the various components look like and can do, which aids in motivation. With it, the physiatrist may try out various devices so the appropriate components can be provided when the permanent prosthesis is ordered. A temporary prosthesis not only helps solve medical difficulties, but also permits the patient to apply earlier for financial and vocational aid.

Stump and skin care

Once the wound has healed satisfactorily, the skin should be kept as nearly normal as possible. This requires exposure to the air and prevention of maceration by minimizing sweating. Astringents and rubbing alcohol should not be applied to the stump, since they dry the skin and cause it to flake. Cornstarch and unscented talcum powder are excellent lubricants that leave the skin supple, smooth, firm, and dry. The powder is used in the socket, as well as after the evening bath.

For patients who prefer softer skin, lanolin or cocoa butter can be used; liquid skin emollients and petrolatum jelly should be used cautiously, since they predispose to skin maceration. These substances should be used only after bathing in the evening and should be washed off in the morning.

The use of any prosthetic or orthotic device requires toughening of the skin that comes into contact with the device. This toughening is best done by progressive use of the device.

Prostheses invariably interfere with the normal functions of the skin. They may cause skin lesions through maceration, occlusion of the sweat glands, excessive pressure suddenly or over a prolonged period, friction and shear forces, and stress concentration.

Prostheses interfere with the temperature-regulating function by inhibiting evaporation of perspiration. Since the use of an artificial limb requires an increased energy cost, sweating is accelerated. Accumulation of moisture promotes maceration of the skin, which predisposes the patient to infection and makes the skin more susceptible to injury by outside forces. Maceration of the skin can be minimized by using porous materials, employing perforated construction for artificial limbs, and selecting stump socks made of absorbent natural (rather than synthetic) fibers. Sweating can be diminished through use of antiperspirants or by iontophoresis with very dilute copper sulfate or formalin solutions.

The occlusion of hair follicles and sweat glands can cause folliculitis, boils, abscesses, and sebaceous cysts. Atrophy of subcutaneous fat and muscle usually results from pressure from a prosthesis. When pressure of a prosthesis is distributed over a relatively large area, the complications from pressure are less manifest because the pressure per unit area is less.

A pressure sore heals if the cause for it is removed. In the case of an open, draining skin lesion, the limb should not be worn until healing has taken place. When the sore is caused by a prosthesis, the device must be modified to eliminate points of excessive pressure. Only rarely is additional surgery on the stump necessary, for example, removal of a sharp bony ridge or spicule. Topical application of a bland cream (vitamin A and D ointment, for example) promotes healing only if the pressure is removed. In rare instances a bypass device is necessary, when it is decided that a socket cannot be worn by the patient until wound healing is complete.

Friction on the stump may be reduced by wearing a thin nylon or porous polyamide sheath under the stump sock. If a friction lesion persists, either the prosthesis must be redesigned to improve its suspension or a slip or gel socket is required. In the gel socket there is a double-layered liner with a gel-like substance encased between the layers. The inner layer fits snugly on the stump and is very flexible. It moves with the skin. Movement is in the gel, rather than between the liner and the skin. In the slip socket the stump socket layer is separate from the outer structural layer. The inner stump layer is held to the stump skin by elastic bands, springs, a tennis ball, or other device during swing phase while the outer layer drops by gravity.

Skin normally moves freely over the underlying tissue. When it is adherent to underlying bone in a stump, stress concentration occurs with stretching and weakening of the skin and frequently with deposition of hemosiderin at the juncture between flexible and adherent skin.

The total contact socket helps reduce stress concentration on a delicate stump by distributing weight bearing more evenly over the entire skin of the stump.

Splinting and bed posture

After amputation there is often a muscle imbalance; some muscles have been weakened or inactivated by surgical removal of all or part of the insertion, whereas their antagonists remain intact. This is the rule in short above-knee amputations, but it may also occur elsewhere. Muscle imbalance may lead to contracture that impairs prosthesis use. To counteract this tendency, splinting is used in the early postoperative period while the limb is still painful.

Skin traction has been recommended to help position the limb in proper alignment, but this is ineffective. When skin traction is applied parallel to the long axis of the bed, the patient usually moves into a comfortable position with the trunk at an angle to the line of force so the stump again assumes a poor position, particularly in above-knee amputees. The usual traction device has its pulley at least 6 to 8 inches above the mattress, which predisposes to flexion contractures at the hip.

Instead of splinting and traction, in my institution we exercise the patient to counteract the tendency toward contractures. We prescribe physical therapy three times a day, a very firm mattress, and periodic sleeping and lying in the prone position. We keep pillows from under the patient's knee or thigh. Except in cases of orthopnea, we do not permit more than one small pillow under the head, nor do we allow the head of the bed to be elevated. We do not allow prolonged sitting in bed or a chair. If the stump is moved through a full range of motion three or four times a day, contractures can usually be prevented, but the best way to avoid contractures and to build up the stump is the early use of a temporary articulated prosthesis.

Exercise

Exercise of the remaining limb is necessary to maintain full range of motion and the muscle power required to operate the prosthesis. Exercise equipment operated alone is useful for only a small percentage of patients, since most of them do not exercise unless the therapist is present. Patients exercise better in a supervised group, where there is mutual encouragement and competition.

Muscular efficiency varies with the angle of flexion of the joint. An efficient method of exercising all of the muscle fibers throughout the range of joint flexion is to use manual resistive exercises except when there is a very short stump. The therapist resists the patient maximally in each part of the arc of the range of motion, whether by isotonic, isometric, isokinetic, or proprioceptive facilitation techniques. If isometric exercises are used, they should be done at different angles of joint excursion. Exercises of the weaker muscle groups should be encouraged most. I believe that proprioceptive neuromuscular facilitation is most valuable in combating joint contractures.

Exercise equipment is helpful as a supplement to manual resistive exercises. The strength and range of motion of the amputated limb must be increased to their maximum. The stability of the artificial limb depends on stabilizing musculature throughout the rest of the body, for unless the base is stable, the muscular prime movers are not effective. In an upper limb amputee the shoulder girdle must have considerable strength and a normal range of motion. Since the conventional prosthesis is activated by pulling on a harness fixed by the opposite shoulder, the muscles of the latter must be strengthened.

For lower limb amputees, balancing exercises are needed to stabilize the superposed trunk on the prosthetic socket. Strong abdominal, paraspinal, and hip muscles are needed for this action. Since the lower limb amputee has to walk using crutches at various times in his or her life, and certainly in the early phases of prosthetic use, crutch walking, preceded by standing, balancing, and walking in parallel bars, is necessary. The use of crutches requires strength not only in the shoulder girdle and arms, but in the trunk as well, so general conditioning exercises should be prescribed. The exercise program and the energy cost in beginning to use a prosthesis place considerable demand on the cardiorespiratory system. The therapist must report to the physician any shortness of breath, undue fatigue, or chest pain.

Massage

Massage of the stump lessens the patients' almost universal fear of handling it. Amputees dislike looking at their stumps and avert their eyes. They respond to massage well because they see that the therapist is not disgusted by the sight of their stumps. Encouraging the patient to massage the stump is helpful. Massage also helps reduce edema and improve circulation. Friction massage helps prevent adhesions that develop during healing period. Since the prosthesis exerts considerable friction on the skin, adhesions between the skin and subcutaneous tissues and underlying structures are detrimental. Maintenance of skin mobility is therefore important. Until the wound heals, the therapist should hold one side of the wound with the thumb and the other side with the fingers and move the skin on both sides of the suture line as a unit. This technique prevents skin adhesions without disturbing wound healing. If the skin is adherent to the underlying tissues and the wound is healed, friction massage helps to free it.

PROSTHESIS PRESCRIPTION PRINCIPLES
Patient evaluation

Prosthetic prescription depends first on the patient's goals, which must be reasonable and attainable. Basic life goals need not be changed after limb ablation, but the methods used to achieve them require reconsideration because the means available have been altered. The psychologic adjustment to a prosthesis depends on a patient's realization that the prosthesis is a tool for performing certain activities. The efficacy of any tool depends on its appropriateness for the job the patient wants done and the skill with which it is used.

Since the prescription of a prosthesis requires the knowledge of many facets of the life and disability of the amputee, it is achieved best through the team effort described earlier. The leader of the team must make the final decision, but unless he or she takes all suggestions seriously, the other team members will lose interest. Patients frequently do not express themselves adequately in front of a group. Different members of the team get different stories from the same patient. For that reason each professional should see the patient individually. In each instance it must be decided whether a part of the team or the entire team needs to meet to discuss the patient, once the data have been collected.

The information gathered before prescription determines whether the patient really wants a prosthesis or is being pressured into it. If there is no real patient desire for a prosthesis, its use will be poor. If the amputation was necessitated by a malignant tumor that has shortened life expectancy to less than 1 year, providing a permanent functional prosthesis may be inadvisable. The training program is time consuming and prevents the patient from enjoying the last days of life with family and interests. A cosmetic prosthesis is sufficient, and then only if desired by the amputee. In some instances a provisional functional limb is ordered for psychologic reasons. Immediate or early postoperative prostheses are advisable for these patients.

The preliminary examination determines the nature of the patient's stump, the general physical condition and any special physical, emotional, or vocational problems. The general medical condition is seldom the reason for not prescribing an artificial arm, but in patients with severe cardiorespiratory involvement a lower limb prosthesis may be contraindicated. Psychologic factors frequently determine whether a limb should be prescribed, and its nature. The condition of the stump is important, but it can usually be modified by surgery or by physical therapy. The socket can be adapted to it in almost all instances, but it may require ingenuity. The noneconomic and economic costs of surgery may be less than the costs of "conservative" care. A cost-benefit evaluation may be indicated in difficult cases.

The patient must decide whether to use the prosthesis for heavy or light work and recreation. For an arm amputee, for example, if light duty is all that is needed, a figure-of-8 or figure-of-9 harness with lightweight components is usually adequate. If the patient plans to do heavy work, the shoulder saddle–chest strap harness should be used and heavy duty components such as elbows, wrist units, cables, and terminal devices should be provided. If the patient needs to perform mechanical work, the "utility hook," with or without a locking mechanism, should be used for holding farm or industrial tools. Heavy duty work usually requires the use of steel rather than aluminum components. If the patient works in a damp area or where there are petroleum lubricants, rubber bushings should not be used. The patient may need more than one limb, each for a defined purpose.

Except in elbow and knee disarticulations, single-wall sockets are seldom used. If the patient lives far from a prosthetic center, only durable components that do not require much maintenance should be used.

The patient's hobbies may also determine which devices are provided. A leg amputee who plays golf may benefit from a dual or universal axis ankle. For an arm amputee,

a set of different terminal devices or limbs may be given for each of the different things the person wishes to do. This is analogous to owning a station wagon for the family and a sports car to go to work.

For the leg amputee the prescription depends on many factors in addition to stump length. The prescription also depends on the amount of stump shrinkage, the range of motion and the strength of the stump, any scarring or "dog ears" (tags of excess skin), and so on. Special adaptations are sometimes necessary. The climate and the person's culture should modify the prescription. The precise (rather than general) nature of the work and hobbies should be factors in component choice. The individual's preferences should be taken into account.

The rehabilitation team must ensure that the activities the patient seeks to perform can be done by the leg or arm provided and that the patient has been adequately trained to use it. If not, another device must be used, further training is needed, or as a last resort, the job must be changed.

The primary purpose of an artificial leg is to diminish functional disability in standing, walking, climbing stairs and hills, pulling, carrying, working, running, and jumping. The specific disability a patient finds most inhibiting may not be one the prosthetic team envisions. Since the team's efforts are to restore the individual to his or her subculture in optimal condition, they must know and modify the patient, the environment, and the human-machine interface between them. This requires, as a minimum, the combined efforts of the surgeon, physiatrist, physical therapist, rehabilitation nurse, and psychologist to work primarily with the patient. The family, social worker, vocational counselor, employer, and clergyman work mostly with the environment, and the prosthetist and physical and occupational therapists work mainly with the human-machine interface.

Treatment may sometimes be complex and long term, requiring the knowledge and skills of many specialists at varying times. Limb provision is one step, but the surgical and training phases must be integral in concept and execution.

The basic principle in devising a machine to enable an amputee to walk is that the patient's center of gravity must be over the base of support to prevent falling. The essence of walking is that the patient falls off one leg and catches himself or herself on the other. This alternating process of propulsion (acceleration) and reception (deceleration) is basic. Both mobility and stability of the limb depend on muscular activity, gravity, and inertia. The joints are stable when they are inhibited from further motion in one direction, and the center of gravity is so located that it moves the joints in that direction, usually with little or no muscular activity.

Few people can be restored to the same physical performance level at which they functioned before amputation. This is possible only when the patient was inactive before amputation. Most people can achieve partial restoration; they are self-sufficient in the activities of daily living at home and can work. No artificial limb can perform the functions of the ablated limb, nor will it ever feel normal. Each person requires a degree of assistance peculiar to his or her own disability and capability. The assistance may include a prosthesis, canes, crutches, wheelchair, and self-help devices.

Although, in the past, age alone was considered a limiting factor in successful prosthetic use, I have many patients well into their nineties who walk, eat, and dress themselves successfully with a prosthesis. Physical factors are important, but the emotional factors associated with the amputation and aging are most crucial.

Work must be done to activate a prosthesis. Work equals force times distance. The distance depends on the joint range, and the force depends on the strength of the appropriate muscles. Range, muscle power, and endurance are therefore crucial. A patient whose stump is painful will not be able to tolerate the prosthesis.

Prosthetic prescription

The most important determinant in the prescription of a prosthesis is the length of the stump. Functional stump length is different from actual stump length. Functional stump length is determined by the length of the residual bone in relation to the circumference and firmness of the stump. The socket should gain a stable purchase on the stump; close fit is necessary. An immediate or early temporary prosthesis is useful for the upper extremity amputee, since it prevents the patient from becoming one handed and gives an opportunity to become accustomed to the prosthesis early and to evaluate the advantages and disadvantages of different terminal devices. It also provides the staff with guidelines for effective prescription of components. If the patient is expected to have maximum function with an upper extremity prosthesis, a hook should be prescribed. If no function is expected, a purely cosmetic passive arm is sufficient. If function and appearance are both important, a hook and a functional hand with cosmetic glove should be prescribed. The power source is a secondary consideration.

Most upper limb amputees have only unilateral involvement and can be trained to be completely independent in the activities of daily living, regardless of the length of the stump on the amputated side. The higher the amputation, the greater the prosthetic functional loss. If there is one normal limb, the stump with or without a prosthesis is an assistive limb for stabilizing and holding an object for the normal limb to manipulate. A prosthesis is rarely used if a sensate, prehensile part of the body can be used instead.

In a bilateral arm amputee or a unilateral amputee with damage to the remaining upper limb, the problem is more complicated. Neither side is good enough for skilled manipulation. The person spontaneously chooses the less damaged or longer side as the dominant side. Bilateral upper extremity amputees at any level should be fitted conventionally with wrist flexion units added on at least one side.

If both sides are amputated above the elbow or higher, externally powered devices should be obtained if available. If they are not available, conventional provisional fitting for function should be tried. If the patient has an above-elbow amputation on one side and a shoulder or forequarter disarticulation on the other, unilateral functional fitting on the above-elbow side should be attempted. A cosmetic arm should be prescribed for the other side. If the patient has a very short above-elbow stump, surgery should be attempted to lengthen the stump by means of a tube graft with secondary insertion of a fibular bone graft or internal prosthetic device. Use of the feet for prehension and manipulation should be encouraged for all bilateral upper extremity amputees.

Body build is important. An obese individual uses an artificial appliance less well than a wiry person. The socket is farther from the bone that must control it. A patient with flabby muscles activates a prosthesis less well than someone who is muscular. A patient's coordination must also be good. The patient's opposite leg may determine whether the patient can and should walk with an artificial leg.

Walking with crutches without an artificial leg puts the entire body weight on the remaining leg. If the vascular supply of this leg is poor, serious consideration must be given to replacing walking with wheelchair use. Walking stimulates new vessel proliferation. The use of an artificial limb diminishes the workload on the remaining limb. This may be an important factor in deciding whether to have the patient use a wheelchair and thus preserve the remaining limb, while at the same time diminishing the patient's ability to get around in the world. The other choice is to permit the patient to use crutches with or without a prosthesis, which places increased demand on the patient's sound leg, increasing the potential for damage to that leg. This allows the patient to function better but may accelerate the time when amputation will be needed. In my experience the provision of a prosthesis is usually best, since it benefits the patient both physiologically and psychologically. It bolsters the patient's self-respect, permits greater mobility, and decreases the workload on the family.

A number of patients want an artificial leg despite their inability to use it for walking. Cosmesis is a form of function. In rare cases, leg cosmesis is an important vocational need. The economic costs are generally overshadowed by the emotional and social advantages. In such cases the use of an endoskeletal prosthesis with a thin-walled socket and a soft, foam, shaped cover is indicated. The shaping should be superior. The soft compressible material does not make noise when the patient bumps the leg into a hard object. Third party payors may not cover the costs without a detailed justification.

Where cost is a factor, the legs used to model stockings in store windows may be purchased for attachment to the wheelchair. Clothing dummies are relatively cheaper than artificial legs. Nonfunctional cosmetic shells that cannot be used for walking may also be used when the team fears that the patient may attempt to walk, despite advice that it is unsafe.

Cost of the prosthesis

Although the cost of an artificial limb is high, it is only equivalent to the cost of about 5 additional days of hospitalization waiting for the stump to shrink. The monetary saving enhances the importance of early fitting. Preparatory prostheses may be of the reusable or custom type. The latter are better but more expensive. Changing the socket shape and size is less costly than keeping the patient in the hospital. Prospective payment to hospitals precludes delays.

For above-knee and higher levels of amputation, the difficulty in using prostheses usually precludes them for patients with senility, psychosis, mental retardation, or severe brain damage. These are not contraindications for those with ablations below the knee. Only use of a provisional limb for evaluation can ascertain whether a patient is able to use the limb. Prescription is largely a matter of judgment based on the experience of the clinic team. Evaluation by use of a temporary prosthesis with interchangeable parts for trial is of real value.

If a patient lives far from a prosthetic facility, more complex devices requiring much maintenance should not be ordered.

It is a real tragedy when a middle-aged or elderly person falls because of the lack of stability in a prosthesis. Such a fall may cause a fracture, immobilizes an elderly person, and results in the additional insult of decompensation of the cardiovascular, respiratory, and muscular reserves. This restricts their activities far more than if a prosthesis had not been ordered. It is no favor to prescribe a more functional but less stable device if the amputee falls with it. One fall a month is 12 chances a year of sustaining a fractured hip.

Parts of a prosthesis

The socket is the part of the prosthesis that partially encloses the stump to form a union between it and the artificial limb. Its function is to provide stability and to transmit forces as accurately as possible between the device and the patient's body.

The prosthesis must be held on by some form of suspension. The suspension mechanism may be suction (atmospheric pressure), a strap, condylar suspension by socket design, a rubber sleeve, or muscular grasp. For young, agile, above-knee amputees, suction suspension may be used if a one-way valve is incorporated into the socket. Another method of suspending the prosthesis is condylar clamping, in which part of the socket or a strap goes above prominent bony structures. Friction is generally not considered a suspension mechanism, but in many instances it is the prime force suspending the prosthesis. It is increased when the patient perspires. Another inadequately investigated suspension method is muscular grasp. As the patient walks,

the muscles contract and bulge. If the socket is designed for muscular grasp, there is room for muscular expansion. The patient does not lose the prosthesis during swing because the bulge of the muscles into the predesigned spaces precludes further slippage of the prosthesis. Various straps may be used over bony prominences, over the shoulders, or around the waist. Garter belt and corset suspension may be advisable in special circumstances.

The terminal device is the part of the artificial limb that contacts the environment. In the arm it is the hook or hand; in the leg it is the foot.

The activating force for the prosthesis is usually muscular power, but external power is used in arm prostheses and experimentally in leg prostheses. Control over the prosthesis may be transmitted from body power over cables through harnessing, or by electrical or mechanical switches.

Length of the prosthesis is gained by structural elements, either internal or external. They are referred to as endoskeletal or exoskeletal.

One important aspect of prosthesis fabrication is alignment, the relationship of parts of the prosthesis to one another. The alignment of the different components strongly influences the patient's comfort and ability to use the prosthesis. In the leg the knee joint must be at or behind a vertical line through the center of gravity or the patient's knee buckles. Faulty alignment may be a fabrication error, but just as frequently it is due to the patient's loss of range of motion. Flexion contractures of the hip and knee in particular may thwart the achievement of successful alignment.

Alignment varies with the heel heights of shoes. All the patient's shoes must have the same heel heights. If a young woman wishes to change from low heels to high heels for social occasions, the prosthetist must be informed of this fact before fabricating the prosthesis so the artificial feet can be made interchangeable. Two or more pairs of removable prosthetic feet are required, fitted to the shoes the patient wishes to wear. The alignment needs to take into account this anticipated change.

Evaluation of the prosthesis

When the prosthesis is completed, it must be inspected for fulfillment of the prescription, workmanship, fit, size, and alignment. This evaluation is done by the prosthetist. It is then reevaluated in the gymnasium if a leg, or in occupational therapy if an arm, first by the therapist and then by the physiatrist. A complete evaluation cannot be done when the prosthesis is delivered, since the patient had no training with it. The alignment given first is an approximation.

I find it useful to have a gentlemen's agreement with the prosthetist. I give automatic tentative approval with the understanding that any adjustments needed, other than major changes in prescription, will be corrected without additional charge. The prosthetist thus is paid promptly, and the prosthesis can be judged according to the patient's needs rather than as an isolated object. I insist that prosthetists guarantee the components and workmanship for 1 year.

If there is a question of whether the socket is truly total contact in nature or whether the fit is appropriate, xeroradiography of the patient's stump inside the socket with and without weight bearing settles the issue. This technique is invaluable because it accentuates margins and interfaces and clearly shows the edges of the bony structures, muscles, skin, stump socks, and both soft and hard parts of the prosthetic socket.

PROSTHESES FOR THE LOWER LIMB
Foot and ankle mechanisms

An artificial foot may be rigid or have an ankle that allows motion in one or more planes. Those that allow motion in one plane are called single-axis ankles. They move in the vertical plane with the axis of rotation parallel to the floor and at 105 degrees to the line of progression (the direction of travel of the center of gravity). The dual-axis ankle has freedom in two directions: flexion-extension and inversion-eversion. A universal ankle allows rotation about all three axes.

The advantages of a rigid ankle are low cost, minimal maintenance, ease of walking, light weight, ease of installation, and good appearance, both static and in walking. The major disadvantages are the inability to adjust the resistance to plantar flexion, the short balance surface for standing, and the toe-up appearance in sitting when the leg is in front of the chair. Rubber artificial feet are water resistant and have no moving parts, but they are heavy and most people have difficulty putting socks over them.

SACH foot

The principle of the solid ankle-cushion heel (SACH) foot was discovered in 1861. It has a rigid ankle, with all of the advantages mentioned previously, and a solid keel that is angled and rounded. This gives a rollover gait, as with a rocker bottom. The heel is compressible, resulting in a plantar flexion equivalent, after which the patient rolls over the solid keel, which gives a type of heel-off. The heel is resilient in all directions at heel strike, so there is no stability at that point. A SACH heel can be made more compressible by drilling holes through the resilient heel pad and less compressible by inserting firmer rubber plugs.

The front of the keel has a corded material with some springiness to prevent dropoff at heel-off. There is no absorption of the torque forces generated at toe-off. The foot is surrounded by a rubberized material, which gives a natural shape to the foot while making it water resistant. By means of a slight change in the shape of the keel or central core, the gait pattern can be changed. If the amputee wishes to change back and forth between high and low heels, the single bolt attached to the shank makes it easier, provided

the prosthetist is advised of the need for this option before fabrication. It is almost as difficult to apply a sock to a SACH foot as it is to a rubber foot, especially for older amputees. The foot is light. For a debilitated patient who does not take long steps and always uses a soft heel, it is an excellent device. SACH feet provide long service. They are prescribed more than any other ankle-foot combination. They are used almost universally for below-knee limbs, and for most other limbs as well.

Single-axis foot

The single-axis ankle and foot may be made of wood or plastics, with metal joints. It can be made with a flexible front hinge to provide imitation of toe-off, or it can have a rubberized flexible front that resembles the SACH foot. The advantages of this type are low cost, easy maintenance, control in attaining the foot flat position, ease of standing, lateral stability, light weight (but heavier than the SACH), and ease of installation. The single-axis ankle has an anterior and a posterior bumper, usually made of rubber in varying degrees of compressibility. The bumpers permit adjustment of the amount of resistance to dorsiflexion and plantar flexion. The anterior dorsiflexion bumper takes over the function of the normal triceps surae muscle, since its resistance to compression determines the ease of dorsiflexion of the foot at push-off. The posterior bumper determines the amount of resistance to plantar flexion at heel strike and thus is analogous to the tibialis anterior muscle.

A patient who is just learning to walk and steps very cautiously on the prosthesis does not compress a hard single-axis heel bumper. Thus a soft posterior bumper should be used at first to permit a fairly safe gait. As the patient becomes more adept in the use of the prosthesis and steps out more, putting more weight on the prosthesis at heel strike, a firmer and less compressible heel is needed. This change is made easily and quickly with a single-axis ankle.

The single-axis ankle and foot is useful for a middle-aged or elderly amputee who has some hesitation in stepping out on the prosthesis at the beginning and usually learns to walk with a more rapid gait as he or she becomes more secure. A young amputee should have a SACH foot of medium or firm consistency, since such a patient rapidly learns to compensate for the hard heel and soon needs it. A firm heel should be prescribed a young amputee, a softer heel for an older amputee, and a single-axis ankle for a middle-aged or elderly patient and a bilateral amputee. Even the bilateral amputee can sometimes use a SACH foot. The disadvantages of the single-axis ankle are that it may be damaged by water, it provides no lateral motion, and the prosthetist must adjust heel height for women. Its weight is a disadvantage to weak patients.

Double- and multiple-axis ankles

The advantage of double-axis ankles is that they adapt to uneven ground. They are expensive, frequently become noisy, require adjustment, and weigh more than simple ankle mechanisms. Their lateral motion permits more latitude in foot placement but requires that the patient have good balance.

The same disadvantages are present in the "functional" or multiple-axis ankles. Their appearance is often poorer than that of other ankles mentioned. Multiple-axis ankles adapt to uneven ground best and provide both axial and lateral motion, so they absorb the torque forces generated at toe-off. This is of considerable importance in some patients with skin problems, since the rotation of the socket on the stump generated by these forces, which are not absorbed by other types of foot-ankle mechanisms, can cause severe frictional stump problems. Multiple-axis ankles have a built-in rotator unit. Rotator units may be added to SACH feet.

The artificial foot may be as simple as a peg leg (still useful for climbing rocky hills and use in underbrush, as well as in areas where poverty does not permit purchase of a prosthetic foot). For soft, boggy terrain a wide peg leg called an elephant boot may be useful.

When ability to move the ankle is increased, stability is decreased. The precise trade-off made depends on the patient's individual needs. Patients who walk on uneven terrain may want a dual- or triple-axis ankle, despite its noisiness, heavy weight, expense, and need for frequent repairs. The dual-axis ankle is prescribed most often for golfers who need the wide stance. Athletes often desire these more sophisticated ankles.

Newer feet are coming on the market. The Seattle foot and the Flex foot allow some push-off by storing energy and releasing it later in the stance phase of gait. The SAFE and Carbon Copy II feet are lighter and said to be more functional than present SACH feet. The precise indications and contraindications for these newer feet have yet to be clarified.

Shank and thigh materials

There are two basic designs for thighs and shanks. The more traditional is the exoskeletal or crustacean design in which a hard external skeleton supports the body's weight. An old and recently revived construction method is the endoskeletal technique in which a central member goes from the socket to the ankle and supports the body's weight. This member may or may not have joints or be surrounded by a soft cosmetic cover mimicking the shape of the missing body part. Endoskeletal limbs when coated with a soft cosmetic cover have a more pleasant feel and are quieter when accidentally struck. They are more expensive and more fragile. They are not shiny, as are many limbs made with exoskeletal methods. Exoskeletal legs are stronger and more durable. It has been said that they are heavier, but this is not necessarily the case with proper fabrication. Exoskeletal legs may be made of willow or balsa wood, which is strong and light and may be covered with laminated plastic or painted rawhide for a better appearance.

Sockets

The socket of the lower limb prosthesis is used to transmit the body weight and may also be used to suspend the device. It transmits stump muscular forces as expressed through bony motion to the artificial limb, and the environmental forces of inertia, floor reaction, and gravity to the stump. The socket is the most important single determinant of comfort and thus must be properly shaped, fitted, and aligned. The excellence of the fit determines the pressure distribution between the patient's body and the device, as well as the control the patient will achieve over the device. The most commonly used socket materials are plastic laminate and wood, either willow or balsa.

The shape of the socket must support the body and transmit the forces without discomfort or damage to the body. This depends on the specific characteristics of the body part to which the socket is fitted. If detrimental stump factors exist, special modifications are required. Even "normal" stumps have areas that are pressure sensitive or pressure resistant. Weight must be borne proportionally by those most tolerant of pressure. Because of the nature of the tissues below the knee, all comfortable sockets bear weight in the same general locations. Some sockets have partial or full weight bearing at the end of the stump, but most depend for the majority of their body weight support on proximal support areas. Total distal contact is more often used to support the distal tissues than for a significant amount of support of the body weight except in the Syme amputation and knee disarticulation.

Sockets are designed according to special criteria from a cast of the residual limb. When a nonsuction socket is fabricated, an interface material is planned for and fabricated where necessary. This may be stump socks or a plastic resilient interface material. Stump socks of various thicknesses are used for resilience and to occupy space when the stump shrinks. They may be removed entirely if the patient has swelling of the stump. Friction-reducing socks are also used.

The usual technique is to make a plaster of paris cast of the stump, with the stump held in its proper attitude. The initial female cast may be modified by the prosthetist's hands or a casting jig. A male model of the stump is made from the female cast. The male model is modified to bear weight in places on the stump tolerant to pressure, such as the patellar tendon, and medial tibial flares, or ischium. Material is added to the socket model to spare areas intolerant to pressure, such as the tibial crest and fibular head. The insert, if any, is made over this male mold. The socket is made over the insert.

The interface may be cotton, wool, or artificial fiber stump socks to decrease friction and absorb perspiration. These materials vary in thickness and may be added as needed to preserve the fit of the prosthesis to the patient's stump. In the below-knee amputation an insert of plastic or leather may be used between the stump sock and the socket. In the above-knee amputee, insert liners are rarely used.

Partial foot amputation

For patients who have had toe excision, either no prosthesis or a simple cotton felt filler for the forepart of the shoe is usually all that is needed. If the first toe has been amputated, the shoe may become deformed and toe-off is somewhat disturbed. In this case a long steel shank, a rigid leather sole, or a foot orthosis may be used to improve toe-off. The same devices are used for patients with transmetatarsal amputation.

Patients who have had some of the metatarsal bones amputated with extensive narrowing of the foot, especially with scarring on the sole, often have impaired balance. To increase the patient's stability and comfort, a custom-made shoe orthosis should be fabricated. The basic principle is that a shock-absorbing and friction-diminishing interface is placed between the foot and the shoe, increasing the surface area available for weight bearing and sensory feedback. The under side should be made from a silicone rubber material, reinforced by nylon threads for toughness and resilience. Over that is a silicone gel layer, covered by flexible leather.

Syme amputation

The Canadian Syme socket is a partially end-bearing socket held on by friction and shape. The proximal brim of the socket must relieve pressure on the distal end of the stump by a patellar tendon–bearing bar, since prolonged total end bearing is seldom tolerated. The patellar tendon–bearing area may be hard or soft. Over the distal shank is a trapdoor, which, when closed, acts as a condylar suspension clamp over the malleoli. It is padded and holds the narrow part of the patient's stump firmly. It allows the bulbous distal end of the stump to enter the prosthesis. No suspension is needed other than the trapdoor, which usually opens medially. An elastic inner wall may replace the trapdoor. Some Syme amputees have the bulbous terminal end of the stump removed, and the opening may then be omitted.

The socket may have a hard weight-bearing surface or a soft resilient pad of felt, Silastic, or rubber. The distal pad supports at least half of the patient's weight. This socket needs a special, low-profile SACH foot.

Below-knee amputation

The socket for a below-knee amputee is now usually made of plastic-impregnated cloth but may be made of metal, wood covered with rawhide or laminate, or plastic. The shape of the socket determines its name and weight-bearing characteristics. The material of which it is made affects strength and weight.

"Conventional" below-knee socket

The now rare but formerly usual "conventional" below-knee socket was usually carved from a block of wood from the inside by eye and so required the attention of an experienced prosthetist. The socket must be fitted so it does not exert pressure over the distal anterior end of the tibial stump, the fibular head, or the tibial crest. Although a superior prosthetist can make a wood leg in the patellar tendon–bearing shape, most are inadequate. By definition, the conventional socket anterior brim ends below the patella and supports the leg on the patellar tendon. It may be fabricated as a molded socket for patients who must kneel often and then is as comfortable as a patellar tendon–bearing limb.

The shank of the prosthesis is carried forward in rapid gait by inertia and in slow walking by pressure of the tibia activated by the quadriceps muscle. The conventional socket requires the use of external knee joints and a thigh lacer for support and stability, except in its molded version. Since it is almost impossible to scoop out the wood in a conventional socket with as close a fit as can be done with a molded socket, the thigh lacer serves the important function of removing part of the body weight from the socket by friction against the skin of the thigh. The socket is customarily left open at the bottom, and for those with perspiration problems this makes evaporation easier. Skin irritation from friction and stump "choking" from constriction of the superior portion of the socket while the bottom is left open is fairly common.

Patellar tendon–bearing socket

The patellar tendon–bearing socket is usually made of plastic laminate over a mold of the patient's stump held at 15 degrees of knee flexion (less for a long stump, more for an ultrashort one). It bears weight primarily on the patellar tendon area on a molded bar and on the medial tibial flare. A popliteal prominence holds the stump forward on the patellar bar. Relief must be provided for the fibular head, hamstrings, and tibial crest. The socket comes to the middle of the patella anteriorly with the sides at the same level or higher, by definition.

To ensure that weight is borne on the proper location, counterforce must be used, keeping the patellar tendon on the patellar tendon bar of the socket. This is done by the shape and size of the posterior wall of the socket, which usually has a popliteal bulge to perform this function. For some patients the bulge may be flattened or even eliminated.

Since this socket is molded, it is easier to make than the conventional socket and is used more often. The patellar tendon–bearing socket may be used with a plastic liner to give resiliency to the weight-bearing areas on ambulation. The soft cushion insert may be omitted, and many amputees prefer the hard socket used with wool stump socks. The socket is commonly used with a suprapatellar cuff suspension. Any of the suspension mechanisms may be used with this type of socket.

Shrinkage of the stump is more rapid with the patellar tendon–bearing socket than with the conventional socket, and adjustments must be anticipated. They can usually be added between the socket and the liner. Ordinarily the socket is total contact, but a small airspace may be built into the bottom. The patellar tendon–bearing prosthesis cannot be used if the distal circumference of the stump exceeds the proximal circumference.

The liner may be soft or semisoft and fabricated, poured, or foamed. The total contact socket is used in young people and in those with sensitive skin to provide even pressure distribution over as much of the stump area as possible. It is also useful in patients with impaired proprioception. The total contact socket may also be of value in diminishing phantom limb sensation and edema. Persons who have cerebellar or vestibular imbalance are aided by wearing the total contact socket. The recent amputee must wait until the stump has shrunk sufficiently to be fitted with a total contact socket or must accept frequent socket change. In my experience the socket design that provides most of the advantages of the patellar tendon–bearing socket without the disadvantage of painful kneeling is a molded conventional socket with high sides.

Slip socket

In patients with skin lesions caused by friction between the socket and the skin, a slip socket may be used. It has the two layers of a double-wall socket separated rather than joined. The inner or stump layer is kept near the stump by elastic suspension, a ball, or a spring, while the outer, structural, or cosmetic layer pistons owing to gravity during swing. It is useful and too rarely considered.

Bent or kneeling prosthesis

For those with extremely short stumps with flexion contractures, the bent-knee or kneeling-knee prosthesis may prove useful. The knee provides an excellent weight-bearing surface. The patient's knee is flexed 90 degrees, and a socket is formed to bear all of the weight on the tibia and knee. Since the stump protrudes behind the rest of the leg, it is uncosmetic for women wearing skirts, and if long, it interferes with the leg of trousers. The external knee hinges damage clothing. Friction knee joints have not been developed. The problems are that the thigh is longer than the normal thigh when the patient is sitting, the knees give a mediocre gait, and posterior protrusion of the stump is unsightly.

Other socket modifications

Total contact sockets using water and air cushion sockets are ways of reducing edema, as well as giving slight support for the tissues of the stump. They may take a small amount of weight bearing.

Below-knee suspensions

Many below-knee socket designs have features for suspension that modify the name but do not modify the weight-bearing characteristics of the socket. The suprapatellar cuff is the most common below-knee suspension. It is a strap of any material and design that goes from the prosthesis to above the patella and around the thigh. It should suspend the limb during swing to minimize pistoning and prevent constriction of the tissues during knee flexion. Conventional sockets may be used with a suprapatellar cuff suspension as is the patellar tendon–bearing socket.

Thigh corset

The thigh corset with side joints has been called an old "suspension," but that is a misnomer. It is really a weight-bearing, partial weight bypass device that has some suspension features, especially if the side bars are curved in over the femoral condyles. It gives mediolateral stability for patients with knee instability. The weight-bearing capacity is important for patients who are obese, have an arthropathy of the knees, are athletes, climb, or lift and carry weights. It may be a valuable addition despite its cumbersome nature, its tendency to cause thigh atrophy, and the wear on clothing that ensues. If a patient has a short below-knee stump and needs assistance with weight distribution, a double-axis knee joint should be used with the thigh corset.

Wedge suspension

The KBM socket uses a wedge condylar clamp to provide suspension. Removable wedges are most common, but a removable medial wall with a wedge built in is excellent. Flexible walls may also give condylar clamping.

Suprapatellar-supracondylar suspension

The suprapatellar-supracondylar suspension (PTS) incorporates the features of supracondylar clamping and has a high anterior wall that cups over the superior pole of the patella for suspension during swing phase.

Muscular grasp suspension

Making a socket with "pockets" for the bellies of contracted muscles for suspension is experimental. It increases friction in muscular limbs. Furthermore, it sometimes depends for success on voluntary muscular contraction, so the limb may be lost during emergencies.

Other suspensions

Shoulder or waist belts and corset suspension are occasionally used for patients with ostomies, abdominal scarring or masses, or gross obesity. Suction suspension has been attempted below the knee but has not proved successful, especially in amputees who have worn a prosthesis for a long period of time and have atrophied, bony stumps. Elastic sleeves of latex or neoprene are useful to maintain atmospheric pressure suspension. Good skin hygiene is mandatory.

Bypass prostheses

For patients who have lesions in the remaining shank, knee, or in the femur, with the distal part of the leg amputated, complete weight-bearing bypass may be needed. In these cases an ischial weight-bearing socket prosthesis with an open end is required. The knee is locked during stance phase but may be bent when the patient sits. A limited action ankle such as the SACH foot is helpful, and a rocker or patten bottom is essential. In the case of only a distal lesion, an open patellar tendon–bearing socket with brace bars and a patten may be sufficient.

Knee disarticulation prosthesis

The through-knee prosthesis is composed of either a socket that ends below the ischium, with a thin flexible brim if all of the weight can be taken by the femoral condyles, or an ischial weight-bearing socket if not. Ancillary suspension is not required because an anterior trapdoor is used to provide condylar clamping, as well as allowing entry. Alternatively, for the knee disarticulation as for the Syme, an expandable inner sleeve may be used so the bulbous condylar end of the bone can expand the liner while it is pushed down into the socket. Then the liner contracts, gripping the femur above the condyles and preventing displacement in swing. The foot and shank are the same as for the below-knee amputee. A knee articulation is required.

The older knee unit consisted of external hinge joints. A drop lock was sometimes incorporated. The disadvantage of external joints is that they wear clothing severely, they are wide and unsightly, and the axis of rotation accentuates the length discrepancy between the artificial limb and the sound knee. During ambulation there is no friction so only one cadence can be used. This usually leads to excessive heel rise and excessive terminal swing impact during walking.

In recent years a number of polycentric knee units have been developed that allow the knee to retract in flexion so the length discrepancy in sitting is less severe than with external knee joints. This is a marked cosmetic improvement. In addition, these units have stance phase stability during walking. A hydraulic resistance mechanism, if added to the polycentric knee joint, allows variation in cadence.

Above-knee prostheses
Above-knee sockets

The socket for the above-knee amputee is designed to bear weight on the body parts that tolerate it best and distribute it so each area is stressed below its level of tolerance. The above-knee stump is essentially circular when seen relaxed. To mimic that shape, sockets were originally conical. That shape is referred to as a "plug fit" socket. The thigh takes a markedly different shape during ambulation when the muscles contract, especially in young, muscular individuals. Newer sockets take into account the form of the active thigh muscles. A number of different socket designs are now used for function and comfort. Each design serves well for certain individuals, so the prescription must suit individual patient needs.

In the "plug fit socket" the pressure is distributed evenly from the socket by friction to the entire skin surface through the stump sock during stance phase, with the friction pushing the skin proximal relative to the bone of the stump. This often causes irritation at the end of the stump. If the bottom of the socket is open, edema and skin irritation at the terminal end from "choking" may cause considerable difficulty. If the scar adheres to the bone, pulling on the suture line with skin breakdown is frequent. The tissues are displaced proximally and form an uncomfortable and unsightly roll of flesh over the medial socket brim, called an adductor roll.

The "plug fit" socket has generally been abandoned because the adductor roll causes hydradenitis suppurativa. There are still indications for prescribing a plug fit socket. Patients who have irregular, tender, adherent postoperative scars or masses in the femoral triangle may be unable to withstand the pressure and friction over the scar from the femoral triangle bulge of a quadrilateral socket. If this is the case, a plug fit socket may be desirable. Patients who have used a plug fit socket satisfactorily for many years should not have their socket modified to another socket design, except at their insistence. A patient needs a minimum of 6 months to become accustomed to a new socket design and almost that long to get used to any other new component.

The most common design for the socket is an ischial weight-bearing quadrilateral shape, which is modified to relieve pressure over the muscles and tendons that are sensitive to pressure. The patient bears weight on a hard or padded ischial seat. The patient's ischium is held on the ischial seat by means of counterforce through the femoral triangle bulge on the anteromedial wall. With this type of socket the patient sits in his socket during stance rather than pushing his stump into the plug fit socket.

The socket has a rounded anteromedial corner to form a channel for conjoint tendon of the adductor longus and gracilis muscles, and a similar posteromedial one for the tender hamstring tendons. Relief for gluteus maximus and rectus femoris muscles is provided by large, hollowed-out areas on the posterior and anterior walls, respectively. If the ischial seat is too thick, the patient will have discomfort while sitting because it will stretch the skin of the gluteal crease. If the ischial seat is too thin, it will cut into the stump during weight bearing. The anterior and lateral walls are classically 5 cm higher than the medial and posterior walls to keep the stump on the ischial seat and to provide stability for the abductor muscles. Variations reflect stump conditions. The external posterior surface of the socket should be flat and parallel to the floor in sitting so the leg hangs vertically.

Since the abductor muscles of the femur are intact whereas the adductor muscles have been sectioned during the amputation, the abductors are relatively stronger. This gives an abducted gait and a limp. The socket must be aligned in adduction. This places the abductors on stretch to prevent a Trendelenburg lurch. Adduction of the socket reduces the bell-clapper motion of the femoral stump relative to the socket, since it displaces the soft tissues medially, reducing the distance between the femur and the lateral socket wall. Inadequate socket adduction is a common fabrication fault.

Planned initial flexion is also provided to allow sufficient extension range for normal stride. Since muscles contract best at a slightly elongated length, and since there is some false motion between the skeletal system and the socket, the initial flexion provides adequate strength and range for the hip extensors to extend the thigh in stance. This is an important consideration with mechanical knee joints, since the prime force causing knee extension is extension of the thigh on the pelvis. It also compensates for hip flexion contracture.

If the socket is too snug at the brim, the stump tends to swell distally. Relief of the socket distally only increases the edema. If the socket is tight anteromedially, the patient walks with his leg externally rotated to relieve the pain. If the anteroposterior dimension is too great, the ischial tuberosity falls inside the socket. If the patient's stump is too far into the socket for any reason, he will have pain over the ramus of the ischium and his adductors. There are many variants of the "quadrilateral socket" depending on manufacturer, stump characteristics, and other factors.

In Germany the older triangular socket is making a comeback. Marquardt avers that his patients are far more comfortable using a triangular socket than a quadrilateral socket.

The contoured adducted trochanteric controlled alignment method (CAT-CAM) socket is said to be more comfortable and functional. It is one of a series of experimental socket designs with a narrow mediolateral dimension and a longer anteroposterior dimension. There is no ischial seat, but the ischium sits inside an indentation in an attempt to prevent lateral socket movement. There is no Scarpa's femoral bulge. The design is still evolving; the newer socket is the SCAT-CAM. It is useful for those with scars or internal prostheses in the Scarpa's triangle. Present costs far exceed the cost of the quadrilateral socket. There is great stress properly placed on socket adduction. The adduction is just what is lacking in proper quadrilateral fabrication.

Another experimental design, from which the CAT-CAM was derived, is the normal shape, normal alignment (NSNA) limb. It is also markedly adducted and has a narrow mediolateral dimension.

Flexible sockets have been proposed for many years (and prescribed by Russek and me) so that changes in stump shape during activity can be reflected in socket shape. Newer materials such as carbon filament reinforcement for structural strength of a supporting frame (Icelandic–Swedish–New York, or ISNY, socket) combined with inserts of flexible polyethylene are now being used. The materials have made the concept much easier to achieve. Flexibility makes the socket more comfortable in standing, walking, and sitting. The expense is one drawback.

Further work in socket design is required before the indications and contraindications of each design are finalized.

Total contact sockets

The total contact socket may have any shape. It contacts the stump all over its surface. The socket end may be hard, soft, or semirigid. The design distributes the pressure over as great a surface of the stump as possible, which helps to control some skin problems. Sensory input is improved and thus assists prosthesis control. In patients who feel a shortened phantom, the total contact socket tends to restore the length. It controls peripheral edema. Recent amputees should not use a total contact socket, since the rapid changes in stump size change the pressure relationships. Distal bearing becomes excessive when the stump shrinks.

Knee units for the above-knee prosthesis

An above-knee prosthesis may have no joint at all, or a joint that is locked while standing but may be unlocked for sitting. These are single-axis, mechanically locking joints. Locked joints are used for patients who are infirm and unstable or are just starting to use an artificial leg. Some experimental joints lock during stance hydraulically, electrohydraulically, or electrically.

Knee locking during stance may be obtained by a weight-activated knee lock, often called a safety knee. It inhibits buckling at heel strike. The safety knee is useful for workers who must carry weights and for patients who are middle aged and need extra stability.

Knee units are generally single axis in construction. Joint stability is determined by the location of the knee axis in relation to the weight line. The farther behind the weight line the joint is located, the more stable the knee is (and the harder it is to flex for heel- and toe-off). For the knee disarticulation amputation, to improve cosmesis while sitting, polycentric knee units are used. They raise the instantaneous axis of rotation to nearer to the hip joint and thus markedly improve stance phase stability during walking. They are used in both the above-knee and the knee disarticulation limb but are noisier, heavier, and more expensive than single-axis knee units.

Extension aids are devices added to a prosthesis to reduce heel rise at the beginning of swing phase. They accelerate the shank after toe-off. They may employ elastic, flexible wood hickory sticks, coiled and wrapped springs, compressed air, or a hydraulic fluid.

A friction mechanism reduces excessive heel rise in early swing and reduces terminal swing impact at the end of swing. The friction may be constant or variable. Variable friction improves the cosmesis of swing phase more than constant friction. The friction may be provided mechanically, by compressing air, by restricting the flow of a hydraulic fluid, or even, experimentally, by electromagnetic forces.

Hydraulic and pneumatic knee units that are cadence responsive improve the cosmesis of swing phase. They are prescribed for young, active, muscular individuals who want to walk at different speeds. Older persons and others who walk at a single speed do not need these heavy, expensive units.

As is apparent from the foregoing, each component must be chosen with care and matched to the patient's ability to use them and the desired type of function. Any combination of the options described previously can be obtained.

Suspension mechanisms

One suspension for the above-knee amputee is a plastic or metal pelvic band. The band has a joint over the ipsilateral greater trochanter, which is near the hip axis of rotation in the sagittal plane. The lower bar is attached to the socket. There is a molded, T-shaped, leather-covered upper bar from the joint contouring the pelvis; the strap goes between the greater trochanter and the iliac crest on the contralateral side. This is used for elderly and very unstable individuals. Since it pinches the abdominal fat during sitting and is restricting, it should be avoided unless experience with the Silesian band shows the latter to be inadequate for the individual.

A more comfortable but less stable suspension is a Silesian bandage. It is a flexible Dacron or nylon webbing attached to the lateral side of the above-knee socket. It is brought across the patient's back and over the contralateral pelvis between the iliac crest and the greater trochanter and attached anteriorly. A variant is a waist belt that goes over the iliac crest. Another is a neoprene sleeve.

Still less stable but much more functional, especially when used in young, agile individuals, is the suction suspension. A spring valve placed in the lower part of the socket allows air to be expelled when the patient puts weight on the stump but does not allow air reentry during swing. When worn without a stump sock, the limb is held on by atmospheric pressure during swing. A slight positive pressure during stance minimizes distal edema.

The donning of the suction socket is difficult in terms of balance and hand strength required, since the patient must bend at the waist to 90 degrees and pull the stump into the socket with the stump stockinette while inserting and withdrawing the stump alternately. Such a maneuver should not be attempted by elderly or infirm patients or by patients with poor balance such as some patients with neurologic impairment.

The suction socket also cannot be used by many patients with severely scarred stumps or by patients whose stump varies in volume because of weight gain or loss, treatment for malignancy with use of chemotherapeutic agents and adrenocorticosteroids, cardiac or renal edema, or other factors. Use of a suction socket by a new amputee is very expensive because of rapid stump shrinkage. Use of partial suction with a thin stump sock, together with a Silesian bandage for suspension, is an excellent way to treat young individuals soon after amputation.

Hip disarticulation prostheses

The hip disarticulation socket is casted to bear weight on the ischial tuberosity, and encloses the ilii for control. The hemipelvectomy socket bears weight on the remaining soft tissues and the lower rib cage. The socket is attached to a thigh piece by means of a Canadian hip joint that is parallel to the ground, transverse to the line of progression, and anterior to the socket. When the patient stands, the body weight is entirely behind the hip joint. A posterior stop permits stability of the pelvic socket on the prosthetic femoral segment. The center of gravity is aligned anterior to the knee joint to provide knee stability. Any of the prosthetic feet may be used, but lightness is important, so a lightweight SACH foot is the usual choice. The prosthesis is activated by active pelvic tilt or, less advisedly, by trunk rotation.

Bilateral hip disarticulation or hemicorporectomy

A hemicorporectomy patient must bear weight on the rib cage to sit. A sitting bucket that allows the patient to sit in a wheelchair is required. Cosmetic legs that are not suitable for ambulation are best for the elderly. A young, very active, muscular patient may try to use lockable articulated prostheses for ambulation with a two-point gait similar to that of a paraplegic patient. Since this is extremely energy consuming, most patients abandon walking after a short time and use a wheelchair.

Amputee training

After delivery of the initial temporary limb, stump hygiene is taught first, since it is the most important factor in preventing skin problems. The patient is taught to wash the skin with a bland soap and water at night so it has time to dry before the socket is donned in the morning. The stump must be rinsed thoroughly and dried by patting rather than by vigorous rubbing. The patient should apply lanolin at night and cornstarch or talc in the morning.

The stump socks should be washed daily with a mild soap in lukewarm water. They must be rinsed thoroughly, allowed to dry flat (not hung up), and put aside 3 or 4 days before being worn again. The rest prolongs their life. The inner surface of the socket must be cleansed each evening with a warm, soapy cloth. The soap must be removed thoroughly with many applications of a clean, damp cloth. The socket should be dried with a towel and allowed to dry overnight. If there is a soft insert, the prosthetist should be asked whether it can be cleansed in this manner without absorbing water.

After delivery of the prosthesis, the patient is taught to don and doff it. Crutch walking is continued, but this time the patient wears the prosthesis. A forearm crutch is desirable to prevent axillary pressure. The crutch should be open on the lateral side in climates where topcoats are worn. The patient is taught to hop, since this is used in the home to go to the toilet and lessens the fear of falling. The patient must learn to balance on each leg, since walking is a matter of systematic, rhythmic losing and regaining of balance on alternating legs. The patient must learn to appreciate the difference in sensation between proper and improper gait. Trunk movement to compensate for poor balance should be minimized.

Unless the patient will need a walker permanently for safety, gait training should not include the use of a walker. It is impossible to walk with equal step lengths using a walker, and walker use gives a habitually abnormal gait pattern. Thus gait training should proceed in the parallel bars, immediately followed by crutches and/or canes. A walker with front wheels lessens the gait abnormality while increasing safety.

An above-knee amputee learns balancing and weight shifting more slowly and with more difficulty because the patient does not have proprioception in the artificial knee. The patient must learn active prosthetic adduction and ab-duction, as well as flexion and extension, to understand how the leg is manipulated and to become familiar with the amount of muscle movement and range-of-motion change required to raise the foot off the ground and to swing the artificial leg.

The patient is then taught to step forward and backward with the good leg, bearing weight on the limb. Mirrors and television instant replay are useful learning techniques so the patient can see his or her gait pattern and correct it. The step length and the weight borne with each leg should be equal.

After level walking is safe, the patient should be taught to ascend and descend curbs, steps, ramps, and irregular terrain. An above-knee amputee ascends ramps and steps with the normal leg first and the prosthesis later. In de-scending, the patient keeps weight on the sound leg and moves the prosthesis first. Some below-knee amputees ascend and descend step-over-step, whereas others use the above-knee method.

Learning to walk with a prosthesis requires adequate com-munication between the therapist and the patient. Some patients have difficulty in learning. Athletic, well-coordi-nated patients generally learn to use an artificial limb more quickly than those less agile. It is important that the physical therapist report back to the physiatrist if the patient is not safe in ambulation after seemingly adequate training. There is then a need for further study of the problem.

Every patient must understand and accept that all amputee gait is somewhat abnormal. Few people can be restored to their previous physical activity level except for the seden-tary.

Prosthetic use depends on many factors including the patient's body build, strength, agility, cardiovascular re-serve, attitude, coordination, desire for cosmesis and func-tion, and intellect. Some other factors influencing the result are the patient's ability to pay for sophisticated devices, repairs, the terrain on which the patient walks, and the climatic conditions. The limb is a tool with which the patient tries to achieve personal goals in life.

Gait

The force of gravity acts on the body and its component parts at all times. For the purpose of gait analysis, body weight can be considered as concentrated at its center of gravity, which for the normal individual is a point slightly anterior to the second sacral vertebra in the midline of the trunk. Work must be done to lift the body's center of gravity. The work is equal to the body mass times the vertical height over which it is lifted.

In ambulation, movement of the body and limb segments, effected by contraction of muscles, is converted into trans-latory motion. The energy requirement for this translatory motion is proportional to movement of the center of gravity in the vertical plane and to correct kinematics, added to the basal metabolic cost, and the inefficiencies in the system. The least energy is needed when the center of gravity during ambulation traces a path most nearly parallel to the ground. In normal gait the path progression follows a smooth rec-tified helical curve of low amplitude (about 5 cm in each direction). During the gait cycle the speed of movement of limb segments varies, and as a result muscle energy is also expended in acceleration and deceleration of various parts of the body.

Gait cycle

The gait cycle is defined as the sequence of events in the body, as well as the lower extremities from the heel strike of one foot during ambulation to the next heel strike of the same foot. It is subdivided into the stance phase and the swing phase. The stance phase, comprising 60% of the gait cycle in walking, is the time when the foot is touching the ground. The swing phase, comprising the remaining 40% of the gait cycle, is the time when the foot is off the ground swinging through toward the next heel strike. During this period, of course, the opposite foot is in the stance phase.

Between the stance and swing phases is a moment, called double support, when both feet are on the ground supporting the body weight. This moment becomes progressively shorter as the speed of walking is increased. Running is defined as locomotion without double support. In running neither foot is touching the ground during part of the cycle, a period called double float.

The gait cycle starts at heel strike at 0% of the cycle; the foot becomes flat on the ground at 10%; the heel lifts off and the knee bends in preparation for forward acceleration of the leg at 45%; and the toe lifts off at 60%. During the swing phase both the hip and knee are flexed and the foot is dorsiflexed for the toes to clear the ground. Acceleration, midswing, and deceleration are the phases of swing. At 100% the gait cycle is completed as the heel strikes again.

Determinants of gait

The center of gravity traces a path in all planes during the gait cycle. This path can be represented by a helical low-amplitude curve, the amplitude of which is less than 2 inches (5.08 cm). To understand how this is effected, one must consider the six traditional determinants of gait:

1. *Pelvic rotation* consists of 4 degrees of alternating rotation (total range of 8 degrees) with right and left hip advancement. This rotation effectively lengthens the leg segments at the lowest position of the center of gravity, when both feet are on the ground. By such means, this "lowest position" is raised by approximately ⅜ inch (0.95 cm).

2. *Pelvic tilt* during stance consists of tilting 5 degrees downward toward the side of the swinging leg, at the time when the center of gravity is at its highest position. As a result, the position of the center of gravity is about ³⁄₁₆ inch (0.48 cm) lower than it would be otherwise.

3. *Knee flexion during stance* occurs when, from the fully extended position at heel strike, the knee immediately flexes about 15 degrees. Flexion effectively shortens the length of the supporting limb during stance and lowers the center of gravity when it is normally at its highest position (midstance) by about ⁷⁄₁₆ inch (1.11 cm).

4. *Foot and ankle motion* after heel strike is plantar flexion of the ankle to its lowest position so the entire foot is on the ground. When the heel lifts off, the ankle arcs up to its highest position at toe-off. During swing the ankle does not influence the center of gravity. Ankle motion smooths out the abrupt changes in direction of the center of gravity at the lowest and highest portions of the curve, thereby reducing deceleration and acceleration.

5. *Ankle and knee motion* is synchronization of ankle and knee motion.

6. *Pelvic movement* is lateral movement of the pelvis producing horizontal displacement of the center of gravity. Since weight is shifted from one foot to the other when walking, equilibrium is maintained by moving the center of gravity alternately over each foot during stance. If the long bones of the lower extremity formed a straight line from the hip to the foot, the lateral shift of the center of gravity would be considerable; however, the angle between the femoral neck and shaft and the femoral-tibial angle reduce the amplitude of this displacement. In women the femoral-tibial angle is greater ("physiologic knock-knees") because the pelvis is wider.

In summary, on right heel strike at the start of double support, the center of gravity is in the midline and at its lowest point in the vertical plane. At about 25% of the gait cycle, when the weight of the body is entirely on the right foot, the center of gravity is at its highest point in the vertical plane and at its maximal lateral shift to the right.

Any change in kinematics alters the determinants of gait and affects the path traced by the center of gravity, by an increase in amplitude or by more rapid acceleration and deceleration of limb segments, which increases energy consumption.

During the gait cycle there is also axial rotation of each segment of the lower extremity, the extent of which is dependent on the speed of walking. At a normal rate of walking the total rotation is about 23 degrees, but at a faster rate it may exceed 35 degrees. The total rotation is divided as follows: 5 degrees of pelvic rotation, 9 degrees of rotation of the femur, and 9 degrees of rotation of the tibia. During stance phase progressive axial internal rotation occurs from the externally rotated foot that contacts the ground. Between heel-off and toe-off a sudden reversal into axial external rotation occurs just as the foot is about to leave the ground. That is what causes the circular mark on a waxed floor. In addition, the subtalar angle moves toward eversion during the first third of the stance phase and reverses toward inversion of the foot during the latter part of the stance phase; the total angular change in eversion and inversion is approximately 6 degrees.

Muscle activity

Muscle activity powers the gait cycle. During the gait cycle most muscles work only intermittently, allowing restoration of blood flow during relaxation and recovery of energy sources for further contraction. Eccentric lengthening contractions are more common than concentric shortening contractions during walking. They are less energy consuming. During running and climbing, concentric contraction is more common.

The pretibial muscle group, the dorsiflexors of the foot, primarily the tibialis anterior and toe extensors, contract maximally from heel strike to foot-flat. They let the foot down gradually by a lengthening contraction, which functions much like a shock absorber. During the rest of the stance phase there is minimal activity of these muscles, which also serve to invert the foot, providing mediolateral stability at the ankle. There is also minimal activity of the pretibial group during the swing phase, especially during walking on rough ground, where a concentric contraction provides toe pickup to prevent stumbling.

The calf muscles, primarily the gastrocnemius and soleus, are active maximally during push-off, contracting to prevent ankle dorsiflexion after midstance so the weight is transferred to the metatarsal heads. The body pivots over the forefoot. In rapid walking and running, the calf muscles provide strong plantar flexion of the foot, which lifts the body and propels it forward.

The deep compartment muscles of the calf (flexor hallucis longus, tibialis posterior, and flexor digitorum longus) also prevent dorsiflexion during push-off. During stance they act as invertors of the foot, providing mediolateral stabilization.

The peroneal muscles, the peroneus longus and brevis, are the prime evertors of the foot. They control the attitude of the foot during swing and help balance the body over the foot during stance. Their activity can be seen best when one observes a woman walking in high-heeled shoes from behind.

The quadriceps muscle group is active twice during the gait cycle for relatively short periods of time. The peak of activity occurs at heel strike. The muscle allows the knee to flex approximately 15 degrees through a controlled lengthening contraction, acting largely as a shock absorber. The second peak of quadriceps activity occurs at the end of the stance phase when the rectus femoris contracts, producing hip flexion and forward acceleration of the leg. The leg would otherwise lag behind with an excessive heel rise.

The hamstring muscles also have a double peak of activity. The first occurs just before heel strike, when their contraction decelerates the forward swing of the leg. The second occurs right after heel strike, when their contraction prevents flexion of the hip. These muscles, serving together with other muscle groups as a shock absorber, control the downward and forward movement of the body.

The gluteus maximus muscle shows its peak activity during heel strike, controlling excessive flexion at the hip. A second peak occurs inconsistently after heel-off during walking. It is more consistent during rapid walking or running. During the last part of stance in running, the full leg including the hip is extended to lift the body weight and propel it forward. At this time the muscle works together with the knee extensors for the same purpose.

The hip abductor muscles, such as the gluteus medius and gluteus minimus, act during early stance to limit downward pelvic tilt on the swing side to 4 degrees. Minor activity in these muscles continues through most of midstance to stabilize the pelvis on the femur.

Information on the function of the hip adductor group is limited. A portion of the adductor magnus is functionally a hamstring muscle. The main activity of the adductor groups occurs right after heel strike and at the very end of the stance phase, at which time it contributes to the forward swing of the leg since it is a hip flexor. This muscle group may help stabilize the pelvis. It may also contribute to the first peak of internal rotation of the limb segment in a closed kinetic chain, whereas at the end of the stance phase it may act as an external rotator in an open kinetic chain. However, none of these interpretations has been verified through research.

The erector spinae muscles show peak activity right after heel strike and act to prevent flexion of the trunk. A second peak of activity in these muscles occurs at the very end of stance just at heel strike of the other leg. The muscles also stabilize the trunk on the pelvis.

Analysis of forces

Another consideration in the analysis of normal gait is the effect of gravity and inertia on the body. It is logical to consider locomotion through the forces it produces against the ground. These forces are most commonly measured by a force plate and consist of the following: vertical loading, anterior and posterior shear, medial and lateral shear, and torque.

Because of deceleration on the reception foot, the vertical loading force is increased immediately after heel strike. During the moment of double support, part of body weight is borne by the opposite foot. The vertical loading exceeds body weight by approximately 10% at foot-flat position as a result of shock absorption. As inertia carries the body forward, vertical loading during midstance is reduced by approximately 10%. During push-off the body is actively accelerated upward and forward, and the vertical load is approximately 20% greater than body weight. After this peak the vertical load decreases as the other foot touches ground and both feet support the body weight, following which the weight is shifted entirely to the other foot.

Anteroposterior shear force varies as follows. At early heel strike there is a small amount of posterior shear, said to be due to contraction of the hamstring muscles decelerating the forward swing of the leg. During the rest of heel strike there occurs a marked forward shear. Thus on slippery ground the foot slides forward out from under the person walking. During midstance the shear returns to neutral, and during push-off a large posterior shear force occurs as the body weight is lifted up and propelled forward.

The small medial shear force is brief and occurs during initial heel strike. During the rest of stance, lateral shear force prevails. This is primarily due to contraction of the gluteus medius and minimus muscles.

Measuring forces on the foot during walking using small pressure transducers gives additional information. The transducers may be used on the bare foot or in footwear with or without orthoses. They are placed on both sides of the heel, the first, second, and fifth metatarsal heads, the hallux, and wherever dysfunction is suspected.

Abnormal prosthetic gaits

It is important that an abnormal gait be analyzed systematically. Snap judgments must not be made from superficially similar patterns. For any deviation from normal it is important to determine not only what the deviation is and what parts of the body it involves, but also at what point it occurs during the gait cycle. A limp is an asymmetric gait. An abnormal gait may also be symmetric.

First the examiner must make a general appraisal of gait, observing symmetry of movements of all body parts in all phases of the gait cycle (length of stride, armswing, movement of trunk), smoothness of movements (staggering, loss of balance, incoordination), width of gait, and presence or absence of pain.

Each part of the body should then be observed systematically. The head and shoulders are watched to see whether they dip or are elevated, depressed, protracted, retracted, or rotated. Particular attention is paid to armswing, noting any asymmetry in abduction or motion. The trunk is checked for any forward or backward lurch, list to either side, or absence of normal lumbar motion. The pelvis is observed for anterior or posterior tilt, hiking of the hip, and whether the sides stay level or drop. The hips are checked for motion in extension, flexion, rotation, dropping, circumduction, abduction, and adduction. The stability, flexion, and extension of the knees are noted. The ankles and feet are evaluated for dorsiflexion, plantar flexion, eversion, and inversion, during both swing and stance.

The observations are best made from the front, back, and the side by videocamera with slow motion and stop frame capability.

Gait deviations

Gait deviations may be caused by many factors. They may be medical, surgical, prosthetic, psychologic, or due to inadequate training. It is easiest to classify them by when they occur during the cycle.

Below-knee gait deviations

HEEL STRIKE DEVIATIONS. Excessive knee flexion at heel strike is usually due to an overly stiff heel cushion in the SACH foot (or heel bumper in a single-axis foot). A socket that is too far anterior to the foot results in this problem. The patient may not adequately resist knee flexion because of discomfort over the distal tibia. The patient may also have weak quadriceps muscles or have received poor training.

The opposite faults cause inordinately delayed knee flexion at heel strike. A patient may put the center of gravity forward at heel strike by bending at the waist, which is commonly due to pain over the distal end of the tibia or to weakness of the quadriceps.

MIDSTANCE DEVIATIONS. During midstance the basic deviations are a medial or lateral thrust of the knee. This is usually due to misplacement of the prosthetic foot relative to the socket.

Excessive knee flexion at midstance may be due to foot dorsiflexion, anterior tilt of the socket, or anterior displacement of the socket over the prosthetic foot.

PUSH-OFF DEVIATIONS. In push-off deviations between midstance and toe-off, the major deviations are abrupt knee flexion or extension. Abrupt knee flexion is usually due to excessive anterior tilt of the socket, the socket being too far forward over the foot, or the foot set in too much dorsiflexion. Abrupt knee extension at toe-off is caused by the opposite faults.

Above-knee gait deviations. Deviations similar to below-knee deviations may occur in above-knee amputees and may have similar or different causes. The different causes are described in this section.

GAIT DEVIATIONS IN STANCE

Heel strike deviations. At heel strike the major deviation is that the toe of the prosthetic foot rotates when the heel strikes the ground. This is generally due to a flabby stump, excessive soft tissues, or inadequate fit of the socket. It may occur when the prosthetic heel is too stiff. Occasionally a patient attempts to increase knee stability by intentionally rotating the prosthetic foot, since the knee of the prosthesis cannot flex unless its axis is perpendicular to the line of progression.

Foot-flat deviations. The major foot-flat deviation is knee instability, excessive flexion of the prosthetic knee. This happens when the knee joint is too far forward relative to the weight line. The patient's weight line should be in front of the axis of rotation of the knee. Knee stability depends on proper alignment for the particular patient. If the knee instability is at heel strike, it may be because the SACH foot is excessively firm or because the patient forgot to actively use the hip extensors to lock the knee. The progressive increase of a hip flexion contracture may predispose to this problem.

Midstance deviations. The major gait deviations during midstance are lateral trunk bending and excessive lordosis. Lateral trunk bending occurs when there is discomfort in the crotch or at the distal lateral aspect of the femoral stump. Less commonly it occurs when there is an abduction contracture. If the prosthesis is functionally too short because the patient is sinking into the socket, the patient bends the trunk laterally. A patient who is insecure or has poor balance does the same.

Excessive lordosis at midstance is generally due to a hip flexion contracture. Other causes may be weak hip extensors or weak abdominal muscles. The ischial tuberosity may not be well seated on the ischial seat because of insufficient support from the femoral triangle bulge. All bilateral above-knee amputees have excessive lumbar lordosis.

Push-off deviations. The major deviation at heel-off is the whip. A whip is a rotation of the heel in either direction. It is most commonly due to flabby musculature. The patient may have put on the prosthesis in an incorrect direction, especially if using a Silesian bandage suspension. More rarely the whip may be due to poor alignment or poor contouring of the socket.

The major deviation at toe-off is inability to flex the prosthetic knee. This is due to excessive plantar flexion of the foot.

GAIT DEVIATIONS IN SWING. The major deviation occurring during swing phase is an uneven step length with an uneven armswing. These occur because the patient has a fear of falling or pain when committing weight to the limb. The patient takes an excessively long brief step with the prosthesis (which may be compounded because of a hip flexion contracture) and a short prolonged step with the sound leg. This may occur because of an incorrect amount of knee friction for the patient's cadence.

Acceleration deviations. One swing deviation occurring at acceleration is excessive heel rise. The artificial foot rises high as the patient walks. This is generally due to inadequate extension aid or inadequate knee friction. Another deviation, called vaulting, is an elevation of the entire body by excessive plantar flexion of the sound foot on push-off. The patient does this to avoid stubbing the toe. Stubbing is due to a functionally long limb with excessive downward movement of the limb because of inadequate tightening of the suspension. Less commonly the limb is functionally too long because weight gain or edema has made the patient's stump larger or the patient has put on too many stump socks. Other causes are that the extension aid is too tight or the knee friction is too high. Vaulting happens when the patient attempts to walk very fast.

Midswing deviations. The most obvious midswing fault is an abducted gait (the patient keeps the prosthesis farther lateral from the line of progression than the sound leg but parallel to it). This also occurs when the prosthesis is functionally too long. Rarely is it due to fabrication errors. Another cause is pain in the groin from the medial brim of the socket, especially if the patient has an adductor roll, or if the stump has shrunk and extends too far into the prosthetic socket. Inadequate adduction of the lateral wall causes this abnormality. Alignment of the prosthetic foot too far from the midline, a pelvic joint that is abducted, or a contracture of the hip in abduction may also cause this deviation. Insecurity and inadequate gait training are other causes.

Related to an abducted gait is a circumducted gait. In this gait, stance is relatively normal. The patient swings the leg through in a semicircular fashion because the prosthesis is too long for the patient. It may also be a residual training fault.

Deceleration deviations. The major deviation during deceleration is an excessive terminal swing impact. This is a loud jarring accompanied by noise as the knee goes into full extension right before heel strike. The shank strikes the bumper very hard. This is due to insufficient friction at the knee or to excessive extension aid. Occasionally it occurs because the knee bumper has fallen out, but more frequently it is a habit established when the patient is insecure. The patient attempts to dig the heel into the ground to ensure knee extension before committing weight to the prosthesis.

Metabolic requirements of ambulation. The energy cost of ambulation after amputation progressively increases with higher levels of amputation. For a given walking speed on level ground, patients with a below-knee prosthesis expend from 10% to 40% more energy than normal subjects. Pa-

tients with an above-knee prosthesis require 65% to 100% more energy expenditure.

The physiologic importance of functioning knee joints is evident from the finding that patients with bilateral below-knee prostheses expend only 41% more energy in walking than normal individuals, whereas persons with a unilateral above-knee prosthesis expend at least 65% more energy. Persons with bilateral amputations using one below-knee and one above-knee prosthesis average a 75% increase over normal values, whereas those using two above-knee prostheses average a 110% increase, more than double the normal energy cost for ambulation. A patient with a hip disarticulation, or hemipelvectomy, uses 75% to 150% more energy.

The energy cost of crutch walking for the patient who has had an amputation of a lower limb and is not wearing a prosthesis averages 60% above normal. This validates the clinical rule of thumb that a patient who does not have the energy for crutch walking will probably not be able to walk well with an above-knee prosthesis. The energy cost of wheelchair mobility averages only 9% above normal walking. Thus the wheelchair is an energy-saving alternative to ambulation for patients who do not have the cardiovascular capacity for ambulation with a prosthesis.

A person walking with a prosthesis usually does not expend more energy per minute than normal subjects; the person simply slows down to keep energy expenditure within tolerable limits. A person with an above-knee prosthesis walks at an average speed of 1.5 mph (2.4 km per hour), while a normal adult walks at 3 mph (4.83 km per hour). At these comfortable speeds of ambulation for each group the rates of energy expenditure are about the same. For a patient with cardiac disease who before the amputation could not tolerate ordinary levels of exertion, the increased energy cost of ambulation even at a slow speed with an above-knee prosthesis may exceed the cardiac reserve. With a below-knee prosthesis the patient should be able to manage ambulation almost as well as before the operation. This underscores the importance of saving the knee joint if feasible at the time of amputation, especially in a patient with limited cardiopulmonary reserve.

All the previously mentioned determinants and forces are subject to the strength and endurance of the person walking. For most people, 70 to 75 meters per minute is a comfortable walking speed. If the calories required to walk 1 meter are prorated per kilogram of body weight, energy consumption is minimal at this rate. That energy requirements per kilometer are higher at slower speeds is probably due to the longer time it takes to walk 1 kilometer at slower speed, so basal metabolism is prolonged. The amount of stabilization required is increased, just as in bicycle riding it is easier to ride quickly than slowly. The natural frequency of pendulum swing for the lower extremity is from 70 to 75 per minute. As the speed of walking increases above the self-chosen rate, energy requirements also increase. For walking at 75 meters per minute, approximately 59 cal/min/kg are required or 0.79 cal/M/kg. Thus the average energy cost of walking, for a 60 kg person, is 2.5 cal/min.

Walking up and down inclines and steps and on irregular surfaces is proportionately more energy costly for the limbless than for the normal. Accurate studies under these conditions have not yet been done.

Prognosis for lower limb amputees

The survival of patients after amputation caused by vascular disease of the legs is short; 30% of patients die within a year after amputation. One of four patients loses the other lower extremity before death; a patient who has not learned to walk with a prosthesis by the time of the second amputation is unlikely to succeed in ambulation with two prostheses.

These figures emphasize the importance of providing a temporary prosthesis in the early postoperative period. The provision of a definitive prosthesis should be delayed until the patient can walk well with the temporary leg. The patient will probably require a new prosthetic socket within from 3 to 6 months. At that time it is most cost effective to provide the definitive limb. The cost of a new socket is approximately equal to two additional days in the hospital and should not be used to justify a long delay in prescribing a prosthesis. Physicians should use their influence in the community to eliminate administrative delays by health insurance companies or state agencies.

UPPER LIMB PROSTHESES

The upper limb can be considered as a mechanism for holding its terminal device, that is, the hand, in such a position in space relative to the body that it can function. The hand is not just a prehensile organ but an intricate mechanism serving many functions; for example, it is a sense organ, a weapon, an organ of expression, and a radiator of heat that assists in temperature homeostasis.

Artificial arms are primarily to achieve prehension. They cannot mimic all of the different types of prehension.

Prehension can be classified into major types. In palmar pinch the palmar surfaces of two fingers grasp an object as does a pair of pliers. It is used to pick up a coin from the edge of a table. The three-jaw chuck type of grasp permits grasp between the thumb and the second and third digits. It is the type of grasp used to hold a pencil or a drill bit. In lateral pinch the ball of the thumb presses against the lateral side of the index finger. This is the type of grasp used to pick up a sheet of paper. Hook grasp relies on fingers other than the thumb and is the method used to carry a briefcase. In cylindric grasp the thumb opposes the four digits to form a circle around an object, such as a hammer handle. Spherical grasp is used in holding a ball. Fingertip pinch is used to pick up a straight pin.

No artificial hand has sensation except for that minimal sensory feedback transmitted through the socket and harness. As an organ of expression the artificial arm is poor. As a weapon it is all too efficient. Since the hand is the most important part of the upper limb, the greatest attention should be given to the prescription of the terminal device.

Loss of part of a hand is usually best treated by reconstructive hand surgery. Surgery is preferable to the best prosthesis because sensation can usually be preserved. If the patient is sensitive about appearance, the reconstructed part can be covered with a cosmetic glove for social occasions.

Before prescribing an artificial arm, the physician must determine whether the patient needs and will wear it. In children with bilateral upper amelia (absence of both arms), the need for artificial arms seems obvious and immediate. However, this is an error. Such children learn from the beginning to use their feet for manipulative and prehensile functions, and this suffices for a lifetime in most individuals. Prostheses may be an option for some who wish cosmesis more than function. The feet are sensate as well as prehensile, whereas prostheses are only prehensile. Acquired bilateral amputation in adults requires limb fitting in most cases.

Parts of the prosthetic system

The parts of a prosthetic system for the absent upper limb are similar to those for a lower limb, including a socket, a suspension, joints, a terminal device (in this case a hand or hook), and a source of activation. The power source for an artificial leg is always body power. For the arm it is most often body power, but on occasion it is external power.

Terminal devices

The terminal device is always chosen first, since it is the most crucial part of the prescription. Two types exist: prehensile and cosmetic. Prehensile terminal devices are of two types. The first is a hook or other nonanatomic shape, and the second is a hand-shaped device that is thus partly cosmetic. Purely cosmetic devices serve many useful purposes, especially for unilateral arm amputees, and are thus also functional.

Prehensile devices are designed to either open or close voluntarily. The voluntary-opening device opens when the wearer uses some body motion transmitted through a cable and harness to open the hook or hand. Closure is by elastic or springs that hold without voluntary exertion. These devices are simple, inexpensive, and almost maintenance free. Since they operate in only one or two fixed ranges of pressure, they may crush delicate objects unless the amputee holds the prosthesis partially open, which can become very tiring.

In voluntary-closing devices the fingers close when the patient reaches for the object. If a lock is included, the device locks only on humeral relaxation. In such devices the pressure is adjustable at will. Sensory feedback of the pressure exerted is learned. Devices made to lock at any desired point are more complex, heavier, and more expensive. In addition, when attempting to release an object, the patient must exert a slight amount of additional pressure, and this may crush a delicate object unless it is done with care.

Hooks

The hook most commonly used is the canted hook, which has one straight, fixed "finger" with a rounded, hooklike extension. The movable finger of the hook is more rounded throughout its entire length. The movable finger has a "thumb" as part of it, to which the cable is attached. The distal ends of the two hooks meet flat near the tip. The hook fingers are offset in shape and tilt so it is difficult to hold cylindric objects. The fingers may be made of aluminum, steel, or plastic and may have rough or smooth inner surfaces. The opposing surfaces may be bare or covered with neoprene rubber or Plastisol.

The lyre-shaped hook has mirror-image fingers of identical size and shape. There is a rounded space between the proximal parts of the fingers to hold cylindric objects. This type comes in both metals and may have either a voluntary-opening or a voluntary-closing mechanism. Studies have shown that the lyre shape is more effective for grasping activities.

There are special hooks of different sizes and shapes, with and without locking mechanisms, for heavy-duty use and for children, as well as for other special purposes.

The most popular voluntary opening hooks are closed by rubber bands. The amount of prehensile force is controlled by the number of rubber bands placed on the proximal part of the fingers. All children's terminal devices are voluntary opening.

Another voluntary opening hook is the Northrup Sierra two-load hook. It has lyre-shaped fingers and closes by a steel spring. A switch determines whether the pinch force will be about 7 pounds or half that much. There is no locking.

The major voluntary-closing hook is the Army Prosthetics Research Laboratory (APRL) hook, which has a spring to keep the fingers open. When the Bowden cable on the harness is pulled, it moves the thumb. A transfer mechanism closes one finger against the other, and the hook locks in the position it is in at the time the cable is released. When the cable is next pulled, the hook unlocks and the finger opens fully. The hook can afterward be closed and locked again. The prehensile force is adjusted at will by the amputee and depends solely on the amount of power transmitted to the thumb. Manipulation of a small button on the hook permits the fingers to spread apart to 3 inches to pick up wide objects, such as a water glass, or to a small opening of $1\frac{3}{8}$ inches, or disengages the lock to permit free wheeling for rapid grasp and release. Since the movement of the thumb transmits work to the fingers, there is more me-

chanical advantage when holding the fingers close together. Less effort is required to obtain the same amount of prehensile force. The T.R.S. Company makes two kinds of voluntary closing hooks, one of which has a lock.

Artificial hands

Artificial hands may be purely cosmetic, or prehensile as well. Cosmesis is important and should not be denigrated. Cosmetic hands and gloves can be off-the-shelf or custom made. True cosmesis does not exist, but the better prostheses are much less noticable. All dyes reflect light of varying wavelengths differently, so the hands look different in daylight, fluorescent light, and incandescent light. Some amputees have different gloves for different seasons, and for daytime or nighttime use.

Functional hands are voluntary opening or voluntary closing. All children's hands are voluntary opening. The size of the hand should be the circumference of the patient's remaining hand measured at the metacarpophalangeal joints in partial flexion. The cosmetic or functional hand should be slightly smaller than the normal hand so it will be less noticeable. Functional hands are rarely used by bilateral amputees, but if they are, the size is estimated.

The APRL in cooperation with the Sierra Company produces hands for children and adults. The device has a three-jaw chuck prehension with the second and third digits moving against a positionable thumb to provide opening for small and large objects. The Dorrance Company manufactures hands for children 5 years or older. They are functional, cosmetic, relatively lightweight, and easy to operate. The thumb and second and third digits all open simultaneously. After outgrowing the size 1 hand, the child can be fitted with sizes 2, 3, or 4, which operate in the same manner. Two ranges of prehensile force are available, but these must be installed by the prosthetist. They cannot be varied by the patient.

Another voluntary-opening hand that combines good appearance and function, with all the fingers meeting a stationary thumb, is the Robin-Aids. As a full hand it is heavy and hard to open. Because the mechanism is in one finger and not in the palm, some of the fingers are removable. It is thus suitable for transmetacarpal or partial hand amputations where other hands are not.

The major body-powered voluntary-closing hand is the APRL. It locks in any position and is released by a second pull on the cable. The second and third digits move to the thumb, giving a three-jaw chuck closure. For grasping wide objects such as a water glass, the thumb has a second position that is uncosmetic. In this position the second and third digits do not touch the thumb at maximum closure.

Hooks versus hands. Prehensile hooks are far more useful tools than any artificial hand. They are the most effective devices that can be used by a bilateral upper extremity amputee. Since a high-level amputee must use a long prosthesis, the weight of the terminal device at the end of the long lever is very important. Aluminum hooks are light. The hook can reach into pockets and corners, which the hand cannot. The artificial hand obscures vision while the hook allows visual control. The hook is better for picking up papers, coins, and other small objects. The hand is better for cylindric objects.

Cosmetic gloves over functional hands are nicer looking than hooks but less attractive than purely cosmetic hands. Cosmetic coverings over functional hands provide friction for holding objects. The use of cosmetic hands is important psychologically for patients who value appearance highly. For a patient with a very high unilateral arm amputation, who should not have an externally powered prosthesis, the purely cosmetic prosthesis is desirable because of its light weight. Cosmesis is denigrated by some therapists, but for the unilateral arm amputee it is often the most important "function" we can restore. It is important for self-image and in many jobs. I offer a hand-shaped device for almost all unilateral patients. I often prescribe both a hook and a hand.

Sockets

The major function of the socket in an upper limb prosthesis is to transmit as accurately as possible the movements of the bones. It does this poorly, which is especially damaging in below-elbow amputees who lose considerable pronation and supination, even with the most accurately constructed socket.

Sockets are now invariably made of plastic. They may be single or double walled. The outer wall gives length and shape. It is used alone in a single-wall socket. The inner wall, called the stump layer, accurately fits the soft tissues and supports them. Since it should closely approximate the bone, its fit determines the efficiency of bony movement transmission. In children a third wall may be used to allow room for growth. For elbow or wrist disarticulation, a single-wall prosthesis is used to diminish the overall length of the socket so the appearance of the limb is more natural. Prosthetic comfort is primarily determined by socket design.

The conventional below-elbow socket is more or less tubular and is custom fitted to the stump. By contrast, the wrist disarticulation socket has its end "screwdriver shaped" around the wrist bones to harness pronation and supination. The dorsal surface is longer than the volar. The opening of the socket is oval.

The Muenster below-elbow socket is used for patients with short below-elbow amputations; it goes above the epicondyles and fits closely around the biceps tendon and olecranon. It is self-suspending, so a simpler control cable can be used, or a self-contained myoelectric system is feasible. The opening is irregular. It can be used only for unilateral amputees, since it inhibits both extension and flexion. It is used more often for short stumps than the previously used split socket attached to an elbow step-up hinge, since it provides more stability and elbow lift. The Muenster suspension may be combined with a preflexed socket of the forearm if getting to the mouth is vital with that limb.

Above-elbow sockets are usually made to just below the acromion to provide increased stability unless there is difficulty in getting into the socket. Anterior and posterior Muenster "wings" should be placed on the socket if there is a problem with rotation. As with all sockets, many variations exist.

For the shoulder disarticulation and the forequarter amputee, a body jacket is necessary and is best made with large fenestrations to allow perspiration to evaporate. Conventional prostheses are often inadequate for this type of amputation, but this type of socket is used for externally powered prostheses as well. If no prosthesis is to be used for the forequarter, a shoulder cap should be used to fill out the jacket shoulder.

Joints

Wrists. The terminal device is connected to the forearm by a wrist unit that comes in different types. The function of the wrist unit is to attach the hook or hand and allow its positioning or locking. For each activity the hook must approach the object to be grasped from a different angle. The approach angles are limited, so the angle of the hook must be decided and the hook turned before the prosthesis is moved toward the object to be picked up. All wrist units must permit positioning.

In manual-friction wrist units a rubber washer acts as a friction gasket that allows pre-positioning but resists rotation of the hook when picking up objects. The resistance to rotation varies with the compression of the washer. This varies with hook position, since the hook is attached by means of a screw thread. Turning the hook increases or decreases the compression of the rubber gasket. When an amputee attempts to do heavy work, a compromise must be reached between the amount of resistance to positioning and the amount of torque that can be resisted by the terminal device.

A constant-friction wrist unit is used when constant friction in all positions is desired. It has a nylon or Delrin gasket that is compressed onto the bolt of the terminal device by a small screw. The tension of the gasket is the same, irrespective of the position of the hook.

A number of manual-lock wrist units are available. These units have a series of serrations that lock the hook in different positions. One type, the quick disconnect wrist, allows a rapid change between a hook and a hand. This wrist was designed for patients who do heavy, dusty work. Since dirt often accumulates in the serrations, it does not always meet the need ideally.

Amputees with limited use of their contralateral extremity should be considered functionally as bilateral amputees. They should be furnished with a passive wrist flexion unit that can change the angle of hook approach when the release switch is activated and then locks on release of the switch. All bilateral amputees should be fitted with two wrist flexion units. Some patients find one adequate and prefer to use extra "body English." Some externally powered arms have powered wrist flexion and rotation (which can be a functional substitute).

Elbows. For below-elbow suspension, flexible elbow hinges, made of simple leather or webbing and extending from a triceps pad or humeral cuff to the socket, may be used. If the below-elbow stump is short or needs lateral stabilization for heavy work, metal or plastic single- or multiple-pivot, rigid hinges may be used with or without hyperextension stops. In a short stump with its tendency to slip out of the socket, polycentric hinges or the Muenster socket may be required.

For an above-elbow amputee, the needs are elbow flexion and locking in place against load. For very young children a passive elbow with friction resistance is best. For older children and adults, elbows that can be locked by a ratchet are used. The lock can be unlocked with the contralateral hand or by motion of distal body parts. The forearm is then flexed by distal part motion, humeral flexion, passive motion by the contralateral hand, leaning against a table, and so on. The reciprocating lock is then locked. Rotation of the forearm is needed to get the elbow close to the body. Passive friction turntables are routine at the upper part of elbows.

External power arms for the above-elbow limb and higher usually have powered elbows, often with automatic locks. Rotation is passive.

Shoulders. Except when certain external power devices are used, the most common shoulder joint is a passive flexion-extension joint. Setting the shoulder in slight abduction, or using a joint that has passive abduction, facilitates donning clothing. For the shoulder disarticulation the socket provides suspension and the chest type of suspension and control is used. The elbow unit is operated by shoulder hiking or lateral trunk flexion, since the elbow lock unit is ordinarily attached to a waist band or a perineal or thigh strap. Very few shoulder amputees receive adequate function from conventional prostheses. A purely cosmetic prosthesis is preferred for the unilateral amputee. Externally powered devices are preferred for bilateral amputees at this level if available.

Harnesses and controls

The harness serves the purpose of suspension. The harness distributes the weight of the prosthesis and any objects carried for comfort and stability.

The position of the socket serves to position the terminal device in a functional location but does not contribute in any way to the use of the terminal device, which must be activated by some other means. In conventional prostheses the motive power must be transferred from one set of muscles through a cable system to operate the terminal devices. In the use of external power sources, switches or the electrical potentials associated with muscle contraction control the source of power.

Cineplastic control. Biceps cineplasty may be used for patients with below-elbow amputation to minimize harnessing and to provide some sensory feedback through tension on the biceps tunnel, but it is indicated only for persons who are intelligent, observe rigid personal hygiene, and will cooperate fully in the surgical and training programs. This type of control provides only moderate strength for the terminal device. The tunnel breaks down frequently. However, pectoral cineplasty may become useful to control external power prostheses in the future.

A goal is power activated by inconspicuous body motions ordinarily associated with the action desired. There should be minimal energy loss. The harness should be easy to doff and don without help and should be removable from the prosthesis for cleaning.

In the below-elbow amputee a triceps cuff helps to provide suspension and acts as an attachment point for the cable housing and joints. The most common type of harness for an amputee not doing heavy manual work is the figure-of-8 harness. It consists of a webbing strap made of washable, nonstretchable material, such as Dacron or nylon, with the axillary closed loop for the normal side covered by a plastic protective tubing. The cross of the "8" is positioned 5 to 8 cm below the seventh cervical vertebra and slightly to the unamputated side of the spinal column.

The anterior strap of the open part of the "8" goes over the patient's ipsilateral shoulder in the deltopectoral groove. It is attached to a webbing inverted-Y suspensor. This ends on the triceps pad and suspends it. The posterior strap of the open end of the figure-of-8 is the control cable–activating strap; the Bowden cable is linked to it. For a bilateral below-elbow amputee the same type of harnessing is used except that both parts of the "8" end in an open loop.

The Bowden control cable is plastic or braided metal inside a flexible coil housing. The cable housing can be bent without decreasing the efficiency of cable pull, since the housing acts like a series of pulleys over which the cable moves. The arm can be moved without such movements affecting the overall length relationship of the operating ends of the cable, so terminal device operation is not dependent on arm position.

For patients using a Muenster below-elbow socket, where the suspensory function of the harness is unneeded, the anterior strap and inverted-Y suspensor are eliminated and the harness is called a figure-of-9 harness.

A shoulder-saddle chest strap suspension is used for heavy work and wherever the axillary loop might be uncomfortable, such as in patients with excessive perspiration, a contralateral radical mastectomy, or a burn scar. The terminal device is activated by a control strap to the posterior part of the chest strap. The University of Michigan design allows the best range of motion.

Above-elbow figure-of-8 harnessing is approximately the

same as for below-elbow amputees. The front support strap has an elastic suspensor mechanism attached parallel to an elbow lock nonelastic strap called the elbow lock billet, which in turn is attached to a hanger loop secured to the elbow lock cable, whose activation locks and unlocks the elbow mechanism. It is the relative length of the elastic suspensor and the inelastic elbow lock billet that determines whether the cable is moved. When the patient extends and abducts the arm, the inelastic elbow lock billet is tightened while the elastic suspensor stretches, and the elbow is unlocked. When the humerus is brought back into its neutral position, the cycle is complete: pull to unlock, release to neutral, pull to lock, release to neutral, and pull to unlock.

The posterior part of the harness for control is the same as in a harness for a below-elbow amputee. Since suspension of the socket is sometimes difficult, a lateral support strap may be used. It usually goes from the nonamputated side of the harness ring, or cross of the harness, to the lateral part of the socket. A cross back strap to help hold the two ends of the figure-of-8 below the seventh cervical vertebra may be added by using a strap between the axillary loop and the control attachment strap posteriorly.

In above-elbow amputees when active elbow flexion is desired, the cable housing is cut (leaving the cable intact) and attachment points are added, which attach the cable housing to the limb. When the elbow joint is locked, the cable activates the terminal device. When the elbow is unlocked, any pull first flexes the elbow to the maximum before transmitting any force to the terminal device. The control activating strap should be at the lower third of the scapula for maximum excursion.

The above-elbow shoulder saddle chest strap harness is the same as the below-elbow except that the elbow lock billet must be attached to the anterior part of the shoulder saddle and the elastic suspension must be parallel with it, as in the figure-of-8 harness. In addition, there is a lateral loop suspensor both anteriorly and posteriorly to help suspend the limb unless the socket is over the shoulder. A webbing shoulder saddle may also be used. It has the same general configuration except that the straps are sewn to each other instead of to a leather shoulder saddle.

Triple control harness for above-elbow prosthesis. If very strong terminal device operation is required, separate from elbow flexion, a triple control harness can be used. The posterior part is like a figure-of-9 harness with an attachment at the posterior chest strap. The cable operates the terminal device by scapular abduction. The control strap from the shoulder saddle operates forearm flexion. Extension of the humerus locks and unlocks the elbow unit. This harness can be operated only by an amputee with wide, strong, mobile shoulders. Since it requires three separate cables, some amputees have difficulty isolating the required movements.

In a patient with shoulder disarticulation, a socket on the chest and a chest strap provide the suspension.

Training of an upper limb amputee

The range of motion, muscle strength, and endurance of the stump, the trunk, and the remaining limbs of an upper limb amputee should be made optimal.

Some authors say that any amputee can be motivated to learn to use a prosthesis well. However, certain individuals reap financial or social gain from not using a prosthesis well or at all. Their failure may be manipulative. To prevent this, I ask amputees about their goals in life and then point out what they must do to meet those goals. I tell them that amputees can do many jobs with or without a prosthesis, if they have sufficient intellectual and physical skills. I point out that the only thing anyone has to offer a potential employer is the work of mind or body. I tell them that after they have learned to use a prosthesis we can evaluate them vocationally and tell them what kind of jobs they may be able to do. We cannot promise amputees that we will train them for jobs that will give them money, pleasure, and self-respect. Most people cannot find such jobs. I point out that before learning a trade and going to work amputees must first learn to feed themselves, dress themselves, and take care of themselves in the washroom, not only at home but in the workplace. To do this, amputees must use prostheses well and therefore should participate in preprosthetic exercise programs. They need to care for themselves whether or not they return to work.

In each training session the patient should be left with a sense of success. For adults, independence in the activities of daily living, with and without the prosthesis, is the most important thing to learn. Training in the use of the controls should be started immediately after the adult patient learns how to put on the prosthesis. Use training follows. Children must be trained in the use of the prosthesis and not the controls. Patients who desire the best-appearing result will be motivated to perform less awkward and conspicuous motions.

Patients who wish to return to work or to learn to do new things try very hard. A desire to please the therapist is of great help. The patient must be given clear instructions and immediate and frequent feedback concerning proficiency. This requires a one-to-one training relationship with the therapist, at least part of the time. Group training alone is inadequate for most amputees. Mental deficiency, psychosis, and senility interfere with training and may contraindicate fitting. A long period of time without a prosthesis mitigates against successful fitting and training. If the patient has worn a prosthesis for a long time and has developed poor habits, these are difficult to correct.

Orientation

The longer stump in a bilateral amputee or the remaining normal limb is the dominant side. The patient must be informed that no device will be as good as the arm that was lost. An artificial limb provides grasp to hold objects that are manipulated with the normal arm.

Some upper limb amputees prefer cotton to nylon stump socks because they absorb perspiration, provide some padding, and feel less clammy, especially in the winter. Patients rarely request wool socks. The socks should be changed and washed daily. Prostheses should be wiped daily with a moist sponge with mild soap and rinsed with a damp sponge. They should never be immersed in water. Harnesses should be provided in pairs so the prosthesis can be worn while one harness is being washed. To prevent local irritation to the skin and axillary hair follicles and to absorb perspiration, the use of an under-blouse in women and a T-shirt in men is advised.

Patients determine the amount of prehensile force they wish to use. At the beginning, minimal force with only a small number of rubber bands should be used; this facilitates success and builds up tolerance with the least fatigue and discomfort. Rubber bands used for closing voluntary-opening hooks do not provide the same amount of closing force with hooks of different sizes, and in time they lose elasticity because of use and exposure to heat, solvents, and sunlight.

Controls training

The first thing a patient must learn is how to put on and take off the prosthesis. A unilateral below-elbow amputee finds it easiest to don the prosthesis by holding the terminal device or socket in the good hand and inserting the stump under the Y strap and in front of the triceps pad, after making sure the harness is not twisted. The patient then raises the stump with the prosthesis on it overhead and slips the hand through the axillary loop, which is hanging behind the patient's back. A shrug of the shoulders settles the harness into place; it is much like putting on a jacket. To doff the prosthesis, the amputee raises both arms overhead, grasps the socket, withdraws the stump, and slips the arm out of the axillary loop.

A patient who has difficulty donning the prosthesis as described may find it easier to put it on like a pullover sweater by placing the stump in the prosthesis and the good arm through the axillary loop and then raising both arms above the head.

If the above-elbow stump is short, the amputee may don the limb by inserting the arm through the axillary loop first and putting the axillary loop into its final correct position. By leaning toward the amputated side, the patient can insert the stump. A shrug of the shoulders settles the harness into place. To remove the prosthesis, the amputee raises both arms overhead, grasps the socket, withdraws the stump, and slips the arm out of the axillary loop.

For shoulder disarticulation and forequarter prostheses, the remaining arm places the prosthesis on the stump. The patient then leans against a wall to maintain the shoulder cap in proper position or uses the chin for the same purpose. The chest strap is grasped from behind and fastened in front.

A bilateral below-elbow amputee has little difficulty putting on the stump sock and then the prosthesis, but for patients with higher amputation, the stump socks tend to fall off. For a bilateral amputee both stump socks can be connected by a strap that goes across the back. Such an amputee can use a "shrug," a T-shirt cut open like a bolero jacket, with prosthetic socks attached to the sleeves.

For bilateral above-elbow amputees, the prosthesis may be put on over the head or from behind the back. The sweater method of the below-elbow amputee is used, except that the shorter stump is inserted into its prosthesis first, while the longer stump stabilizes the device. When the longer stump is in its socket, both prostheses are raised so the harness slides over the head. If the appliances are put on like a suit jacket, the longer stump goes into the socket first. The stump is then elevated, and the amputee leans toward the side of the shorter stump, which is then inserted into its socket.

Taking off all prostheses is the reverse of putting them on.

The control motions are taught next. The first motion is flexion of the humerus to operate the terminal device. It is helpful to explain that in actuality the cable is not pulled. One end of the cable is connected to the axillary loop on the contralateral side. It does not move. The hook thumb is attached to the other end of the cable. Since the cable does not stretch, the thumb stays where it is. When the person flexes the humerus, the prosthetic socket is pushed forward. The cable housing is connected by means of attachment plates to the socket. The housing thus moves forward relative to the cable. This is the mechanical equivalent of cable pull but is in reality cable housing push. True cable pull is used for fine work when the patient wants to keep the hook steady while opening it. Contralateral scapular abduction is used.

To teach the amputee the control motion without excessive and unsightly motions, the therapist should stabilize the shoulder on the amputated side and grasp the prosthetic forearm in his other hand. The patient should be told to stabilize the opposite shoulder against the pull of the harness but not to contract it. With the patient's elbow at 90 degrees and the humerus vertical, the patient should be made aware that the cable is slack. The therapist should bring the prosthesis forward until tension develops in the control cable. The amputee should appreciate the tension in the harness. If the opposite shoulder is not stabilized, it should be held firmly against a wall so the patient learns to recognize the tension. The terminal device then opens. Humeral flexion on the amputated side should be no more than necessary to produce a comfortable reaching-out motion, without excessive scapular abduction.

In an above-elbow amputee the control motion is the same, but more humeral flexion is needed to open the terminal device when the elbow is locked. Humeral flexion is also used for elbow flexion when the elbow is unlocked. That motion flexes the elbow before opening the hook. When we teach humeral flexion to an amputee, we shield the patient's face so that the patient does not accidentally hit himself or herself if misjudging the amount of force required.

The elbow is locked by a combined humeral extension, abduction, and shoulder protraction. This motion pulls on the elbow lock billet, which locks the elbow, and stretches the elastic suspensor. Relaxation resets the mechanism. A repetition of the motion unlocks the elbow. The motion is difficult to learn and must be demonstrated to the patient repeatedly. After the patient learns it with the forearm vertical, the next step is to flex the forearm and then use the motion to lock the elbow. It is best to first teach humeral extension and abduction and to add shoulder protraction later. Each of the additional motions reduces the amount of humeral extension required.

Functional fitting of a patient with unilateral shoulder disarticulation or forequarter amputation is rarely of benefit unless external power is used. Since these patients have only scapular abduction and shoulder elevation for power sources, harnesses consist of a chest strap, a waist band, and occasionally a perineal strap. No active functional shoulder joint is available, and scapular abduction must be used for terminal device operation and elbow flexion. The waist band or perineal strap is usually employed to lock the elbow with shoulder elevation or lateral trunk flexion.

MYOELECTRIC CONTROL. Besides the body-powered prostheses mentioned, externally powered limbs have been developed, especially since World War II. There have been pneumatic, electric, and hydraulic limbs, but most externally powered limbs are now battery powered. The electric motors are of many types, as is the power transmission.

The motors may be activated by switches of many types. The most popular "switch" is myoelectric control, that is, the use of the electrical potentials generated during muscle activity to turn on the motor. The control may be on-off or proportional to the electromyographic potential (or the difference between opposing potentials).

A new generation of arms has thus come into being. Most are hand shaped and therefore appealing. A few limbs are for above elbow and higher amputees. They are very expensive. More than 90% of the limbs provided are below elbow in type. Their functional advantage is questionable, but their appearance in the unilateral patient is a plus. They can exert great prehensile force. For workers wanting a strong tool, the Otto Bock Company makes a hook, the Greifer, that can be interchanged with the hand.

The patient must be taught to contract the muscle to activate the limb. For a below-elbow prosthesis it is a brief process if the muscles are normal. For patients with higher amputations the muscles used are not associated with grasp, so learning is slower. These persons must learn not only to grasp and release, but also to flex and extend the elbow, and sometimes to pronate and supinate.

Use training

Children must be taught what can be done with a prosthesis to stimulate their interest before they are shown how it works. They learn the mechanics intuitively. Use training for an adult follows controls training. Controls training teaches the basic body movements and coordination necessary for efficient, graceful use. Once having mastered the required motions, the adult learns to use the prosthesis for the activities of daily living and possibly for vocational and avocational tasks. In the early stages of prosthetic use the device may be more of a hindrance than a help, and the patient who fails to become proficient will discard it. Without pleasurable use there is little motivation for continuing to wear a heavy, hot, constricting device.

Pre-positioning. The first thing to teach is pre-positioning. Pre-positioning is anticipatory placement of the terminal device in a position where it can function optimally once the hook is brought to the object it is to prehend. When reaching for an object, a normal person automatically positions the humerus, forearm, hand, and fingers in such a way as to grasp or handle the object effectively without excessive motions of the joints. The compensatory movements are integrated, coordinated, and simultaneous. Any final adjustments that may be required when the hand approaches the object are easily made by slight motions of the wrist or fingers.

The terminal device has only limited patterns of grasp. These are lateral pinch and hook in the hook and three-jaw chuck, cylindric, and hook grasp in the hand. If the axis of prehension of the object does not correspond to the axis of the terminal device, the object cannot be prehended. The terminal device must be realigned by pronation and supination at the wrist, elbow rotation, abduction of the shoulder, or use of "body English." To avoid this inefficient and graceless activity, the amputee must learn to pre-position.

The hand is worn so the fingers approach the object from the side, with the thumb closest to the body. This is so the dorsum does not obscure the object. If the object axis does not permit this approach, the hand is used thumb down. The hook is used rotated in any convenient position, with the fingers facing in any direction. A useful drill in pre-positioning is to hold a ruler in space at different angles and ask the patient to grasp and release.

To teach the patient approach, grasp, release, and selective opening, we first use simple objects, such as small cubes of wood, pegs, coins, and nails, and then progress to rounded objects. The patient should grasp a piece of foam rubber, a fragile ice cream cone, and a paper cup with and without water until he or she learns to keep a slight amount of tension on the cable to avoid crushing with voluntary-opening devices. A voluntary closing device requires a slightly greater force to unlock than to lock. The amputee should be taught to use no more force than is absolutely necessary.

Activities of daily living

The activities of living should be taught first. In a unilateral amputee the prosthetic side should be used for bimanual activities only, and the remaining arm, if normal, should be used for all other activities.

Grooming

Most unilateral amputees are able to wash themselves, bathe, and go to the toilet without the use of the prosthesis. Bilateral amputees may find brushing teeth a problem. The brush is held in the hook, and the head is moved against the brush. The electric toothbrush, for which holders are available, has lessened this problem. Shaving is easy for a unilateral amputee, but for a bilateral amputee it is preferable to use an electric razor with a leather or plastic holder. The surface must be high-friction rubber or plastic. It is useful to cover the washbowl with a folded towel to minimize breakage of razors.

For a bilateral arm amputee, cleaning the anal region is extremely difficult because it is hard to hold the toilet paper in the proper position for use and because the patient cannot see or feel where he reaches. Cleansing the vulva is usually not a problem. If one arm is amputated below the elbow, the toilet paper can be held in the hook on that side. For bilateral above-elbow amputees, several layers of toilet tissue may be spread across the toilet seat or the edge of a bath tub or chair. A moist surface or Dycem will help stabilize the paper. The patient then sits so the buttocks straddle the seat or chair edge and shifts the pelvis from side to side. This is difficult and not very efficient.

If the patient is able to kneel, the toilet tissue can be placed over the heel and a fore and aft motion of the pelvis does the wiping. Many repetitions are needed. Toilets such as the European bidet cleanse the perineum, and some dry the perineum with a stream of warmed air. Such toilets are preferable but are expensive and not portable. If the methods mentioned are not available, special reaching devices patterned to the individual need are required.

Clothing selection is probably the most difficult part of toileting for the amputee. Women may wear underpants in which the crotch is split and refinished with binding so the garment does not need to be removed for urination. Some "unionsuits" incorporate this feature. The opening should close when the patient is erect. When the patient sits on the toilet seat, with the trunk flexed on the thighs and the lower limbs abducted, the opening is sufficiently wide to prevent soiling of the garment. Some women avoid wiping after urination.

Women amputees usually find tampons superior to sanitary napkins during menstruation. If insertion by hook is a problem, insertion aids can be used. Sanitary pants can be modified to hold the sanitary napkin in a pocket in the correct location.

Eating

A unilateral amputee holds the fork in the prosthesis, and cuts with the normal hand. The amputee puts down the knife and switches the fork to the normal hand. The fork tines should be held downward. The fork should be held at the wide part and not on the handle. The "thumb" stabilizes the handle. Amputees prefer a serrated knife that saws rather than cuts. The knife can be used in the prosthesis with the hook fingers pointed downward and the handle resting on the "thumb." Most one-handed patients prefer the use of a rocker knife. The hook is prepositioned to hold the fork parallel to the plate and the knife vertical to the plate. Arm abduction and elbow internal rotation are usually required. The elbow must be locked in flexion.

To prevent slipping of the plate on the table, a moist paper towel, a flat sponge, a suction cup, or a Dycem pad can be placed between the two. Bilateral amputees find a plate guard helpful to prevent the food from slipping off the plate. Patients who have difficulty eating with a spoon may use a swivel spoon or a "spork." When food slips around the plate, especially round items such as peas and beans, bilateral amputees may use a "pusher." A cup is usually grasped with the fingers of the hook held over the top rim of the cup. Some cups can be held by the handle. A sandwich is difficult for a bilateral amputee to manipulate unless a special sandwich holder is used.

Dressing

In trousers for a unilateral amputee, the terminal device stabilizes the fabric at the bottom or top of the zipper. The zipper is preferable to buttons, hooks, or snaps, but even these may be manipulated with practice. For above-elbow amputees the forearm is flexed and locked and the elbow turntable is rotated internally. For shirts and blouses, buttons are nice but may be replaced with Velcro. The buttons may be sewed on for appearance. It is advisable to have the patient practice on different hooks, buttons, and zippers, shoelaces, and other clothing fastenings on a "prop" board. Other "props," such as locks, switches, doorknobs, and faucets, are also useful.

To unbutton a shirt cuff on the unamputated side, the patient stabilizes the edge of the cuff near the button by pressing one edge of the cuff between the third and fourth digits and the thenar eminence. The hook grasps the other side of the cuff near the button; the cuff may be pulled off the button. Shirtsleeves should be long enough to allow this activity. Some prefer a cuff that is so wide that buttoning becomes unnecessary. A unilateral amputee can learn buttoning without devices; the button hook is an inexpensive appliance that helps greatly. For a bilateral amputee a button hook is necessary. Elastic thread for buttons or cuff links may simplify matters.

For women a front-opening brassiere is useful. If a favorite style is not available commercially, a brassiere can

be made by sewing the back together and closing the front with Velcro. Usually, women prefer to close back-opening skirts and brassieres in front and then twist them around.

Skirts, jackets, and sweaters may be put on by first inserting the prosthesis all the way into the sleeve. The sound extremity can be manipulated into the other sleeve, and the garment is then shrugged into place. Covering the cosmetic glove with a handkerchief decreases friction. For above-elbow amputees, after one side is in, the elbow should be flexed to more than 90 degrees and locked to prevent the sleeve from sliding off again.

Socks are not difficult to put on, but occasionally aids are used. It is advisable to teach a unilateral amputee one- or two-handed shoelace tying. For most amputees, elastic gores, elastic shoelaces, spring closures, or even Velcro closures are preferred. Obese people experience difficulty in tying shoelaces, since vision is necessary. The abdomen gets in the way. To tie the shoes, the patient should be taught to use a stool, a chair, or the semikneeling position. Because the shoelace frequently slips out of the hook, an extra loop should be taken around the stationary hook finger to pull it tight. An amputee can tie a necktie quite easily by stabilizing the narrow end with the prosthesis. For bilateral amputees the problem is solved by the use of pretied and elastic neckties.

Clothing for amputees. Clothing for amputees should be as similar in style as possible to the clothing worn by non-amputees. It should be looser than usual for donning, since the limbs are frequently bulky. Loose clothing also helps to dissipate body heat, which is an almost universal need. Whenever clothing comes in contact with a hard surface, it wears out more quickly than when in contact with the resilient flesh, especially where there are metal parts and hard plastics. The problem is most serious where clothing is stretched, as over joints. The interposition of a softer substance, such as leather on the posterior thigh or over metal parts, may solve the problem.

A prosthetic shoe worn by a unilateral amputee wears much less than the shoe on the normal side, since the remaining leg does more of the work. The latter bears more weight and has a push-off function that is accentuated in an above-knee amputee. Shoes may be purchased from a dealer who stocks split sizes so the shoe on the normal side may be replaced by buying a spare single shoe of the same color and design as the good shoe on the amputated side. A worn heel on the ablated side makes ambulation unstable and changes the pressure areas and alignment. Amputees with vascular disease in the remaining leg should wear undyed socks. Socks should be washed a few times before wearing to avoid contact dermatitis and irritation. In women, when plastic laminates are used to cover a leg, the objectionable shine observable through nylon stockings can be eliminated if the leg is covered with a cotton lisle stocking under the nylons. Prostheses covered with rawhide painted a dull color are preferable.

In amputees the principle of minimal fastening should be applied. Clothing openings should be in front or rarely at the side. They should never be in the back if the patient must close them. If closure is needed, elastic or Velcro closures are desirable. If shirt cuffs are not wide enough, elastic thread for the button or a button hook may be used. In women who are bilateral amputees, closures only to the waist are often insufficient. The opening should be extended to below the waist to prevent excessive wear. If the patient has a very short below-elbow amputation, with the stump-activated elbow lock, a wide sleeve is mandatory both on the shirt and on the suit jacket.

Driving

In driving a car, a Northrup Sierra steering ring may be dangerous, since in trying to turn a sharp corner the fingers of the hook may catch in the ring. The regular swivel steering wheel knob is much safer for amputees than the driving ring. Regardless of which device is used, it should be placed at either the 9 o'clock or the 3 o'clock position. In driving, control modifications are frequently desirable. The turn signal control can be operated by the patient's knee. Any of the switches may be relocated to meet the needs of a given patient. Power steering and automatic transmission are necessary. Lower limb bilateral amputees need hand controls for driving. Right above-knee amputees need the pedals moved left.

Training time

The duration of training varies with the type of amputation and the physiologic and mental age of the patient. If it continues while the patient is using the temporary articulated prosthesis, it is rarely needed for the final prosthesis. The occupational therapist must provide instruction not only in routine activities, but also in specific needs at home and at work, correcting inefficiencies in the prosthesis, in activities, and in appearance. A new unilateral below-elbow amputee requires at least 5 hours of training, whereas an above-elbow needs at least 10 hours. The very young and the aged need much more time; bilateral amputees need more than twice the time mentioned. The patient should return to the amputee center to discuss with the team members any problems encountered at home, at work, or in school. The patient must be taught the care of the device. For those who are still growing, follow-up observation should occur at least every 3 months.

ACCEPTANCE OR REJECTION OF PROSTHESES

The acceptance and use of a prosthesis reflects the patient's evaluation of its relative advantages and disadvantages. The advantages of the leg are that it improves appearance and the patient's body image, frees the hands from crutches, and permits easier transfer, standing, and ambulation. The prosthesis does not increase the speed of walking

or decrease energy expenditure in comparison to crutch walking. Ambulation with an above-knee prosthesis is considerably slower and more laborious than propelling a wheelchair.

The disadvantages of a prosthesis include discomfort, heaviness, difficulty in donning and doffing, somewhat ungainly appearance, noise in operation, and disagreeable texture to touch. The discomfort cannot be eliminated but can be diminished by proper fit and stump conditioning. The prosthesis usually weighs about half as much as the body segment it replaces, from 3 to 7 pounds (1.18 to 3.18 kg) for a below-knee and from 7 to 12 pounds (3.18 to 5.45 kg) for an above-knee prosthesis. Lightweight prostheses are available, but there is usually a tradeoff in strength, durability, and cost. The patient often complains of prosthetic "dead weight," which is not due to a defect in fabrication.

The lower limb prosthesis gives a somewhat unnatural gait pattern, which is not cadence responsive, except for the hydraulic and pneumatic swing phase units. All units present difficulties when the amputee tries to go up or down inclines or steps. The higher the amputation, the greater the energy cost. This has many implications, including vocational ones.

The upper limb prosthesis is heavy, has no ability to manipulate, is mediocre in grasp, and has no sensation. Conventional upper limb prostheses give insufficient power to perform certain tasks. The artificial arm cannot be used above the head or behind the back because of the harnessing, nor can it be used where there is no vision.

All prostheses are hot, expensive, and unnatural, have mediocre cosmesis, and cause skin irritation and sweating.

The extent to which the rehabilitation team can minimize the disadvantages and maximize the advantages of a prosthesis determines acceptance by the patient. The patient evaluates the limb by weighing the costs against the benefits. Costs include economics, comfort, time lost from work and play, and appearance. The team should seek the help of successfully rehabilitated patients as volunteer patient counselors.

In our enthusiasm for prosthetic fitting, we should not delude the patient into believing that he or she will be "almost normal" after fitting and training with an artificial limb.

PROSTHESIS MAINTENANCE AND REPAIR

The prosthesis is a tool that may be damaged if used incorrectly or for an inappropriate purpose, such as a hammer or pry bar. Artificial limbs are expensive, and their maintenance is important. The joints should be lubricated every 2 or 3 weeks with a silicone spray after the lint is cleaned off. Harnesses should be washed weekly. A good-quality saddle soap should be used to clean the leather parts at least weekly. The stump and prosthesis should be washed every night so each may dry before wearing. When voluntary

opening hooks are used, the patient should change the rubber bands as needed with the band applier. Patients should not attempt to repair deteriorating or breaking parts but should return the limb to the prosthetist for adjustment.

PROBLEMS OF AMPUTEES AND THEIR TREATMENT
Skin problems

The human skin has complex functions and extraordinary abilities to adapt to changes in the demands placed on it. The skin regulates body temperature by heat loss through those body parts with the greatest exposed surface area. The amputation of digits puts an extra strain on all of the remaining sweat glands. In an amputee the remaining body parts are responsible for heat dissipation to control body temperature. Perspiration therefore is increased over the rest of the body, which is annoying but not detrimental. Sweating of the stump is also excessive and causes maceration, since the stump is covered by an impervious socket. The maceration allows the growth of bacteria and fungi. The socket and other prosthetic materials dissolve in the sweat and as solutes may act as antigens and cause allergic problems in the stump. Skin is fairly resistant to abrasive action, but this resistance decreases when the skin is moist. The function of the skin as an exchanger of gases and as a sensory organ is impaired by the perspiration and the socket. The sense organs accommodate rapidly, and sensation diminishes.

Weight bearing in the socket causes many mechanical stresses on the skin, such as intermittent stretching and friction. Friction on the skin gives both abrasion and heat, both of which are destructive. Mechanical stresses are highest at the junction of a rigid and flexible part of an object; skin problems are most severe where the edge of the socket holds the skin in a rigid manner, while the skin immediately adjacent to and not enclosed in the socket has a great amount of flexibility. The same problem occurs inside the socket where the latter is not in total contact with the skin.

Tight proximal brims, especially in suction sockets, may cause engorgement of the small blood vessels of the skin with resultant rupture and extravasation of blood. The dark pigmentation frequently seen at the end of the stump is the result of such bleeding.

Blockage of the eccrine temperature-controlling sweat glands by the socket or by keratin, especially when the patient perspires profusely, may cause rupture of the sweat ducts. Superficial duct ruptures result in small blisters on the skin; somewhat deeper ones lead to prickly heat, and still deeper ones cause papules. Sweating is under autonomic control and can sometimes be controlled with anticholinergic agents. When general perspiration diminishes too much, the temperature control of the body may be compromised. Local excessive perspiration may be diminished after copper sulfate or formalin ion transfer.

Apocrine glands are important only in the groin and axilla where the former may be irritated by the socket in an above-knee amputee and the latter may be irritated in crutch walking. These adrenergic glands respond to painful stimuli and anxiety. Their involvement may cause a stubborn disease of the skin called hidradenitis suppurativa, which is characterized by a foul discharge from painful cysts. The emotional state of the amputee is therefore also of physical importance.

Sebaceous glands seldom cause skin problems, since the back pressure of the sebum usually stops further production. Epidermoid cysts may occur when small keratin plugs develop in the skin of the adductor region of the thigh at the upper edge of the prosthesis. They may become infected and prevent the wearing of the device. Infections, primarily those caused by staphylococci, occur most frequently during the summer. Good stump hygiene diminishes the incidence of this condition, which is treated in the traditional manner when it does occur.

Allergic manifestations of the skin are common in amputees and may be due to the plastics and resins used in finishing the prosthesis. Sometimes a new cleansing agent (cream or lubricant) or the use of a foam rubber cushion or plastic-covered pad in the bottom of the socket results in contact dermatitis. Incompletely cured epoxy resins may produce an irritation dermatitis. The pink Pelite often causes irritation, but the white never does.

A fungus infection resulting from excessive perspiration is manifest as a reddish brown incrustation with weeping. The socket should be washed with 5% formalin and rinsed with alcohol. Fungicidal solutions, powders, or ointments such as Tinactin, Desenex, and Astero should be used on the stump. Applying liquid medication at night and powder in the morning is the best regimen. Measures to decrease perspiration should be taken.

Ingrown or infected hair follicles can be treated by plucking. Sometimes the infection is so severe that it requires antibiotics along with incision and drainage of the abscess. If this is a recurring problem, the prosthesis should be checked for excessive piston action. If it persists, epilation, either chemical or electrolytic, should be performed. Any sebaceous cysts interfering with socket fit should be removed. If they become infected, they should be treated with incision and drainage. If they recur, excision is the treatment of choice. Chafed areas suggest piston action or poor socket fit.

If the stump has had split-thickness skin grafts, either because of extensive burns or for surgical considerations, insensitivity or hypersensitivity of the skin may be a problem. Pressure should be avoided over such areas, but surgical reconstruction such as replacement after skin expansion may become necessary. Occasionally the use of an elastic garment or pressure from an Unna dressing whenever the limb is not worn helps. Friction reduction with polyamide sheaths, gel inserts, cornstarch, or "Second Skin" may be of value.

Atrophy

Pressure on the stump causes atrophy of the subcutaneous fat. Lack of the use of the musculature of the stump causes muscle atrophy. Bypassing weight bearing through the remaining skeletal system, such as ischial weight bearing in an above-knee prosthesis, causes osteoporosis. The remaining periosteum may develop bony spurs.

Neuromas

The cut end of every nerve becomes a neuroma, which is usually painless if adequately protected. Neuromas exposed to pressure may be painful and require revision. Capping of the nerve ends is of occasional benefit. Burial in bone and injection of the nerve with destructive chemicals are of no use.

Phantom sensation

Phantom sensation is a normal occurrence after amputation of a limb. This is the sensation that the amputated part is present. It may be accompanied by not unpleasant tingling. At first the phantom sensation can be so deceptive that the patient may attempt to scratch with the absent hand or to walk on the missing leg. With time, phantom sensation usually diminishes in a manner that has been described as "telescoping into the stump," but occasionally it persists for decades. The last sensations to disappear are those seeming to originate from the missing thumb or index finger, or from the great toe, which may be perceived as directly attached to the stump.

Almost all amputees except young children and those with brain damage have phantom sensation. Patients who have congenital limb deficiencies or have had a surgical or traumatic amputation before 4 years of age do not usually experience phantom sensation. The phantom sensation assists some patients in learning to use prostheses.

A number of theories have been proposed for the phenomenon. A limb is an integral part of the body, continuously bombarding the sensory cortex with tactile, proprioceptive, and occasionally painful stimuli, which are remembered largely subconsciously as part of the body image. After amputation these remembered perceptions produce phantom sensation, which may even include the feeling of a ring, wristwatch, or bracelet worn on the phantom hand or wrist. Deformity of a limb present before amputation usually continues to be perceived in the phantom. Anesthetic limbs leave no phantom after amputation, and gradual loss of an extremity, as in leprosy, usually is not associated with phantom sensation. However, surgical amputation of a body part in leprosy gives rise to phantom sensation of the whole part even after partial resorption has not resulted in a phantom.

Pain

Pain may occur in a number of forms. If it originates in the stump itself, it is called local pain. It may appear to be in the stump or in the absent part but be referred pain. There

also may be phantom pain. In addition, pain in other areas may interfere with prosthetic use.

Local pain may be due to pressure on an unprotected neuroma. Desensitization by tapping and socket relief generally alleviate this pain, but injections and ultrasound are required occasionally. Rubbing, tapping, and massaging should be continued. If these measures are not successful, acupressure, transcutaneous electrical nerve stimulation, or nerve blocks may be used. Surgical revision may be necessary to excise the neuroma and place the residual nerve in a more protected location. Adherent scars and bone spurs may be tender. Socket modifications or surgical revision by plastic or orthopedic surgery may be required. Skin and bone pain, as well as ischemic pain, may occur.

Some pain felt within or outside the stump is referred from a proximal organ. A patient who has a herniated intervertebral disc feels pain in the lateral side of the calf and in the toes, even though some of those parts may have been removed. Pain may be perceived in stump or limb areas innervated by the same spinal root where other irritated nerve fibers originated (perhaps in an internal organ).

Pain from pelvic congestion may be referred to the leg, stump, or phantom leg. Pain in the hip joint, caused by arthritis in the hip or merely biomechanical problems, may be referred down the leg. The etiology of the referred pain must be determined by investigation. This is not phantom pain. The problem is treated as though the patient were not an amputee.

Biomechanical pain in joints, muscles, tendon, and ligaments away from the amputated limb must also be considered. This pain is due to biomechanical abnormalities that develop from walking with a prosthesis. The abnormal gait should be evaluated to see whether it is due to a problem in the patient, in the prosthesis, or in the training. Improving prosthetic alignment and beginning an exercise program may clarify the problem and help to determine the proper treatment. Careful examination by a physician skilled in both prosthetic use and back and biomechanical pain problems is necessary to identify and correct the problem.

Phantom pain

Phantom pain must be distinguished from phantom sensation, stump pain, and referred pain. If the sensation of the absent limb is painful and disagreeable, with strong paresthesias, it is referred to as phantom pain. Phantom sensation seems normal; phantom pain is not. Phantom pain is more commonly associated with parts that have been crushed and those in which ablation has been delayed than with those removed promptly for nonpainful conditions. Phantom pain may be constant or intermittent and may be of any degree of severity.

One third to one half of amputees complain of phantom pain at some time. It is severe early in 5% to 10% of patients who undergo amputation. At that stage it is hard to determine whether the pain is stump pain referred distally or is phantom pain. Phantom pain is variously described as cramping, crushing, burning, or shooting and may be continuous or intermittent, frequently waxing and waning in cycles of several minutes' duration. It is localized in the phantom, not the stump. It is often perceived as a painful twisting or distortion of the part, as for example a clenching of the fist with the fingernails digging into the palm. Phantom pain remains severe in less than 1% of amputees, but in those it may be destructive of the entire personality.

Phantom pain may be precipitated or intensified by any contact, not necessarily painful, with the stump or with a trigger area on the trunk, contralateral limb, or head. A neuroma may occasionally be tender in the stump, but 80% of patients with phantom pain have no detectable abnormality of the stump. Phantom pain may also be triggered by urination, defecation, sexual intercourse, angina pectoris, or cigarette smoking.

Phantom pain has often been associated with emotional disturbance, but it has been difficult to determine whether the emotional disturbance preceded or resulted from the phantom pain. Some studies indicate that after amputation the incidence of neuroses is no greater among patients with phantom pain than among those without such pain. Amputations necessitated by war wounds or other trauma are less likely to be followed by phantom pain than amputations for other reasons, even though the emotional trauma understandably might be greater in the former group.

Nevertheless, psychogenic factors may be suspected in patients who experience phantom pain immediately after amputation, who complain bitterly about their physical disfigurement, or who have excessive difficulty learning to use or who refuse to use their prostheses. Reports of phantom pain from patients who are chronically maladjusted at home and in society or who complain of increased pain after discussion of disturbing events, contact with other patients who have had amputations, or an interview with a staff member concerning some significant conflict or interpersonal relationship are also suspect. In these patients the phantom pain may represent an emotional response to the loss of the limb, which may be helped by skillful psychiatric management.

Despite considerable research the cause of phantom pain remains elusive. The most likely explanation, consistent with recent understanding and theories of pain and of the structure and function of the central nervous system, relates phantom pain to the loss of inhibitory influences normally initiated through the afferent impulses from the limb and their associated central connections. The spinothalamic tract was thought to be the principal pathway to the sensory cortex for the afferent impulses from the limbs. However, recent information suggests that the multisynaptic afferent system (MAS) carries much more afferent information through the spinal cord to the brain than the oligosynaptic spinothalamic tract. The bilateral MAS crosses and recrosses the midline, eventually ending in the reticular formation of the brainstem.

Melzack proposed a model to explain phantom limb pain consistent with these considerations and the gate control theory of pain. He believed that a portion of the brainstem reticular formation acts as a "central biasing mechanism" by exerting a tonic inhibitory influence, or bias, on transmission at all synaptic levels of the somatic projection system. When a large proportion of sensory fibers is destroyed by amputation of a limb, thereby decreasing the amount of input into the reticular formation, the inhibitory influence decreases. This results in self-sustaining activity at all neural levels that can be triggered repeatedly by the remaining fibers. Pain occurs when the output of the self-sustaining neuron pools reaches or exceeds a critical level. This model helps to explain not only the failure of surgical interruption in producing lasting relief of phantom pain, but also the frequent temporary success of therapeutic procedures that influence the central excitatory state of the nervous system at different levels.

Phantom pain can be more easily understood and treated if classified into different categories. In my experience four common types exist, with variants.

The most common type is a cramping sensation, pain similar to that of muscle spasm. The patient says that the fist or foot remains in an uncomfortable position and that it would be comfortable if it could just be moved. This pain seems to be relieved by simultaneous bilateral exercise of the phantom and of the contralateral normal limb. Occasionally, surging sinusoidal electrical stimulation of the stump assists voluntary exercise and relieves the pain. In addition, massage of the stump may help relieve the pain. Muscle relaxants and heat application are occasionally helpful. Percussion of the stump by the fingers or by a rubber mallet or mechanical vibrator may also be used to desensitize the part. Proponents of the osteomyoplastic amputation insist that cramping phantom pain is much less common after that surgical method than after other procedures.

The second type of phantom pain is an electric shock–like discomfort in the phantom limb that lasts for a few seconds and then disappears. It is lancinating and episodic, superimposed upon either painless sensations or some other type of phantom pain. It appears to be a neuritic pain. If the pain is due to the pressure of a poorly fitting prosthesis, in which case correcting the fit or alignment will relieve it, it is not phantom pain. If injection of the neuroma with a steroid is helpful, again it is stump pain and not phantom pain. Desensitization by "therapeutic abuse" and prosthesis use are both helpful in true phantom pain. The application of cold with ice packs or by ethyl chloride spray decreases the central excitatory state of the pathways in the spinal cord. Ultrasound over the nerve trunk may offer some relief from this type of phantom pain. Since the pain lasts a short time, narcotics should not be used. Systemic analgesics are pointless for a pain that lasts only a few seconds and comes intermittently. Most patients can ignore it.

The third and most severe type of phantom pain is a burning, agonizing discomfort throughout the stump and the phantom limb. The stump generally feels hot but may feel cold. It may look normal, red, or cyanotic. It is exquisitely tender. Clothing or a gust of air touching the stump can trigger the pain. The patient often wraps the stump in protective clothes or towels to avoid irritation. The pain often occurs after crushing or stretching trauma to the nerves. This is the same type of pain described by patients with causalgia.

Conservative treatments as for causalgia are indicated. Early temporary blockade of the autonomic nervous system by injection is desirable. Other treatments include anticholinergic and nonnarcotic analgesics, TENS, acupuncture, electrical stimulation, and the physical measures for desensitization. This pain is ameliorated by measures that increase the central excitatory state in the central nervous system. Such measures are rubbing, tapping, heating, or cooling the stump or spraying with ethyl chloride spray. Gradually increasing prosthetic use may be helpful. Sympathectomy may be effective. Because the condition may become increasingly severe, it has been treated with drastic surgical procedures such as rhizotomy and even prefrontal lobotomy, the value of which is doubtful. Since most surgical methods of treatment are unsuccessful, they should be used only when suicide is anticipated.

The fourth type of phantom pain is a squeezing, wrenching, "hot poker" sensation, not as easily classified as the other three. All of the measures used in the other three types of phantom pain should be tried for relief.

Management of a patient with phantom pain

Treatment for phantom pain should proceed from simple noninvasive to more complex or invasive measures and be based on general principles of good management. One should not consider destructive surgical procedures until simpler methods have failed to provide lasting relief. The following points summarize a practical program of management:

1. The patient should be prepared before surgery by being told that phantom sensation is normal after amputation.
2. After the surgery the stump should be examined regularly, with checks of its appearance and function. The words "stump" and "residual limb" should be used in conversation to get the patient used to both terms.
3. Postoperative care is as important as surgical technique in healing of the incision. Any evidence of infection should be treated vigorously.
4. When the wound is sufficiently healed, the therapist should instruct the patient in massaging the stump with an emollient lotion and afterward applying tincture of benzoin to toughen the skin. The patient may also be instructed in gentle pounding or slapping of the stump and in use of a mechanical vibrator, taking care not to traumatize the scar.
5. The patient should exercise the stump muscles

through imaginary movement of the phantom limb (for example, peddling an imaginary bicycle using the stump and good leg in reciprocal fashion or rowing an imaginary boat using the stump and good arm simultaneously).

6. Both a functional and a cosmetic prosthesis should be provided as soon as possible, since this can often prevent or relieve phantom pain. Immediate postoperative fitting of a temporary prosthesis is used to reduce the incidence of phantom pain.

7. A number of measures may be tried to relieve phantom pain: ethyl chloride spray, local procaine injection of sensitive areas in the stump, procaine peripheral nerve or dorsal nerve root blocks (which although providing only temporary anesthesia can be followed by long-lasting relief), ultrasound, and hypertonic saline injection to interspinous ligaments. If temporary nerve blocks prove effective, phenol blocks are indicated.

8. Many neurosurgical procedures have been advocated, but none give permanent relief. Probably the best results reported have been with anterolateral cordotomy. A new development is electrostimulation of the dorsal column in the spinal cord by subdural implanted electrodes activated by a radiofrequency receiver-stimulator buried in the subcutaneous tissues of the chest wall. The long-term value is still debated. Frustratingly, pain recurs after section of peripheral nerves or dorsal nerve roots and even after amputation of the limb at a higher level. Neurosurgical procedures on the spinal cord may provide initial relief but often are followed by late recurrence of phantom pain, even after bilateral high thoracic or cervical cordotomies. Surgical ablation of the cerebral somatosensory cortex and injury to this area of the brain have been observed to abolish both phantom pain and phantom sensation.

9. Psychiatric treatment may be necessary in some cases. Hypnosis, distraction conditioning, imagery, and psychotherapy have been used.

10. When any procedure results in relief of phantom pain, the patient should resume handling and normal movement of the stump, prescribed exercises, massage, and use of the prosthesis to decrease the likelihood of recurrence of phantom pain.

Edema

Stump edema immediately after amputation is usual. It may be controlled by elastic bandaging, a plaster cast, air bags, or other means. During prosthesis wear, stump edema usually means that there is proximal constriction of the stump and space for the stump to expand below the prosthetic brim. Constriction blocks the return of venous and lymphatic fluids, causing distal swelling. This usually is due to the patient's stump sinking into the prosthesis. The amputee can increase the number of stump socks worn to compensate for stump shrinkage. The atrophy is not uniform, so venous return is compromised. Edema may be caused by excessive suction or lack of total contact between socket and stump, cardiac or renal failure, or use of chemotherapeutic agents for malignancy. A patient's weight gain may have a similar effect.

The socket must be modified to fit the stump properly. Total contact should be ensured to prevent edema. The edema may proceed to ulceration if not corrected early, but usually it causes an indurated, red mass that progresses to chronic eczema and a fungoid lesion. A well-fitted total contact socket is the cure.

Ulceration

Prostheses invariably interfere with the normal functions of the skin. They may cause skin ulceration through maceration, excessive pressure over a prolonged period, friction and shear forces, and stress concentration. A pressure sore heals if the cause for it is removed. When it is caused by a prosthesis, modification of the device is necessary to avoid points of excessive pressure. Additional surgery on the stump, such as removal of a sharp bony ridge or spicule, is only rarely necessary. Topical application of a bland cream (vitamin A and D ointment, for example) to the pressure area promotes healing once the cause is gone. In the case of an open, draining skin lesion, the limb should not be worn until healing has taken place. In rare instances a "bypass" device will be necessary, for example, an above-knee socket for a below-knee stump when it is decided that the patient cannot wear a below-knee socket for the time being.

Wearing a thin nylon or porous polyamide sheath under the stump sock reduces friction. If a friction lesion persists, either the prosthesis must be redesigned to improve its suspension or a slip socket or gel socket is required. In the gel socket there is a double-layered flexible liner with a gel-like substance encased between the layers. The inner liner fits snugly on the stump.

Skin normally moves freely over the underlying tissue. When it is adherent to underlying bone in a stump, stress concentration occurs with stretching and weakening of the skin and frequently with deposition of hemosiderin at the juncture between flexible and adherent skin. The total contact socket helps reduce stress concentration on a delicate stump by distributing weight bearing evenly over the entire skin of the stump. Pulling the stump into the socket rather than pushing it in also helps. Friction massage helps loosen the skin attachment. If ulceration recurs, friction-reducing measures are indicated.

Ulceration of the skin of the stump may be due to chronic edema, excessive pressure, or shear, especially to insensate or partial-thickness graft or adherent skin. The prosthesis should not be used while an open ulceration exists.

Contractures

Joint contractures usually occur before or immediately after an amputation. Fibroblasts function continuously. For this reason every limb requires a full joint range of motion at least four times a day. Even in the presence of pain and severe injury, most limbs can be moved passively with care. Not only involved joints but also uninvolved joints must be moved for prevention of contractures, which is easier than treatment. Hip contractures are generally in flexion and abduction, and knee contractures are usually in flexion. It is extremely difficult to walk with one or both of these contractures. The patient's ability to walk is markedly diminished if they are allowed to develop and are not corrected.

For correction, serial casting, progressive passive or dynamic splinting, proprioceptive neuromuscular facilitation-inhibition of antagonist stretching, and traction are useful. Surgery is a last resort.

Infections

Careful daily cleansing of the residual limb, prosthetic sock, and socket generally prevents infection of the stump unless ulceration occurs. Open stump infections require antibiotic treatment, and closed ones must be opened along with associated antibiotic treatment.

Accumulation of moisture promotes maceration, which predisposes to infection. Skin maceration can be minimized by using porous materials and perforated construction for artificial limbs and braces and by selecting stump socks made of absorbent natural (rather than synthetic) fibers. Sweating can be diminished through use of antiperspirants or by iontophoresis with very dilute copper sulfate or formalin solutions.

The occlusion of hair follicles and sweat glands can cause folliculitis, boils, abscesses, and sebaceous cysts.

Bony overgrowth

The most common type of bony overgrowth is associated with production of bone spurs from remnants of periosteum left in the stump at surgery. Generally socket modifications can compensate for the bone and reduce its irritation. On occasion a pull-in type of socket rather than a push-in type is needed. Surgical removal of the spur and periosteum is sometimes required. Xeroradiography of weight-bearing stance and non-weight-bearing swing with the prosthesis shows the relationship of the spur to the socket and skin and exactly how "total contact" the socket really is.

After an amputation through a long bone in a patient who has not reached bony maturity, endosteal and periosteal growth of bone increases the bone length while the skin does not grow as much. The bone end becomes pointed and pushes through the skin. When feasible, skin traction is the preferred treatment to prevent stump shortening. If surgery is required, the technique of Marquardt in which the spur is removed and replaced by a fragment of cartilage or epiphysis is best. This obviates the need for repeated surgery to shorten the bone.

Scoliosis

In patients who have unequal leg lengths, either anatomically or functionally, scoliosis may occur. Usually this is a functional scoliosis that can be corrected by attention to leg length discrepancies. The scoliosis may become fixed if attention is not paid to this possible complication. Trunk exercises, especially for range of motion, are advised for a growing child. Although some say that absence of one arm without the weight replacement of a prosthesis may cause scoliosis, this has never been proved.

Other complications and associated problems

Any artificial limb has an unstable attachment to the skeletal system. The soft tissues between the bone and the socket lead inevitably to socket instability. Any artificial limb feels heavier than the limb it replaces.

Patients with peripheral vascular disease, with or without diabetes, have vascular disease in the arteries of both legs, the heart, the brain, and the eyes. Thus these amputees may have cardiac, cerebral, mental, and visual problems in addition to their amputations. Patients may also have pulmonary or cardiac disease incidental to their amputations. Degenerative or inflammatory arthritis limits a patient's ability to use a prosthesis. Malignant tumors may be both the cause and a complication of amputation.

VOCATIONAL ASPECTS

Prospective employees have only two things to sell: the work of their minds and the work of their bodies. After amputation the work of the mind is not impaired. For a lower extremity amputee, varying amounts of difficulty are manifest, depending on the level of amputation and the adequacy of prosthetic fit, as well as the person's general physical condition. Any vocation requiring prolonged standing or walking, carrying of heavy loads, and running presents some difficulty. A lower extremity amputee can perform any type of physical work with the exception of those requiring fine balance. Thus construction work at high altitudes is contraindicated, even if just part of the foot is missing, since the fine balance adjustments necessary for high-altitude work require intact neuromuscular and skeletal systems. With higher levels of amputation, such as the Syme and the below knee, heavy work can frequently be performed provided the prosthesis is adequate for the patient's need.

With above-knee amputations, the ability to walk for long distances and to carry weights is diminished. Sedentary jobs are always possible for such patients. In bilateral lower extremity amputations the problems are much more than merely additive.

A unilateral upper limb amputee must be considered as being one handed. The amputated side should be thought of as an assistive extremity whose ability depends on the form and level of amputation. A partial hand amputee with some pinch is almost as able vocationally as if both upper limbs were normal. With higher levels of amputation, all fine function is performed with the remaining upper extremity and the prosthesis is used to hold and stabilize objects.

In bilateral upper limb amputees the loss of function increases rapidly with each higher level of amputation. Bilateral above-elbow amputees have an enormous problem vocationally. Work that is primarily intellectual is not made impossible by such an amputation. For amputations at a still higher level, the only effective devices are externally powered and can perform only light work. Work requiring rapid opening and closing, as well as pronation and supination, is very difficult for an upper limb amputee. The only test of work is the job itself or a suitable substitute example; vocational evaluation should use the job sample technique.

Unilateral arm amputees find little difficulty in doing most clerical tasks. Writing can be done by the remaining arm. The prosthesis acts mainly as a paperweight. The hook or hand may be used to carry a briefcase. The stump or prosthesis may be used to carry objects in the flexed elbow or the axilla. If there is one normal hand, the patient should learn to type with it alone, since this permits faster typing than with one good hand and one artificial device. For use of the telephone, the terminal device can usually hold the phone while the other hand is used for note taking.

In a bilateral arm amputee who must write with a hook, rubber tubing may be slipped over the stationary finger of the hook to increase friction on the writing implement, which is laced behind the thumb for stability. The rubber helps to turn pages, open jars, and so forth. The paper must be stabilized by the weight of the prosthesis or held in a clipboard. The use of shoulder telephone rests found in many business offices frees both prostheses. Typing may be done directly with the fingers of the hook or with the eraser end of a pencil held in the artificial hand. Bilateral amputees prefer electric typewriters. A prosthetic hand with cosmetic glove should not be used for typing, since it is almost impossible to remove carbon paper pigment from the glove. Bilateral amputees find it convenient to use dictating machines and other work-saving devices in the office.

Most amputees who were doing manual work before the limb loss change to sedentary or managerial work. Others retire. Only a few continue to do manual work, and most of those need many job modifications.

The role of the vocational counselor is to identify the medical, psychologic, and social needs of the client as related to work. Among the valuable tools available to the counselor are interest and aptitude testing, job restructuring, counseling, and client advocacy. The specific tasks performed by the client in the previous job must be thoroughly analyzed to determine the extent to which the disability reflects a real vocational impediment.

Some characteristics that can be considered prognostic for successful rehabilitation in disabled persons are the following: male; under 45 years of age; high educational level; engaged in skilled, sales, clerical, or professional occupation before being disabled; married, with children; acceptance of disability and "realistic" ambitions; employed full time with satisfactory work record before disability; mild or moderate disability; high degree of functional performance; no other health problems; and free of psychiatric symptoms.

In the United States in 1962 there were more than 400,000 people who had had an amputation. In a recent national survey of 1654 persons with amputations, males outnumbered females by 2.5:1. There were seven times as many males as females among those whose amputation was necessitated by trauma. There was no significant difference in incidence between right and left side amputation in either upper or lower extremities for either sex. In the age group of greatest interest to vocational rehabilitation counselors (from 21 to 50 years old), in 59% the cause of amputation was trauma; this group comprised 23% of all individuals with amputations in the survey and 80.5% of all those with traumatic amputation.

Many individuals between 21 and 50 years of age who undergo amputation because of trauma probably have a number of characteristics prognostic for success in rehabilitation. Although they must make many adjustments as a result of their disability, including acceptance of changed body image, their previous physical and psychologic health provides an excellent basis for rehabilitation. In addition, it is fairly easy for persons in this age range to return to their previous work if this is not precluded by the amputation. Employers are more likely to rehire good former employees who have become disabled than to take a chance with an unproved individual.

Less fortunate are adults with missing limbs since childhood, whether from congenital limb deficiency, trauma, or disease. Research with children from 5 to 12 years of age showed that they considered classmates with amputations as "least-liked, not good-looking, the least fun to play with, and the saddest children in the class." These individuals probably have difficulty developing a positive self-image and are unable to participate fully in normal childhood activities. Some, with counseling and strong parental support, may overcome the prejudice they encounter, but for others the disability becomes the primary focus of their lives. This latter group can present almost unsurmountable problems to the vocational counselor and to the rehabilitation team as a whole. For them, careful psychologic testing and counseling, as well as development of vocational skills and attitudes, are imperative.

Ease of reemployment is strongly influenced by the type of work formerly done. The duties of the professional, managerial, and executive group depend primarily on intellect and personality (ability to think, speak, write, persuade, or make decisions), whereas those in the unskilled group depend primarily on manual resources (carry, push, pull, walk, stack, or load).

When professionals, managers, or executives suffer an amputation, there are probably few significant threats based on economic considerations. However, those who earn their livelihood primarily by the performance of physical activities involving the use of arms and legs and who do not have intellectual and personal resources for training in other fields suffer a severe economic handicap as a result of amputation. They are no longer able to compete with their full-bodied peers. The cosmetic losses of amputation may be a vocational handicap irrespective of the functional loss. An artificial arm is often a detriment to a person who must meet the public. A limp is a handicap in a job interview, even for a job not requiring ambulation.

The unskilled group particularly needs vocational evaluation, supportive vocational guidance, job retraining, further education where indicated, and job-seeking skills. The job market often precludes employment despite the best efforts of vocational counselors. Employers choosing between potential candidates choose the nondisabled person except where the characteristics of the amputee are clearly superior.

An amputee who receives good medical care and follow-up monitoring, has a healthy stump and is trained in how to use a properly fitted prosthesis, and has access to vocational and psychologic counseling should be independent in daily activities and be able to handle a wide variety of jobs, presupposing good general health.

Of individuals under 50 years of age who have had a single extremity amputated, 75% should be able to return to their former occupations. Even in extreme types of amputation, such as hemicorporectomy, in which the lower half of the body is surgically removed above the bony pelvis, successful vocational rehabilitation is possible. Although vehicle operations would intuitively seem to be a poor vocational choice for persons with amputations, one study found no evidence that those who passed regular driver's license tests had any greater frequency of accidents than unimpaired persons in operating highway transport equipment. Using vehicle simulators, they found that with appropriate power assists, unilateral amputation should not impair driving performance.

It is easier to change a prosthesis than a person's job. After training with a prosthesis, an amputee should be tried on a simulated job in his or her previous occupation to determine whether a return to the former work with or without modifications is possible. An amputee who has spent a long time doing one type of work finds it difficult to switch to an entirely different field. The economic and emotional impact of having worked oneself up from the ranks to a position of some experience or authority, and then starting over as a beginner in a new trade, is immense. When a job change is unavoidable, it should be done only after a job sample evaluation.

JUVENILE AMPUTEES

Amputation in children is usually congenital or traumatic but may be due to malignant disease. The major difference in treatment from that of adult amputees is the growth factor. Growth occurs not only in size, but also in intellectual capacity and neuromusculoskeletal maturation. Emotional problems are found in congenital amputees if feelings of guilt and inadequacy of the parents are transmitted to the youngster. The child is usually unconcerned with appearance until the age of social consciousness, starting school, and puberty, but parents are frequently very concerned with appearance.

In most aspects of growth and development, a limb-deficient child is similar to normal children. At first the child with congenital amputation does not miss the absent limb. The lack of an arm becomes bothersome at 3 to 4 months of age, and the problem increases when the child begins to sit, sometime between the ages of 6 and 9 months. If a mechanical replacement for the missing part is not available at 4 months of age, the child develops ingenious substitution patterns that are difficult to break. The artificial limb inhibits sensory exploration with the stump but permits two-handed activities. A prosthesis should be used only part time so sensory exploration is not precluded.

Between the ages of 9 and 15 months the child usually begins to stand. A child with a congenital lower limb deficiency uses the stump and the normal lower limb, if there is one, for pulling up and standing. If before the age of 9 months, an artificial limb of adequate length and stability is provided, the child starts to walk with it. At no subsequent age does either an upper or lower limb amputee learn to use a device as well.

The child's personality is developed to a greater degree during the first year than at any time thereafter. For this reason the parents should be given informed help so they will accept the limb-deficient child as an integral part of the family and so a relationship will develop between the patient, the family, and the clinic team. Prostheses need frequent adjustments in the first year or two. The second major growth spurt occurs between the ages of 11 and 13 years in girls and 13 and 14 years in boys. During periods of rapid growth, frequent visits to the clinic are necessary to adjust the length and form of prostheses.

Evaluation and prescription

Evaluation of a juvenile amputee is even more difficult than that of an adult. Since the child has difficulty in communication, rapport may be more difficult to establish. Whereas an adult can frequently be evaluated in one session, the young amputee commonly requires many sessions to develop the relaxation and cooperation needed for a determination of ranges of motion, muscle tone, and strength. While congenital amputees frequently have coexisting anomalies, other abnormalities may be attributed to the limb absence itself. A congenital scoliosis may develop in an otherwise normal child, but it is far more common in patients with unilateral limb anomalies or deficiencies. In the absence of a lower limb, if the growth of the normal limb is not compensated for by frequent prosthetic adjustments, a compensatory scoliosis may develop and become permanent.

Flexion contractures following traumatic amputation are almost unknown in young amputees, but in a congenitally limb-deficient child there is a relatively high incidence of joint contractures and deformed limbs that need correction by casting, stretching, or dynamic splinting. Slow, steady stretching should be aided by manual stretching on an intermittent basis.

Surgical correction of anomalous limbs is beyond the scope of this chapter. If surgical correction can give a prehensile function to a sensate stump, it should be done. Surgical ablation should be deferred if possible, since the amputated extremity tends to grow at a slower rate than the congenitally deformed limb would have done. Thus a long above-knee amputation in a young child, performed for deformity at the knee, becomes a short above-knee stump by the time of skeletal maturity. The longer the amputation can be deferred, the better the physical end result in many instances. To avoid early amputation of the lower limb, special ischial weight-bearing prostheses may be constructed even for patients with an abnormal femur, tibia, and foot. Some cases of femoral abnormality with a telescoping false joint may be treated with full or partial end bearing in the prosthesis. Ablation of the foot early in focal deficiency of the proximal femur may be advisable to fit a more cosmetic limb for the future. Tibial hemimelia is another frequent indication for early amputation.

Overgrowth of the bone of the stump, primarily of the humerus and tibia, with lack of compensatory lengthening of the skin and subcutaneous tissues, is common in juvenile amputees and may require surgical intervention. Conservative treatment by traction at night and in the prosthesis is advised. Marquardt uses epiphysis or cartilage implanted at the bone end to correct the problem, with much success.

The removal of abnormal digits in the lower limb is of little significance. The removal of terminal skin tabs is advisable if they interfere with prosthetic fit. In the upper limb the early removal of any digit that contains bone is usually not advisable; prosthetic adjustments are preferable. If the patient has a useless small nubbin that does not contain bone, removal may be helpful. In a young child, small digits with bone may seem nonfunctional, but later function may be induced. This is of considerable importance in high amputations, since the slightest function of a digit in an upper limb may be an important control source for externally powered devices.

The prosthetic need is the key to the prescription. Some patients with upper limb amputations function better without artificial devices. This is especially true if phocomelic hands can reach the mouth. Children would rather use any part of their body with sensation than a prosthesis. Thus, in the patient who is severely disabled by bilateral upper extremity absence, training with the feet is important.

The principles of preprosthetic care are the same as those for adults. Active involvement in childhood activities should be encouraged. Bilateral prehension is needed for many activities and should be encouraged using prostheses, the feet, and other parts of the body. Games and sports, especially swimming, should be urged. It is possible and desirable for patients with bilateral upper limb amelia to learn to swim. Active exercises prevent contractures. Positioning to prevent contractures is of less benefit in an active child than in an adult.

Prostheses and components

Most prosthetic devices have been designed for adult war casualties. Children's prostheses are often small models of adult prostheses and are usually far from optimal. They do not take into account the immature neuromusculoskeletal system of the child with its limited sources of power for transfer, the limited ability to learn control techniques, or the growth of the child, which requires frequent prosthetic changes and annual replacements. In an adult, shrinkage of the stump requires frequent changes in the socket, but in a child, although there is considerable loss of subcutaneous fat from pressure of the socket, most of this loss is replaced by muscular bulk increase. The proportionally greater amount of soft tissue around the bone and the stump predisposes to instability. Harnessing is also more difficult because of the soft tissue. Growth may necessitate checks every 1 to 3 months to ensure that the socket and harnessing still fit.

Adolescent lower limb amputees may be fitted with adult-type conventional prostheses. A below-knee amputee may be fitted with a standard or modified patellar tendon–bearing prosthesis with suprapatellar cuff suspension and SACH foot. The SACH foot has been a boon to children's prosthetics. The energy-storing feet are still better. The use of a thigh corset is advised for young children with below-knee amputations, since many have genu recurvatum after prolonged use of a cuff suspension.

For an above-knee amputee, conventional prostheses can be used. Suspension is usually by Silesian bandage. Although true suction suspension is rarely possible before 7 years of age because of rapid changes in size, ancillary suction may make prosthetic use more effective. Children quickly learn to use lower limb prostheses. For patients with deformed lower limbs, the foot may be able to take some weight bearing even with a false joint proximally. Gluteal weight bearing is often a great assist. True ischial weight bearing is difficult for a young child because of baby fat, but it should be attempted. Patients with very short lower limbs or absence of both lower limbs can be taught to walk in bucket sockets with short, stubby legs, without knee joints. These can be lengthened as the child grows, changing to the Canadian-type hip disarticulation design and modifications thereof. Unilateral hip disarticulation amputees are managed the same as adults. The younger the child when fitted, the better the result.

An upper limb amputee should be fitted with passive prostheses as early as possible, preferably before the age of 6 months. The reasons for early fitting are to stimulate bilateral function, help the child and parents accept the prosthesis for function or cosmesis, incorporate the prosthesis into the child's body image, improve balance, get the child used to normal length of the limb, prevent scoliosis and other skeletal abnormalities caused by asymmetry, make the child aware of prehensile function, and promote eye-hand control.

The passive mitt, which was supposed to provide better appearance, has been abandoned. For some parents who cannot tolerate anything but a hand-shaped device, a cosmetic hand may be a psychologic necessity. They are not safer than hooks, nor is the abandoned wafer hook. At the age of 8 months the patient may be fitted with a passive artificial arm whose terminal device is usually a Dorrance 12P steel Plastisol-covered hook. At this age the cables are usually omitted. The parent operates the hook to allow the child to observe prehension by the hook. The object to be held is placed in the hook for manipulation by the child. The child eventually pulls objects from the hook.

Depending on the child's intellectual and neuromusculoskeletal maturity, at 18 to 24 months of age the terminal device is connected to a cable and harness. This is operated by humeral flexion on the amputated side by both a below-elbow and an above-elbow amputee and permits the child to perform more complex bimanual activities than merely grasping in the pat-a-cake manner. Later the child drops a held object when the hook opens accidentally and then learns to open the hook to let go of the object. Eventually the child opens the hook to put things in.

At approximately 4 years of age the child is provided with a larger hook to match his or her longitudinal growth. The 10P hook is similar in design to the canted 12P hook. The hooks used later are of aluminum without plastic covering, beginning first with the 10X hook, then the 99X, and finally the 88X. These are durable hooks and provide more secure grasp and finger manipulation because of the neoprene lining. Hooks are provided for all children because they are functional. Hands to be worn in public may be provided to please the parents.

Prosthetic hands for children are voluntary opening and are supplied more to satisfy parents who are looking for cosmesis than because of the function of which they are also capable. A small number of children's hands of different weights, sizes, and mechanisms are available. The smallest APRL hand (No. 1) fits a child of about 6 to 7 years of age. For a large child it may be used 1 or 2 years earlier, but a small child may not use it until later. Unfortunately, a size intermediate between the No. 1 and the adult hand is not available. The APRL child's hand operates so that the second and third digits move in opposition to the thumb. As in the adult hand, the thumb can be positioned in two ranges of flexion to permit grasping of small and large objects. The hand is voluntary opening, in contrast to the adult APRL hand, and tends to cut the cosmetic glove at the finger joints.

The excellent child's hands made by the Dorrance Company come in sizes 1 to 4. They are easy to operate, relatively lightweight, functional, and fairly good looking. Unfortunately, the smallest (No. 1) cannot be used by a normal-sized child until about 7 years of age.

The Robin-Aids hand provides flexion of the four digits at the metacarpophalangeal joints against an immovable thumb. Although it is not always suitable, it is the only hand useful for a transmetacarpal or partial-hand amputee. For such an amputee, an opposition post, a device against which the remaining digits or palm can oppose, may be useful.

Smaller hands are now available from England and Scandinavia but are used mainly with myoelectric prostheses. Myoelectric prostheses for children are fairly attractive but prohibitively expensive for most unsubsidized patients. The gloves are fragile, and replacement is costly for active children. Most parents prefer them to hooks, but children who have a hook first usually would rather keep it. Parental pressure generally determines what the child will wear. Most myoelectric limbs are for below-elbow amputees, who usually have enough strength to use the conventional body-powered limb well.

Standard socket designs are used for children and usually fit poorly because of the large amount of soft tissue in a child. In addition to standard sockets for below-elbow amputees, a "preflexed" socket set in an initial degree of flexion has been developed to help get the hook to the mouth. A bent banana-shaped forearm also helps getting to the mouth and groin. The Muenster device fits snugly above the epicondyles. It prevents full extension and flexion and affords excellent stability, especially for amputees with very short stumps. In a bilateral amputee with a limited range of motion, a split socket may be necessary so the terminal device can be brought to the mouth. Like adults with bilateral upper extremity amputations, children need wrist flexion units; since these increase the length of the forearm, smaller hooks or a shorter forearm must be used.

Suspension may be the figure-of-8 harness, usually with the Northwestern ring-type cross. In the presence of baby fat the chest strap design occasionally proves more useful. The shoulder saddle is usually of the web type rather than leather.

Children with amputation above the axilla obtain little function from conventional prostheses. Our experience with conventional prostheses at the shoulder disarticulation and forequarter levels has convinced us that unilateral amputees do not use externally powered devices effectively because they can use the normal upper limb and feet for manipulation. A bilateral shoulder disarticulation amputee must have externally powered devices to function well, although minimal function is obtainable with conventional prostheses. Foot use is required for all bilateral upper extremity amputees.

The training of a juvenile amputee is done with games in both physical and occupational therapy. Since children have difficulty doing rote exercise, attempts to teach a child how to use the controls of a prosthesis are unrewarding. When the child wants to play, we assist him or her in using the limb to perform the desired activity. A child who learns how the prosthesis can help in function is willing to learn to use it. Thus, for the child, training for use precedes controls training.

To ensure proper fit of the first prosthesis and give some initial intensive training, when a child receives the first active device, he or she may be admitted as an inpatient for a few weeks, after which the training is continued on an outpatient basis. A better method is to have the parents stay in a motel or trailer with the child, who spends all day in the training center as an outpatient. If prostheses are applied early and properly, the child incorporates the prosthesis into his or her self-image.

A check of the prosthesis fit is necessary every 3 months, and monthly during periods of rapid growth. Children are hard on prostheses; they may use them improperly, for example, as destructive tools. Parents must be told to prevent such activities, just as they would prevent the child from breaking fine china.

SUMMARY

I have said that the prosthesis is merely a tool to help the patient accomplish goals in life. This concept is crucial to understanding the place of the prosthesis. It is a means of returning the patient to society and its activities: walking, driving a car, working, and playing. It is merely a part of the therapeutic armamentarium. One artificial limb may not suffice; patients get legs for special purposes such as work or play in a wet environment or sports such as golf, mountain climbing, skiing, and swimming. The patient must be encouraged to participate socially and vocationally in the community. Rehabilitation must be an integral process from prevention of amputation through amputation surgery and postoperative care, provision of a prosthesis, and restoration of the person to an optimal place in the environment.

The patient as a whole must be considered in treatment. We treat the person, with his or her joys and sorrows, and not a stump.

All too often we put our faith in a prosthetic mechanism to solve the problems of the individual who has had a limb removed. It is the human-machine combination, working in harmony, that determines performance. Even that performance is but one aspect of the person's success or failure in meeting goals in life.

The patient's success is our reward.

SUGGESTED READINGS

American Association of Orthopaedic Surgeons: Atlas of limb prosthetics, St. Louis, 1981, The CV Mosby Co, pp 277-314.

Bowker, JH, and Thompson, RG: Management of musculoskeletal complications, In American Association of Orthopaedic Surgeons: Atlas of limb prosthetics, St. Louis, 1981, The CV Mosby Co.

Ducroquet, R, Ducroquet, J, and Ducroquet, P: Walking and limping—a study of normal and pathological walking, Philadelphia, 1968, JB Lippincott Co.

Friedmann, LW: Rehabilitation of amputees. In Licht, S, editor: Rehabilitation and medicine, New Haven, Conn, 1968, E Licht, Publisher.

Friedmann, LW: Lower limb prosthetics, New York, 1975, New York University Post-Graduate Medical School.

Friedmann, LW: The psychological rehabilitation of the amputee, Springfield, Ill, 1978, Charles C Thomas, Publisher.

Friedmann, LW: The surgical rehabilitation of the amputee, Springfield, Ill, 1978, Charles C Thomas, Publisher.

Friedmann, LW: Amputation. In Stolov, WC, and Clowers, MR, editors: Handbook of severe disability, Washington, DC, 1981, US Department of Education, Rehabilitation Services Administration.

Gonzalez, EG, Corcoran, PJ, and Reyes, RL: Energy expenditure in below knee amputees: correlation with stump length, Arch Phys Med Rehabil 55:111, 1974.

Inman, VT, Ralston, J, and Rodd, F: Human walking, Baltimore, 1981, Williams & Wilkins Co.

Klopsteg, PE, and Wilson, PD: Human limbs and their substitutes, New York, 1968, Hafner Publishing Co.

Levy, SW, et al: Skin problems of the leg amputee, Arch Dermatol 85:65, 1962.

Murdoch, G, editor: Prosthetic and orthotic practice, London, 1970, Edward Arnold, Publishers.

Traugh, GH, Corcoran, PJ, and Reyes, RL: Energy expenditure of ambulation in patients with above knee amputations, Arch Phys Med Rehabil 56:67, 1975.

CHAPTER 42 | # Hand rehabilitation

ANN H. SCHUTT AND JOACHIM L. OPITZ

The goal of hand rehabilitation is to maximize the residual functional capacity of persons with injured, operated, or diseased hands or upper extremities. Hand rehabilitation is organized as a team effort. One member is the physician who evaluates the patient and prescribes and coordinates the physical, psychosocial, and vocational interventions of other health professionals. The physical measures are provided by specially trained physical therapists, occupational therapists, and orthotists. The emotional, social, and vocational needs of the patient are addressed by social workers, psychologists, vocational counselors, and, at times, qualified rehabilitation consultants of insurance companies. A well-coordinated team effort is essential for the efficient and effective rehabilitation of the person with acute or chronic upper extremity impairment.[63]

Hand therapy may be required for various reasons. Injuries to the hand or upper extremity include fractures, tendon injuries, crush injuries involving all tissues, amputations, or combinations of any of these. Patients with arthritis frequently require hand rehabilitation. Rehabilitation of the upper extremity is an essential component after procedures such as carpal tunnel release, replacement arthroplasties of the digital joints or wrist, tendon transfers or repairs, tumor excision, and reconstruction of congenital defects. Patients are often referred shortly after completion of the procedure and essential postsurgical care and while the patient's limb is in a cast. Therapy can and should be initiated at this stage.

Some other conditions that may require hand rehabilitation include the muscular dystrophies, primary myopathies, congenital deformities, and neuropathic lesions that involve the upper extremities (for example, traumatic brachial plexitis).

EVALUATION OF THE HAND

Many techniques are used to evaluate the functional status of the upper extremity and hand, but all require a precise knowledge of anatomy, kinesiology, and physiology of muscle, tendon, nerve, and joint functions. Measurements have to be well defined and precisely executed in a standardized fashion to ensure reproducibility by multiple evaluators.* A specially devised measurement tape and a volumeter are used to measure the circumference of digits and edema volume. In addition to standard tools, small rulers and small, specially adapted goniometers are used to measure the active and passive ranges of motion. The data must be recorded accurately. Special forms and graphs are available to facilitate perception of the patient's progress. Range of motion and grip strength should be reevaluated and measured at least weekly during the initial period of treatment. Reproducibility of measurements is usually more accurate for active range of motion than for passive range of motion.

Specific techniques are used to measure range of motion for digital flexion and extension lags, thumb flexion, extension reposition, abduction and opposition, and wrist flexion and extension.† Strength can be measured with a dynamometer for opposition pinch (tip pinch), apposition pinch (lateral pinch), and grip. Sensation is tested for touch, moving touch, two-point discrimination, proprioception, temperature perception, and vibration.[8,9] Nylon filaments of various diameters, two-point calipers,[39] needles, tuning forks, vibrometers,[10,19] and test tubes of various temperatures are used to test the sensations of the hand and upper extremity.

There are many functional evaluations for activities of

---

*References 14, 15, 24, 27, 30, 40, 51.
†References 14, 15, 24, 25, 31, 40, 51.

daily living and homemaking.[26,29,44,54] Prevocational assessments have been standardized and are regularly used in occupational therapy departments and are applicable to hand rehabilitation.[6,29,30,40] Hand and upper extremity function tests and standards are available.[7,12,39] Work simulators with at least 20 different tool attachments have been developed and tested for vocational evaluation, treatment, and work hardening in the person with impaired function of the upper extremity.[7] Completeness and proficiency in evaluating hand function are essential for developing optimal treatment programs and for modifying and remodifying these programs. The effects of treatment are thereby observed and recorded during the initial and follow-up examinations.

GOALS OF THERAPY

Priorities of treatment goals need to be established because shotgun-type prescriptions usually overwhelm the patient and make the therapies inefficient. They frustrate the patient and the team alike.

The sequence of steps in a treatment program usually relates to the redevelopment of comfort, normal motor behavior, posture, and comfortable functional residual capacity of the hand or upper extremity. Once this goal has been accomplished, increasing the range of motion and redeveloping functional use of the extremity may be addressed using acceptable motor patterns. Once light functional activities are performed smoothly and consistently, more resistive engagements of the upper extremity may be pursued for strengthening purposes. The patient generally may resume work activities once the reconditioning allows for pain-free use with coordinated motor patterns.

The specific goals of hand therapy are prevention and decrease of edema; assistance in tissue healing; relief of pain; assistance in relaxation; prevention of misuse, disuse, and overuse of the muscle; desensitization of areas of hypersensitivity; and redevelopment of acceptable and conscious purposeful performance by reeducation of motor and sensory function. At the appropriate time, measures are taken to maintain and increase range of motion, improve independence and endurance in performing daily functional activities, increase strength, and protect the hand from deforming forces, thermal injuries, or other injuries to which the insensitive hand is particularly susceptible.

Certain complications of hand injuries can be prevented by early evaluation and treatment. These include edema, pain, loss of range of motion, loss of strength, adhesions, hypersensitivity, and misuse and disuse of the extremity. Overuse of the extremity during rehabilitation therapy may be harmful and counterproductive.

PREVENTION AND TREATMENT OF EDEMA

Edema is commonly present after injury or operation, and its prevention and treatment are essential to effective hand rehabilitation.

The effects of lasting edema, resulting from reduced venous and lymphatic dynamics, are often due to immobilization of the hand and loss of the muscle pump in moving the lymph from the hand.[5,6,16,22,46] After releasing a tourniquet used during operation, for example, the lymph channels, particularly on the dorsum of the hand, may be overwhelmed by the rapid return of circulation and by the results of secondary hyperemia.[48] If edema is allowed to persist and become chronic, it tends to cause fibrosis of the joints, muscles, moving planes, vessels, and nerves. Chronic edema also promotes infection. Elevation and early range of motion of the limb are effective preventive measures. Range of motion should be started in the joints that can be moved postoperatively or after trauma. Even small amounts of motion can be helpful. When the extremity is elevated with the elbow above the level of the shoulder and the hand above the level of the elbow, the circulation time is two-thirds less than when the elbow and arm are held at waist level.[57] The patient should be instructed to keep the hand elevated whenever possible.

Postoperatively, edema is prevented initially by bulky dressings to provide gentle, even compression while the hand and wrist are splinted.[56,57] The hand is usually splinted in the position of function, and the fingers are separated by layers of fluffy gauze. The exceptions to this position are when the hand is positioned in an intrinsic-plus position to protect intrinsic repairs or, in cases of tendon transfer, tendon repair, or nerve repair, when the hand is splinted in a position to protect the tendon or nerve from traction at the site of the anastomosis.[28] The extremity is elevated for at least 3 to 5 days postoperatively if edema is present.

Decongestant massage is helpful to treat edema.[34] The extremity is massaged from distal to proximal to facilitate movement of edema fluid proximally out of the fingers and hand. Elastic wraps such as Coban, dental rubber dam, or thick string placed around the fingers from distal to proximal can also temporarily help to decrease edema.[55] Ace wraps have also been helpful (Figure 42-1). These materials are inexpensive and effective for reducing edema. The wrap is applied slowly in immediately adjacent loops distally to proximally, and it is overlapped at each turn by one-half the width of the wrap. It is left in place for 5 to 15 minutes. The wraps can be applied several times a day.[63]

Active range-of-motion exercises are done during and after wrapping the hand to help reduce the swelling through the pumping action of active muscle contractions.[46-48,60] Elastic gloves (Aris-Isotoner Glove, Aris Gloves, Inc., New York) or elastic sleeves also can be used to control or reduce the swelling.[25,55]

Decongestant massage, as previously described, should be used before applying an elastic glove or garment. The glove has a built-in pressure gradient from high to low, progressing distally to proximally (Jobst Glove, Jobst Institute, Inc., Toledo). It helps to reinforce the fluid dynamics.[16,48,54,55] The glove should be worn during activities of daily living. The intermittent pneumatic compression pump

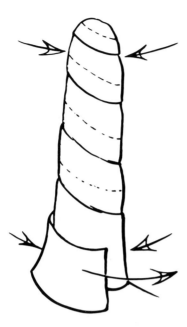

Figure 42-1. Elastic paper wrapping begins at tip of finger and wraps in spiral direction toward base of finger. Each turn is overlapped by one-half width of wrap. Pressure should be firm but not painful and should decrease as one wraps toward base of finger.

is useful in cases of edema caused by soft tissue injury, reflex sympathetic dystrophy if the extremity is not painful, dependent edema, and chronic edema, such as postmastectomy lymphedema. Use of an elastic garment, glove, sleeve, or Ace wrap after the pumping helps to maintain the reduction.[63]

The intermittent pneumatic compression device can be applied evenly by placing the patient's hand in a plastic bag of Styrofoam beads and inserting it into the pneumatic sleeve of the pump.[55,60] The sleeve is intermittently inflated to approximately 50 mm Hg and deflated as tolerated for 30 to 60 minutes at a time. Controlling edema is a vital element in accelerating tissue healing.

TISSUE HEALING

Tissue healing may be promoted by hydrotherapy, such as whirlpool or contrast baths. Contrast baths are relaxing and cleansing and tend not to produce edema as frequently as whirlpool treatments. The whirlpool can be used for removal of dried secretions and superficial necrotic debris and for cleansing of open wounds. A moderate temperature of 34° to 36° C helps to minimize the formation of edema. Because dependency of the extremity in the water may promote edema, the submerged hand should be elevated in the water. Active motion augments the fluid dynamics and helps to counteract the edema formation that is favored by the dependent position. Edema formation is also minimized if the duration of hydrotherapy is kept as short as possible.

Careful manual debridement in the water, with particular attention to blood vessels and nerve, may be a helpful adjunct to the healing process. Active motion during secondary wound healing is most important for optimal formation of scars, particularly in burns and postoperative hand infections and after release of Dupuytren's contracture.

PAIN MANAGEMENT

Pain is a common problem in hand rehabilitation. It can occur after injury, for a short time postoperatively, or in cases of neuropathy or arthritis. Pain can cause motor incoordination. Many types of therapy are used for the relief of pain. It is important not to increase edema by inappropriate use of heat.[65] Contrast baths can be performed in cycles of 10 minutes in warm water, 1 minute cold, 4 minutes warm, and 1 minute cold, for a total of approximately 30 minutes. The temperature of the water may be adjusted downward to prevent edema. The usual temperatures of contrast baths are 43.7° C for the warm water and 18.3° C for the cold. Occasionally the temperature of the contrast bath is modified to 40.6° C for the warm water and up to 21° C for the cold. These values are helpful. For example, edema occurs with a higher temperature, and Raynaud's phenomenon may be precipitated by a lower temperature of the cold water. Whirlpool baths at a temperature of 35° to 37° C (at skin temperatures) are used to prevent or minimize the formation of edema yet relieve pain.

Other forms of thermal therapy such as radiant heat, hot packs, ultrasound, paraffin baths, or fluidotherapy (Figure 42-2) have been used before massage to foster relaxation and to decrease pain. The tissue temperature of the hand is most effectively increased by the use of paraffin baths or fluidotherapy.[3,4] However, in many cases the use of heat can promote edema and therefore may be contraindicated.

The use of transcutaneous electrical nerve stimulation before or during active exercise should be considered. It is helpful in the patient with pain and hypersensitivity.[17,37,59] It is also helpful for relief of pain in causalgia and reflex sympathetic dystrophy.[37] Relief of pain with the use of a transcutaneous electrical nerve stimulation unit may depend on variables such as the shape, duration, and frequency of the pulse wave.[37]

A deep sedative massage is also helpful for pain relief.[34] If the pain is unrelieved by these techniques and treatment devices, further investigation is required. Other therapies, such as nerve blocks and operation, may be needed.[1,31,49]

TREATMENT OF LOSS OF RANGE OF MOTION
Muscle reeducation

The purpose of muscle reeducation is to reestablish purposeful, voluntary, acceptable motor behavior, as in range-of-motion exercises when abnormal motor patterns are present. (Muscle misuse, disuse, and overuse are discussed in

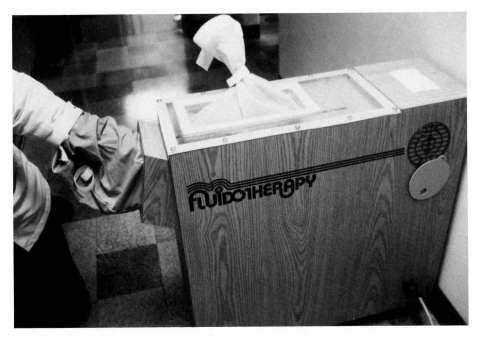

Figure 42-2. Fluidotherapy unit, used at temperature of 48.9° C for 15 to 30 minutes for pain management.

the next section.) Muscle reeducation is often an important part of hand rehabilitation and frequently requires much of a therapist's time before the actual range-of-motion exercises may be started. A classic method of muscle reeducation was described by Sister Elizabeth Kenny for the treatment of poliomyelitis.[32] The course of treatment progresses from passive relaxed range of motion to active range of motion followed by strengthening. If a desired exercise cannot be done in an efficient and acceptable fashion, this specific technique for redevelopment of motor skills must be used regularly before the therapeutic exercise is initiated. Neuromuscular reeducation ensures that the patient's performance during therapeutic exercise is acceptable. The patient must concentrate and be aware of the desired action of the muscle by feeling the muscle tendon with the contralateral hand and observing the muscle's action.

Augmentation of proprioceptive feedback from the contracting muscle enhances motor control. This can be effected by pressure with the patient's uninvolved contralateral hand if a gentle, prolonged stretch is desired. This assistance must be specified in the therapeutic prescription. Auditory or visible feedback from a contracting muscle may also be used to maintain active, gentle, prolonged stretching, and gentle bipolar electrical stimulation of the prime movers may result in favorable prolonged contractions. The duration of the electrical stimulation initially may be 10 seconds, and it can be increased to several minutes or longer. Whatever form is used, the patient may tolerate only a few minutes of active stretch initially, but the time then can be increased.

Electrical stimulation (Figure 42-3) and electromyographic biofeedback can be used to enhance awareness of the action of the muscles.[11,12,17] Physician, patient, and therapist must be aware of and try to prevent misuse, disuse, and overuse of the affected muscles and the other muscles of the extremity during the course of muscle reeducation.

Muscle misuse, disuse, or overuse

Misuse is the use of an extremity in an abnormal motor pattern, such as substitution, inappropriate co-contraction, and guarding. Abnormal motor patterns are characterized by unreasonable use of stabilizing or antagonistic muscle groups or both.[50,51] They can also involve lack of spontaneous relaxation and coordination after a completed task and a protective quivering, trembling, shaking, guarding, and tightening in the muscles or parts of the extremity during motion. Misuse leads to tension myalgia, muscle attachment pains, unnecessary compression or jamming of the joints, and unnecessary traction of the soft tissues during motion. It can lead to pain and swelling in the joints and pain at the attachments of the muscles. Misuse is fatiguing and painful and makes range-of-motion exercises irritating and inefficient. In our experience, compulsive persons who practice exercises despite persistent misuse are prone to develop shoulder-hand syndromes and increased pain syndromes. The treatment for misuse is neuromuscular reeducation, including teaching use of the extremity in acceptable motor patterns.

Disuse of muscles is the insufficient use of the involved extremity, which leads to atrophy of the tissues and to in-

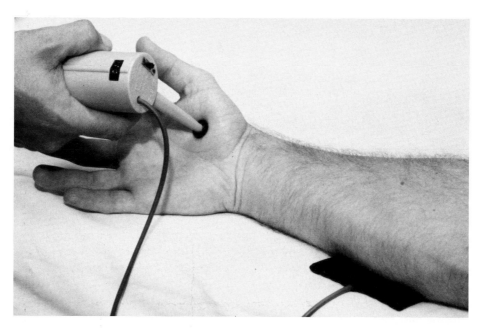

Figure 42-3. Hand-held electrical stimulator.

secure and inefficient performance of the muscles.[52,53] Disuse is avoided by incorporating functional hand activities in a supervised treatment plan as soon as smooth, basic hand function has been redeveloped. Early reintroduction of reasonable activities of daily living by regular use of the involved extremity with an acceptable motor pattern and within its comfortable work capacity can be helpful for preventing disuse. Progressively increasing the use of the hand within a comfortable and safe limit is also helpful. Determining a patient's habits by observing the extremity during typical activities of daily living and then modifying the habits to the advantage of the involved extremity can be helpful and important.

Overuse of muscles involves excessive activity that is too fast or too forceful.[50,51] Overuse is often associated with misuse. Patients may attempt to return to their normal preinjured level of activity too quickly; this results in intensified misuse, swelling, pain, hypersensitivity, guarding, limited range of motion, and eventually severe deconditioning of the extremity.

Careful monitoring and guidance in the progression from light to moderate to heavy activities are part of the hand therapy of each patient. The speed of performance should be consistent with the level of coordination achieved by the injured or rehabilitated part. Adequate time must be invested in intermittent relaxation and use of the extremity. The extremity should be kept relaxed when it is not in use. A static splint can be used at night or part time during the day to promote rest and relaxing of the extremity.

Active range-of-motion exercise and stretching

Loss of range of motion is a frequent complication of hand trauma, arthritic diseases, neuropathy, or operation.[61]

Appropriate, early hand therapy is imperative. The loss of range of motion can be due to several mechanisms. Edema interferes mechanically with the function of the fingers, joints, and muscles of the hand, and its progression to fibrosis causes swelling and stiffness to persist or become permanent. Capsular or ligamentous tightness after immobilization of the joints is another cause of loss of range of motion. At times a joint must be immobilized to allow for healing of bones or soft tissue structures that have been repaired. For any joints that do not require immobilization for healing, range-of-motion exercises should be started without delay as soon as the bones and structures that have been repaired can safely be mobilized. Gentle active assisted range-of-motion exercises should be initiated without forcing. With the loss of muscle power or innervation, tightness and contracture can result.

The shoulder has a tendency to become stiff and painful when the patient is unable to use the hand because it is not used in a normal way to place the hand where it is needed. Specific range-of-motion exercises are needed to help the patient use the shoulder and to maintain its range of motion. These exercises can be done with the patient supine. The shoulder is moved by active-assisted or by passive relaxation exercises. These exercises are performed until the patient can comfortably do the shoulder motions actively and correctly. Likewise, the elbow, forearm, and wrist should have range-of-motion exercises applied when appropriate and possible.

Active range-of-motion exercise is the most commonly used to maintain and increase the motion of the extremity, although other forms of range-of-motion exercises are also used. The degrees of permissible range of motion may be limited and must be identified by the surgeon on the basis

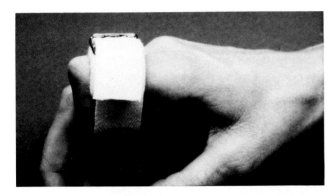

Figure 42-4. Web wrapping, used to prolong stretching of proximal interphalangeal and distal phalangeal joints.

of the type of operative procedure and the structural results that are achievable and necessary. Careful review of the operative reports therefore is essential. Questions about the description of the operation or the tendon repairs, ligament or capsular repairs, or stability of the bone fractures[33] should be clarified with the surgeon before proceeding with hand therapy.

Passive range of motion, in which an external force is applied to produce the motion, may be used postoperatively in cases of neurologic lesions or muscle weakness. The movement required can be provided by the therapist, the patient's contralateral hand, a family member, continuous passive range-of-motion machines, or dynamic splints. For passive range-of-motion exercises, the patient's muscles must be fully relaxed. These exercises do not imply stretching. They are done slowly to increase the available range of motion as far as is indicated but with maintenance of full relaxation.

In active-assisted range-of-motion exercises, the patient moves the part as much as possible while maintaining an acceptable motor performance. An external force then completes the movement through the available range, again without stretching. Active-assisted range-of-motion exercise therefore combines passive movement and coordinated active muscle contraction by the patient; it increases or maintains the available range of motion slowly without muscle misuse, disuse, or overuse.

In active exercise the range of motion is produced in a coordinated, muscle contraction by the patient through the available range; its purpose is to increase the arc of motion slowly. Active, general, prolonged stretching is used when adhesions of the tendons or moving planes restrict the proximal motion of the tendon. An example of this type is digital extension from a flexed position. In such a circumstance, no external force can efficiently mobilize an adherent tendon proximally. Therefore gentle, prolonged muscle contraction is the only force capable of moving the adherent tendon proximally, gradually increasing the active extension range of the digit.

Stretching exercise

A gentle, prolonged, passive stretch by an external force for as long as 20 minutes four times a day can be prescribed (Figures 42-4 and 42-5). Stretching is usually contraindicated until 6 weeks postoperatively because connective tissue needs this interval to regain adequate tensile strength. For the elongation of shortened soft tissue, the application of a gentle stretching force over a prolonged period is much more effective and safe than is the use of a high deforming force over a short time. The procedure involves a progressive increase in the number of repetitions with appropriate rest periods. The patient should be able to tolerate the frequency

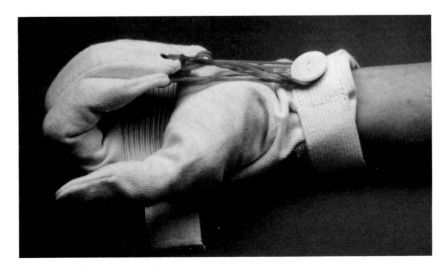

Figure 42-5. Flexion glove, used for long periods to flex joints of digits to provide prolonged stretching.

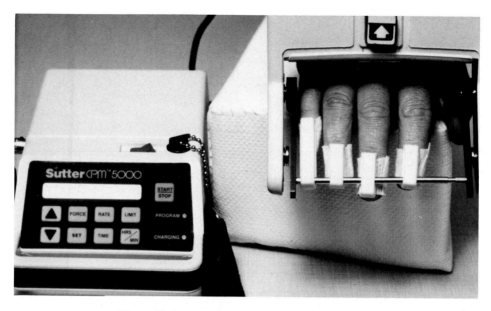

Figure 42-6. Sutter passive range-of-motion machine.

without pain, swelling, or fatigue. Various prolonged passive range-of-motion devices such as the Sutter (Figure 42-6), Richards, and Striker mobile limbs can be helpful if they are fitted properly, and they ensure proper alignment while moving the extremity through a comfortable, relaxed range of motion.

Adjunct treatments to range-of-motion exercises

Application of heat, such as a whirlpool bath, hot packs, radiant heat, fluidotherapy, or paraffin baths during and before treatment, may make movement easier.

Joint mobilization techniques performed by the therapist may be used to gain full joint movement or capsular motion. These delicate procedures require knowledge of specific techniques that do not cause overstretch or injure important joint capsular structures.

Friction massage can be helpful to improve a range of motion if the scar tissue or skin is tight over an area.[34] Friction massage softens scar tissue in preparation for range-of-motion exercises. The use of Lubriderm lotion, Eucerin Creme, Alpha Keri lotion, white Vaseline Intensive Care lotion, lanolin creams, or cocoa butter during massage can be helpful. Constant firm pressure by elastomer pads, iodoform pads, or elastic wraps or garments can also help to soften scars.

Adjunct treatments to stretching

Ultrasonographic therapy with passive or active gentle, prolonged stretching can be applied across the restricted part to enhance the process.[35,36] For adhesions about the tendon between moving planes and in restricted joints and for adhesions of the skin to the deeper tissues, ultrasonographic therapy can be applied under water. Ideally the ultrasound

wattage is set to cause periosteal pain within about 5 minutes of use. Severe periosteal pain should be avoided. At the onset of periosteal discomfort the tissue being treated has reached a temperature of approximately 45° C and has become more stretchable. The wattage is then reduced slightly to a level of comfort, and the stretching is continued for another 5 to 10 minutes. Ultrasound phonophoresis can also be used with 10% cortisone in Aquasonic or Aquaphore and is especially helpful for tendinitis and epicondylitis. Iontophoresis can also be used to infiltrate localized areas with cortisone or other drugs.[18]

Other devices that help to increase range of motion are finger trapping, web strapping (Figure 42-4), flexion gloves (Figure 42-5), and rubber band strapping for stretching.

Joint jacks, knuckle benders, and reverse knuckle benders may be effective for stretching joint contractures or directing joint motions in a correct arc. These devices should fit the patient well, have an efficient angle of pull, and not cause undue pressure or compromise in adjacent joints or circulation.

ORTHOSES

Orthoses of many types are frequently used in hand rehabilitation. They can be made for individual joints, entire areas, such as the elbow, hand, and wrist, or a portion of the extremities. The orthoses are fabricated from special thermoplastics, metal, or light cast material. Prefabricated splints of plastic, thermoplastic, or canvas are available, but they are not usually helpful and do not fit as well as custom-made hand orthoses.[43]

The duration that an orthosis must be used depends on the specific lesion. When an orthosis must be worn con-

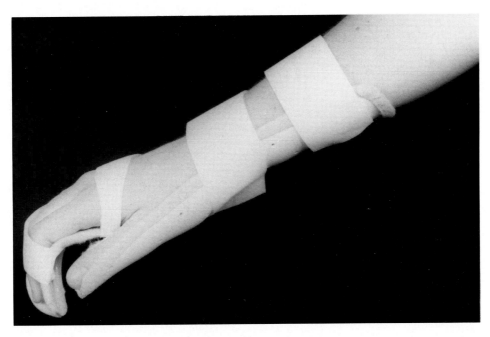

Figure 42-7. Resting hand-wrist-thumb orthosis. (From Department of Physical Medicine and Rehabilitation; Department of Occupational Therapy: Static and dynamic splinting of the upper extremity, Rochester, Minn, 1985. By permission of the Mayo Foundation.)

stantly, it should be specifically fabricated to avoid damage to the underlying parts, such as pressure areas or insensitive skin, and to avoid compression of digital arteries or nerves. Precise fitting is necessary to avoid damage, especially when prolonged healing of tendons or fractures is necessary.[33] Orthoses should be worn according to a schedule set by the physician and tolerable to the patient, and the duration and frequency they are worn should be gradually increased.

The two basic types of orthoses are static and dynamic. A static orthosis for the hand and wrist is used to protect from overstretching, to prevent contractures, to support digits that have recently been surgically repaired, and to facilitate healing of soft tissues and fractures. Static splints do not allow for movement.[38,43,52]

Static orthoses prevent deformities and may maintain increases achieved in the range of motion when they are serially adjusted. Also, they provide rest and promote healing. They may splint each of the interphalangeal joints alone or in combination. These are used in such conditions as posttraumatic tendon injury, hyperesthetic or anesthetic fingers, proximal interphalangeal joint deformities (for example, boutonnière deformities and swan-neck deformities), claw hands from burns, scleroderma, or nerve injuries. Static splinting of the thumb can be either hand based or wrist based. A large C-bar splint holds the thumb in abduction and opposition to obtain a web space between the thumb and index finger (Figure 42-7). Static wrist orthoses support the wrist and may be used in combination with static splint-

ing of the metacarpophalangeal and proximal interphalangeal areas or to allow freedom of the use of the fingers and thumb. A static wrist cock-up orthosis can be used to support the hand with weak or paralyzed wrist extensors. Static wrist orthoses may provide attachments for writing and eating and other assistive devices.

After nerve repair the extremity is splinted about 7 to 10 days postoperatively in such a way as to prevent traction on the repaired nerve.[61] The Kleinert splint, used after nerve repair of the wrist, has the appearance of a shepherd's crook (Figure 42-8). This splint is well molded around the bony prominences and padded as needed to prevent pressure on insensitive areas. If tendon repair is also needed, hooks can be added to the fingers and rubber bands attached to the wrist for dynamic passive flexion of the fingers. In the case of median or ulnar nerve repair at the wrist, this splint leaves the fingers free for touching and massaging. Elbow splints can be made for repairs above the wrist and around the elbow. The repair is protected in the splint for about 6 weeks.

Dynamic orthoses allow for movement. Dynamic splints may be made with hinges or external joints and usually have a source of power, such as rubber bands, electric motors, other muscles, springs, or compressed gas that provides movement. Dynamic orthoses may be used to align, resist, assist, or simulate movement. They allow for mobility of a joint with a specific directional control provided by forces that substitute for weak or absent muscle power. They can also be used to assist movement of the interphalangeal joints, metacarpophalangeal joints, and the first carpal-metacarpal

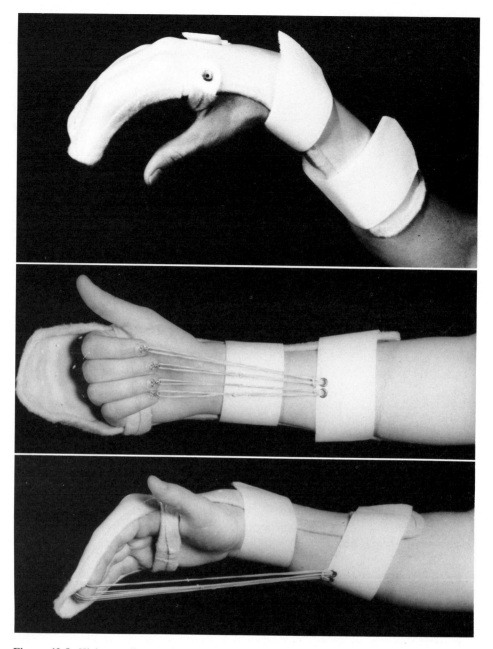

Figure 42-8. Kleinert splint, used to protect finger flexor tendons and nerve repairs at wrist and digits. (From Department of Physical Medicine and Rehabilitation; Department of Occupational Therapy: Static and dynamic splinting of the upper extremity, Rochester, Minn, 1985. By permission of the Mayo Foundation.)

joints and thumb (Figure 42-9). These joints may be assisted in flexion or extension by outrigger supports, hooks applied to the nails, rubber-band devices, or springs with slings. The elastic pull should be gentle and not cause pain or swelling. The orthoses are used to assist the wrist in flexion or extension and the elbow in flexion, extension, pronation, or supination, and they may increase the range of motion. Dynamic splints can be fabricated to provide a prolonged,

gentle stretching and can be worn for a prescribed duration, such as a half hour or four times a day.

Alignment is important in both the resting and the dynamic orthosis. It is especially important in arthritic patients and for protecting repaired tendons and periarticular tissues. The orthoses may resist abnormal or undesirable movements; for instance, they prevent a patient from putting tension on a newly repaired tendon, yet they allow mild

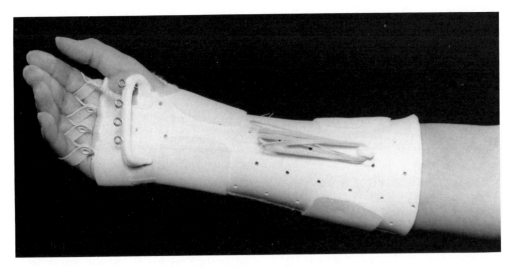

Figure 42-9. Dynamic metacarpophalangeal flexion orthosis. (From Department of Physical Medicine and Rehabilitation; Department of Occupational Therapy: Static and dynamic splinting of the upper extremity, Rochester, Minn, 1985. By permission of the Mayo Foundation.)

gliding of the tendon, such as with the Kleinert splint (Figure 42-8).

Special orthoses that simulate functional movement have a source of stored energy, which can be activated by the patient's own muscles (myoelectric splints) or by an external power source. An example of this type is the shoulder-operated hand orthosis.

STRENGTHENING AND ENDURANCE

Once full range of motion has been accomplished, muscle strength and endurance are gradually increased. Manual resistance exercises play an important part in this strengthening. The patient can use the contralateral hand as the resistive force and to monitor the force. Progressive resistive exercises of gradually increasing weight or gradation of resistance by the unaffected hand can be helpful. These exercises can be isotonic, isometric, or isokinetic.[7] Several devices that have proved helpful in a graded program of exercise are the hand helper, hand exerciser, various spring-resistive devices, weight devices, therapeutic putty, and elastic straps; functional activities of progressively increasing difficulty and resistance are also useful.[7] Machines such as the Cybex isokinetic machine (Cybex Division of Lumex, Ronkonkoma, New York) and the Baltimore Therapeutic Equipment Work Simulator (Baltimore Therapeutic Equipment Company, Baltimore, Maryland) are helpful for strengthening and endurance training.

Endurance is increased by slow and gradual increments of exercise. The patient may do activities of daily living or special functional activities and may gradually increase the time spent on these activities from day to day (for example, as little as 1 minute twice a day and increasing up to 1 hour a day). The activities or exercises must not cause pain, unusual muscle discomfort, or signs of overuse. Assistive devices may be prescribed to perform the activities of daily living or to improve the patient's ability to perform. Reeducation techniques to train the nondominant hand to take over activities from the dominant hand have been helpful for patients with permanent disabilities. Assistive devices may be prescribed as needed. In a severely injured patient, follow-up, especially of long-term rehabilitation, is vital.

HAND PROTECTION

Specific diseases may require joint protection and the prescription and training in the use of self-help devices. Some examples of these conditions are rheumatoid arthritis, psoriatic arthritis, systemic sclerosis, acrosclerosis, carpal tunnel syndrome, and degenerative joint disease of the hand. Several books evaluating equipment helpful for joint protection are available from the Arthritis and Rheumatism Foundation.[41,45]

For a patient with scleroderma the hands must be well lubricated with cream or oil to help maintain the moisture balance and suppleness of the skin and to prevent chapping and cracking. Among the recommended lotions, oils, or creams are cocoa butter, Lubriderm, mineral oil, Alpha Keri, Vaseline, Eucerin, or petrolatum jelly. These can be applied three to four times a day, especially after washing the hands or after having been outdoors in the sun, wind, or cold. The skin should be patted damp dry after washing and the lotion applied to the slightly damp skin. Friction massage to the skin can help maintain elasticity and reduce swelling. The hand can be massaged after the cream is applied. If dryness of hands or skin is a problem, it is helpful to apply the cream and wear loose white gloves and flannel pajamas to bed. Basis or superfatty soap is suggested for bathing. It is important to protect the hands from cuts, scratches, and bruises. Cuticles should be cared for meticulously to prevent hangnails. Cuticles can be kept soft by applying cream or using a cotton-tipped swab soaked in a cuticle remover. Sharp objects should not be used to push the cuticles back. If a hangnail should develop, it should not be pulled off but instead carefully cut off. The nails should be cut in a rounded fashion to the tip of the fingers, with care taken not to cut the skin.

For protecting the skin of a patient with scleroderma from the cold, gloves or mittens (preferably down mittens or extra-large, fur-lined mittens) should always be worn outside during cold weather. Mittens are preferable to gloves, but if gloves are worn, they should be extra large and fur lined. Electric mittens and socks are available from hunting or athletic supply stores. Exposure to excessive heat and sunburn should be avoided.

When working with frozen foods or removing objects from a refrigerator, patients should wear insulated mitts. Ice cubes should not be handled with bare hands, and skin contact with cold water should be avoided. The use of insulated cups when drinking hot or cold beverages is important. In cold weather, preheating the car before getting into it helps avoid acrosclerosis. Large fur- or pile-lined boots and warm socks (wool) should be worn. Tight shoes or boots should be avoided.

Large rubber gloves should be worn when washing dishes. The gloves should protect the hands from extremes of water temperature and from accidental cuts on a knife or other sharp utensils. Nondetergent dishwashing soap, such as Ivory, should be used. The patient should avoid bumping the arms, hands, legs, and feet against low furniture and counters. When one handles hot foods or works around the stove, care must be taken to prevent burning the skin. The patient should avoid hand sewing or using a tight grasp on small objects (for example, crochet hooks and knitting needles). Also, the use of coarse threads or yarns should be avoided and extreme care taken not to stick fingers with pins or needles. To avoid trauma to the fingertips, a patient with scleroderma should not type on a manual typewriter or play the piano or guitar.

It is important to maintain skin elasticity and full range of motion of all the joints, including the web spaces. Exercises for the face, feet, ankles, fingers, and thumbs to maintain mobility are important.

Carpal tunnel syndrome results from the entrapment of or pressure on the median nerve at the wrist. The median nerve and the tendons of the finger flexors share a common tunnel at the wrist. Any process that decreases the space in the tunnel may result in the symptoms associated with carpal tunnel syndrome. The following suggestions are intended to decrease stress on the carpal tunnel area and to lessen the symptoms of this syndrome. The patient should avoid flexing and extending the wrist. During sleep a splint may be used. Trying to use the hand in a neutral position is recommended. Instead of flattening the palm of the hand when using it, the patient should use it in a cupped position. A hard grip should be avoided when scrubbing, driving a car, or carrying items. The patient should avoid prolonged holding of items, such as a steering wheel, paintbrush, pen, rake, newspaper, or book. The grip should be relaxed frequently when these items are held. Pinching activities, such as needlework or writing, should be avoided, performed only for short periods, or adapted to decrease stress. Some ways to adapt are to use an enlarged object, use a felt- or nylon-tipped pen, and relax the hand for several minutes before resuming an activity. The patient should avoid repetitive pounding, such as stapling or hammering.

TREATMENT OF HYPERSENSITIVITY

Neurologic involvement is often complicated by heightened responses to painful or sensory stimulation. The excessive state may be associated with bizarre responses. The treatment of the hypersensitivity that occurs after nerve injury must precede sensory reeducation.[13,21,23,53,67] Patients usually have varying degrees of hypersensitivity or dysesthesias, which must be desensitized early in the rehabilitation program. The only contraindications to desensitization techniques are open wounds and infection in the affected areas. The best results are achieved with early intervention.

Massage is one technique of desensitization that applies materials of different textures—smooth, coarse, and rough. The material is rubbed gently over the area for 1 to 2 minutes, rubbed more vigorously for 1 to 2 more minutes, and then rubbed softly again for 1 to 2 minutes. The treatment is repeated as needed and is based on the concept of increasing the pain threshold of the nerve. Treatment begins at the patient's level of tolerance with the softer, less irritating material. Force, duration, and frequency are increased with a more irritating material as desensitization occurs.

Tapping lightly or heavily over the area to decrease sensitivity may also be done.[53] The patient must not bruise the part being desensitized. Mechanical vibrators or tappers for percussion used for 10 minutes and up to 30 minutes once or twice a day have been suggested. In another approach the patient immerses the sensitive areas in such materials as soft Styrofoam balls, rice, beans, or popcorn. The stimulation should be repetitive and constantly performed 20 to 30 minutes at a time two or three times daily. Desensitization treatment is started in the less hypersensitive regions and progresses to the more hypersensitive areas as tolerated. The patient should be able to remain relaxed at all times during treatment.

Pain relief in the hypersensitive hand can often be attained with transcutaneous electrical nerve stimulation, contrast baths, and whirlpool baths. It is helpful to apply oil or lanolin cream to hold the moisture in the skin of the hand and prevent scaling and cracking. Massaging the cream or oil into the hand can assist in desensitization while simultaneously promoting awareness of altered sensibility patterns.

SENSORY REEDUCATION

Sensory reeducation is a technique used to redevelop conscious perception and proper interpretation of distorted or insufficient sensation in a patient with impaired sensory perception.[11,12,21,58] Sensory reeducation is important when the hand sustains damage or undergoes surgical repair of peripheral nerves.

Sensory reeducation has several training prerequisites.[11,12,20,65,66] The training area should be free of distractions, and the extremity should be pain free. The patient and therapist should have good rapport, and adequate time must be allotted for the treatment. Education of the patient is paramount for treatment. The patient should understand the objectives of the treatment and what participation in treatment entails. The patient must have the abilities to comprehend the instructions and participate actively in the program and be adequately prepared to interpret the sensation. The learning involved in sensory retraining requires perception, recognition, retention, and recall.

The patient must prevent further injuries to the insensitive areas and the areas with decreased sensitivity. These injuries generally occur by doing things automatically; therefore the patient must be constantly vigilant and should be instructed in protecting the insensitive hand when, for example, holding cigarettes, grabbing a frying pan handle, or working near a hot stove or in a freezer. The insensitive hand should not be placed in water that is too hot and should be protected in cold weather. The patient should even be told to avoid taking toast from a toaster or touching or bumping a hot pan or popcorn popper. The insensitive hand should not be placed over a steaming pot or on a hot automobile motor.[25,42]

Wynn Parry's sensory reeducation program is based on the pattern theory,[62-66] which involves the following concepts:

1. The skin is reinnervated at random, and the patient must learn new patterns of sensation.
2. The more skilled the patient and the more the limb is used, the more likely the patient is to maintain the improvement gained with training.
3. Sensory exercises should begin after protective sensation is recovered, that is, when the patient can recognize pain and temperature.

In the first part of the exercise program the patient is given several wooden blocks of various shapes, sizes, and weights; the blocks are hidden from the patient behind a screen or the patient is blindfolded. The patient moves a block slowly around in the hand, assessing the corners and different surfaces. If the object is not recognized within 60

seconds, the patient is asked to look at the object and to move it in the hand at the same time. In this way the patient relates what is felt with what is seen, building up a tactile visual image. The intervals until recognition are noted for comparison at a later date. As progress is made, the shapes are varied to avoid a training effect.

The second part of retraining involves the recognition of textures. Again, recognition times are recorded and the textures are varied as recognition is mastered. Retraining for localization of touch is done by blindfolding the patient and then touching the hand in various areas. The patient is asked to point to the spot that was touched. Failure is noted if the patient does not identify the spot in 60 seconds. This process is repeated with the blindfold off so that the patient starts to learn correct localization.

The final stage of retraining involves recognition of everyday objects. First large objects (such as tennis balls, matchboxes, and pegs) and later finer objects (such as safety pins, keys, matches, and dominoes) are recognized. The patient slowly explores each object, assessing its size, weight, density, texture, and temperature and putting together clues to identify the object. The affected hand does in slow motion what the normal hand does automatically with speed. The training sessions are as short as 10 to 15 minutes and take place several times a day. These sensory training methods seem to be based not only on the pattern theory of sensation but also on the concept that most external stimuli require motor participation.

If only the median nerve is involved, a thick leather glove or covering can be placed on the fingers and palm in the areas innervated by the ulnar nerve to allow the areas innervated by the injured median nerve to relearn the meaning of the stimuli and not rely on the ulnar nerve areas.

External stimuli can be divided into two types: those that are passively impressed and those that require active movement for sensory discrimination. Passive stimuli are rarely encountered in normal life. After sensory retraining, patients can achieve good sensory function despite poor two-point discrimination.

The sensory reeducation program of Dellon and Curtis[8,9,11,12] is based on the neurophysiologic subdivision of the large, myelinated sensory fibers (group A-beta fibers) into those that adapt quickly and those that adapt slowly to mechanical stimuli. This is the specificity theory of sensory reeducation. The quickly adapting fibers can in turn be subdivided into a group maximally responsive to 256 cycles/sec of vibratory stimuli and a group maximally responsive to 30 cycles/sec. The slowly adapting fibers mediate the perception of constant touch, and the quickly adapting fibers mediate the perception not only of vibrations of 30 cycles/sec and of 256 cycles/sec but also of moving touch. These investigators thought that the time to begin the reeducation program is determined by the pattern of recovery of sensation. Typically the pattern of sensory recovery would be perception of pain (pinprick), 30 cycles/sec of vibration, moving touch, constant touch, and finally 256 cycles/sec of vibration. During recovery, if a stimulus of 30 cycles/sec is perceived only in a proximal part of the hand, it is appropriate for the patient to begin sensory exercises specific for moving touch in that area. The exercises are simple, repetitive, and manageable by the patient at home. In the early phase, when the patient can appreciate 256 cycles/sec at the fingertips but cannot perceive moving or constant touch, the patient is asked to touch any blunt object (such as another finger or a pencil) on the given area of the patient's fingertips with varying pressure. The quickly adapting fibers are reeducated by moving the blunt object across the given area. In the later phase, when perception of constant or moving touch has been recovered at the fingertips, the exercises use shaped nuts and bolts.

For reeducation of constant touch, patients are initially asked to discriminate between largest and smallest nuts; with improved discrimination, this task is made more difficult.

For reeducation of moving touch, the patient is asked to discriminate between a square nut and a hexagon nut, each of which is rolled across the finger. The patient is first asked to distinguish these with eyes open, observing the stimulus, and then with the eyes shut, concentrating on the stimulation evoked by the stimulus.[8,11,12]

Carter added to these exercises a program of sensory bombardment and the differentiation of an object from a background medium such as sand, rice, or beans.[25] Special boards used for sensory reeducation allow the hands to be used for screwing nuts and bolts while the patient's vision is obstructed. Another suggestion is to use various black boxes and screens to obstruct vision while the patient attempts to use the hand to distinguish objects.

The goals of sensory reeducation are to teach responses to the sensation of pain (sharp, dull), temperature (hot, cold), shape (sphere, cube), size (large, small), length (long, short), texture (rough, smooth), consistency (hard, soft), material (wood, cotton, nylon), and weight (heavy, light).

After nerve injury, function of the upper extremity generally tends to improve slowly over 12 months or more.[2,13,21,27,30] Regular reexaminations with the development of updated home programs and practicing of updated home programs before dismissal are essential.

Whenever possible before major operative intervention, the patient should be advised that a regular home program of exercise must be carried out for several months, that regular reexamination may be needed, and that reinstruction may at times necessitate treatments several days a week or twice a day on an outpatient basis. A full understanding of the rehabilitation program is important.

Rehabilitation of hand disabilities may require a long time, but much can be accomplished. Delays in referral can result in slow or less than optimal recovery. Cooperation and communication among the patient, hand surgeon, physician, therapists, and other health professionals must be fully developed, maintained, and practiced. These relationships are the core of the system leading to maximal benefits and recovery for the patient.

REFERENCES

1. Atkinson, L: Upper dorsal sympathectomy, Med J Aust 1:267, 1975.
2. Borrell, RM, et al: Fluidotherapy: evaluation of a new heat modality, Arch Phys Med Rehabil 58:69, 1977.
3. Borrell, RM, et al: Comparison of in vivo temperatures produced by hydrotherapy, paraffin wax treatment, and fluidotherapy, Phys Ther 60:1273, 1980.
4. Bosarge, J: Finger replant patient undergoing rehabilitation, J Rehabil 42:29, 1976.
5. Casley-Smith, JR: The structural basis for the conservative treatment of lymphedema. In Clodius, L, editor: Lymphedema, Stuttgart, 1977, Georg Thieme Verlag.
6. Clodius, L: Lymphedema, Stuttgart, 1977, Georg Thieme Verlag.
7. Curtis, RM, and Engalitcheff, J, Jr: A work simulator for rehabilitating the upper extremity—preliminary report, J Hand Surg 6:499, 1981.
8. Dellon, AL: The moving two-point discrimination test: clinical evaluation of the quickly adapting fiber/receptor system, J Hand Surg 3:474, 1978.
9. Dellon, AL: Evaluation of sensibility and re-education of sensation in the hand, Baltimore, 1981, Williams & Wilkins Co.
10. Dellon, AL: The vibrometer, Plast Reconstr Surg 71:427, 1983.
11. Dellon, AL, Curtis, RM, and Edgerton, MT: Reeducation of sensation in the hand after nerve injury and repair, Plast Reconstr Surg 53:297, 1974.
12. Dellon, AL, and Jabaley, ME: Reeducation of sensation in the hand following nerve suture, Clin Orthop 163:75, 1982.
13. Dykes, RW, and Terzis, JK: Reinnervation of glabrous skin in baboons: properties of cutaneous mechanoreceptors subsequent to nerve crush, J Neurophysiol 42:1461, 1979.
14. Fess, EE, et al: Evaluation of the hand by objective measurement. In Hunter, JM, et al, editors: Rehabilitation of the hand, St. Louis, 1978, The CV Mosby Co.
15. Fess, EE, and Moran, C: Clinical assessment of recommendations, Indianapolis, 1981, American Society of Hand Therapists.
16. Foldi, M: Physiology and pathophysiology of lymph flow. In Clodius, L, editor: Lymphedema, Stuttgart, 1977, Georg Thieme Verlag.
17. Fried, T, Johnson, R, and McCracken, W: Transcutaneous electrical nerve stimulation: its role in the control of chronic pain, Arch Phys Med Rehabil 65:228, 1984.
18. Gangarosa, LP, et al: Conductivity of drugs used for iontophoresis, J Pharm Sci 67:1439, 1978.
19. Frohring, WO, et al: Changes in the vibratory sense of patients with poliomyelitis as measured by the pallesthesiometer, Am J Dis Child 69:89, 1945.
20. Frykman, GK, and Waylett, J: Rehabilitation of peripheral nerve injuries, Orthop Clin North Am 12:361, 1981.
21. Gelberman, RH, et al: Digital sensibility following replantation, J Hand Surg 3:313, 1978.
22. Guyton, AC, Granger, HJ, and Taylor, AE: Interstitial fluid pressure, Physiol Rev 51:527, 1971.
23. Hardy, MA, Moran, CA, and Merritt, WH: Desensitization of the traumatized hand, Va Med 109:134, 1982.
24. Heck, CV, Hendryson, IE, and Rowe, CR: Measuring and recording of joint motion, Chicago, 1965, Committee for the Study of Joint Motion, American Academy of Orthopedic Surgeons.
25. Hunter, JM, et al: Rehabilitation of the hand, St. Louis, 1978, The CV Mosby Co.
26. Jebsen, RH, et al: An objective and standardized test of hand function, Arch Phys Med Rehabil 50:311, 1969.

27. Jones, JM, Schenck, RR, and Chesney, RB: Digital replantation and amputation—comparison of function, J Hand Surg 7:183, 1982.

28. Jones, RF: The rehabilitation of surgical patients with particular reference to traumatic upper limb disability, Aust NZ J Surg 47:402, 1977.

29. Kellor, M, et al: Hand strength and dexterity, Am J Occup Ther 25:77, 1971.

30. Kellor, M, et al: Technical manual of hand strength and activity test, Minneapolis, 1971, Kenny Rehabilitation Institute.

31. Kleinert, HE, et al: Post-traumatic sympathetic dystrophy, Orthop Clin North Am 4:917, 1973.

32. Knapp, ME: The contribution of Sister Elizabeth Kenny to the treatment of poliomyelitis, Arch Phys Med Rehabil 36:510, 1955.

33. Knapp, ME: Aftercare of fractures. In Krusen, FH, editor: Handbook of physical medicine and rehabilitation, ed 2, Philadelphia, 1971, WB Saunders Co.

34. Knapp, ME: Massage. In Krusen, FH, editor: Handbook of physical medicine and rehabilitation, ed 2, Philadelphia, 1971, WB Saunders Co.

35. Lehmann, JF: Diathermy. In Krusen, FH, editor: Handbook of physical medicine and rehabilitation, ed 2, Philadelphia, 1971, WB Saunders Co.

36. Lehmann, JF, et al: Effect of therapeutic temperatures on tendon extensibility, Arch Phys Med Rehabil 51:481, 1970.

37. Mannheimer, JS, and Lampe, GN: Clinical transcutaneous electrical nerve stimulation, Philadelphia, 1984, FA Davis Co.

38. Long, C, and Schutt, AH: Upper limb orthotics. In Redford, JB, editor: Orthotics *etcetera*, ed 3, Baltimore, 1986, Williams & Wilkins Co.

39. Markley, JM, Jr: The preservation of close two-point discrimination in the interdigital transfer of neurovascular island flaps, Plast Reconstr Surg 59:812, 1977.

40. Mathiowety, V, et al: Grip and pinch strength: normative data for adults, Arch Phys Med Rehabil 66:69, 1985.

41. Mayo Clinic Occupational Therapy Department: Joint protection for the arthritic person, Rochester, Minn, 1985, Mayo Foundation.

42. McQuillen, MP: Practical approaches to managing peripheral neuropathies, Geriatrics 30:109, 1975.

43. Meier, RH, III, et al: Prosthetics, orthotics, and assistive devices (syllabus), ed 2, Chapter J, Self-Directed Medical Knowledge Program, Chicago, 1984, American Academy of Physical Medicine and Rehabilitation.

44. Moberg, E: Objective methods for determining the functional value of sensibility in the hand, J Bone Joint Surg (Br) 40B:454, 1958.

45. National Arthritis Foundation: Self-help manual for patients with arthritis, 3400 Peachtree Road Northeast, Atlanta, GA 30326.

46. Olszewski, W: Pathophysiological and clinical observations of obstructive lymphedema of the limbs. In Clodius, L, editor: Lymphedema, Stuttgart, 1977, Georg Thieme Verlag.

47. Olszewski, WL, and Engeset, A: Intrinsic contractility of leg lymphatics in man: preliminary communication, Lymphology 12:81, 1979.

48. Olszewski, WL, and Engeset, A: Intrinsic contractility of prenodal lymph vessels and lymph flow in human leg, Am J Physiol 239:H775, 1980.

49. Omer, GE, Jr, and Thomas, SR: The management of chronic pain syndromes in the upper extremity, Clin Orthop 104:37, 1974.

50. Opitz, JL: Reconstructive surgery of the extremities. In Kottke, FJ, Stillwell, GK, and Lehmann, JF, editors: Krusen's handbook of physical medicine and rehabilitation, ed 3, Philadelphia, 1982, WB Saunders Co.

51. Opitz, JL, and Linscheid, RL: Hand function after metacarpal phalangeal joint replacement in rheumatoid arthritis, Arch Phys Med Rehabil 59:160, 1978.

52. Parkes, A: Some thoughts on examination of the hand, Hand 7:104, 1975.

53. Russel, WR: Percussion and vibration. In Licht, SH, editor: Massage, manipulation and traction, West New Haven, Conn, 1960, SH Licht.

54. Sensory rehabilitation of the hand (editorial), Lancet 1:135, 1981.

55. Stillwell, GK: Treatment of postmastectomy lymphedema, Mod Treat 6:396, 1969.

56. Stillwell, GK: Therapeutic heat and cold. In Krusen, FH, editor: Handbook of physical medicine and rehabilitation, ed 2, Philadelphia, 1971, WB Saunders Co.

57. Stillwell, GK: The law of Laplace: some clinical applications, Mayo Clin Proc 48:863, 1973.

58. Terzis, JK: Sensory mapping, Clin Plast Surg 3:59, 1976.

59. Thorsteinsson, G, et al: Transcutaneous electrical stimulation: a double-blind trial of its efficacy for pain, Arch Phys Med Rehabil 58:8, 1977.

60. Tinkham, RG, and Stillwell, GK: The role of pneumatic pumping devices in the treatment of postmastectomy lymphedema, Arch Phys Med Rehabil 46:193, 1965.

61. Weeks, PM, and Wray, RC: Management of acute hand injuries: a biological approach, ed 2, St. Louis, 1978, The CV Mosby Co.

62. Wynn Parry, CB: Painful conditions of peripheral nerves, Aust NZ J Surg 50:233, 1980.

63. Wynn Parry, CB: The Ruscoe Clarke Memorial Lecture, 1979. The management of traction lesions of the brachial plexus and peripheral nerve injuries in the upper limb: a study of teamwork, Injury 11:265, 1980.

64. Wynn Parry, CB: Sensory rehabilitation of the hand, Aust NZ J Surg 50:224, 1980.

65. Wynn Parry, CB: Rehabilitation of the hand, ed 4, London, 1981, Butterworths.

66. Wynn Parry, CB, and Salter, M: Sensory reeducation after median nerve lesions, Hand 8:250, 1976.

67. Yerxa, EJ, et al: Development of a hand sensitivity test for the hypersensitive hand, Am J Occup Ther 37:176, 1983.

PART VI

PAIN SYNDROMES

CHAPTER 43

Chronic pain

EVALUATION AND TREATMENT

MARTIN GRABOIS

Chronic pain is difficult and frustrating to control, and patients who experience it are often viewed as undesirable. At the same time, medical students, house officers, and practitioners often inadequately understand this clinical problem and its management.[16] From a clinical standpoint the complexity of the painful sensation is exacerbated by the absence of objective scales for the character and quality of pain, psychosocial factors influencing pain, and inconsistency of the responses to treatment techniques. In spite of these problems, however, a clear understanding of pain syndromes, an appreciation of the evaluative techniques available, and treatment programs geared to the individual patient help in the management of this frustrating problem. Specifically, this chapter addresses the chronic pain problem from six perspectives:

1. Magnitude of the problem
2. Concept of chronic pain from the physical, psychologic, and social point of view
3. Concept of the pain clinic
4. Evaluation of the patient with chronic pain
5. Treatment approaches and the techniques available
6. Expected results

Perhaps the best way to define chronic pain is to compare and contrast it to acute pain:

Acute	Chronic
Physician trained in evaluation and diagnosis	Physicians less interested and less trained
Short evaluation and treatment course	Long evaluation and treatment course
Pain is a biologic symptom	Pain is a disease
Pain plus anxiety	Pain plus depression
Medications as needed	Nonnarcotic analgesics, antidepressants
Little addiction concern	Polyaddiction concern
Diagnosis easy	Diagnosis complex
Cure likely	Cure usually not achieved

In chronic pain the original causes are blurred by subsequent complications of multiple procedures, medication dependency, compensation factors, and psychosocial behavioral changes. Therefore, when examining the patient with chronic pain, one cannot consider the typical medical model in which the symptoms or illness is controlled by an underlying pathologic event.[16] Chronic pain often cannot be explained by a specific organic or psychogenic cause. A more appropriate model must take into account the behavioral component and its chronicity. Finally, pain should be viewed as a spectrum of nociceptive events ranging from pathogenic pain to learned pain with considerable overlapping along this spectrum (Figure 43-1).

Accurate statistics on the incidence and cost of chronic pain are not easy to find.[14] Available figures, however, indicate that the incidence and cost of chronic pain in human suffering and economic loss is staggering.[2] It is estimated that 75 million Americans suffer from some kind of pain at a total cost of about $57 billion per year.[2] Brena[2] noted this

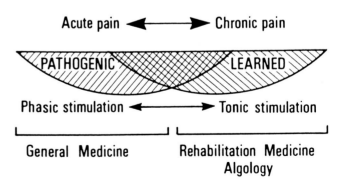

Figure 43-1. Nociceptive spectrum. (From Brena, SF, and Chapman, SL: Management of patients with chronic pain, New York, 1983, SP Medical & Scientific Books.)

may be an underestimate and emphasized that the incidence of chronic pain is growing faster than the rate of population growth. He further observed that a significant number of individuals should be able to return to gainful employment compatible with their age, education, previous work history, and work skills if they are properly managed medically and vocationally.[2]

CHRONIC PAIN MANAGEMENT PROGRAMS

Swanson[21] remarked that when pain becomes chronic it increases in complexity and the patient becomes more resistant to treatment. The origins of the pain, as noted earlier, are often masked by subsequent complications of multiple surgical procedures, medication dependency, compensation factors, and psychosocial behavioral changes (Figure 43-2). It is widely accepted that the continuation of the sequential outpatient-inpatient approach will not be successful for the typical chronic pain patient.[9]

The following are typical characteristics of a chronic pain patient:

1. 35 years old
2. Low back pain for 3 years after injury at work
3. Has not worked for 3 years
4. Depressed, irritable
5. Multiple hospitalizations, physicians, and surgical procedures
6. Currently taking oxycodone (Percodan), diazepam (Valium), and flurazepam (Dalmane)
7. Inactive physically and socially

Since chronic pain is a complex problem with medical and psychosocial aspects, it requires a comprehensive and interdisciplinary approach in evaluation and treatment.[9] Chronic pain therefore must be considered similar to disabilities such as alcoholism, stroke, and spinal cord injury if the patient is to reach the highest functional goals possible within his or her medical and psychologic limitations.[7] Pain programs have attempted to accomplish this by an interdisciplinary comprehensive approach to evaluating and treating patients with chronic pain.

Programs for chronic pain management, like those for physical medicine and rehabilitation, are relatively new developments and began during World War II.[8] First started by Alexander and popularized by Bonica,[1] these programs have multiplied in the past decade and by 1986 numbered approximately 2000. This increased interest in a pain clinic concept results from many factors, including the trend toward combining medical and psychosocial approaches, renewed interest in pain research, and realization of the economic impact of chronic pain.[1] Careful evaluation of a pain management program's appropriateness for each patient with chronic pain is, of course, essential.

Ideally a pain clinic should be comprehensive and interdisciplinary and offer a wide range of treatment techniques. Provision for inpatient and outpatient clinical facilities combined with a commitment to education and research is optimal. In the organization of a typical pain clinic (Figure 43-3), the director provides overall leadership, and the coordinator is responsible for day-to-day management. The patient's manager is the attending physician. In smaller programs these positions may be combined into one or two positions.

The clinical team consists of a core group of personnel who regularly evaluate patients, set goals, treat patients, and evaluate treatment outcomes. These core personnel include a physician, psychologist, physical therapist, vocational counselor, occupational therapist, social services counselor, pharmacist, and rehabilitation nurse. They attend regular team conferences that select patients and monitor their progress. The physician leads the team, coordinates the program, and provides overall medical management to the patient. The psychosocial vocational team, consisting of the psychologist, social worker, and vocational counselor, provide leadership in the evaluation and treatment of the behavioral changes that are a result of chronic pain and provide appropriate vocational intervention. The therapy team, consisting of nursing, pharmacy, physical therapy, and occupational therapy personnel, provide daily therapy to control medical level, modulate pain level, and increase activity. Additional subspecialties are available on a consultative ba-

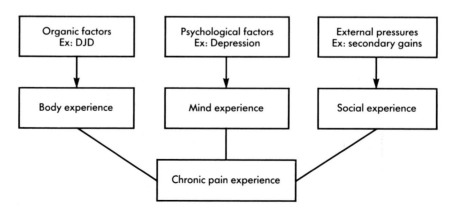

Figure 43-2. Chronic pain: interaction of organic, psychologic, and social factors.

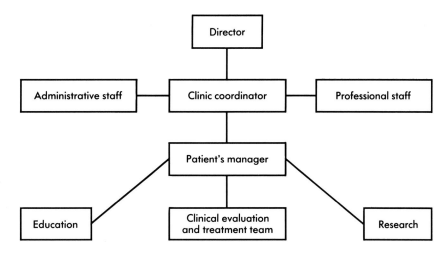

Figure 43-3. Organization of multidisciplinary pain clinic. (From Grabois, M: Ann Acad Med [Singapore] 12:430, 1983.)

sis; they include representatives from anesthesiology, neurosurgery, physical medicine and rehabilitation, psychiatry, recreational therapy, dietary, and biomedical engineering. The flowchart of patient care in a typical pain management program is depicted in Figure 43-4.

Referrals are accepted from medical and nonmedical sources. Appropriate past medical information must be supplied, and the patient should complete a pain evaluation form. Appropriate patients are those who demonstrate chronic pain, who are motivated to participate in the program, who do not have secondary gains that will make improvement unlikely, and who accept the concept and goals of the program.

EVALUATION

A comprehensive medical and psychosocial evaluation is necessary for every patient. It includes the following:

1. History—pain, drug, occupational, social, medical, psychologic
2. Physical examination—functional, musculoskeletal, neurologic
3. Psychologic—interview and Minnesota Multiphasic Personality Inventory (MMPI)
4. Special studies—radiographs, vascular studies, computerized tomographic (CT) scan, thermograms, electromyography and nerve conduction velocities (EMG/NCV), specialty consultation

Functional abilities and behavioral responses to pain must be fully evaluated. This type of evaluation is integrated into the usual model of history taking, examination by physician, ordering and assessing appropriate diagnostic tests, and formulating a diagnosis.[18] The evaluations should be as objective and quantitative as possible. As noted earlier, the patient's medical records must be obtained and reviewed, preferably before the evaluation. It is vital not to repeat

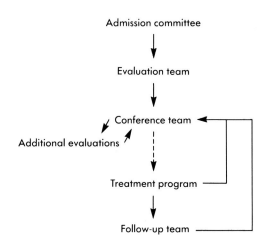

Figure 43-4. Pain clinic: patient flowchart.

evaluations already appropriately performed or to use evaluation techniques that have not proved effective. A pain questionnaire completed by the patient and reviewed before the examination is a helpful tool in the evaluation procedure.

The clinical history of the chronic pain patient should concentrate on the following: pain description (location, radiation characteristics, time sequence, what makes it worse and better, and activity level); pain evaluations (physicians, hospitalizations, and diagnostic tests performed); and past treatment (medical, surgical, and rehabilitative). The psychosocial evaluation should emphasize behavioral responses to pain, adjustments to impairment and disability, and motivation factors. The MMPI is the most frequently used psychologic test for evaluating the psychophysiologic components of the pain syndrome.[7] The typical chronic pain patient tends to have an increase in hypochondriasis, depression, and hysteria scales (Figure 43-5). Diagnostic studies should be considered an extension of the clinical evaluation. If appropriate studies have already been performed and eval-

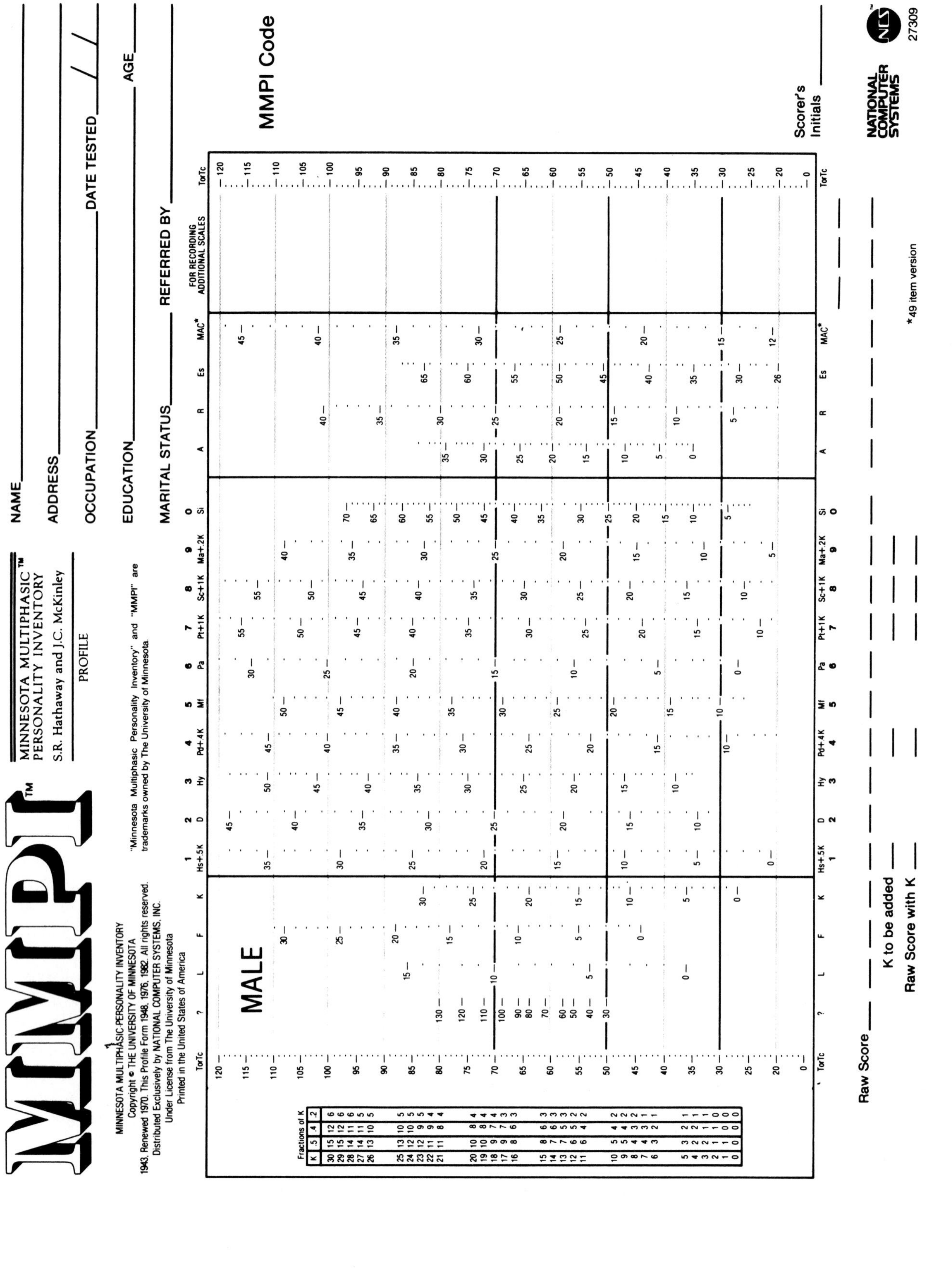

MMPI

MINNESOTA MULTIPHASIC
PERSONALITY INVENTORY

S.R. Hathaway and J.C. McKinley

PROFILE

"Minnesota Multiphasic Personality Inventory" and "MMPI" are
trademarks owned by The University of Minnesota.

MALE

NAME

ADDRESS

OCCUPATION ___ DATE TESTED __ / __ / __

EDUCATION ___ AGE ___

MARITAL STATUS ___ REFERRED BY

MMPI Code

FOR RECORDING
ADDITIONAL SCALES

Scorer's
Initials

Raw Score

K to be added

Raw Score with K

Fractions of K

*49 item version

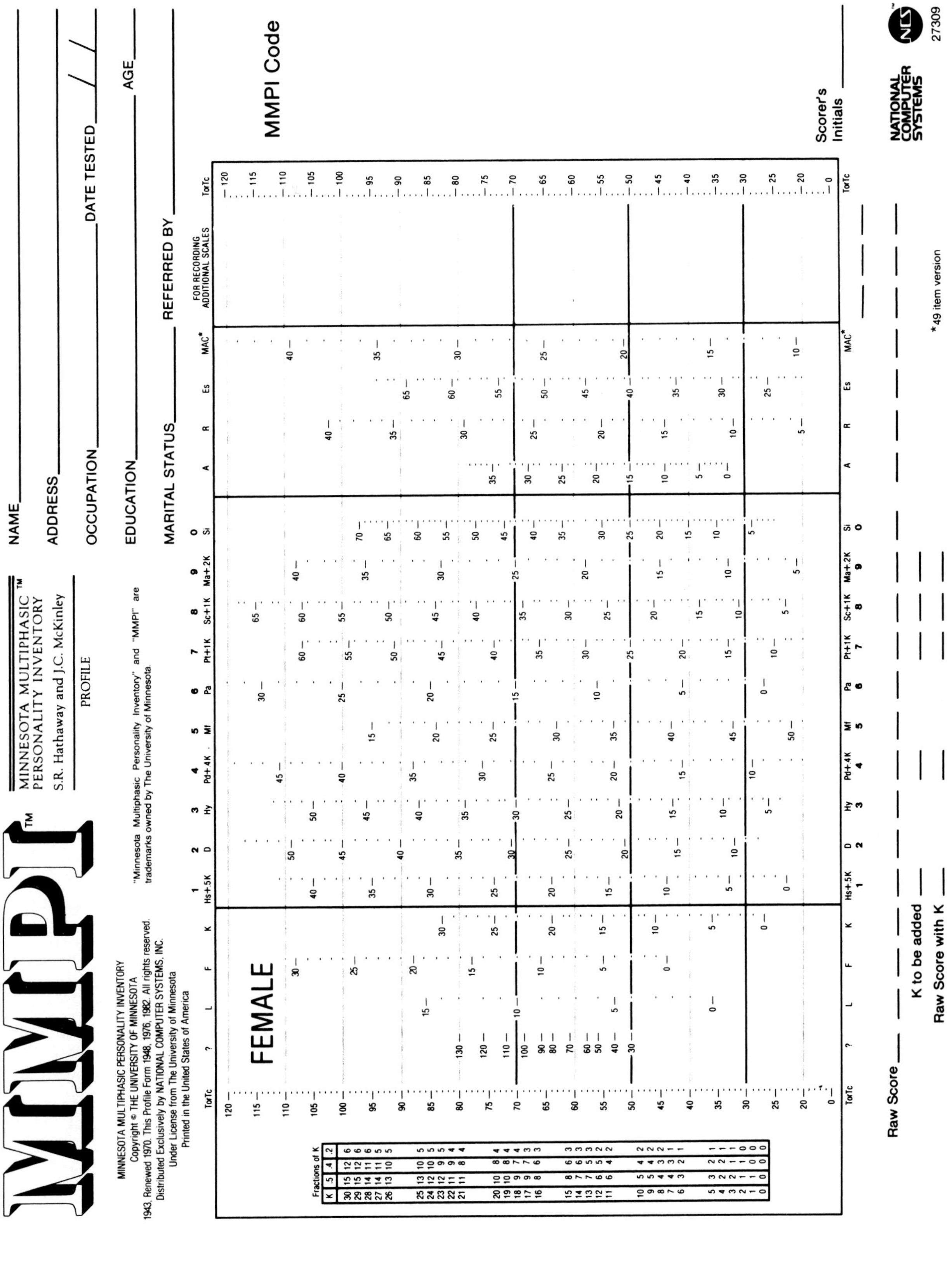

Figure 43-5. Minnesota Multiphasic Personality Inventory (MMPI) of typical chronic pain patient.

uated, it is rare to require additional testing unless there has been a change in the clinical evaluation.

PAIN MEASUREMENT

It is Reading's opinion that pain measurement is vital in the diagnosis and evaluation of the treatment techniques[15]; such procedures to quantify pain are critical if there is to be therapeutic and scientific progress. Without adequate methods for measurement, pain treatment will continue to be adopted and used without proper scientific evaluation. In addition, as pain clinics become more numerous and the evaluation and treatment of chronic pain more costly, the concept of cost effectiveness becomes more important. Scientifically established and proven assessment techniques are vital in evaluating alternative techniques for treating chronic pain that are less invasive, less extensive, and therefore less costly.[15]

Measurement of induced acute pain is easier than measurement of chronic pain. In laboratory-induced acute pain there are no emotional or cognitive factors, and the quantity of the pain stimulus is easily controlled. In the measurement and assessment of chronic pain, unfortunately, we do not have an acceptable laboratory model. A clear linear relationship between amount of noxious input and intensity of pain experience is not apparent in chronic pain. It is difficult to capture what is a very private sensory experience. Many times, all we have are the patients' words, their recollections of their experience, and the behavior exhibited when they have this private experience.

Sternbach and co-workers[20] noted that pain is a complex experience; evidence confirming it involves variation of several dimensions that depend on changing states and that are continuously influenced by a multitude of extrinsic and intrinsic stimuli. Fordyce described four main components of pain: nociceptive, sensation, suffering, and behavioral reactions.[4]

Using Sternbach's and Fordyce's concepts, three components of chronic pain measurement are noted: subjective, physiologic, and behavioral. The interaction between these components is dynamic and involves a balanced appraisal of sensory input and the degree to which this is modulated by psychologic factors, including other determinants of verbal and overt behavior. Of course, any scale must meet a few basic criteria, including ease of administration and scoring, potential for accurate use by a variety of health care professionals, high interrater reliability, and validity.

The subjective component of chronic pain measurement is reflected by rating scales, questionnaires, and diary cards. The Picaza Scale is an example of a rating scale used to measure chronic pain:

Limitation of activity	0->100
Waking hours with pain	0->100
Intensity of pain	0->100
Effect of pain on mood	0->100
Drug type and dosage	0->100

Questionnaires have gained wide acceptance. The McGill Pain Questionnaire is the best known and most popular.[12] It evaluates three major classes of word descriptions—sensory, affective, and evaluative—that patients use to specify the subjective pain experience and has a built-in intensity scale. Multiple reports in the literature evaluate this method of pain measurement, and it has been used extensively in clinical evaluation and treatment trials. Melzack and others[11] believe it provides a quantity of information that can be treated statistically and that is it sufficiently sensitive to detect differences among pain relief methods. Although physiologic techniques such as cortical evoked potential, muscle tension, vasodilatation, heart rate, and blood pressure have a firm scientific basis and have been used to measure pain in the laboratory, they have not been scientifically evaluated in the clinical setting.

Behavioral measurements of pain frequently advocated by Fordyce are logical techniques to measure pain, since people in pain must engage in behavior indicative of their state.[5] Most behavior measurement techniques use three categories of behvior: somatic intervention, impaired functional capacity, and pain complaints. The University of Alabama behavioral measurement of pain is based on 10 behaviors such as vocalization and the frequency and intensity of these expressions.[17] Although theoretically this technique is more ideal than the others noted, there are problems with correlation between behavior and other rating techniques and methods of collection of data (indirect versus direct). Although interobserver reliability is good, many trained observers and many observations are needed to obtain appropriate information.

Clearly there is no ideal method to evaluate and measure chronic pain and its treatment techniques. Measurements that reflect subjective, physiologic, and behavioral components with independent and direct monitoring are most appropriate. Reading[15] has said that behavioral indexes may assume greater importance as chronicity increases, since the question of how much the patient is able to do rather than how much it hurts may be the more important question in a chronic pain management setting. This is especially true when considering the cost effectiveness of pain management programs.[15]

TREATMENT APPROACHES

If the concept of chronic pain as previously described is accepted, the Fordyce model of behavioral modification becomes very appealing.[3] The goal in these patients is not to cure the individual of the pain but to interrupt the pain behavioral reinforcement cycle by rewarding healthy behavior and appropriate goal setting that the patient must achieve. The emphasis of the program is to reduce medication, modulate pain response, increase activity, and modify pain behaviors.[7]

Medication management

Physicians and the patients they serve have a long history of inappropriate medication use (Figure 43-6), particularly with narcotic medications. Studies show that patients are usually inadequately treated for acute pain syndromes and overtreated for chronic ones.[16] In addition, some physicians mistakenly think that giving medication as needed will result in less addiction. Lastly, physicians tend to incorrectly place placebo responders in the nonorganic category of pain.

The goal in the medication management of a patient with chronic pain is to reduce and eliminate narcotics, tranquilizers, and hypnotic medications. This approach usually requires an in-hospital or day-hospital program. No injectable medications are allowed; patients are switched to an oral preparation as soon as possible. Patients are initially allowed to take their current oral medications on as needed basis with strict record keeping. No new narcotics, tranquilizers, or hypnotics should be prescribed. Once the 24-hour baseline requirement for the individual is obtained over a few days, a "pain cocktail" approach is used on a time-contingent basis, and the active ingredient is gradually reduced (Table 43-1). The pain cocktail consists of metradone or a similar preparation in an equivalent dose equal to the currently used narcotic medication in a masking vehicle (for example, cherry syrup). The cocktail is given around the clock at an interval the patient has already demonstrated is required. Gradual reduction of the active ingredient with equal increase in the masking vehicle is carried out over 3 to 6 weeks; decrements are made slowly so as not to elicit withdrawal signs and symptoms. Figure 43-7 compares the pain cocktail approach with the medication as needed method. When the individual is receiving the masking vehicle only, the cocktail is discontinued. All information is shared with the individual before the program begins, except the time when the active ingredients will be reduced. This approach can also be used for tranquilizers and hypnotics as well as for narcotic medications.

Chronic nonmalignant pain is frequently accompanied by depression, and therefore antidepressants have been reported to be effective when this association exists.[6] Although not well defined, the mechanism of action may involve blockade of the pain-anxiety-depression pain sequence seen in patients with chronic pain.[16] It has also been suggested that these medications can act synergistically with current pain medication; in addition, one can take advantage of their sedative

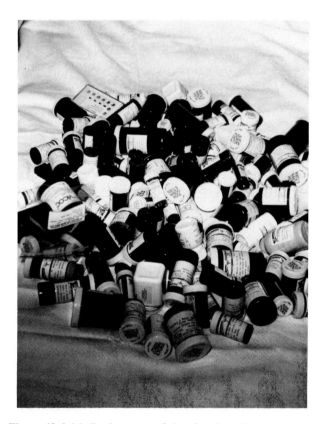

Figure 43-6. Medication usage of chronic pain patient over 1-year period.

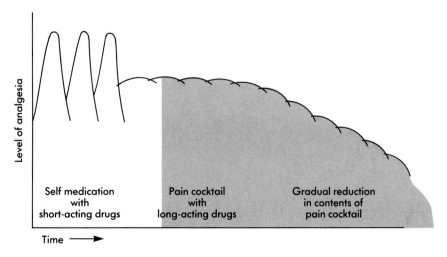

Figure 43-7. Pain cocktail approach: comparison of as needed and around-the-clock approaches.

Table 43-1. Sample pain cocktail regimen

Inpatient days		Pain cocktail format
1-6	*Baseline:*	Patient reports preadmission pattern of "one or two of the 50 mg tablets of Demerol two or three times a day, as needed, at home."
		Physician orders to nurse: "May have Demerol, *prn* pain, not to exceed three 50 mg tablets every 3 hours. Carefully record amount taken."
		Analysis of baseline data: Patient averaged 600 mg of Demerol per 24-hour period, averaging of 3- to 4-hour intervals between requests.
7-9 *First cocktail*		
	℞ *to pharmacists:*	Demerol, 1920 mg
		Bevisol, Plebex, or other liquid B complex, 12 ml; cherry syrup qs 240 ml
	Sig:	Pain cocktail, 10 ml po q3h, day and night, *not prn*
	Nursing order:	Pain cocktail, 10 ml po q3h, day and night, *not prn*

Since contents of the pain cocktail are not on the label, a copy of the prescription must be kept in a separate pain cocktail book.

10-12		Decrease each daily total by 64 mg, ¹⁄₁₀ or original amount. A 3-day ℞ is decreased by 64 × 3 or 192 mg.
	℞ *to pharmacists:*	Demerol, 1728 mg
		Bevisol, Plebex, or other liquid B complex, 12 ml; cherry syrup qs 240 ml
	Sig:	Pain cocktail, 10 ml po q3h, day and night, *not prn*
	Nursing order:	Pain cocktail, 10 ml po q3h, day and night, *not prn*
13-15	℞ *to pharmacists:*	Demerol, 1536 mg
		Bevisol, Plebex, or other liquid B complex, 12 ml; cherry syrup qs 240 ml
	Sig:	Pain cocktail, 10 ml po q3h, day and night, *not prn*
	Nursing order:	Pain cocktail, 10 ml po q3h, day and night, *not prn*
16-18	℞ *to pharmacists:*	Demerol, 1344 mg
		Bevisol, Plebex, or other liquid B complex, 12 ml; cherry syrup qs 240 ml
	Sig:	Pain cocktail, 10 ml po q3h, day and night, *not prn*
	Nursing order:	Pain cocktail, 10 ml po q3h, day and night, *not prn*
19-21	℞ *to pharmacists:*	Demerol, 1152 mg
		Bevisol, Plebex, or other liquid B complex, 12 ml; cherry syrup qs 240 ml
	Sig:	Pain cocktail, 10 ml po q3h, day and night, *not prn*
	Nursing order:	Pain cocktail, 10 ml po q3h, day and night, *not prn*
22-24	℞ *to pharmacists:*	Demerol 960 mg
		Bevisol, Plebex, or other liquid B complex, 12 ml; cherry syrup qs 240 ml
	Sig:	Pain cocktail, 10 ml po q3h, day and night, *not prn*
	Nursing order:	Pain cocktail, 10 ml po q3h, day and night, *not prn*
37-39	℞ *to pharmacists:*	Demerol 0 mg
		Bevisol, Plebex, or other liquid B complex, 12 ml; cherry syrup qs 240 ml
	Sig:	Pain cocktail, 10 ml po q3h, day and night, *not prn*
	Nursing order:	Pain cocktail, 10 ml po q3h, day and night, *not prn*

(Maintain patient on vehicle for 2 to 10 days; if all is going well, inform patient and ask if continuation of vehicle is desired.)

From Fordyce, WE: Behavioral methods for chronic pain and illness, St. Louis, 1979, The CV Mosby Co.

side effects by ordering their administration at bedtime as substitutions for hypnotic medication. Dosages smaller than those used to treat pure depressive states are often effective. Kanner[10] believes that judiciously used, these agents, particularly the tricyclic antidepressants, can lead to a smoother course for the patient with chronic pain. Nonsteroidal anti-inflammatory drugs and muscle relaxants can be used if necessary during and after the pain management program.

Pain modulation

Pain modulation or reduction rather than pain elimination is a more realistic goal in treating chronic pain patients. Although a few appropriately treated patients eliminate their pain complaints, such occurrences are rare. Obviously, a procedure or technique that has this potential benefit should be presented to the patient and a trial should be attempted before involvement in a behavioral modification pain management program.

Guidelines for using methods that modulate chronic pain are the ability of the patient to use it in the home setting, an active rather than passive nature, and use for the shortest time possible with gradual decrease in the interval it is used.

Two of the most frequently used modalities that fall within these criteria are transcutaneous electrical nerve stimulation (TENS) and biofeedback. TENS stimulates the afferent peripheral nerves to modify the pain sensation level (Figure 43-8). This result may be caused by a direct effect on the electrical current of the afferent stimulated peripheral nerve, modulation of pain in the dorsal horn of the spinal cord, or activation of the supraspinal inhibition system by the gate or endorphin theory of pain. Patient selection criteria for TENS follow:

I. Type of pain
   A. Best response
      1. Neurogenic (peripheral)
      2. Musculoskeletal
      3. Neurogenic (central)
   B. Least response—psychogenic
II. Duration of pain—best results obtained when TENS begins soon after the onset of pain, especially in peripheral nerve lesions
III. Effect of other therapy—best results reported when the patient has had minimal prior intervention
IV. Psychologic factors
   A. Best response
      1. No psychopathologic signs
      2. Reactive decompensation
      3. Situational problems
      4. Pathologic personality
   B. Least response—mental illness

Contraindications in placement of the stimulators include over the carotid sinus, pregnant uterus, eye, and anterior chest wall in patients with cardiac problems and patients with cardiac pacemakers. In a number of instances skin may be irritated by electrical, chemical, allergenic, and mechanical stimuli. Guidelines for the use of the TENS units include an appropriate education in its usage and a trial period before purchase (Table 43-2). TENS effectiveness decreases significantly over time, and a high placebo effect has been noted in the literature.[23]

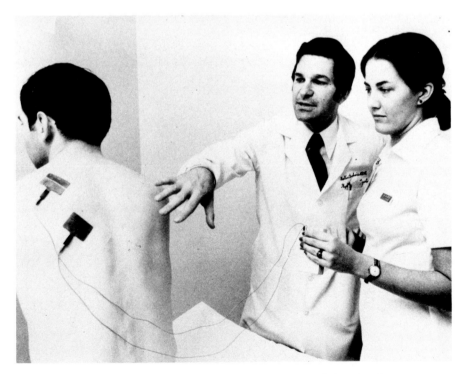

Figure 43-8. Transcutaneous electrical nerve stimulation (TENS).

Table 43-2. Guidelines for using TENS

	TENS mode		
	Conventional	**Low rate**	**Brief, intense**
Modulation mode	Modulated rate	Burst	Modulated amplitude
Pulse frequency	High (50 to 100 pps*)	Low (1 to 5 pps)	High (100 to 150 pps)
Pulse width	Narrow (30 to 200 μs)	Wide (200 to 500 μs)	Wide (250 to 500 μs)
Pulse amplitude	10 to 40 mA	50 to 100 mA	50 to 100 mA
Treatment duration	As needed (but not recommended during sleep)	30 min	15 to 30 min
Onset of relief	Less than 10 min	20 to 40 min	Less than 5 min
Duration of relief	Minutes to hours	Hours to days	Less than 30 min
Clinical applications	All types of pain (especially musculoskeletal pain); acute soft tissue injury; postoperative surgical pain; headaches/temporomandibular joint pain; lumbar/cervical spondylosis; osteoarthritis; radiating pain; tendinitis/bursitis; fibrositis/myofascial pain syndrome	Chronic pain; deep structural pain; fibrositis/myofascial pain syndrome; reflex sympathetic dystrophy; muscle spasms	Temporary analgesia before joint mobilization or therapeutic exercise

From Bechtel, T, and Fan, PT: Musculoskel Med, November 1985, p 41.
*pps, Pulses per second.

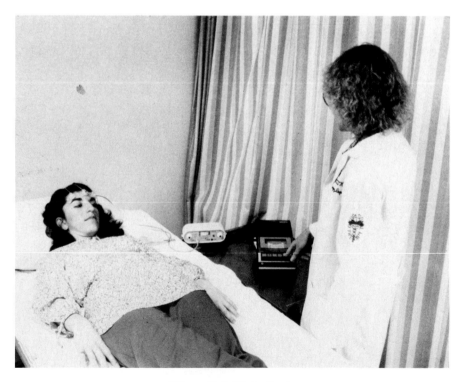

Figure 43-9. Biofeedback.

Biofeedback techniques have been increasingly used in the management of chronic pain because research has shown that the information feedback is powerful enough to teach humans autonomic and somatic control (Figure 43-9).[16] This technique has modified the pain response by assisting the patient in reducing anxiety, in learning to use self-control, and in learning about the mind-body relationship.[13] Biofeedback works by augmenting relaxation or altering specific physiologic functions by providing the patient with instantaneous feedback of a physiologic function, which is then presented to the patient as visual or auditory feedback. Results of treatment vary from individual to individual and are most likely secondary to compliance, course of disease, influence of secondary gains, and length of follow-up.[13] The most successful responders seem to be individuals with tension headache, neck pain, and Raynaud's disease. Biofeedback has also been suggested to promote better sleeping patterns with subsequent reduction of hypnotic medication.

A number of other modalities have been suggested to help patients with chronic pain:
1. Nerve blocks
2. Trigger point injections and spray and stretch techniques
3. Acupuncture—hyperstimulation
4. Hypnotherapy—learned state of selective concentration
5. Mobilization/manipulation
   a. Stretch muscle tendons
   b. Alteration of lumbar articular facets
6. Surgical treatment—rhizotomy to cordotomy

If they can help break an acute pain symptom superimposed on the chronic pain problems, and make it possible to begin an appropriate treatment program, or both, they may have some value.

Increased activity

Patients with chronic pain generally exhibit varying degrees of immobilization and resultant deconditioning. Appropriate exercises that are specific for the area involved with pain (Williams' flexion exercises for low back pain), and general conditioning exercise such as bicycling, ambulation, and swimming are indicated. Fordyce[3] noted that to be appropriate in a behavior modification program the exercise must be pain relevant or limitation relevant, quantifiable, visible, and accessible. A baseline of appropriate exercises is achieved by asking the patient to exercise to tolerance (until pain, weakness, or fatigue necessitates stopping) over a few days.[3] Once the baseline has been established, the initial goal is programmed within the patient's tolerance and then gradually increased, with new goals being set every few days (Figure 43-10). Rewards and reinforcement are given for accomplishing the established goals without pain behavior. In some patients, however, it is important to reduce excessive activity levels by teaching them to pace themselves more appropriately.

Behavior modification and management of psychosocial and vocational issues

The psychosocial and vocational component of the behavioral management program involves the individual, family, employer, and pain management team. Depression, if present, should be treated with appropriate antidepressant medication, involvement in an active program, and psychotherapy if necessary. Pain behavior is managed by a

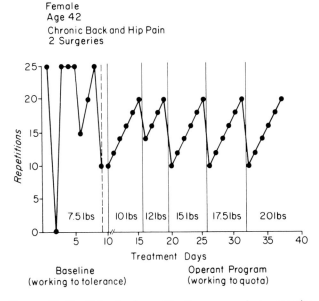

Figure 43-10. Behavioral modification approach to exercise. (From Fordyce, WE: Behavioral methods for chronic pain and illness, St. Louis, 1976, The CV Mosby Co.)

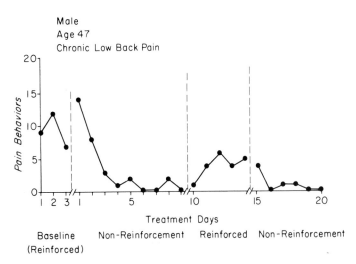

Figure 43-11. Pain behavior: modification by nonreinforcement. (From Fordyce, WE: Behavioral methods for chronic pain and illness, St. Louis, 1976, The CV Mosby Co.)

neutral response to it and a positive response to well be-havior (Figure 43-11). This often involves developing an insight into the patient's behavioral or coping mechanisms and modifying them to increase the rate of desired behavior change. The behavior should be followed systematically by effective positive reinforcement such as praise and rewards when the patient's behavior is positive.[16] To decrease un-wanted behavior, the principle of extinction by withdrawing attention and sympathy for unwanted behavior can be used.[16]

RESULTS

In discussing the results of the pain management program it is important to measure them in objective and quantifiable terms. These measurements include medication, walking distance, strength, flexibility, sitting tolerance, pain behav-iors, vocational placement, and use of health care resources. In addition, in comparing one program to another, it is important to evaluate each program in terms of type of patient accepted, type of treatment offered, criteria for im-provement, and follow-up time. Patients who are ideal can-didates can achieve an 80% to 90% success rate. As the incidence of psychosocial problems and secondary gain is-sues increase, however, this rate is reduced to 40% to 50%, and with major psychiatric or secondary gains, the success rate drops to 20% or less.[8] Steig and co-workers[19] have devised a limited but useful model for determining and dem-onstrating the cost benefit of a pain management program. The cost to the insurance carrier of supporting the patient now and in the future is compared with the cost of the pain management program and the saving to be achieved by de-creased use of health-care personnel, facilities, and medi-cation and by returning to work.

SUMMARY

If one understands the concept of chronic pain and its physical and behavioral components, a program that uses an interdisciplinary comprehensive team concept with a be-havioral modification approach becomes a realistic method of treatment. However, one must perform a complete eval-uation of the individual and treat appropriately contributing causes of the chronic pain syndrome. The goal of the pro-gram presented here is to keep patients' sickness and pain from being the central point of their lives. By emphasizing well behavior the program teaches patients to live with pain rather than merely exist with it.

REFERENCES

1. Bonica JJ: Preface. In Ng, LKY, editor: New approaches to treatment of chronic pain: a review of multidisciplinary pain clinics and pain centers, Rockville, Md, 1981, National Institute on Drug Abuse Re-search Monograph 36.
2. Brena, SF: Pain control facilities: roots, organization and function. In Brena, SF, and Champman, SL, editors: Management of patients with chronic pain, New York, 1983, Spectrum Publications, Inc.
3. Fordyce, WE: Behavioral methods for chronic pain and illness, St. Louis, 1976, The CV Mosby Co.
4. Fordyce WE: The validity of pain behavior measurement. In Melzack, R, editor: Pain measurement and assessment, New York, 1983, Raven Press.
5. Fordyce, WE, et al: Pain measurement and pain behavior, Pain 18:53, 1984.
6. Getto, CJ, Sorkness, CA, and Howell, T: Anti-depressants and chronic non-malignant pain: a review, Pain Symptom Manage 2:9, 1987.
7. Grabois, M: Comprehensive evaluation and management of patients with chronic pain, Cardiovasc Res Center Bull 19:113, 1981.
8. Grabois, M: Pain clinics: role in rehabilitation of patients with chronic pain, Ann Acad Med (Singapore) 12:428, 1983.
9. Greehhott, JD, and Sternbach, RA: Conjoint treatment of chronic pain, Advan Neurol 4:595, 1974.
10. Kanner, R: Psychotropic drugs in the management of pain, Curr Con-cepts Pain 1:11, 1983.
11. Melzack, R: Measurement of the dimensions of pain experience, in, Bram EV, editor: Pain measurement in man: neurophysiological cor-relates of pain, New York, 1984, Elsevier Science Publishers.
12. Melzack, R: The McGill pain questionnaire: major properties and scoring methods, Pain 1:277, 1975.
13. Pawlicki, RE, and Hovanitz, C: Biofeedback. In Raj, PP, editor: Practical management of pain, Chicago/London, 1986, Year Book Medical Publishers.
14. Raj PP: Epidemiology of pain. In Raj, PP, editor: Practical manage-ment of pain, Chicago/London, 1986, Year Book Medical Publishers.
15. Reading, AE: Testing pain mechanisms in persons in pain. In Wall, PD, and Melzack, R, editors: Textbook of pain. Edinburgh, London, Melbourne, and New York, 1984, Churchill-Livingstone.
16. Reuler, J, Girard D, and Nardone, D: The chronic pain syndrome: misconceptions and management, Ann Intern Med 93:588, 1980.
17. Richards, JS, et al: Assessing pain behavior: the UAB pain behavior scale, Pain 14:393, 1982.
18. Savitz, D: Medical evaluation of the chronic pain patient. In Aronoff, GM, editor: Evaluation and treatment of chronic pain, Baltimore/Munich, 1985, Urban & Schqarzenberg.
19. Steig, RL, Williams, RC, and Gallagher, LA: Multidisciplinary pain treatment centers, J Occupat Med 23:94, 1981.
20. Sternbach, RA, et al: On the sensitivity of the tourniquet pain test, Pain 3:105, 1977.
21. Swanson, DW, Floreen, AC, and Swenson, WM: Programs for man-aging chronic pain. II. Short term results, Mayo Clin Proc 51:409, 1979.
22. Swanson, DW, et al: Program for managing chronic pain. I. Program description and characteristics of patients, Mayo Clin Proc 51:401, 1976.
23. Thorsteinsson, G, et al: The placebo effect on transcutaneous electrical stimulation, Pain 5:31, 1978.

CHAPTER 44

Muscle pain

HANS KRAUS

The four distinct problems with muscle that involve pain can be differentiated as spasm, tension, muscle deficiency (stiffness and weakness), and trigger points. Proper treatment depends on recognizing the clinical aspects of each of these four groups.

SPASM

Muscle spasm is most frequently characterized by acute onset, painful involuntary contraction that limits motion, great intensity, and incapacity to function. The affected muscles may be tender to the touch, although tenderness is not necessarily localized. Any attempt to move increases pain.

Since immobilization relieves pain, at least temporarily, muscle spasm has often been called "protective," and management has consisted chiefly of immobilization or traction. The rationale, especially in the case of injury, was that immobilization would not only relieve pain but also enhance healing.

This theory was contradicted in 1932 by Kowalski, an athletic coach who would send his patients with fractures to our institution but never those with muscle strain, minor ligament tear, or sprain, for he had learned that immediate motion would restore function more quickly and effectively than immobilization. He used to wrap the injured extremity or joint in an alcohol-soaked towel, expose it to live steam, and take advantage of the ensuing numbness and insensitivity to initiate active motion. When this process was repeated several times a day and combined with rest, the patient experienced immediate relief without the then customary prolonged immobilization.

When we tried this procedure on two young men who had sprained their ankles skiing, we were surprised to note how rapidly and completely function was restored. We then started experimenting with various coolants. Ethyl chloride proved to be the most effective agent for producing temporary anesthesia of a joint or muscle.[10-12,23] Although we tried other coolant sprays such as Fluorimethane, ice,[24] and ice massage,[25] ethyl chloride was superior and far easier to handle. Although ethyl chloride is flammable and a general anesthetic when inhaled, our patients never experienced any untoward effect. In fact, we frequently gave or prescribed ethyl chloride to patients for home use with the proper exercise.

In recent experiments with rabbits, Salter and co-workers[20] showed that an injured knee healed most quickly when the joint was moved passively without weight bearing. Rabbits that were neither immobilized nor treated fared less well, but not as poorly as those whose joints were immobilized. The latter lost a significant degree of function and suffered severe cartilage degeneration. Dovelle and Heeter[4] described speedier and more complete recovery early with controlled mobilization after extensor tendon repair.

Essential to this approach is controlled exercise. Spray or ice makes movement possible by relieving pain. The combination of pain relief with exercise is crucial to a desirable result.

Ruskin[18] has been successful in breaking muscle spasm by the cocainization of the sphenopalatine ganglion. Here again, the relief of pain makes normal function possible and eliminates the need for immobilization.

Details of exercises are mentioned later in the chapter in connection with muscle deficiency. Exertion must be avoided. Weight bearing is not permitted. For spasm of the upper extremity, the patient can wear a sling and remove it frequently for exercise periods. For pain in a lower extremity, the patient can use crutches until able to walk without pain or limping.

The indications for treatment are any muscle spasm not caused by major pathology, ligament tears not resulting in instability, and back and neck muscle spasm of muscular origin (these represent a majority of back pain injuries). Strains to muscles of the extremity, such as calf muscle, hamstring, deltoid, and triceps, respond well.

Icing with compression and elevation is less effective because it does not allow mobilization. Mobilization—movement—should commence as soon as possible. Early mobilization is especially important for the patient with an acute back injury or an acute "stiff neck" for whom rest, braces, or collars are still the most common methods of treatment. We try to keep patients ambulatory. A patient with acute back pain, for instance, may come in for treatment and then go home or even return to work if the problem is not severe. Otherwise, the patient may need to use a coolant, preferably ethyl chloride, several times a day, do simple limbering and relaxing exercises, and return for treatment daily.

The average back pain usually responds within a week. Then the patient should be evaluated and examined carefully, especially in chronic cases in which muscle stiffness and weakness, tension, and trigger points are frequently present and the acute attack is usually one of several episodes. At this time it is necessary to take a thorough history of the patient's activities, sports, hobbies, and emotional and situational stresses to help establish the original causes of the problem. A patient who has a stiff neck from squeezing the telephone between neck and ear several hours a day never escapes recurrence unless this habit is abandoned (by using a speaker or earphones).[11] A runner who never warms up or relaxes and stretches before running will strain the calf or hamstring muscles if he or she continues to ignore proper preparation and cool-off.[12]

The effect of ethyl chloride and gentle controlled motion can be greatly enhanced by using 10 minutes of tetanizing current to fatigue the muscle and then 10 minutes of sinusoidal current to restore the muscle's ability to contract and relax. For injuries of the extremities we apply sinusoidal current only.

The general indications for treatment with ethyl chloride and controlled mobilization are as follows:

1. Sprains
   a. Ankle
   b. Knee
2. Strains
   a. Low back
   b. Neck
   c. Upper and lower extremities
3. Fractures
   a. Thoracic and lumbar spine
   b. Pelvis (os pubis)
   c. "Intraboot" fractures
   d. Tip, external malleolus
   e. Head of humerus, imp.
   f. Metacarpals

A time-honored way to relieve muscle spasm is with hot packs, most commonly Kenny packs. A towel soaked in boiling water should be wrung out and applied to the painful area. Gentle exercises must follow to make this procedure worthwhile. We do not apply heat or hot packs for injuries of the extremities, especially in acute or subacute cases, because the influx of blood may produce further swelling. Heat can be applied, however, in the chronic phase.

TENSION

The modern way of life forces people to suppress the fight-or-flight response[1] with its instinctive tensing of muscles to get ready for action. When the fight-or-flight response has no outlet, especially among sedentary people, hypokinetic diseases result, for example, ulcers, high blood pressure, and obesity[15] (in addition to tension—of prime interest here).

People who typically experience tension are those in hectic occupations with deadlines, those whose sedentary work forces them to remain in one position for long periods of time, and those who are beset by constant irritants. Patients with emotional problems may experience tension syndromes without external situational or activity stresses. Most frequently physicians see a combination of both: people who are emotionally unstable or under emotional strain and who are also exposed to outside stresses. One of the most common producers of stress is the automobile; tension in the neck or upper back can often be traced to driving, particularly in heavy traffic.

Tension can be treated by alleviating stress, by medication, or by relaxation exercises (see "Muscle Deficiency"). The physician should explore and correct, where possible, situational and postural stress. Tension pain, as in tension headache, neck, and back, responds readily to tranquilizers. Muscle spasm does not respond to tranquilizers or other medication, which only masks pain. Relaxation exercises are essential in beginning any exercise program or warm-up and stretching program for an active or athletic person. More injuries occur when stretching exercises are done without adequate prior relaxation than the stretching actually can prevent. Relaxation exercises are meant to teach the patient how to "let go."

Relaxation exercises are of various types. In the Jacobson exercises, for instance, the patient is asked to make a movement, such as lift the hand and let it drop, to acquire the feel of relaxing a muscle.[9] We usually employ a supine breathing and relaxing program. We have the patient lie comfortably supine, with pillows under the knees. The patient is asked to take a deep breath and slowly exhale, draw up the shoulders to the ears and let go, drop the head left and then right and let go, let go of one arm and then the other, and let go of one leg and then the other. With the eyes closed, the patient concentrates on breathing, slowly inhaling and exhaling. This exercise requires at least 5 to 10 minutes and sometimes longer.

An excellent way to teach relaxation is by hypnosis, pro-

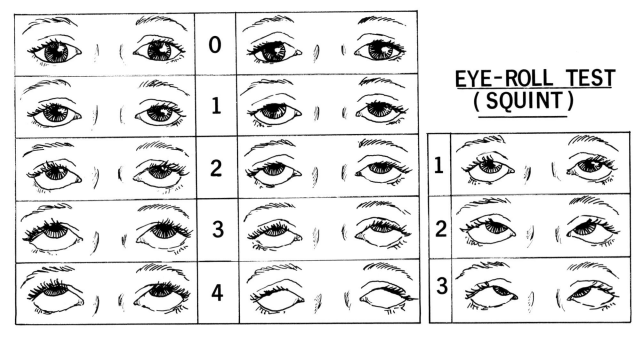

Figure 44-1. Eye-roll test for hypnotizability. (From Spiegel, H, and Spiegel, D: Trance and treatment: clinical uses of hypnosis, New York, 1978, Basic Books.)

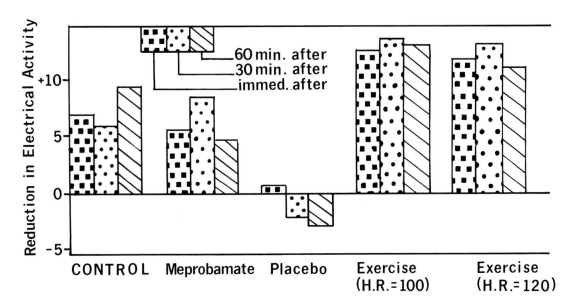

Figure 44-2. Electromyographic comparison of effect of single doses of exercises and meprobamate on muscle relaxation. (From DeVries, HA, and Adams, GM: Am J Phys Med 51:130, 1972.)

vided the patient is hypnotizable. We test all patients for hypnotizability with Spiegel's eye-roll test (Figure 44-1).[22] The hypnotizable patient can often reduce tension in the middle of the day by self-inducing a trance. This trance may last for just a minute or two and can be produced almost anywhere without being obvious. Brief as the interruption may be, the patient may begin tensing again when he or she returns to activity.

If local tension pain is not present or has been relieved, physical activity is an excellent way to alleviate general tension. We can think of it as a vicarious physical outlet that we are denied in our daily stressful occupations. DeVries and Adams[3] have shown that a sprint that raises the pulse rate to 100 or 110 beats per minute is far more relaxing than meprobamate (Figure 44-2).

Sainsbury and associates[19] demonstrated that tension caused by a stressful interview can in turn cause pain that registers on the electromyogram (EMG) in areas such as the frontalis muscle in the forearm group. It was obvious that pain set in when the interview caused the patient enough stress to respond with tension. Administering a tranquilizer resulted in relief lasting 2 or 3 hours.

Tension frequently accompanies an acute episode and can lead to muscle spasm. If spasm is associated with tension, administering a tranquilizer to the patient before the spasm is treated can be extremely effective. Although patients should not be given tranquilizers for extended periods, temporarily prescribing one may be necessary.

MUSCLE DEFICIENCY

Muscles perform in only two ways: they contract or they relax. Both aspects of muscle function are equally important. The inability to contract a muscle constitutes weakness. The inability to "decontract," or relax, a muscle signifies tightness and stiffness. Muscles that are weak or stiff, that lack strength or flexibility, are considered deficient (Table 44-1).[11] Certain conditions interfere with a muscle's ability to decontract. Prolonged contraction, often resulting from immobilization or maintaining a fixed position for an inordinate time, produces contracture, or permanent shortening of the muscle.

Beyond its physiologic ability to relax, a muscle can yield to passive stretch; however, such stretching may be ineffective and even traumatic if the muscle is not actively relaxed first.

Muscle deficiency itself can be a source of pain. For example, weakening of abdominal muscles through pregnancy can bring on back pain. Premature walking after immobilization of the lower extremity or premature exertion after immobilization of the upper extremity may cause pain by overloading the extremity and overstretching tight muscles.

The remedy for muscle deficiency is therapeutic exercise. Before prescribing an exercise program, the physician must

Table 44-1. Basic qualities of muscle function

Physiology	Dysfunction	Therapy
Strength Total elasticity	Weakness	Strengthening exercises
Physiologic elasticity	Spasm	Local relaxing exercises and relief of pain
	Tension	General relaxing exercise and relief of sources of tension
Physical elasticity	Contracture	Stretching exercises

determine the type and degree of muscle deficiency. Strength of extremities is graded in percentile of expected normal strength. Contracture is measured in degrees short of full range.

For back problems we use the Kraus-Weber Minimum Muscular Function tests (Figure 44-3) to determine exercises during the acute phase. Basic rules are as follows[11,13,14]:

1. Do not start an exercise program for back, neck, or extremities without first relaxing the patient and especially the affected area.

2. Begin with general relaxation exercise. Have the patient lie down with a pillow under the knees and with eyes closed. Ask the patient to breathe deeply and exhale slowly through the mouth, pull up the shoulders and let loose, drop the neck to the left and then to the right, and let the whole body go limp. Then have the patient make a fist, tighten one arm, and let go, repeat with the other arm, and then tighten each leg and let go (relaxation by contrast). Continue these relaxation techniques as long as necessary to put the patient in a reasonably relaxed state (Figure 44-4).

3. Follow with limbering movements, that is, movements within easy range. In a knee joint that requires stretching of the flexors, before beginning to stretch have the patient gently bend and extend to the present range without attempting to exceed that range. Have a patient with back pain lie supine with both knees flexed and then bend and extend the knee well within easy range. Then have the patient perform the same movement, again well within easy range, while lying on one side.

4. After these limbering exercises, add gentle strengthening exercises as a warm-up. When strengthening is the main objective, these gentle strengthening exercises should be gradually increased with incremental small loads until they approach the patient's maximum potential. If stretching is indicated, follow only gentle strengthening exercises. Ballistic stretching should be

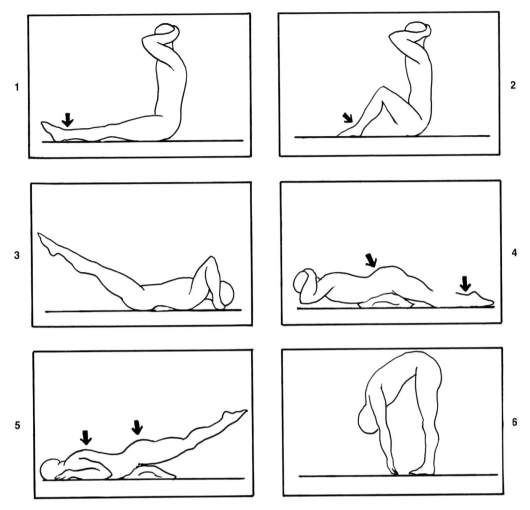

Figure 44-3. Tests to evaluate minimum muscular fitness. **1,** Sit up from prone position, hands behind head, legs straight, and ankles held down. **2,** Repeat, same position with knees flexed. **3,** Raise both legs straight to 30-degree angle and hold for 10 seconds. **4,** Lie prone with pillow under hips, keep trunk raised, hands behind neck, hold for 10 seconds. **5,** Lie prone with pillow under hips. Raise both legs. **6,** With knees straight, slowly reach toward floor. Arrows indicate point at which individual's body is stabilized by another person.

avoided. The stretch movement should slightly exceed the patient's present range. Although it may be uncomfortable, the movement should not be painful. Active stretches, that is, stretches performed by the patient, should start the program. This step is followed by stretches that involve resisting the antagonist of the tight muscles (reflex and relaxation). Finally, a gentle, passive stretch at the extreme range is added.

After maximum stretching, the program should be performed in reverse order, ending with relaxation exercises.

Since multiple repetitions stiffen and tire muscles, they should be avoided. We prefer three or four repetitions of each movement at a time. If more are required to produce strength and stretching, we repeat the entire procedure sev-

eral times, working back and forth until the patient begins to tire. We do not push for fatigue, and we add both resistance and stretching gradually. A program that follows this approach, *The Y's Way to a Healthy Back,* has achieved high success, with improvement among 82% of 12,000 participants.[14]

Movements should be slow and deliberate through the full available range. A brief instant of complete relaxation should occur between movements. Manual resistance should be provided whenever possible. For homework, that is, work between treatments, weights may be used.[11] These weights can be increased gradually but should not exceed present potential. A slight overload brings about increased strength[8] and a slight overstretch affords greater flexibility, but too

Figure 44-4. Basic back exercises for acute episode of back pain. Use exercises 1 to 4 at first, then add 5 and 6.

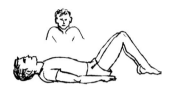

Exercise 1
Take a deep breath, then exhale slowly. Now, shrug and breathe in. Exhale as you let go of the shrug.

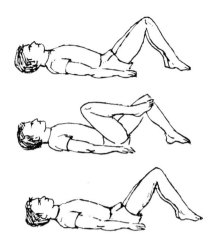

Exercise 2
Position yourself comfortably with your back on the floor and both knees bent. Close your eyes. Take a deep breath and exhale slowly. Slide your right leg forward and then slide it back. Slide the left leg forward and then back. Take another deep breath. Tighten both fists, then let go.

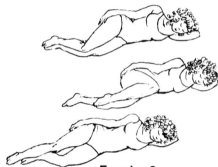

Exercise 3
Lie on your left side with your head resting comfortably on your arm. Keep both knees flexed and hips slightly flexed. Slide your right knee as close to your head as is comfortably possible, then slowly extend the leg until it is completely straight. The leg is dead weight; you do not lift your right leg, slide it on the left leg. Do the exercise three times, then turn to your right side and repeat the exercise with your left leg. Remember, *the top leg is dead weight*.

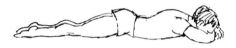

Exercise 4
Lie on your stomach. Let your head rest comfortably on your folded hands and point your toes inward. Now, tighten your seat muscles. Hold that position for two seconds, then let go.

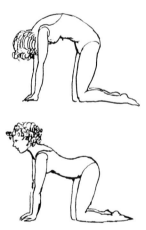

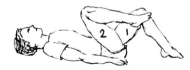

Exercise 5
Lie on your back and flex both knees. Pull both knees up to your chest. Then, lower your legs gradually to the floor in the flexed position. Do not raise your hips off the floor.

Exercise 6
Assume a kneeling position, resting on your hands and knees. Arch your back like a cat and drop your head at the same time. Now, reverse the arch by bringing up your head and forming a "U" with your spine.

much fatigues the patient, causing pain and stiffness.

Frequent mistakes leading to unnecessary and prolonged disability are using excessive overloads to increase strength, ballistic stretching, stretching without prior relaxation, and relying on machines. Exercise machines do not permit frequent change of motion from one muscle to another. They do not provide relaxation, and if used properly, they require as much of the therapist's time as good resistance exercises. We have found Nautilus machines especially dangerous in a therapeutic setup. Many of our patients can trace pain in the back or extremities to Nautilus machines, whereas the old Universal machine has not produced any injuries known to us.

Present interest in physical fitness has encouraged many people to start fitness programs on their own. Unnecessary strains and sprains have resulted. Participants fail to relax, limber, and stretch before warming up to a workout and also neglect cool-off. We have treated many joggers, participants in exercise programs and spas, and especially people who follow exercise tapes.

In summary, an exercise program should consist of the following[11,13]:

1. Relaxation
2. Limbering
3. Gentle strengthening (warm-up exercises)
4. Stretching
5. Heavier strengthening exercises
6. More stretching
7. A reverse to relaxation

Multiple repetitions must be avoided. It is important to relax after each movement and to take a brief intermission before starting the next.

TRIGGER POINTS

Max Lange,[16] an orthopedic surgeon, first described trigger points in 1932 in an excellent book, *Myogelosen (Muscle Hardening)*. Defining trigger points as well-defined hard knots in the muscle, Lange measured the pressure resistance of trigger points in a cadaver and found them discernible

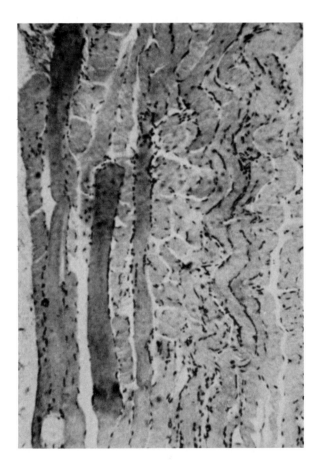

Figure 44-5. Biopsy study of trigger point, showing several darker, straightened-out, club-shaped muscle fibers and relative increase of nuclei. (Formaldehyde, paraffin, hemalum-erythrocin stain; ×80.) (From Glogowski, G, and Wallraff, J: Z Orthop 80:237, 1951.)

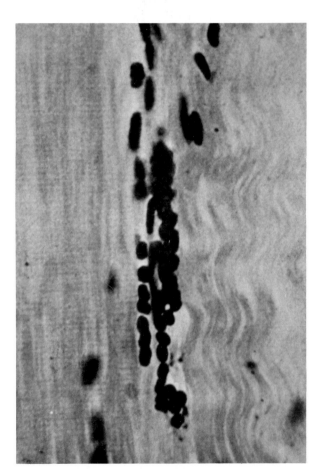

Figure 44-6. Biopsy study of trigger point, showing heaps of nuclei between muscle fibers. Nuclei appear thickened and shrunken. (Formaldehyde, paraffin, hemalum-erythrocin stain; ×560.) (From Glogowski, G, and Wallraff, J: Z Orthop 80:237, 1951.)

from normal tissue. He experimentally produced trigger points in animals and described their histologic characteristics. Lange noted Froriep's reference, as far back as 1881, to tiny "rheumatic" nodules. Lange's students, Glogowski and Wallraff,[7] performed biopsies of trigger points (Figures 44-5 and 44-6). So did Miehlke and co-workers[17] who discovered normal tissue in biopsies of the trapezius muscle of persons experiencing spasm and tension but found that trigger points, which are small areas of degenerated muscle tissue, developed after a prolonged history of pain.

Diagnosis

Trigger points can often be diagnosed on the basis of the history alone.[11,13,24] Patients may point to and describe the distribution and radiation of pain in typical local areas.

Localized tenderness can be felt on palpation. Patients frequently respond to pressure in these areas by moving away.[6] In the acute phase, when the whole muscle is tender, trigger points cannot be identified, so we do not inject into the muscle spasm but treat the pain with ethyl chloride spray, electrotherapy, and gentle motion.

The following are typical patterns:

1. Suboccipital trigger point producing posterior headache
2. Sternomastoid trigger point causing dizziness
3. Posterior neck trigger point causing neck stiffness
4. Trapezius trigger point radiating to neck and arm
5. Scalenus trigger point resulting in peripheral entrapment of cervical plexors and simulating disc disease
6. Trigger point in infraspinatus radiating to posterior aspect of arm and curtailing inward rotation (This condition is often misdiagnosed as bursitis.)
7. Pectoral muscle trigger points, left and right, leading to arm pain and suggesting angina
8. Trigger points near humeral condyles, mostly lateral and usually medial, tennis elbow, radiating to form and frequently combined with trigger point in forearm muscle
9. Interscapular trigger point causing upper back pain (round back)
10. Trigger point in sacrospinal muscles radiating toward upper back (same effect produced by trigger points in quadratus)
11. Trigger points in gluteus maximus radiating to posterior aspect of thigh
12. Trigger point in gluteus medius tensor frequently radiating to lateral aspect of thigh and causing entrapment of nervus cutaneus femoris lateralis
13. Trigger point in origin of rectus femoris radiating to patella
14. Trigger point in vastus intermedius radiating to patella and patella femoral ligament
15. Trigger point in piriformis causing true sciatic nerve compression (peripheral nerve entrapment), which is frequently misdiagnosed as disc disease
16. Trigger point in vastus lateralis and fascia lateralis causing knee pain
17. Trigger point in head of triceps surae causing knee pain and radiating toward heel
18. Trigger point in soleus radiating toward heel; often misdiagnosed as Achilles tendonitis
19. Trigger points in interossei muscles; most often misdiagnosed as neuroma
20. Trigger point in masticatoris muscle; frequently caused by temporomandibular joint problem

Trigger points can occur in any muscle. A patient may have trigger points in a subacute phase. These cannot be differentiated from spasm, tension, or muscle deficiency until the last three conditions have been treated. During the course of treatment, when local areas of tenderness persist, they can eventually be identified as trigger points and injected.

Fischer[5] developed a pressure gauge (Figure 44-7) that quantifies the amount of discomfort the patient feels when presure is applied. This gauge can demonstrate considerable difference between the pressure threshold in a trigger point and that of the contralateral side.

Once trigger points have been identified, we inject them in order to mechanically destroy these nodules. We use lidocaine, or if the patient is sensitive to lidocaine, saline. After marking the spot with a scratch in the skin, we select a needle according to the size of the muscle; needle sizes range from 25 gauge, 1 to 2 inches in length, for muscles of the neck or hands to 19 gauge, 3 inches, for large muscles such as the gluteus maximus. For the area of the buttock or lower back, we prefer spinal needles. Since trigger points are usually found at the insertion of the muscle (Figures 44-8 to 44-10), proceeding in a full circle from the point of local tenderness is not sufficient. It is important to inject and needle both insertion and origin of the affected muscle.

Treatment must not be stopped at this point. We ask the patient to return for at least 3 days in succession to relax the muscle and to relieve postinjection pain with sinusoidal current, ethyl chloride spray, and gentle exercise—much as we would treat the muscle in spasm. In checking on postinjection tenderness with Fischer's pressure gauge, we have seen that the pressure threshold immediately after injection increases dramatically. The following day the threshold is sometimes lower than before injection. After several days it reaches or exceeds normal.

Injection of trigger points, like treatment of muscle spasm, is only the beginning of rehabilitation. Therapeutic exercises must be prescribed as needed. The cause of the muscle problem must be identified and controlled.

Muscle pain is often the leading, if not the only, symptom causing the patient to see a physician.

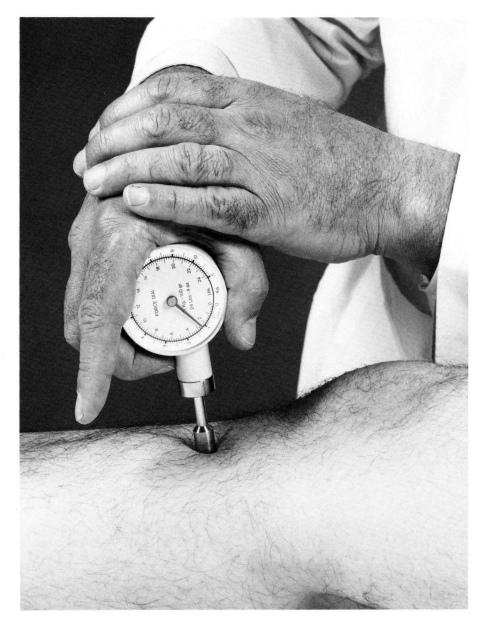

Figure 44-7. Fischer's pressure gauge.

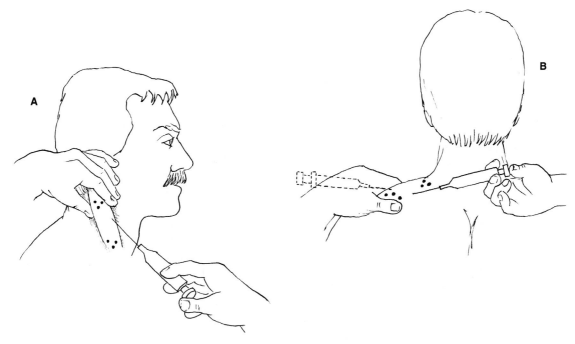

Figure 44-8. Injection into trigger points in sternocleidomastoid muscle and upper trapezius. Dots indicate entry of needle. **A,** Sternocleidomastoid muscle is grasped firmly with one hand and held firmly while other hand directs needle cranially, then caudally. **B,** Upper trapezius is grasped between thumb and index finger to avoid puncturing apex of lungs. Needle is directed medially and then laterally, or vice versa.

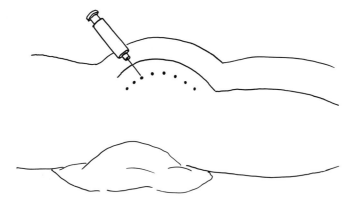

Figure 44-9. Injection of trigger point in gluteal muscle.

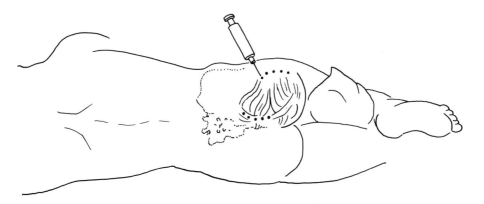

Figure 44-10. Injection of trigger point in piriform muscle.

MASSAGE

Generalized tenderness can be caused by tenderness of the subcutaneous tissue—fibrositis—and is usually distributed over the lower back and sometimes the upper back and the lateral aspect of the thighs. Fibrositis occurs more often in women than in men.

Fibrositis responds well to rolling or pinching massage. Other forms of massage are helpful in treating muscle pain. Kneading massage is useful in the phase described by the Germans as Muskelhärten (muscle hardening). Deep point massage may give temporary relief of trigger point pain; however, such massage is uncomfortable and does not eliminate real trigger points, which may act up even more after deep point massage.

We frequently use massage and exercise as preliminary treatment when trigger points cannot be definitely identified or are too numerous, especially in patients whose disorder has been tentatively diagnosed as an endocrine problem and who are being examined by an endocrinologist.[21] Exercise and massage for several weeks before trigger point injection are very helpful in chronic cases. Patients learn how to relax, some of their muscle deficiency can be corrected, and some of the tender areas actually yield to deep point and kneading massage.

CONCLUSION

Muscle pain or muscle deficiency is a part of most orthopedic problems; it is often the sole cause of disability and pain. An orthopedic examination is incomplete if it does not include a thorough examination of the muscles involved. This is especially true of neck and back pain and of athletic and work-related injuries. Much suffering and unnecessary surgery could be avoided if more attention were paid to neglected skeletal muscles.

REFERENCES

1. Cannon, WB: Bodily changes in pain, hunger, fear, and rage, ed 2, College Park, Md, 1970, McGrath Publishing Co.
2. DeLorme, TU, and Watkins, A: Progressive resistance exercises, New York, 1951, Appleton-Century-Crofts.
3. DeVries, HA, and Adams, GM: Electromyographic comparison of single doses of exercises and meprobamate as to effects on muscular relaxation, Am J Phys Med 51:130, 1972.
4. Dorelle, S, Hecter, P, and Killis: Early controlled mobilization following extensor tendon repair in zone V-VI of the hand, Preliminary Report, Contemp Orthop, vol 11, 1985.
5. Fischer, A: Advances in documentation of pain and soft tissue pathology, Med Times, p. 24, Dec 1983.
6. Gillette, HF: Office management of musculoskeletal pain, Tex J Med 62:47, 1966.
7. Glowgowski, G, and Wallraff, J: Ein Beltrag zur Klinik und Histclogie der Muskelharten (Myogelosen), Z Orthop 80:237, 1951.
8. Hillebrandt, FA: Application of the overload principle to muscle training in man, Am J Phys Med, vol 37, 1958.
9. Jacobson, E: Progressive relaxation, ed 2, Chicago, 1938, University of Chicago Press.
10. Kraus, H: Use of surface anesthesia in the treatment of painful motion, JAMA 116:2582, 1941.
11. Kraus, H: Therapeutic exercise, Springfield, Ill, 1949, Charles C Thomas, Publisher.
12. Kraus, H: Evaluation and treatment of muscle function in athletic injury, Am J Surg 98:353, 1959.
13. Kraus, H: Clinical treatment of neck and back pain, New York, 1970, McGraw-Hill Book Co.
14. Kraus, H, Nagler, W, and Melleby, A: Evaluation of an exercise program for back pain, Am Fam Physician, p 153, Sept 1983.
15. Kraus, H, and Rabb, W: Hypokinetic disease, Springfield, Ill, 1961, Charles C Thomas, Publishers.
16. Lange, M: Die Muskelharten (Myogelosen), Munich, 1931, JF Lehmann.
17. Miehlke, K, Schulze, G, and Eger, W: Clinical and experimental studies on fibrositis syndrome, Z Rheumaforsch 19:310, 1960.
18. Ruskin, AP: Current therapy in physiatry, Philadelphia, 1984, WB Saunders Co.
19. Sainsbury, P, and Gibson, TG: Symptoms in anxiety and tension and the accompanying physiological changes in the muscular system, J Neurol Neurosurg Psychiatry, vol 17, Aug 1954.
20. Salter, RS, et al: The biological effect of continuous passive motion on the healing of full thickness defects in articular cartilage, J Bone Joint Surg 1974.
21. Sonkin, L: Myofascial pain in metabolic disorder, Med Times, p 43, April 1983.
22. Spiegel, H, and Spiegel, D: Trance and treatment: clinical uses of hypnosis, New York, 1978, Basic Books.
23. Travell, J: Ethyl chloride spray for painful muscle spasm, Arch Phys Med 33:291, 1952.
24. Travell, J, and Simons, D: Myosfascial pain and dysfunction: the trigger point manual, Baltimore, 1983, Williams & Wilkins.
25. Waylonis, GW: The physiological effects of ice massage, Arch Phys Med 48:37, 1967.

CHAPTER 45

Myofascial pain syndrome due to trigger points

DAVID G. SIMONS

This chapter will interest anyone whose patients complain of the remarkably common myofascial pain that originates in muscle. Pain and tenderness are characteristically referred from myofascial trigger points located in muscle remote from the site of the pain. This is confusing to the patient and misleading to the practitioner. Despite its cryptic origin, referred pain from trigger points can be devastatingly severe. Fortunately, pain from myofascial trigger points can be identified by careful history taking and skillful physical examination; it is quickly responsive to physical medical management in the absence of serious perpetuating factors.

We all owe Janet G. Travell, M.D., an enormous debt of gratitude for her lifelong dedication to our understanding of myofascial trigger points.[134] The recent surge of research interest in the elucidation of muscle pain syndromes is now reducing the confusion and doubts surrounding the pathophysiology of trigger points. Many of these studies are considered here.

Skeletal muscle is the largest organ of the body; it makes up nearly half of body weight. Muscles are the motors of the body. They work with and against the ubiquitous spring of gravity. With cartilage, ligaments, and intervertebral discs, they serve as the body's mechanical shock absorbers. Each of the approximately 500 skeletal muscles is subject to acute and chronic strain. Each muscle can develop myofascial trigger points and has its own characteristic pattern of referred pain.[133,134]

Acute cases of myofascial pain syndrome (MPS) in a single muscle can often be treated readily and effectively when the specific muscle harboring the trigger point responsible for the pain is promptly recognized. Prompt resolution of an acute single-muscle MPS prevents the needless persistence of disabling pain. Perpetuating factors can increase irritability of muscles, leading to the propagation of trigger points and increasing the distribution and severity of pain. This progression leads in time to the complex disaster of chronic pain.[51]

DEFINITIONS

A myofascial trigger point is defined clinically as "a hyperirritable spot, usually within a taut band of skeletal muscle or in the muscle's fascia, that is painful on compression and that can give rise to characteristic referred pain, tenderness, and autonomic phenomena."[134]

The term "myofascial pain syndrome" is used here with either a specific or a collective meaning. A single-muscle MPS refers to the signs and symptoms caused by active trigger points in one specific muscle. Generically, MPS as used in the title refers to the diagnosis and the signs and symptoms associated with one or many single-muscle myofascial pain syndromes resulting from trigger points.

Trigger points in other tissues such as skin, fat pads, tendons, joint capsules, ligaments, and periosteum are not considered myofascial. These trigger points in other tissues apparently do not produce referred pain patterns that are as consistent and characteristic of specific sites or origin as are the patterns from trigger points in muscles. The referred tenderness and autonomic phenomena associated with myofascial trigger points are also an important and common source of confusion.

Through the years many different terms have been used to describe the specific myofascial pain syndromes generated by trigger points in muscles throughout the body. Previous literature was extensively reviewed for muscle pain syndromes by Simons[105] and for fibrositis by Reynolds.[93] Confusion developed over the past century because successive authors recognized different, often overlapping, aspects of pain from myofascial trigger points and sometimes included features of other conditions. Many authors used general terms applicable to the whole body, such as fibrositis (which has accrued multiple meanings through the years),[93] fibromyalgia,[144] muscular rheumatism (used in Europe for nearly a century),[80] nonarticular rheumatism,[24] myogeloses (muscle gelling),[54,63] Muskelhärten (muscle hardenings) in Germany,[63] interstitial myofibrositis in America,[1] myalgia or myalgic spots in England,[40] and osteochrondrosis in Russia.[87,88]

Other authors used terms applicable to one region of the body without noting its muscular origin or its commonality with other parts of the body. Examples include occipital neuralgia,[102] tendinitis, tennis elbow,[16] chest wall syndrome,[23] scapulocostal syndrome,[78] lumbago,[56,69] and sciatica.[46,125] Each of these terms may be used to identify at least two conditions, one of which is often MPS caused by trigger points.

INCIDENCE

A meaningful interpretation of incidence must distinguish between active trigger points that cause pain, either at rest or in relation to muscular activity, and latent trigger points. A latent trigger point may show all the diagnostic features of an active trigger point except that it causes pain only when the trigger point is examined by palpation.

Latent trigger points afflict nearly half the population by early adulthood. Among 100 male and 100 female 19-year-old asymptomatic Air Force recruits, Sola and associates[122] found focal tenderness in shoulder-girdle muscles indicative of latent trigger points in 54% of the women and 45% of the men. Pain referred from the trigger point to its reference zone was demonstrable in 5% of these subjects.

Recent reports from chronic pain treatment centers showed that myofascial syndromes were the cause of pain in over half of the patients. Among 283 consecutive admissions to a comprehensive pain center, the primary organic diagnosis was myofascial syndromes in 85% of cases.[30] A neurosurgeon and a physiatrist made this diagnosis independently, based on physical examination for soft tissue findings as described by Travell.[113,133] In another study the diagnosis was tabulated for 296 patients referred to a dental clinic for chronic head and neck pain of at least 6 months' duration.[37] In 164 (55.4%) of these patients the primary diagnosis was MPS from active trigger points. The pain of another 21% was ascribed to disease of the temporomandibular joint.[37]

Acute myofascial pain syndromes caused by trigger points are relatively common in general medical practice. In an internal medicine group practice, 10% of 61 consecutive consultation or follow-up patients for all causes had myofascial trigger points that were primarily responsible for their symptoms. Of patients with a pain complaint, myofascial trigger points caused the pain in 31%.[117]

Many health professionals who have learned how to recognize myofascial syndromes are impressed with how common they are. Only when one looks for them routinely with a skilled examination technique does the true magnitude of this source of musculoskeletal pain become apparent. Mounting experimental evidence is now confirming that most chronic pain and much acute pain for which patients seek relief is referred pain. Thus the source of the pain is most likely *not* where the patient complains of pain. To add to the confusion, the site of referred pain often exhibits referred tenderness.

PATHOPHYSIOLOGY

Seven clinical features of MPS caused by trigger points[134] require explanation:

1. The exquisite local tenderness of the trigger point
2. The referral of pain, tenderness, and autonomic phenomena to areas some distance from the trigger point
3. The nature of the electrically quiet palpable band associated with a trigger point in a muscle that exhibits restricted stretch range of motion
4. The nature of the local twitch response that is uniquely characteristic of a trigger point in a palpable band
5. The perpetuation of trigger points by only slight compromise of the muscle's energy supply or of its energy enzyme systems
6. The remarkable therapeutic effect achieved by stretching the involved muscle
7. The weakness without atrophy and the increased fatigability[44] of muscles afflicted with myofascial trigger points

Clinical and research evidence indicates that the trigger point phenomenon begins primarily as a neuromuscular (histochemical) dysfunction resulting from muscle overload. Active trigger points then progress at an unpredictable and variable rate to a dystrophic phase with demonstrable pathologic changes.[88,134]

Sensitization of nerves at the trigger point

The exquisite local tenderness of the trigger point is well explained by sensitization of the nerve endings of group III and group IV muscle nociceptors. Mense[77] reported in his doctoral thesis on the muscle nociceptors in mammalian (cat) muscles that nociception (response to stimuli of tissue-damaging intensity) is mediated by group III, small myelinated (A-delta) fibers and by group IV, unmyelinated (C) fibers. He found little response to algogenic substances from the larger myelinated group I and II fibers serving muscle spindles and musculotendinous receptors.[76] Sensitization is clearly one mechanism responsible for the tenderness and pain associated with tissue injury and inflammatory processes.[86] Sensitization of an afferent nerve, such as a C-fiber polymodal nociceptor, causes the nerve to respond at a reduced threshold and to increase its response to a given stimulus; thus sensitization may induce spontaneous firing in a nerve that was not spontaneously active.[85] Substances known to sensitize tissues include potassium, bradykinin, prostaglandins, histamine, serotonin, substance P, and leukotrienes. Mense and co-investigators[76] found that the group III and IV muscle nociceptors are most responsive to bradykinin[33] and less responsive to serotonin, histamine, and potassium in that order.[31,59] These small fibers are also responsive to prostaglandin[77] and essentially unresponsive to the metabolic products phosphate and lactate.[60] A clinical study by Frost[38] specifically implicates prostaglandin as a sensitizing agent in trigger points. He found that injecting a prostaglandin inhibitor, diclofenac, into myofascial trigger points provided more relief than lidocaine. The role of leukotrienes as a sensitizing agent is controversial,[136] and substance P appears unlikely to be a major sensitizing agent in trigger points.[34]

Awad[1] performed biopsies of tender nodular areas in muscles (trapezius, triceps brachii, or quadriceps femoris) of 10 subjects. Electron microscopic examination showed discharging mast cells and large clusters of blood platelets, each of which is the source of a sensitizing agent, histamine and serotonin, respectively.

Referred pain

Sensitized group III and IV nociceptor muscle afferents are capable of generating nerve action potentials that are misinterpreted by the brain and projected as referred pain and tenderness. Neural input from this source may also account for referred autonomic phenomena such as coryza, scleral injection, and tearing caused by trigger points in the sternocleidomastoid muscle. The nerves that mediate local pain at the trigger point may or may not be the same nerves that initiate referred phenomena.

Appreciation of the ubiquitousness of referred pain is critical to the successful diagnosis and management of myofascial pain syndromes. The source of the pain is rarely where the patient feels pain.

Four known physiologic mechanisms can explain referred pain from trigger points: convergence-projection, convergence-facilitation, peripheral branching of primary afferent nociceptors, and activity of sympathetic nerves. The first two, and to some extent the fourth, mechanisms depend on central nervous system pathways.

When pain is referred by the convergence-projection mechanism, a single cell in the spinal cord receives nociceptive (pain) input via nerves from an internal organ and via other nerves from the skin, muscle, or both. The brain has no way to distinguish whether the nociceptive signal originates from the somatic structure or from the visceral organ. According to this mechanism the brain interprets any such messages as coming from the skin or muscle nerves rather than from the internal organ. Convergence of visceral nociceptive fibers and skin and/or muscle nociceptive fibers onto pain projection neurons in the thoracic spinal cord has proved to be the rule in cats[32] and monkeys.[81] In the case of myofascial trigger points, the visceral (originating) input

arises from the muscle and the somatic (reference zone) nerves originating in the skin and subcutaneous tissues of the reference zone.

Clinically, both the convergence-projection and the axon branching mechanisms explain how blocking the zone of referred pain with a local anesthetic could have no effect on the perception of pain originating from a visceral or muscular source. Convergence-projection is the rule, not the exception, for mammalian visceral nociceptors[32] and is very common for mammalian muscle nociceptors.[81]

Many sensory nerves have a resting background activity that is greatly exceeded when they respond to a noxious (tissue-damaging) stimulus. When pain is referred by the convergence-facilitation mechanism, the effect of this background signal from the reference zone on the ascending (spinothalamic tract) neuron is greatly enhanced (facilitated) by the augmented activity arriving from a visceral source (or from a trigger point). Clinically, when pain is mediated by the convergence-facilitation mechanism, blocking the sensory pathways from the reference zone with cold or other local anesthetic would be expected to provide relief for the duration of the anesthesia.

With axon branching of one sensory nerve to separate parts of the body, the brain could easily misinterpret the source. Impulses actually originating from a nerve ending is one part of the body could easily be interpreted as coming from another part. Evidence for peripheral branching of unmyelinated nerves has been observed in anatomic studies as high as root level in spinal nerves.

Experiments have demonstrated that anesthesizing the reference zone sometimes provides relief and sometimes does not.[134] Apparently several of these mechanisms cause clinical referred pain.

Sympathetic nerves may mediate referred pain originating in trigger points by releasing substances that sensitize primary afferent endings in the region of referred pain.[90] Alternatively, sympathetic activity may cause pain by restricting blood flow in vessels that nourish the sensory nerve fiber itself.[95]

Torebjörk and associates[127] demonstrated clearly that action potentials in nearly one third of the nociceptive median nerve fascicles supplying muscles distal to the elbow generate the perception of referred pain. Experimental subjects felt pain proximally in the arm and chest wall. This experiment did not identify which model of referred pain applied.

There is no longer reason to doubt the ubiquitousness of referred pain from muscle. The pertinent question remaining is, "Which of several mechanisms is responsible for the patient's referred pain?"

Palpable band

The palpable taut band is characteristic of myofascial trigger points and is very helpful in identifying a trigger point when examining superficial muscles. The absence of electrical activity in a taut band in resting muscle restricts possible mechanisms to ones that do not involve the usual excitation-contraction mechanism mediated by action potentials. This eliminates muscle spasm of central origin as a mechanism. The absence of a taut band helps to distinguish a tender point from a myofascial trigger point.

The palpable characteristics of the taut band are best explained by shortening, in the region of the trigger point, of the sarcomeres of the muscle fibers comprising the taut band.[112] The local twitch response (LTR) is uniquely characteristic of the taut band associated with a myofascial trigger point. The LTR is not known to occur under any other circumstances and therefore is a valuable objective clinical identifier of myofascial trigger points. The nature of the palpable band is discussed under the headings "Shortened Sarcomeres" and "Local Twitch Response."

Shortened sarcomeres

The ropy sensation produced by rubbing the tip of the palpating finger across the muscle fibers of a palpable taut band at the trigger point can be explained by contracture (shortening of the sarcomeres without electrical activity).

Palpation of the muscle reveals increased muscle tension from tautness of the palpable band.[61,83] This increased muscle tension has been a prominent feature in past descriptions of muscular rheumatism and myogelosis.[105] Early in this century the increased consistency was identified as a fibrositic "nodule"[126] and later as a ropy band.[61] Some authors described both nodules and ropiness.[99,100] Most patients with myofascial trigger points show ropiness; occasionally one encounters a more circumscribed nodular sensation on palpation.

Motor neurons supplying muscles in the reference zone show increased spontaneous background activity and increased excitability during voluntary activity. This can be considered a form of spasm. In addition, other muscles, whose function parallels that of the afflicted muscle, are likely to exhibit protective splinting (spasm) that is also measurable as electromyographic activity.

To compensate for the shortened sarcomeres at the trigger point, the sarcomeres distant from the trigger point near the musculotendinous junction would become longer than the average-length sarcomeres in a normal fiber, as illustrated in Figure 45-1. Considering the serial arrangement of sarcomeres in one muscle fiber, and the marked change in sarcomere strength with change in length, normal muscle function depends strongly on all sarcomeres remaining the same length throughout the length of a fiber. Involvement of sarcomeres through a limited distance could explain the sensation of a nodule instead of a band. Both clinical and histologic evidence exists for shortened sarcomeres in the region of the trigger point.

Clinically, the patient experiences pain whenever tension on the fibers of the taut band is increased by passive stretch beyond the slack position of the muscle, by strong voluntary contraction of that muscle, or by pressure applied to the

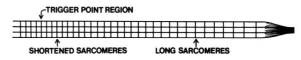

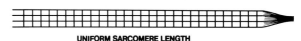

Figure 45-1. Schematic of sarcomeres that are of equal length in normal muscle fibers compared with likely distribution of unequal sarcomere lengths in fibers of palpable taut band passing through trigger point. Shortened sarcomeres in region of trigger point would increase tension in fascicles of taut band and restrict stretch range of motion of muscle.

trigger point area. Attempts to rapidly stretch the muscle passively or actively to its full range of motion result in so much pain that the individual cannot tolerate it.

In a recent study the tender, tense areas in the muscles of 26 myofascial pain patients were massaged 30 to 45 minutes for 10 treatments.[19] Among the 21 patients who responded to massage, the plasma myoglobin concentration more than doubled 2 hours following the first massage. This myoglobin release progressively subsided with subsequent treatments along with progressive relief of pain, resolution of the local induration, and reduction of local tenderness.

All 13 patients in a preceding study responded.[18] These results indicate that massage caused leakage of myoglobin from the muscle fibers and that the palpable tenseness of the muscle involved the contractile elements of muscle fibers, not just connective tissue elements.

Sarcomere shortening also explains why leaving the muscle in a shortened position for a prolonged period (for example, while sleeping at night) may convert a latent trigger point to an active one. Patients sometimes report initial awareness of a severe single-muscle MPS when awakening in the morning.

Additional clinical evidence for shortened sarcomeres is seen when an LTR is elicited by snapping palpation of a trigger point. The greatest movement through the skin is seen along the line of taut band fibers at a distance from the trigger point where the fibers approach the musculotendinous attachment. This movement is in the region of lengthened sarcomeres that have the greatest potential for change in length (Figure 45-1).

Several histologic observations support the presence of increased fiber tension and shortened sarcomeres in the taut band of a trigger point; however, in each study there is ambiguity as to whether the findings apply to tender points of fibrositis or fibromyalgia, to myofascial trigger points, or to both. Under electron microscopy, biopsy specimens of tender points in the upper trapezius muscle in 11 of 12 fibromyalgia patients showed papillary projections of the sarcolemmal membrane at locations corresponding to Z bands.[55] Two of the 11 patients with papillary projections also had narrowing of the I band, which raises the possibility that the projections were the sarcomeres of hypercontracted segments.

Fassbender[24] examined tender areas in the muscles of patients with nonarticular rheumatism by electron microscopy. He reported fibers with "moth-eaten" I bands, which appeared as degeneration of the actin close to the Z band. These disrupted actin filaments may reflect degeneration caused by prolonged, unrelieved mechanical tension on the sarcomeres; they may reflect disintegration of the sarcomeres from metabolic distress; or they may reflect both processes.

Contraction knots seen by light microscopy may be part of the trigger point process. A knot involves one muscle fiber and appears as severe maximal shortening of 100 or so adjacent sarcomeres with compensatory elongation of the sarcomeres on either side. Occasionally only an empty sarcolemmal tube remains on either side of the contracted sarcomeres; the contractile elements have torn loose. This phenomenon was clearly described and illustrated by Simons.[111] In a 1960 study of 77 biopsies of involved muscles, the muscles most severely afflicted with muscular rheumatism showed these "knotty distentions," hyperchromicity, and emptying of the sarcolemmal sheaths of muscle fibers.[80] An earlier study by Glogowski and Wallraff[39] of 24 muscle biopsies is accompanied by illustrations that include contraction knots in "myogelotic" muscles.

It is difficult to determine the relative in vivo sarcomere length from histologic techniques because all fixation techniques are prone to cause muscle contraction with sarcomere shortening during fixation.

Two well-known physiologic mechanisms could account for the shortening of sarcomeres without electrogenic activity (physiologic contracture). McArdle's disease serves as a model for one mechanism and rigor mortis for the other. The McArdle's disease model appears more likely. Employing it, the following hypothesis explains the clinical phenomena associated with myofascial trigger points.

Contraction of striated skeletal muscle depends on forceful interaction between actin and myosin filaments. The contraction process is normally activated by ionic calcium that is released from the sarcoplasmic reticulum in response to an action potential. Contractile activity persists until the calcium is returned to the sarcoplasmic reticulum. The calcium pump that returns the calcium to the sarcoplasmic reticulum is driven by the high-energy phosphate, adenosine triphosphate (ATP).[48]

Absence of phosphorylase (McArdle's disease) or phosphofructokinase (Tarui's disease)[97] results in the clinical symptoms of painful muscle contracture with exercise. This contracture is remarkable for the absence of electrogenic activity. In McArdle's disease the temporary contracture of the muscle fibers is attributed to depletion of ATP in the sarcoplasmic reticulum compartment, causing failure of its calcium pump and loss of calcium uptake. This ATP depletion must be specific to the sarcoplasmic reticulum compartment because there is no generalized depletion of ATP in the diseased muscle either at rest or in the contractured state.[96] A comparable deficit of ATP in the sarcoplasmic compartment because of the energy crisis in the region of a trigger point might produce a similar, localized contracture.

Rupture of the sarcoplasmic reticulum from stress overload of the muscle could release calcium with no immediate mechanism for recovering it. The calcium would initiate an uncontrolled localized contracture of the muscle, comparable to that of McArdle's disease.[96,97] Such localized severe shortening in a group of muscle fibers can be expected to cut off local circulation of the capillaries in the TP zone just as strong voluntary contraction produces severe ischemia in an entire muscle. If the local ischemia were to prevent restoration of ATP to the sarcoplasmic reticular compartment and the muscle fiber contracture were to continue to consume large amounts of energy, the ATP-dependent calcium pump of the sarcoplasmic reticulum would still be unable to recover ionized calcium after the rupture repaired itself.

This mechanism explains why sustained voluntary contraction, especially in the shortened position, or too frequent repetitive contraction without adequate intervening rest periods is likely to convert latent trigger points to active ones and to perpetuate active trigger points. The energy crisis also explains the more rapid onset of fagitue in muscles afflicted with active trigger points than in muscles that are free of them.

The other model of contracture without electrogenic activity is rigor mortis. After a myosin head locks into position onto actin, it is released only by ATP. In the absence of ATP, the cross bridges are fixed in place and the muscle becomes stiff.

Either contracture mechanism might account for the observation by Schade[101] that in four patients following death, the palpable bands remained palpable until they were indistinguishable from surrounding fibers stiffened by rigor mortis.

Local twitch response

The LTR is a transient contraction of essentially only those muscle fibers in a taut band associated with a trigger point. The LTR may be seen as a transient twitch or dimpling of the skin near the musculotendinous attachment of the fibers, or during injection it may be felt through the skin with the examining hand. The LTR is clearly demonstrable electromyographically.[36] It is valuable clinically to confirm the presence of a myofascial trigger point. Studies to date[20,49] do not resolve to what extent this response is propagated from the trigger point through the muscle fibers in the taut band and to what extent the response is mediated through the central nervous system reflex arc. There is experimental evidence for both mechanisms.[49] The clinical observations of projected LTRs (when palpation of a taut band in one muscle elicits an LTR in a different but nearby muscle) strongly implicates a spinal reflex mechanism in those responses.

Metabolic distress

The trigger point is a region of metabolic distress that is already deficient in energy. The metabolic dysfunction could account for the local generation of sensitizing agents. Further clinical compromise of the muscle's energy supply or energy enzyme systems would aggravate the metabolic distress reinforcing the trigger point mechanism.

Several lines of experimental evidence, both specific and nonspecific, point to the trigger point as a region of metabolic distress because of the combination of increased energy demand and impairment of oxygen and energy supply, probably because of locally restricted circulation. This combination could produce a self-sustaining cycle (Figure 45-2).

Any compromise of muscle energy pathways appears to sensitize a muscle to the development of trigger points and to aggravate and perpetuate existing trigger points. Clinically, compromises of this kind include vitamin inadequacies (B_1, B_6, B_{12}, folic acid), anemia, and inadequate thyroid function.

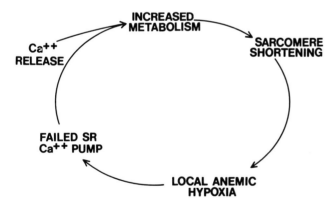

Figure 45-2. Schematic of cycle of events that could maintain sarcomere shortening. Process would begin with release of ionized calcium from ruptured sarcoplasmic reticulum. Vigorous contractile activity increases local metabolic demand. Vigorous local sarcomere shortening compromises local circulation producing anemic hypoxia, which could compromise adenosine triphosphate (ATP) energy supply of sarcoplasmic reticular compartment. Resulting failed calcium pump of sarcoplasmic reticulum (SR) would leave ionized calcium free to maintain spontaneous contractile activity.

Experimental evidence

Bengtsson and associates[9] found nonspecific evidence for metabolic distress in a recent light microscopic biopsy study of 77 muscles from 57 patients with primary fibromyalgia. They compared these patient biopsy specimens with 17 control biopsy specimens from nine healthy subjects. Of the 77 biopsy specimens, 41 were taken from the upper trapezius muscle. Of those 41 trapezius specimens, 31 were taken from a tender point (local pain on compression). Often these biopsy sites were identified as "trigger points" (radiation of pain on compression). Nearly half of the patient specimens showed significant pathologic changes, most conspicuous of which were ragged red fibers and moth-eaten fibers. Neither of these changes are seen in most normal skeletal muscles; however, the trapezius muscle showed changes in both patient and control specimens. Ragged red fibers are commonly seen in mitochondrial myopathies, muscles that also are suffering from metabolic compromise; both ragged red fibers and moth-eaten fibers can be induced by experimental hypoxia.[9]

Biopsy specimens of upper trapezius muscles in patients with soft tissue rheumatism that were studied by electron microscopy showed swollen capillary organelles and enlarged mitochondria and were interpreted as indicating hypoxia and that disturbed metabolism.[24]

An earlier light microscopic study of 77 biopsy specimens from mostly upper trapezius muscles in patients with muscular rheumatism identified four groups based on the presence or absence of palpable changes in the muscle and the severity of symptoms.[80] The authors identified no histologic abnormality in the tender muscles of those who had pain but no palpable findings (probably a fibrositis group). Among those with no pain complaint but with tender palpable hardenings in the muscle (probably a group with latent trigger points), the authors noted consistent microscopic fat accumulation, "fat dusting," which was attributed to an oxygen deficit. Muscles of patients with palpable findings and serious pain complaint (probably a group with active trigger points) showed nonspecific dystrophic pathologic changes, but the fat dusting was not always present. The same authors also identified a disproportionate deficit of aldolase compared with lactic acid in the 59 biopsy samples studied histochemically.[80] This finding was interpreted as a failure of oxidative disposal of lactic acid that was caused by hypoxia.

Experimental studies specifically of trigger points also point to increased metabolic activity in the presence of impaired circulation. The temperature of a trigger point measured with a needle thermocouple by Travell[129] was greater than surrounding muscle. A radioisotope study reported by Popelianskii and associates[88] indicated slowing of perfusion in the region of the muscular lesion. These observations are consistent with the trigger point being a source of more metabolic heat than surrounding muscle or local reduction of heat removal by decreased blood perfusion.

Using an oxygen electrode, Lund and associates[70] recently measured oxygenation directly in the subcutaneous tissue and at eight points on the surface of the muscle overlying "trigger points" in trapezius and brachioradialis muscles. The total mean subcutaneous oxygen pressure in seven patients was 45 mm Hg, which was significantly lower ($p > .01$) than the 65 mm Hg observed in six controls. The surface of the muscle overlying 14 trigger points in 10 patients produced abnormal oxygen test results, indicating subnormal oxygenation, probably because of disturbed vascular control, as compared with normal results in seven of eight normal control subjects. The muscle oxygenation was abnormally low in the region of trigger points in these fibromyalgia patients. The authors identified the trigger point as an area of such intense pain on compression that the patient often jumped and that produced radiation of pain.[70] No palpable changes were required.

In a companion biopsy study, Bengtsson and associates[8] found a significant decrease in high-energy phosphate levels coupled with an increase in low-energy phosphate and creatine levels. This strong evidence of energy depletion was found in biopsies of the trapezius muscles of 15 patients when compared with samples of nonpainful anterior tibial muscles in six patients and with samples of the trapezius muscle from eight healthy controls. Together, these last two studies strongly confirm the previous evidence that a trigger point (or tender point?) is a region of metabolic distress.

In shortened sarcomeres where ionized calcium is still present, the actin and myosin filaments continue to interact and consume energy as long as ATP is available. However, if the sarcomere is fully stretched, few if any of the myosin heads can reach active sites on the actin filaments; contractile metabolic activity would cease and the vicious cycle (Figure 45-2) would be broken.

Value of stretch

Stretching the contracted sarcomeres to their full length would be difficult but immediately therapeutic because the use of ATP would cease, the contractile tension would be released, and normal metabolic equilibrium would return. If the metabolic stress generated sensitizing agents such as prostaglandins that were responsible for the hyperirritability of the trigger point, normalization of metabolism would remove the source of sensitization and hence eliminate local tenderness and referred phenomena. Some prostaglandins have half-lives of seconds or less and would disappear rapidly with normalization of metabolic activity in the region of the trigger point.

The metabolic distress previously described could explain what caused the severe dystrophic changes observed in patients who had the most severe pain and dysfunction in the study by Miehlke and associates.[79]

The need to equalize the length of individual sarcomeres throughout the entire length of each muscle fiber also explains why athletes find muscle-stretching exercises so valuable before and after sporting events. This need also explains the importance of following any myofascial therapeutic procedure with full range of motion to both the totally lengthened and totally shortened positions to reestablish normal muscle function.

Weakness and fatigability

The increased fatigability and weakness observed in patients with trigger points may be due to the reduced circulation and hypoxia observed in afflicted muscles.[70]

Weakness and increased fatigability of the adductor pollicis muscle were demonstrated in patients with fibromyalgia and many trigger points. The changes were interpreted as being central in origin.[7] This weakness could also be due to inhibition of a reflex nature that was initiated by afferent impulses from an active trigger point.

DIAGNOSIS

Each of the individual myofascial pain syndromes is caused by trigger points in a specific muscle.[134] The symptoms and signs are strongly muscle oriented. In the absence of diagnostic laboratory and imaging tests, the recognition of a myofascial syndrome depends on a history that identifies referred pain patterns and a physical examination that includes palpation of the muscles for myofascial trigger points. One *must* look for trigger points to find them.

History and pain patterns

The recognition and management of acute single-muscle syndromes can be remarkably simple. Successful management of chronic multiple-muscle pain syndromes complicated by perpetuating factors intertwined with pain behaviors is challenging and time consuming. Specific details of the mechanical stresses associated with the acute initial onset of myofascial pain helps greatly to identify the muscles most likely involved. In motor vehicle accidents the direction of impact provides guidelines as to which muscles are most likely to have developed active trigger points.[3] To distinguish acute from insidious onset, one can ask the patient, "Can you remember the day that you were first aware of the pain?" If the patient remembers the moment of onset of pain, it is important to find out exactly what the patient was doing: what position or movement and what stress or trauma were associated with the onset.

In the absence of perpetuating factors and with normal daily activities that stretch the muscle, active trigger points tend to revert to latent ones. Latent trigger points do not cause clinical pain complaints but may have all the other diagnostic signs of active trigger points.

The pain and tenderness referred by a trigger point are usually projected to a distance, much as pressure on the trigger of a gun causes the bullet to impact elsewhere. The pain is usually aching (dull or intense) and variable from hour to hour and day to day. Pain intensity is often strongly related to posture and muscular activity. Pain experienced only with movement indicates a lesser degree of trigger point irritability; pain at rest indicates more severe involvement. It is not unusual for patients to suffer activation of a latent trigger point for several days or weeks with gradual spontaneous recovery followed by subsequent recurrence. Increasingly frequent recurrences with progressively greater severity and more widespread and severe myofascial pain, whether of acute or insidious onset, strongly suggest serious perpetuating factors that require resolution.

The referred pain pattern is usually the key to diagnosis. A precise drawing that includes all of the patient's pain patterns is essential. Each area of pain should be delineated by the patient with one finger on the body and should be drawn by the examiner; the drawing is then corrected or confirmed by the patient. When pain involves several parts of the body, it is useful to number the pain areas in the sequence of their appearance, distinguishing which pains are experienced together and which occur at different times in association with different movements and positions. The known pain pattern of each muscle (see "Treatment") is then applied in reverse to identify which muscle or muscles are most likely to be causing the patient's pain. The importance of obtaining a complete and accurate pain drawing at the initial as well as subsequent patient visits cannot be overemphasized.

Examination

Overall patient examination concentrates on the observation of antalgic movements and postures and the identification of restricted range of motion.

Restricted stretch range of motion is identified by noting protective and substitute movements and by screening tests. An involved muscle may cause pain both when passively stretched and when voluntarily contracted,[71] especially in the fully shortened position. Range is painfully restricted in the direction of stretch.[71] Merely holding an involved muscle in the shortened position, and especially contracting it when shortened, are likely to further activate its trigger points.

Testing for strength reveals a "ratchety" or "breakaway" weakness that may reflect conscious or unconscious limitation of effort to avoid pain. If the test produces pain, the severity and location of the pain is important. Pain may be local or referred from active trigger points in the muscles being tested or from trigger points in remote muscles that stabilize the movement.

Examination of a muscle suspected of harboring active trigger points begins by palpation with the fingertip rubbed gently across the long axis of muscle fibers in the region of the suspected trigger points. Successive palpations along the taut band identify the most sensitive spot—the trigger point. Pressure at the trigger point causes a "jump sign," with grimacing or vocalization by the patient. Eliciting a local twitch response of the taut band by rapid snapping palpation of the trigger point confirms the presence of the

trigger point, most likely an active one. Occasionally an additional remote twitch response may appear simultaneously in a taut band of a nearby but anatomically independent muscle.

Quantification of the sensitivity of a trigger point is now possible using recently developed algometers.[28,29,52,53,91] Algometry is one effective way to impress the patient with the exquisite sensitivity of the trigger point area. Patients assume that the examiner is pressing harder on the trigger point, not that the trigger point is so sensitive. Pressure threshold measurements help to document the extent and severity of trigger point involvement and to quantify the progress achieved by treatment. The patient's pain symptoms may be relieved with only partial elimination of the abnormal trigger point sensitivity; a latent trigger point remains.

The final confirmation of the trigger point source of pain to both the patient and clinician is reproduction of the patient's pain complaint by pressure on the trigger point. Identification of a trigger point pain syndrome sometimes can be as simple as recognizing the pain pattern, placing a finger directly on the predictably sensitive trigger point, and reproducing the patient's pain. However, simply finding one trigger point that reproduces the pain does not eliminate the possibility of active trigger points in other muscles that refer pain to the same area.

Laboratory findings

At this time no laboratory or imaging test is diagnostic of myofascial pain syndromes caused by trigger points. However, many systemic perpetuating factors are identified by laboratory abnormalities. When perpetuating factors are present, their identification and resolution are essential for lasting pain relief. Two new imaging tests, thermography and magnetic resonance imaging, are promising.

Thermograms are obtainable using electronic radiometry or films of liquid crystals. Recent advances in infrared radiation (electronic) thermography with computer analysis make it a powerful new tool for the visualization of cutaneous reflex phenomena characteristic of myofascial trigger points. The less expensive contact sheets of liquid crystals have many limitations that make reliable interpretation difficult.

Any thermogram measures the temperature of the skin surface only to a depth of a few millimeters; it effectively measures changes in the circulation of blood within, but not beneath, the skin. Sympathetic nervous system activity is usually the endogenous cause of these changes. A thermographic picture is similar in meaning to changes in skin resistance and sweat production, but electronic radiation thermography is superior in convenience and in spatial and temporal resolution.

At this point, electronic thermography alone is not sufficient to make the diagnosis of myofascial trigger points; however, it appears to be a very useful way to document myofascial trigger points that have been identified by history and physical examination. Early human thermographic studies noted that myofascial pain is associated with disc-shaped hot spots that are 5 to 10 cm in diameter and are located over the trigger point.[25] Whether this spot is actually over the referred pain zone rather than the trigger point is unclear from the literature to date. Some papers avoid this issue[145]; another paper indicated that a reduced pressure threshold reading at the hot spot proved it is a trigger point.[26] However, the local tenderness at the hot spot could be referred tenderness in the pain reference zone rather than tenderness of the trigger point itself. Other papers specifically relate the hot spot to the area of pain complaint,[25,27,139] which is usually the zone of referred pain, not the location of the trigger point. The referred pain zone has been variously referred to as hot,[27] as hot or cold,[25] and as cold.[134] Failure to clearly distinguish whether observed thermal changes are located over the trigger point itself or over its referred pain zones is a potential source of much confusion in the interpretation of thermographic changes caused by trigger points.

With sufficient resolution, magnetic resonance imaging has promising potential for imaging changes in the phosphorus (ATP) concentrations in the vicinity of active myofascial trigger points.

DIFFERENTIAL DIAGNOSIS

Referred pain of muscular origin can readily be confused with pain of neurologic or rheumatic-inflammatory origin. In addition, one must consider pain of skeletal, vascular, tumor, or psychogenic origin. Pain of muscular origin characteristically waxes and wanes in relation to posture and muscular activity. This pain frequently relates to the use of one specific muscle group. Other sources of pain are usually not so closely related to muscular function.

Myofascial pain from trigger points is one of three common musculoskeletal dysfunctions that are frequently overlooked and deserve serious attention. The other two are fibrositis-fibromyalgia and articular dysfunction. At this time none of the three conditions can be evaluated by a diagnostic laboratory or imaging test; they depend on diagnosis by history and physical examination alone. All three diagnoses are likely to be missed on routine conventional examination. In each case the examiner must know precisely what to look for and how to look for it and must be considering the diagnosis.

Pain of neurologic origin is likely to be associated with neurologic deficits such as loss of or change in sensation, electrodiagnostic abnormalities, and deficits that match a peripheral nerve or root distribution. These characteristics do not apply to "central" pain of central nervous system origin.

The signs and symptoms of multiple joint involvement help greatly to identify rheumatic articular disease. Fibrositis-fibromyalgia as identified by rheumatologists is dis-

cussed separately in the following section. Inflammatory conditions such as bursitis and tendinitis can present symptoms that are easily confused with those of myofascial trigger points.

In contrast to well-recognized skeletal conditions that show clearly on radiographs and computerized tomography scans, the articular dysfunctions that require mobilization or manipulation for restoration of normal joint function are considered controversial by many physicians. A recent study reveals that although many patients with musculoskeletal backache do seek aid from those who practice joint mobilization, the patients are most likely to experience only temporary relief.[58] This compilation of the experience of 492 backache patients with various health care providers was conducted by a patient and gives some insight into where patients go for help and how much help they receive. Of those studied, 86% saw a chiropractor and 87% an orthopedist. For both providers, one fourth of the patients experienced moderate or dramatic long-term relief; however, 28% seeing a chiropractor, but only 9% of those seeing an orthopedic surgeon, also experienced short-term relief. The chiropractor was ineffective in 33% of cases and 61% found the orthopedist ineffective.

Interestingly, although only 6% of those studied[58] went to a physiatrist, one third of them experienced dramatic long-term relief and over half received moderate long-term help. Only 7% found this approach ineffective. Lewit[67] emphasized that a significant number of patients experience lasting relief only if both the joint dysfunction and the muscle dysfunction from trigger points are relieved. Each type of dysfunction requires a different examination and different treatment techniques.

Pain of vascular origin is likely to have a stocking-glove distribution or be pulsatile—synchronous with the heart beat. Tumors generally produce pain through direct mechanical pressure or indirectly through pressure on nerves.

Purely psychogenic pain is rare.[51] Anxiety and frustration facilitates the development and perpetuation of myofascial trigger points and intensifies the suffering caused by the pain[89]; psychologic stress, in turn, is augmented by the uncertainties and limitations imposed by persistent pain, the cause of which is obscure and which responds poorly to the efforts of health-care providers.

Fibrositis-fibromyalgia

An MPS is distinguished from fibrositis-fibromyalgia by the presence of trigger points. A trigger point is a focal lesion in a muscle; it occurs equally often in men and women.[122,134] The presence of perpetuating factors blurs the distinction between the syndromes.

A recent 2-day symposium summarized current concepts of fibrositis-fibromyalgia.[11] A short monograph is also available that summarizes fibrositis and MPS.[13] Their relationship is addressed in a current text on soft tissue rheumatic pain[104] and in a recent chapter.[110]

Much evidence indicates that fibrositis-fibromyalgia is a systemic disease of unknown origin with a 5:1 preponderance of females.[141] Only supportive treatment, aimed at factors that modify the condition, is available to date.[11,13] Its systemic nature is substantiated by widespread bilateral pain,[141] subcutaneous IgG deposits at the dermal-epidermal junction,[14,15,22] and muscle destruction not specific to tender points or trigger points.[5] To distinguish between fibrositis-fibromyalgia and MPS, at this time it is essential to distinguish between tender points and trigger points.[109] Only trigger points have palpable taut bands with local twitch responses, and trigger points are more likely to produce referred pain on palpation. How much more likely has yet to be resolved.

Over the last two decades, rheumatologists generally have adopted a redefinition of fibrositis. In 1981, Smythe,[119] who initiated this redefinition, listed his updated diagnostic criteria for fibrositis: widespread aching of more than 3 months' duration, local tenderness at 12 or more of 14 specific sites, skin roll tenderness over the upper scapular region, and disturbed sleep with morning fatigue and stiffness. Other authors have slightly modified these criteria as to the number of tender points and the associated clinical symptoms.[10,141,142] Based on extensive studies, Wolfe[141] requires seven tender points at 14 prescribed sites to make the diagnosis of fibrositis. In 1982, Yunus and associates[144] introduced the term "fibromyalgia" to replace "fibrositis" because the latter is a misnomer with a long history of multiple confusing definitions.[93] They reduced the required number of tender points to three and further modified the definition for fibromyalgia to include patients with increased tiredness and fatigue, anxiety, and depression. These patients also sometimes experience increased symptoms when exposed to cold or humid weather, fatigue (physical or mental), and physical inactivity. Characteristic physical findings included normal joints and normal strength, three or more tender points, muscle spasm, tender "fibrositic nodules," and erythema over the palpated tender points.

These definitions clearly distinguish fibrositis-fibromyalgia from myofascial trigger points in patients with an acute single-muscle MPS because of the short duration and the presence of trigger point phenomena in the latter. However, in patients with chronic pain in multiple regions, the distinction between fibrositis-fibromyalgia and a patient who has multiple trigger points with perpetuating factors becomes blurred unless the taut bands, local twitch responses, and reproduction of referred pain patterns of trigger points are carefully considered. In 1960 Miehlke and associates[80] found that in biopsy specimens of patients with soft tissue rheumatism, tender muscles without palpable changes (tender points?) showed no fat dusting but that biopsy specimens of muscles with palpable indurations (taut bands at trigger points?) consistently had this finding. Clinically, the presence of taut bands may be the most useful characteristic to distinguish trigger points from tender points.

To date, treatment of fibrositis-fibromyalgia is aimed at educating the patient about the condition and modifying factors that influence severity, including sleep disturbance, overuse syndromes, mechanical stress, psychic stress, and unnecessary concern about the prognosis.[11,13] Management of an MPS, on the other hand, is aimed at eliminating the cause of the pain (myofascial trigger points) and their perpetuating factors.[134] Many patients having either MPS or fibrositis-fibromyalgia are probably misdiagnosed as having the other, and some patients have both conditions.

Articular dysfunction

Articular dysfunction is identified by examining the joint for loss of normal mobility and range of motion, not only in its kinesiologic planes of voluntary motion but also for "joint play." This joint play is motion not obtainable by voluntary muscular action.[72,75] The classic techniques for joint mobilization or manipulation have been well described.[12,21,45,73,82] Lewit[66,67] emphasizes the previously recognized[82] importance of releasing muscular tightness in conjunction with joint mobilization. The need for joint mobilization is established by skilled examination of the joint specifically for loss of mobility in all its planes of motion.

Common pain diagnoses

Many common pain conditions are misdiagnosed because the examiner is not aware of referred pain patterns characteristic of myofascial trigger points and fails to examine the muscles for them. Some commonly misdiagnosed conditions are listed in Table 45-1 and discussed below.

It is now becoming clear that tension headache is usually due to myofascial trigger points[42] and that frontal headache is probably due to trigger points in the clavicular division of the sternocleidomastoid muscle (Figure 45-3, *C*).[134]

Face pain of enigmatic origin is likely to be called atypical facial neuralgia by physicians[131] and commonly identified by dentists as temporomandibular joint dysfunction or myofascial pain dysfunction.[134] The latter diagnosis is often at least partly due to myofascial trigger points in the lateral pterygoid (Figure 45-3, *G*) or masseter (Figure 45-3, *E*) muscles. It is critically important when dealing with chronic masticatory muscle pain and dysfunction to inactivate trigger points in cervical musculature that refer pain to the face.

The sternocleidomastoid (Figure 45-3, *C* and *D*) and upper trapezius (Figure 45-3, *A*) muscles commonly cause pain referred to the face and secondarily activate and perpetuate trigger points in the masticatory muscles, which likewise refer pain to the face and sometimes to the teeth.

Otolaryngologists are frequently deeply frustrated by patients who complain of earache caused by referred pain from the deep masseter muscle (Figure 45-3, *E*). Many dentists are familiar with this syndrome and manage it well.

Pain diagnosed as occipital neuralgia has been demonstrated often to be caused by trigger points in the posterior neck muscles (Figure 45-4, *A* and *B*).[41]

Table 45-1. Common pain diagnoses frequently unrecognized as originating from myofascial trigger points in specific muscles

Common diagnosis	Muscle origins	References
Tension (migraine) headache	Sternocleidomastoid	42, 134 (Ch. 7)
	Upper trapezius	43, 134 (Ch. 6)
	Posterior cervicals	134 (Ch. 16)
	Splenius capitis and cervicis	134 (Ch. 15)
	Temporalis	134 (Ch. 9)
Atypical facial neuralgia	Sternocleidomastoid (sternal division)	131, 134 (Ch. 7)
	Facial muscles	134 (Ch. 13)
Myofascial pain dysfunction	Lateral pterygoid	134 (Ch. 11)
	Masseter	134 (Ch. 8)
Earache, normal drum	Deep masseter	134 (Ch. 8)
	Sternocleidomastoid (clavicular division)	134 (Ch. 7)
Occipital neuralgia	Splenius capitis and cervicis	41, 134 (Ch. 15)
	Multifidus, semispinalis	134 (Ch. 16)
	Suboccipital muscles	98, 134 (Ch. 17)
Acute stiff neck	Levator scapulae	128, 134 (Ch. 19)
	Sternocleidomastoid	134 (Ch. 7)
	Upper trapezius	134 (Ch. 6)
Postdural puncture headache	Posterior cervical muscles	50, 134 (Ch. 16)
Arthritis of shoulder	Infraspinatus	92, 134 (Ch. 22)
Subdeltoid bursitis	Infraspinatus	137, 134 (Ch. 22)
	Deltoid	134 (Ch. 28)
	Supraspinatus	134 (Ch. 21)
Thoracic outlet syndrome	Scaleni	43, 98, 134 (Ch. 20)
	Pectoralis minor	98, 134 (Ch. 43)
Epicondylitis, "tennis elbow"	Supinator	134 (Ch. 36)
	Wrist extensors	134 (Ch. 34)
	Triceps brachii	134 (Ch. 32)
Angina	Pectoralis major, minor	134 (Ch. 42, 43)
	Sternalis	134 (Ch. 44)
Upper back pain	Scaleni	134 (Ch. 20)
	Lavator scapulae	134 (Ch. 19)
	Rhomboids	134 (Ch. 27)
	Latissimus dorsi	134 (Ch. 24)
	Serratus posterior superior	134 (Ch. 45)
	Thoracic paraspinals	134 (Ch. 48)
Low back pain	Quadratus lumborum	108, 114, 121, 135 (Ch. 4)
	Thoracolumbar paraspinals	134 (Ch. 48)
	Gluteus maximus and medius	115, 135 (Ch. 7, 8)
	Rectus abdominis	134 (Ch. 49)
	Iliopsoas	114, 135 (Ch. 5)
Appendicitis	Rectus abdominis	103, 134 (Ch. 49)
	Iliocostalis	134 (Ch. 48)
Pelvic pain	Coccygeus and levator ani	115, 118, 135 (Ch. 6)
Arthritis of hip (hip pain)	Tensor fasciae latae	135 (Ch. 12)
Meralgia paresthetica	Tensor fasciae latae	135 (Ch. 12)
	Sartorius	
Sciatica	Posterior gluteus minimus	115, 135 (Ch. 9)
	Piriformis	46, 135 (Ch. 10)
Arthritis of knee	Rectus femoris	135 (Ch. 14)
	Vastus medialis	135 (Ch. 14)
	Vastus lateralis	135 (Ch. 14)
	Gastrocnemius	135 (Ch. 21)
Trochanteric bursitis	Vastus lateralis	135 (Ch. 14)
	Tensor fasciae latae	135 (Ch. 12)
	Quadratus lumborum	115, 135 (Ch. 4)
Heel spur	Soleus	115, 135 (Ch. 22)

An acute stiff neck is usually of myofascial origin,[128] in contrast to the neurogenic or psychogenic chronic torticollis.[134]

What is first assumed to be postdural puncture headache may arise from trigger points in the cervical paraspinal muscles during the postpartum period following a delivery in which spinal block was used.[50]

Pain referred to the shoulder from the infraspinatus muscle (Figure 45-4, *G*) is likely to be ascribed to arthritis because the pain usually is perceived deep in the shoulder joint.[92,134]

Rather than coming from subdeltoid bursitis, pain and tenderness in the acromial and middle deltoid area of the shoulder are often referred from myofascial trigger points.

The myofascial origin of thoracic outlet syndrome is entrapment of the lower trunk (mostly ulnar nerve fibers) of the brachial plexus by taut bands in the anterior or middle scalene muscles (Figure 45-4, *C*).

A common underlying cause of epicondylitis or tennis elbow—which has many other names, including "briefcase elbow"—is referred pain and tenderness from trigger points in the supinator muscle (Figure 45-5, *F*) and also from the wrist extensor muscles (Figure 45-5, *G*) near the lateral epicondyle. In such cases the lateral epicondyle is tender to thumping palpation. Examination for trigger points and referred pain from trigger points in these muscles quickly establishes the true origin of the pain. Occasionally, the triceps brachii (Figure 45-5, *E*) contributes to tennis elbow pain.

Pain mimicking angina, but poorly correlated with the duration and intensity of exercise or activity, may arise from trigger points in the pectoralis major or minor muscles (Figure 45-6, *C*).

The most common source of upper back pain in the region of the upper vertebral border of the scapula is from trigger points in the scalene muscles (Figure 45-4, *C*), with trigger points of the levator scapulae (Figure 45-4, *D*) running a close second. The latissimus dorsi (Figure 45-5, *A*) may be responsible. When the rhomboids[134] are involved, the large pectoralis major muscles are often shortened by latent trigger points. Even though the pectoral trigger points are not causing pain, the shortened pectoral muscles overload the rhomboids. Serratus posterior superior trigger points are covered by the retracted scapula and usually produce a pain deep in the chest (Figure 45-6, *F*). Upper thoracic paraspinal muscles are common offenders; trigger points in their superficial layers are easily identified by palpation.

The most common muscular source of low back pain is trigger points in the quadratus lumborum muscle (Figure 45-6, *G*). The iliopsoas is often involved in conjunction with the quadratus lumborum and occasionally is involved by itself. Paraspinalis muscles (Figures 45-6, *H,* and 45-7, *A* to *D*) frequently harbor trigger points that, except in the deep multifidi and rotatores muscles, are readily identified by palpation. The gluteus maximus and gluteus medius trig-

ger points commonly refer pain to the region of the buttock and sacrum. Pain referred from the rectus abdominis is distinctively horizontal and generally at either the midthoracic or low lumbar level corresponding to trigger points in the upper and lower ends of the rectus abdominis muscle.

Many patients who were found to have a normal appendix at surgery for appendicitis may have had a misdiagnosed myofascial pain syndrome of the rectus abdominis (Figure 45-7, *H*) or iliocostalis (Figure 45-7, *A*) muscles.[103]

A muscular source of enigmatic pelvic pain may be located by intrarectal palpation of the coccygeus, levator ani, obturator internus, and sphincter ani muscles for trigger point tenderness and taut bands.[115,118]

Pain simulating arthritis of the hip is referred by the tensor fasciae latae muscle[135] deeply into the hip joint, comparable to the pain referred by the intraspinatus muscle into the shoulder joint; patients with arthritis of the hip or pain referred from the tensor fasciae latae muscle find weight bearing painful.

The neurologic pain of meralgia paresthetica may be due to entrapment of the lateral femoral cutaneous nerve by involved sartorius or tensor fasciae latae muscles.

The pain commonly attributed to sciatica is rarely due to a demonstrable neuropathy of the sciatic nerve. This pain is much more likely to be referred from trigger points in the posterior section of the gluteus minimus (Figure 45-8, *B*) or in the piriformis (Figure 45-8, *C*) muscles.[115]

The pain of arthritis of the knee or knee pain from known hip disease is mimicked by active myofascial trigger points in the rectus femoris (Figure 45-8, *E*) and vastus medialis (Figure 45-8, *F*) muscles, which cause knee pain in the region of the patella; trigger points in the upper end of the vastus lateralis (Figure 45-8, *I*) and the gastrocnemius (Figure 45-9, *B*) muscles refer pain to the back of the knee.

The pain and tenderness of trochanteric bursitis is emulated by trigger points in the vastus lateralis (Figure 45-8, *G*) or tensor fasciae latae[135] muscles.

When there is a heel spur, the spur is easily misidentified as the source of heel pain that actually is referred from trigger points in the soleus muscle (Figure 45-9, *A*). In this case the asymptomatic contralateral side often has an equally large and innocuous heel spur.

One simple way of confirming that myofascial trigger points are the cause of the patient's symptoms is to inactivate the trigger points and relieve the pain and tenderness.

TREATMENT

Single-muscle myofascial pain syndromes can be refreshingly simple to manage, whereas complex chronic myofascial syndromes driven by severe perpetuating factors can be enormously difficult to resolve. (The latter are discussed under "Perpetuating Factors.") Uncomplicated single-muscle syndromes may persist but are nonprogressive. If the muscle is relieved of strain for several days, the trigger points may revert from active to latent, relieving pain.

The key to treating an acute MPS is to identify the specific muscles harboring the active trigger points. The muscles needing therapy are identified by a detailed history of the onset of pain, knowledge of myofascial referred pain patterns, and confirmation of the location of active trigger points responsible for the pain by examining the muscles. Palpation with one finger tip is used to look for the tender trigger point with its taut band and local twitch response. Modification of the patient's sensation in the pain reference zone by pressure on the trigger point provides diagnostic confirmation.

Lasting success in treatment depends on educating the patient while inactivating the responsible trigger points by stretch and spray of the involved muscles or by injection of the trigger points, often by both. These techniques are used to restore full range of motion with pain-free function. Often the most difficult part of treatment is locating and correcting perpetuating factors. It is critically important to teach the patient a home self-stretch program[62] that is tailored to prevent and manage recurrences and to train the patient how to safely use, not abuse, the involved muscles.[134]

Specific myofascial trigger point therapies include stretch and spray, postisometric relaxation, injection, specific kinds of massage, and ultrasound or electrical stimulation applied to the trigger point. Since stretch and spray usually is the initial treatment of choice, the principles underlying its use are identified first and then its application to individual muscles is presented with each muscle's pain pattern.

Stretch and spray

The stretch and spray method of treatment is one of the simplest, quickest, and least painful ways to resolve a single-muscle MPS; it is frequently used immediately after trigger point injection to ensure inactivation of all trigger points in that muscle. It is also valuable for complex cases where many muscles in a region of the body are involved.[107] Since muscles within one functional group interact strongly, this technique can release several closely related muscles at one time.

The purpose of stretch and spray is to inactivate the trigger point or points by restoring the muscle to its full stretch range of motion with minimal discomfort and without exciting reflex spasm. Voluntary relaxation of the muscle being stretched is essential. The alarming cutaneous stimulation generated in the reference zone by the vapocoolant spray helps to block reflex spasm and pain,[130] permitting gradual passive stretch of the muscle and inactivation of the trigger point mechanism.

A jet stream of vapocoolant spray is applied to the skin in unidirectional parallel sweeps. If the skin is cold to the touch, it is too cold for application of vapocoolant. Excessive cooling evidenced by frosting of the skin is avoided. Fluori-Methane (Gebauer Chemical Co., Cleveland) is preferred to ethyl chloride because the latter is a potentially

lethal general anesthetic, is flammable and explosive, and is colder than desirable. Parallel sweeps of Fluori-Methane spray are applied slowly at 10 cm (4 inches)/sec over the entire length of the muscle in the direction of and including the referred pain zone. The bottle is held about 45 cm (18 inches) from the skin to permit the room-temperature vapocoolant in the bottle to cool as it passes through the air before it hits the skin. The stream of spray is most effective if it impacts the skin at an angle of about 30 degrees.[134]

Complete relaxation of the muscle to be stretched is essential. To obtain this relaxation, the patient should be positioned comfortably with all limbs and the back well supported. Initially one or two sweeps of spray should precede the stretch to inhibit the pain and stretch reflexes. Then, during each sweep of spray, the operator maintains gentle, smooth, steady tension on the muscle to take up any slack that develops, carefully avoiding force strong enough to produce pain. Jerky and rapid rocking motions activate trigger points and should also be avoided.

Stretch is facilitated by asking the patient to slowly take a deep breath and then slowly exhale through pursed lips, fully exhaling. During this long, slow exhalation, the muscles tend to relax and are more easily stretched. Inspiration is facilitated by having the patient look up, and exhalation by having the patient look down toward the feet.[67] Thus, looking down and exhaling together further facilitate relaxation. The Lewit stretch technique,[68] which is discussed later, may be combined with stretch and spray or used as an alternate method of stretching the muscle without spray.[68] Following stretch and spray the skin should be rewarmed with moist heat by dry hot packs or a wet-proof moist heating pad, and then the muscle should be moved through the full active range of motion. A more detailed description of the stretch and spray procedure is available.[134]

Head and neck pain

A number of neck muscles, including the upper trapezius, sternocleidomastoid, splenii, and suboccipital muscles, refer pain strongly to the head. These muscles frequently are responsible for headache, especially when it has been diagnosed as "tension" headache or "muscle tension" headache.[42] Masticatory muscles are likely to cause temporal, maxillary, and jaw pain, as well as earache and toothache; trigger points in cutaneous muscles of the head and neck sometimes contribute to facial pain.[134]

The primary masticatory muscles for closing the jaw include the masseter, temporalis, medial pterygoid, and upper division of the lateral pterygoid; their antagonists are the digastric and lower division of the lateral pterygoid muscles, which primarily open the jaw. When ear pain, temporal headache, and hypersensitivity of the teeth to pressure, heat, and cold are present, the masseter and temporalis muscles are most likely involved. Pain referred from myofascial trigger points to a normal tooth has resulted in the extraction of a healthy tooth because the myofascial origin of the pain was not identified. When pain, dysfunction, or both include the temporomandibular joint, the lateral pterygoid muscle often is involved.

A simple test for normal range of jaw opening is the ability to insert a tier of the first three knuckles of the nondominant hand between the incisor teeth.[134] Masticatory muscles respond best to stretch therapy when the patient is supine or when the head is tilted backward, nearly horizontal. The upright seated position is less effective.

Upper and lower trapezius

The upper trapezius is the muscle generally considered most likely to develop myofascial trigger points. These trigger points project pain up the back of the neck and to the temporal region (Figure 45-3, *A*).[120,133] Upper trapezius trigger points are sometimes activated, and often perpetuated, by lack of support for the elbows when sitting; support for the elbows is critical when a person's upper arms are so short that the elbows fail to reach the chair's armrests. Many

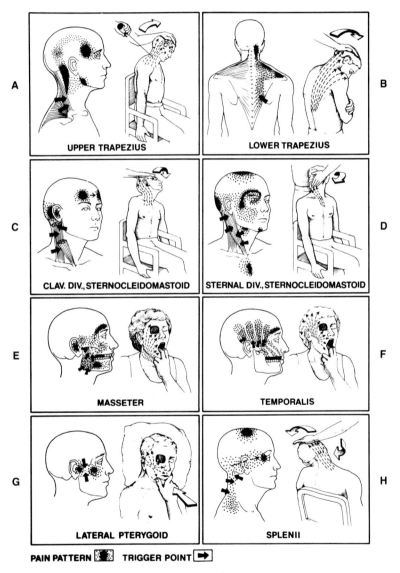

PAIN PATTERN ▓ **TRIGGER POINT** ➡

Figure 45-3. Location of trigger points *(solid arrows)* and pain patterns *(black stipples)*, stretch positions and spray patterns *(dashed arrows)* for muscles that cause head and neck pain. Curved white arrows show direction of pressure applied to stretch each muscle, and dashed arrows trace the path of parallel sweeps of vapocoolant spray to release tension and permit stretch of each muscle. In **H,** broken arrow in pain pattern deep to ear indicates pain deep in head radiating to back of eye. (From Simons, DG: Myofascial pain syndromes. In Basmajian, JV, and Kirby, RL, editors: Medical rehabilitation, Baltimore, 1984, Williams & Wilkins Co.)

daily activities encourage persistent shoulder elevation.

For treatment of the upper trapezius, the patient should be seated and relaxed, while the shoulder on the side to be stretched is anchored by having the patient grasp the chair seat with the hand. The spray pattern extends upward from the acromion over the upper trapezius muscle covering the posterolateral aspect of the neck, behind the ear, and around to the temple (Figure 45-3, *A*). The head is tilted passively toward the opposite side with the face turned to the same side, putting the muscle on maximum stretch. For most effective self-stretch, the patient must place the head in the same position and use the hand on the opposite side to gently but firmly add stretch tension.

The lower trapezius trigger point (Figure 45-3, *B*) is usually located at the inferior margin of the lower trapezius muscle near where it crosses the vertebral border of the scapula. This trigger point refers pain and tenderness to the region of the upper trapezius muscle and can induce satellite trigger points in it. Satellite trigger points like these rarely clear until the primary trigger point, in this case the lower trapezius, has first been inactivated.

The spray pattern for the lower trapezius muscle is primarily upward over the muscle to the acromion and continuing upward over the upper trapezius to cover the posterior cervical referred pain zone. Stretch is conveniently applied in the seated position as indicated by the curved white arrow in Figure 45-3, *B*. The operator grasps the patient's arm and brings the elbow across the chest while lifting slightly to fully protract and elevate the scapula in order to maximally stretch the lower trapezius fibers. This stretch is smoothly coordinated with unidirectional parallel sweeps of spray. The patient can perform this by self-stretch as illustrated in Figure 45-3, *B*.

Sternocleidomastoid

The clavicular and sternal divisions of the sternocleidomastoid muscle have distinctively different pain patterns, refer different autonomic phenomena, and require different stretch positions. Myofascial trigger points of the clavicular division refer pain bilaterally across the forehead (one of the few muscles that refers pain across the midline), deep in the ear, and also close behind the ear (Figure 45-3, *C*).[120,134] The trigger points in this division also may cause postural instability, spatial disorientation, and dizziness when the patient suddenly changes neck muscle tension by flexing the neck, looking up, or turning over in bed.

The stream of vapocoolant is directed upward from the clavicle covering the muscle and occiput to the vertex. This division is stretched by having the patient anchor the hand under the chair seat and by cradling the patient's head against the operator's torso to reassure the patient of support. The operator gradually extends the head backward and sidebends it (curved white arrow in Figure 45-3, *C*) to swing the mastoid process as far from the clavicular attachment of the muscle as possible.

The sternal division refers pain to the occiput, the vertex of the head, and the cheek, around the eye, and to the throat (Figure 45-3, *D*). Its lowermost trigger points may refer pain downward over the sternum. These trigger points may cause narrowing of the palpebral fissure, distressing coryza, scleral injection, and lacrimation on the same side as the trigger point.

After initial sweeps of spray, stretch of the sternal division is performed gently by rotating the face to the same side as the muscle to be treated and finally tipping the chin to the acromion for maximum stretch. As this maneuver slowly proceeds, the spray sweeps along the length of the muscle from the sternum to the mastoid process and over the back of the head (dashed arrows in Figure 45-3, *D*). It helps for the operator to direct sweeps just above the eye, being careful to cover the patient's eye with an absorbent pad and making sure that the patient closes the eye tightly. Spray in the eye can be extremely painful for about 2 minutes but causes no permanent damage. A stream of spray that accidentally hits the eardrum is startling and sometimes painful.

Masseter and temporalis

The trigger points in the superficial masseter refer pain to the face and upper or lower molar teeth (Figure 45-3, *E*), whereas trigger points in the temporalis may refer pain to any of the upper teeth and over the temporal bone and eyebrow in fingerlike projections (Figure 45-3, *F*). Deep masseter trigger points can cause ipsilateral tinnitus.

It is convenient to stretch and spray the masseter, temporalis, and medial pterygoid muscles together by combining the spray patterns (dashed arrows of Figure 45-3, *E* and *F*). The spray begins just below the jaw and continues in parallel sweeps upward and covers the cheek, temporal region, eyebrow, and area behind the ear. Self-stretch by having the patient pull the jaw forward down and sideways may be more effective than the operator's stretch and helps the patient to learn the technique of self-stretch for a home program.

Lateral pterygoid

The lateral pterygoid (Figure 45-3, *G*) is difficult to stretch because its main action is to protrude the jaw for opening. Retrusion of the jaw to stretch that muscle is severely limited by the articular fossa of the temporal bone. It is inaccessible to ischemic compression. Alternate treatment techniques such as injection or ultrasound are usually necessary.

Splenii

Myofascial trigger points in the splenii refer pain upward to cause a deep-seated headache (Figure 45-3, *H*) that concentrates behind the eye and often extends to the vertex.[120] Stretching the splenius capitis and cervicis muscles requires the combination of head and neck flexion with sidebending of the head and rotation of the face toward the opposite side, as illustrated in Figure 45-3, *H*. The arm must be anchored—usually by the patient's hand holding the chair seat or by the patient's sitting on the hand. The procedure is usually more effective if relaxation is facilitated by the patient slowly exhaling with the eyes directed down.

Posterior cervical muscles

Semispinalis cervicis and capitis trigger points project pain to the occiput and along the side of the head to the temporal region (Figure 45-4, *A*). Multifidus trigger points most commonly are found deep in the paraspinal mass at the C5 and C6 levels; they refer pain to the suboccipital area and downward to the scapula medially. When these pain patterns are combined, the pain covers much of that side of the head and the back of the neck. The multifidus trigger points are likely to incite satellite trigger points in the suboccipital muscles.

To stretch these muscles for treatment, the head and neck are flexed against the chest as parallel sweeps of spray are directed upward over the occiput and along the side of the head. Then a down pattern of spray sweeps across the lower neck and over the thoracic paraspinal muscles to cover the longissimus as shown in Figure 45-4, *A*.

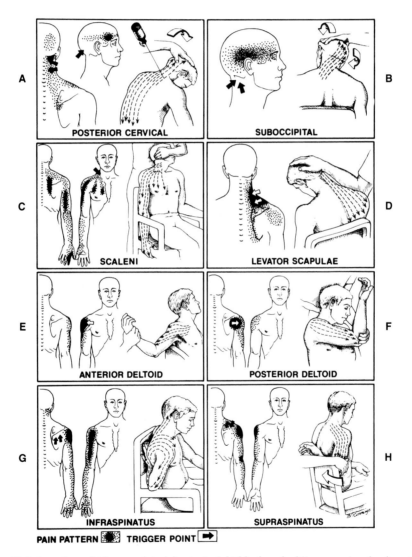

Figure 45-4. Location of trigger points *(short, straight black and white arrows)* and pain patterns *(stipples),* stretch positions and spray patterns *(dashed arrows)* for two muscles producing head and neck pain (**A** and **B**) and six muscles causing shoulder and upper extremity pain (**C** to **H**). Curved white arrows identify directions of pressure applied to stretch muscle. The dashed arrows trace impact of the stream of vapocoolant spray applied to release the muscular tension during stretch. (From Simons, DG: Myofascial pain syndromes. In Basmajian, JV, and Kirby, RL, editors: Medical rehabilitation, Baltimore, 1984, Williams & Wilkins Co.)

Suboccipital muscles

The trigger points of suboccipital muscles project pain along the side of the head to the upper face (Figure 45-4, *B*) and are responsive to stretch and spray and also to massage and pressure therapy.[98] They are not injected because of proximity to the external loop of the vertebral artery, nor should the vertebral artery itself be compressed.

The stream of spray is applied upward over the muscles and over the head (dashed arrows in Figure 45-4, *B*). Stretch of the medial suboccipital muscles is achieved by a combination of flexion of the head on the neck with rotation of the face to the opposite side (curved arrows, Figure 45-4, *B*). The lateral suboccipital muscles are stretched by flexion of the head while tilting the head on the neck to the opposite side. Neck movement does not stretch suboccipital muscles; only head movement on the cervical post stretches them.

Shoulder and upper extremity pain

Myofascial pain is referred to upper extremity and shoulder regions from trigger points in the ipsilateral neck, shoulder-girdle, and upper extremity muscles. Myofascial trigger points are a common cause of persistent posttraumatic shoulder pain[94] following trauma, such as a dislocated shoulder, fracture, and other injury in falls.[134]

Marked restriction of sidebending of the neck is most likely caused by scalene or upper trapezius trigger points or both. The levator scapulae restricts rotation more severely than does the sternocleidomastoid muscle. Severe muscular restriction of abduction of the arm at the shoulder is often due to subscapularis trigger points. Moderate restriction of abduction may be caused by trigger points in the more vertical thoracic and abdominal fibers of the pectoralis major muscle or in the triceps brachii muscle. The latissimus dorsi is a long, slack muscle; its trigger points minimally restrict forward flexion of the arm. Internal rotation at the shoulder is restricted by trigger points in the posterior deltoid, infraspinatus, teres minor, and teres major muscles.

Scaleni

All three scalene muscles can refer pain to the anterior, lateral, and posterior shoulder-girdle regions, as well as down the length of the upper extremity to the index finger (Figure 45-4, *C*).[108,133] In addition, tension resulting from trigger points on the anterior and middle scalene muscles can entrap the lower trunk of the brachial plexus, producing neurapraxia of the ulnar nerve.

To initiate treatment, a stream of vapocoolant spray is swept downward over the scalene muscles and over the entire referred pain pattern, including the hand and upper back. The stretch position for stretch and spray requires sidebending of the head and neck to the opposite side. The face position in Figure 45-4, *C*, places maximum stretch on the posterior scalene; rotating the face to the same side emphasizes stretch of the anterior scalene; simply sidebending the head and neck to the opposite side stretches

chiefly the middle scalene. A self-stretch program and correction of mechanical perpetuating factors are usually critical for sustained relief from active trigger points in the scalene muscles.[134]

Levator scapulae

A "stiff neck" is most commonly due to active trigger points in the levator scapulae muscle, which severely restricts rotation of the neck.[128] This muscle is a common source of pain referred to the base of the neck and along the vertebral border of the scapula and to the shoulder posteriorly (Figure 45-4, *D*).[121,134]

The spray pattern is downward, in the direction of the referred pain pattern, and requires three simultaneous functions with the operator's two hands. The operator must press the shoulder down and back to stabilize it, press the head forward and to the opposite side, and apply sweeps of spray at the same time. Placing the spray bottle in the same hand as the one that is applying the shoulder pressure may be easier for some operators than the technique illustrated in Figure 45-4, *D*. Stretch is achieved with the patient seated and requires flexion with sidebending and rotation of the head to the opposite side.

Deltoid

The free borders of the anterior and posterior deltoid muscle are common sites of active myofascial trigger points. Occasionally, the middle deltoid also becomes involved. As in the gluteus maximus, the referred pain from these trigger points is referred locally (Figure 45-4, *E* and *F*).

The sweeps of spray are applied distalward over the muscle and then over the pain pattern for trigger points in the anterior, middle, or posterior deltoid. The stretch position for the anterior deltoid (Figure 45-4, *E*) requires both horizontal extension and external rotation of the arm for maximum stretch. The stretch position for the posterior deltoid (Figure 45-4, *F*) brings the elbow as far across the chest as possible. Additional stretch may be obtainable by adding internal rotation rather than the external rotation illustrated in Figure 45-4, *F*.

Infraspinatus

The infraspinatus muscle commonly develops active trigger points. Pain referred from these trigger points is distinctive for its penetration deep into the shoulder joint (Figure 45-4, *G*).[92,121] Satellite trigger points in the anterior deltoid are sometimes activated by their location in the zone of pain and tenderness referred from trigger points in the supraspinatus muscle.

The sweeps of spray (dashed arrows in Figure 45-4, *G*) progress laterally over the muscle and extend downward over the upper extremity and also upward over the occipital area pain patterns. For stretch, the seated patient reaches behind the back as high as possible, then leans back against the chair, and relaxes as spray is applied. The arm is progressively repositioned as long as range of motion increases until full range of motion is achieved; chilling of the skin is avoided.

Supraspinatus

The supraspinatus muscle projects pain and tenderness to the middeltoid region and to the elbow (Figure 45-4, *H*), which the infraspinatus and scaleni patterns usually skip.

The spray path (dashed arrows in Figure 45-4, *H*) extends laterally over the supraspinatus muscle and downward over the upper extremity pain pattern to the wrist. Obtaining full stretch is difficult because the body obstructs full adduction.

It helps to adduct the arm alternately behind and in front of the torso to stretch all fibers of the muscle as much as possible.

Latissimus dorsi

Myofascial trigger points in the latissimus dorsi (Figure 45-5, *A*) are particularly obnoxious because no positioning of the arm seems to relieve the pain referred by these trigger points and they are so commonly overlooked; the muscle is long and slack. Pain from trigger points in both the latissimus dorsi (Figure 45-5, *A*) and serratus posterior superior (Figure 45-6, *F*) is referred to the scapular area. Pain re-

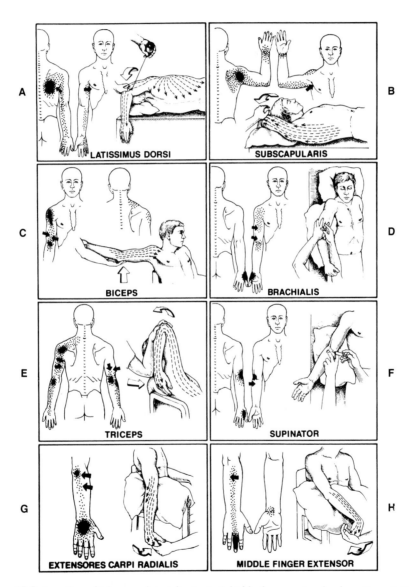

Figure 45-5. Location of trigger points *(short, straight black arrows)* and pain patterns *(stipples),* stretch positions and spray patterns *(dashed arrows)* for eight muscles responsible for shoulder and upper extremity pain. Curved white arrows identify directions of pressure applied to stretch muscle. Dashed arrows trace impact of stream of vapocoolant spray applied to release muscular tension during stretch. (From Simons, DG: Myofascial pain syndromes. In Basmajian, JV, and Kirby, RL, editors: Medical rehabilitation, Baltimore, 1984, Williams & Wilkins Co.)

ferred to the posterior scapula from trigger points in the serratus posterior superior tends to be more cephalad and feels deep in the chest, sometimes through the chest. This depth is not characteristic of pain referred from the latissimus dorsi.

Because of the complex pain pattern referred by the latissimus dorsi muscle, vapocoolant is directed from the trigger point in the direction of the pain pattern, covering the entire muscle, including its attachments on the crest of the ilium and to the lumbar and thoracic spine; sweeps of spray also course upward over the upper half of the muscle covering the pain pattern on the dorsum of the upper extremity to the tips of the ulnar fingers (Figure 45-5, *A*).

Full stretch can be attained seated, but stretch and spray is usually more satisfactory when the patient is in the supine position. Effective stretch requires full arm flexion and external rotation (Figure 45-5, *A*) in essentially the same position as for the subscapularis (Figure 45-5, *B*). If the subscapularis is involved, full stretch of the latissimus dorsi is not attained until the subscapularis is released.

Subscapularis

A frozen-shoulder syndrome often develops because of trigger points (thick black arrow in Figure 45-5, *B*) in the subscapularis muscle.[116,134] Active trigger points in this muscle severely restrict both abduction and external rotation of the arm. The severely restricted range of motion predisposes to trigger points in numerous other shoulder-girdle muscles, which leads to a frozen-shoulder syndrome. The pain referred from the subscapularis muscle is focused on the back of the shoulder and frequently includes a "band" of pain and tenderness around the wrist. The chief complaint may be this pain and tenderness of the wrist with restricted range of shoulder motion.

Treatment begins with the application of upsweeps of spray covering the side of the chest and axilla as in Figure 45-5, *B*, covering all of the scapula, including its vertebral border. Sweeps continue until they cover the wrist. The stretch position requires gentle, progressive abduction and external rotation of the arm at the shoulder.

Biceps brachii

The biceps referred pain pattern covers the anterior shoulder and sometimes extends to the elbow (Figure 45-5, *C*). Bicipital tendonitis may require inactivation of trigger points in the long head of the biceps brachii for prompt, lasting relief.

The stream of vapocoolant is directed upward over the entire length of the muscle in parallel sweeps to include the referred pain pattern at the shoulder. The long head of this muscle crosses two joints and requires both elbow extension and horizontal extension of the arm at the shoulder for full stretch as in Figure 45-5, *C*. The doorway stretch is an important part of the patient's home program.[134]

Brachialis

The pain referred from the brachialis muscle is remarkable for its strong projection to the base of the thumb (Figure 45-5, *D*), to which the supinator (Figure 45-5, *F*), brachioradialis,[116] and adductor pollicis[116] muscles also refer pain and tenderness. The stream of spray progresses downward over the muscle to cover the thumb as in Figure 45-5, *D*. Stretching the brachialis muscle requires extension of the forearm at the elbow. Brachialis trigger points are readily palpated by pushing aside the distal biceps; they respond well to injection.

Triceps brachii

The three heads of the triceps muscle have five trigger point locations that refer separate pain patterns.[134] The five patterns are combined in Figure 45-5, *E*. The long head is a two-joint muscle; trigger points in it restrict flexion both at the elbow and at the shoulder. The long head of the triceps is commonly involved with other shoulder-girdle muscles and is a frequently overlooked cause of shoulder dysfunction. The taut bands of the long head trigger points are readily felt by pincer palpation of the belly of the long head just above midarm adjacent to the humerus. The muscle is examined for taut bands as the muscle fibers slip between the fingertips that start palpating outward from the groove between the muscle and the humerus.[134]

The spray is applied in parallel sweeps over the muscle or muscles harboring active trigger points in the direction of the pain pattern, which may be upward over the arm or distalward over the forearm to the hand. Full stretch requires simultaneous flexion at the elbow and at the shoulder (Figure 45-5, *E*).

Supinator

For patients with tennis elbow, or epicondylitis, trigger points in the supinator muscle are often the key to resolving their distress. This muscle refers pain to the dorsal web space of the thumb and to the region of the lateral epicondyle (Figure 45-5, *F*), which becomes tender to finger taps.

The stream of vapocoolant sweeps downward over the muscle, swings back to cover the lateral epicondyle, and then proceeds distalward over the dorsum of the forearm and thumb. Stretch is achieved by combined extension at the elbow and pronation of the hand. Injection of the most common trigger points in the medial (radial) portion of the muscle is sometimes required (Figure 45-5, *F*). The radial nerve passes through a more lateral portion of the muscle and should be avoided when injecting.[134] The finger and wrist extensors, which form the extensor muscle mass attached to the lateral epicondyle, frequently also develop trigger points as part of the tennis elbow syndrome. These trigger points are readily located by palpation of the extensor muscles for taut bands and local twitch responses.

Extensores digitorum and carpi radialis

The hand and finger extensor group of muscles is essential for strong grip. Patients with trigger points in these muscles frequently develop a painful hand grip and an impaired sense of grip strength; a cup or a glass unexpectedly drops from their grasp. Active trigger points in the extensor carpi radialis refer pain to the lateral epicondyle and dorsum of the hand (Figure 45-5, *G*). The trigger points in the finger extensor muscles refer pain specifically to the dorsal surface of the corresponding finger, as exemplified by the middle finger extensor in Figure 45-5, *H*.

The stream of spray covers the dorsal forearm, wrist, hand, and fingers. The stretch position of the extensor digitorum muscle requires full flexion of the wrist and fingers (Figure 45-5, *H*). This positioning also stretches the wrist extensors except for the addition of ulnar or radial deviation of the wrist.

Flexores digitorum

No distinction is made in the distribution of pain referred from the flexores digitorum sublimis and profundus. Pain from their trigger points refers to the finger that corresponds to the muscle involved as, for example, the third finger flexor (Figure 45-6, *A*). Patients with trigger points in this

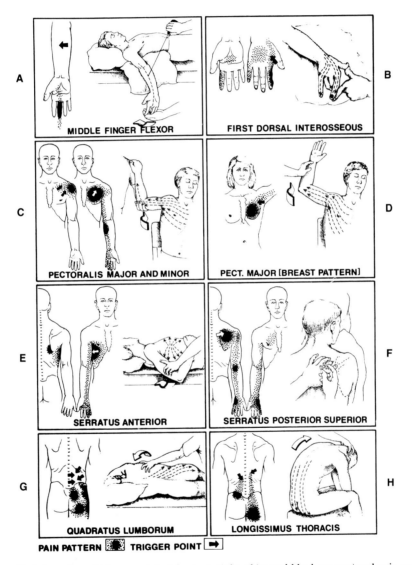

Figure 45-6. Location of trigger points *(short, straight white and black arrows)* and pain patterns *(stipples)*, stretch positions and spray patterns *(dashed arrows)* for two muscles producing shoulder and upper extremity pain (**A** and **B**) and six muscles causing trunk and back pain (**C** to **H**). Curved white arrows identify directions of pressure applied to stretch muscle. Dashed arrows trace impact of stream of vapocoolant spray applied to release muscular tension during stretch. (From Simons, DG: Myofascial pain syndromes. In Basmajian, JV, and Kirby, RL, editors: Medical rehabilitation, Baltimore, 1984, Williams & Wilkins Co.)

muscle usually feel that the pain is projected to the very tip of the finger, and occasionally beyond.

The stream of vapocoolant spray is directed distalward over the forearm flexor surface of the forearm and to the fingertips. Since this muscle produces flexion across multiple joints, all of those joints must be extended simultaneously for a full stretch (Figure 45-6, *A*).

Interossei of hand

Myofascial trigger points in the interossei are not uncommon, and those in the dorsal interossei are readily palpable against the metacarpal bones. These trigger points refer pain primarily along the side of the digit that corresponds to the distal attachment of that interosseus muscle. The first dorsal interosseus muscle also projects pain across the hand and into the little finger (Figure 45-6, *B*).

The stream of vapocoolant spray is applied distalward from the wrist to the ends of the painful digits while the fingers are separated to stretch the dorsal interosseus muscle that lies between them as in Figure 45-6, *B*. Frequently, injection is more satisfactory because the metacarpophalangeal joints of many patients have limited lateral mobility.

Trunk and back pain

Myofascial trigger points in muscles of the chest and abdomen exhibit viscerosomatic and somatovisceral interactions. Viscerosomatic influence is demonstrated by the satellite trigger points that develop in the pectoralis major muscle in the zone of pain referred from an acute myocardial infarction or from recent myocardial ischemia.[134] Similarly, trigger points in the external oblique muscle of the abdomen may develop in response to the pain referred to that region by gastrointestinal ulcer disease.[74]

Conversely, an example of somatovisceral interaction is the cardiac arrhythmia associated with the "arrhythmia trigger point" in the right pectoralis major muscle.[134] These interactions suggest feedback loops within the central nervous system among trigger points, visceral structures, and their referred pain zones.

Pectoralis major and minor

Myofascial trigger points in the more horizontal sternal division fibers of the pectoralis major and in the pectoralis minor muscle can refer pain that closely mimics cardiac ischemia (Figure 45-6, *C*).[120,134] Trigger points in the lateral, nearly vertical, thoracic fibers of the pectoralis major refer pain and tenderness to the breast (Figure 45-6, *D*). These trigger points may cause a degree of breast hypersensitivity that in either sex makes clothing contact with the nipple intolerable.

For both pectoral muscles, the vapocoolant is first directed upward and laterally over the muscle fibers on the chest. The path of the stream continues over the arm to include, for the pectoralis major, the lateral side of the hand (Figure 45-6, *C*).

Stretch is applied to the sternal division fibers of the pectoralis major by horizontal extension of the arm and to the pectoralis minor by retraction of the scapula with backward traction on the arm (curved white arrow in Figure 45-6, *C*). The nearly vertical thoracic fibers along the lateral border of the pectoralis major are stretched more effectively by full abduction and flexion of the arm at the shoulder than by the partial stretch position shown in Figure 45-6, *D*. The fully flexed position of the arm also stretches the latissimus dorsi. The application of spray should also include that muscle, as in Figure 45-5, *A*, to ensure that it is not restricting full stretch of the pectoralis major.

The head-forward, round-shouldered posture that maintains the pectoral muscles in the shortened position usually requires correction for lasting inactivation of pectoral trigger points. This poor posture is spontaneously improved without muscle strain by providing comfortable lumbar support with a roll or small pillow whenever the patient sits and by assumption of the weight-on-toes posture with full lumbar lordosis when standing.[134]

Serratus anterior

This muscle is not generally considered a muscle of accessory respiration,[134] but active trigger points in it decrease maximum chest expansion and cause the patient to feel short of breath. Pain is referred over the side of the chest and to the lower vertebral border of the scapula (Figure 45-6, *E*), not far from the focus of pain characteristic of latissimus dorsi trigger points (Figure 45-5, *A*). Pain from both muscles may extend down the arm to the hand.

The stream of vapocoolant is directed in radial sweeps that start at the trigger point, cover the muscle, and include the entire pain pattern, ensuring coverage of the lower half of the scapula. The serratus anterior is stretched with the patient either supine as illustrated in Figure 45-6, *E*, or seated in an armchair. For a self-stretch, the patient can sit and reach backward with the arm, retracting the scapula and using the uninvolved arm to reach behind the body and grasp the humerus of the involved arm distally to assist the stretch. In either position the elbow is progressively moved posteriorly to strongly retract the scapula.

Serratus posterior superior

The pain produced by this muscle can be a tantalizing joker. It is threateningly deep, frequently projecting into and through the chest, suggesting visceral disease. It is enigmatic because positioning of the arm or shoulder may have little effect on it. The serratus posterior superior trigger points are not palpable unless the scapula is fully protracted, uncovering the muscle laterally.[134] These trigger points are identified by palpating through the trapezius and rhomboid muscles against the ribs for their exquisite sensitivity, taut bands, and reproduction of pain pattern. Trigger points in this muscle respond well to ischemic compression. Because these serratus fibers run between the ribs and the spinous processes, stretch is frequently unsatisfactory, so the trigger points may require injection (Figure 45-6, *F*). However, one must be very careful to direct the needle nearly parallel to the skin surface and not let it penetrate between the ribs, causing a pneumothorax.

Quadratus lumborum

The quadratus lumborum muscle is probably the most common source of myogenic back pain[114,120,145] and is all too commonly overlooked.[121] Quadratus lumborum trigger points project pain to the sacroiliac joint, lower buttock, and lateral hip regions (Figure 45-6, *G*).[123] These trigger points are prone to generate satellite trigger points in the posterior gluteus minimus muscle, producing a secondary sciatica-like pain pattern (Figure 45-8, *B*) that further misleads the diagnostician. Bilateral quadratus lumborum involvement is likely to produce pain that extends across the sacroiliac region.

A complete examination of the quadratus lumborum muscle requires that the side-lying patient be positioned to provide adequate space for palpation between the twelfth rib and the crest of the ilium. The space is realized by elevating the rib cage and dropping the pelvis on that side. This examination position is similar to the stretch position of Figure 45-6, *G*, but with the upper leg behind the lower leg and with the upper knee resting on the examining table.[108,114,135]

To release these trigger points, the stream of vapocoolant is directed downward, covering all of the lumbar area and all aspects of the buttock, particularly the sacral and sacroiliac joint region. Two stretch positions may be needed to release trigger points in all parts of this complex triple muscle.[135] The leg-forward stretch position in Figure 45-6, *G*, tilts the pelvis away from the ribs and rotates the pelvis forward with respect to the chest; the leg-back position[108,135] places the upper leg behind the lower leg, reverses the twist on the thoracolumbar region, and also stretches the iliopsoas muscle. To ensure that tightness of the iliopsoas muscle is not blocking stretch of the quadratus lumborum, spray is directed downward over the abdomen beside the midline to the inner thigh. This releases iliopsoas muscle tightness.

Injection of trigger points of this muscle is remarkably effective but requires careful technique and appreciation of the anatomy involved.[108,135]

Quadratus lumborum trigger points are often perpetuated by a short leg, a small hemipelvis, or both. Both are readily correctable with lifts, which are often essential for lasting relief of myofascial low back pain.[134,135]

Thoracolumbar paraspinal muscles

In the midthoracic region the most medial paraspinal muscle group is the spinalis, which lies close to the spinous processes. Next laterally is the longissimus, which is one of the longest muscles in the body; it covers most of the paraspinal space in the thoracic and lumbar areas. The il-

iocostalis fibers are the most lateral paraspinal muscles and attach to the ribs. Bilaterally, the deeper paraspinal muscles form an inverted V; the deeper they lie, the shorter they are and the more diagonal their course. The deepest and shortest rotatores connect adjacent vertebrae at nearly a 45-degree angle. Therefore, to stretch the deeper fibers, one must either mobilize the adjacent vertebrae by spinal mobilization techniques or strongly rotate as well as flex the spine.

Taut bands in the longissimus fibers are readily palpated and course parallel to the axis of the spine. Myofascial trigger points in these bands refer pain distalward, usually at least several segments removed; pain from longissimus trigger points may project to the distal buttock (Figure 45-6, *H*).

Lower thoracic iliocostalis trigger points may refer pain anteriorly to the abdominal wall at approximately the same dermatomal level, as well as caudally (Figure 45-7, *A*). Upper lumbar iliocostalis trigger points refer pain lower to the midbuttock (Figure 45-7, *C*). The deeper multifidus muscles refer pain more locally (Figure 45-7, *D*). The short rotatores often refer pain to the midline at the same segmental level so the pain pattern alone may not identify on which side these trigger points lie.[134]

The spray pattern for all thoracolumbar paraspinal muscles is caudalward and covers all of the muscle fibers of the involved muscle, which, for the longissimus and iliocostalis muscles, extends the length of the spine below the trigger points and includes the buttocks (Figures 45-6, *H*, and 45-7, *B*). Multifidus trigger points require a less extensive spray pattern, which is angulated somewhat laterally (Figure 45-7, *D*).

The stretch position for the longissimus is simple flexion, most effectively performed with the patient seated with the legs spread widely apart, feet on the floor. The arms dangle; the patient must allow the neck, hands, and elbows to flex in a relaxed manner as the fingers reach the floor. The spray must also be extended downward to cover the gluteus maximus (Figure 45-6, *H*), which is stretched by hip flexion in this position. Stretch of the iliocostalis can be augmented by having the patient rotate the face and chest to the opposite side while flexing the spine.

For stretch of the multifidi the patient rotates toward the same side and flexes the spine at the same time (Figure 45-7, *D*). Strong rotation is essential. Injection may be more effective for these deep diagonal muscles. Care must be exercised in the thoracic region to direct the needle medially toward the deep rotatores to avoid injecting too laterally— between the ribs—thus producing a pneumothorax.

Abdominal muscles

Myofascial trigger points in an external abdominal oblique muscle may refer pain that is nearby, or the pain may extend into adjacent areas and cross the midline (Figure 45-7, *E*).[120,134] Those trigger points close to the thoracic or pelvic attachment of the rectus abdominis are likely to refer

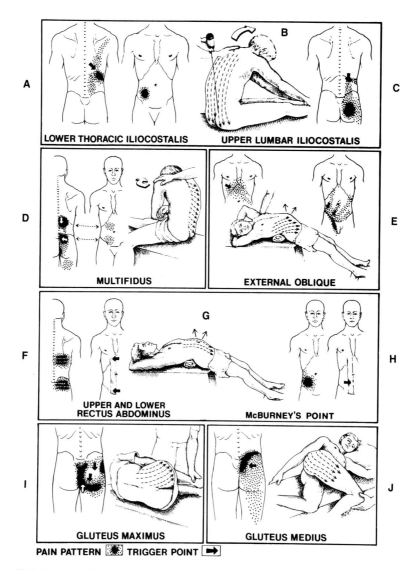

Figure 45-7. Location of trigger points *(short straight black and white arrows)* and pain patterns *(stipples)*, stretch positions and spray patterns *(dashed arrows)* for five muscles producing trunk and back pain (**A** to **H**) and two muscles responsible for lower extremity pain (**I** and **J**). Curved white arrows identify the directions of pressure applied to stretch a muscle. Dashed arrows trace impact of vapocoolant spray applied to release muscular tension during stretch. (From Simons, DG: Myofascial pain syndromes. In Basmajian, JV, and Kirby, RL, editors: Medical rehabilitation, Baltimore, 1984, Williams & Wilkins Co.)

pain horizontally across the back at approximately the same level as the trigger point (Figure 45-7, *F*). A trigger point in the lower right quadrant of the rectus abdominis may convincingly simulate the pain of appendicitis (Figure 45-7, *H*). Having the patient tense the abdominal muscles by elevating the feet while lying in the supine position easily differentiates a source of pain in the viscera from one in the abdominal wall. Tensing the abdomen augments tenderness of the musculature and protects the underlying viscera from the pressure of palpation.[118] If the patient also has a complaint of back pain, one must exercise caution to avoid

overstrain with this test. Instead, the examiner could elicit contraction of the supine patient's abdominal muscles by resisting with one arm the patient's effort to extend downward his or her upper limbs while palpating with the other hand.

The spray pattern for trigger points in the abdominal muscles is essentially downward over the entire abdomen, including any additional referred pain patterns. Stretch of the abdominal wall muscles is achieved by having the patient lie supine with the hips over the end of the table and the feet resting on a chair seat; a towel or roll is placed under the lumbar spine to hyperextend it (Figure 45-7, *G*). The patient then protrudes the abdomen by taking a deep breath, holding it, and contracting the diaphragm while relaxing the abdominal wall muscles as parallel sweeps of spray are applied downward over the entire abdomen. A twisting movement is added for the external oblique (Figure 45-7, *E*) that is not required for the rectus abdominis (Figure 45-7, *G*).

Lower extremity pain

With a few exceptions, trigger points in lower extremity muscles refer pain locally, distally, or both. Since the gluteal regions are often identified by patients as part of the low back, gluteal muscle trigger points often contribute to "low back pain" syndromes.[115]

Gluteus maximus

As in the deltoid muscle, trigger points in the gluteus maximus are easily palpated for taut bands, usually have eloquent local twitch responses, and produce relatively local referred pain patterns that concentrate along the sacrum and inferior surface of the buttock (Figure 45-7, *I*).

For treatment the patient is placed in the side-lying position, as illustrated in Figure 45-7, *I*. Vapocoolant spray is directed distally over the buttock to the upper thigh as the thigh is progressively flexed, bringing the knee to the chest. Gluteal trigger points are commonly associated with tight hamstring muscles that also must be released (see Figure 45-8, *H*) for return of full function and lasting relief.

Gluteus medius

The trigger points in the gluteus medius muscle (Figure 45-7, *J*) refer pain along the crest of the ilium and over the sacrum and may project downward across the buttock to include the upper thigh.

To inactivate these trigger points, a stream of vapocoolant spray is directed from the crest of the ilium downward over the buttock and upper half of the thigh in parallel sweeps as illustrated in Figure 45-7, *J*. The thigh is flexed 90 degrees and, since this muscle is primarily an abductor, the thigh is progressively adducted as the sweeps of spray are applied. It is often helpful to have an assistant pull backward on the anterior superior iliac spine region to anchor the pelvis for more effective stretch. The Dudley J. Morton foot configuration (disproportionately long second metatarsal bone) is a perpetuator of these trigger points and should be corrected.[134,135]

Gluteus minimus

Myofascial trigger points in the anterior and posterior portions of the gluteus minimus muscle have distinctively different pain patterns. The anterior trigger points project pain primarily along the lateral thigh that may extend to the lateral ankle and also to the lower buttock (Figure 45-8, *A*); posterior gluteus minimus trigger points refer pain over a sciatic distribution that concentrates on the buttock, posterior upper thigh, and upper calf (Figure 45-8, *B*). This pattern is suggestive of an S1 radiculopathy; the patient may have a combination of active gluteus minimus trigger points and a radiculopathy that perpetuates them.

Sweeps of spray for treatment of the anterior portion of the gluteus minimus are applied along the anterior portion of the muscle belly and downward over the lateral thigh and leg to the ankle, including a detour to cover the lower buttock (Figure 45-8, *A*). The stretch position for this muscle requires the patient to be side lying with progressive extension and adduction of the thigh at the hip. The knee may be bent (Figure 45-8, *A*).

The direction of spray for the posterior gluteus minimus is downward from the crest of the ilium over the posterior buttock and thigh to include most of the calf. To stretch this muscle the patient is placed on the edge of the table with the shoulders flat against the table; the thigh being treated is flexed slightly, placed forward over the other leg, and moved into adduction (Figure 45-8, *B*). Care must be taken to include the gluteus maximus muscle with sweeps of spray to eliminate any restricting trigger points in that muscle.

Piriformis

An active piriformis trigger point restricts the combination of adduction and internal rotation of the thigh at the hip. Trigger point tenderness is palpable both rectally and externally.[115] Piriformis trigger points refer pain to the buttock laterally and sometimes medially to the sacrum (Figure 45-8, *C*).

The stream of vapocoolant is applied distally over the lateral and posterior hip and thigh to the knee as the muscle is stretched in the side-lying patient. The thigh is flexed at the hip to nearly 90 degrees and internally rotated by elevating the ankle as the knee is lowered gently to increase adduction at the hip, as seen in Figure 45-8, *C*.

The gluteus maximus muscle should be included in the spray pattern; it, too, is being stretched and may harbor restricting trigger points.

Tension caused by taut bands of trigger points in the piriformis muscle may entrap the peroneal part or all of the sciatic nerve, depending on anatomic variations of how the nerve passes under or through the muscle.[115]

Adductores longus and brevis

In addition to the pain pattern represented in Figure 45-8, *D*, pain from the adductores longus and brevis may refer upward throughout the groin[116,133] or downward to the anteromedial aspect of the thigh just above the knee; referred pain may extend down to the ankle (Figure 45-8, *D*). Active trigger points in this muscle markedly restrict abduction of the thigh and are a common source of groin and distal anterior thigh pain above the knee. To treat these muscles, the stream of vapocoolant is applied in upward sweeps across the anteromedial thigh and over the inguinal region, and then in downward sweeps across the lower anteromedial thigh and medial knee and over the pain pattern covering the anteromedial leg to the ankle. As the spray is applied, the muscle is gradually stretched by placing the patient's foot against the opposite knee and slowly abducting the thigh at the hip as indicated by the white arrow in Figure 45-8, *D*.

Quadriceps femoris

Rectus femoris trigger points are usually located at the proximal end of the muscle near its musculotendinous junction (solid black arrow, Figure 45-8, *E*) and refer pain distalward to the knee cap and sometimes the distal half of the anterior thigh. The vastus intermedius trigger point (small white arrow, Figure 45-8, *E*) is deeper than and distal to the rectus femoris trigger point; it refers intense pain locally and distally over the upper part of the thigh.

The vastus medialis trigger points (Figure 45-8, *F*) refer pain to the medial aspect of the knee. The distal (more anterior) trigger points of the vastus lateralis (solid black arrow in Figure 45-8, *G*) are frequently multiple and difficult to eliminate; they refer pain intensely and extensively over the lateral thigh, sometimes including the lateral buttock. The proximal (and more posterior) trigger points of the vastus lateralis (small white arrow, Figure 45-8, *H*) usually refer pain only to the vicinity of the trigger point.

To release trigger points in the rectus femoris muscle, the patient is placed with the knee flexed and the hip extended in the side-lying position. The stream of vapocoolant is applied distalward from the anterior inferior iliac spine region over the muscle to and including the knee cap (Figure 45-8, *E*). For release, trigger points in the vastus medialis require distalward sweeps of spray from the hip over the muscle to the knee (Figure 45-8, *F*). However, the proximal referral pattern of the vastus lateralis calls for upward sweeps of spray (dashed arrows, Figure 45-8, *G*).

Of the four quadriceps muscles, only the rectus femoris crosses two joints, the hip and knee. Therefore only that muscle requires hip extension as well as knee flexion for full stretch; the three vasti require only knee flexion. The latter are stretched by bringing the heel to the buttock, a position that also stretches the posterior portion of the vastus lateralis muscle.

Biceps femoris

Pain referred from trigger points in this hamstring muscle (solid black arrow, Figure 45-8, *H*) is projected to the back of the knee and sometimes extends over the proximal calf.

Vapocoolant spray is applied in parallel sweeps distalward from the hip over the posterior thigh and knee to include the calf. Stretch can be obtained by slowly performing a straight leg raising maneuver as vapocoolant is applied (Figure 45-8, *H*). Usually, effective stretch is obtained more quickly by initially abducting the thigh at the hip without raising the foot and applying the spray upward over the

adductor magnus and inguinal region to release it. This massive adductor muscle is an important extensor of the thigh. The foot is then elevated to bring the thigh from the abducted to the 90-degree flexed position, applying parallel sweeps of spray over the length of the thigh; the spray should be applied progressively more laterally as more lateral muscles are stretched by gradually moving the flexed thigh into adduction.[135]

Gastrocnemius

Myofascial trigger points in the superficial, two-joint gastrocnemius muscle are usually found along either the medial or the lateral border of the muscle at the level indicated by the solid black arrow in Figure 45-9, *B*. These trigger points commonly refer pain over the calf and to the instep of the foot.[121,135] Active trigger points in this muscle make walking uphill painful and commonly cause nocturnal calf cramps.

For treatment the patient is placed in a prone position with the feet hanging over the end of the treatment table and with the knees straight (Figure 45-9, *B*). The stream of spray is directed distally over the back of the thigh downward over the calf and heel covering the sole. The foot is strongly dorsiflexed using the operator's knee for powerful leverage (curved white arrow, Figure 45-9, *B*).

The patient is taught to self-stretch this muscle by standing with the involved leg behind the other and moving the pelvis and body forward, bending the forward knee while keeping the knee of the affected leg fully extended and the heel solidly on the floor. Moving the pelvis and body forward dorsiflexes the foot and with the knee straight stretches the gastrocnemius muscle.[135]

Soleus

Myofascial trigger points in the second-layer, single-joint soleus muscle frequently are the cause of heel pain and tenderness that is mistakenly attributed to a heel spur (Figure 45-9, *A*). Occasionally, trigger points in this muscle project pain to the area of the sacroiliac joint on the same side.[115,135]

A stream of vapocoolant is directed distally in parallel sweeps covering the calf, the heel, and most of the sole. The stretch position (Figure 45-9, *A*) is flexion of the knee with the patient prone. Progressive downward dorsiflexion pressure is applied to the ball of the foot to stretch this muscle (curved arrow, Figure 45-9, *A*). The patient should be taught self-stretch by standing and progressively bending the knee while keeping the heel on the floor. Progressive dorsiflexion at the ankle with the knee bent selectively stretches the soleus but not the gastrocnemius muscle. To take up the slack as the tight soleus muscle releases, the patient slowly increases ankle dorsiflexion by further flexing the knee, while keeping the heel firmly on the floor.

Tibialis anterior

The tibialis anterior muscle dorsiflexes and helps to invert the foot. Its trigger points occur at the proximal end of the muscle (Figure 45-9, *C*). They refer pain downward along

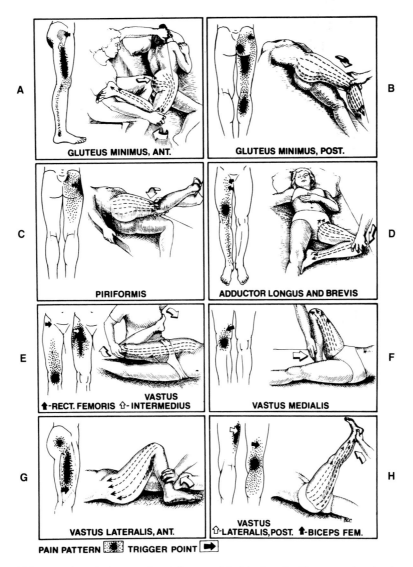

Figure 45-8. Location of trigger points *(short straight black and white arrows)* and pain patterns *(stipples)*, stretch positions and spray patterns *(dashed arrows)* for 10 muscles causing lower extremity pain. Curved white arrows identify the directions of pressure applied to stretch the muscle. Dashed arrows trace impact of stream of vapocoolant spray applied to release muscular tension during stretch. (From Simons, DG: Myofascial pain syndromes. In Basmajian, JV, and Kirby, RL, editors: Medical rehabilitation, Baltimore, 1984, Williams & Wilkins Co.)

the course of the muscle and its tendon to the medial aspect of the foot, concentrating on the great toe.[116,121,133]

To release anterior tibial trigger points, a stream of vapocoolant is applied distalward over the muscle and its pain pattern on the shin, the dorsum of the ankle, and the large toe. To stretch this muscle, the end of the foot is grasped firmly and simultaneously plantar flexed and slowly everted (white curved arrow, Figure 45-9, *C*) to pick up the slack as the spray helps to release muscle tension.

Peroneus longus and brevis

The peroneus longus and brevis are adjacent muscles that generally have indistinguishable referred pain patterns. The trigger points in the peroneus longus are usually a few cen-

timeters distal to the common peroneal nerve as it passes over the fibula and under the peroneus longus muscle just distal to the fibular head (Figure 45-9, *D*).

Referred pain from the peroneal muscles projects behind the lateral malleolus and may extend distally over the lateral aspect of the leg and over the lateral aspect of the dorsum of the foot (Figure 45-9, *D*).

Treatment is initiated by applying vapocoolant spray distalward over the lateral aspect of the leg, ankle, and dorsum of the foot to the toes. The foot of the supine patient is strongly dorsiflexed and inverted (curved white arrow, Figure 45-9, *D*) to slowly take up the slack that develops as the muscle releases in response to the vapocoolant spray.

The tension produced by taut bands associated with trigger points in the peroneus longus can entrap the deep peroneal nerve against the underlying fibula, producing characteristic loss of sensation and a degree of dorsiflexion weakness (footdrop). Inactivation of the trigger points promptly relieves neurapraxia of the peroneal nerve caused by the taut bands. Trigger points in these muscles are perpetuated by the stress of walking on the "knife-edge" produced by a long second metatarsal bone (D.J. Morton foot configuration).[134]

Extensores digitorum and hallucis longus

The trigger points of the extensores digitorum hallucis longus, like those of the peroneal muscles, refer pain that includes the dorsum of the foot laterally (Figure 45-9, *E*). In addition, this pain may extend part of the way up the leg or downward to include the toes.

With the patient supine, vapocoolant is applied distally over the length of the muscles from the knee over the anterolateral aspect of the leg and over the pain reference zones on the ankle, dorsum of the foot, and the toes. These toe extensors are stretched together by simultaneously plantar flexing the foot and all toes, as illustrated in Figure 45-9, *E*.

Interossei of the foot

As in the hand, active trigger points in the dorsal interossei of the foot are not rare. These trigger points refer pain distally to the side of the toe corresponding to the attachment of the involved muscle (Figure 45-9, *F*). However, in the foot, interosseous trigger points are commonly associated with hammer toe and, if not too long standing, this joint restriction can be alleviated by inactivating the trigger points. The taut bands are exquisitely tender. The dorsal interosseous trigger points are readily palpable against the metatarsal bones and, once localized, easily injected. Stretch and spray is not reliably effective in these muscles. Full stretch may be difficult to achieve.

Patient education

Characteristically, one stress activates a trigger point and other factors or conditions perpetuate it. To effectively manage an acute MPS that has persisted and propagated into

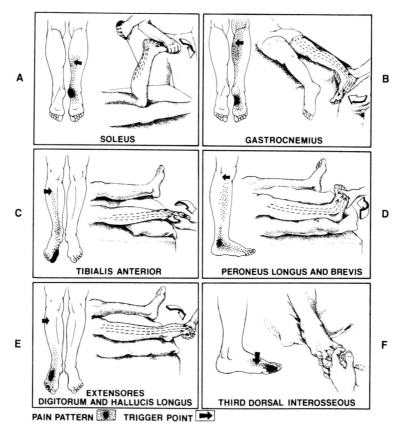

Figure 45-9. Location of trigger points *(short, straight black arrows)* and pain patterns *(stipples),* stretch positions and spray patterns *(dashed arrows)* for eight muscles producing lower extremity pain. Curved white arrows identify directions of pressure applied to stretch muscle. Dashed arrows trace impact of vapocoolant spray applied to release muscular tension during stretch. (From Simons, DG: Myofascial pain syndromes. In Basmajian, JV, and Kirby, RL, editors: Medical rehabilitation, Baltimore, 1984, Williams & Wilkins Co.)

widespread chronic involvements, one must clearly distinguish perpetuating factors from the stress or stresses that initially activated the trigger points.

Acute single-muscle myofascial syndromes are much less likely to recur and become chronic if the patient understands the myofascial origin of the pain. The patient then learns what muscle caused the pain and what movements can overload that muscle. Acute onset is often associated with an accident or fall, when specific muscles are overloaded by lengthening contractions used to cushion impact. Sometimes the trigger points were initiated by muscle overload stress resulting from a specific movement or positioning that the patient should learn to avoid. This is particularly true when the muscle is commonly used in a repetitive movement that would also perpetuate its trigger points.

A patient who has a clear-cut MPS must understand that the pain is of muscular origin and not due to nerve damage or bone changes. When shown the exact position of the part of the body being moved before and after stretch, the patient can see the increase in range of motion, experience the increase in function, and relate these to the reduction in pain. Emphasizing that the treatment that provided relief changed only the muscles and did nothing to the nerves or bones helps convince the patient that the pain originated in the muscles.

Reproduction of the patient's pain by pressure on a trigger point convinces both the patient and the operator that the trigger point is responsible for at least part of the patient's pain complaint. Frequently, patients with chronic pain are as concerned about its origin and prognosis as about the pain itself. Learning the muscular cause of the pain and how to relieve it is profoundly reassuring.

Not uncommonly patients return discouraged because they still have pain and therefore feel that their last treatment was of no help. When an accurate detailed drawing is made of their current pain patterns and compared with their previous drawing, it often becomes apparent that the pattern of pain has changed significantly; the pattern of pain produced by those muscles treated previously is gone. These patients are aware only that they still have pain but had not noticed precisely where it was located and thereby overlooked their progress. Many times, a previous pain emerges from less irritable trigger points that are now uncovered— like peeling off the outer layer of an onion.

Whenever possible, patients are encouraged to continue their accustomed activities but in a manner that avoids overloading vulnerable muscles. Patients learn to use, not abuse, their muscles. Correction of an anatomic or postural perpetuating factor frequently requires change in patient behavior; unless patients fully understand the relationship between that perpetuating factor and the cause of their pain, they quickly revert to previous behavior and then wonder why the pain has returned.

Other stretch techniques

Muscle stretch can be achieved in several ways: by stretch and spray, which was described previously; by postisometric relaxation; by ischemic compression; and by deep friction massage. Additional modalities can be helpful. Low-intensity ultrasound applied directly to the trigger point is valuable when the trigger point is otherwise inaccessible. Some find electrical stimulation over the trigger point helpful; high-voltage galvanic stimulation is usually effective.

Postisometric relaxation

Use of voluntary contraction alternated with passive stretch for releasing tight muscles has been identified by many names. Physical therapists frequently refer to contract-relax or rhythmic stabilization. Osteopathic physicians are likely to speak of muscle energy techniques and myofascial release.

Postisometric muscular relaxation, as described by Lewit and Simons,[68] is simple and effective. It combines nicely with the stretch and spray technique and is most valuable when used by the patient for self-treatment at home. The muscle is gently stretched to the onset of resistance (take up the slack) and held there isometrically. For the next 3 to 7 seconds, either the operator or the patient exerts fixed resistance against which the muscle gently contracts in that position at approximately 25% of maximal effort. While the same position is passively maintained, the patient "lets go" (relaxes the contracting muscle). Only after the patient has thoroughly relaxed is the muscle slowly, gently, and passively extended, taking up the slack that developed. This contract-relax cycle is repeated three to five times. Full release of tension may not occur until after the second or third cycle. Relaxation is facilitated after the patient slowly takes a full (complete) breath and while slowly exhaling through pursed lips, empties the lungs to maximal exhalation. The patient concentrates on total relaxation of the muscle to be stretched.[68] Additional relaxation and release may be achieved by downward gaze during exhalation.[67]

Ischemic compression

Ischemic compression, or "thumb therapy," is noninvasive and effective but painful.[106] This technique may be applied by the operator or as self-treatment by the patient. Pressure is applied directly on the spot of greatest tenderness (the trigger point) with a steady moderately painful (tolerable) pressure. As the pain eases, the pressure is increased to maintain approximately the same level of discomfort. When the trigger point is no longer painful (after 15 seconds to 1 minute of pressure), the pressure is released and full active range of motion performed.

Immediately after release, blanching of the skin is followed by reactive hyperemia at the site of pressure. Very likely the same hyperemia is present in the muscle itself and is part of the benefit. Some therapists apply less pressure for a shorter time but with repeated applications on successive days until trigger point tenderness is obliterated and the referred pain disappears.

Massage

Deep muscle massage (deep friction, or stripping massage) can effectively inactivate trigger points. Stripping massage requires lubrication of the skin and the application of firm bilateral thumb pressure by sliding the thumbs slowly and progressively along the length of the taut band. The band is firmly compressed between the thumbs. The slowly progressive "milking" action relieves the sense of induration at the trigger point after several repetitions and releases the tautness of the palpable band. This technique is painful but effective in superficial muscles. A confirmation and extension[19] of an earlier study[18] found that repeated massage of tender tense areas in the muscles of myofascial pain patients effectively relieved their pain and eliminated the areas of abnormal tenseness in 21 of 26 patients. Elevation of serum myoglobin levels following massage decreased as the amount of remaining induration decreased with successive treatments.[18,19]

Injection and stretch

Treatment by injection of trigger points is selected initially when the trigger points are inaccessible to stretch therapy or because of mechanical restriction of joint motion. It is used on trigger points unresponsive to the foregoing noninvasive methods. Dry needling[65,92,134] and isotonic saline injection[134] also are effective; without a local anesthetic, dry needling is likely to be more painful. Isotonic saline for injection usually contains 0.9% of the preservative and local anesthetic, benzyl alcohol. The flushing effect of the injected fluid on sensitizing agents is probably also important.

Needle penetration of the skin can be painless if the needle is inserted rapidly with a flick of the wrist after the antiseptic alcohol has dried. Stretching the skin until it is tight reduces skin sensitivity to needle prick. Alternatively, the site may be chilled for 6 to 8 seconds with a stream of Fluori-Methane applied in a figure-of-eight pattern with the crossover at the point of needle penetration.[134,138] The site of injection is chilled just short of frosting the skin.

The rationale of needle therapy depends primarily on the disruption of the self-sustaining trigger point mechanism. This approach requires precise localization and penetration of the trigger point with the needle. Injection of 0.5% procaine in isotonic saline *without epinephrine* reduces the severe, sometimes devastating, pain of trigger point penetration. It preserves the tenderness to palpation of the remaining trigger points and thus permits detection of any trigger points that were overlooked. The local analgesic effect of the 0.9% concentration of benzyl alcohol preservative in the saline for injection permits its substitution for procaine in those few patients who are allergic to procaine. Half percent lidocaine also is less desirable than procaine but can

be used if necessary. Long-acting local anesthetics are avoided because they temporarily obliterate all local trigger point tenderness and produce muscle necrosis.[134]

When injecting muscles next to the ribs, the needle must not penetrate between the ribs, which easily produces a pneumothorax.

Before an injection the tender trigger point and its taut band are localized between the fingers. The needle is then directed precisely into the trigger point.[134] Contact with the trigger point is confirmed by a jump response of the patient and a local twitch response of the taut band in the muscle. Probing should continue until a response has been obtained or the region has been fully explored with the needle. Tenderness to palpation must be relieved. Pressure is applied during and after injection to ensure hemostasis.

Procaine injection is followed by stretch and spray to release any trigger points that were missed by the needle. Application of moist heat by a hot pack or wet-proof heating pad for 5 minutes immediately after injection helps to avoid postinjection soreness that otherwise may last for 2 or 3 days. The patient should be warned of this possible soreness; aspirin relieves it. The moist heat is immediately followed by several cycles of active full range of motion in both the shortened and stretch positions of the treated muscles to reestablish normal function. Passive self-stretch range-of-motion exercises at home are instituted routinely. This stretching helps to maintain the increased range of motion obtained by treatment.

Perpetuating factors

The presence or absence of perpetuating factors determines the answer to the question, "How long should the effect of specific myofascial therapy last?" In the absence of perpetuating factors, relief should last indefinitely until the trigger point is reactivated, as in the beginning, by another overload stress. In the presence of perpetuating factors, relief is temporary; lasting relief depends on eliminating perpetuating factors[35,42,134] so that response to therapy is cumulative.

The muscles can become so hyperirritable because of perpetuating factors that any attempt at specific myofascial therapy aggravates the pain. The perpetuating factors, in these cases, must be addressed first. Perpetuating factors are usually multiple.

A significant perpetuating factor may have caused no symptoms before activation of the trigger points. A leg-length discrepancy of 6 mm (¼ inch) may have caused no pain or discomfort throughout most of a lifetime; on activation of quadratus lumborum trigger points by another stress, the discrepancy becomes a potent perpetuator of the distressing quadratus lumborum trigger points.

Perpetuating factors are identified as mechanical or systemic. Mechanical perpetuating factors are ubiquitous, and systemic perpetuating factors are common. Elimination of one or several, but not all, of the factors may provide only modest improvement in the therapeutic response until the remaining factors are resolved. The more thoroughly all significant perpetuating factors are managed, the more effective and longer lasting the treatment becomes.

Mechanical perpetuating factors

Table 45-2 lists specific mechanical perpetuating stresses juxtaposed beside the muscle or muscles most likely to be affected by each stress. Systemic perpetuating factors may relate to any or all skeletal muscles. Mechanical perpetuating factors include anatomic variations, seated and standing postural stress, life-style, and vocational stress.

Anatomic variations. One common anatomic variation is a short leg or small hemipelvis or both,[134] which must be corrected by a heel lift or buttock lift for lasting relief of low back[114] and sometimes head, neck, and shoulder pain caused by myofascial trigger points.

The relatively common phenomenon of short upper arms is frequently an unrecognized perpetuator of trigger points in the shoulder elevator muscles. This variation is corrected by providing elbow rests or pads that modify the furniture to fit the individual.[134]

Table 45-2. Muscles most likely to be affected by specific mechanical perpetuating factors

Stress	Muscles	References
Anatomic variations		
Short leg and/or small hemipelvis	Quadratus lumborum	134 (Ch. 4), 135 (Ch. 4)
	T-L paraspinals	134 (Ch. 48)
	Shoulder-girdle and neck-righting*	134 (Ch. 7, 19, 20)
	Masticatory	134 (Ch. 8-12)
Short upper arms	Levator scapulae	134 (Ch. 4, 19)
	Upper trapezius	134 (Ch. 6)
	Rhomboids	134 (Ch. 27)
Long second metatarsal (D.J. Morton foot configuration)	Peroneus longus	134 (Ch. 4), 135 (Ch. 20)
	Vastus medialis	135 (Ch. 14)
	Gluteus medius	135 (Ch. 8)
Seated postural stress		
Hard smooth mat	Long toe flexors	135 (Ch. 25)
	Foot intrinsics	135 (Ch. 27)
Heels dangling	Hamstrings	135 (Ch. 16)
	Soleus	135 (Ch. 22)
Back unsupported	Quadratus lumborum	114, 135 (Ch. 4)
No backrest contact	T-L paraspinals	134 (Ch. 48)
No lumbar support	Pectoralis major	134 (Ch. 42)
No scapular contact	Rhomboids	134 (Ch. 27)
Standing postural stress		
Head-forward posture	Pectoralis major and rhomboids	134 (Ch. 42)
	Posterior cervicals	134 (Ch. 16)
Canted running surface	Quadratus lumborum	114, 135 (Ch. 4)
	Scaleni	134 (Ch. 20)
Vocational stress		
Shoulder elevation	Upper trapezius	134 (Ch. 6)
	Levator scapulae	134 (Ch. 19)
Arm abduction	Supraspinatus	134 (Ch. 21)
	Deltoid	134 (Ch. 28)
Hand supination	Supinator	134 (Ch. 36)
Grasp	Finger extensors	134 (Ch. 35)
	Finger flexors	134 (Ch. 38)
Systemic factors		
Any muscular function	All muscles	134 (Ch. 4)

*Neck-righting muscles include scalene, sternocleidomastoid, and upper trapezius muscles.

The long second metatarsal, or D.J. Morton foot configuration, throws the foot off balance because of the knife-edge effect during toe-off that disturbs gait and overloads lower extremity muscles. This is corrected by inserting a toe pad under the head of the first metatarsal bone.[134,135]

Seated postural stress. Seated postural stress on the muscles may be induced by a hard smooth mat under an office chair, a chair seat too high for heels to reach the floor, the lack of a firm back support, and persistent head-forward posture.

A hard, smooth mat, such as Plexiglas, makes the office chair with free casters glide readily whenever its occupant changes position or exerts the slightest pressure against the desk. This causes the intrinsic foot muscles to try to grasp the slick floor; the effort overloads and perpetuates trigger points in these muscles.

Another seated postural stress is caused by a chair seat too high for that individual's leg length, leaving the heels dangling off the floor. This causes under-thigh compression of the hamstrings and chronic shortening of the soleus muscle. Both effects are perpetuating factors for trigger points and can be avoided by providing a suitable footrest (book, pillow, or small footstool).

Sitting in a chair with the back unsupported may be caused by a seat that is too long from front to back, that is flat and provides no lumbar support, or that supplies no scapular contact or whose backrest has inadequate backward angulation. In a seat that is too long from front to back, the backs of the knees solidly engage the front of the seat before the buttocks reach the backrest. The backrest should be contoured to support a normal lumbar lordosis. This also corrects the head-forward posture by correcting the thoracic kyphosis induced by an abnormally flattened back, thereby balancing the head erect over the shoulders without muscular effort. Scapular contact with the backrest and backward angulation of the backrest help to carry the weight of the head and shoulders and to stabilize the spine, relieving the quadratus lumborum and paraspinal muscles.

Standing postural stress. The head-forward posture is also induced by weight bearing on the heels and relieved, when standing, by shifting the center of gravity forward onto the balls of the feet. This weight distribution augments lumbar lordosis and permits the person to hold the head erect, balanced over the shoulders without muscle strain. It elevates the chest and restores normal postural relations by swinging the scapulae backward to their normal resting position and thus relieving the persistent shortening of the pectoral muscles.[134] This improved posture takes a major load off the posterior cervical muscles, which in the head-forward posture must hold the weight of head against the pull of gravity. To many neck and shoulder-girdle muscles the head-forward posture is a powerful perpetuating factor that requires a major change in patient behavior.

A canted running surface is common on the slanted beach of the seashore or a slanted circular track. It produces the same effect as a short leg[134] that tilts the pelvis. The tilt must be compensated by the quadratus lumborum, paraspinal muscles, or both, causing a persistent overload that perpetuates trigger points in these muscles.

Vocational stress. Sustained shoulder elevation commonly overloads the upper trapezius and levator scapulae muscles, perpetuating their trigger points. Typists and other workers using their hands in a relative fixed elevated position are prone to maintain their shoulders in a shrugged position to help elevate the hands to the level of their work. The work should be lowered or the patient's body raised.

Prolonged arm abduction similarly overloads the supraspinatus and deltoid muscles. Elbow support should be provided. In one study workers developed myofascial syndrome of the supraspinatus and upper trapezius muscles from frequent repetitive movements stressing those muscles.[44] When tested, these painfully involved muscles had less endurance and more rapid onset of electromyographic evidence of fatigue than nonpainful muscles. The author related these findings to alteration in muscle metabolism resulting from ischemia.

Overload of hand supination as when playing tennis or using a screwdriver readily overloads the supinator muscle. The symptoms produced by active trigger points in the supinator muscle are frequently labeled epicondylitis, or tennis elbow. The arm should not be fully extended at the elbow when playing tennis, since that eliminates the forceful supinator function of the triceps brachii muscle.

Strong grasp overloads the finger extensors because the extensors function vigorously as an essential part of grasp. Active trigger points in these muscles tend to cause a painful and weak grip. Items are likely to slip out of the grasp unexpectedly due to unpredictable reflex inhibition. The supinator, the wrist, and finger extensor muscles are commonly involved together.

Systemic perpetuating factors

Systemic perpetuating factors can aggravate trigger points in any muscle and increase the irritability of all skeletal muscles, rendering them more vulnerable to the development of secondary and satellite trigger points.[134] Systemic factors include enzyme dysfunction, metabolic and endocrine dysfunction, chronic infection or infestation, and psychologic stress.

Correction of a significant perpetuating factor reduces irritability of the muscles, which results in less pain, improved responsiveness of the muscles to specific myofascial therapy, or both.

Muscle is an energy engine. It converts the energy of a high-energy molecule, ATP, to mechanical movement by converting it to a lower-energy molecule, adenosine disphosphate (ADP). Understandably, anything that interferes with energy metabolism of the muscle tends to compromise this function and thereby increases both muscle irritability and susceptibility to trigger points.

Enzyme dysfunction. The nutritional inadequacies that most commonly perpetuate myofascial trigger points are lack of B-complex vitamins, particularly B_1, B_6, B_{12}, and folic acid. The metabolic enzymatic functions and congenital deficiencies of each of these vitamins has been reviewed in detail.[134] Low electrolyte levels, potassium, and calcium may be critical, and minerals such as calcium, copper, and iron are essential. Vitamin deficiency is signaled by abnormally low laboratory values and by clinical symptoms that are ascribable to a lack of that vitamin. Vitamin inadequacy is a suboptimal level that may produce only a partial picture of deficiency or simply impair muscle function by increasing its irritability and tendency to develop trigger points.

The prevalence of unrecognized vitamin deficiency is remarkably high, especially in hospital patients. Among 120 hospital patients, 88% had abnormally low levels in one or more of 11 vitamins.[4] Despite this high prevalence, the history of dietary intake was inadequate in only 39%. More than half of the patients were deficient in two or more vitamins. Serum folate, the most common vitamin deficiency, was low in 45% of these patients. Symptoms of vitamin deficiency were clinically apparent in only 38% of these patients.[4] How many more of these patients had a vitamin inadequacy was not determined.

Clinical experience shows that the lower the serum value within the lower quartile of the "normal" range, the more likely that this degree of vitamin inadequacy is contributing significantly to increased muscle irritability and that it will require correction for lasting relief of the patient's chronic trigger point pain.

Vitamin dependence is observed in a few babies who are born with severe congenital deficiency of an enzyme that requires that vitamin as its coenzyme. Such defects require the ingestion of pharmacologic megadoses of the vitamin to sustain life; the specific enzyme defects and their chemical recognition have been summarized for each of the B vitamins considered here.[134] Unexplored, however, is the prevalence of milder degrees of such congenital enzyme deficiencies that could multiply by many times the minimum vitamin requirement of individuals who have become increasingly deficient in that one enzyme. The serum vitamin level might appear safely in the normal range. The wide range of individual variation in the requirements for essential nutrients including vitamins is well established[140] and should be considered.

All of the B-complex vitamins and vitamin C are water soluble. They have remarkably low toxicity because an excess is quickly excreted in the urine.

The common assumption that adequate dietary ingestion ensures an adequate metabolic supply of a vitamin does not consider the many causes of vitamin insufficiency. They include not only inadequate ingestion of the vitamin but also impaired absorption, inadequate utilization, increased metabolic requirement, and increased excretion or destruction within the body.[143] In addition, the usual selection process for individuals who serve as controls to establish normal values does not screen out individuals with marginal insufficiency, including many who show chemical evidence of vitamin deficiency and depletion of stores.[2] One should expect therefore that published normal values are not optimal values. This helps to explain why, clinically, the lower quartile of "normal" is often a zone of inadequacy for muscle metabolism.

A characteristic neurologic finding in vitamin B_1 inadequacy is increasingly severe loss of vibration sense at progressively more distal sites on the upper and lower extremities. By comparing the time of loss of sensibility at successively more proximal levels following one activation of a long-period tuning fork, one can demonstrate progressively lower thresholds of response at successive proximal sites on the extremities.

The recommended daily allowance (RDA) for thiamine (vitamin B_1) is dependent on the daily energy expenditure. The requirement for vitamin B_1 is greatest when carbohydrate is the source of energy. It is an essential enzyme for the entry of pyruvate (end product of anerobic metabolism) into the Krebs' cycle for oxidative metabolism (the chief source of energy in muscle).[64] The critical symptoms of severe thiamine deficiency are recognized as wet beriberi (heart muscle failure) or dry beriberi that includes severe skeletal muscle weakness and serious central and peripheral nervous system dysfunction.[84]

Pyridoxine (vitamin B_6) is an impressive jack-of-all-trades—an essential coenzyme to more than 60 enzymes in human metabolism. It is essential for the metabolism of numerous amino acids, including the methionine-to-cysteine pathway, blockage of which leads to homocystinuria. It plays an important conformational or structural role in the enzyme phosphorylase. This enzyme is essential for the release of glucose from glycogen, which is a necessary first step for all anaerobic (glycolytic) metabolism in skeletal muscle. Pyridoxine is essential to the synthesis or metabolism of nearly all neurotransmitters. This correlates with the deterioration of mental function seen in experimental pyridoxine deficiency. It is required for the synthesis of nucleic acids, which are required for messenger ribonucleic acid (RNA) and therefore essential for normal cell reproduction. It is critical in the synthesis of at least 10 hormones, including insulin and growth hormone.[17,134] This list is by no means complete.

Symptoms of vitamin B_6 deficiency include skin symptoms of dermatitis, glossitis, and stomatitis and nervous system symptoms of convulsion, connective tissue swelling (carpal tunnel syndrome), and peripheral neuritis. Severe compromise of erythropoiesis has been clearly demonstrated as hypochromic anemia in experimental animals.[17] Several classes of drugs are well known to increase the demand for vitamin B_6. They include antitubercular drugs, oral contraceptives, the chelating agent penicillamine, anticonvulsants, corticosteroids, and excessive alcohol consumption.[134] Severe depletion of vitamin B_1 is well recognized in chronic alcoholism and is not uncommon in the heavy social drinker. Laboratory tests for serum levels of vitamins B_1 and B_6 unfortunately are expensive and sometimes difficult to obtain but often provide critically important information.

Both thiamine and pyridoxine are widely distributed in nature but in modest amounts. Vitamin B_1 is rapidly destroyed by heat in neutral and alkaline solutions. It is stable in acidic solutions but only to boiling temperature. Vitamin B_1 is quickly leached out of food during washing or boiling. Pyridoxine suffers substantial losses during cooking and is quickly destroyed by ultraviolet light (sunlight) and oxidation (when held on a steam table). Riboflavin (vitamin B_2) and ascorbic acid (vitamin C) are destroyed in milk in clear plastic bottles by fluorescent light at the grocery store.

Both cobalamin (vitamin B_{12}) and folate play an essential role in the synthesis of deoxyribonucleic acid (DNA) that is required for the maturation of erythrocytes and therefore for oxygen transport. Vitamin B_{12} is also essential for fat and carbohydrate metabolism; this may account for its importance to the integrity of the peripheral and spinal nervous system.[47]

Both vitamin B_{12} and folate deficiency characteristically cause megaloblastic anemia, but only vitamin B_{12} produces serious peripheral nervous system deficits. Many clinicians have been accustomed to basing vitamin therapy on the response of the patient's hematopoietic system. If the anemia is caused by vitamin B_{12} deficiency but the patient is being treated with folic acid, the hematologic picture reverts to normal with no improvement in, or even exacerbation of, the neurologic deficits. This approach has led to permanent neurologic damage. For this reason the Food and Drug Administration limits nonprescription folic acid to 400 μg per dose.

There is no need to guess about deficiencies of vitamin B_{12} and folate. Laboratory tests for serum levels of these vitamins are readily available and usually leave no doubt as to what needs correction. Every patient with chronic myofascial pain deserves these tests.

The metabolic interdependence of vitamin B_{12} and folate produces a reciprocal therapeutic effect. An example is the methyl folate trap in which folate metabolism is blocked for lack of vitamin B_{12}.[47] Folate may actually accumulate to unexpectedly high serum folate levels. Administration of vitamin B_{12} can precipitously drop the serum folate level and deplete what may initially have seemed to be an adequate reserve. A reverse effect may also be seen: a 20% or 30% drop in the serum vitamin B_{12} level with oral supplementation of badly needed folic acid.

Vitamin B_{12} is rarely deficient in the diet except in strict vegetarians. This vitamin is synthesized by bacteria and obtainable only in food products that have been contaminated by or affected by bacterial action. Useful foods include practically all animal products and some legumes.[47]

An adequate serum cobalamin level is dependent on adequate ingestion, gastric secretion of intrinsic factor, adequate intestinal absorption (which is compromised by ileal disease), reabsorption of much of the vitamin B_{12} that is secreted in the bile, and adequate amounts of transport transcobalamines in the gut wall. Normally, daily ingestion of 3 to 5 μg of cobalamin is sufficient.

Conversely, folates are widely distributed in many foods in modest amounts, particularly leafy green vegetables (foliage), and are readily destroyed by processing and cooking. Folate is highly vulnerable to destruction by heat and oxidation; generally, 50% to 95% of the folate in food is destroyed in processing and preparation. Folate deficiency is the most common vitamin deficiency, especially in the elderly and those eating institutional cafeteria meals. Consistently over a period of years, three fourths of the select group of patients referred to a chronic myofascial pain clinic had inadequate levels of vitamin B_{12} or folate (within the lower quartile of "normal" or lower).

Supplementation with 1 to 3 mg of folic acid administered orally each day should bring the folate level to at least the midnormal range within 2 or 3 weeks. A 1 mg (1000 μg) daily oral supplement of vitamin B_{12} usually restores it to midrange within 4 to 6 weeks, thus avoiding the necessity for injection. This dose is several hundred times the RDA but totally innocuous. The administration of vitamin B_{12} or folic acid alone can be hazardous because of their reciprocal relationship, unless the serum level of the other is safely above the midnormal range. One cannot predict one vitamin inadequacy based on another, but the demonstrated inadequacy of one or several vitamins should increase suspicion. The administration of a balanced B-complex supplement of at least several times RDA should ensure that minor problems of diet, absorption, and increased demand are met. Also, adverse interactions caused by excessive administration of one vitamin are avoided. This philosophy of providing an excess is not applicable to the fat-soluble vitamins A, D, and E. Quite the contrary, one source of increased muscular irritability appears to be above-normal serum vitamin A levels. Chronic MPS patients taking a total of more than 30,000 IU (including dietary intake) of vitamin A daily should have the serum level of this vitamin tested.

For different reasons, ascorbic acid (vitamin C) is important to MPS patients. It is essential for hydroxylation of the amino acids lysine and proline to form the protocollagen molecule. Without it, the integrity of the connective tissue is compromised. In the absence of vitamin C to provide the collagen needed for strong vessel walls, the patient experiences marked capillary fragility and easy bruising. Capillary fragility leads to ecchymoses following injection of trigger points. Ecchymoses are unsightly and irritating to the muscle.

Smoking greatly increases the oxidation of vitamin C, rapidly depleting it. One should beware of injecting trigger points in smokers unless they have taken at least 1 g (preferably 3 or 4 g) of timed-release vitamin C daily for a week before treatment.

Vitamin C is also of clinical importance to the muscles because 500 mg of timed-release vitamin taken at the time of excessive muscular activity can reduce postexercise muscle soreness and stiffness.

Metabolic and endocrine dysfunction. The metabolic factors of gout, anemia, low electrolyte levels, and hypoglycemia increase muscle irritability and symptoms from trigger points, as do the endocrine disturbances of hypometabolism and estrogen deficiency.

The monosodium urate crystals of gout are less soluble in the acidic media of injured tissues than in blood and hence are deposited in areas of tissue injury and metabolic distress such as trigger points. Patients with a gouty diathesis respond better to treatment when the hyperuricemia is under control and generally respond better to injection than to stretch and spray. Vitamin C in relatively large amounts (1 to 4 g per day) is an innocuous and effective uricosuric agent.[57] The hyperirritability of trigger points in the muscles of some patients with serum uric acid levels in the high normal range subsides remarkably with uricosuric therapy.

From the muscle's point of view, anemia of any cause is a serious metabolic problem because the muscle depends on oxygen to sustain oxidative metabolism essential for meeting the bulk of its energy needs.

Abnormally low electrolyte levels of ionized calcium and potassium seriously disturb muscle function and increase muscle irritability, apparently because of their critical roles in the contractile mechanism. Serum ionized calcium is the essential measure. The total calcium ordinarily obtained on a blood chemistry profile correlates poorly with the ionized calcium.

The occurrence of hypoglycemia intensifies the metabolic distress of the muscle, and it clearly aggravates myofascial trigger points. Stretch or injection therapy should be deferred in patients while they are hypoglycemic; treatment during hypoglycemia is likely to aggravate rather than relieve their symptoms. A packet of gelatin prepared as a drink is a handy source of available carbohydrate with enough protein to prevent a subsequent hypoglycemia bounce.

Evidence of hypometabolism is found in some treatment-refractory patients with persistent active myofascial trigger points. Their serum folate levels are normal; this is important because folate inadequacy can cause symptoms resembling those of low thyroid function. Confusion arises because findings of laboratory tests of thyroid function are usually low normal and said to be within normal limits. These patients have marginally low T_3 uptake and low to midrange T_4 by radioimmunoassay (RIA). In these patients, insufficient thyroid function is revealed by a low basal metabolic rate[124] or a low basal body temperature,[6] by elevation of the serum cholesterol level, and by the response to thyroid supplementation.[124] The latter is evidenced by reduced irrita-

bility of the muscles and restoration of normal energy and stamina.

The basal temperature is obtained with an ovulation thermometer placed in the axilla by the patient each morning for 10 minutes before arising after sleep. Normally the basal temperature averages more than 36.1° C (97° F). The farther the basal temperature is below this value, the more vulnerable the patient is to hyperirritable trigger points in the muscles and often to depression. Basal temperature in ovulating women is reached immediately after menses.

Sonkin[124] demonstrated that with thyroid therapy those patients needing supplemental thyroid consistently recovered their energy and positive outlook on life and had an increased basal metabolic rate with a decreased serum cholesterol value. Their muscles became less vulnerable to myofascial trigger points and were more responsive to specific trigger point therapy. Travell[131] corroborated these observations.

Thyroid supplementation is contraindicated in patients with known cardiac arrhythmias or known myocardial disease that compromises cardiac reserve. Thyroid medication increases vitamin B_1 and estrogen requirements and may increase blood pressure. Overmedication causes symptoms of hyperthyroidism. Adjustment of dosage in these patients is dependent largely on clinical judgment and responses of basal metabolic rate and basal temperature. The site of metabolic dysfunction is apparently at the level of cellular utilization and is poorly reflected in serum hormone levels.

Thyroid supplementation for those patients who meet the criteria described by Sonkin[124] remains controversial among endocrinologists but of critical importance to patients in whom this is a major perpetuating factor for severe myofascial pain.

Chronic infection and infestation. Viral disease, bacterial infection, and parasitic infestation can perpetuate MPS. During a systemic viral illness, including the common cold or attack of flu, the irritability of myofascial trigger points increases markedly. One of the most common sources is an outbreak of herpes simplex virus type 1; however, neither herpes simplex virus type 2 (genital herpes) nor herpes zoster is known to aggravate MPS. Herpes virus type 1 can cause the common aphthous mouth ulcer, canker sore, or cold sore. It may also appear on the skin of the body or extremities as isolated vesicles filled with clear fluid. Lesions have been reported in the esophagus, and the symptoms of vomiting and diarrhea strongly implicate gastrointestinal involvement comparable to that of the mouth.

No drug is known to cure herpes simplex virus type 1, but a multipronged attack can greatly reduce the frequency and severity of recurrences. A daily dose of 300 to 500 mg of niacinamide reinforces mucous membrane resistance. Three tablets (or 1 packet) of viable lactobacillus, two or three times daily for at least a month, helps to reestablish the normal intestinal bacteria, reducing the chance of an intestinal viral outbreak. Local therapy is applied by rubbing an antiviral ointment into the skin or mouth lesions three times daily, which accelerates resolution of the lesion.

Any bacterial infection tends to exacerbate muscle irritability. A chronic infection such as an abscessed tooth, infected sinus, or chronic urinary tract infection can be a persistent perpetuating factor. Chronic sinusitis may arise from both infection and allergy. Normal erythrocyte sedimentation rate and C-reative protein tests help to eliminate the possibility of chronic infection.

A parasitic infestation is of concern as a likely perpetuator of myofascial pain in travelers exposed to conditions of poor sanitation and among active homosexuals. The worst offender is the fish tapeworm; next is giardiasis, and occasionally amebiasis. The first two tend to impair absorption of or consume vitamin B_{12} and the amebae may produce myotoxins that are absorbed. The diagnosis of infestation is investigated by three stool examinations for occult blood, ova, and parasites.

Posttraumatic hyperirritability syndrome. The group of myofascial pain patients with posttraumatic hyperirritability syndrome suffer greatly, are poorly understood, and are difficult to help. They respond to strong sensory stimuli much differently than most patients. Following a major impact to the body, head, or both, the muscles exhibit marked hyperirritability of trigger points and a distressing vulnerability to strong sensory stimuli. The trauma has usually been an automobile accident or fall that was sufficiently severe to have inflicted some degree of damage to the sensory pathways of the central nervous system. These patients describe constant pain that is easily augmented by any strong sensory input, including severe pain, a loud noise, vibration, prolonged physical activity, and emotional stress. It may take days or weeks to recover from a degree of trauma or noise that to most people would be inconsequential. From the date of onset, coping with pain has suddenly become the focus of life for these patients, who previously paid no particular attention to pain. Their function is impaired by a marked increase in pain and fatigue if they exceed their restricted limit of activity.

One of the distinguishing characteristics of the posttraumatic-hyperirritability syndrome is the loss of tolerance to what are to most people inconsequential mechanical stresses such as jarring, vibration, loud noises, and mild bumps or thumps. Exposure to such a stimulus immediately produces an increase in the pain level. The stimulus also causes a markedly increased sensitivity to subsequent stimuli so they suddenly become much more vulnerable to further aggravation of their misery. This increased arousal of the sensory system subsides slowly. It may take hours, days, or weeks, depending on the intensity of the stimulus required for this increased excitability of the sensory system to subside to its previous state. A strong sensory input appears to modulate the excitability of the arousal system. This increased excitability is paralleled by a corresponding increase in irritability of all of that patient's myofascial trigger points in the involved region.

The target area of trigger points and pain tends to concentrate in the somatic distribution of the brainstem, cervical cord, or lumbosacral cord. A few unfortunate individuals seem to have involvement of several regions. These patients are highly vulnerable to reinjury by additional trauma. It takes much less subsequent impact to exacerbate the process than in the initial accident.

The most effective treatment has been to inactivate all identifiable trigger points and to correct perpetuating factors. On occasion it may be necessary to reset the system by suppressing central nervous system excitability. To date, barbituates have been found most effective.

Psychologic stress. It is generally agreed that among chronic pain patients, malingering is rare.[51] Much controversy surrounds the question: "Is the chronic pain an expression of the patient's psychologic dysfunctions, or is the pain driving the patient crazy?" Patients who experience a serious chronic MPS that is undiagnosed and untreated are strongly impacted psychologically. They are confronted with a severe inescapable pain of unknown origin and of uncertain prognosis that is devastating their vocational, social, and private lives. The future is an ominous, impenetrable dark cloud. The ensuing depression aggravates the pain and reinforces the uncertainty and sense of hopelessness.[51] The most important service to these patients is the unambiguous, clear diagnosis of treatable MPS. They learn self-treatment and self-management techniques that give them control of the pain, rather than the pain controlling their lives and victimizing them.

As a positive prognostic factor for patients in chronic pain rehabilitation programs, continued employment as a productive member of society is usually a significantly more important factor than whether their case is in litigation or not.[51] Most patients initially would prefer to be well and earn their living. Eventually, if work is too painful and treatment ineffective, they turn to compensation. When patients reorient their primary focus of attention from being productive members of society to being pain patients, they develop a new self-image that shifts from function orientation to sickness orientation. Psychologically it is of utmost importance to preserve the patient's vocational activity, if possible.

PROGNOSIS

The initial prognosis when seeing a patient with MPS depends primarily on the number of perpetuating factors that must be identified and resolved and on the competence with which the active trigger points are located and inactivated.

The disability produced by a latent trigger point may persist throughout a lifetime. The limitation in range of motion caused by a latent myofascial trigger point has persisted for decades in many individuals. Stretch and spray after that length of time may nevertheless inactivate the trigger points and within minutes restore normal, pain-free, full range of motion.[132] Following inactivation of clinically active myofascial trigger points, the patient experiences pain relief and recovery of full range of motion, but careful examination often reveals some residual trigger point tenderness and a taut band. In this case, an active trigger point has been converted to a latent trigger point but remains a potential locus of reactivation whenever that muscle is subjected to overload or perpetuating factors develop.

It is not clear whether a muscle harboring an active myofascial trigger point, with the best of treatment, reverts completely to its previous normal state. Some trigger points appear to resolve completely with specific myofascial therapy; others clearly remain latent.

Some individuals are more prone to develop trigger points than others and have greater difficulty keeping them inactivated. These patients should be more conscientious in their daily stretch program to prevent the muscles from shortening and redeveloping trigger point tightness. For these individuals it appears that myofascial trigger points accumulate throughout their life and that they must learn to correct perpetuating factors and to avoid the overloads that convert latent trigger points to active ones.

ACKNOWLEDGMENT

I express deep indebtedness to Janet G. Travell, M.D., for the great reservoir of wisdom that she has so generously contributed to this chapter and to both her and Lois Simons, R.P.T., for review of the manuscript.

REFERENCES

1. Awad, EA: Interstitial myofibrositis: hypothesis of the mechanism, Arch Phys Med 54:449, 1973.
2. Azuma, J, et al: Apparent deficiency of vitamin B_6 in typical individuals who commonly serve as normal controls, Res Commun Chem Pathol Pharmacol 14:343, 1976.
3. Baker, BA: The muscle trigger: evidence of overload injury, J Neurol Orthop Med Surg 7:35, 1986.
4. Baker, H, and Frank, O: Vitamin status in metabolic upsets, World Rev Nutr Diet 9:124, 1968.
5. Bartels, EM, and Danneskiold-Samsoe, B: Histological abnormalities in muscle from patients with certain types of fibrositis, Lancet 1:755, 1986.
6. Barnes, B: Basal temperature versus basal metabolism, JAMA 119:1072, 1942.
7. Bengtsson, A, et al: Primary fibromyalgia, a clinical and laboratory study of 55 patients, Scand J Rheum 15:340, 1986.
8. Bengtsson, A, Henriksson, K-G, and Larsson, J: Reduced high-energy phosphate levels in painful muscle in patients with primary fibromyalgia, Arthritis Rheum 29:817, 1986.
9. Bengtsson, A, Henriksson, K-G, and Larsson, J: Muscle biopsy in primary fibromyalgia, Scand J Rheumatol 15:1, 1986.
10. Bennett, RM: Fibrositis: misnomer for a common rheumatic disorder, West J Med 134:405, 1981.
11. Bennett, RM: The fibrositis/fibromyalgia syndrome: current issues and prospectives, Am J Med 81(suppl 3A):1, 1986.
12. Bourdillon, JF: Spinal manipulation, ed 3 (edited by W. Heinemann), London, New York, 1983, Appleton-Century-Crofts.
13. Campbell, SM, and Bennett, RM: Fibrositis, DM 32:653, 1986.
14. Caro, XJ: Immunofluorescent detection of IgG at the dermal-epidermal junction in patients with apparent primary fibrositis syndrome, Arthritis Rheum 27:1174, 1984.
15. Caro, XJ: Immunofluorescent studies of skin in primary fibrositis syndrome, Am J Med 81(suppl 3A):43, 1986.
16. Cyriax, J: Textbook of orthopaedic medicine, ed 5, vol 1, Baltimore, 1969, Williams & Wilkins.
17. Danford, DE, and Munro, HN: Water-soluble vitamins: the vitamin B complex and ascorbic acid. In Gilman, AF, Goodman, LS, and Gilman, A, editors: The pharmacological basis of therapeutics, ed 6, New York, 1980, MacMillan Publishing Co, Inc.
18. Danneskiold-Samsoe, B, et al: Regional muscle tension and pain ("fibrositis"): effect of massage on myoglobin in plasma, Scand J Rehab Med 15:17, 1983.
19. Danneskiold-Samsoe, B, Christiansen, E, and Anderson, RB: Myofascial pain and the role of myoglobin, Scand J Rheum 15:154, 1986.
20. Dexter, JR, and Simons, DG: Local twitch response in human muscle evoked by palpation and needle penetration of a trigger point, Arch Phys Med Rehabil 62:521, 1981.
21. Dvoràk, J, Dvoràk, V, and Schneider, W: Manual medicine, 1984, Berlin, 1985, Springer-Verlag.
22. Eneström, S, Bengtsson, A, and Lindström, F: Attachment of IgG to dermal collagen in patients with primary fibromyalgia. Submitted for publication.
23. Epstein, SE, Gerber, LH, and Borer, JS: Chest wall syndrome, JAMA 241:2793, 1979.
24. Fassbender, HG: Non-articular rheumatism. In Pathology of rheumatic diseases, New York, 1975, Springer-Verlag.
25. Fischer, AA: Diagnosis and management of chronic pain in physical medicine and rehabilitation. In Ruskin, AP, editor: Current therapy in physiatry, Philadelphia, 1984, W.B. Saunders Co.
26. Fischer, AA: The present status of neuromuscular thermography, Academy of Neuro-muscular Thermography Clinical Proccedings, Postgraduate Medicine, Custom Communications, March 1986.
27. Fisher, AA: Correlation between site of pain and "hot spots" on thermogram in lower body, Academy of Neuro-muscular Thermography Clinical Proceedings, Postgraduate Medicine, Custom Communications, March 1986.
28. Fischer, AA: Pressure threshold meter: its use for quantification of tender spots, Arch Phys Med Rehabil 67:836, 1986.
29. Fischer, AA: Pressure tolerance over muscles and bones in normal subjects, Arch Phys Med Rehabil 67:406, 1986.
30. Fishbain, DA, et al: Male and female chronic pain patients categorized by DSM-III psychiatric diagnostic criteria, Pain 26:181, 1986.
31. Fock, S, and Mense, S: Excitatory effects of 5-hydroxytryptamine, histamine and potassium ions on muscular group IV afferent units: a comparison with bradykinin, Brain Res 105:459, 1976.
32. Foreman, RD, Blair, RW, and Weber, RN: Viscerosomatic convergence onto T2-T4 spinoreticular, spinoreticular-spinothalamic, and spinothalamic tract neurons in the cat, Exp Neurol 85:597, 1984.
33. Franz, M, and Mense, S: Muscle receptors with group IV afferent fibres responding to application of bradykinin, Brain Res 92:369, 1975.
34. Fricton, JR: Unpublished data, 1987.
35. Fricton, JR, and Schiffman, LS: The craniomandibular index: validity, J Prosthet Dent 58:222, 1987.
36. Fricton, JR, et al: Myofascial pain syndrome: electromyographic changes associated with local twitch response, Arch Phys Med Rehabil 66:314, 1985.
37. Fricton, JR, et al: Myofascial pain syndrome of the head and neck: a review of clinical characteristics of 164 patients, Oral Surg 60:615, 1985.
38. Frost, A: Diclofenac verus lidocaine as injection therapy in myofascial pain, Scand J Rheumatol 15:153, 1986.
39. Glogowski, G, and Wallraff, J: Ein beitrag zur Klinik und Histologie der Muskelhärten (Myogelosen), Z Orthop 80:237, 1951.
40. Good, MG: Rheumatic myalgias, Practitioner 146:167, 1941.
41. Graff-Radford, SB, Jaeger, B, and Reeves, JL: Myofascial pain may present clinically as occipital neuralgia, Neurosurgery 19:610, 1986.

42. Graff-Radford, SB, Reeves, JL, and Jaeger, B: Management of chronic headache and neck pain: effectiveness of altering factors perpetuating myofascial pain, Headache 27:186, 1987.

43. Grosshandler, SL, et al: Chronic neck and shoulder pain, Postgrad Med 77:149, 1985.

44. Hagberg, M, and Kvarnström, S: Muscular endurance and electromyographic fatigue in myofascial shoulder pain, Arch Phys Med Rehabil 65:522, 1984.

45. Haldeman, S: Modern developments in the principles and practice of chiropractic, New York, 1980, Appleton-Century-Crofts.

46. Hallin, RP: Sciatic pain and the piriformis muscle, Postgrad Med 74:69, 1983.

47. Hillman, RS: Vitamin B₁₂, folic acid, and the treatment of megaloblastic anemias. In Gilman, AG, Goodman, LS, and Gilman, A, editors: The pharmacological basis of therapeutics, ed 6, New York, 1980, MacMillan Publishing Co, Inc.

48. Hoyle, G: Excitation-contraction coupling. In Muscles and their neural control, New York, 1983, John Wiley & Sons, Inc.

49. Hong, C-Z, Simons, DG, and Statham, L: Electromyographic analysis of local twitch responses of human extensor digitorum communis muscle during ischemic compression over the arm, Arch Phys Med Rehabil 67:680, 1986.

50. Hubbell, SL, and Thomas, M: Postpartum cervical myofascial pain syndrome: review of four patients, Obstet Gynecol 65(suppl):56S, 1985.

51. Institute of Medicine: Pain and disability: clinical, behavioral and public policy perspectives, Washington, DC, 1987, National Academy Press.

52. Jaeger, B, and Reeves, JL: Quantification of changes in myofascial trigger point sensitivity with the pressure algometer following passive stretch, Pain 27:203, 1986.

53. Jensen, K, et al: Pressure-pain threshold in human temporal region: evaluation of a new pressure algometer, Pain 25:313, 1986.

54. Jordan, HH: Myogeloses: the significance of pathologic conditions of the musculature in disorders of posture and locomotion, Arch Phys Ther 23:36, 1942.

55. Kalyan-Raman, UP, et al: Muscle pathology in primary fibromyalgia syndrome: a light microscopic, histochemical and ultrastructural study, J Rheumatol 11:808, 1984.

56. Kelly, M: Lumbago and abdominal pain, Med J Aust 1:311, 1942.

57. Kelley, WN: Gout and other disorders of purine metabolism. In Isselbacher, KJ, et al, editors: Harrison's principles of internal medicine, ed 9, New York, 1980, McGraw-Hill Book Co.

58. Klein, AC, and Sobel, D: Backache relief, New York, 1985, Random House.

59. Kniffki, K-D, Mense, S, and Schmidt, RF: Mechanisms of muscle pain: a comparison with cutaneous nociception. In Zotterman, Y, editor: Sensory functions of the skin, (Wenner-Gren vol 27), Oxford, 1976, Pergamon Press.

60. Kniffki, K-D, Mense, S, and Schmidt, RF: Responses of group IV afferent units from skeletal muscle to stretch, contraction and chemical stimulation, Exp Brain Res 31:511, 1978.

61. Kraft, GH, Johnson, EW, and LeBan, MM: The fibrositis syndrome, Arch Phys Med Rehabil 49:155, 1968.

62. Kraus, H: Clinical treatment of back and neck pain, New York, 1970, McGraw-Hill Book Co.

63. Lange, M: Die Muskelhärten (Myogelosen), Müchen, 1931, JF Lehmann's Verlag.

64. Lehninger, AL: Biochemistry, New York, 1970, Worth.

65. Lewit, K: The needle effect in the relief of myofascial pain, Pain 6:83, 1979.

66. Lewit, K: Manipulative therapy in rehabilitation of the motor system, Boston, 1985, Butterworths.

67. Lewit, K: Postisometric relaxation in combination with other methods of muscular facilitation and inhibition, Manual Med 2:101, 1986.

68. Lewit, K, and Simons, DG: Myofascial pain: relief by post-isometric relaxation, Arch Phys Med Rehabil 65:452, 1984.

69. Lindstedt, F: Zur Kenntnis der Aetiologie und Pathogenese der Lumbago und ähnlicher Rückenschmerzen, Acta Med Scand 55:248, 1921.

70. Lund, N, Bengtsson, A, and Thorberg, P: Muscle tissue oxygen pressure in primary fibromyalgia, Scand J Rheumatol 15:165, 1986.

71. Macdonald, AJR: Abnormally tender muscle regions and associated painful movements, Pain 8:197, 1980.

72. Maitland, GD: Peripheral manipulation, ed 2, London, Boston, 1977, Butterworths.

73. Maitland, GD: Vertebral manipulation, ed 4, London, Boston, 1977, Butterworths.

74. Melnick, J: Trigger areas and refractory pain in duodenal ulcer, NY State J Med 57:1073, 1957.

75. Mennell, JM: Joint pain, Boston, 1964, Little, Brown & Co.

76. Mense, S: Nervous outflow from skeletal muscle following chemical noxious stimulation, J Physiol 267:75, 1977.

77. Mense, S: Muskelreceptoren mit dünnen markhaltigen und marklosen afferenten fasern: receptive Eigenschaften und mögliche Funktion [Muscle receptors with thin myelinated and unmyelinated afferent fibers: receptive characteristics and possible function], doctoral thesis, Physiologisches Institute der Universität Kiel (D-2300 Kiel 1), Kiel, West Germany, 1978.

78. Michele, AA: Scapulocostal syndrome—its mechanism and diagnosis, NY State J Med 55:2485, 1955.

79. Miehlke, K, and Schulze, G: Der sogenannte Muskelrheumatismus, Internist 2:447, 1961.

80. Miehlke, K, Schulze, G, and Eger, W: Klinische und exerimentelle Untersuchungen zum Fibrositissyndrom, Z Rheumaforsch 19:310, 1960.

81. Milne, RJ, et al: Convergence of cutaneous and pelvic visceral nociceptive inputs onto primate spinothalamic neurons, Pain 11:163, 1981.

82. Mitchell, FL, Jr, Moran, PS, and Pruzzo, NA: Evaluation and treatment manual of osteopathic muscle energy procedures, Valley Park, Mo, 1979, Mitchell, Moran & Pruzzo Associates.

83. Müller, A: Der Untersuchungsbefund am rheumatisch erkrankten Muskel, Z Klin Med 74:34, 1912.

84. Neal, RA, and Sauberlich, HE: Thiamin. In Goodhart, RS, and Shils, ME, editors: Modern nutrition in health and disease, ed 6, Philadelphia, 1980, Lea & Febiger.

85. Perl, ER: Sensitization of nociceptors and its relation to sensation. In Bonica, JJ, and Albe-Fessard, editors: Advances in pain research and therapy, vol 1, New York, 1976, Raven Press.

86. Perl, ER: Unraveling the story of pain. In Fields, HL, et al, editors: Advances in pain research and therapy, vol 9, New York, 1985, Raven Press.

87. Popelianskii, I, Bogdanov, EI, and Khabirov, FA: [Algesic trigger zones of the gastrocnemius muscle in lumbar osteochondrosis (clinico-pathomorphological and electromyographic analysis)] (Russian), ZH Nevropatol Psikhiatr 84:1055, 1984.

88. Popelianskii, I, Zaslavskii, ES, and Veselovskii, VP: [Medicosocial significance, etiology, pathogenesis, and diagnosis of nonarticular disease of soft tissues of the limbs and back] (Russian), Vopr Revm 3:38, 1976.

89. Price, DD, Harkins, SW, and Baker, C: Sensory-affective relationships among different types of clinical and experimental pain, Pain 28:297, 1987.

90. Procacci, P, et al: Cutaneous pain threshold changes after sympathetic block in reflex dystrophies, Pain 1:167, 1975.

91. Reeves, JL, Jaeger, B, and Graff-Radford, SB: Reliability of the pressure algometer as a measure of myofascial trigger point sensitivity, Pain 24:313, 1986.

92. Reynolds, MD: Myofascial trigger point syndromes in the practice of rheumatology, Arch Phys Med Rehabil 62:111, 1981.

93. Reynolds, MD: The development of the concept of fibrositis, J Hist Med Allied Sci 38:5, 1983.

94. Reynolds, MD: Myofascial trigger points in persistent posttraumatic shoulder pain, South Med J 77:1277, 1984.

95. Roberts, JT: The effect of occlusive arterial diseases of extremities on the blood supply of nerves; experimental and clinical studies on the role of the vasa nervorum, Am Heart J 35:369, 1948.

96. Rowland, LP, Araki, S, and Carmel, P: Contracture in McArdle's disease, Arch Neurol 13:541, 1965.

97. Rowland, LP: Inherited diseases (of muscle and neuromuscular junction). In Wyngaarden, B, and Smith, LH, Jr, editors: Cecil textbook of medicine, Philadelphia, 1985, WB Saunders Co.

98. Rubin, D: An approach to the management of myofascial trigger point syndromes, Arch Phys Med Rehabil 62:107, 1981.

99. Rueff, S: Ein Beitrag zur Frage der Myogelosen, Wien Arch Inn Med 23:139, 1932.

100. Ruhmann, W: Über das Wesen der rheumatischen Muskelhärte, Dtsch Arch Klin Med 173:625, 1932.

101. Schade, H: Beiträge zur Umgrenzung und Klärung einer Lehre von der Erkältung, Z Ges Exp Med 7:275, 1919.

102. Schultz, DR: Occipital neuralgia, J Am Osteopath Assoc 76:335, 1977.

103. Schwartz, RG, Gall, NG, and Grant, AE: Abdominal pain in quadriparesis: myofascial syndrome as unsuspected cause, Arch Phys Med Rehabil 65:44, 1984.

104. Shoen, RP, Moskowitz, RW, and Goldberg, VM: Soft tissue rheumatic pain, ed 2, Philadelphia, 1987, Lea & Febiger.

105. Simons, DG: Muscle pain syndromes, I and II, Am J Phys Med 54:289, 1975; 55:15, 1976.

106. Simons, DG: Myofascial pain syndromes. In Basmajian, JV, and Kirby, RL, editors: Medical rehabilitation, Baltimore, 1984, Williams & Wilkins Co.

107. Simons, DG: Myofascial pain syndromes due to trigger points. I. Principles, diagnosis, and perpetuating factors, Manual Med 1:67, 1985.

108. Simons, DG: Myofascial pain syndromes due to trigger points. II. Treatment and single-muscle syndromes, Manual Med 1:72, 1985.

109. Simons, DG: Fibrositis/fibromyalgia: a form of myofascial trigger points? Am J Med 81(suppl 3A):93, 1986.

110. Simons, DG: Myofascial pain syndromes of head, neck and low back. In Dubner, R, Gebbhart, GF, and Bond, MR, editors: Pain research and clinical management, vol 3. Proceedings of the Fifth World Congress on Pain, Hamburg, August 1987, Amsterdam, 1988, Elsevier Science & Publishers.

111. Simons, DG, and Stolov, WC: Microscopic features and transient contraction of palpable bands in canine muscle, Am J Phys Med 55:65, 1976.

112. Simons, DG, and Travell, JG: Myofascial trigger points, a possible explanation, Pain 10:106, 1981.

113. Simons, DG, and Travell, JG: Myofascial origins of low back pain. I. Principles of diagnosis and treatment, Postgrad Med 73:66, 1983.

114. Simons, DG, and Travell, JG: Myofascial origins of low back pain. II. Torso muscles, Postgrad Med 73:81, 1983.

115. Simons, DG, and Travell, JG: Myofascial origins of low back pain. III. Pelvic and lower extremity muscles, Postgrad Med 73:99, 1983.

116. Simons, DG, and Travell, JG: Myofascial pain syndromes. In Wall, PD, and Melzack, R, editors: Textbook of pain, London, 1984, Churchill-Livingstone.

117. Skootsky, S: Incidence of myofascial pain in an internal medical group practice, presented to the American Pain Society, Washington, DC, November 6-9, 1986.

118. Slocumb, JC: Neurological factors in chronic pelvic pain: trigger points and the abdominal pelvic pain syndrome, Am J Obstet Gynecol 149:536, 1984.

119. Smythe, HA: Fibrositis and other diffuse musculoskeletal syndromes. In Kelley, WN, et al, editors: Textbook of rheumatology, vol 1, Philadelphia, 1981, WB Saunders Co.

120. Sola, AE: Treatment of myofascial pain syndromes. In Benedetti, C, et al, editors: Advances in pain research and therapy, vol 7, New York, 1984, Raven Press.

121. Sola, AE: Trigger point therapy. In Roberts, JR, and Hedges, JR, editors: Clinical procedures in emergency medicine, Philadelphia, 1985, WB Saunders Co.

122. Sola, AE, Rodenberger, ML, and Gettys, BB: Incidence of hypersensitive areas in posterior shoulder muscles, Am J Phys Med 34:585, 1955.

123. Sola, AE, and Williams, RL: Myofascial pain syndromes, Neurology 6:91, 1956.

124. Sonkin, LS: Endocrine disorders, locomotor and temporomandibular joint dysfunction. In Gelb, HG, editor: Clinical management of head, neck and TMJ pain and dysfunction, Philadelphia, 1977, WB Saunders Co.

125. Steindler, A: The interpretation of sciatic radiation and the syndrome of low-back pain, J Bone Joint Surg 22:28, 1940.

126. Stockman, R: Rheumatism and arthritis, Edinburgh, 1920, W Green.

127. Torebjörk, HE, Ochoa, JL, and Schady, W: Referred pain from intraneural stimulation of muscle fascicles in the median nerve, Pain 18:145, 1984.

128. Travell, J: Rapid relief of acute "stiff neck" by ethyl chloride spray, J Am Med Wom Assoc 4:89, 1949.

129. Travell, J: Introductory comments. In Ragan, C, editor: Connective tissues: transactions of the fifth conference, 1954, New York, 1954, Josiah Macy, Jr, Foundation.

130. Travell, J: Myofascial trigger points: clinical view. In Bonica, JJ, and Albe-Fessard, D, editors: Advances in pain research and therapy, vol 1, New York, 1976, Raven Press.

131. Travell, J: Identification of myofascial trigger point syndromes: a case of atypical facial neuralgia, Arch Phys Med Rehabil 62:100, 1981.

132. Travell, JT: Unpublished data, 1986.

133. Travell, J, and Rinzler, SH: The myofascial genesis of pain, Postgrad Med 11:425, 1952.

134. Travell, JG, and Simons, DG: Myofascial pain and dysfunction: the trigger point manual, Baltimore, 1983, Williams & Wilkins Co.

135. Travell, JG, and Simons, DG: Myofascial pain and dysfunction: the trigger point manual, vol II, Baltimore, Williams & Wilkins Co. In press.

136. Wall, PD: Cancer pain: neurogenic mechanisms. In Fields, HL, et al, editors: Advances in pain research and therapy, vol 9, New York, 1985, Raven Press.

137. Weed, ND: When shoulder pain isn't bursitis, Postgrad Med 74:97, 1983.

138. Weeks, VD, and Travell, J: How to give painless injections. In AMA Scientific Exhibits, New York, 1957, Grune & Stratton.

139. Weinstein, G: The diagnosis of trigger points by thermography, Academy of Neuro-muscular Thermography Clinical Proceedings, Postgraduate Medicine, Custom Communications, March 1986.

140. Williams, RJ: Physicians handbook of nutritional science, Springfield, Ill, 1975, Charles C Thomas, Publisher.

141. Wolfe, F: The clinical syndrome of fibrositis, Am J Med 81(suppl 3A):7, 1986.

142. Wolfe, F, and Cathey, MA: Prevalence of primary and secondary fibrositis, J Rheumatol 10:965, 1983.

143. Wood, B, and Breen, KJ: Clinical thiamine deficiency in Australia: the size of the problem and approaches to prevention, Med J Aust 1:461, 1980.

144. Yunus, M, et al: Primary fibromyalgia, Am Fam Physician 25:115, 1982.

145. Zohn, DA: The quadratus lumborum: an unrecognized source of back pain, clinical and thermographic aspects, Orthop Rev 15:87, 1985.

PART VII | **ALLIED THERAPIES AND TECHNOLOGY IN REHABILITATION**

CHAPTER 46

Principles of occupational therapy

SOPHIA CHIOTELIS AND MURIEL ZIMMERMAN

Occupational therapy is defined as "the art and science of directing man's participation in selected tasks to restore, reinforce and enhance performance, facilitate learning of those skills and functions essential for adaptation and productivity, diminish or correct pathology, and to promote and maintain health."[31]

The treatment paradigm incorporates purposeful, goal-oriented activities in several treatment approaches to effect change in the performance capacity of individuals impaired by disease, injury, congenital disability, or the aging process. In the rehabilitation process the roles and functions of the occupational therapist include the following:

1. Assess and evaluate the individual's performance components.
2. Establish immediate and long-term goals for treatment.
3. Formulate and implement a treatment plan with the appropriate frame of reference.
4. Reevaluate the individual periodically to measure response to treatment and identify the need to modify goals and alter treatment.

PATIENT EVALUATION

To formulate and implement an appropriate and individualized treatment program, the therapist focuses patient evaluation in several major categories[4]:

1. Daily living skills and performance
2. Therapeutic adaptations, for example, assistive equipment, orthotics, and prosthetics
3. Sensorimotor skills and performance components, for example, neuromuscular and sensory integration
4. Cognitive skills and performance components, for example, orientation, conceptualization, and cognitive integration

Data and information related to these aspects of function are obtained through several procedures, such as activity performance checklists, standardized tests and measurements, and special evaluations, as well as clinical observations and judgment. Although not all test procedures are standardized or have a high test reliability and validity, the results gleaned from the combination of evaluation procedures assist the therapist to establish treatment goals and to determine the frame of reference for treatment. Evaluation results provide a baseline of function-dysfunction by which the therapist can measure change and functional outcome.

Sensory integrative evaluation

Sensory integrative skills are assessed for their development and coordination of sensory input, motor output, and sensory feedback. These skills include obtaining information on the status of exteroceptive, proprioceptive, and cortical sensations from the neurologic examination. Some specific test procedures as they apply to the practice of occupational therapy are described in Trombley and Scott.[36] In addition to sensory awareness, the status of visual awareness and body integration are also obtained to understand the impact on motor function and the implications for treatment.

Neuromuscular evaluation

The neuromuscular status is assessed by evaluating strength, range of motion, coordination, reflex integration and endurance.

Gross strength and range of motion

The Functional Motion Test (Figure 46-1) is a standardized test used for patients with lower motor neuron disability to measure upper extremity motion strength, limitations in joint range, and coordination. This test, developed by Zimmerman,[39,40] is based on an analysis of motions used for several important activities of daily living (Table 46-1).

**The Rusk Institute
of Rehabilitation Medicine
New York University Medical Center**

OCCUPATIONAL THERAPY

FUNCTIONAL MOTION TEST REPORT

Date: _____

Therapist: _____   4/77 - PS-490

Name: _____

Address: _____

Age: _____   Chart No. _____

Disability
Onset:
Occupation:
Dr.:

Summary of Findings:

Activity Limitations or Problems

GOALS

  Immediate

  Long Range

Recommended Program

Recommended Devices (if any)

Figure 46-1. Functional Motion Test, a tool for measuring motion strength in patients with lower motor neuron lesions.

OCCUPATIONAL THERAPY FUNCTIONAL MOTION TEST REPORT
PAGE 2

10/73

LEFT (dominant)													RIGHT (dominant)												
								Examiner's Initials															
								Date															
Extent of Spasticity			loss of R.O.M.			Strength							Strength			loss of R.O.M.			Extent of Spasticity		
								SHOULDER															
								Abduction															
								Adduction															
								Flexion															
								Extension															
								Int. Rotation															
								Ext. Rotation															
								ELBOW Flexion															
								Extension															
								FOREARM Supination															
								Pronation															
								WRIST Flexion															
								Extension															
								Radial Deviation															
								Ulnar Deviation															
								HAND Flexion MCP															
								Flexion PIP															
								Flexion DIP															
								Extension MCP															
								Extension PIP															
								Extension DIP															
								Finger Abduction															
								Finger Adduction															
								Thumb Abduction															
								Thumb Adduction															
								Thumb Flexion															
								Thumb Extension															
								Thumb Opposition															
								Prehension-palmar															
								Prehension-lateral															
								Gross grasp															

BREATH PRESSURE: maximum (regular/sustained)

Positive _____ Negative _____

SCAPULAR & NECK MOTIONS

Sh. Elevation _____ Sh. Depression _____

Sh. Protraction _____ Sh. Retraction _____

Neck Flexion _____ Neck Extension _____

Neck Lateral   R _____   L _____

OTHER: _____

Trunk Balance _____ Sitting Posture _____

Endurance _____ Sensibility _____

Visual Problems _____ Yes _____ No

Auditory Problems _____ Yes _____ No

Edema _____

Motivation/OT _____ good _____ poor _____ hopeful

CODING KEYS:

Strength:
O - zero   F - fair
T - trace   G - good
P - poor   N - normal

ROM/Control:
1 - minimal
2 - moderate
3 - maximum
Pain - *

Color:
red - O to F-
black - F to N

Activities Performed	Potent.	Equ.	Asst.	Actual	Equ.	Asst.
Eating						
Bathing (upper)						
Grooming:						
Shaving						
Teeth						
Cosmetics						
Dressing						
Communications:						
Writing						
Typing						
Telephone						
Reading						
Wheelchair						
Manipulation						

KEY: G=Good   F=Fair;   P=Poor;   O=Zero;   NA=Not Applicable

Sample of
Patient's Signature _____

NYU 4/77 - PB-490

Table 46-1. Findings and summary of analysis of motion (eating, combing hair, writing, typing, turning pages)

	Motion	Active motion	Holding motion	Total
Shoulder	Abduction	0	0	0
	Adduction		5	5*
	Flexion	3	2	5†
	Extension	3		3*
	External rotation	4		4‡
	Internal rotation	4		4*
Elbow	Flexion	3	2	5†
	Extension	3		3*
Forearm	Supination	3		3‡
	Pronation	3	2	5*
Wrist	Flexion	1		1*
	Extension	1	4	5†
Hand pinch§	Palmar	1		1
	Lateral		3	3
	Hook	1		1

*Gravity aided.
†The most frequently used arm motions not aided by gravity are shoulder flexion, elbow flexion, and wrist extension.
‡Next important are shoulder external rotation and forearm supination.
§Some type of hand function (with or without splints) is mandatory.

From the test results one can assess the patient's actual performance, predict potential performance, and develop a rationale for selecting assistive devices to improve performance. The grades and deficiencies of motions that impair function indicate the need for devices. When strength is tested, a grade of zero to fair-minus in any antigravity arm or hand motion indicates the need for a device, which can then be selected according to the purpose for which that motion is necessary. Moderate to severe losses in range of motion also indicate a specific need according to which motion is limited, as does loss of coordination. Examples of selection of equipment for improving performance are as follows:

1. Loss of hand function (zero to poor-minus strength). Use ADL cuff, C-clip, or swivel ADL cuff with vertical holder for various utensils (Figure 46-2). A prehension orthosis, wrist activated, also may be selected to provide function.
2. Loss of hand function (poor to fair-minus strength). Use adapted equipment, such as universal built-up handle for spoon, fork, buttonhook, toothbrush, and adapted cup handles (see Figure 46-2).
3. Loss of wrist dorsiflexion (zero to poor-minus wrist strength). Obtain stabilization for maintaining a neutral or slight cock-up position through use of a wrist orthosis (Figure 46-2).
4. Loss of forearm supination (moderate to severe loss of range of motion). Use swivel fork and spoon.

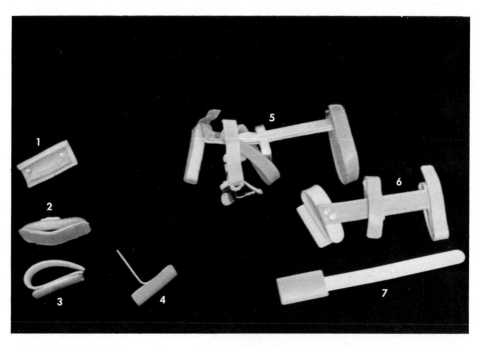

Figure 46-2. Universal components used to assist in daily living skills such as eating, writing, and grooming. *1,* Universal built-up handle; *2,* ADL cuff; *3,* universal C-clip swivel ADL cuff; *4,* universal vertical holder; *5,* combined ADL–long opponens splint; *6,* dorsal wrist splint; *7,* universal folding extension handle.

5. Loss of shoulder and elbow flexion (zero to poor-minus strength). For early stages of recovery select counterbalance overhead slings (Figure 46-3). For permanent use of regressive condition select a balanced forearm orthosis.

In addition, the grades and deficiencies of motions provide the basis for planning the treatment program.

Hand strength and function

The hand is evaluated as a coordinated structure of sensations, muscle control, and strength. There are methods by which one can measure specific hand strength; however, a more accurate assessment of hand function considers the use of the hand in conjunction with the proximal use of the arm.

Grasp strength. Using the Jaymar dynamometer instrument, gross hand strength can be measured in pounds and kilograms. Standard procedures for testing and recording are described by Kellor and associates.[25] Norms are available for adult males and females.

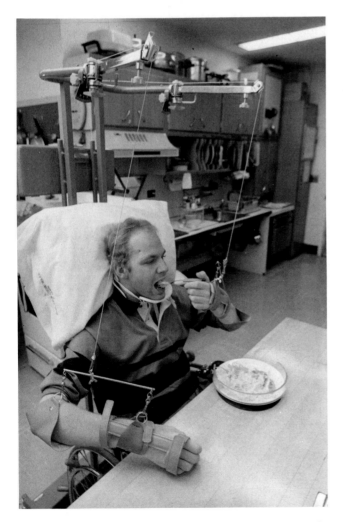

Figure 46-3. Counterbalance assistive overhead sling allows early participation in eating for quadriplegic patient.

Pinch. The OSCO pinch meter is a reliable calibrated instrument used to measure strength of palmar, three-point, and lateral pinch. Testing and recording procedures are described by Kellor and co-workers.[25] Norms are available.

Hand function. The Jebsen-Taylor Hand Function Test[21] consists of seven subtests, which are based on motions used in seven basic daily living skills. This test evaluates hand function with the hand in various positions. The test is easy to administer, and norms are available by age and sex.

Endurance

Endurance is assessed through observation of performance and by measuring the length of time a patient can sustain activity before fatigue sets in. Fatigue is an important factor influencing work capacity[10] and has many implications for occupational therapy treatment. With an understanding that the level of strength correlates with energy output and has an inverse effect on endurance, the occupational therapist prioritizes the treatment activities. Activities are most beneficial if they are scheduled when the patient is less fatigued to promote success in achieving some component of the activity. This not only reinforces the patient's motivation but may also lead to reaching a functional level of independence sooner. It is important for the rehabilitation team to adjust activities and exercise continually in a sequence that considers the patient's changing endurance and fatigue levels.

Motor control

For patients who exhibit upper motor neuron lesion disability, it is essential to be cognizant of the influence of sensation on motor function. Assessment is done of muscle tone, integration of primitive reflexes, righting and equilibrium reactions, and positive supporting reactions. Specific testing procedures are described in Abreau[1] and Trombley and Scott[36] as they apply to the practice of occupational therapy.

Daily living skills and performance

There are a few valid and fairly reliable standardized tests that measure functional performance in self-care such as eating, grooming, bathing, personal hygiene, and toileting activities. These standardized tests can also be used to quantify functional outcome and to indicate the effectiveness of the rehabilitation program. Several activities of daily living (ADL) scales described in the literature include the Klein-Bell ADL Scale,[22,26,33] the Barthel Index,[30] PULSES,[16] the Revised Kenney Self Care Evaluation,[20] and the Katz Index.[23] The Klein-Bell Scale, for example, is an objective and valid measurement of six self-care skills—dressing, bathing, elimination, mobility, eating, and emergency telephone use. Each behavior is broken down into component parts, which makes it possible to monitor the individual's progress as different levels of the same activity are achieved.

The use of performance checklists (Figure 46-4), which

OCCUPATIONAL THERAPY SERVICE

DAILY LIVING SKILLS PERFORMANCE

Patient: _____ Age: _____
Disability: _____
Therapist: _____

SCORING KEY

1 = Independent
2 = Supervision/verbal cuing
3 = Minimal assistance/contact guarding
4 = Moderate assistance/set-up
5 = Dependent - can instruct
    c̄ = With assistive devices

6 = Dependent
X = Not applicable
Y = Insufficient information
Z = Not assessed
P = Projection of outcome
    s̄ = Without assistive devices

	c̄ / s̄	1	2	3	4	5	6	X	Y	Z	P	1	2	3	4	5	6	X	Y	Z	c̄ / s̄	Date

INITIAL _____ Date   **DISCHARGE** _____ Date

EATING/DRINKING
    Chews food
    Swallows food/liquids
    Uses utensils
    Sets-up food for eating
    Finger feeds

PERSONAL HYGIENE
    Washes hands
    Washes face
    Oral hygiene
    Applies deodorant
    Inspects for pressure
    Manages urinary appliances

GROOMING
    Care of hair
    Care of nails
    Shaving
    Applies make-up

DRESSING/UNDRESSING
    Upper garments
    Lower garments
    Fastenings
    Socks/stockings
    Shoes
    Accessories
    Orthoses
    Prosthesis

WHEELCHAIR MOBILITY
    Positioning
    Operates controls
    Maneuvers inside
    Maneuvers outside
    Manages parts & accessories

Figure 46-4. Checklist to evaluate patient's daily living skills performance. (Courtesy Occupational Therapy Department, Rusk Institute of Rehabilitation Medicine, New York University Medical Center.)

OCCUPATIONAL THERAPY SERVICE

Patient:_____   Therapist:_____

SCORING KEY

1 = Independent ————————————————————▶   6 = Dependent

	INITIAL											DISCHARGE										
								Date														c̄/s̄	Date
c̄/s̄	1	2	3	4	5	6	X	Y	Z	P	1	2	3	4	5	6	X	Y	Z		

FUNCTIONAL COMMUNICATION
Use of writing equipment
Telephone
Reading
Typewriter
Computer

HOME MANAGEMENT
Meal planning
Meal preparation
Open/close containers
Clean-up
Laundry
Bedmaking
House cleaning

OBJECT MANIPULATION
Controls
Switches
Money
Keys

ADAPTIVE SKILLS
Initiates
Integrates information
Transfers learning
Problem solves

YES	NO	X	Y	Z		YES	NO	X	Y	Z

**ACCESSIBILITY/MANAGEMENT
OF ENVIRONMENT**
Accessible
Recommend relocation
Modifications recommended
Manages environmental controls
Manages accessories

PREVENTION (is aware of)
Safety
Energy conservation
Joint protection
Body mechanics

EDUCATION
Home program
Family instruction

LEISURE INTERESTS: _____

include a comprehensive list of functional activities, is a more subjective method of documenting performance. Initial and final status is checked and is usually ranked on a gross four-point scale: dependent, with assistance, with supervision, and independent. These checklists are not sensitive to changes of performance because activities are not usually broken down into component parts and usually do not include endurance or speed of performance. Most activity checklists do describe whether the activity was completed with or without assistive devices. In recent years, health care delivery system costs have risen and cost containment has become an important issue. Reimbursement groups, as well as licensing bodies, are demanding documentation that reflect functional outcome and the effectiveness of rehabilitation. Standardized methods for measuring performance in daily living skills and functional outcome are a major concern for the occupational therapist.

GENERAL PRINCIPLES OF TREATMENT

Underlying any frame of reference for treatment are two basic principles for using activities: Activities must be purposeful and are analyzed for their performance components.

The occupational therapist does not have to compromise a functional paradigm of treatment when attempting to improve basic organic dysfunctions. Remediation of basic deficits is a prerequisite for the acquisition of functional skills. When purposeful activities are integrated with remediation techniques, the patient is at an optimum advantage for improvement. Purposeful activities sustain interest, increase output, and are a key element for intrinsic motivation.[34] Gliner[15] viewed purposeful activity as a necessary prerequisite for the formation of coordinated structures, the basis for skilled movement. He suggested an ecologic approach to motor learning where the patient and the task are considered together, that is, the therapist is aware of the patient's limitations, as well as the demands of the task, and is ready to intervene to assist the patient to form appropriate coordinated structures.[15]

Selecting appropriate therapeutic activities requires a thorough analysis of the components of the activity and their relationship to the goals of treatment. The theoretic basis for improvement of specific deficits has to be translated into activities appropriate for that individual.[36] The usual method to analyze an activity is by observing the sequences of performance, with attention given to all sequences of activity and their influence on muscles, joints, and the lever system (see Tables 46-3 and 46-4). It would be ideal to have electromyography (EMG) available because this modality is the most accurate. Basmajian's text, *Muscles Alive, Their Functions Revealed By Electromyography,*[6] is an excellent reference for muscle activity analyses. One such EMG study was conducted by Trombley[36] on several hand activities and their influence on four different hand muscles: the extensor digitorum, flexor profundus, interosseus dor-

salis, and abductor pollicis brevis. Unfortunately, not many such studies have been completed for the numerous activities used by occupational therapists.

Rationale for treatment approaches

In the rehabilitation of individuals with dysfunction, occupational therapy uses two major frames of reference in clinical practice: biomechanical and neurobehavioral. A combination of these two approaches may be required for some conditions.

Biomechanical approach

As described in Trombley and Scott[36] and Abreau,[1] this frame of reference is used for treating patients with dysfunction of the musculoskeletal system, peripheral nervous system, and cardiopulmonary system. The central nervous system is intact. The techniques and activities used are based on mechanical principles of kinetics and kinematics to restore movement and are selected to improve strength, increase joint range of motion, and increase endurance. The activities and therapeutic exercises are analyzed for components that will effect the desired change. Remediation of deficits in joint range of motion requires activities that can provide active stretch and minimal resistance. Muscle strengthening requires activities and exercise that have qualities allowing for gradation of resistance, as well the ability to promote specific muscle contraction, such as isotonic or isometric. Activities to improve endurance should be gradable for duration and for resistance.

Neurobehavioral approach

The neurobehavioral frame of reference is used for management of patients with disabilities from upper motor lesions of the central nervous system. Treatment is based on developmental, neurophysiologic, and motor learning theories that are incorporated in specific treatment techniques to promote change in behaviors.[1] The basic assumption is that the spinal cord and peripheral neural pathways are intact, allowing for transmission of sensory stimuli to the brain. The sensory integrated processes of the central nervous system are responsible for effecting changes in abnormal behavior and learning new behaviors.[1] The sensorimotor, postural, and cognitive behaviors most often impaired are intrinsic to daily living skills, and in light of this the occupational therapist uses intervention strategies for remediation of deficits in these behaviors. An eclectic approach is used based on theories promoted by Rood,[31] Bobath,[7,8] Brunnstrom,[9] and Knott and Voss.[28] All of these techniques promote the concept that sensation, repetition for learning, and sequential development are necessary to improve muscle control and postural reflexes. All stress the influence of sensation on motor function. Major differences in the theoretic basis of techniques is whether movement is promoted through conscious attention or is reflex elicited.[36] These techniques remain controversial and continue to require systematic study as new theories evolve in neurophysiology.

When occupational therapists apply neurobehavioral techniques in treatment, they are integrated with purposeful activities. Huss[19] emphasized that motor output can be retained more effectively and built upon by the central nervous system when the patient can respond to sensory input in a meaningful way.[19] The occupational therapist is in a position to select, analyze, and incorporate purposeful activities from a large repertoire basic to the clinical practice. Activities are selected according to the specific goals of treatment and should have components that promote stability or mobility responses, are facilitory or inhibitory, can influence desired reflex activity, and can provide sensory stimulation. It is important that the therapist coordinate treatment with that of other disciplines so there is consistency in the management of these problems.

Functional approach

Management of the brain-injured person requires an interdisciplinary approach to provide consistency, so essential to treating deficits in cognition such as confusion, memory deficits, inattention, inability to solve problems, impaired judgment, and difficulties with integration. Treatment focuses on teaching the patient strategies for processing information in an effort to ameliorate problems. When successful, these learned strategies provide the patient with skills that can be generalized in other activities. Occupational therapy is task oriented, and the therapist can draw from a large repertoire of activities such as daily living skills, games, computer programs, and physical activity to stimulate the learning process. The activities chosen can be adapted to the individual needs, level of ability, and desired response.

In the treatment process the therapist can manipulate activities to meet specific requirements and goals determined by the team. Activities have the potential of being regulated according to amount of structure needed, stimulation provided, duration, complexity, and familiarity. Because distractibility is predominant early on, it is essential to treat patients within their optimal coping powers. Some management strategies to facilitate attention and inhibit distraction are to present the patient with short and achievable tasks, increase duration of activity as attention can be sustained, reinforce information processing and encourage focusing on a task by having the patient verbalize steps of activity, use both demonstration and verbal directions, and give constant positive feedback.

Memory deficits, a common and mostly short-term encoding deficit, are difficult for the patient, leading to frustration and interference with the learning process. Teaching patient strategies that can help him get through the daily program is an approach the team plans together to maximize consistency. Strategies may be taught to family members so reinforcement is consistent to facilitate improvement. A common problem is remembering people, places, and events. Examples of strategies are the following:

1. Establishing the use of a daily journal with entries that are important for the patient to remember. This becomes an important cue system for the patient and gives him some control and responsibility for the program. Entries can be made by team members and family.
2. Posting wall charts at bedside that provide a similar cue system to which the patient can refer on waking in the morning
3. Initially providing familiar activities so the patient can rely on old learning. Gradation of activities is made as the patient improves by pairing new learning with old learning
4. Using several sensory modalities that reinforce learning, that is verbal, as well as demonstrated, and visual
5. Providing consistent repetition
6. Reducing distractions in the environment
7. Using photographs as cues for remembering newly met people

As the patient gradually integrates learning, these skills can be generalized to most situations. The reader should consult the references for specific and systematic systems of intervention of cognitive deficiencies.

• • •

Whereas these approaches use specific techniques to remediate basic physical and cognitive deficits that underlie pathology, the restoration of the human processes still is often incomplete. The residual impairments impinge on the patient's potential for participation in human activity. In rehabilitation, occupational therapy follows a functional paradigm of treatment by applying compensatory and adaptive measures to maximize the patient's performance for independent living. The use of occupations for the rehabilitation of patients toward human activity is central in treatment. Keilhofner and Burke[24] describe occupation as a major human activity, made up of different occupational behaviors that are interrelated. These occupational behaviors refer to daily living activities, work, and play, which are the major concern in occupational therapy treatment. Daily living activities refer to self-care activities, home management, and travel. Work refers to productive activities, such as homemaking, school, and prevocational training. Play-leisure refers to a continuum of activities in which we participate from childhood to a mature age. Occupation is fundamental for human adaptation, and when disruption occurs owing to trauma or disease, the occupational behaviors need to be replaced or reorganized. The use of occupation becomes itself an effective tool for reorganizing dysfunctions.[24]

The goal of teaching and training the patient in occupational tasks is to achieve optimum performance for independent living appropriate to age, life-space, and disability. The level of functional outcome often depends on the degree of improvement the patient has made in the sensorimotor cognitive components of behavior and how effectively these skills are transferred to occupational tasks (daily living skills).

THERAPEUTIC ADAPTATION

Therapeutic adaptation, an important aspect of occupational therapy, is a strategy for maximizing independence in patients with residual or permanent loss of function. It is the selection, fabrication, or modification of special equipment to achieve the following goals:

1. Provide more dynamic treatment measures
2. Permit early independence and the active participation of the patient in the treatment program
3. Maximize independence in daily activities despite partial or total loss of function
4. Help build self-esteem and achieve either partial or complete economic independence

Therapeutic adaptation[4] includes not only the provision of special equipment, but also training and instruction in their use. Categories include the following:

1. Technical aids—self-help and assistive devices, electronic systems, wheelchair modifications, and environmental modifications
2. Orthotics—dynamic and static splints, slings, and braces
3. Prosthetics—conventional or myoelectric upper extremity artificial limbs

Technical aids

Technologic development has provided a proliferation of technical aids, from the simplest assistive device to sophisticated electronic systems. They give the disabled person more options for increasing independence for productive living. For example, the Abledata System (National Rehabilitation Information System, Washington, D.C.) is a national computerized databank containing information about rehabilitation products, including more than 40,000 commercially available aids and equipment that are useful to the disabled person. Product information data include name, manufacturer, cost, description, comments, and formal evaluation of the product. The product data are disseminated through information brokers by telephone or printout. Other similar database systems are listed in the references.

Technical aids can be prescribed for the following purposes:

1. To provide positioning and support to help maintain body alignment against weakened segments, thus preventing either permanent loss of power in overstretched and overfatigued muscles and to prevent possible permanent deformity
2. To encourage early motion and function to prevent atrophy from diseases, thus maintaining muscle strength, and to prevent loss of range of motion of joints
3. To increase function of residual muscle power and skill involved in various motions
4. To replace function totally and permanently lost either from muscle weakness or from loss of range of motion
5. To assist in control of incoordination, spasm, or spasticity
6. To substitute for loss of special senses (for example, sight, voice) or body part when prosthesis is not recommended
7. To minimize the amount of assistance needed from other persons when complete independence is not possible

Criteria for selection

Factors that determine selection of technical aids are physical requirements for use, the patient's acceptance of equipment, and the impact the equipment will have on functional independence.

Motion analysis of activities. As discussed earlier in this chapter, the functional motion test provides an expedient method for developing a rationale for the selection of technical aids to enhance function. Many clinicians, however, use the more traditional approach of completing a motion analysis of specific activities to determine deficiencies and their solutions.

Tables 46-2 and 46-3 illustrate the analysis of motion required for eating and writing. Both activities are performed with one extremity. The motion of each segment of the arm is observed and recorded separately with compensatory actions used for the deficiencies. This method of analysis can be applied to most daily living skills, such as shaving, brushing teeth, combing hair, typing, and using the telephone. The analysis of these two activities deals only with the main event of the skill. One must also consider other elements in addition to the analysis given in Tables 46-2 and 46-3 such as use of the other hand for stabilization, handling other equipment, relationship of table height, position in bed, and sitting position.

When motion and positioning of the whole body are involved in an activity, such as dressing, and when a variety of garments adds to the complexity, one begins by analyzing actions, such as putting on and fastening clothing and then by observing these actions as used for each type of clothing. A sample motion analysis involving one garment only is found in Table 46-4.

Other factors. Other factors to be considered for selecting equipment include these:

1. Duration of disability (congenital, acquired, subacute, or chronic)
2. Extent of disability (mild, moderate, or severe)
3. Prognosis of disability (static, progressive, or improving)
4. Age as contributory factor
5. Type of activity to be performed
6. Other physical limitations (for example, pain)
7. Cultural factors

Table 46-2. Analysis of motions used in eating (limited to use of one arm and one process only, in sitting erect position)

Body part	Motion	Purpose	Substitution	Loss	Technical aids used to compensate
Hand	Pick-up Palmar prehension	Pick up	1. Lacing spoon between fingers 2. Adduction of fingers	Minimal	1. Utensil interlaced in fingers (some shaping may be necessary) 2. Moleskin or tape over handle to prevent slipping
	Holding Lateral prehension to middle finger (modified lateral pinch)	Hold utensil	3. Hook grasp	Moderate	3. Built-up handle 4. Grip-shaped handles 5. Handle with horizontal and vertical dowels (pegged handle) 6. Handle with finger rings
				Severe	7. Short opponens with C-bar and utensil attachment
				Complete	8. ADL (universal) cuff 9. Universal C-clip, swivel ADL cuff 10. Universal vertical holder 11. Prehension orthosis, manually or power operated
Wrist	Stabilization (slight flexor and extensor or radial and ulnar deviation normally used depending on whether grasp is hook or pinch)	Positioning of hand for optimal function (to prevent wrist flexion)	1. Use of finger or thumb extensors	Partial stability	1. ADL wrist support, dorsal 2. Wrist support with flexible or adjustable assist (spring wire, etc.) 3. Universal combined ADL–long opponens orthosis 4. Cock-up splint, rigid, palmar
Forearm	Pronation	Pick up food on utensil	1. Shoulder abduction and internal rotation	Partial or complete	1. Swivel spoon/fork 2. Universal vertical holder
		Keep utensil level while putting food in mouth to avoid spill	1. Shoulder adduction and external rotation		1. Swivel spoon 2. Placing fork or spoon over thumb; use thumb extensors
Elbow	Flexion of forearm	Provides position and assists in raising hand to level of mouth	1. Shoulder abduction 2. Trunk flexion 3. Rock forearm on edge of table	Partial or complete	1. Balanced forearm orthosis 2. Overhead sling with balancer attachment 3. Overhead counterbalance sling 4. Balanced forearm orthosis (BFO) 5. Functional arm orthosis

Continued.

Table 46-2, cont'd. Analysis of motions used in eating (limited to use of one arm and one process only, in sitting erect position)

Shoulder	Stabilization against hyper-extension and internal rotation in position of slight flexion, slight abduction, plus slight active flexion and extension	Provides position and assists in raising hand to level of mouth	1. Trunk flexion 2. Prop elbow on table 3. Prop elbow on thigh and flex hip	Partial or complete	1. Pillow behind upper arm 2. Overhead sling with balancer 3. Overhead counterbalance sling 4. Balanced forearm orthosis (BFO) 5. Functional arm orthosis with hyperextension stop

Table 46-3. Analysis of motions for writing (with right hand only)

Method and position	Body part	Motion	Purpose	Technical aids used to compensate
Commonly used method	Hand	Opposition of thumb to index finger and lateral opposition to middle finger (modified palmar prehension)	Provides grasp	1. Built-up pencils, diameter increased 2. Clothespin holder with pegs 3. Three-finger loop holder (orthoplast etc.)
Sitting with arm on writing surface		Flexion and extension of middle phalangeal	Moves pencil	4. Vertical ADL holder (used in ADL cuff) 5. C-clip writing device 6. Prehension orthosis: manually operated; power operated
	Wrist	Slight flexion and extension or	Moves pencil	1. Universal dorsal wrist support, plain or with palmar C-clip with ADL pocket
		Stabilization in neutral or slight cock-up position	Provides positioning	2. Universal combined ADL–long opponens orthosis
	Forearm	Stabilization in approximate midposition	Provides positioning	1. Supination assist
	Elbow	Stabilization in approximately 90-degree flexion	Provides positioning	1. Overhead sling 2. Balanced forearm orthosis 3. Functional arm orthosis
		Alternating action of Flexors	Lift weight of arm from writing surface	1. Overhead sling
		Extensors	Provides pressure during writing	1. Soft lead pencil (needs less pressure) 2. Certain pens, ball-point pens, felt-tip pens

Table 46-3, cont'd. Analysis of motions for writing (with right hand only)

Method and position	Body part	Motion	Purpose	Technical aids used to compensate
		Slight flexion and extension	Moves hand across paper	1. Powder on board or surface
		with		2. Ball caster support
				3. Teflon-covered elbow cuffs
	Shoulder	Slight internal and external rotation	Moves hand across paper	1. Overhead sling
				2. Rotation mechanism on functional arm orthosis
		Stabilization in position of slight flexion and abduction	Provides positioning	1. Overhead slings
				2. Balanced forearm orthosis (BFO)
		Minimal synergistic action of shoulder girdle muscles	Minimum motion and pressure	3. Functional arm orthosis

Table 46-4. Clothing analysis (one garment only)

Type of garment	Problem	Disability	Solution
Short-sleeved and cardigan blouses	Putting on and taking off	Loss of motion of shoulder and elbow	Loose armholes, such as raglan, kimono, or dolman; action back pleats; vertical-style dress (divided into two pieces); stick with closet hook on end (to remove garment from shoulders)
	Fastening front	Weakness of both hands Use of only one hand	Vertical rather than horizontal button holes; larger buttons, size at least ⅝ inch; flat buttons; snaps instead of buttons; slip-over blouse or sweater; button hook (regular or wire loop), Velcro fastening
Long-sleeved blouses and shirts	Same as others with addition of fastening cuffs	Use of only one hand	Large enough cuff to let hand pass through; elasticized or knit cuff; elasticized thread on button; elastic loop over button
Both of above	Keeping shirt or blouse tucked in	Weakness of hands and arms	Long tails; latex gripper inside skirt or trouser band
	Wear of underarm from crutches		Knitted gusset piece under arms
			Action pleat at armhole in blouse back
		Weakness or loss of use	Material with stretch (such as jersey); action back pleats (center back or at armhole)
	Tear or binding when wheeling chair		Three-quarter length sleeves (to prevent soiling cuffs)

Not least important are the cosmetic factors of devices. They should be as inconspicuous as possible, simulate function as near normally as possible, be cosmetically acceptable, and be easy to use, handle, and maintain.

Mechanical considerations. When constructing or purchasing commercial technical aids, general principles of concern include the following:

1. Proper fit and function
2. Universality of use
3. Adaptability to the patient's progress
4. Simplicity of construction
5. Durability
6. Cost
7. Design and properties of material

A comprehensive and excellent discussion of special equipment for the cervical spinal cord–injured patient is presented by Zimmerman in *Rehabilitation Approaches in Spinal Cord Injury.*[41] Figure 46-2 shows a variety of universal components that can be used for substitution of function for some self-care activities, such as eating, writing, and grooming.

Electronic technical aids

With the rapid growth and advancement of electronic technology, the severely disabled person has many more possibilities for improving quality of life. The availability of electronic technical aids, such as environmental control systems, mobility systems, telephone units, computer access, and robotic devices, is contributing to a more productive and independent life for the severely disabled consumer at home and in the community. It has become essential for the rehabilitation professional to keep abreast of these advancements, as well as to be knowledgeable regarding the satisfactory use and application of these systems. Dickey's manual, *Electronic Technical Aids for Persons with Severe Physical Disabilities,*[11] is an excellent source of information. The manual includes a detailed description of several categories of electronic equipment, such as environmental control units, page turners, and telephone units. Each device in the manual is described by name, labeled picture, type of system, cost, general function, standard component list, specifications, available accessories, interfaces, mode of operation, feedback, and some advantages and disadvantages. For the severely disabled person who has minimal to no function, electronic aids are an option to increase independence, particularly through environmental control units and electronically powered mobility systems.

Criteria for selection

Major factors for consideration when selecting electronic systems are the following:

1. Types and requirements of interfaces for operation by patient
2. Mode and requirements of operation of interface
3. Extent or volume, as well as type of peripherals that can be controlled
4. Location or goal of use of electronic aids

Because this area of devices is experiencing rapid growth and expansion, only basic principles and concepts for selection of such equipment are presented.

Interfaces. All types of controls or switches used by the disabled to activate various equipment or systems require some body function, whether it be minimal movement of body parts or use of the vocal, visual, or respiratory systems. The auditory system may also be employed, but it is used primarily to augment the others, especially during the operation process.

TYPES AND REQUIREMENTS OF INTERFACES. Types and requirements for switches using body functions are microswitch, capacitance, pneumatic, photocell, or audio switches:

1. Microswitch—body movements
   a. Range: touch to 1¼ inches
   b. Force: 0.01 to 4 ounces
2. Capacitance switch—body movements
   a. Range: trace to 6 inches
   b. Force: none
3. Pneumatic switch—breath
   a. Positive pressure: 0.05 to 8 mm
   b. Negative pressure: 0.05 to 10 mm
4. Photocell—eye (ocular movements)
   a. Full range
5. Audio switch
   a. Tone or pitch (sounds, whistle)
   b. Actual voice commands

MODE OF OPERATION OF INTERFACES. Depending on the type of interface, the patient's disability (weakness, incoordination, loss of range of motion), and the body function being used to activate the device, the following factors must be considered and the total situation evaluated before final selection of equipment:

1. Force (pressure) of body movements. This may need to be as little as mere touch or can be up to 4 ounces. For incoordination, higher values may be of more benefit. When breath is used to create pressure, it has been found that positive pressures can be obtained comfortably up to 8 mm, and negative pressure up to 10 or even 12 mm. When the patient is unable to move away from the switch, it has been found best to keep the level at no less than 3 mm of pressure to avoid accidental tripping.
2. Travel (range) of body movements. Range may require ⅛ to ¼ inch, up to 1½ inches, depending on force. Generally, with incoordination, range is no problem; rather, the direction of the travel may be important. In cases of both weakness and incoordination, stability of the switch is necessary to take advantage of minimal travel and force. With eye movements, usually the

extreme ranges are required so as not to interfere with normal visual needs.

3. Intermittent or sustained activation depends on force, travel, types of interface, type of peripheral, and patient's residual abilities. Some switches are easier or preferable if intermittent. Sustained activation is more difficult generally but may offer more speed.

4. Sequential or direct selection depends on the number of peripherals to be operated and whether only on-off activation is sufficient. For the wheelchair, direct signals are a necessity to achieve efficiency and practicality.

5. Simple or complex codes depend on the patient's ability and the need of the peripheral being operated. A typewriter, for example, requires a code to achieve the desired number of outputs with the minimal number of inputs.

Types and number of peripherals. Many types of peripherals or equipment can be operated by remote control such as television, telephone, and radio; environmental devices (also known as comfort and communication devices); electric beds; window drapes; heat; and fan; and mobility aids, such as the power-driven wheelchair. These provide more freedom of operation.

Environmental controls. This area is perhaps the least demanding and the most flexible because it can use a variety of interfaces and modes of operation, from the simple on-off switch for one piece of equipment up to the most complex. However, it still requires evaluation of patient and equipment to ensure the proper or best selection (Figures 46-5 and 46-6).

Mobility controls. These controls are a necessity for most severely disabled individuals, as mobility is a vital part of today's culture. For example, the details of operation are important when breath is used as one type of interface. The timing required for sustained inputs can be critical. In tests with a standard Everest and Jennings power-driven wheelchair, pressure must be held for a maximal time of 8 to 10 seconds to turn the chair one complete revolution during low speed (when the chair is fully charged and with batteries fully energized). The highest speed takes only 2½ to 3 minutes.

Location or goal of use. When equipment is used in various locations, such as hospital room (in bed), home (indoors or outdoors), or at work, other considerations are necessary:

1. Noninterference with other electrical equipment
2. Easy installation with minimum of wires and parts
3. Total amperage of peripherals within limits of each individual circuit
4. Safety factors, such as meeting fire regulations, emergency calls, emergency cutoff switches
5. Reliability of basic control units to eliminate frequent time-consuming and costly repairs, to provide uninterrupted independence, and to prevent frustration and psychologic rejection
6. Ease of handling (by attendant or family)
7. Minimum space allocation for practicality

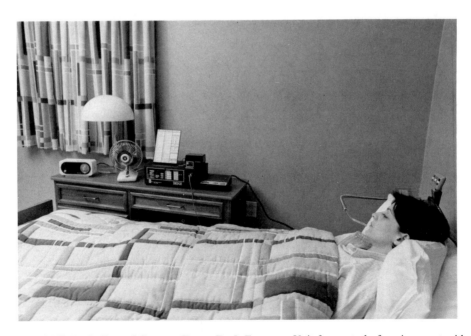

Figure 46-5. Du-It Control System. Deuce Du-It Economy Unit for control of environment with integrated display and BSR remote control receiver. Sip and puff pneumatic switch operates peripherals, that is, bed, radio, light, and fan. BSR can control up to 16 functions.

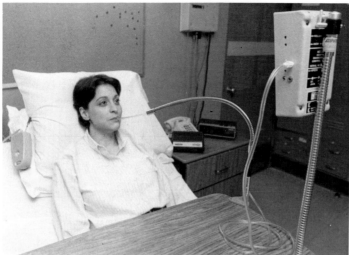

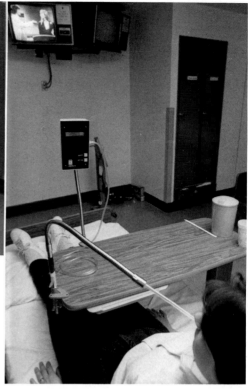

Figure 46-6. Prentke-Romich Hospital Environmental Control System (HECS-3) allows control of electric bed, nurse call bell, television, telephone, and two other user-selected functions.

Electronic equipment has been able to provide a considerable amount of independence for the severely disabled. It has also placed more demands on the design of equipment being operated. For example, with the tremendous increase of computer use in industry and the business world, and their potential vocational or educational value to the disabled person, access to computers has been an important development. Tash Inc. (Markham, Ont.) has available several options including keyboard emulators, keyboard adaptions, and keyboards of various sizes and methods of key activation. Micro-Dec, one environmental control unit, has been designed to accept additional control function that allows keyboard bypass to the Apple IIe computer (Figure 46-7). Such design developments provide increased options for independence for the disabled consumer.

Wheelchairs

The wheelchair, as a mobility system, requires careful and individualized assessment of the disabled person's needs if it is to offer maximal comfort, safety, and easy access for social, recreational, and vocational participation. Wheelchair design is constantly improving, and today there are many choices of type, size, and accessories. Wheelchair manufacturers have excellent catalogs, illustrating and describing the many types of chairs and accessories, as well as offering guidelines on fit and care.

Criteria for wheelchair selection

Types

STANDARD WHEELCHAIRS. For the person who is able to propel the chair independently, three types of chairs are available: the standard outdoor chair, which has the large wheels in back with the casters in front; the amputee chair, for the patient with lower extremity amputations, which has the axle located behind the large wheels to accommodate the weight of the patient distributed in the rear of the seat, thus preventing tipping; and a one hand–driven chair, which is available for a triplegic patient. The hand rims are both located on one side, thus controlling both wheels simultaneously. A patient who has the use of one side of the body (for example, a hemiplegic) gains mobility with a standard chair with lower seat and one foot pedal removed. A wheelchair may be selected by weight according to the needs of the patient. There are heavy-duty chairs, as well as a large variety of lightweight chairs for the sports participant. The reader is referred to wheelchair catalogs for the descriptions and evaluation of specifications of the various wheelchairs available.*

SIZES. Wheelchairs are available in adult, narrow adult,

---

*Everest and Jennings Inc., 3233 East Mission Oaks Blvd., Camarillo, CA 93010; Medical Equipment Distributors Inc., Catalog 1987, Rehabco, 2811 Qulette Ave., Bronx, NY 10461.

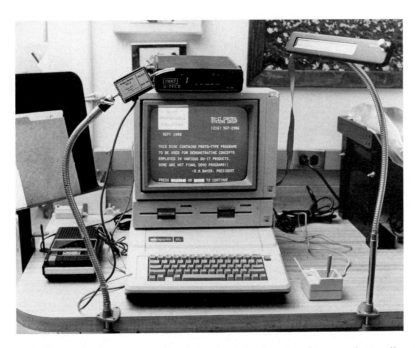

Figure 46-7. MED Micro-Dec II; microprocessor-based distributed environmental controller; allows keyboard bypass to Apple IIe computer.

slim adult, junior, growing chair, tiny tot-hi, tiny tot-low, and preschool pediatric sizes. Each of these chairs has specifications measured by inches and centimeters for seat width, depth, and height; arm height; and back height. Patient measurements are compiled according to these specifications, and the wheelchair size is determined according to the patient's dimensions. For proper fit and comfort, precise measurements must be taken. In the selection of a wheelchair the user's needs and life-style is evaluated. The vocational, social, and recreational activity of the wheelchair user influences other characteristics of the chair chosen.

Accessories

LARGE WHEELS. Wheels vary in size from 20 to 26 inches according to the type of chair selected. Tires may be pneumatic, semipneumatic, or of polyurethane. Again, choice of tires depends on the user's activity.

HAND RIMS. Hand rims may be aluminum or plastic coated. Some have vertical projections to aid maneuvering for patients with hand dysfunction.

CASTERS. Casters may be 8 or 5 inches; 8-inch casters are preferable because they give the chair a larger base and therefore more stability. This makes propelling the chair over small obstacles easier.

ARMRESTS. Armrests can be fixed or detachable. Detachable armrests are preferred for close approach. Desk arms have a cutout front section, which permits access to desks and tables without removing the armrest. Armrests can also be adjustable in height, accommodating the patient for optimal leverage in transfer activities when pushed up and for

trunk stability. They are upholstered for comfort. Locks are available for detachable armrests.

FOOTRESTS. Footrests may be stationary or detachable. Detachable footrests are preferred as they allow close approach for all front transfer activities. Another advantage is that by removing footrests, the overall length and weight of the chair is reduced. This facilitates storage and placement in an automobile. Footrests should be adjustable in length to accommodate the distance between the foot and the knee. Heel loops prevent the patient's feet from slipping backward. Toe loops are also available.

Elevating footrests are indicated if the knee cannot be flexed, the legs need to be elevated with a reclining chair, or edema is present. Elevating footrests should be adjustable and detachable.

BACKRESTS. Backrests are chosen according to the patient's dimensions and type of wheelchair selected. The standard backrest reaches approximately to the shoulder blades. Additional postural support may be added with a hook on the headrest if needed. A wheelchair or full reclining backrest may be needed for patients who have restriction at the hip joint or difficulty maintaining the vertical position. A wheelchair with reclining backs always has elevating footrests with legrests.

SEAT CUSHIONS. Wheelchair cushions are used to relieve pressure and to stabilize the body for balance and comfort. The anatomic risk areas of the seated person include ischial tuberosities, coccyx, sacrum, and the trochanters. Seat cushions can be subcategorized into dynamic and static de-

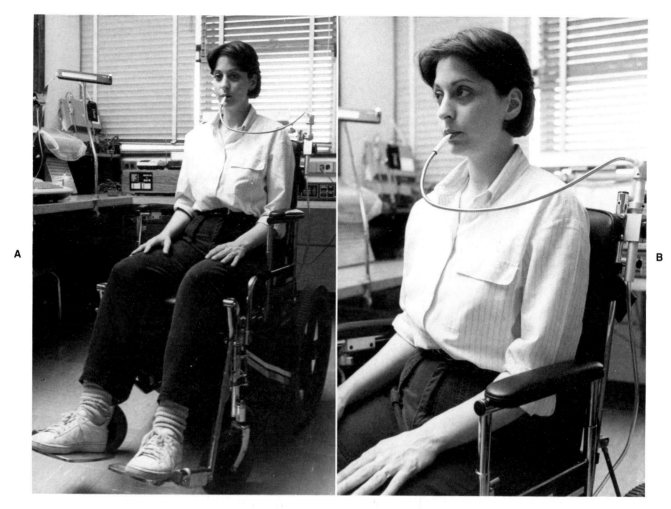

Figure 46-8. A, Everest and Jennings 5M Power Premier Electric Chair. **B,** Dufco Sip and Puff Pneumatic Control System.

vices.[13a] Dynamic systems depend on external power for activation to relieve pressure cyclically; they are cumbersome and limit mobility. Static systems for relieving pressure may be air filled (for example, Roho dry flotation cushion); flotation type, either gel or filled, which adjust to the body's movement, and polymer foam, the most versatile for sizing and shaping. Foam cushions are least expensive and are lightweight; however, they are difficult to clean and their life span is limited in comparison to the other types. Seating position for comfort and stability remains a challenge for the severely disabled patient with deformities. Molded inserts of many varieties are available. Consideration must be given to the materials used, that is, their desirability and their characteristics for adjustment. Many seating systems are commercially available and may be located via a database (Abledata System, National Rehabilitation Information System, Washington, D.C.).

Electric wheelchairs. For the severely disabled person who is unable to propel standard wheelchairs, power chairs offer independent mobility. Many control systems are available, and selection depends on the residual functions of the patient. The simplest version is not unlike a standard wheelchair but with a power device control box located on the user's armrest. Access to control may be simply a drive stick T or an on-off switch extension. Other control systems available are sip and puff pneumatic control, short throw switch controlled by chin or tongue, rocker controls and slot controls for gross motor ability (Figure 46-8).

Electronic controls provide patients optimal independence in mobility. Most systems are used to start, stop, steer, and change speed. Some controls offer acceleration and deceleration control to ensure smooth mobility. Through use of command modules, some systems can access computer systems and environmental control devices (Figure 46-9). Strict considerations of many factors are involved in electronic wheelchair selection.

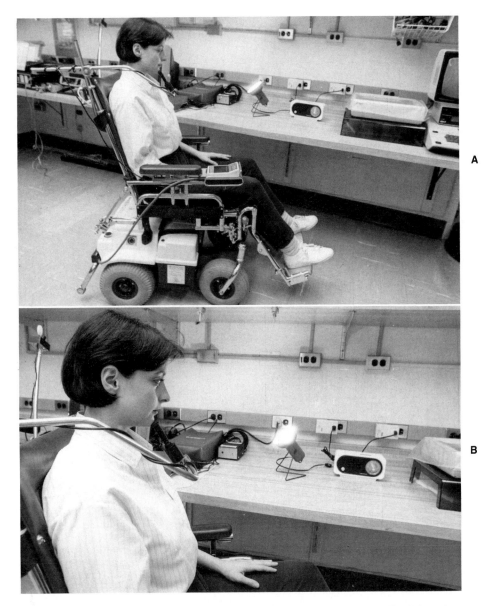

Figure 46-9. A, Fortress Scientific 655FS power base with fully reclining seat. **B,** Chin-activated short throw joystick gives patient remote access of four separate peripherals: light, radio, computer, and telephone.

Wheelchair prescription

A customized fit can be accomplished easily. A wheelchair prescription form is an efficient method for preparing the information before ordering the chair. Figure 46-10 is an example of a form used for a power chair prescription.

User training

Any system, equipment, or device will be only as good as the amount of time and efforts spent in practice to acquire skill and proficiency. The patient's understanding of the function of complex systems is equally important, and a major portion of training should include a thorough education of the equipment parts and their maintenance.

TRAINING IN DAILY LIVING SKILLS

Training the patient to perform daily living skills is an individualized process. The level of functional outcome depends in part on the residual physical and cognitive function, how effectively these functions can be transferred, and the patient's motivation for gaining some level of independence. It is preferable that these activities be accomplished with

```
        The Rusk Institute              Name: _____
     of Rehabilitation Medicine
 New York University Medical Center     Address: _____
 OCCUPATIONAL THERAPY DEPARTMENT        Age: _____ Chart No. _____
         TECHNICAL AIDS
                                        Diagnosis/Disability: _____

 Therapist: _____ Date: _____     Dr's. Signature: _____
```

POWERED WHEELCHAIR PRESCRIPTION

BRAND & TYPE

__ E&J 5M 24V Proportional
__ Fortress FS655
__ Fortress Add-on FS-1000
__ Meyra 1482
__ Invacare Arrow

CONTROL

__ Control Box: rt./lt.
__ OTHER

__ Sip & Puff
__ Chin control __
__ Prentke Romich System
   MCB___   DLT___
   WCP 1 ___   WCP 2___
   Chin___ Joy Stick___

CONTROL ACCESS

__ Drive Stick "T"
__ On/Off Switch Exten.
__ OTHER

FRAME TYPE & SIZE

__ Standard Adult 18"x16"
__ Narrow Adult 16"x16"
__ 4 Post
__ Goldwater Frame
__ OTHER

BACK STYLE

__ Standard 16½"
__ Raised-Height____
__ Sectional-Height____
__ Handles Welded/Round
__ Upholstry Front/Back
__ Semi reclining
__ Fully Reclining
__ Fully Reclin. Motorized
      Type:_____
      Activation:_____
__ OTHER

BACK ACCESSORIES

__ Headrest Extension
    Size: _____
__ Reclining Headrest
    Type:_____
__ Headrest Cushion
__ Back Cushion
    Type:_____
    Size:_____
__ Reinforced Upholstry
__ Solid Back Insert
    Type:_____
    Size:_____
__ OTHER

ARMREST

__ Removable Desk/Full
__ Remove. Adj. Desk
__ Remove. Adj. Full Lgth.
__ Trough Arm Pad
__ Retract. Trough/Reg.
__ OTHER

LEG REST STYLE

__ Standard Footrest
__ Elevating Legrest
__ Below Seat Pivot
__ #1 foot Plate
__ #2 Foot Plate
__ Adj. Angle Ft. plate
__ OTHER

LEG REST ACCESSORIES

__ Heel Loops
__ Toe Loops
__ Calf Straps
__ quad Release
__ Trough Legrest Panels
__ OTHER

CASTERS & ACCESSORIES

__ 8"x1" Solid Rubber
__ 8"x1¼" Pneumatic
__ 8"x1 3/4" Semi Pneu.
__ OTHER

__ Davis Forks
__ Caster Guides

REAR WHEELS

__ Hard Rubber
__ Pneumatic 20"x1"
__ Pneumatic 20"x2
__ Extra Tubes, tires
__ OTHER

SEAT ACCESSORIES

__ Foam cushion
    Size:__
    Type:__
__ Roho
__ Solid Seat Insert
__ OTHER

MISC. ACCESSORIES

__ Auto Seat Belt
__ Velcro Seat Belt
__ Brake Extensions
__ Lapboard
    Type:_____
    Size:_____
__ Lateral Trunk supp.
    Type:_____
    Size:_____
__ Lateral Trunk Supp.
    Type: MED
          E&J
          Invacare
__ Deep Cycle Batteries
__ OTHER

__ COLOR

Figure 46-10. Electric wheelchair prescription form. (Courtesy Occupational Therapy Department, Rusk Institute of Rehabilitation Medicine, New York University Medical Center.)

the minimal use of assistive devices and equipment; however, this depends on the disability and residual function. Several excellent references describe in detail techniques for teaching activities of daily living. The reader is referred to Lawton's *Activities of Daily Living*[29] and Ford and Duckworth's *Physical Management for the Quadriplegic Patient*[13] for an in-depth study of specific techniques used for training. The following general principles apply to all patients and all activities.

General principles

All daily living skills have fundamental similar motions in common: changing position, sitting balance, moving in the seated position, reaching, grasping, standing, and walkins.[29] In addition to the physical requirements, these motions require cognitive integrative skill.

An analysis of the patient's attempt to perform the skill determines what deficits prevent completion of the task. The initial standard of performance is documented and becomes the reference point for measuring improvement.

Having determined the patient's limitations, the rehabilitation program focuses on improving or restoring dysfunctions to facilitate later success in performance. It is paramount that the patient's treatment program be structured to remediate specific motions that relate to the demands of activities of daily living. As the patient goes through the restorative process, it is important to introduce daily living skills, within the patient's capabilities. Sometimes the patient is able to complete one or two components of an activity, and every effort should be made to assist and involve the patient in this participation. To sustain the patient's motivation and prevent frustrations and encourage feelings of competency, the therapist may need to assist the patient. For example, in training a quadriplegic patient in eating, the therapist may need to don the patient's equipment and arrange the food, such as opening packages and applying the utensils to the assistive device. The patient's energies will then be reserved for the food intake sequence. This approach for training is usually more gratifying for the patient, who experiences a sense of control.

The therapist monitors the patient's improvement and reduces the amount of assistance given, until the patient can achieve the activity as independently as possible. This principle applies to most of the skills the patient is to perform.

As the patient's physical improvement levels off, teaching compensatory techniques becomes another focus of treatment. It requires teaching the patient how to use the body intelligently, including how to use the forces of gravity advantageously (Figure 46-11), how to protect joints by avoiding stresses and deforming forces, how to use good body mechanics and leverages to compensate for weakness, and how to use stabilization techniques to reduce uncoordination.[36] Patients with sensory losses are at risk of injury and must be made aware of alternative approaches, as well

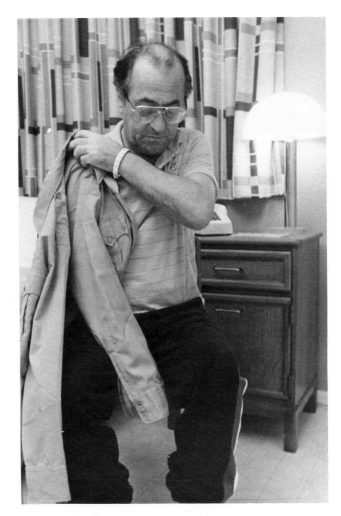

Figure 46-11. Dressing activity incorporates controlled position of impaired upper extremity to inhibit shoulder retraction and elbow flexion in hemiplegic patient.

as precautions to prevent injury. When performing activities in homemaking and bathing, the patient must learn strategies to prevent injury caused by burns and cuts.

For patients with cognitive or perceptual motor dysfunction, one can structure the activity into component parts and use a repertoire of cues—visual, auditory, and tactile—that can guide and validate the patient's performance. As the patient demonstrates improvement in attention, memory, and problem solving, one can begin to reduce the structure and lessen the cueing system.[12] This technique has been systematically researched with the brain-damaged population for the remediation of memory and neglect. Since attention is an important requirement for relearning, training should begin with activities the patient views as most important. In this way the patient's own interest sustains motivation, which can be an additional reinforcement for performance improvement.

Independent living experience

The ideal condition for training patients in daily living skills is in a homelike setting. This can be a training apartment, where the patient can engage in an entire day's sequence of activity as a final evaluation of skills in daily living. The Rusk Institute of Rehabilitation Medicine's Horizon House is such an environment. Horizon House is an example of accessible housing for the disabled and is used as the setting for an independent living experience program. Patients are assigned for a day or overnight experience in the Horizon House with their care partner. This experience takes place without direct supervision of professional staff. The objectives are the following:

1. To provide a realistic educational experience in independent living for patients and their care partner before discharge home
2. To provide the patient and family member the experience of shared responsibilities
3. To better prepare the patient and family members for the patient's discharge by determining from this experience whether the patient has acquired maximal skill in management of activities of daily living

After the day's experience an exit interview is conducted with the patient and the family. The information gathered assists the team in modifying the patient's program to meet specific needs before discharge.

Horizon House was remodeled in 1982 with the assistance and support of the Whirlpool Corporation. The interior of the house has functional design features that provide solutions of access for the disabled person and incorporate a design for the nondisabled members of the family (Figure 46-12).

Home management retraining

The rehabilitation of the homemaker took on significant importance when in 1956 the Office of Vocational Rehabilitation recognized homemaking as a vocation and provided funds for the rehabilitation of the disabled homemaker. The goal of homemaker retraining is to return the disabled homemaker to her work environment so she can resume her place as a manager of her home. Home management retraining is not limited to women, for it is not uncommon to see role reversals in today's family. A disabled man who cannot return to work may be trained to take over some household duties to free his wife for employment outside the home.

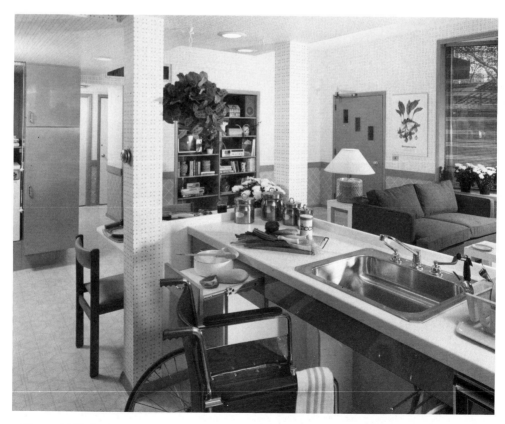

Figure 46-12. Horizon House at Rusk Institute of Rehabilitation Medicine, New York University Medical Center, incorporates functional design for use by disabled and nondisabled members of family. (Courtesy Whirlpool Corporation, Benton Harbor, Mich.)

Goals

The goals of training in home management are these:

1. Retraining or, if necessary, initial training in basic household skills
2. Reducing fatigue and amount of energy and time expended through work simplification techniques
3. Providing therapeutic exercise and use of prosthetic and orthotic equipment through functional home management tasks
4. Providing psychologic benefits and motivation through satisfactory performance
5. Planning for modifications of the home, if necessary, to maximize the disabled person's independence in the home

Evaluation

An intake interview covers issues related to the individual's role in the family as a homemaker before the disability. The interview can also reveal the patient's readiness to accept the idea of learning new methods for performing previous responsibilities. Having the patient participate in a simple procedure sometimes helps to alleviate doubts and fears, and at the same time the therapist can note the patient's performance in terms of physical limitations, use of equipment, adeptness and ingenuity, concepts of work (haphazard and careless or careful and meticulous), mental and emotional reliability (such as judgment as opposed to confusion), ability to follow direction, visual perceptual deficits, and safety.

Training area

Training the patient in all aspects of home management is ideally achieved in a homelike or apartment setting. Only then can one simulate the homemaker's work environment. If that is not possible, one arranges a training unit that provides a standard-height work area, as well as a work area modified to accommodate the wheelchair user. This type of training area offers the patient an opportunity to succeed in activities under optimal conditions from the wheelchair and then progress to the standard unit, once confidence and skills are achieved (Figure 46-13).

Training program

The actual steps or plan of a treatment program should never be routine but should be determined according to individual needs. Experience has shown, howver, that it is usually more acceptable to the patient to start with familiar routine tasks, especially those of immediate concern. Several comprehensive publications on training the disabled homemaker are available.[3,27,35] The basic goals of a training program are practice to gain assurance of competent performance, retraining in new techniques, development of one-handed skills, selection and use of proper or suitable tools and equipment, testing of work heights and arrangements, testing and selection of various kinds and types of storage units, use of energy-saving methods evolved through work simplification and management planning techniques, and planning for modification of the patient's living situation.

Basic skills

A patient's basic skills are determined first of all by individual responsibilities on returning home. Activities such as food preparation, washing dishes, making beds, and ironing are the usual basic skills. Teaching work simplification techniques to the disabled homemaker is most important and is basic to training. Techniques include the following[32]:

1. Use both hands in opposite and symmetric, smooth flowing motions.
2. Arrange work areas within normal reach.
3. Slide; do not lift or carry objects.
4. Arrange work areas and tools for different tasks, such as preparation and clean-up areas, mixing and baking center.
5. Eliminate any unnecessary motions or processes.
6. Avoid holding—use clamps and stationary equipment.
7. Use the assistance of gravity where possible.
8. Locate switches and controls within easy reach.
9. Sit—don't stand—whenever possible.
10. Use proper work heights, according to the job and the individual.
11. Use good working conditions—proper light and ventilation, pleasing colors, comfortable clothing.

Management, although a separate and unique process, is another way in which energy is ultimately saved.[14,17] It is economy of human resource, accomplished by the planning of work, through evaluation of the various jobs and the decisions and choices involved. Management involves not only the homemaker but also her entire family and the use of their skills, income, and possessions. It includes the buying of furnishings, food, and equipment. It means scheduling of tasks and supervision of work done by others. If severe limitations rule out the actual accomplishment of household tasks by the homemaker herself, the role of manager may provide a place and a need for those remaining skills that involve only mental processes. Actually, management in any home, as well as in business, is a keynote to the smoothness and efficiency with which tasks involving physical effort are accomplished.

Selection and use of equipment

The variety of household tools available usually makes it possible to manage with standard equipment. However, the ability to evaluate the different designs in terms of various problems may save a lot of frustration and wasted energy. Some of the factors to look for are as follows:

1. Possibility of operating with only one hand. Items such as one-handed whisks and eggbeaters, long-handled dustpans and brushes, and clip-around aprons are available.

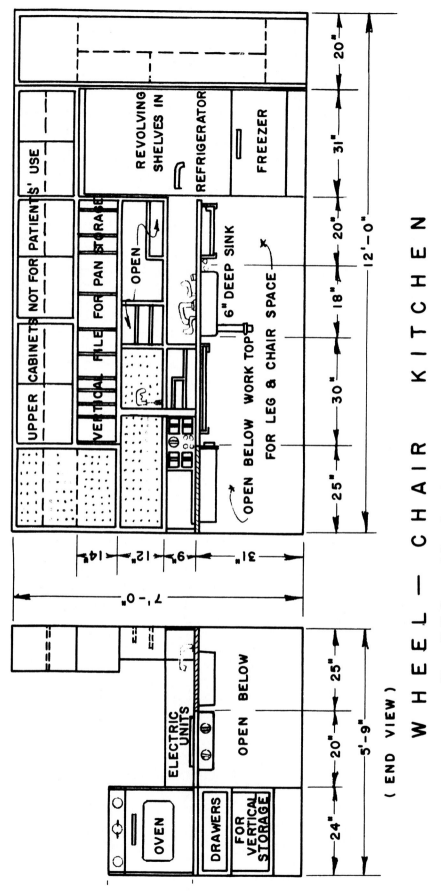

Figure 46-13. Suggested dimensions of wheelchair kitchen. (Courtesy Occupational Therapy Department, Rusk Institute of Rehabilitation Medicine, New York University Medical Center.)

2. Stabilization of tools and appliances
3. Placement and shape of handles and knobs determine the type of grasp necessary, positioning of arms during reach and use, safety, and extent of energy required.
4. Use of electric equipment to eliminate manual operation. Articles such as electric mixers, can openers, blenders and food processors, and carving knives can facilitate work. New cordless appliances are lightweight and easy to use.
5. Weight, size, shape, durability, and ease of care of utensils
6. Selection of containers and jars for easier opening

There may be times when no standard equipment is adequate and when some adaptations are necessary. One of the most common is the cutting board with nails to stabilize vegetables and fruits (Figure 46-14).

When considering the purchase of any equipment, either standard or adapted, in addition to the selection factors previously listed, one should be guided by the following general principles:

1. The device should be really necessary.
2. It should save time.
3. It should save energy or prevent overuse of weak muscles.
4. It should provide for safety.
5. It must meet the requirements applicable to all equipment as to durability, cleansability, ease of maintenance, and enough use to justify storage and cost.

Work areas and storage

Every job in the home has a work area, but perhaps none is so detailed or confined within such a small space as those in the kitchen (Figure 46-15). Much has already been done toward the planning of good kitchens; these guides should be used as basic criteria, with adjustments and adaptations planned as needed for the individual's physical limitations.[27] Refer to the additional readings at the end of the chapter for sources.

The two factors that most frequently need changing are work height and the placement and type of storage units. Proper work height, either for standing or for sitting on a stool or in a wheelchair, improves posture and lessens fatigue. Depth of the counter should also be considered, especially when one is confined to a wheelchair. Heights of storage cupboards and arrangement of equipment within these areas may be a major factor in achieving independence (Figure 46-16).

Vertical filing, revolving shelves, pullout bins, and racks all bring utensils within easier reach and eliminate unnecessary lifting and bending. The addition of extra storage arrangements by means of a midway cabinet or pegboard is an invaluable help in storing utensils at the area where they are first used.

If standard items cannot be altered, the use of substitute equipment may be helpful. Such equipment includes microwave ovens to replace surface burners and ovens or dropleaf tables to provide lower working surfaces.

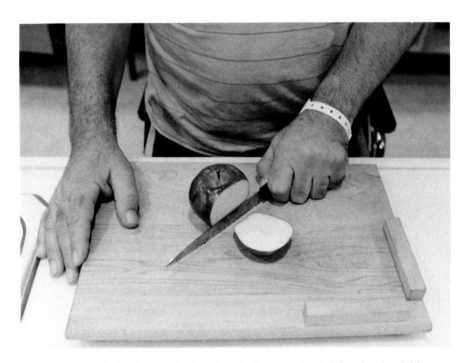

Figure 46-14. Cutting board adapted to facilitate one-handed functional activities.

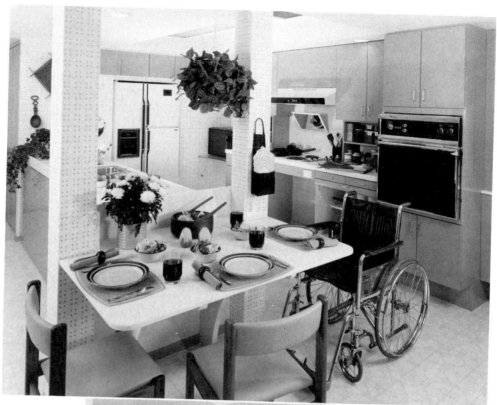

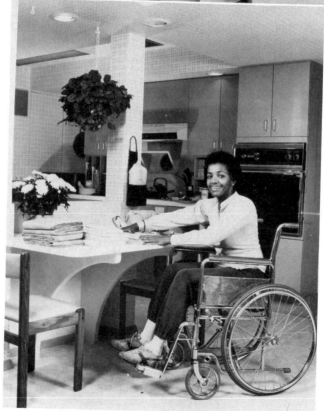

Figure 46-15. Kitchen space designed to serve as both eating and working area. Counter height of 30 inches serves several functions. (Courtesy Whirlpool Corporation, Benton Harbor, Mich.)

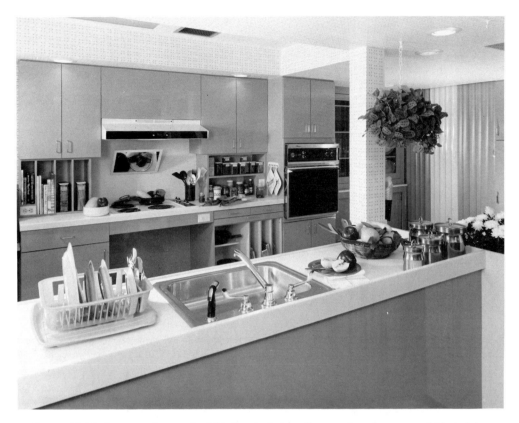

Figure 46-16. Features of a standard kitchen include pullout work surfaces at variable heights, vertical and accessible storage, and open spaces under appliances for wheelchair access.

Child care

Although child care is not an area involving every homemaker, many have infants and preschool children who demand their attention and care. Standard guidance on child care and development should be provided if it is not already available. Training in early independence is rewarding to both mother and child and is a practical help to the disabled mother.[38]

Some areas in which special information and help are frequently needed are selection and adjustment of clothing, bathing and lifting of infants, feeding techniques, and provision for and participation in play activities.[5]

ELIMINATING ENVIRONMENTAL BARRIERS

Rehabilitation of the disabled person is complete only when consideration is given to home, work, and community environmental barriers. Several facets to be considered in such a program are site and type of dwelling, ecology of housing, and architectural design features.

Site and type of dwelling

Level areas are most desirable and eliminate modifications to accommodate changes in ground rises. Sidewalks and curbs (removal at intersections or crosswalks) must be given attention. The type of dwelling depends on the needs of the occupants. Most desirable is a single dwelling or apartment located within the nondisabled community. To make this practical, access to public facilities (stores, bank, post office, library, church) must also be suitable for the disabled and aged.

Apartment complexes, partially or totally designed for the disabled, can include these facilities, as well as recreation or workshop areas. Total "villages" may be desirable to provide the ultimate in independent living for the severely disabled (such as Het Drop in Arnhem, Netherlands).

Ecology of housing

Ecology of housing is a specialized derivative of the field of sociology in which the consumer takes part in a personal environmental design.[37] It expands the concept of human ecology, defined as the consideration of spatial aspects of the symbiotic relations of people and institutions. This includes not only the social, psychologic, and economic aspects of family living, but also the world of designing, construction, and industrial production. The two fields must be interrelated and their effects on each other considered. More study of human activities, their relationships with each other, and their needs for space and form requirements will force architects to plan with both design and function in mind; by nature these two aspects should go hand in hand.

Architectural design features

Architectural design features and requirements for elimination of those features that create barriers for the disabled, with consideration of ecologic and architectural demands, can be classified into three areas relating to function as follows:

1. Features providing access or egress to various areas (doors, sills, stairs, ramps, curbs, elevators)
2. Features that contribute to space enclosure (floors, walls, windows, lights, heating, ventilation)
3. Features relating to various activity work areas (kitchen, bedroom, bathroom, including fixtures and furniture)

Access or egress features

Stairs (for the ambulant). Risers should not be more than 6 inches. Nosings should not be abrupt or square. There should be rails on both sides, extending beyond both the top and bottom, with ends curving out of the way.

Ramps. Ramps should not exceed 1 foot rise in 12 feet of length (5 degrees) and should be at least 36 to 40 inches in width. There should also be a level entrance area extending approximately 2 feet beyond the opening side of the door. Rails should be available on ramps. Portable ramps may be necessary.

Sills. All indoor sills should be eliminated, and all outside ones should be confined to a minimum.

Doors. A door width of 36 inches is preferred but may be less, depending on the width of the hall or entrance area and the amount of turning space availalbe. For small rooms, some arrangement such as a sliding door is needed to allow room for a chair and for closing the door behind the chair. Sliding or folding doors are best for closets.

Elevators. Elevators should be 3 feet in width by 4 feet in depth—the minimum interior space. The height of the operating controls should be approximately 30 to 36 inches from the floor. Doors should be self-closing, but with a time lag.

Curbs. Curbs should be cut or ramped. Warning features for the blind should be incorporated.

Space enclosures

Floors. Floor should be nonskid, such as terrazzo with Carborundum chips or vinyl tile. They must not be waxed. Carpets should be eliminated in favor of woven mats or other coverings of firm surface.

Walls. Washable paint or vinyl coverings should be used on the walls; all surfaces should be smooth.

Windows. Casement or awning-type windows are generally easiest to open. Crank or push-bar type controls require less force and range of motion to operate. The height of the sill should not exceed 32 inches. Clear access to the window and controls should be provided.

Lights. Wall switches should be no higher than 36 inches, and electrical outlets should be placed no less than 24 inches from the floor. Placement should be near doors and sometimes be controlled by master switches. For persons with minimal strength, some special electronic switches requiring only touch are available.

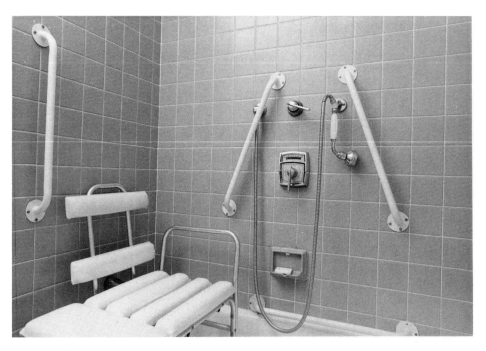

Figure 46-17. Vertical grab bar at outside end of tub provides assistance for safe transfer to tub. Removable Lumex tub bench permits wheelchair-to-tub transfer.

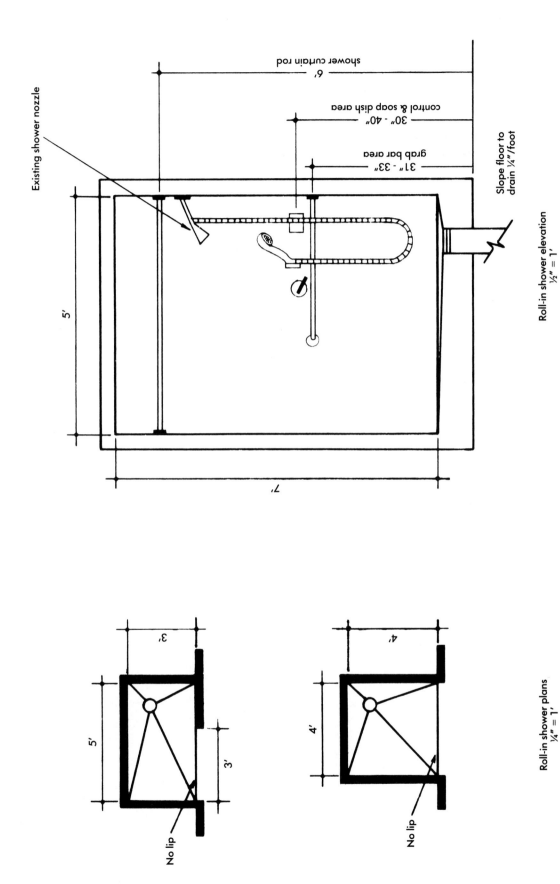

Existing shower nozzle

shower curtain rod
6'

control & soap dish area
30" - 40"

grab bar area
31" - 33"

Slope floor to
drain ¼"/foot

5'

7'

Roll-in shower elevation
½" = 1'

3'

5'

3'

No lip

4'

4'

No lip

Roll-in shower plans
¼" = 1'

Figure 46-18. Scale drawing for roll-in shower. (Courtesy Occupational Therapy Department, Rusk Institute of Rehabilitation Medicine, New York University Medical Center.)

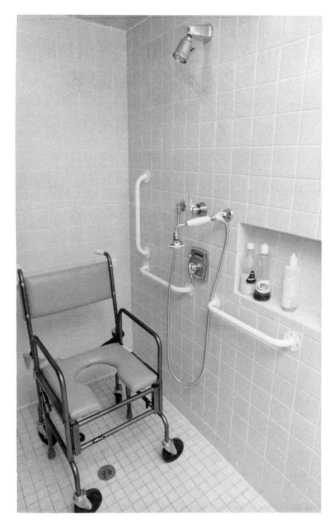

Figure 46-19. Roll-in shower with thermostat control for water temperature, accessible water controls, and shower commode chair.

Activity or work areas

Living, dining, and family rooms. The size of rooms depends on the number of family members and their living patterns. Arrangement should allow space for easy maneuvering of wheelchairs or use of crutches and at the same time should eliminate distances traveled to and from each area. A study of movements within these spaces (similar to a work flow chart) should result in a truly functional space design. If the design is well done, hallways, doorways, and separating walls are kept to a minimum. The wheelchair user requires a turning circumference of 4½ to 5½ feet.

Furniture should be selected according to heights of seats and of top surfaces. Chair seats should be no less than 18 inches in height and should be firm yet comfortable. Crossbars on chairs and tables are best eliminated or kept to a height of 10 inches above the floor. Sharp edges should be avoided on all pieces of furniture.

Kitchens. For specifications for kitchen designs, refer to Figure 46-13. The area may include some space for eating. Otherwise, open wall areas or pass-throughs help to minimize the transport of food.

Bedrooms. Size and location depend on family living patterns and on the type and extent of disability. Beds, especially if double sized, should have free access to both sides. Storage drawers can be wall hung or recessed into walls. Closets should be no deeper than 24 inches and are best when provided with sliding doors; rods should be no higher than 48 inches.

Bathrooms. Grab bars at tub and toilet are essential. Heights of 26 to 30 inches are generally suitable. Bars are best if horizontal and vertical, rather than diagonal. Toilet bars may need to be the fold-up or swing-away type. Tub bars should provide for standing transfer, transfer to tub seats, or transfer directly into the tub (Figure 46-17).

The basin should be wall mounted in a countertop not more than 30½ inches top height. The depth of the counter should allow close approach by wheelchair. It is frequently desirable to have the basin installed next to the toilet so bathing can sometimes be managed from this position. This arrangement is also helpful for persons with a colostomy.

Many individuals prefer showers, which are easier to manage for the more severely disabled. Sills and enclosures (except for curtains) should be avoided. A back drain and slight floor slope to the drain prevent water from running over the bathroom floor (Figure 46-18).

Water controls should be placed on the wall adjoining the spray and within reach of the occupant. A thermostat for controlled temperature is desirable for all and essential for some. The shower spray should be adjustable in height or should convert to a hand-held spray and is best if an on-off control is also on the handpiece (Figure 46-19).

Tub or shower seats should be wheelchair height to facilitate transfer. The fold-up or easily removable types permit use of the equipment by others not desiring seats (Figure 46-17).

There are many sources to guide one in creating barrier-free environments with functional architectural design features (see the references at the end of this chapter).

Procedures and approach for elimination of architectural barriers in the home

Planning for elimination of architectural barriers to the disabled person's environment includes the following procedures:

1. Proper timing for introduction of patient to planning. This depends on the patient's (and family's) attitudes; however, the need for planning should be introduced as early as possible during the rehabilitation program.
2. Method of acquiring information. A rough sketch of the floor plan should be obtained from the patient or family member's description; if possible, blueprints of their living quarters should be requested. A home

visit is recommended whenever possible.

3. Assessment of individual needs and changes. The home visit is used to make accurate measurements of present architectural features (entrances, widths of doorways, layout of bathroom, kitchen, and living spaces). Taking instant photos of major problem areas is helpful during the planning stage.

4. Translation into scale drawings. Once the necessary data are collected, a scale drawing and elevations with the recommended solution to problems can be produced for use by family, the architect, or contractor (Figure 46-18). The family must be an integral part of the planning process.

5. Financing. Financial assistance may be available through agencies such as the Office of Vocational Rehabilitation (OVR), insurance companies, and local citizens' organizations. It is important for the professional to indicate justification for costly modifications, including their impact on the individual's quality of life and the vocational implications of these changes.

Since the enactment of the Architectural Barrier Act of 1968, federal legislation has established standards for accessibility through the American National Standards Institute (ANSI), which are available to individuals and facilities.[2] Among the many excellent references to educate the reader on designs that provide access for the disabled person is the Guide and System, available from the Information Development Corporation[18]; this source provides information on accessibility, survey evaluations, and product information.

REFERENCES

1. Abreau, B: Physical disabilities manual, New York, 1981, Raven Press.
2. American National Standard: Providing accessibility and usability of physically handicapped people, New York, 1986, American National Standards, Inc.
3. Anderson, H: The disabled homemaker, Springfield, 1981, Charles C Thomas, Publisher.
4. Bair, J, and Gwin, C, editors: A productivity systems guide for occupational therapy, Rockville, Md, 1985, The American Occupational Therapy Association Inc.
5. Bare, C, Boettke, E, and Waggoner, N: Self-help clothing for handicapped children, Chicago, 1962, National Society for Crippled Children and Adults.
6. Basmajian, JV: Muscles alive, their functions revealed by electromyography, ed 4, Baltimore, 1979, Williams & Wilkins.
7. Bobath, B: Abnormal postural reflex activity caused by brain lesions, ed 2, London, 1971, Heineman Medical Books.
8. Bobath, B: Adult hemiplegia: evaluation and treatment, ed 2, London, 1978, Heineman Medical Books.
9. Brunnstrom, S: Movement therapy in hemiplegia, New York, 1970, Harper & Row.
10. Delateur, BJ, et al: Mechanical work and fatigue: their role in the development of muscle work capacity, Arch Phys Med Rehabil 57:319, 1976.
11. Dickey, R: Electronic technical aids for persons with severe physical disabilities, New York, 1986, Rusk Institute of Rehabilitation Medicine, New York University Medical Center.
12. Diller, L, et al: Studies in cognition and rehabilitation in hemiplegia, rehabilitation monograph, No 50, Rusk Institute of Rehabilitation Medicine, New York, 1974, New York University Medical Center.
13. Ford, J, and Duckworth, B: Physical management for the quadriplegic patient, ed 6, Philadelphia, 1987, FA Davis Co.
13a. Garber, S: Wheelchair cushion; a historical review, Am J Occup Ther 39:453, 1985.
14. Gilbreth, L, et al: Management in the home, New York, 1954, Dodd, Mead & Co.
15. Gliner, JA: Purposeful activity in motor learning theory: an event approach to motor skill acquisition, Am J Occup Ther 39:28, 1985.
16. Granger, C, Albrecht, G, and Hamilton, B: Outcome of comprehensive medical rehabilitation: Measurement by pulses profile and the Barthel Index, Arch Phys Med Rehabil 60:145, 1979.
17. Gress, JH, and Crandall, EW: Management for modern families, New York, 1963, Appleton-Century-Crofts.
18. The guide to disabilities and barriers and facilities evaluation survey; and Product Information System, Division of Information Development Corporation, 1985 (The Guide), 360 St Alban Ct, Winston-Salem, NC.
19. Hopkin, HL, and Smith, HO, editors: Willard and Spackman's occupational therapy, ed 6, Philadelphia, 1983, JB Lippincott Co.
20. Iverson, IA: The Revised Kenny Self-Care Evaluation. Publication 722, Sister Kenny Institute, Minneapolis, Abbot, Northwestern Hospital.
21. Jebsen, R, et al: An objective standardized test of hand function, Arch Phys Med Rehabil 50:311, 1969.
22. Kanny, EM, Bell, B, and Klein, RM: Occupational therapy evaluation: Klein Bell Activity of Daily Living Scale (videotape), Seattle, 1980, Division of Occupational Therapy, University of Washington.
23. Katz, S, et al: Studies of illness in the aged. The index of activities of daily living. A standardized measure of biological and psychosocial function, JAMA 185:914, 1963.
24. Keilhofner, G, and Burke, JP: A model of human occupation. I. Conceptual framework and content, Am J Occup Ther 34:572, 1980.
25. Kellor, M, et al: Technical manual, hand strength and dexterity tasks, Minneapolis, 1971, Sister Kenny Institute.
26. Klein, RM, and Bell, B: Self-care skills: behavioral measurement with the Klein-Bell ADL Scale, Arch Phys Med Rehabil 63:335, 1982.
27. Klinger, JL: Mealtime manual for people with disabilities and the aging, ed 2, Ronks, Penn, 1978, Campbell Soup Co.
28. Knott, M, and Voss, DE: Proprioceptive neuromuscular facilitation, patterns and techniques, ed 2, New York, Harper & Row, 1970.
29. Lawton, EB: Activities of daily living for physical rehabilitation, New York, 1963, McGraw-Hill Book Co.
30. Mahoney, FI, and Barthael, DW: Functional evaluation, the Barthel Index, Md State Med J 14:61, 1965.
30a. Occupational therapy: its definition and function, Am J Occup Ther 26:204, 1972.
31. Rood, MS: Neurophysiological mechanisms utilized in treatment of neuromuscular dysfunction, Am J Occup Ther 10:220, 1956.
32. Rusk, HA, Judson, J, and Zimmerman, M: A manual for training the disabled homemaker, Rehabilitation Monograph VIII, New York, 1961, Rusk Institute of Rehabilitation Medicine.
33. Smith, R, et al: The effects of introducing the Klein-Bell ADL Scale in a rehabilitation service, Am J Occup Ther 40:420, 1986.
34. Steinbeck, TM: Purposeful activity and performances, Am J Occup Ther 40:529, 1986.
35. Strebel, MB: Adaptations and techniques for the disabled homemaker, Publication #710, Minneapolis, 1980, Sister Kenny Institute, Department Research and Education.
36. Trombley, CA, and Scott, AD: Occupational therapy for physical dysfunction, ed 2, Baltimore, 1983, Williams & Wilkins Co.
37. Van Leewwen, H: Ecology of habitat, Wageningen, Netherlands, 1968, Department of Home Economics, Agricultural University.
38. Waggoner, NR, and Reedy, GW: Child care equipment for physically handicapped mothers, suggestions for selection and adaptation, School of Home Economics, Storrs, 1961, University of Connecticut.

39. Zimmerman, ME: Devices: development and direction, Proceedings of the Annual Occupational Therapy Association Conference, Los Angeles, 1960.

40. Zimmerman, ME: The Functional Motion Test as an Evaluation Tool for Patients with Lower Motor Neuron Disturbances, Am J Occup Ther 23:9, 1969.

41. Zimmerman, ME: The role of special equipment in the rehabilitation of the spinal cord injured. In Cull, JG, and Hardy, RE, editors: Physical medicine and rehabilitation approaches in spinal cord injury, Springfield, Ill, 1977, Charles C Thomas, Publisher.

ADDITIONAL READINGS

Abreu, B: Perceptual—cognitive rehabilitation: An occupational therapy model, Physical Disabilities Special Interest Newsletter, American Occupational Therapy Association 3, 1985.

Abreu, B, and Toglia, J: Cognitive rehabilitation, ed 5, New York, 1985, E Village Copy Center.

Abreu, B, and Toglia, J: Cognitive rehabilitation: a model for occupational therapy, Am J Occup Ther 41:439, 1987.

Auchincloss, A, and Youdin, M: A know how manual on electricity for the severely disabled and their families, Rehabilitation Monograph, No 65, New York, 1982, Rusk Institute of Rehabilitation Medicine, New York University Medical Center.

Ayers, AJ: Integration of information in the development of sensory integration theory and practice, In Henderson, A, et al, editor: The development of sensory integration theory and practice, Dubuque, Ia, 1974, Kendell Hunt Publishing Co.

Baum, CM: Independent living: a critical role for occupational therapy, Am J Occup Ther 12:34, 1980.

Baum, CM: Growth, renewal, and challenge: an important era for occupational therapy, Am J Occup Ther 39:778, 1985.

Bell, J: Sensibility evaluation. In Hunter, JM, Schneider, LH, and Mackin, TH, editors: Rehabilitation of the hand, St. Louis, 1978, The CV Mosby Co.

Brandenburg, S, and Vanderheiden, G: Rehab/education technology, resource book series, Boston, 1986, College Hill Press, Little Brown & Co.

Cary, JR: How to create interiors for the disabled, New York, 1978, Pantheon Books.

Clark, PN: Human development through occupation: theoretical framework in contemporary occupational therapy practice, Am J Occup Ther 33:505, 1979.

Coloin, ME, and Korn, TL: Eliminating barriers to the disabled, Am J Occup Ther 38:748, 1984.

Delong, G: Independent living: from social movement to analytic paradigm, Arch Phys Med Rehabil 60:435, 1979.

Designs for Independent Living, Appliance Information Service, Whirlpool Corporation, Administrative Center, Benton Harbor, Mich.

DiJoseph, LM: Independence through activity, mind, body and environment interaction in therapy, Am J Occup Ther 36:740, 1982.

Eastern Paralyzed Veteran's Association, 432 Park Avenue South, New York (Accessibility Brochures).

Eggers, O: Occupational therapy in the treatment of adult hemiplegia, Rockville, Md, 1986, Aspen Systems Corp.

Jacobs, MJ: Development of normal behavior, Am J Phys Med 46:41, 1967.

Johnson, J: Old values—new directions: competence adaptation, integration, Am J Occup Ther 35:589, 1981.

Kielhofner, G: Health through occupation, theory and practice in occupational therapy, Philadelphia, 1983, FA Davis Co.

Kottke, FJ: From reflex to skill: the training of coordination, Arch Phys Med Rehabil 61:551, 1980.

Kottke, FJ, Stillwell, GK, and Lehmann, JF: Krusen's handbook of physical medicine and rehabilitation, ed 3, Philadelphia, 1982, WB Saunders Co.

Laurie, G: Housing and home services for the disabled, New York, 1977, Harper & Row.

Levy, R: Interface modalities of technical aides used by people with disability, Am J Occup Ther 37:761, 1983.

Lifchez, R, and Winslow, B: Design for independent living, the environment and physically disabled people, New York, 1979, Watson-Guptill Publications.

Logigian, MK, et al: Clinical exercise trials for stroke patients, Arch Phys Med Rehabil 64:364, 1983.

Lowman, E, and Klinger, J: Aids to independent living, self-help for the handicapped, New York, 1970, McGraw-Hill Book Co.

Mathiowitz, V, Bolding, D, and Trombly, C: Immediate effects of positioning devices on the normal and spastic hand measured by electromyography, Am J Occup Ther 37:247, 1983.

May, EE, Waggoner, NR, and Hotte, EB: Independent living for the handicapped and the elderly, Boston, 1974, Houghton-Mifflin Co.

McCullogh, H, and Farnham, M: Space and design requirements for wheelchair kitchens, agricultural experiment.

McNeny, R: Deficits in activities of daily livng. In Rosenthal, M, et al, editors: Rehabilitation of the head injured adult, Philadelphia, 1983, FA Davis Co.

Mosey, A: Occupational therapy, configuration of a profession, New York, 1981, Raven Press.

Nestadt, ME: Occupational therapy goals for adults with developmental disabilities, Am J Occup Ther 40:672, 1986.

Occupational therapy in practice, vol 1: 1978-1983, Rockville, Md, The American Occupational Therapy Assoc, Inc.

Panikoff, LB: Recovery trends of functional skills in the head injured adult, Am J Occup Ther 37:735, 1983.

Pederson, E: Management of spasticity on neurophysiologic basis, Scand J Rehabil Med [Suppl] 7:68, 1980.

Rashko, BB: Housing interiors for the disabled and elderly, New York, 1982, Van Nostrand Reinhold, Inc.

Rehabilitation Institute of Chicago: A manual of behavior management strategies for traumatically brain-injured adults, Chicago, 1983.

Rosenthal, M, et al: Rehabilitation of the head injured adult, Philadelphia, 1983, FA Davis Co.

Rushworth, G: Some pathophysiological aspects of spasticity and the search for rational and successful therapy, Int Rehabil Med 2:10, 1980.

Sargent, JV: An easier way handbook for the elderly and the handicapped, Ames, 1981, Iowa State University.

Self help manual for patients with arthritis, Atlanta, 1980, The Arthritis Foundation.

Spinal cord injury, a guide to functional outcomes in occupational therapy, Rehabilitation Institute of Chicago, Gaithersburg, Md, 1986, Aspen Publishers, Inc.

Technology for independent living source book, RESNA, Washington, DC, 1988.

Tools for independent living, Appliance Information Service Whirlpool Corporation, Administrative Center, Benton Harbor, Mich.

Tracey, DJ: Joint receptors and the control of movement, Trends in Neuroscience 29:253, 1980.

Webster, JG, et al: Electronic devices for rehabilitation, New York, 1985, John Wiley & Sons.

Wheeler, VH: Planning kitchens for handicapped homemakers, Rehabilitation Monograph #27, New York, 1966, Rusk Institute of Rehabilitation Medicine, New York University Medical Center.

DATABASES FOR REHABILITATION

ABLEDATA, The National Rehabilitation Information Center, Washington, DC.

Accent on Information, Bloomington, Ill.

Assistive Device Resources Center, California State University, Sacramento.

Job Accommodations Network (JAN), Morgantown, West Va.

CHAPTER 47

Physiology and therapeutics of exercise

CHARLES D. CICCONE AND JUSTIN ALEXANDER

Exercise plays a fundamental and invaluable role in virtually every aspect of rehabilitation. In its broadest sense, therapeutic exercise includes any body movement used to prevent or correct a physical impairment. Current use of exercise in rehabilitation has narrowed this definition to the implementation of specific exercise protocols to achieve specific goals. That is, depending on the individual needs of the patient, exercise can be used to achieve beneficial effects, such as increased flexibility and range of motion, increased muscle strength and endurance, or increased cardiovascular fitness. A fairly high degree of specificity exists between the different exercise regimens designed to achieve different goals. For example, exercises designed to improve muscular strength may have little effect on the overall cardiovascular fitness of the individual. Consequently, exercise programs must be carefully designed and implemented to meet the specific needs of the patient in order to ensure optimal results.

Because of the wealth of information available on this subject, it would be impossible to chronicle completely the history and changes of different exercise strategies and their implementation in a rehabilitation setting. The purpose of this chapter is to review briefly some basic concepts in therapeutic exercise. Also, some relatively recent advances in the role of exercise in therapeutics are discussed, especially in the area of technologic advances in exercise equipment. Finally, application of exercise training in selected patient conditions is presented.

TRADITIONAL EXERCISE CONCEPTS
Exercises to increase flexibility and joint range of motion

Adequate mobility of the synovial joints and flexibility of the associated soft tissues is a prerequisite for normal function. Active and passive range-of-motion exercises must be routinely performed to maintain flexibility and joint integrity.[6,64,69,99] In terms of passive physiologic motion, several different types of continuous passive motion (CPM) machines have been introduced that can be preset to provide passive motion throughout the joint range. Preliminary reports on the use of these CPM devices in maintaining motion and flexibility have been favorable in a number of situations, including the immediate postoperative mobilization after joint reconstruction and replacement.[22,96,112] Of course, with any external device, caution should be used in applying the apparatus, and the patient must be monitored periodically. Improper use of any type of external force, either in magnitude or duration, could have disastrous effects on the patient's progress. However, CPM machines do offer the advantage of providing range of motion for extended periods of time, which would not be practical if treatment were rendered directly by a therapist.

Stretching exercises are essential in maintaining normal flexibility and range of motion. Soft tissues, such as muscle, connective tissue, and skin are usually stretched by applying some type of force when the tissues are already at or near their greatest available length. The magnitude of the stretching force is dependent on patient tolerance and the underlying disorder. Obviously, a joint with normal but tight supporting tissues can be stretched much more vigorously than an arthritic joint or a joint with inflamed soft tissues.

The method of applying the stretching force has been the subject of some debate, but it is now generally accepted that the use of a relatively low-load, long-duration (static) stretch is preferable to high-load, repetitive-bouncing (ballistic) maneuvers.[64,69,73,99] Although several investigations have shown that both static and ballistic stretching increase flexibility in normal tissues,[21,30] static stretching is the method of choice for several reasons. With a static stretch, there is less chance of overstretching the affected tissues and inducing additional pain and trauma. In cases of increased muscle tone or spasticity, there is also a diminished risk of activating the myotatic reflex with static stretch.[6,51]

Static stretching also seems to be more consistent with several established concepts in the lengthening of the collagenous fibers present in various forms of connective tissue. Stretching of collagen has been proposed as being essential for inducing permanent lengthening of connective tissue.[69,72,119] It appears that collagen fibers are lengthened most effectively with application of a prolonged, sustained stretch, whereas high-intensity, short-duration forces predominantly affect elastin fibers.[99,118] Consequently, static stretching should be more efficacious in producing more long-term increases in tissue extensibility and joint flexibility.

Static stretching may be enhanced with the use of thermal agents or neuromuscular facilitation techniques.[53,77,93,118,119] External devices may also be employed to provide static stretch. Various weight and pulley systems can be used to apply the stretching force.[11,73] Commercial products, such as the Dynasplint (Dynasplint Systems, Inc., Baltimore, Md.) are designed to provide a low-load, prolonged stretch to the affected soft tissues.[55] Serial casting has also been described as an extremely effective method of providing a prolonged static stretch, especially in cases where soft tissue shortening has been present for extended periods.

Caution should be exercised when using any external device (including the CPM machines) with regard to contact with the patient's skin and the potential for skin breakdown. Proper skin care and frequent inspection are essential to prevent any adverse effects from prolonged contact with the device.

Exercises to increase muscle strength: general principles

Virtually every technique used to induce an increase in muscle strength uses some type of overload on the muscle's contractile component. That is, to increase in strength, a muscle must develop tension repeatedly or for prolonged periods of time, and the tension developed must be on the order of some critical level of the muscle's maximal contractile capacity. Despite years of intensive research, the exact mechanism by which this increased tension induces changes in contractile force remains unclear. Increased tension has been shown to have an anabolic effect by stimulating muscle protein synthesis with a subsequent increase in muscle fiber size.[20,43,75,83] Increased contractile protein content would certainly allow greater tension development and a stronger muscle. However, strength gains are often seen in the absence of any morphologic changes, and increments in strength usually precede any overt or proportional increase in muscle size.[83,89] Clearly, however, tension development remains the common denominator by which strength gains are mediated. This is evidenced by the fact that even inactive or immobilized muscle retains its size and contractile strength to a greater extent when placed in a

lengthened position so the tension on the musculotendinous unit is maintained.[44,63,115]

Increases in muscle strength are generally accomplished by having the muscle develop tension against a large resistance for only a few repetitions. This idea of high load, low repetition is a fundamental concept of most training protocols in which increases in muscle strength are the primary goal. During the course of strength training, progressively larger resistances must be employed to continue to achieve strength gains. The use of progressive increments in resistance, or progressive resistance exercise (PRE), was first formally proposed by Delorme.[28] Since that time, many strength-training programs have capitalized in some way or another on the original concept of PRE and the overload principle. Variations in different strength training regimens based on the use of different muscle contraction techniques and training protocols have been proposed from time to time. In addition, recent technologic advances in exercise equipment have revolutionized the field of strength training. Because of the abundant information and recent changes in this area, further attention is directed toward the various modes of strength training later in this chapter.

Exercises to increase muscular endurance

Whereas muscular strength is the ability of the muscle to generate tension or force, muscular endurance can be described as the ability of the muscle to continue to do work or perform a task for prolonged periods of time. More simply stated, endurance is the ability of the muscle to resist fatigue. Although increases in muscular strength and endurance are both frequently goals of rehabilitation, it has long been understood that some degree of specificity exists between exercises that attempt to increase muscular strength and those increasing endurance.[46] Just as using a high-load, low-repetition regimen increases muscular strength, low-load, high-repetition training increases endurance in individual muscles. In other words, the same resistive exercise used to promote strength in individual muscles can be adapted to increase endurance by decreasing the load (or percentage of maximal tension developed per contraction) and increasing the number of consecutive repetitions performed. This increase in endurance of specific muscles described here differs from the overall increase in cardiovascular endurance achieved through a more generalized conditioning program. The latter form of exercise is discussed later in the chapter.

The specificity of strength versus endurance training does not mean that some increments in both parameters may not occur during resistive exercise training. For instance, performing isotonic exercise with moderate loads that permit a moderate number of repetitions induces changes in both strength and endurance. However, the strength increments are not as great as if the traditional high-load, low-repetition protocols were used; likewise, optimal endurance benefits may not be achieved by this approach. In addition, studies by de Lateur, Lehmann, and Fordyce[27] suggest that some transfer of training may occur if subjects exercise to fatigue during each training session rather than for a preset number of repetitions. Groups who trained to fatigue using high loads were compared with an analogous group training with low loads, and it was found that strength and endurance gains were ultimately similar between the two groups. However, it is unknown if the strength and endurance gains achieved in that study were as great as they would have been had the subject trained more specifically for one type of activity versus the other.

The physiologic mechanisms responsible for increased endurance in individual muscles seem to be complex and undoubtedly involve local changes in blood flow and substrate utilization, as well as morphologic changes in the contractile element.[45,59,61,94] In addition, fatigue that occurs during certain types of repetitive tasks may occur at a site within the central nervous system.[108] This suggests that the resistance to fatigue seen in individual muscles after endurance training may also be due to changes in central synaptic transmission. However, the exact role of central factors in muscular fatigue remains to be determined.

Exercises to increase cardiovascular fitness

The concept of specificity of training is best illustrated by the difference between exercises used to promote cardiovascular conditioning and those exercises used to increase strength or endurance in individual muscles. Exercises used to increase cardiovascular fitness should be "any activity that uses large muscle groups, that can be maintained continuously, and is rhythmical and aerobic in nature, e.g. running-jogging, walking-hiking, swimming, skating, bicycling, rowing, cross-country skiing, rope skipping and various endurance game activities."[3] The term "aerobic exercise" is commonly used to describe these and other activities for cardiac training. In reality, this term refers to performing these activities at a submaximal level so that the major form of substrate utilization is via mitochondrial metabolic pathways, which employ oxygen, rather than strictly glycolytic (anaerobic) pathways. In addition to the type of activity, parameters of excercise intensity, duration, and frequency should be well defined for both the healthy, asymptomatic individual and the rehabilitation patient.

Basic guidelines for these parameters (known collectively as the exercise prescription) have been established and are summarized in Table 47-1. It should be noted that these are only guidelines; the specific characteristics of each individual must be considered.

The physiologic changes that occur during aerobic training are extensive and have been well documented.[9,33,59,98,102] Basically these changes involve increases in the oxygen delivery system and the metabolic pathways involved in substrate use. These changes and several other beneficial effects are summarized in the following list:
1. Cardiovascular adaptations
   a. Increased maximal oxygen consumption (VO_2 max)[9,102]

Table 47-1. Guidelines for exercise to improve cardiovascular fitness

Parameter	Guideline
Frequency of training	3-5 days per week
Intensity of training	60%-90% of maximum heart rate (or) 50%-85% of maximum oxygen uptake
Duration of training	15-60 minutes of continuous aerobic activity
Mode of activity	Rhythmic activities using large muscle groups (running, swimming, cycling, etc.)

From American College of Sports Medicine Position Statement: Med Sci Sports 10:vii, 1978.

   b. Increased maximal cardiac output (owing to increased maximal stroke volume)[9,33]
   c. Resting bradycardia[33,102]
   d. Lower heart rate at submaximal workloads[33,102]
   e. Increased systemic vascular conductance[9]
2. Skeletal muscle adaptations
   a. Increased oxidative enzyme capacity[59]
   b. Increased mitochondrial volume[59]
   c. Increased myoglobin concentration[59]
   d. Increased capillary density[60,61]
3. Other beneficial effects
   a. Decreased body fat[8]
   b. Improved plasma lipid profile[52]
   c. Possible decrease in blood pressure in certain patient subgroups[104,116]

Specialized exercises for other goals

Several other exercise protocols have been established to achieve specific goals. For example, exercises that stress the repeated performance of a motor task can be used to increase coordination of the task.[67,68] Balance and vestibular training activities are employed to increase these skills.[34,117] Relaxation exercise protocols have been developed that attempt to promote physiologic and behavioral improvements.[57] The development of these and other specialized protocols is an ongoing process mediated by the creativity of the clinician and the needs of the patient.

STRENGTH TRAINING MODES

In general, strength training regimens are described according to the type of muscular contraction and/or the resistance encountered, that is, either isometric, isotonic or isokinetic. Isometric exercise occurs when tension is developed in the muscle with no appreciable change in muscle length. Isometric exercises are also termed "static" because muscle length remains essentially constant, whereas isotonic and isokinetic exercises are referred to as "dynamic" because muscle length changes during the contraction. In isotonic exercise, the muscle changes length as it develops tension in either a shortening (concentric) or lengthening (eccentric) fashion. However, the load applied to the skeletal lever remains fixed during isotonic exercise. The key feature of isokinetic exercise is that the applied load varies as the muscle develops tension, either concentrically or eccentrically. Each of these primary modes of resistive exercise is discussed in the next section.

Isometric exercise

After the initial experiments of Hettinger and Muller in the 1950s, a great deal of interest was generated in the idea that substantial gains in muscle strength could be achieved by brief isometric contractions of skeletal muscle. Originally it was suggested that maximal isometric strength gains in various muscle groups could be achieved by performing one maximal isometric contraction for 1 or 2 seconds once each day.[58] Subsequent studies have generally not been able to produce as dramatic strength gains using these exercise parameters, and several other investigators have attempted to establish optimal training parameters for obtaining maximal isometric strength gains. McDonagh and Davies[83] have reviewed different isometric training studies, and the results of several pertinent investigations are presented in Table 47-2. From their review of the parameters of intensity, duration, and frequency of contractions, they concluded that isometric training regimens are most effective when maximal contractions are used and the product of the contraction duration and number of contractions per day is large. That is, iso-

metric contractions of longer duration can be performed less frequently, and contractions of shorter duration must be performed more times each day to induce optimal isometric strength gains.[83]

Isometric strengthening regimens have been criticized for several reasons. First, there is evidence that strength gains achieved during an isometric contraction at a specific joint angle may induce strength increments in the muscle only when the joint is in the position in which the isometric training took place.[40,74] Training the elbow flexors isometrically at 90 degrees of elbow flexion may induce an increase in strength when the elbow is at 90 degrees but not when it is at 45 or 125 degrees. A second major criticism of isometrics has been the acute effect of isometric exercise on the cardiovascular system. The consensus of information seems to suggest that isometrics may cause a rapid and sudden increase in blood pressure, with the magnitude of the pressor response being dependent on factors such as contraction intensity, age of the patient, and muscle mass being exercised.[91,97]

Thus isometric exercise has received a great deal of attention, both favorable and unfavorable, over the years. Of course from a clinical perspective, isometrics have always been used and will continue to be used in various situations where joint motion is either undesirable or impossible (for example, after surgery or during cast immobilization). It seems reasonable to assume that this type of strength training should be part of some rehabilitation programs but should be used with some caution regarding the cardiovascular implications and with the awareness of the limitations of these techniques in producing optimal strength gains.

Table 47-2. Effect of training using maximal voluntary isometric contractions on maximal voluntary contraction (MVC) strength

Author	Duration of contraction (sec)	Contractions/ day	Product column 1 × column 2	Number of training days*	MVC increase (%)†	MVC % day‡	Muscles
Ikai and Fukunaga 1970	10	3	30	100	92	0.9	Elbow flexors
Komi et al. 1978	3-5	5	15-25	48	20	0.4	Quadriceps
Bonde-Petersen 1960	5	10	50	36	16	0.4	Elbow flexors
Bonde-Petersen 1960	5	1	5	36	0	0	Elbow flexors
Davies and Young 1983	3	42	126	35	30	0.86	Triceps surae
McDonagh et al. 1983	3	30	90	28	20	0.71	Elbow flexors
Grimby et al. 1973	3	30	90	30	32	1.1	Triceps

From McDonagh, MJN, and Davies, CTM: Eur J Appl Physiol 52:139, 1984.

*Days on which training was actually performed.

$$†MVC\ increase = \frac{Post\text{-}training\ force\ -\ pretraining\ force}{Pretraining\ force} \times 100$$

$$‡MVC\ \%\ day = \frac{MVC\ increase\ \%}{Number\ of\ training\ days}$$

Isotonic exercise

Isotonic exercises use a fixed amount of weight to overload the muscle as the muscle develops tension to move the load throughout a given range of motion. Some of the earliest formal training regimens using this form of exercise were developed by Delorme[28] and later modified by Delorme and Watkins.[29] Delorme based his training regimen on the principle of using large loads that can be lifted only a few repetitions before fatigue occurs. He suggested the use of a load sufficient to be lifted exactly 10 times by the subject. This load is identified as the 10 repetition maximum (10 RM). As strength increases, the load is progressively increased so the maximum number of repetitions always remains constant at 10. This technique of progressive increments in load is generally termed progressive resistance exercise (PRE).

Most isotonic training is still performed according to Delorme's original guidelines or some modification of them. Many studies have been performed by other investigators in an attempt to determine the most effective method of PRE. For instance, studies by Berger[7] suggested that 4, 6, or 8 RM rather than 10 RM may be the optimal training load. The number of bouts or "sets" of repetitions also must be considered, as well as the frequency of training in terms of number of days per week. Surprisingly, this latter parameter has never been adequately researched, and some PRE programs advocate daily training sessions whereas others intersperse days of rest between training sessions.

It is not possible at this time to describe all of the variations in isotonic strength training protocols. In general, most protocols are based on the premise that if increased muscle strength is desired, maximum resistance must be overcome. The number of repetitions, rest periods between sets, number of sets, frequency of training sessions, and speed of motion vary among the different techniques. For a more detailed description of different isotonic training protocols, the reader is referred to excellent reviews.[18,83]

Isotonic strengthening programs have several limitations. Primary among these is that the load lifted by the muscle remains constant, whereas the ability of the muscle to produce tension varies during the range of motion (Figure 47-1).[122] That is, owing to the interaction of mechanical and physiologic factors, a muscle is typically able to generate more force at some points in the range than at others. Since the muscle produces variable amounts of force but the load remains constant, the chance exists that the muscle will not be maximally stressed throughout the range of motion. For example, the maximum amount of weight that can be moved through a given range during a concentric contraction may be limited by the muscle's ability to lift the load at the "weaker" points in the muscle's range.

This problem is actually more complex because one must consider the torque generated around the joint, as well as the loading factor. That is, even though the load remains fixed, the torque imposed on the joint changes in accordance with the perpendicular distance of the load from the joint axis. Still, it is unlikely that the torque imposed by the load during isotonic exercise will exactly match the ability of the muscle to generate force at each point in the range. In fact, the highest imposed torque could occur when the muscle is at the lower limits of its ability to generate tension sufficient to overcome the imposed torque. In Figure 47-2 the closed circles represent the relative torque produced by the knee extensors of a normal individual during a concentric isokinetic contraction. If the same individual were performing isotonic exercise while seated with a weight attached to the foot or ankle, the torque imposed by the weight would occur in a pattern represented by the open circles. Note that the pattern of torque generated by the extensor muscles varies dramatically from the torque imposed by this particular isotonic load. The relative maximal torque that the musculature is able to generate occurs at a point in the range of motion when the imposed torque is fairly small. Con-

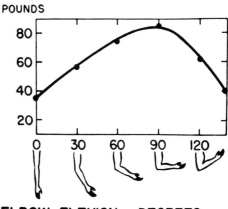

ELBOW FLEXION : DEGREES

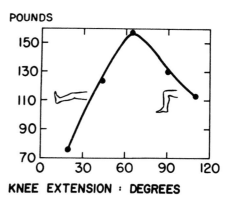

KNEE EXTENSION : DEGREES

Figure 47-1. Isometric torque curves for elbow flexion and knee extension in college men. Muscular force generation varies depending on joint position. (Reprinted from Williams, M, and Stutzman, L: Phys Ther Rev 39:145, 1959, with permission of the American Physical Therapy Association.)

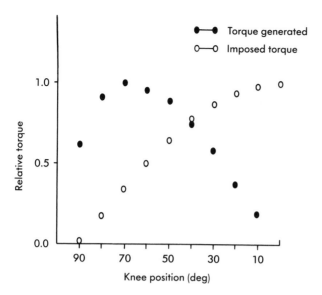

Figure 47-2. Pattern of torque produced during isokinetic contraction of the knee extensors *(closed circles)* versus the pattern of torque that would be imposed by weighted boot during isotonic knee extension performed while seated *(open circles)*. Torque values are expressed as fraction of maximal torque that would be either produced or imposed. See text for further discussion.

versely, the maximum torque imposed by the load occurs when the muscular torque production is declining. This "mismatch" of imposed torque on muscular force could have detrimental effects if the muscle is excessively weak or in the early stages of rehabilitation, since the maximum imposed torque occurs at a point at which the muscle is least able to generate tension to overcome the load.

Isotonic exercises have been used successfully for many years and will undoubtedly continue to be a viable and popular method of strength training. However, to use them safely and to their optimal capacity, one must give careful consideration to the progressive increase in the applied load, as well as the manner in which the load imposes torque on the exercising muscle and joint. The latter point emphasizes the need for the therapist to have a working knowledge of biomechanics and applied anatomy to ensure the optimal use of these techniques.

Isokinetic exercise

The basic goal in isokinetic exercise is to vary the resistance during a dynamic contraction so resistance changes in direct proportion to the ability of the muscle to produce force. This is usually accomplished through the use of an isokinetic machine, which maintains the speed of the exercising limb at a predetermined constant value (the term "isokinetic" refers to movement performed at a constant speed). Changes in muscular force normally used to accelerate the limb are now met as resistance by the isokinetic machine. In effect, the muscle contracts against maximal

resistance at each point in the range of motion. This allows an optimal training effect in terms of matching the imposed resistance with the muscle's ability to produce force.

Training velocity is the key variable to be considered in isokinetic exercise. For concentric isokinetic contractions, muscle tension varies inversely with contraction velocity in accordance with the classic force-velocity relationship of skeletal muscle.[66] Consequently, isokinetic strength training has led to the concept of "specificity of speed." That is, the speed at which the training takes place may have a profound influence on the nature of the strength gains achieved. Early studies suggested that isokinetic training at a relatively high speed (108 degrees/sec) produced an increase in muscle force at all speeds at and below the training speed, whereas training at a relatively slow speed (36 degrees/sec) was associated with increments only at the slow speed.[87] Subsequent investigations have suggested that this specificity of speed may be even more confined, with strength gains at fast-velocity training (300 degrees/sec) overlapping only into medium fast velocities (180 degrees/sec) but not into slow velocities (speeds less than 180 degrees/sec).[23] For practical purposes it must be assumed that a fairly high degree of specificity of speed does exist in isokinetic training, and training sessions should include a variety of training speeds if strength increments are desired over a wide range of contraction velocities.[23,106]

CURRENT USE OF EXERCISE EQUIPMENT

Several recently developed devices warrant particular attention in the field of exercise and strength training. Different machines have been developed in an attempt to use the basic concepts previously described to effectively exercise skeletal muscle. Two of the more popular types of commercially available devices are discussed.

Isokinetic machines

Isokinetic exercise machines provide variable resistance by maintaining the speed of movement at a constant rate. The prototypic device of this type is the Cybex II (Cybex Division of Lumex Inc., Ronkonkoma, N.Y.) (Figure 47-3). The functional unit of the Cybex II and similar devices is an electromechanical dynamometer, which maintains the speed of movement at a preset level. Depending on the manufacturer, other devices use a hydraulic or electromagnetic mechanism in an attempt to achieve this effect. The subject is attached to an input arm; by changing the subject's position, location and angle of the input arm, and its specific configuration and length, different joints and muscle groups can be exercised. Some devices are designed to exercise several isolated joints, whereas others are designed to exercise only one specific joint or movement in a specific plane (for example, trunk flexion-extension).

Recently several manufacturers introduced isokinetic machines with varying features and capacities to test different

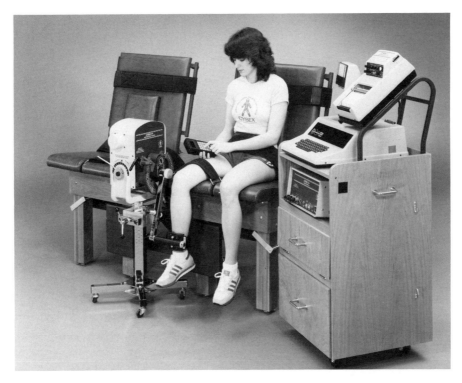

Figure 47-3. Isokinetic dynamometer. Axis of input arm is aligned with anatomic axis for knee flexion-extension. Other joints and muscle groups may be exercised on this device by varying patient's position and mechanical attachments to dynamometer. (Courtesy Cybex, Division of Lumex, Inc.)

joints. Some devices such as the Kin-Com (Chattecx Corp., Chattanooga, Tenn.) and Biodex (Biodex Corp., Center Moriches, N.Y.) have the capacity to exercise muscles eccentrically and perform continuous passive motion. An individual given the opportunity to acquire isokinetic equipment is now faced with several different options. Considering the rather high cost of these devices, it is certainly worthwhile to take the time to examine all the features of each device to ensure the choice of a machine (or machines) that most closely suits the facility's needs.

Since their inception, isokinetic machines have been used extensively in the rehabilitation of musculoskeletal injuries and are classically associated with increasing strength after trauma, surgery, and immobilization. In addition, these devices have been used in the rehabilitation of a wide variety of nonorthopedic problems. A more detailed discussion of the clinical use of isokinetic machines occurs later in this chapter.

Cam-weight systems

As with isokinetic devices, cam-weight machines may be used to vary the resistance in proportion to the ability of the muscle to generate force throughout the range of motion. Rather than maintaining the speed of movement constant, these devices use a variation on the weight and pulley system

by including an asymmetrically shaped cam along the course of the pulley (or cable/chain as the case may be) (Figure 47-4). The function of the cam is to vary the resistance imposed on the exercising muscle by altering the mechanical factors of the weight-pulley system. Different machines are specifically designed for different functional muscle groups. Each machine has a cam designed to vary the resistance according to established norms for the muscle group being exercised.

Several manufacturers have capitalized on the concept of the cam-weight system. Some examples include Nautilus (Nautilus Sports/Medical Industries Inc., DeLand, Fla.), Eagle (Cybex Division of Lumex, Ronkonkoma, N.Y.), and Polaris (Ironco, Spring Valley, Calif.). These machines have long been popular in athletic training and recreational use by individuals in health clubs. However, many cam-weight systems are being used in the rehabilitation of athletic, as well as nonathletic, injuries. They actually provide strengthening programs similar to the traditional isotonic regimens but tend to offer better stabilization and control of the movement pattern than free weights. Also, they allow a fairly close match of resistance to muscle force. It must be remembered, however, that these machines are designed based on averages, and that individual variations in force production within the range of motion will not be compensated for by the machine.

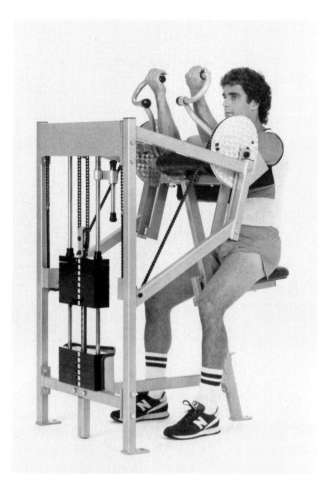

Figure 47-4. Cam-weight system. (Courtesy Nautilus Sports/ Medical Industries, Inc.)

CLINICAL USE OF ISOKINETIC EQUIPMENT
Isokinetic machines as a testing device

An important feature of isokinetic machines is the opportunity to objectively measure and document muscle strength. The use of these machines in joint testing has been invaluable in evaluating the patient's initial status and progress during rehabilitation. These machines have been used to evaluate muscle strength and endurance in a variety of disorders including musculoskeletal injuries and neurologic problems, such as hemiplegia and multiple sclerosis.[4,48,76,120] Isokinetic testing has also been used to establish norms for muscle strength in specific populations, such as normal adults, children, and individuals with specific disorders.[1,47,88] The reliability and validity of these devices have been the subject of many investigations, with the general consensus being that they tend to have a fairly high degree of accuracy when used properly as an evaluative tool.[36,62,80,88]

Use of isokinetic machines in musculoskeletal injuries

Isokinetic devices have been found useful in the rehabilitation of musculoskeletal injuries. Since these devices offer resistance that exactly matches the muscle's ability to generate tension at each point in the range, there is minimal chance of overstressing the muscle and its related joint. This is especially advantageous in an orthopedic patient recovering from surgery or trauma because there is little chance of reinjuring the joint because of an excessive load or a "mismatch" of the imposed torque on the muscle and joint similar to what was described earlier during isotonic exercise. Depending on the type of injury or surgical procedure, isokinetic programs are initiated when dynamic contractions against resistance are permitted at least through part of the range of motion. Specific training programs vary according to the individual patient. In general, training is performed at a variety of speeds, and a maximal pain-free effort is encouraged at all times.[76,106] After unilateral musculoskeletal injury, isokinetic training is usually continued until the strength of the involved extremity is equivalent to the noninvolved side.

Use of isokinetic devices in nonorthopedic conditions

The extensive use of isokinetic devises in musculoskeletal injuries tends to obscure the application of these machines in the rehabilitation of other problems. For instance, isokinetic exercise machines have been used in the treatment of neurologic disorders, such as hemiparesis. In cases of muscular weakness secondary to stroke or head trauma, isokinetics can be used to facilitate and strengthen movement patterns. The variable resistance offered by the isokinetic machine will allow contraction of stronger muscles to recruit weaker muscles in the same associated movement pattern, a concept consistent with several facilitation techniques such as those developed by Brunnstrom[15] and the proprioceptive neuromuscular facilitation (PNF) principles of Knott and Voss.[117] The variable resistance supplied by the machine mimics the accommodating resistance normally supplied by the therapist. Isokinetic machines can be used in the involved extremity or in the noninvolved side to invoke associated reactions in the contralateral, involved extremity. When they are used in the involved extremity, the variable resistance encountered by the patient also provides additional proprioceptive input considered essential for restoration of normal motor function.[51,117]

Of course, no machine is a substitute for the fine control over all joints in the movement pattern that an experienced therapist offers. However, isokinetic machines can be used in selected patients to allow longer, more intense workouts than would be practical in most clinical settings. In addition, use of an isokinetic machine on either the involved or the noninvolved side can act as an "extra" pair of hands, enabling the therapist to try other facilitation techniques such as tapping, stroking, or icing while resistance is supplied by the machine.

When a machine is to be used in the hemiplegic patient, some creative modifications of the typical patient setup may be desirable.[16] For instance, some therapists have devised methods of aligning the patient to the machine so upper and

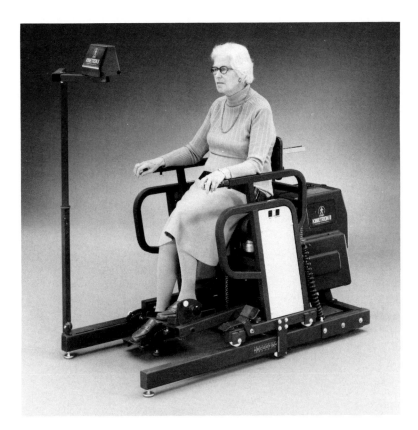

Figure 47-5. Bilateral, reciprocal isokinetic device (Kinetron) used for lower extremity exercise. (Courtesy Cybex, Division of Lumex, Inc.)

lower extremity movements are performed in the diagonal patterns advocated by the PNF techniques. In this way the variable resistance is encountered in a manner similar to the diagonal patterns that are suggested to be functionally more important than movement in the cardinal planes.[117]

The use of isokinetics as a tool in neuromuscular facilitation may help to restore the normal muscle balance between agonist and antagonist groups. In cases where the agonist is weak at the expense of an antagonist with increased tone, maximal contraction of the agonist through a dynamic contraction inhibits the antagonist through reciprocal innervation while strengthening the weaker group.[51,117] Repeatedly performing this movement pattern against maximal resistance reinforces the appropriate agonist-antagonist relationship. Also, the need to switch agonist-antagonist relationships at the extremes of the movement pattern can be enhanced with isokinetic machines. The patient performing elbow flexion against isokinetic resistance must contract the biceps while relaxing the triceps and then reverse this situation and actively contract the triceps against resistance to extend the elbow. The ability of the therapist to preset the speed of movement dictates how quickly this reversal must occur.

Isokinetic machines can be used to increase the speed of muscle contraction. To encounter resistance, the patient must at least meet the preset speed of the machine. Using higher angular velocities forces the patient to recruit the agonist more rapidly in order to encounter resistance. Many machines offer some form of visual analog (such as a torque dial, chart recorder, or computerized representation), which may act as a form of biofeedback in helping the patient recruit the agonist effectively. Also, some machines allow a differential speed setting between agonist and antagonist. That is, movement in one direction can be set at a slower speed than movement in the opposite direction. Therapists can use different speed settings to encourage strength increases or functional recruitment, depending on their specific goals for each patient.

One isokinetic device that has proved useful for the rehabilitation of neurologic patients is the Kinetron (Cybex Division of Lumex Inc., Ronkonkoma, N.Y.) (Figure 47-5). This machine is designed to exercise both lower extremities in a reciprocal fashion, thus mimicking a normal gait pattern. Variables, such as the speed of movement of each lower extremity, the amount of weight bearing, and range of motion, can be adjusted for each patient. Preliminary reports on the use of this device in hemiplegic patients have suggested that functional improvements in the gait pattern were facilitated by the use of this machine.[42,121] Improvements in other neurologic problems, such as Parkinson's disease, may also be possible with isokinetic devices that exercise the patient in a reciprocal and functional manner. The Kinetron has been suggested for other nonneurologic conditions involving functional gait training (such as prosthetic training in lower extremity amputees).[100]

An interesting approach to the use of isokinetic resistance in neurologically involved patients has been reported by Harris.[50,51] In a study involving cerebral palsied children, variable accommodating resistance was applied to the neck musculature through a device originally intended to stabilize a child's head during dental procedures. When resistance was applied in this fashion, even for a short period, head control improved and tremors and the incidence of large-amplitude erratic head movements decreased. The author attributed the beneficial effects to a prolonged increase in proprioceptive feedback from the resisted musculature.[50] It was also suggested that this principle of reciprocal variable resistance could be applied to other body parts to achieve similar results in cases involving tremor and athetoid-like movements.[51]

EXERCISE IN SPECIFIC CONDITIONS
Back pain
Flexion versus hyperextension exercises

Perhaps no two approaches differ as much as the exercise techniques currently used in the conservative treatment of low back pain. For years, treatment of back pain secondary to lumbar disc disease incorporated a series of exercises that tended to decrease the lumbar lordosis and increase flexion.[123] Commonly termed Williams' flexion exercises for their originator, these maneuvers were based on the rationale that flexing the low back reduces pressure on the posterior aspect of the lumbar spine, including the spinal nerve as it exits the intervertebral foramen. More recently McKenzie[85,86] advocated the use of exercise protocols that primarily involve hyperextension of the low back with an effort to restore or maintain the lumbar lordosis. The basic theory behind the McKenzie approach is that increasing the lumbar lordosis helps move the intervertebral disc anteriorly away from the pain-sensitive structures of the posterior region of the spine. Extension programs are also used in cases of extension dysfunction, as well as derangement of the intervertebral disc. There are advocates of both flexion and hyperextension protocols, but the latter approach has been gaining popularity in many clinical settings.

Preliminary reports of clinical studies comparing these two different approaches have suggested that the hyperextension approach of McKenzie may be more efficacious in treating low back pain of disc origin. Ponte, Jensen, and Kent[92] treated 10 patients with Williams' flexion exercises and 12 patients with the McKenzie protocol. Their results indicated that the hyperextension group showed significant improvements in pain-free sitting time, forward flexion, and

amount of passive straight leg raise, as well as an overall decrease in subjective pain. Hyperextension regimens may also be advantageous over flexion exercises in their apparent ability to induce less trauma in the vertebral body. A study of postmenopausal women with back pain found fewer vertebral compression fractures in women performing extension exercises than in those performing flexion exercises or flexion combined with extension.[109]

Most of the research currently available that compares flexion and hyperextension protocols uses fairly small patient groups and takes place over a relatively short period of time. Additional research using large populations will be needed to assess adequately the long-term effects of hyperextension protocols. Also, future studies should investigate any potential adverse effects of hyperextension protocols, such as damage to the lumbar facet joints, when these exercises are used for extended periods.

Strength and flexibility in back pain

In contrast to the controversy over flexion and extension exercises, there is general agreement that adequate flexibility and muscular support of the low back facilitate normal, pain-free movement. For instance, even hyperextension protocols advocate the use of some flexion activities as treatment progresses so adequate mobility is maintained in both directions.[86] In terms of muscle strength, it has long been held that the trunk musculature is important in providing extrinsic support and stability to the spine.[90] Consequently, strengthening of the trunk musculature should be incorporated at the appropriate point in the rehabilitation of back problems. New developments in isokinetic machines are currently being used to test and strengthen the trunk musculature in order to provide adequate support to the vertebral column.[25,71,111] Preliminary reports indicate that these devices may be extremely useful as part of a comprehensive back program.[79,81,82]

Scoliosis

In idiopathic scoliosis, exercises are generally used in an attempt to stretch the shortened musculature on the side of the concavity and strengthen the overstretched musculature on the convex side of the scoliotic curve.[37,64] However, considerable doubt exists as to whether exercises are beneficial in treating scoliosis. It is generally accepted that exercise alone does not halt the progressive nature of this condition.[10,64,113] Some clinicians go so far as to say that exercises offer no benefit whatsoever.[17] Still, exercises are routinely prescribed as an adjunct to other forms of management, such as bracing, electrical stimulation, and surgical intervention. The greatest value of exercise in scoliosis, as summarized by Cailliet,[17] is to improve posture, flexibility, muscle strength and balance, and respiration. Ultimately, the decision of whether to include an exercise regimen in the treatment of scoliosis is left to the clinician.

Upper motor neuron disorders
Spasticity

The overall function of exercise in spasticity is to restore normal muscle balance by inhibiting tone in the tight agonist while strengthening (if possible) the weakened antagonistic group.[49,51] There are of course numerous facilitative techniques to achieve this goal. More recently, it has been suggested that general aerobic exercise may decrease the overall electrical activity in skeletal muscle via some decrease in the activation level of the alpha motor neuron.[31,32] This so-called tranquilizer effect has been documented in normal subjects as a residual attenuation of the electrical activity of the resting muscle, as well as a decrease in the evoked reflex activity after an aerobic exercise bout. These findings are consistent with the reported observation that physical exertion tends to produce a general relaxation in spasticity in cerebral palsied patients.[51] This suggests that patients capable of performing some type of aerobic activity may experience the favorable effect of a subsequent reduction in spasticity. Further study is necessary to determine the exact mechanism of this tranquilizer effect, as well as the practical application of this principle in decreasing spasticity in various patient populations.

Cortical and cerebellar involvement

In cases of cortical lesions that result in motor loss, exercises initially focus on the need to maintain joint integrity and range of motion. Facilitation of motor return is initiated using any number of techniques that attempt to promote optimal motor function. If motor return is present, resistive exercises are ultimately incorporated in some way to increase muscle strength. Cerebellar involvement that results in ataxia necessitates the use of coordination exercises, such as those originally developed by Frenkel.[68] Typically these involve the active repetition of specific functional motor patterns. Additional proprioceptive input is often provided during the motor task by using maximal resistance or external weights. The goal is not necessarily to increase strength, but to provide additional input in an attempt to reestablish the role of the cerebellum as a "comparator" in modulating sensory input with the intended motor output. Patients may be encouraged to look at the moving extremity to track the motion. Visual tracking may be decreased in patients whose proprioceptive sensation is increased; others may be forced to look always at the extremity to know where it is in space. Other forms of visual input may be gained by performing the exercises in front of a mirror.

Lower motor neuron and primary muscle disease

In virtually all stages and types of problems involving the alpha motor neuron, neuromuscular junction, or muscle cell itself, maintenance of normal flexibility and joint range is essential in preventing joint contractures and the pain and spasm that ensue. Passive and active exercises in combination with splinting and bracing are used to prevent these detrimental effects. Strengthening exercises have a variable role, depending on the type and severity of the disorder. Resistive exercises may help limit pain and spasm in certain conditions by promoting increased muscle metabolism and blood flow, as well as by helping to restore muscle balance in weakened groups. Sister Kenny stressed the importance of exercises (in conjunction with moist heat) to reduce spasm, minimize muscle shortening and imbalance, and reeducate paralyzed muscles.[19] Knapp stated that in such disorders as amyotrophic lateral sclerosis and Charcot-Marie-Tooth disease, efforts to increase muscle strength are impractical because the disease becomes progressively worse despite treatment.[65] Although this is true, gentle conditioning exercises can be used in the earlier stages of these and similar diseases to prolong useful function as long as possible. If we may include muscular dystrophy in this category, it was long held that strengthening exercises of any kind were counterproductive owing to the possibility of causing residual or "overwork" weakness.[65] Although this is certainly true if the duration and intensity of the exercise are extreme, several studies have shown that submaximal strengthening programs can be used effectively in muscular dystrophy without any ill effects.[26,39,103]

In other lower motor neuron disorders that are nonprogressive or show signs of recovery, resistive exercise also serves the obvious role of helping regain muscle strength. Again, exercise should be monitored closely to avoid fatigue. In peripheral neuropathies, Herbison, Jaweed, and Ditunno[56] summarized the goals of exercise as the maintenance of joint motion, reeducation of skilled activities, and optimizing strength recovery. These authors also warned against the potential damage to partially denervated muscle after exhaustive exercise and recommend that exercise levels be limited.

Cardiopulmonary exercises
Cardiac conditioning

A wealth of information is available that describes the benefits of cardiac conditioning exercise, both as a means of maintaining cardiovascular fitness in asymptomatic adults and in the rehabilitation of patients with coronary artery disease. In both situations the use of specific exercise parameters (type, intensity, frequency, and duration) must be instituted and followed. In patients recovering from myocardial infarction, more structured protocols are often employed according to the status and course of recovery of the patient.[5,124] Periodic reports of the danger of sudden death in "healthy" individuals and recovering patients must be tempered with the bulk of evidence in favor of cardiac conditioning. This last point emphasizes the importance of appropriate medical supervision and periodic examination to diminish the chance of any adverse episodes in the use of cardiac conditioning protocols.

Peripheral vascular disease

Exercise may help to alleviate specific peripheral vascular conditions. Several studies have documented a substantial increase in walking tolerance in patients with intermittent claudication after a supervised program of walking, jogging, dynamic exercises, and stretching.[13,24,35,95] The exact mechanisms responsible for this increase in work capacity remain unclear, although changes in blood flow resistance and muscle metabolic activity have been suggested as possible factors. Other investigators have found similar results in the benefits of exercise training programs in various peripheral vascular conditions, especially if exercise is used in conjunction with vasoactive drug therapy.[70,107] It appears that exercise may be beneficial in the early stages of some peripheral vascular diseases and that consideration should be given to exercise training as a possible therapeutic intervention in certain situations.

Pulmonary therapy

Exercise training programs in pulmonary therapy can be roughly categorized as either general (systemic) in nature or focused directly on the respiratory musculature (specific). General exercises can be any of a variety of aerobic activities, such as jogging, cycling, or organized games; whereas specific exercises, such as diaphragmatic breathing or incentive spirometry, are used to increase strength and endurance of the ventilatory muscle groups.[12,78,105,110]

The use of general training programs in chronic obstructive pulmonary disease (COPD) has been shown to produce favorable improvements in several cardiovascular parameters, such as increased maximal oxygen consumption and decreased resting heart rate. However, considerable debate exists as to the efficacy of training on improved pulmonary function. Most investigations have failed to document objective improvements in lung function after either a general or a systemic exercise training program.[2,12,14,105] However, other favorable changes in patient mood and attitude have been reported in COPD patients after general conditioning programs.

Exercise training in individuals with asthma has received a great deal of attention. The ability of an acute exercise bout to induce an asthma attack is well known.[41] However, evidence exists that systemic exercise training may help decrease the incidence of asthmatic attacks and the need for antiasthma drugs.[54,84,101,114] In addition, physical training may improve dynamic pulmonary function, as well as several other physiologic and psychologic factors, particularly in young asthmatic patients.[78] Although many different modes of exercise have been used, swimming may be preferential as a means of training for several reasons. Evidently, swimming offers advantages of increased humidity of inspired air, exercise being done in a horizontal position, more coordinated breathing control, and a smaller increase in body temperature during and after exercise.[38,78] Regardless of which mode of exercise is used, training protocols should be tailored to the specific needs of each individual.

SUMMARY

Exercise has always played a prominent and crucial role in rehabilitation. Throughout the years, techniques have been refined through the information obtained from countless basic and clinical research studies. We now recognize the need for specific exercise protocols to obtain specific goals in rehabilitation. In addition, technologic advances in exercise equipment have been important in helping the patient obtain maximal benefits from an exercise program, as well as providing an objective and reliable method of assessing patient progress. Finally, physical activity and exercise training can be employed in a variety of patient problems, including some situations where exercise was once thought useless or even harmful to the patient. The need for the clinician to be aware of all the possible applications and the safe implementation of training regimens is an essential part of the rehabilitation process.

ACKNOWLEDGMENT

We gratefully acknowledge the assistance of Suzanne Babyar, Amira Ranney, Andrew Robinson, and Gary Sforzo in reviewing this chapter.

REFERENCES

1. Alexander, J, and Molnar, GE: Muscle strength in children: preliminary report on objective standards, Arch Phys Med Rehabil 54:424, 1973.
2. Alison, JA, Samios, R, and Anderson, SD: Evaluation of exercise training in patients with chronic airway obstruction, Phys Ther 61:1273, 1981.
3. American College of Sports Medicine: The recommended quantity and quality of exercise for developing and maintaining fitness in healthy adults, Med Sci Sports Exerc 10:vii, 1978.
4. Armstrong, LE, et al: Using isokinetic dynamometry to test ambulatory patients with multiple sclerosis, Phys Ther 63:1274, 1983.
5. Atwood, JA, and Nielsen, DH: Scope of cardiac rehabilitation, Phys Ther 65:1812, 1985.
6. Beaulieu, JE: Developing a stretching program, Phys Sports Med 9:59, 1981.
7. Berger, RA: Optimal repetitions for the development of strength, Res Q Exerc Sport 33:334, 1962.
8. Bjorntorp, P: Physiological and clinical aspects of exercise in obese persons, Exerc Sport Sci Rev 11:159, 1983.
9. Blomqvist, CG, and Saltin, B: Cardiovascular adaptations to physical training, Annu Rev Physiol 45:169, 1983.
10. Blount, WB, and Bolinske, J: Physical therapy in the non-operative treatment of scoliosis, Phys Ther 47:919, 1967.
11. Bohannon, RW, et al: Effectiveness of repeated prolonged loading for increasing flexion in knees demonstrating post-operative stiffness, Phys Ther 65:494, 1985.
12. Booker, HA: Exercise training and breathing control in patients with chronic airway limitation, Physiotherapy 70:258, 1984.
13. Boyd, CE, et al: Pain free physical training in intermittent claudication, J Sports Med Phys Fitness 24:112, 1984.
14. Brown, HB, and Wasserman, K: Exercise performance in chronic obstructive pulmonary diseases, Med Clin North Am 65:525, 1981.
15. Brunnstrom, S: Movement therapy in hemiplegia, New York, 1970, Harper & Row.
16. Buccieri, K, et al: Creative use of isokinetics in the rehabilitation population, paper presented at S.M. Dinsdale International Conference in Rehabilitation, Ottawa, Ontario, May 28-30, 1986.
17. Cailliet, R: Exercises for scoliosis. In Basmajian, J, editor: Therapeutic exercise, ed 4, Baltimore, 1984, Williams & Wilkins Co.

18. Clarke, DH: Adaptations in strength and muscular endurance resulting from exercise, Exerc Sport Sci Rev 1:73, 1973.

19. Cole, WH, and Knapp, ME: The Kenny treatment of infantile paralysis, JAMA 116:2577, 1941.

20. Costill, DL, et al: Adaptations in skeletal muscle following strength training, J Appl Physiol 46:96, 1979.

21. Cotton, DJ, and Waters, JS: Immediate effect of four types of warmup activities upon static flexibility of four selected joints, Am J Corrective Ther 24:133, 1970.

22. Coutts, RD, Toth, C, and Kaita, JH: The role of continuous passive motion in the rehabilitation of the total knee patient. In Hungerford, R, editor: Total knee arthroplasty: a comprehensive approach, Baltimore, 1983, Williams & Wilkins Co.

23. Coyle, EF, et al: Specificity of power improvements through slow and fast isokinetic training, J Appl Physiol 51:1437, 1981.

24. Dahllof, AG, Holm, J, and Schersten, T: Exercise training of patients with intermittent claudication, Scand J Rehabil Med 9(suppl):20, 1983.

25. Davies, G, and Gould, J: Trunk testing using a prototype Cybex II isokinetic dynamometer stabilization system, J Orthop Sports Phys Ther 3:164, 1982.

26. de Lateur, B, and Giaconi, RM: Effect on maximal strength of submaximal exercise in Duchenne muscular dystrophy, Am J Phys Med 58:26, 1979.

27. de Lateur, B, Lehmann, F, and Fordyce, WE: A test of the Delorme axiom, Arch Phys Med Rehabil 49:245, 1968.

28. Delorme, TL: Restoration of muscle power by heavy resistance exercise, J Bone Joint Surg 27:645, 1945.

29. Delorme, TL, and Watkins, AL: Techniques of progressive resistive exercises, Arch Phys Med Rehabil 29:263, 1948.

30. deVries, HA: Evaluation of static stretching procedures for improvement of flexibility, Res Q 33:222, 1962.

31. deVries, HA, et al: Tranquilizer effect of exercise, Am J Phys Med 60:57, 1981.

32. deVries, HA, et al: Fusimotor system involvement in the tranquilizer effect of exercise, Am J Phys Med 61:111, 1982.

33. Dowell, RT: Cardiac adaptations to exercise, Exerc Sport Sci Rev 11:99, 1983.

34. Effgen, SK: Effect of an exercise program on the static balance of deaf children, Phys Ther 61:873, 1981.

35. Ekroth, R, et al: Physical training of patients with intermittent claudication: indications, methods and results, Surgery 84:640, 1978.

36. Farrell, M, and Richards, JG: Analysis of the reliability and validity of the kinetic communicator exercise device, Med Sci Sports Exerc 18:44, 1986.

37. Fidler, MW, and Jowett, RL: Muscle imbalance in the aetiology of scoliosis, J Bone Joint Surg 58B:200, 1976.

38. Fitch, KD, Morton, AR, and Blanksby, BA: Effect of swimming training on children with asthma, Arch Dis Child 51:190, 1976.

39. Fowler, WM, and Taylor, M: Rehabilitation management of muscular dystrophy and related disorders. I. The role of exercise, Arch Phys Med Rehabil 63:319, 1982.

40. Gardiner, G: Specificity of strength changes of exercised and nonexercised limbs following isometric training, Res Q Exerc Sport 34:98, 1963.

41. Ghory, JE: Exercise and asthma: overview and clinical impact, Pediatrics 56(suppl):844, 1975.

42. Glasser, L: Effects of isokinetic training on the rate of movement during ambulation in hemiparetic patients, Phys Ther 66:673, 1986.

43. Goldberg, AL, et al: Mechanism of work-induced hypertrophy of skeletal muscle, Med Sci Sports Exerc 7:248, 1975.

44. Goldspink, DF: Influence of immobilization and stretch on protein turnover of rat skeletal muscle, J Physiol (Lond) 264:267, 1977.

45. Gollnick, PD, et al: Effect of training on enzyme activity and fiber composition in human skeletal muscle, J Appl Physiol 34:107, 1973.

46. Gonyea, WJ, and Sale, D: Physiology of weight lifting exercise, Arch Phys Med Rehabil 63:235, 1982.

47. Goslin, BR, and Charteris, J: Isokinetic dynamometry: normative data for clinical use of lower extremity (knee) cases, Scand J Rehabil Med 11:105, 1979.

48. Griffin, JW, McClure, MH, and Bertorini, TE: Sequential isokinetic and manual muscle testing in patients with neuromuscular disease: a pilot study, Phys Ther 66:32, 1986.

49. Harris, FA: Correction of muscle balance in spasticity, Am J Phys Med 57:123, 1978.

50. Harris, FA: Treatment with a position feedback-controlled head stabilizer, Am J Phys Med Rehabil 58:169, 1979.

51. Harris, FA: Facilitation techniques and technological adjuncts in therapeutic exercise. In Basmajian, JV, editor: Therapeutic exercise, ed 4, Baltimore, 1984, Williams & Wilkins Co.

52. Haskell, WL: The influence of exercise on the concentrations of triglyceride and cholesterol in human plasma, Exerc Sport Sci Rev 12:205, 1984.

53. Henricson, AS, et al: The effect of heat and stretching on the range of hip motion, J Orthop Sports Phys Ther 6:110, 1984.

54. Henriksen, JM, and Nielsen, TT: Effect of physical training on exercise induced bronchoconstriction, Acta Paediatr Scand 72:31, 1983.

55. Hepburn, GR, and Crivelli, KJ: Use of elbow dynasplint for reduction of elbow flexion contractures: a case study, J Orthop Sports Phys Ther 5:269, 1984.

56. Herbison, GJ, Jaweed, MM, and Ditunno, JF: Exercise therapies in peripheral neuropathies, Arch Phys Med Rehabil 64:201, 1983.

57. Hertling, D, and Jones, D: Relaxation. In Kessler, RM, and Hertling, D, editors: Management of common musculoskeletal disorders, New York, 1983, Harper & Row.

58. Hettinger, T: Physiology of strength, Springfield, Ill, 1961, Charles C Thomas, Publisher.

59. Holloszy, JO, and Coyle, EF: Adaptations of skeletal muscle to endurance exercise and their metabolic consequences, J Appl Physiol 56:831, 1984.

60. Hudlicka, O: Growth of capillaries in skeletal and cardiac muscle, Circ Res 50:451, 1982.

61. Ingjer, F: Effects of endurance training on muscle fiber ATP-ase activity, capillary supply and mitochondrial content in man, J Physiol (Lond) 294:419, 1979.

62. Johnson, J, and Siegel, D: Reliability of an isokinetic movement of the knee extensors, Res Q 49:88, 1978.

63. Jokl, P, and Konstadt, S: The effect of limb immobilization on muscle function and protein composition, Clin Orthop 174:222, 1983.

64. Kisner, C, and Colby, LA: Therapeutic exercise: foundations and techniques, Philadelphia, 1985, F.A. Davis Co.

65. Knapp, ME: Exercises for lower motor neuron lesions. In Basmajian, JV, editor: Therapeutic exercise, ed 4, Baltimore, 1984, Williams & Wilkins Co.

66. Komi, PV: Measurement of force-velocity relationship in human muscle under concentric and eccentric contractions. In Cerquiglini, S, Venerando, A, and Wartenweiler, J, editor: Biomechanics III, Basel, 1973, Karger.

67. Kottke, FJ: From reflex to skill: The training of coordination, Arch Phys Med Rehabil 61:551, 1980.

68. Kottke, FJ: Therapeutic exercise to develop neuromuscular coordination. In Kottke, FJ, Stillwell, GK, and Lehmann, JF, editors: Handbook of physical medicine and rehabilitation, ed 3, Philadelphia, 1982, WB Saunders Co.

69. Kottke, FJ, Pawley, DL, and Ptak, RA: The rationale for correction of shortening of connective tissue, Arch Phys Med Rehabil 47:345, 1966.

70. Krause, D, and Dittmar, K: Active therapeutic exercise in combination with vasoactive drugs in intermittent claudication, Munch Med Wschr 120:69, 1978.

71. Langrana, NA, et al: Quantitative assessment of back strength using isokinetic testing, Spine 9:287, 1984.

72. Lehmann, JF, Masock, AJ, and Warren, CG: Effect of therapeutic temperatures on tendon extensibility, Arch Phys Med Rehabil 51:481, 1970.

73. Light, KE, et al: Low-load prolonged stretch versus high-load brief stretch in treating knee flexion contractures, Phys Ther 64:330, 1984.

74. Lindh, M: Increase in muscle strength from isometric quadriceps exercises at different knee angles, Scand J Rehabil Med 11:33, 1979.

75. MacDougall, JD, et al: Biochemical adaptations of human skeletal muscle to heavy resistance training and immobilization, J Appl Physiol 43:700, 1977.

76. Malone, T, Blackburn, TA, and Wallace, LA: Knee rehabilitation, Phys Ther 60:1602, 1980.

77. Markos, PD: Ipsilateral and contralateral effects of proprioceptive neuromuscular facilitation techniques on hip motion and electromyographic activity, Phys Ther 59:1366, 1979.

78. Marley, WP: Asthma and exercise, a review, Am Correct Ther J 31:95, 1977.

79. Marras, WS, King, AI, and Joynt, RL: Measurements of loads on the lumbar spine under isometric and isokinetic conditions, Spine 9:176, 1984.

80. Mawdsley, R, and Knapik, J: Comparison of isokinetic measurements with test repetitions, Phys Ther 62:169, 1982.

81. Mayer, TG, et al: Quantification of lumbar function. II. Sagittal plane trunk strength in chronic low-back pain patients, Spine 10:765, 1985.

82. Mayer, TG, et al: Quantification of lumbar function. III. Preliminary data on isokinetic torso rotation testing with myoelectric spectral analysis in normal and low-back pain subjects, Spine 10:912, 1985.

83. McDonagh, MJN, and Davies, CTM: Adaptive response of mammalian skeletal muscle to exercise with high loads, Eur J Appl Physiol 52:139, 1984.

84. McElhenny, TR, and Petersen, KH: Physical fitness for asthmatic boys, JAMA 185:142, 1963.

85. McKenzie, R: Prophylaxis in recurrent low back pain, NZ Med J 89:22, 1979.

86. McKenzie, R: The lumbar spine, Upper Hutt, NZ, 1981, Wright & Carmen Ltd.

87. Moffroid, M, and Whipple, R: Specificity of speed of exercise, Phys Ther 50:1692, 1970.

88. Molnar, G, and Alexander, J: Objective quantitative muscle testing in children: a pilot study, Arch Phys Med Rehabil 54:224, 1973.

89. Moritani, T, and deVries, HA: Neural factors versus hypertrophy in the time course of muscle strength gain, Am J Phys Med 58:115, 1979.

90. Morris, JM, Lucas, DB, and Bresler, B: Role of the trunk in stability of the spine, J Bone Joint Surg 43A:327, 1961.

91. Petrofsky, JS: Isometric exercise and its clinical implications, Springfield, Ill, 1982, Charles C Thomas, Publisher.

92. Ponte, DJ, Jensen, GJ, and Kent, BE: A preliminary report on the use of the McKenzie protocol versus Williams protocol in the treatment of low back pain, J Orthop Sports Phys Ther 6:130, 1984.

93. Prentice, WE: An electromyographic analysis of the effectiveness of heat or cold and stretching for inducing relaxation in injured muscle, J Orthop Sports Phys Ther 3:133, 1982.

94. Rose, SJ, and Rothstein, JM: Muscle mutability. I. General concepts and adaptations to altered patterns of use, Phys Ther 62:1773, 1982.

95. Ruell, PA, et al: Intermittent claudication: the effect of physical training on walking tolerance and venous lactate concentration, Eur J Appl Physiol 52:420, 1984.

96. Salter, RB, et al: Clinical application of basic research on continuous passive motion for disorders and injuries of synovial joints: a preliminary report of a feasibility study, J Orthop Res 1:325, 1984.

97. Saltin, B, et al: Role of muscle mass in the cardiovascular response to isometric contractions, Acta Physiol Scand 102:79, 1978.

98. Saltin, B, and Rowell, LB: Functional adaptations to physical activity and inactivity, Fed Proc 39:1506, 1980.

99. Sapega, AA, et al: Biophysical factors in range-of-motion exercise, Phys Sports Med 9:57, 1981.

100. Savander, GR: Use of the Kinetron in the training of the below-knee amputee, Phys Ther 52:286, 1972.

101. Scherr, MS, and Frankel, L: Physical conditioning programs for asthmatic children, JAMA 168:1996, 1958.

102. Scheuer, J, and Tipton, CM: Cardiovascular adaptations to physical training, Annu Rev Physiol 39:221, 1977.

103. Scott, OM, et al: Effect of exercise in Duchenne muscular dystrophy, Physiotherapy 67:174, 1981.

104. Seals, DR, and Hagberg, JM: Effect of exercise training on human hypertension, Med Sci Sports Exerc 16:207, 1984.

105. Shaffer, TH, Wolfson, MR, and Bhutani, VK: Respiratory muscle function, assessment and training, Phys Ther 61:1711, 1981.

106. Sherman, WM, et al: Isokinetic rehabilitation after surgery: a review of factors which are important for developing physiotherapeutic techniques after knee surgery, Am J Sports Med 10:155, 1982.

107. Siewert, VH, et al: The effect of interval running exercises in combination with vasodilatory therapy on microcirculation in the lower leg in cases of peripheral arterial circulation disturbances (stage I and II), Z Alternsforsch 38:377, 1983.

108. Simonson, E: Physiology of work capacity and fatigue, Springfield, Ill, 1976, Charles C Thomas, Publisher.

109. Sinaki, M, and Mikkelsen, BA: Postmenopausal spinal osteoporosis: flexion versus extension exercises, Arch Phys Med Rehabil 65:593, 1984.

110. Sinclair, JD: Exercise in pulmonary disease. In Basmajian JV, editor: Therapeutic exercise, ed 4, Baltimore, 1984, Williams & Wilkins Co.

111. Smith, SS, et al: Quantification of lumbar function. I. Isometric and multispeed isokinetic trunk strength measures in sagittal and axial planes in normal subjects, Spine 10:757, 1985.

112. Stap, LJ, and Woodfin, PM: Continuous passive motion in the treatment of knee flexion contractures: a case report, Phys Ther 66:1720, 1986.

113. Stone, B, et al: The effect of an exercise program on change in curve in adolescents with minimal idiopathic scoliosis: a preliminary study, Phys Ther 59:759, 1979.

114. Svenonius, E, Kautto, R, and Arborelius, M: Improvement after training of children with exercise induced asthma, Acta Paediatr Scand 72:23, 1983.

115. Tabary, JC, et al: Physiological and structural changes in the cat's soleus muscle due to immobilization at different lengths by plaster casts, J Physiol (Lond) 224:231, 1972.

116. Tipton, CM: Exercise, training, and hypertension, Exerc Sport Sci Rev 12:245, 1984.

117. Voss, DE, Ionta, MK, and Myers, BJ: Proprioceptive neuromuscular facilitation, ed 3, New York, 1985, Harper & Row.

118. Warren, CG, Lehmann, JF, and Koblanski, JN: Elongation of rat tail tendon: effect of load and temperature, Arch Phys Med Rehabil 52:465, 1971.

119. Warren, CG, Lehmann, JF, and Koblanski, JN: Heat and stretch procedures: an evaluation using rat tail tendon, Arch Phys Med Rehabil 57:122, 1976.

120. Watkins, MP, Harris, BA, and Kozlowski, BA: Isokinetic testing in patients with hemiparesis: a pilot study, Phys Ther 64:184, 1984.

121. Wilder, PA, and Sykes, J: Using an isokinetic exercise machine to improve the gait pattern in a hemiplegic patient, Phys Ther 62:1291, 1982.

122. Williams, M, and Stutzman, L: Strength variation through the range of joint motion, Phys Ther Rev 39:145, 1959.

123. Williams, P: Examination and conservative treatment for disc lesions of the lower spine, Clin Orthop 5:28, 1955.

124. Wilson, PK, Fardy, PS, and Froelicher, VF: Cardiac rehabilitation, adult fitness and exercise testing, Philadelphia, 1981, Lea & Febiger.

CHAPTER 48

Principles of physical medicine

SAMUEL S. SVERDLIK

The therapeutic and diagnostic application of physical energies is described in this chapter. The modalities include thermotherapy (heat and cold), ultraviolet irradiation, electrotherapy, massage, manipulation, stretching, and traction. The chapter concludes with discussions of diagnostic tests and prescription writing.

THERMOTHERAPY
Heat

Biologic processes generate and are affected by physical energies, one of which is heat.

Heat is the most commonly used modality in rehabilitation medicine and is applied before exercises, stretching, or electrotherapy. It is employed for both acute and chronic disorders, and the physiologic effects are the same whatever the source, varying only in the depth of penetration.

Physics

Heat is a part of the electromagnetic spectrum and is a state of particle excitation (entropy). Every atom or molecule above zero degrees Kelvin has excitation and is capable of transmitting energy to another particle either by direct collision or radiation. Energy transfer by collision in solids is *conduction* and in liquids or gases *convection*. It occurs only when the absorbing particle has lower entropy (temperature). Heat can therefore be transmitted only from higher temperature to lower temperature. *Radiation* is the emission of photons (quanta or packets of energy), which cross space and when absorbed increase the particle's excitation state, alter its chemistry, or are reemitted as heat or light (fluorescence, phosphorescence).

The skin is a good reflector, fair radiator, and poor conductor of heat. The heat absorbed by the skin immediately encounters the high concentration of water molecules in the subcutaneous capillary and fat beds, which are subject initially to physical and then to physiologic reactions. The specific heat, the calorie gain or loss needed to change the temperature of 1 g of a substance, is approximately three times greater for water than it is for tissue molecules. The subcutaneous water thus becomes an excellent heat storage reservoir or insulator and significantly contributes to maintenance of relatively constant body temperature.

Heat can also be produced in tissue by conversion of high-frequency electromagnetic waves into microcurrents (short wave or microwave) or into shearing, vibrational, frictional, or compressive mechanical waves. These modalities are described as diathermy and ultrasound, or deep heat. Conductive, convective, or radiant heat penetrates 0.5 to 1 mm beneath the skin and is called superficial heat. Diathermy can reach superficial muscle fascia, and ultrasound reaches deeper.

In summary, heat is electromagnetic energy that is absorbed by a particle having a lower temperature than the source. The absorbed energy raises temperature, produces chemical reactions, is transmitted to another particle, or is reemitted as light or heat.

The skin may reflect or absorb the energy. Absorption is achieved to the greatest extent by water in the subcutaneous fat and capillary beds.

Physiologic effects of heat[22]

Physiologic functions are governed by the energy manipulations of specialized molecules, usually protein within the cell, its membranes, and extracellular compartments. These molecules have inherent mechanical, electrical, and chemical energy that they generate and transfer. Adding thermal energy to this system increases these transduction processes. Thermal energy in the water molecules acts as a driving force for the reactions and may increase oscillating motion and charges or dipole separation or may produce electrical changes. In addition, heat causes hydrogen bonds to be made or broken and causes chemical changes from alterations in molecular configurations. These effects are anabolic or catalytic and function in life as substrate molecules are available.

We may postulate the following sequence resulting from the application of heat to cells: (1) increase cellular catalysis-metabolism requiring (2) energy source molecules (O_2, proteins, fats, carbohydrates) producing (3) vasodilation and increased capillary pressures with (4) transudation and, from alteration of membrane configuration or dynamics, (5) ionic "pumping" of electrolytes, fluids, metabolites, and enzymes.

Continuing application of heat or reduction of temperature may result in protein degradation, creating histamine-like substances or cryoglobulin; leukocytosis and associated immunologic reactions; and concomitant inflammatory or antiinflammatory reactions.

The molecular and structural characteristics of proteins such as collagen are temperature dependent. Such proteins elongate with temperature elevation (viscoelastic effect).[7,17] The chemical energy of dephosphorylation of adenosine triphosphate (ATP) to adenosine diphosphate (ADP), with accompanying mechanical work of shortening muscle fibers, generates heat that may produce changes in the configuration of fiber proteins and in the mechanical characteristics of the sliding filaments. Protein fractions such as histamines or antigens (cryoglobulins) may be released with temperature alterations.

Dynamics of fluids and electrolytes in the membrane, particularly in excitable tissues such as nerve, are temperature dependent. The mechanisms of impulse transmission, including ionic, electrical, thermal, and light energies, are interrelated. Infrared emissions from live crab nerves have been described.[50] The configurations of protein lipoid molecules in end organs and membranes are modified by temperature changes, and secretions of synovial fluids increase with temperature elevation.[35]

Thermal energy therefore affects the structural, chemical, immunologic, and electrical characteristics of molecules; enzyme activity; degradation products; and membrane functions of cells.

Clinical effects of heat

Local skin reactions to heat include the sense of warmth, vasodilation (erythema), sweating, reduction in skin resistance, and increase in local tissue metabolism. If heating is continued beyond 60 minutes, core temperature may be elevated and homeostatic responses of distal vasodilation occur.

Usually temperature, pulse, and blood pressure are unaffected by heat, as are the renal and gastrointestinal systems. Nerve conduction velocities and action potentials may increase. Muscle tone or tension may soften, or the elasticity increase. Ligament and capsular fibers similarly gain elasticity, and the motion of joints increases.

Pain may be relieved by heat. One explanation is that pain relief with heat may be related to spindle gamma afferent release, but there is as yet insufficient evidence to support this.

The anti-inflammatory action of heat includes leukocytosis, increased capillary pressure, and hormonal enzyme effects that act toward suppression of the tissue reaction. Thermolabile reactions of reactive proteins and of other cellular (lymphocyte) components of tissue injury such as bradykinin, prostaglandins, and leukotrienes may be postulated.

The amount, rate, and direction of tissue heat gain or loss depend on the following:

1. The source of heat, its temperature, and duration of application
2. The optical properties of the skin: reflective or absorptive
3. The core/skin temperature gradient, which varies from $5°$ to $10°$ C depending on the sites tested; core temperature averages $37°$ to $40°$ C, and skin temperature $29°$ to $35°$ C.
4. The amount of water and fat in the subcutaneous capillary and fat beds
5. Hypothalamic and skin neural controls that maintain constant temperature, such as reflex vasomotor reactions distal to treated areas
6. Respiratory and excretory mechanisms
7. Ambient temperature and humidity
8. Age (elderly and infants tolerate heat poorly), sex, nutrition, exercise, hydration, sensitivity, and disease

Indications

Heat is indicated primarily for its analgesic effect. The usual applications are for musculoskeletal and neuromuscular disorders such as neuralgias, sprains, strains, articular problems, muscle spasm, trigger points, and problems labeled by a host of terms that attempt to describe the vague problem of muscle pain. In an exhaustive review of muscle pain syndromes, Simons[44] attempted to define the many terms used to describe the problem and reported the pathologic conditions found by many investigators. Although there does not appear to be a clear understanding of the etiology, pathology, or indications for treatment of pain, heat and cold are recommended among many other modalities.

Muscle spasm is an indication for heat treatment. The nature of this condition is included in Simons' discussion[44] but has not been clearly defined. That it is benefited by heat is often noted subjectively and objectively. If possible a diagnosis should be made and aspirin or other anti-inflammatory analgesics prescribed, with rest or splinting, before a program of thermotherapy begins.

Heat before exercise, stretching, traction, or manipulation often enhances their effect and benefits.

Heat as therapy in obliterative arterial or in arteriolar

disease may be helpful but should be employed with great caution.

Wounds and ulcers may benefit from topical heat. Cellulitis and abscesses may be ripened to the point of drainage with hot, wet compresses. Since heat has an evaporative drying and vasodilating effect, it may be beneficial in the treatment of open wounds.

The use of heat in addition to surgery, chemotherapy, and radiation therapy is being favorably reported in the management of cancer. Diathermy or microthermy is applied to the tumor site. Raymond and co-workers[38] reported beneficial effects using microwave diathermy on patients with refractory tumors of the head and neck.

The soporific effect of heat is frequently noted.

Contraindications

Heat, whatever its source, should not be used in acute inflammation or trauma until the initial reaction has subsided, nor in venous obstruction, severe arterial insufficiency, hemorrhagic diathesis, or coagulation defects. In the absence of sensation special care must be exercised.

In the presence of cardiovascular, respiratory, or renal failure, heat should be used sparingly, if at all. Active inflammatory arthritis, particularly with joint swelling, may be worsened by the application of heat because collagenase activity is increased with heating.

Saunas are not advised for pregnant women or for patients with cardiac disease, epilepsy, hypotension, or hypertension. Patients taking tranquilizers, narcotics, or antihypertensive medication should be cautioned about using a sauna.

Sources

Superficial (conductive) heat.[35] Conductive heating is achieved by direct contact with the skin. The sources include solids (electric pad, hot water bottle, sand, peloids [muds], poultices), liquids (water, paraffin wax or packs, whirlpool), and gases (dry or moist air, saunas, fluidotherapy).

The choice is one of convenience and should be based on accessibility of the part, need for movement, availability of the agent, and the patient's and physician's preference. The conductive heat agents most commonly used in rehabilitation are water, hot packs, and paraffin. Hot water bottle, heating pad, moist packs, and tub baths are all readily available at home, making these preferred heat sources.

LIQUIDS.[51] The accessibility, bouyancy, cleansing effect, and ease of temperature control of water makes hydrotherapy one of the most frequently employed heat sources. Although normal heat loss is reduced with immersion, undesirable temperature elevation may occur. Movement of painful joints under water is frequently possible when motion is otherwise inhibited.

The *bathtub, pool, tank,* or *whirlpool* is used for palliation, exercises, or debridement of wounds or ulcers. Soaps, antiseptics, and detergents can be added to the water as appropriate but often are unnecessary. Full body immersion

in tubs or tanks for recent widespread surface burns is used in many centers. Maintenance of neutral temperature is recommended (38 to 41° C). The addition of common salt at the ratio of 0.7 pounds per 10 gallons of water brings the bath to isotonic concentration.

Pool temperature for exercise therapy should be approximately that of the body, 32° C. Therapy may be daily, starting at 10 to 15 minutes and increasing to 20 to 30 minutes. Alternate days for elderly or debilitated patients may be considered.

Tubs, saunas, and steam rooms have been subject to bacterial contamination with *Pseudomonas aeruginosa*. Herpes simplex may also be transmitted in hot tubs without body contact.

The fluidotherapy apparatus used in hand therapy applies heat, massage, and sensory stimulation by using heated organic cellulose particles or polypropylene propelled by a compressor at a hand inserted into the unit. This is equivalent to a dry whirlpool device and is very effective in hand rehabilitation therapy. The pressure and temperature can be adjusted to the desired levels. Exposures of 20 to 30 minutes are usually adequate.

Paraffin wax remains liquid after melting at 49° C. Adding mineral oil lowers the melting temperature. Paraffin, which can be applied directly to the skin, is often prescribed for arthritis of the hand or foot. Its effectiveness for an acute swollen joint is questionable. The oil that remains after removal of the wax makes subsequent massage and stretching easier. Electric heaters or double boilers for melting paraffin are available for home use. Patients applying paraffin at home should use a thermometer to ensure proper temperature.

GASES. Saunas and steam rooms are usually available in recreational facilities and are even found in homes. The steam source is usually water on dry hot stones or on an electric heating element. The specific therapeutic benefits from these units have not been established, but the relaxing effects may be related to the hypotension that follows vasodilation of the skin and subcutaneous capillary bed.

Compresses may be made from turkish towels, strips of felt or wool blankets, or silica gel packs (Hydrocollator). The last retains heat longer when heated to 60° to 71° C. The heat is retained for approximately 30 minutes after application at above 65° C. Patients and families can easily be taught to use packs at home. To prevent burns, placing several layers of terry-cloth towels between the pack and skin is recommended.

Radiant heat. Radiant heat (noncontact, dry heat)[47] is infrared radiation, which has a wavelength of 7700 to 120,000 Å and is above the visible spectrum (3900 to 7700 Å). Its depth of penetration is approximately 1 to 10 mm for near (7700 to 15,000 Å), and 0.05 to 1 mm for far (15,000 to 120,000 Å). Photons at longer wavelengths have less energy and therefore less penetrance (Table 48-1).

The physiologic effects of radiant heat are identical to those of conductive heat.

Table 48-1. Various ranges of the electromagnetic spectrum

Type of radiation	Range of wavelengths (Å)
Long-wave infrared	12,000-1500
Short-wave infrared	1500-770
Visible	770-390
Near ultraviolet	390-290
Far ultraviolet	290-180
Grenz X rays	5-1
Diagnostic X rays	0.3-1.2
Therapeutic X rays	1.2-0.5
Gamma rays	01.-0.2

Sources of radiant heat include luminous or visible infrared bulbs, which emit near infrared, and nonluminous radiators, which are metallic coils or wire covered with refractory materials and emit far infrared. Some light may be visible with the coils and always is with bulbs. Bulbs are available for home use, but caution must be exercised against burns or fire.

Diathermy and ultrasound[12]

Physics

High-frequency currents are generated by an oscillator that in addition to a current source requires a capacitor or condenser and an inductance coil. The patient circuit is coupled to this apparatus. This circuit can produce electromagnetic waves that have frequencies described as short and ultrashort (microwave), as compared to long radio waves. The same basic generator coupled to a piezoelectric crystal (transducer) produces high-frequency sound waves.

The short waves or microwaves create microcurrents in a field that develops between the plates of the coupled capacitor or within an inductance coil.

A piezoelectric crystal placed between capacitor plates will be subjected to expansions and contractions with each oscillating half cycle. Placing a patient between coupled capacitor plates produces capacitor heating, or inductance heating where a wire is either coiled or looped about a part. The "short" wavelengths fixed by the Federal Communications Commission at 27.33 mHz have a length of 12.2 cm.

Microwaves are generated off directors described as A, B (hemispherical—4- and 6-inch diameters) and C and D (dihedral—4.5×5 and 5×21 inches). The directors are connected by a coaxial cable to the oscillator as is the U.S. transducer.

The term "diathermy" is a misnomer because the microcurrents do not go through the body but, like any current, move through a volume conductor along the lines of least impedance (resistance in high-frequency fields) or across its surface. They usually penetrate to the subcutaneous fat where high resistance exists in the water molecules.

Diathermy

The currents generated inside a capacitor field vary according to the capacitor size, the distance between the plates, the material between the plates, and the voltage and frequency applied. The quantification of the current within the field (patient circuit) cannot be accurately measured. Meters on the apparatus only define the "resonance" or tuning of the patient and generator circuits. The patterns of the heating fields are different for condenser pad, inductance coil, and microwave directors, but they all have the effect of developing heat at or slightly below the skin's surface. The depth of penetration varies with the technique or apparatus employed and the thickness of the subcutaneous fat.

Microwaves are applied in a similar manner to an infrared lamp, and some of the energy is scattered, reflected, absorbed, and refracted. The heating patterns vary with different directors and differ according to their size and design.

Because microwaves have greater frequency than short wave diathermy, they penetrate to a greater depth.

Ultrasound[27]

Ultrasound energy is mechanical oscillating waves (800,000 to 1 million cycles/sec and 0.15 cm) that produce vibration, shearing, compression, rarefaction, and frictional forces above the audible range (17,000 cycles/sec). The energy is generated by particle collisions and therefore cannot be generated in a vacuum.

Coupling ultrasound to the body surface by such agents as oil, gel, or water ensures transmission of the energy. A space or gap of air dissipates the energy. The energy absorbed by the tissues is transmitted by conduction. Metallic implants, except those close to the skin, are good conductors and their presence is therefore not a contraindication to therapy because they rapidly transmit the heat and do not reach toxic temperatures. Ultrasound should not be used in the presence of methyl methacrylate (bone cement) because the interface and binding may be broken.

Sound waves, including ultrasound, penetrate deepest of all the diathermy modalities. They can penetrate to depths such as the hip joint or through the body as is the case when listening with a stethoscope.

The primary energy produced by ultrasound is thermal, which can cause alteration of membrane configuration or possible membrane destruction. Trapped gas molecules may expand and coalesce (cavitation) and with the interface reaction contribute to membrane rupture. The compressive-rarefaction phenomenon creates streaming, which may also alter membrane or cellular functions and be beneficial in accelerating diffusion of injected medication.

Equipment and dosage. The generator produces high-frequency alternating current on the piezoelectric crystal. The latter may be quartz or barium titanate, which is in the treatment head. The intensity is expressed as watts/cm², which describes the field of energy under the transducer. It is derived by dividing the maximal total wattage output by the size of the applicator's radiating surface in square centimeters. Thus a machine with 30 watts total output and a radiating surface of 10 cm² has an average intensity of 3 watts/cm². The sound head must be coupled to the area under treatment and moved slowly to avoid local buildup of thermal reactions, which patients usually describe as sharp pain.

The dosage should be at maximal tolerable levels. These levels change along the line of movement of the transducer, and dosage can be corrected by concomitantly modifying the wattage. Tolerance increases during the course of treatment, and greater intensities may be applied. Sessions of up to 20 minutes may be given for acute injuries. Twice daily treatments may resolve acute problems within 3 to 5 days.

Contraindications

Contraindications for diathermy, microtherm, and ultrasound are the same as those mentioned for thermotherapy. Microthermy causes a high temperature concentration in the presence of edema, on adhesive tape or a wet dressing, and over bony prominences. Malignancy is not a contraindication. Short wave diathermy should not be applied over metal implants.

Bryan[6] reported electromagnetic radiation interference with cardiac pacemakers in the microtherm frequencies. He noted this effect from microwave ovens, and this precaution should be observed with microwave diathermy.

Cold[26,45]

Reduction of skin or body temperature is used in rehabilitation for local analgesia, anti-inflammatory effect, control of pyrexia, and possibly control of spasticity.

Physics

The physics of hypothermia is identical to that described for heat. However, the patient and the part treated act as the heat source and the applied agent or ambient temperature absorbs the calories. Lowering body temperature over an extended time period is hypothermia. Cryotherapy uses extremely low temperatures (near or below zero degrees centigrade) for a short time such as seconds to a minute. Heat transmission away from the body or tissues is by conduction or radiation, depending on the agent and the method employed.

Physiology

Reduction in metabolism with lowering of entropy reduces the mechanical, chemical, and electrical energy of molecules. Understandably, intracellular and extracellular dynamics decreases as does that of membranes or end organs. Details of the specific physiologic reactions can be found in the noted references.[36,41] Physiologic reactions to cold are affected by the rate, extent, duration, and degrees of temperature reduction.

The reaction to lower temperature locally is immediate

vasoconstriction and, if the temperature difference is significant (10° to 15° C lower), protein degradation or cryoglobulin precipitation. Reactive hyperemia may follow mild superficial application of cold. Systemic effects of hypothermia are directed toward conserving energy and later creating calories because this may elevate a lowered core temperature. The conservation mechanisms of the skin are vasoconstriction and reduced sweating. The cardiopulmonary mechanisms are bradycardia, hypocapnia, and hypotension.

The most notable energy-creating response to cold is shivering, which creates calories. The inability of infants to shiver contributes to their poor tolerance to hypothermia.

Increased fat metabolism occurs in the liver, the greatest heat generator in the core area. Fifty percent of basal oxygen consumption is in the viscera, and 25% of this is by the liver.[4] Eskimos have hepatomegaly and prefer high-fat diets. The subcutaneous fat acts as an insulator, and when it is absent or deficient as in infants, the elderly, or debilitated patients, the intolerance for hypothermia occurs.

Neuromuscular activity is modified by lowered action potentials and delayed motor conduction velocities. A 1° C drop in temperature reduces conduction velocity by 2.5 to 4 meters per second. Paresis or paralysis may occur when myoneural transmission is compromised at approximately 5° C.

In cold temperatures, muscle tension is increased, which may be due to increased spindle excitability, as well as lowered viscoelastic properties of the fibers. Analgesia occurs because of depressed activity in both end organ and fiber conduction. The cerebral reactions may include lethargy, narcosis, and depression of neurohumoral activities.

Transudation is decreased so that edema formation is reduced. This reaction to hypothermia is very effective in treating acute soft tissue and sport injuries.

The toxic effects of hypothermia or cryotherapy may be tissue death. Before this occurs, ventricular fibrillation and shock as a consequence of hypotension may develop.

When frostbite or severe hypothermia occurs, slow rewarming with systemic fluids, anticoagulants, and appropriate antibiotics is the appropriate procedure. Using temperatures slightly higher than skin or core temperature is recommended for rewarming.

Indications

Anti-inflammatory effect. The application of any object cooler than an inflamed area draws off calories and modifies the progress of the tissue reaction. This applies to acute reactions from trauma, physical agents, acute burns, or infections. Temperature can be lowered in an acute burn by the immediate application of ice and may reduce the degree of tissue damage.[43] Cold is effective for capsular and soft tissue inflammation.

Analgesic effect. Cooling with either vapor or ice reduces pain in soft tissue injuries. Patients can be instructed in icing technique for home programs.

Antipyretic effect. The antipyretic effect of cooling, using cooling mattresses or blankets or a cold tub bath, is often effective for refractory temperature elevation. Quadriplegic and paraplegic patients may have this problem, and cooling augments antibiotic and other medical measures. The failure of their autonomic mechanisms in the affected skin limits their conducting or radiating temperature capacity.

The technique of slow, gradual cooling is equivalent to that described by Simon Baruch in his *Epitome of Hydrotherapy*[2] 60 years ago for the treatment of sun (heat) stroke. He described it as the St. Vincent's Hospital treatment. The patient is covered with wet cool sheets. This is essentially what is currently recommended, with the addition of the supportive measures for possible circulatory failure.

Spasticity.[30,34] Lowering muscle temperature to 32° C affects the sensory motor pathways. Gamma fiber potentials, which initially may be increased by shivering, are slowed after 20 minutes of cooling. Neuromuscular transmission is also slowed and partially blocked.[8] When muscle temperature approaches 12° C, spasticity is reduced or eliminated for several hours.

Burns. The immediate application of ice may reduce the tissue damage in a burn.[43]

Contraindications

Ischemia, with inadequate transport of metabolites to and from tissue, may cause necrosis when cold is applied to areas with obliterative arterial or impaired venous circulation.

Anesthesia of an area may allow longer exposure to be tolerated, with resulting tissue damage.

Patients with vasculitis, dermatomyositis, systemic lupus erythematosus, diabetes, and Raynaud's phenomenon have both vascular and immunologic factors that affect cold sensitivity, thus contraindicating the use of cold.

The aged, infants, or cachectic individuals also tolerate cold poorly. Constitutional reactions with urticaria, purpura, and possibly collapse may occur.

Indolent wounds are compromised by the vasoconstrictive effect of cooling, and healing is further delayed.

Sources

Vapor-coolant or evaporation technique uses ethyl chloride or fluorimethane sprayed on the area to be treated. A modest frost, accomplished by holding the spray container approximately 1½ feet from the area for 15 to 20 seconds, is well tolerated. Repeating this two or three times at short intervals should produce analgesia. Stretching and deep tissue massage for relief of pain in trigger points can then be performed.

Ice packs, bags, or compresses can be applied to an area for 5 minutes or longer in acute sprains.[3] Repeating this at 10-minute intervals two or three times will often be effective.

Immersion of a limb in ice water may be tolerated for only 1 minute. If repeated with intervals similar to those noted for ice packs, it may be equally effective.

Cooling pads, or blankets attached to pumps of cooling liquid such as saline or alcohol, may be applied for several hours and are an effective means of lowering body temperature. This is used at times for spinal cord–injured patients.

Summary

The physiologic effects of superficial heat are subcutaneous vasodilation and elevation of metabolism in cellular and extracellular compartments. Deep heat may elevate muscle temperature. The analgesic, spasmolytic, anti-inflammatory, and soporific effects of heat are the major indications for its use.

Cold is anti-inflammatory, analgesic, antipyretic, and capable of reducing spasticity. It depresses physiologic activity by reducing the heart and respiratory rate and can lead to coma and death.

ULTRAVIOLET RADIATION[50]
Biophysics

Ultraviolet rays range from 180 to 400 nm. The range closest to the visual is identified as UVA (3600 to 4000 Å). Ultraviolet rays have properties similar to those of other electromagnetic waves but differ by having photons of greater energy. The quantum of energy of a photon is directly related to its frequency and is expressed by the equation $E = hn$ or energy in ergs equals Planck's constant h (6.625×10^{-25} erg sec) times the frequency per second. The energy of the ultraviolet photon is therefore several times greater than that of visible light or infrared. Ultraviolet rays penetrate only to the capillary bed of the dermis and cause photochemical changes. Infrared effect is essentially molecular excitation or heat.

Ultraviolet energy varies with different wavelengths. The action spectra indicate the most efficient wavelength for specific biologic effects. These effects are accomplished by either direct or indirect reactions.

Direct reactions occur when the absorbing molecule, such as melanin, changes chemically or a photosensitizer is raised to a higher energy state capable of enhancing the activity of other compounds. Photosensitizers may be foods, drugs, or disease toxins. PUVA therapy (psoralen, a photosensitizer taken by mouth, followed by exposure to ultraviolet irradiation) is recommended for psoriasis.

The indirect effect is the transduction of light energy, such as visible light to photoreceptors in the retina. Neural signals in neuroendocrine pathways and neurotransmitters in the hypothalamus, spinal cord, pituitary, and pineal body can depress the synthesis and secretion of melatonin in the blood and cerebrospinal fluid. This results in elevation of hormonal activity in the pituitary, ovaries, adrenal, and other endocrine glands and can produce estrus.

Physiology[15]

Penetration of ultraviolet rays is approximately 0.1 mm, varying with skin thickness and coloring. The absorbing substances in the skin are proteins or nucleic acid. The photochemical reactions may be erythema, tanning, epithelialization, bactericidal effects, vitamin D_3 synthesis, and neurohumoral effects.

Erythema is noted within several hours after exposure. It is due to direct or thermal effects on capillaries and the possible release of denatured proteins into the prickle layer of the skin. The action spectrum for erythema is 2500 Å to 2970 Å, and none is produced beyond 3300 Å. This response is used for dosage control. The minimal erythemal dose is the minimal time of exposure that gives the faintest reddening effect 4 hours later and clears in 24 hours.

Tanning is the increase of melanin granules in the prickle cell layer, which contains the keratinocytes. Within a few minutes after photo-oxidation, melanocytes divide and secrete melanosome bodies, which contain the melanin granules and deposit them in the keratinocyte layer. This is immediate tanning and reaches a maximum in 1 hour. Delayed tanning, which involves an increase in functioning melanocytes, occurs in 72 hours. Their number, size, and transfer to keratinocytes produce the delayed tanning. The action spectrum is between 3000 and 4400 Å. After 2 to 3 days the tan fades as the keratinocytes slough off. Tanning may provide some protection against later ultraviolet exposure.

Epithelialization or cornification results from accelerated cell division of the epidermis. With excessive exposure, this may progress to desquamation.

Bactericidal effects of ultraviolet rays occur in the 2600 Å range. The energy alters mitosis in some skin pathogens, causing lethal mutations. This effect can be beneficial in treating infected ulcers.

Vitamin D_3 (cholecalciferol) in the skin and subcutaneous tissue is formed when 7-dehydrocholesterol absorbs ultraviolet light. Wurtman[50] described the improved ability of an experimental group of men in a soldier's home to absorb calcium after daily ultraviolet irradiation. Using total body irradiation to modify osteomalacia is supported by other studies described in his article. Its use in geriatric practice should be encouraged.

The neurohumoral action of ultraviolet light is described above. The relationship of this action to the seasonal effects of sunlight on the reproduction cycle is but one example.

Toxic reactions

Burns result from overexposure to ultraviolet light, usually from wavelengths in the 3200 Å (ultraviolet B).

Sunburn may result from ignorance that ultraviolet rays can penetrate light overcast clouds and be reflected from sand, snow, or water. The action spectrum for sunburn is 2500 to 2790 Å. Common complications in addition to the burn are conjunctivitis and photophthalmia. The sensitivity of the conjunctiva and retina to natural and artificial ultraviolet requires eye shields or protective goggles.

It is better to prevent sunburn than to treat it. The application of a sunscreen that filters ultraviolet A reduces the likelihood of burn.

Ultraviolet A (3900 to 3200 Å) tans; ultraviolet B (3200 to 2900 Å) burns. After para-aminobenzoic acid (PABA) is applied topically before exposure, ultraviolet B is essentially blocked. Some broad-spectrum screens additionally contain oxybenzene, which blocks ultraviolet A.

Prolonged or excessive exposure can age skin or cause skin cancer.

Special protection should be exercised for exposure of the eyes, lips, and nipples. The length of time one can tolerate sunlight depends on one's native skin tolerance. Sensitivity, general health, age, medications, and nutrition also affect tolerance. The latitude, time of year, time of day, and weather should be considered, since each affects the ultraviolet radiation intensity.

Dry skin, as occurs after frequent exposure to sunlight and excessive washing, should also be recognized as a possible cause of greater reactions to sunlight. Photosensitizers to ultraviolet light are listed in the box on p. 780.

The effects of overexposure or sensitivity to ultraviolet light are as follows:

1. Pain
2. Edema
3. Bulla formation
4. Fever, chills, weakness
5. Conjunctivitis and photophthalmia
6. Desquamation
7. Infection
8. Shock, possible death
9. Cancer; wavelengths between 2800 and 3400 Å are carcinogenic, particularly with chronic exposure

Sources

The artificial sources of ultraviolet light are carbon or mercury arc lamps where electrons from carbon electrodes or a tungsten cathode ionize gases (argon, krypton, neon, or mercury vapor). These emit wavelengths that have a high concentration in the ultraviolet range. They are either under low pressure (cold quartz) where the electron temperature is higher than the mercury vapor temperature or high pressure (hot quartz) where these are equal.

The envelope may be quartz, fused quartz, high silicate, or calcium phosphate glass. Some are coated with phosphors (tungstates, silicates, borates, or phosphates of magnesium, calcium, cadmium, or zinc). These phosphors fluoresce and reemit ultraviolet wavelengths of broader bands including visible rays. A reflector directs and concentrates the rays.

PHOTOSENSITIZERS OF ULTRAVIOLET LIGHT

I. Diseases
  A. Endocrine
    1. Insulin
    2. Thyroxine
    3. Adrenalin
    4. Pituitrin
  B. Metabolic
    1. Pellagra
    2. Erythropoietic protoporphyria
    3. Porphyria
  C. Vasculitis
    1. Scleroderma
    2. Lupus—systemic, discoid
    3. Polyarteritis nodosa
    4. Polyvinyl chloride
II. Infections
  A. Herpes
  B. Tuberculosis
III. Cardiorenal failure
IV. Dermatologic diseases
  A. Eczema
  B. Urticaria solaris
  C. Hereditary xeroderma
  D. Vitiligo, albinism
  E. Epidermolysis bullosa
V. Drugs
  A. Eosin
  B. Perfumes
  C. Green soap
  D. Coal tar
  E. Antibiotics
    1. Tetracyclines
    2. Riboflavin, griseofulvin, nalidixic acid
    3. Methotrexate
    4. Quinine
    5. Phenylbutazone
  F. Phenothiazines
    1. Chlorpromazine, prochlorperazine (Compazine), trifluoperazine (Stelazine), chlordiazepoxide (Librium)
    2. Barbiturates
    3. Heavy metals: gold, mercury, iron, bismuth
    4. Phenothiazines
    5. Chlorthiazides (Hydrodiuril)
    6. Estrogens and progesterones, cyclamates)
    7. Sulfonylurea (Orinase, Diabinese)

High-pressure hot quartz lamps have a broad spectrum and produce bactericidal effects (2537 Å), erythema (2500 to 2970 Å), or pigmentation (3400 Å). A cooling jacket of circulating air or water (Kromayer lamps) permits close approximation of the lamp to the skin.

Ninety percent of the radiation from cold quartz mercury lamps has a wavelength of 2537 Å (bactericidal). These are used when air sterilization is desired. A sodium barium silicate with nickel oxide glass (Wood's filter), with a low-pressure cold quartz lamp, transmits rays of 3700 to 3800 Å. This causes hair infected with tinea capitis to fluoresce a bright green. Hair with pediculosis capitis or pubis similarly fluoresces.

Professional models are large, gas-filled tubes. They cover greater areas and are used for general irradiation. Narrow tubes, straight or wound into coils, are available for orificial or sinus tract irradiation.

Sunlamps are silica glass tubes coated with phosphors. They are usually several bulbs in a reflector and are available for home or solarium use. They produce a spectrum of 2800 to 3500 Å and cause erythema and mild pigmentation. The use of such lamps without eye protection has caused severe eye problems. These episodes have occurred in commercial tanning facilities where appropriate precautions were not exercised.

Indications

The application of ultraviolet therapy is for bactericidal effect, enhancing calcium metabolism, or treating psoriasis or neonatal jaundice.

Bactericidal effect

Using ultraviolet irradiation adjunctively for routine wound care often helps resolve refractory or indolent wounds, such as decubiti or varicose ulcers. After the areas are cleansed with saline or a medicated whirlpool, local ultraviolet irradiation is applied four or five times daily to reduce bacterial infection and encourage epithelialization. As epithelium develops at the edges of the wound area, the time and frequency of the exposure are reduced. A shield around the edges of the wound to avoid burning the developing epithelium is necessary.

Enhancement of calcium metabolism

The beneficial effects of ultraviolet irradiation on calcium and vitamin D metabolism suggest that general body irradiation in elderly infirm patients should be considered. It is a relatively inexpensive technique and may reduce the problems of osteopenia.

Treatment of psoriasis and icterus neonatorum

Parrish and co-workers[37] described the use of PUVA: a photosensitizer (8-methoxypsoralen) followed 2 hours later by 10-minute exposure to ultraviolet light (3650 Å). After several exposures the psoralen as a photosensitizer enhances lymphocyte chromosomal abnormalities and epidermal reactions such that the skin lesions are cleared. It is more acceptable than the previously employed coal tar ultraviolet treatment.[19]

A modification of this technique employs sunlight filtered through 0.005-inch mylar plastic. Patients are exposed for 3 hours, from 11 AM to 2 PM, 2 days a week. Two to 3 hours before exposure the patient is given 40 mg of 8-methoxypsoralen. Bruce and Walters[5] reported that 22 of 23 patients with histories of the disease for 10 to 24 years had complete clearing of their lesions.

Bilirubin can be bleached and destroyed by ultraviolet light.[9] The mechanism is complex. It is possibly an intermediate reaction of photosensitization of circulating riboflavin to enhance albumin binding the bilirubin. Neonatal hyperbilirubinemia is significantly modified by exposing affected infants to ultraviolet light.

Contraindications

The toxic photosensitizing effects of food, diseases, or drugs are the contraindications for using ultraviolet irradiation.

Prescription

Dosage initially requires establishing the minimal erythemal dose (MED). The MED is usually 15 seconds for a standard high-pressure mercury arc quartz burner. An exposure, usually on the volar surface of the forearm, produces a mild erythema or first-degree erythema after 2 hours. The erythema disappears in 24 hours.

Dosages are in multiples of the MED and are written as, for example, 3 MED or 4 MED. Treatment is usually on alternate days so any concomitant erythema may subside.

Summary

Ultraviolet light produces photochemical reactions in and on the skin. In rehabilitation medicine it is employed for bactericidal and vitamin D_3 production. Its employment in treating psoriasis and hyperbilirubinemia of infancy suggest possibilities for a greater application in clinical medicine using specific photosensitizers.

ELECTROTHERAPY

At present the clinical applications of electrotherapy are for motor disturbances, pain, pacemakers, functional electrical stimulation, biofeedback, electrophoresis or phonophoresis, and diagnosis.

Motor disturbances[46]

Denervated muscle demonstrates histologic changes analogous to atrophy of disuse. These include decrease in fiber diameter, proliferation of sarcolemmal nuclei, loss of striation patterns (late in atrophy), thickening of intramuscular arteries, and venous stasis. Later there is increase in connective tissue and finally, after several years, dissolution of muscle fibers, with residual fat, blood vessel, and connective tissue replacement into the area.

If reinnervation occurs within the first year, a fairly good functional recovery may be achieved. If the atrophy can be retarded, the degree of recovery may be increased.

Medical and surgical management of peripheral neuropathies has improved the prognosis for many patients with lesions previously considered incapable of recovery.

The inclusion of a program of electrical stimulation can enhance recovery and reduce the changes described. Ten to 15 isometric contractions in the muscle under slight tension, using a current delivering 1000 to 2000 cycles/sec and repeating these three or four times daily, 5 days a week, is recommended. Denervated muscles respond to frequencies of 10 to 30 cycles/sec or an interrupted galvanic (DC) current. The treatment is similar for innervated muscles.

Home stimulators are available, and self-treatments should be encouraged, since such programs may extend for many months. However, the benefits of these programs over longer periods is questionable. As a maintenance measure, with its concomitant circulatory and tensing benefit on residual muscle fibers and their attachments, electrotherapy's benefit is still to be proved.

Pain control

Percutaneous high-frequency currents have been used to relieve pain for many years. Applying currents up to 80 milliamperes at frequencies of 80 to 180 Hz over painful areas, dermatomes, or distal sites may suppress pain. Fifteen to 30 minutes of application may be effective for 24 hours of pain suppression.

Melzack and Wall's description of the gate theory with these currents shutting the gate was initially proposed as an explanation.[32,48] Now we are trying to relate the effect on suppression of inflammatory effectors such as the prostaglandins. Another possibility is the effect on neuroendocrines such as enkephalin and endorphins. No comprehensive explanation has been forthcoming. These devices are applied at times for 24 hours. Excoriation of the skin, as well as habituation similar to that observed with narcotics, may occur.

The effectiveness of electrotherapy varies. Success has been claimed in a wide variety of syndromes, but hard data supporting its effectiveness are not yet forthcoming. The technique is no more successful than any other effort, either in acute or chronic pain situations. The decision to use it should be carefully considered, and the patient would probably best be served if it were not prescribed at all.

Artificial pacemakers

Stimulating the phrenic nerve[40] as a respiratory aid and stimulating the bladder detrusor for micturition or anal sphincter for incontinence control have been successful.

These techniques are limited by the tissue tolerance for the electrodes and the problems of power source.

Functional electrical stimulation[21]

Functional electrical stimulation is the stimulation of paralyzed muscles to produce muscular contraction or useful movement. Initially it was employed on paralyzed patients with the objective of restoring lost movement using surface electrodes on leg muscles of patients with hemiplegia and footdrop. This was offered as an alternative to the use of orthoses. At present a multichannel electric stimulation device to mobilize paraplegics is being evaluated.[24] The technique also has been attempted in multiple sclerosis, in cerebral palsy, and for hand functions in selected patients.

The application of functional electrical stimulation requires a trained staff and prolonged training of patients. Adequate maintenance service is required when necessary. These requirements limit application to patients who have the necessary medical and technical services available. The limited tolerance of the skin to the repeated local chemical actions at the electrode site remains a limiting factor. A detailed description of the technique is to be found in the noted reference.[21]

Biofeedback

Biofeedback[25,42] is the training technique that attempts to modify autonomic functions, pain, and motor disturbances by acquired volitional control. It is a form of behavior modification. Using monitors that demonstrate electrical activity on a screen or with audioamplification may help a patient acquire the ability to lower blood pressure; slow pulse rate, respiration, and spasticity; recover or control motor functions; or eliminate pain. Many patients cannot succeed in these efforts. Furthermore, some of these functions are beyond conscious control and limit the use of this technique.

Coupling a patient to an electromyograph so that the sight and sound of action potentials are presented, and using these stimuli to restore conscious control of motor function, is reinforcement or muscle reeducation. When used in treating hysteric paralysis or selected cases of paresis for varied neuromuscular-musculoskeletal disorders, it may enhance recovery.

The staff, equipment, and time required to provide this training restrict it to programs where staff and time are available.

Iontophoresis

Iontophoresis drives molecules into the skin by ion transfer with direct current. The necessity, effectiveness, or value of this technique is limited by the drug's chemical characteristics, ionic charge, and penetrability through the skin. The recent development of drug patches for absorbing medications limits these techniques. Harris' description and critique is recommended to the interested reader.[23]

MASSAGE[11,16]

When intelligently applied, massage is an effective modality for relieving pain or reducing swelling or muscle tightness. It is most frequently employed for soft tissue injuries.

Technique

The manual movements in massage include stroking (effleurage), compression and pretrissage, and percussion (tapotement rhythmically striking the underlying tissue). These movements can be augmented with machines attached to the hand or by machines alone. The pressure and force applied can be varied and should be guided by the diagnosis and tolerances of the patient and the part being massaged.

Physiologic effects[49]

Hyperemia from the frictional effects on the skin is the most notable physiologic effect of massage. An analgesic effect may be related to hypotensive effect of the skin hyperemia.

Pressure on intravascular and extravascular compartments may produce an increased rate of fluid movement. Whether kneading or deep pressure breaks up fibrositic nodules is questionable. Light stroking or fingertip massage over muscle tendon or ligament is often effective in relieving pain and permits subsequent stretching to a greater extent.

The relaxing, soporific effects of massage are widely recognized. This may be an effective means of relieving muscle spasm, tightness, or "tension." The explanation of this effect remains empiric, since such reactions are not universal. Cost containment often forces us to use tranquilizers, relaxants, soporifics, analgesics, or anti-inflammatory drugs where massage might be as effective.

Indications

Soft tissue injuries with pain, stiffness, spasm, and muscle tension are the usual disorders for which massage is ordered. Articular pain, with or without swelling, can also be helped, as can arterial or venous insufficiency. Scars may be loosened. Massage after exercise, stretching, or vigorous activities is often beneficial in relieving pain and stiffness.

Contraindications

Patients with infection, hemorrhagic or clotting disorders, or inflammatory disease of muscle should not receive massage.

MANIPULATION[33]

Manipulation is stretching of periarticular tissues bimanually along the anatomic axis of a muscle or across a joint. It differs from stretching and traction in that it is a brief application of a distracting force with sharp pressure above and below the region treated. Prior application of heat, massage, and rest increases its effectiveness.

The benefit of manipulation in refractory problems of neck and back pain cannot be discounted. When correctly employed on properly selected and prepared patients, the procedure often is very effective.

STRETCHING AND TRACTION[10,28]

Stretching and traction produce a lengthening of periarticular soft tissues, tendons, or muscles by manual or mechanical means. Application in chronic problems where motion is incomplete is the only effective measure, other than surgery, that may restore full arcs of motion. Dynamic splinting of selective areas such as tight finger flexors is often effective as a stretching technique.

The contraindications are acute inflammation, painful sprains or strains, fracture, or other acute painful musculoskeletal, articular, vascular, or skin diseases.

The technique of stretching is the application of a stretching movement, using the patient's body mass as a counterforce. Knowledge of the anatomy of the tight structure, be it muscle, tendon, or joint capsule, defines the desired direction of the forces. Thermotherapy, massage, an analgesic, or anti-inflammatory medication before traction enhance its effectiveness and increase the extent and patient tolerance of the procedure.

Preparation of the patient for traction is similar to that for stretching. A counterforce of up to 50 pounds applied to the neck, or 75 to 100 pounds to the pelvis, is used to stretch periarticular soft tissue.

• • •

Detailed descriptions of the techniques and applications of each of the modalities discussed can be found in available manuals. Referral to registered physical and occupational therapists is recommended, since their skill and training ensure optimal and efficient care. Their role as instructor and supervisor of assistants, aides, family, and patient is invaluable and can save time and reduce costs.[14]

DIAGNOSTIC TESTS

The monitoring of energy transduction requires a sensor that can demonstrate the energy on a visual record or meter. The energy may be from the body's surface as in thermography or dermohmetry or fluorescence as in the ultraviolet effect on the lesions of ringworm, or after injection of a fluorescent material in a limb with circulatory impairment.

Imposing an energy such as ultrasound onto the body provides a technique for sonography where the varying densities of the tissue transmit differently to a sensor that converts these variations to visual records.

Applying heat or cold can affect blood pressure, change

action potentials as in myasthenia gravis, or alter neurologic signs as in multiple sclerosis.

Reactions of nerve and muscle to electrical stimuli of varying strength and duration can be used to establish the strength/duration curve with the chronaxie rheobase values.

Thermography

A thermograph scans the skin and records on film the emitted infrared radiation intensities. The details of the technique are described by Barnes.[1]

The merit of thermography is its safety: the patient is not exposed to any ionizing radiation or invasive component. The ability to visualize vascular and inflammatory reactions not otherwise easily assessed or scaled is another merit of this test. An obliterative lesion can be easily identified without any contrast media required, and repeating the study after therapy can provide a record of results.

Infrared photography is a simpler, less expensive technique that monitors energy at shorter wavelengths.

Dermohmetry[29]

Dermohmetry is an electrical test of skin resistance. The conductivity of the skin is reflected by a change in current flow that occurs with any disorder of autonomic controls. Direct current with constant voltage increases or decreases with a change in skin resistance. When a meter is calibrated for measurement in ohms, dry cold skin averages 1 megohm and moist, warm skin is in the range of 1 to 2000 ohms. The data from the affected area is compared with data from unaffected areas. Dermohmetry is easy to perform, and the equipment is not expensive. Disease, such as peripheral neuropathy, that produces vasomotor change results in elevated skin resistance.

Skin resistance should be lowered by warming and wetting before electrotherapy or testing. The least amperage is then required and discomfort is reduced.

Fluorescence

The employment of the fluorescent effect of ultraviolet through Wood's filter in the diagnosis of ringworm is described above.

The use of intravenous injection of fluorescent dye in diagnosis of vascular disease has been replaced by arteriography and venography. However, its low incidence of local or systemic reactions makes it a method of choice in selected situations.

Temperature changes
Heat

Raising body temperature in a patient with neuromuscular disease alters axonal and end-plate activity. Multiple sclerosis[39] patients have a notable sensitivity to heat and this is used as a provocative test; the patient exposed to heat frequently develops signs such as nystagmus, increased reflexes, or sensory losses that otherwise were not noted.

These reactions are not exclusive to patients with demyelinating disease and are often described by patients with other nervous system disorders.

Cold

The repetitive stimulation test in myasthenia gravis elicits a decrement of the action potentials after the third to fifth stimulus. The potentials are restored by cooling the muscle and are decreased with warming, suggesting that quanta of transmitter substance may be stored with cooling[13] or degradation enhanced with the heat of contraction activity.

Low volt testing[18,31]

Low volt testing records the strength and duration of stimuli that elicit a minimal twitch of a muscle. The stimuli are applied either to the nerve or, in denervation, to the muscle belly.

Recording the values on a graph provides a curve for each with their different values. The details of the method of performing the test are described by Goodgold and Eberstein.[20] The test is somewhat uncomfortable but is relatively simple to perform, readily reproduceable, and noninvasive. It has largely been replaced by electromyographic studies, but there are occasions when it may be employed. When used in the third or fourth week after onset of paralysis, this technique may provide adequate data in pediatric patients with facial palsy and does not require needle insertions.

PRESCRIPTION WRITING
Goals

In all plans for therapy the hierarchy of goals is (1) palliation, (2) prevention, and (3) correction. These goals are equally applicable in medicine, surgery, psychiatry, and physiatry. They are evident when therapy is being prescribed. Often physical therapy precedes the other rehabilitation modalities in any prescription.

The initial goal in any therapeutic endeavor is to palliate. For example, a prescription for physical therapy for postdislocation capsulitis of the right shoulder would read as follows:

Diagnosis: Post dislocation capsulitis (R) shoulder
 ℞: 1. Thermotherapy 20 min. (R) shoulder
   2. Gentle passive stretching (R) shoulder
   3. Active assistive exercise (pulley)
   4. Instruct patient in home program.
    3 × wkly 2 wks, 2 × wkly 3 wks

This example reflects the role of thermotherapy as a palliative measure before the passive stretching and active exercises. Also, the importance of instructing the patient and family in the home program is reflected in this prescription.

The first order in this prescription was deliberately written "Thermotherapy." This allows for either heat or cold to be applied, and heat may be radiant (infrared), diathermy, ul-

trasound, moist packs, or other heating agents. Where specific agents are necessary, they should be spelled out. This might then be written "Ultrasound 10 min. 1.5 watts/cm. sq." or "I.R. at 30 inches for 20 min."

As another example, the following prescription might be written for a patient with radial palsy and wristdrop:

Diagnosis: Radial palsy (post compression), wristdrop
 ℞: (1) Moist packs 10 min. forearm (R)
   (2) D.C. stimulation to wrist/finger extensors 15 min.
   (3) Passive stretch shoulder, elbow, wrist/finger joints
   (4) Cock-up splint
   (5) Shoulder arm sling
   (6) Instruct in (a) home low volt stim technique
        (b) stretching
   (7) Instruct in A.D.L.—writing
    Daily 1 wk, 2 × wkly 2 wks, 1 × wkly 2 wks

The objective of cost containment can be met only when the patient or family is trained to assume responsibility for the daily treatments they can perform.

In this prescription "moist heat" is employed both for palliative purposes and for reduction of skin resistance before application of electrical stimulation to artificially mobilize the paretic muscles. The exercises here are made possible by use of the electrical stimulation. Stretching, splints, sling, and activities of daily living instructions follow the initial palliative and preventive objectives to reduce atrophy, paresis, and contractures.

Diagnosis: S/P below knee amputation (R)
Etiology: Diabetes mellitus, peripheral arterial thrombosis—gangrene. Flexion contracture stump.
 ℞: 1. Radiant heat 30″ 15 min. (R) knee
   2. Gentle passive stretch hamstring
   3. Strengthening exercises quadriceps
   4. Instruct patient in quad setting exercises
   5. Splint to knee to maintain extension range
   6. Crutch walking 20 ft
    Daily 1 wk, 3 × weekly 2 wks, 2 × wkly 3 wks
Caution: Observe skin for any thermal reaction i.e., erythema, blistering. [In all prescriptions, cautions must be noted particularly where anesthetic areas or arterial insufficiency exists. Here the arterial insufficiency and possible hypalgesia of the skin could cause a burn, but this is unlikely to happen because the area being heated can be observed and appropriate reduction of time of exposure made. Were a hot pack employed, this visual monitoring would be denied the therapist.]

All three examples demonstrate the therapeutic goals of palliation, prevention, and correction. They include the application of the modality heat as a palliative or as a means to increase the extensibility of inelastic collagen in tendon or capsule.

The electrical stimulation of paretic muscles retards muscle atrophy and also acts to maintain some kinesthetic sense.

Therefore this is used as a preventive measure.

Correction in the three examples is achieved by exercises and training in self-care. Modalities do not correct any disorder, but stretching, exercises, functional training, and use of appliances or apparatus may correct or substitute for any physical or functional deficiencies imposed by the disorder or physiologic impairment.

The most challenging problem to physicians is that of chronic pain. Acute pain can be dealt with quite effectively by any practitioner, but chronic disabling pain requires the involvement of a team that includes the physiatrist. Modalities such as heat, cold, transcutaneous electrical nerve stimulation, massage, stretching, and exercises are all employed individually or in combination with medications and possibly surgery and counseling. This is described in more detail in Chapter 37.

PRECAUTIONS

The following precautions should be taken before any therapy:

1. Diagnosis. Pathology, age, nutrition, and physiologic problems of cardiopulmonary sensory systems should all be identified and considered when determining the duration, frequency, and number of treatment sessions. Anaesthesia is not a contraindication but requires a careful monitoring.
2. Comprehension. The patient must demonstrate understanding of what the treatment involves and how to signal if discomfort develops.
3. Equipment. All wires, heating elements, bulbs, switches, dials, and timers must be in working state and in the off or zero position when treatment is started and ended. Apparatus should be unplugged when not in use. Only Underwriter's Laboratory approved equipment should be used.

The following general rules apply when ordering physical therapy:

1. Do not use physical therapy if medication, surgery, or psychiatry is more effective.
2. Select the simplest, safest, least complicated modality, requiring the minimal involvement of personnel.
3. Use a device that allows easy observation of the treated part.
4. Use home therapy whenever possible.
5. Have specific goals.
6. Limit the number of treatments, and if no benefits are noted, consider these measures.
   a. Repeating the series
   b. Reviewing the procedure to ensure that it conforms to your order
   c. Changing the dosage or frequency (two or three times daily, 5 or more days a week)
   d. Discontinuing the treatment

REFERENCES

1. Barnes, RB: Thermography and its clinical application, Ann NY Acad Sci 121:34, 1964.
2. Baruch, S: An epitome of hydrotherapy, Philadelphia, 1920, WB Saunders Co.
3. Basur, RL, Shephard, E, and Mouzas, GL: A cooling method in the treatment of ankle sprains, Practitioner, 216:708, 1976.
4. Brauer, RW, et al: The liver in hypothermia, Ann NY Sci 80:390, 1959.
5. Bruce, WW, and Walters, LT: PUVA: using filtered sunlight as an energy source, Cutis 20:59, 1977.
6. Bryan, P, Furman, S, and Escher, DJ: Input signals to pacemakers in a hospital environment, Ann NY Acad Sci 167:823, 1969.
7. Castor, CW: Connective tissue activation: the effects of temperature studied in vitro, Arch Phys Med Rehabil 57:5, 1976.
8. Chatfield, PO: Hypothermia and its effects on the sensory and peripheral motor systems, Ann NY Acad Sci 80:445, 1959.
9. Cremer, RK, Perryman, PW, and Richard, PM: The influence of light on the hyperbilirubinaemia of infants, Lancet 1:1094, 1958.
10. Crisp, EJ: Manipulation of the spine. In Licht, SH, editor: Massage, manipulation and traction, New Haven, Conn, 1960, S Licht & E Licht, Publisher.
11. Cyriax, JH: Clinical application of massage. In Licht, SH, editor: Massage, manipulation and traction, New Haven, Conn, 1960, S Licht & E Licht, Publisher.
12. deLateur, BJ, et al: Muscle heating in human subjects with 915 MHz microwave contact applicator, Arch Phys Med Rehabil 51:147, 1970.
13. Desmedt, JE, and Borenstein, S: Diagnosis of myasthenia gravis by nerve stimulus, Ann NY Acad Sci 274:174, 1976.
14. Downer, AH: Physical therapy procedures, Springfield, Ill, 1974, Charles C Thomas, Publisher.
15. Fischer, F, and Solomon, S: Physiologic effects of ultraviolet radiation. In Licht, SH, editor: Therapeutic electricity and ultraviolet radiation, Baltimore, 1967, S Licht & E Licht, Waverly Press, Inc.
16. Francun, F: Classical massage technique. In Licht, SH, editor: Massage, manipulation and traction, New Haven, Conn, 1960, S Licht & E Licht, Publisher.
17. Gerstein, JW: Effect of ultrasound on tendon extensibility, Am J Phys Med 34:362, 1955.
18. Gilliatt, RW: Nerve conduction: motor and sensory. In Licht, SH, editor: Electrodiagnosis and electromyography, New Haven, Conn, 1961, S Licht & E Licht, Publisher.
19. Goeckerman, WH: Treatment of psoriasis, Northwest Med 24:229, 1925.
20. Goodgold, J, and Eberstein, A: Strength duration curve. In Electrodiagnosis of neuromuscular diseases, Baltimore, 1972, Williams & Wilkins Co.
21. Gracanin, F: Functional electrical stimulation. In Kottke, FJ, Stillwell, GK, and Lehmann, JF, editors: Krusen's handbook of physical medicine and rehabilitation, ed 3, Philadelphia, 1982, WB Saunders Co.
22. Green, DE: A framework of principles for the unification of bioenergetics, Ann NY Acad Sci 227:6, 1974.
23. Harris, R: Iontophoresis. In Licht, SH, editor: Therapeutic electricity and ultraviolet radiation, ed 2, New Haven, Conn, 1967, Elizabeth Licht, Publisher.
24. Reference deleted in proofs.
25. Jacobs, A, and Felton, GS: Visual feedback of myoelectric output to facilitate muscle relaxation in normal persons and patients with neck injuries, Arch Phys Med Rehabil 50:34, 1969.
26. Lehmann, JF, and deLateur, BJ: Cryotherapy. In Lehmann, JF, editor: Therapeutic heat and cold, ed 3, Baltimore, 1982, Williams & Wilkins Co.
27. Lehmann, JF, and deLateur, BJ: Diathermy and superficial heat and cold therapy, ultrasound. In Kottke, FJ, Stillwell, GK, and Lehmann, JF, editors: Krusen's handbook of physical medicine and rehabilitation, ed 3, Philadelphia, 1982, WB Saunders Co.

28. Leslie Doran, DM: Manipulation of joints and extremities. In Licht, SH, editor: Massage, manipulation and traction, New Haven, Conn, 1960, S Licht & E Licht, Publisher.

29. Licht, S: Electrical skin resistance. In Licht, SH, editor: Electrodiagnosis and electromyography, New Haven, Conn, 1961, S Licht & E Licht, Publisher.

30. Lippold, OCJ, Nicholls, JG, and Redfearn, JWT: A study of the afferent discharge produced by cooling a mammalian muscle spindle, J Physiol 153:218, 1960.

31. Lovelace, RE, and Myers, SJ: Nerve conduction and synaptic transmission. In Downey, JA, and Darling, RC, editors: Physiological basis of rehabilitation medicine, Philadelphia, 1971, WB Saunders Co.

32. Melzak, R, and Wall, PD: Pain mechanism: a new theory, Science 150:971, 1965.

33. Mennell, J: Joint manipulation. In Kiernander, B, editor: Physical medicine and rehabilitation, Oxford, Eng, 1939, Blackwell Scientific Publications.

34. Michalski, WJ, and Seguin, JJ: The effect of muscle cooling and stretch on muscle spindle secondary endings in the cat, J Physiol 253:341, 1975.

35. Millard, JB: Conductive heating. In Licht, S, and Licht, E, editors: Therapeutic heat, Baltimore, 1965, Waverly Press, Inc.

36. Nightingale, A: Physics and electronics in physical medicine, New York, 1959, The Macmillan Co.

37. Parrish, JA, et al: Photochemistry of psoriasis with oral methoxsalen and longwave ultraviolet light, N Engl J Med 291:1207, 1974.

38. Raymond, U, et al: Fractionated doses of hyperthermia and radiotherapy in the management of malignant neoplasms, Paper presented at the Third International Symposium: Cancer Therapy, Fort Collins, Colo, June 22-26, 1980, Colorado State University.

39. Rose, AS, et al: Criteria for the clinical diagnosis of multiple sclerosis, J Am Acad Neurol 28:21, 1976.

40. Sarnoff, SJ, Gaensler, EA, and Maloney, JV, Jr: Electrophrenic respiration. IV. The effectiveness of contralateral ventilation during activity of one phrenic nerve, J Thorac Surg 19:929, 1950.

41. Scotts, PM: Clayton's electrotherapy and actinotherapy, London, 1962, Bailliere, Tindall & Cox.

42. Shapiro, D, and Schwartz, GE: Biofeedback and visceral learning: clinical applications, Semin Psychiatry 4:171, 1972.

43. Shulman, AG: Ice water as primary treatment of burns, JAMA 173:1916, 1960.

44. Simons, DG: Muscle pain syndromes, Am J Phys Med 54:289, 1975; 55:15, 1976.

45. Smith, RM, and Stetson, JB: Therapeutic hypothermia. In Licht, S, and Licht, E, editors: Therapeutic heat, Baltimore, 1965, Waverly Press, Inc.

46. Stillwell, GK: Clinical electric stimulation. In Licht, SH, editor: Therapeutic electricity and ultraviolet radiation, ed 2, New Haven, Conn, 1967, Elizabeth Licht, Publisher.

47. Stoner, EK: Luminous and infrared heating. In Licht, S, and Licht, E, editors: Therapeutic heat, Baltimore, 1965, Waverly Press, Inc.

48. Wall, PD, and Sweet, WH: Temporary abolition of pain in man, Science 155:108, 1967.

49. Wood, EC, and Becker, PD: Bear's massage, ed 3, Philadelphia, 1981, WB Saunders Co.

50. Wurtman, PJ: The effects of light on the human body, Sci Am, July 1975, pp 69-77.

51. Zislis, JM: Hydrotherapy. In Krusen, FH, Kottke, FJ, and Elwood, E, editors: Handbook of physical medicine and rehabilitation, Philadelphia, 1966, WB Saunders Co.

CHAPTER 49

Communication disorders

PATRICIA KERMAN-LERNER

If all my possessions were taken from me with one exception, I would choose to keep the power of communication, for by it I would soon regain all the rest.

Daniel Webster

The ability to communicate, and specifically to use speech abstractly and in meaningful and unique contexts, is an integral part of being human. The primary goal of human communication is the accurate and rapid transfer of information through spoken, written, or gestural modes. The ability to share daily experiences, to communicate needs, wishes, and emotions, and to read and write depend on an extensively developed communication system. Since most of us have acquired our native verbal language with little voluntary effort, we are unaware of the complexities of human communication until we attempt to learn a second language or experience a communication breakdown. The beauty, intricacy, and versatility of language are taken for granted; however, if the communication process is impaired or lost, the damage can be devastating.

Communication impairment may involve any aspect of the hearing, language, or speech processes, and discussion of all possible communication disorders in this chapter would lead necessarily to superficial descriptions of each. Therefore only those speech and language disorders having a physical basis, specifically those that have a neurogenic cause and that are often encountered by rehabilitation professionals, are detailed here. Further, the focus is on those speech and language disorders that are not congenital but are acquired and are often seen in the adult population. This chapter is intended to provide the reader with theoretic information central to each major communication disorder, with a summary of traditional treatment approaches and highlights of some current technologic advances in diagnosis and treatment as they affect these communication disorders.

APHASIA AND APRAXIA

The most prevalent acquired language disorder with which the rehabilitation professional can expect to come into contact is *aphasia* (also called dysphasia). It has been estimated that nearly 2 million Americans have suffered a cerebral vascular accident, or stroke[76a]; of these, approximately two thirds are believed to have the resulting language deficit of aphasia.[3] Aphasia may also be a sequela of other neurologic insults including, but not limited to, head trauma, arteriovenous malformation, and tumor.

Aphasia is defined as the inability to express or comprehend language or both as a consequence of known neurologic impairment. It is an acquired impairment of language processes underlying the receptive and expressive modalities and is caused by focal damage, usually in the left cerebral cortex; occasionally it occurs following right hemispheric damage, especially in a left-handed individual. Recently, with the advances in neurodiagnostic procedures, aphasia is also being diagnosed as a result of known subcortical lesions.

Darley defines aphasia as an

impairment, as a result of brain damage, of the capacity for interpretation and formulation of language symbols; multimodality loss or reduction in efficiency of the ability to decode and encode conventional meaningful linguistic elements (morphemes and larger syntactic units); disproportionate to impairment of other intellectual functions; not attributable to dementia, confusion, sensory loss, or motor dysfunction; and manifested in reduced availability of vocabulary, reduced efficiency in application of syntactic rules, reduced auditory retention span, and impaired efficiency in input and output channel selection.*

---

*Darley, F: Aphasia, Philadelphia, 1982, WB Saunders Co.

Classification of aphasia

Rehabilitation professionals use many classification systems. None of these is totally satisfactory, but they are of value in our attempt to understand underlying pathology and linguistic disturbances. These classification systems provide us with additional information concerning language deficits, possible hierarchies of language recovery, and indicators of prognosis. A classification schema may also assist the speech-language pathologist in planning appropriate treatment goals and intervention strategies.

Over the past 125 years of modern aphasia history, aphasiologists have employed different classification systems. When the descriptions of such aphasias and their major subtypes are reviewed, language characteristics and lesion sites of these subtypes appear markedly similar despite their differences in terminology. Benson,[8] in his extensive work on modern aphasia history, summarizes the classification schemas and nomenclature employed by 21 aphasiologists spanning over 100 years. Although a complete description of the systems used by various aphasiologists goes beyond the scope of this chapter, we focus on one schema that gives us information on linguistic disintegration of language, as well as information on possible sites of lesion. Central to this classification is the character of the patient's speech output, which may be viewed as either *fluent* or *nonfluent*.[8,12,36]

In some aphasias, the flow of speech is impaired at the level of speech initiation, finding and sequencing of articulatory movements, and production of grammatical sequences. The resulting speech is limited, uttered slowly with great effort, and often poorly articulated. It is referred to as *nonfluent*. Often the prerolandic, anterior portion of the anatomic speech area—Broca's area—is involved. The contrasting or *fluent* forms of aphasia are marked by facility in articulation and many long strings of words in a variety of grammatical constructions. This fluidity is evidenced, however, in conjunction with word-finding difficulty for substantive nouns and picturable action words. Melody and prosody of the utterance are often preserved. The fluent aphasias are usually due to lesions posterior to the rolandic fissure, which spare Broca's area. The terms "fluent" and "nonfluent" are sometimes used interchangeably with "posterior" and "anterior," respectively, to characterize the major neuroanatomic subdivisions of the aphasias.

In addition to viewing verbal output along a continuum of fluency, other language features are important when identifying and describing specific subtypes of aphasia. The following system described by Goodglass and Kaplan[36] allows the clinician to view language disturbances in a holistic fashion and aids in our understanding of aphasia.

Broca's aphasia

Broca's aphasia is the most common nonfluent aphasia. It is characterized by slow, often awkward articulation; limited vocabulary; simplistic grammatical forms; and relative preservation of auditory comprehension. The patient's system may be telegraphic, containing only the information-bearing words and excluding the syntactic words of an utterance such as prepositions and conjunctions.

Written language is usually impaired at least as severely as speech, whereas reading may be only mildly affected. The patient with Broca's aphasia is often acutely aware of the language deficit.

Wernicke's aphasia

The most prevalent form of fluent aphasia is Wernicke's aphasia. A patient with Wernicke's aphasia may sound like a normal speaker from a distance because of the fluency and the normal melodic contour of his or her speech. The critical features of this syndrome include fluently articulated but paraphasic speech often accompanied by severely impaired auditory comprehension. Sound transpositions (literal paraphasias), such as "benkle" for "pencil," and word substitutions (verbal paraphasia), such as "crayon" for "pencil," may also be evidenced. Speech is usually rather facile in its motor output, but there are typically many errors of word choice and word ordering. Meaningless jargon may be present. Occasionally there is a press of speech with a vocal rate greater than normal. In both verbal and written production there is frequently a lack of substantive nouns and concrete action words. The patient exhibiting Wernicke's aphasia may be unaware of this language disorder.

Conduction aphasia

In conduction aphasia, repetition skills are severely disrupted. Furthermore, the severe impairment of the repetition component is disproportionate to the patient's good spontaneous speech and good auditory comprehension skills. The melodic pattern of the patient's utterance may be considered fluent or semifluent. This is a less commonly seen form of aphasia.

Anomia

The major feature of anomia, another type of fluent aphasia, is the prominence of word-finding difficulty in the context of fluent, grammatically well-articulated speech.

The patient with anomia usually has a less severe language disturbance and usually speaks freely, but with an emptiness of substantive words in oral output. Auditory comprehension is usually good; reading and writing skills are variable.

Global aphasia

Global aphasia, according to Collins,[18] is a severe impairment of communicative ability across all language modalities. Often, no single language modality is strikingly better than another. Nonverbal problem-solving abilities are often severely depressed and are usually compatible with language performance. At times the global aphasic produces stereotyped utterances that may consist of a few real or nonsense words. Some patients emit a continuous output of syllables that employ a limited set of vowel-consonant combinations that make no sense, even though they might be uttered with expressive intonation. Global aphasia usually results from extensive damage to the language zones of the left hemisphere but may also result from smaller subcortical lesions.

Transcortical aphasia

In contrast to conduction aphasia is transcortical aphasia, in which repetition is preserved out of proportion to the other language functions. This disorder has been subdivided into *transcortical motor aphasia, transcortical sensory aphasia,* and *mixed echolalia.* The major characteristic of transcortical motor aphasia is poor verbal output with good comprehension and repetition abilities. In transcortical sensory aphasia, poor comprehension abilities are evidenced with fluent but often irrelevant speech and good repetition skills. Mixed echolalia is characterized by poor comprehension abilities and poor verbal output but with good repetition skills.

Subcortical aphasia

The introduction of more sophisticated radiographic studies such as computerized tomography (CT) brain scans or magnetic resonance imaging has permitted aphasiologists to identify many new aphasias by correlating their predominantly subcortical lesion sites with clusters of speech and language behaviors.[42] Before these procedures became available, these aphasic syndromes often were unclassified because they tended to deviate from traditional speech and language patterns observed in the cortical aphasias.

Within the past few years, several subcortical aphasia syndromes have been described. Among these are *thalamic aphasia* and the *capsular-putamental aphasia,* which has three types—anterior, posterior, and global.[76] Anterior subcortical aphasias are characterized by sparse verbal output concomitant with severely impaired articulation and dysphonic speech. In contrast, a form of fluent aphasia has been observed with posterior subcortical lesions. Extensive subcortical lesions may produce a lasting global aphasia. Goodglass and Kaplan[36] observed that the resultant aphasia closely resembles Wernicke's aphasia. In some cases, repetition and comprehension are seemingly spared, whereas word finding and paraphasia difficulties are pronounced.

Table 49-1 summarizes aphasia classifications and prevailing symptoms.

Classification consistency

Not all aphasias fit neatly into a single classification schema. In fact, as Goodglass and Kaplan state, "depending on the rigor or looseness with which the definitions are applied, estimates of the proportion of cases that can be unambiguously classified range from 30% in some centers to 80% in others."[36] Actually, an exact syndrome is rare. The individual components of the syndrome may have a specific anatomic localization while linguistic variations in performance may exist. The syndromes that are named and described in this chapter represent the most regularly recurring patterns of language behavior secondary to damage within the language area. Variations of these syndromes occur, not only because lesions differ in location and extent, but because the response to the same injury is not fixed among individuals.[36]

Cerebral hemisphere function

The notion of a changing cerebral hemisphere dominance might partially explain the lack of consistency in correlation between site of lesion and aphasia subtype. Most traditional theories about the representation of language in the brain are based on the premise that cerebral dominance for language is specified at birth or completed in the early years of life, certainly by puberty.[60,61,65,115] An alternative possibility, hypothesized by Brown and Grober,[13] is that the lateralization of language continues over the life span. This theory is consistent with age-specific trends in aphasia type that have recently been reported in the literature. Brown and Jaffe,[14] in their review of clinical literature in aphasia, noted an age specificity for certain aphasic disorders.

For example, a lesion in Wernicke's area can produce motor aphasia in a child, conduction aphasia in middle age, and jargon aphasia in late life, suggesting a progressive differentiation of regional specification within the dominant hemisphere language area. Brain representation of language therefore appears to develop gradually from a diffuse, bilateral organization to a focal, unilateral one.

According to this theory, expression may lateralize earlier than comprehension. The more diffuse representation of production mechanisms in younger patients accounts for the occurrence of nonfluent aphasia with more widely distributed lesions. The relative preservation of comprehension abilities in these patients may reflect the contribution of the right hemisphere or of intact portions of the left.[13]

Consistent with the idea of progressive differentiation of brain representation within the life span, it may be noted that fluent aphasia, which usually has a sizable comprehension deficit, rarely occurs in young patients. Statistically, there is a high frequency of occurrence of fluent aphasia in late life. Presumably this reflects the fact that comprehension is becoming more restrictive to the left posterior language zone. Thus the degree of lateralization at the time of brain damage determines not only the occurrence but the type of aphasia. Nonfluent aphasia should predominate in younger patients or in subjects with relatively bilateral diffuse language representation, whereas fluent or jargon aphasia should occur in older patients or in subjects with more lateralized and focal representation. Obler and co-workers[80] found that the patients exhibiting Broca's aphasia tended to be younger, whereas patients with Wernicke's aphasia were frequently in the older age range.

The disorder of aphasia can also evolve from one sub-

Table 49-1. Summary of fluent and nonfluent aphasic language behaviors

Aphasia type	Lesion site	Fluency of spontaneous speech	Comprehension	Naming	Repetition	Paraphasias
Broca's, also known as motor, cortical-motor, verbal-efferent, motor-expressive	Posteroinferior frontal (subcortical white matter extending posteriorly to inferior portion of motor strip)	Nonfluent	Auditory comprehension relatively well preserved	Word-finding difficulty; naming better on confrontation; lexical level best preserved; most preserved in spontaneous speech	Better than self-generated; may do well on short utterance with a model	Semantic level: correct word choice. Phonemic level: awkward, stiff (contextual/associative cues help)
Wernicke's, also known as sensory, syntactic, receptive, acoustic	Posterior portion of first temporal gyrus	Fluent	Auditory comprehension impaired in comparison to fluency; reading comprehension impaired	Word-finding difficulty; naming paraphasic or jargonized; poorest in confrontation; impaired availability of specific names	Poor substitution of key words; intrusion of paraphasias with some neologisms and irrelevant insertions	Semantic level: word substitutions. Phonemic level: transpositions (literal paraphasias), neologisms
Conduction, also known as afferent-motor central	Posterosuperior temporal (supramarginal gyrus); arcuate fasciculus	Fluent	Good	Impaired to same degree as repetition	Very poor; intrusion of paraphasias; grammatical components more difficult	Semantic level: word substitutions. Phonemic level: transpositions
Anomia, also known as nominal, semantic, amnesic	Difficult to localize; temporal-parietal damage; angular gyrus	Fluent	Relatively good	Impaired naming, word-finding difficulty; circumlocutions	Good-normal	Semantic level: word substitutions well articulated; grammatical; circumlocutory
Transcortical motor	Borders Broca's area; supplemental speech area	Nonfluent	Good	May be fairly good	Good	
Transcortical sensory	Borders Wernicke's area	Fluent	Poor	Poor	Good (echolalic)	Like Wernicke's aphasia
Combined transcortical (sensorimotor); isolation	Can occur with above two lesions or central speech zone lesion	Nonfluent	Poor	Poor	Good (echolalic)	
Global	Central; can occur with anterior or posterior lesion	Nonfluent	Poor	Poor	Poor	

classification to another as time after onset increases and severity decreases. Thus the specific aphasia disorder is not always constant. The patient's language functioning may initially be diagnosed as symptomatic of a global aphasia yet may evolve during the first few months after onset toward a Broca's aphasia. Additionally, this patient may show improved auditory comprehension and verbal production abilities following a period of therapeutic intervention and later may evolve toward symptoms of an anomic or conduction aphasia.

Apraxia of speech

A disturbance that often accompanies aphasia is *apraxia* of speech, or dyspraxia. Although an in-depth discussion of apraxia is beyond the scope of this chapter, the following will provide the reader with information regarding the nature of apraxia and its symptoms.

Geschwind[34] defined apraxia as "a disorder of execution of learned movement which cannot be accounted for either by weakness, incoordination, or sensory loss, or by incomprehension of or inattention to commands." The patient with apraxia can hear and comprehend the requested commands and understands that he is physically capable of performing this task, but when he attempts performance, he cannot execute the movement or series of movements required to complete the requested task.

Verbal apraxia results from disturbed volitional, oral movements. Apraxia of speech is usually viewed as a non-dysarthric, nonaphasic sensorimotor disorder of articulation and prosody. Aphasia and dysarthria may coexist with apraxia of speech, but language deficits and impairments of muscle strength or endurance do not account for apraxic errors.[83] When used for reflexive and automatic acts, the apraxic patient's speech musculature does not show significant weakness, slowness, or incoordination. The patient is able to perform most vegetative and reflexive functions, such as coughing and chewing; however, functions needing a higher level of cortical integration, such as the production of sounds or words, are disrupted.

The speech pattern of the apraxic patient is characteristically slow and labored with numerous consonant and vowel articulatory errors. Articulatory errors include omissions, substitutions, distortions, and additions of speech sounds. Articulation tends to be inconsistent across trials; sounds are produced correctly on one occasion and distorted on other occasions.[49] Errors often increase as words increase in length. Errors appear to result from difficulties in motor execution and programming rather than of phonologic selection. The speaker is often aware of errors but is unable to anticipate or to correct them.

Appraisal of language disorders

The appraisal of language disorders with or without a concomitant apraxia includes the collection of data, encompassing medical evaluation, behavioral observations and testing, and linguistic analysis in varying communication contexts.

The collection of such data assists the professional in formulating a diagnosis, projecting a prognosis, and determining a treatment plan. It also provides important data that can validate a decision not to treat a patient. During the past 30 years a large number of formal diagnostic batteries have been devised for the assessment of aphasia. Some of the most frequently used tests for diagnosing aphasia and apraxia are the following.

The Boston Diagnostic Aphasia Examination (BDAE)[36] is a comprehensive battery of language tasks devised to determine overall communicative ability. It was designed to meet three general goals: diagnosis of presence and type of aphasic syndrome, leading to inferences concerning cerebral localization; measurement of the level of performance over a wide range, for both initial determination and detection of change over time; and comprehensive assessment of the assets and liabilities of the patient in all areas as a guide to therapy.[18] The diagnostic battery includes 31 subtests with scoring that is primarily a plus or minus system. An evaluation of conversational speech, an important component of this test, yields seven additional scores of language characteristics (melodic line, articulatory agility, grammatical form, phrase length, paraphasia, word finding, and auditory comprehension). The conversational speech sample is rated on a seven-point, equal-appearing interval scale. Raw scores are converted to percentiles, which allows comparison of subtest scores with the performance of a standardized group. Supplementary tests of the BDAE include assessments for disconnection syndromes, a parietal lobe battery, and a test for nonverbal apraxia.

The BDAE is lengthy and usually must be administered in separate sessions over the course of several days. The clinician may find the BDAE of value, however, as it is considerably more inclusive than other tests of its type.

The Minnesota Test for Differential Diagnosis of Aphasia (MTDDA), developed by Schuell,[92] is an extensive examination of many separate language functions and consists of 47 subtests. The main language areas assessed are auditory disturbances, visual and reading disturbances, speech and language disturbances, visuomotor and writing disturbances, numeric relations and arithmetic processes, and body image. The responses are scored as correct or incorrect. The MTDDA test is specifically designed to classify aphasic patients into one of five categories and two minor syndromes. Schuell contends that a prognosis for language recovery may be determined from the diagnostic findings of this examination.

The Porch Index of Communicative Ability (PICA)[81] samples performance in language behavior across five modalities (speaking, listening, gesturing, reading, and writing). Each of the 18 subtests uses 10 homogeneous items of equal difficulty. Responses are scored with a 16-point, multidimensional binary choice scoring system to reveal subtle differences in performance. The scoring system encompasses aspects of completeness, accuracy, promptness, responsiveness, and efficiency of the patient's attempts at communication. An overall test score, determined from all 180 items, is obtained together with separate scores on verbal, gestural, and graphic subtests. A percentile score can then be determined that indicates how a patient compares with a large standardized sample of aphasic patients. The PICA is often used to measure changes over time, chart standardized test data, and predict recovery patterns.

The PICA takes less time to administer than many other aphasia batteries and can be repeated with high test-retest reliability. The PICA, however, demands extensive training of the clinician in its administration and has an exacting scoring system.

The Western Aphasia Battery (WAB)[59] was composed, in part, from subtests of the BDAE. It assesses communication ability on a variety of relatively heterogeneous language tasks. The WAB has four oral language subtests (spontaneous speech, naming, repetition, and comprehension), from which an aphasia quotient (AQ) is derived. Additional tests of writing, reading, praxis, block design, drawing, calculations, and the Raven's Colored Progressive Matrices can be combined to offer a performance quotient (PQ). AQ and PQ combine to provide a cortical quotient, which can offer insight into the patient's cognitive function. The WAB is relatively easy to administer and score and provides a comprehensive database for most aphasic syndromes.

The Neurosensory Center Comprehensive Examination for Aphasia (NCCEA), developed by Spreen and Benton[100] in 1969, samples a variety of language behaviors. It consists of 20 language subtests that are administered to assess the patient's level of comprehension and expression, ability to retain verbally presented material, and ability to make functional use of reading and writing skills. Four additional subtests of visual and tactile function are included and are designed to detect deficits that might affect performance on the language tests.

Two profiles of patient behavior are obtained through administration of the NCCEA. The first compares the patient's specific areas of deficits with the performance of normal adults. The second profile compares the patient's performance with a "reference" group of aphasic patients previously evaluated at the Neurosensory Center at the University of Iowa. In this manner, ranking of performance can measure dysfunction along a mild-to-severe hierarchy and can serve to distinguish the patient's specific areas of strengths and weaknesses.

A neglected area of appraisal within all of the aforementioned tests is in adequate assessment of the patient's functional language ability. This ability often differs from the patient's ability to perform structured language tasks. Information regarding the aphasic deficit, the residual language, and site of lesion must be supplemented by an as-

sessment of how well the patient functions in communicative activities of everyday life. Two tests have been designed to assess these skills.

The Functional Communication Profile (FCP)[89] was developed for use in nonstructured, conversational situations. While informally interacting with the patient, the clinician rates the patient's ability to use residual communication skills in 45 activities. Five areas are subjectively rated— movement, speaking, understanding, reading, and other— on a nine-point scale, ranging from no ability (0) to normal (9). An overall percentage score, from 0 to 100, of estimated premorbid functional communication can be derived to indicate the general language ability of the patient.

The Communicative Abilities in Daily Living (CADL)[46] was designed to assess communication use in everyday situations. The CADL is a comprehensive assessment of functional language, which has been positively correlated with major formal tests of aphasia. The test content is presented in interview and role-playing situations during which the examiner evaluates the patient's ability to handle 68 communicative tasks involving various levels of listening, reading, writing, and speaking. Responses are rated on a three-point scale from 0 (total communication failure) to 2 (successful communication).

These tests, briefly outlined here, are considered comprehensive in that they sample a variety of communicative behaviors across different language modalities and in varying communication tasks. Administered alone, however, few tests have sufficient breadth to provide a complete assessment of aphasia and related disorders. Many clinicians prefer to administer several complete tests or portions of a number of different tests.

Recovery and prognosis

Spontaneous recovery from aphasia and apraxia occurs most rapidly during the first 3 months after onset of neurologic insult and then, to a lesser extent, continues throughout the next 3 months.[16,19,90] Several central nervous system changes influence this spontaneous recovery phenomenon. During the initial period of posttrauma, cerebral edema, which causes displacement and compression of the brain, begins to diminish. Cerebral blood flow, which is commonly reduced bilaterally following a cerebral infarct, increases during the progression of spontaneous recovery. Finally, abnormal amounts of neurotransmitters, released after an acute cerebral infarction and related to decreased neuronal metabolism, normalize as recovery progresses.[85] After 6 months the patient with aphasia is considered to have a chronic aphasia.[97] At this point, language return is no longer as dependent on central nervous system changes and thus may occur more slowly and with fewer notable increases in function.

Some aphasiologists purport that language recovery follows a particular pattern. In his review of the literature on recovery, Darley[20] highlights studies indicating that improvement in comprehension generally exceeds improvement in expression. In addition, recovery in imitative task performance, for example, repeating or copying, often precedes recovery in language generation abilities. Longitudinal studies of recovery patterns show that as the patient's linguistic performance changes, so does the pattern of performance. As noted previously, the original language diagnosis is not static. With recovery the linguistically impaired patient's aphasia may resolve from one form to another. Kertesz[58] observed that global aphasia may evolve toward Broca's aphasia in the chronic state and that acute Wernicke's aphasia may resolve as anomic aphasia or occasionally as conduction aphasia.

The prognosis for an aphasic patient's recovery depends on many factors, including the location, type, and extent of brain damage; severity of language symptoms; associated impairments such as apraxia or dysarthria; motivation for recovery; error awareness and ability to self-correct errors; frustration threshold; and the amount of time since the onset of the brain damage. More specifically, the existence of hemorrhagic insult rather than nonhemorrhagic infarct may further complicate recovery time and prognosis. Of lesser importance is the patient's age and amount of formal education. Since judgment of prognostic factors in any patient's recovery has a large subjective component, speech-language pathologists often recommend that aphasic patients, regardless of the severity and duration of symptoms, receive the benefit of a trial period of treatment.

Neurophysiologic status has direct bearing on recovery of language function. In general, the larger the cerebral lesion, the poorer the prognosis for eventual recovery. This is particularly true if the lesion is larger than 6 cm^3 and involves the frontal, temporal, and parietal language zones, especially if the posterior temporal gyrus is involved.[18] Furthermore, small, strategically placed subcortical lesions can produce a severe, persisting aphasia. In summation, patients with small lesions, a single lesion, and lesions that avoid the temporoparietal cortex generally have better prognoses than those with large lesions, multiple or bilateral lesions, and damage to the temporoparietal cortex. Kertesz[58] supports this view in his finding of a statistically significant positive correlation between recovery of language comprehension and lesion size.

Aphasia treatment

Language rehabilitation must be geared to meeting the patient's daily communication needs. The goals of aphasia treatment should be to maximize the patient's functional communication abilities in daily life situations. It would be unrealistic to expect a severely impaired aphasic person to regain all the language abilities he or she had before the brain injury. A more manageable goal might be for the patient with severe aphasia to regain some functional language which, along with the use of gestures, forms the basis of an adaptive method of communication.

The specific plan for remediation depends on the nature and severity of the language disorder. To illustrate, a patient with severe auditory comprehension deficits and no functional verbal expression would have very different treatment goals from an aphasic patient with good auditory comprehension but severe word-finding difficulty. In the former situation, short-term treatment goals might focus on improved auditory comprehension within daily communication situations and initiation of simple expressive acts, whether through verbalization or gestures. In the latter, treatment goals might emphasize word retrieval and facilitation strategies such as visual imagery and semantic associations. The patient would also be provided with alternate methods for expressing needs should verbal communication breakdowns occur. These compensatory strategies might include use of a picture or word board or use of residual written language or gestures.

Throughout the decades, theories of aphasia treatment have abounded. Some therapeutic approaches are based on a theoretic framework of what the aphasic language deficit represents. There has been the traditional stimulus-response approach of Wepman,[107] the operant conditioning approach presented in the early works of Holland[45] and Sarno and co-workers,[91] and the language stimulation approach of Schuell and associates.[93] Wepman[107] and more recently, the Base-10 Programmed Stimulation approach of LaPointe[63] emphasized a relearning or reeducational approach to language therapy. Operant approaches spring from an underlying conception of aphasia as a loss of language abilities and therefore the rehabilitation process emphasizes relearning linguistic skills through a programmed hierarchy. Schuell and associates,[93] in contrast, developed and refined a stimulation-facilitation approach to treatment that is a more cognitively based treatment mode. Their treatment is based on the theoretic construct of a reduction, not loss, of language after the onset of aphasia. If aphasia is not viewed as a loss of language, treatment cannot be viewed primarily as a reeducation process. Instead, aphasia is viewed as an interference with normal language processing. In treatment, therefore, intensive, multimodality stimulation of residual language processes is used to facilitate the recovery of disturbed language functions.

Even for patients exhibiting similar disorders, no one treatment approach can be uniformly applied. Some methods, such as Schuell's stimulation approach[93] and the Language Oriented Treatment (LOT) approach of Shewan and Bandur,[95] were designed to be used with many types of aphasia. The Language Oriented Treatment methodology is the newest attempt to integrate treatment procedures into a hierarchy of tasks based on knowledge of language processing. The LOT activities are directed toward auditory and visual processing, gestural-verbal communication, and oral and graphic expression.

In recent years certain treatment approaches for particular deficits have evolved and are worth noting. For example,

Melodic Intonation Therapy (MIT), first described by Albert, Sparks, and Helm,[2,98,99] is suggested only for patients who meet certain language criteria, in this case patients with severe nonfluent aphasia. Melodic Intonation Therapy is based on the spoken prosody of verbal utterances. MIT uses high-probability phrases and sentences that are intoned in a slow and rhythmic manner using a clinician-determined melodic structure. The rhythm and stress of the utterance is exaggerated during treatment. The theoretic basis of MIT is its utilization of the usually spared right brain functions of prosody and melody.

In contrast, Visual Action Therapy (VAT),[43] a nonverbal treatment method, is used in the remediation of severely aphasic patients. All instructions, reinforcements, and treatment units are nonverbal. This thereby encourages the patient to use nonverbal strategies to achieve a basic means of symbolizing needs through gestures or any other nonverbal mode. VAT may also be regarded as treating the apraxic component so often found in severe aphasia while improving such skills as attention, visual scanning, and visual discrimination.

In recent years, another approach has been to use facilitation techniques as a therapeutic strategy for language reacquisition. Patients with severe expressive aphasia often respond to an individualized therapeutic regime based on facilitation of language units using a variety of priming techniques.[56] The patient is encouraged to attempt verbal retrieval of linguistic symbols using available primes or cues to aid in recall. These cues can be semantic, syntactic, visual, graphic, or gestural. When successful retrieval of the language unit has been achieved, the clinician-directed primes are gradually withdrawn while the patient is encouraged to internalize appropriate cues so further language output may be facilitated without assistance. The patient may then use these new verbal utterances in a variety of linguistic and environmental contexts.

As functional communication has become a primary focus in aphasia rehabilitation, clinicians have devised techniques that focus on maximizing communication in any understandable way. The pragmatics of language, that is, the use of language in interactive contexts, has taken on new importance. Therapy goals target not only the achievement of a set of language skills, but also the generalization of these skills to the patient's daily communicative environment. Techniques such as Promoting Aphasics' Communicative Effectiveness (PACE)[24,25] have been developed to meet this need. PACE is designed to use aspects of natural conversation where the goal of the patient-clinician interaction is to convey messages consisting of new information. Messages can be transmitted through linguistic, (oral or written) or nonverbal signals and symbols that convey intentions and meanings. Since persons with aphasia often have limited ability to generate intent verbally, the burden for conveying messages is shifted to other modes of expression.[24,25]

A mode of therapeutic remediation that has recently gained widespread enthusiasm has been in the use of microcomputers with the language-impaired adult. Therapeutic intervention with this population has recently become more efficacious and innovative with the addition of microcomputer-assisted treatment regimens. The microcomputer offers the speech-language pathologist a means of expanding the treatment options available to the adult with aphasia given appropriate software, user time, and motivation. Additionally, clinical management may be rendered and mediated through computer software packages designed to facilitate improvements in reading abilities,[54] sequencing skills, memory, auditory comprehension, visual-perceptual organization, and cause-effect relationships.

Microcomputer assessment and treatment have been incorporated into aphasia rehabilitation quite easily, as evidenced by the abundance of available software packages presently available (for example, Volin and Groher, Language Stimulation Software 1-6, Aspen Publishers Inc., Gaithersburg, Md.). These software packages are oriented toward improving reading abilities, although corollary gains have been noted for auditory comprehension skills and semantic and syntactic organization. A treatment protocol may prove illustrative. A computer-based supplemental treatment hierarchy for facilitating reading skills has recently been implemented with moderately to severely impaired aphasic adults and found to be successful.[44] Tailored to meet patient's individual needs, this hierarchy includes an introduction to the microcomputer environment, beginning with a letter-to-letter matching task. Following achievement of this skill (90% criterion achievement), word-to-picture matching (Weiner, Functions Pictures, Parrot Software, State College, Penn.) may be initiated and eventually followed by an associative word-to-picture matching program (Weiner, Association Pictures, Parrot Software, State College, Penn.) (Figure 49-1). Syntactic learning is also incorporated into computer treatment with the addition of programs that require the patient to complete simple sentences (Major and Wilson, Computerized Reading for Aphasics-Closure, College Hill Press, San Diego, Calif.) and programs requiring the patient to make judgments regarding the accuracy of grammar usage (Volin and Groher, Language Stimulation Software No. 3, Aspen Publishers Inc., Gaithersburg, Md.).

Recent software by Mills and Thomas (Brain-Link Software, Ann Arbor, Mich.) has offered alternative suggestions for incorporating microcomputer intervention with adults. The authors developed a software treatment package using digitized speech, an artificial speech replica produced by the computer. The software provides practice drills for patients in selecting a pictured response from a field of four pictures following auditory cues produced by digitized speech. A case study of the efficacy of this mode of treatment showed that an aphasic adult demonstrated improved performance as measured by the PICA, following computerized treatment.[73]

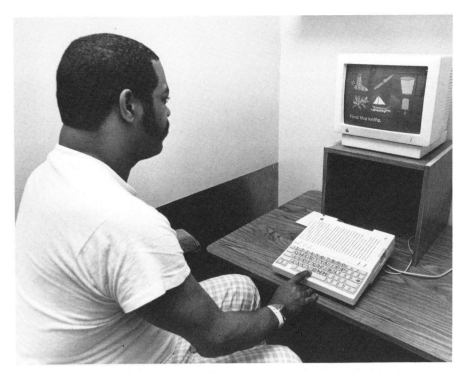

Figure 49-1. Patient working on Apple IIc computer with word-to-picture matching program for treatment of severe reading comprehension deficit.

Individual patient objectives therefore can be enhanced through microcomputer-assisted intervention. For most patients it can be safely purported that microcomputer-based treatment helps to increase motivation, acceptance, and goal-directed behaviors.[33] Additionally, through carefully designed treatment programs suited to the specific needs of each patient, task protocols can be programmed to ensure that the patient achieves certain levels of success while receiving continuous and consistent reinforcement. In this manner the patient is able to exert control over the immediate environment (for example, responding when ready or self-correcting responses) while still working toward goal achievement.

Other inherent advantages of microcomputer intervention are also notable. For example, the provision of supplementary computer-assisted treatment allows the clinician to provide consistent presentation of stimuli over extended periods of time to individual patients. In this manner, drill and reinforcement are provided to the patient within treatment tasks designed to facilitate goal achievement and eventual attainment of discharge criteria. At the same time the computer records the patient's responses according to predetermined criteria to accurately and objectively measure changing performance. This hard copy allows the clinician more time to interpret and analyze his or her findings and provides necessary documentation of patient performance.

The inherent advantages of microcomputer-based treatment within speech and language intervention programs therefore appear empirically warranted. Actual reported efficacy, however, is at present minimal owing to difficulties in establishing treatment paradigms. One clinical study was recently completed at Goldwater Memorial Hospital, New York University Medical Center. Through the incorporation of microcomputer technology into the rehabilitation process, this study examined efficacy of treatment and quantity of improvement in reading skills with adults who exhibit dyslexia secondary to acquired aphasia. Aphasic subjects were assigned to experimental or control groups with all patients receiving a combination of traditional language remediation plus supplemental treatment. Treatment was rendered for a total of 8 hours a week for a minimum of 3 months. Control subjects received traditional reading remediation using paper and pencil tasks, whereas experimental subjects received microcomputer-delivered reading treatment. Preliminary analysis suggests that while most subjects made gains, the experimental subjects exhibited significantly more improvement in their reading performance than the control subjects. The microcomputer and its accompanying software were effective and efficient tools in the remediation of reading deficits.[57]

Other recent applications have included the use of microcomputers in treating cognitive impairments secondary to head trauma. Hartley software (Dimondale, Mich.) provides a series of diskettes aimed at improving patient's categorization skills, sequencing abilities, and memory abilities. With gains in these specified areas, additional gains in orientation and attention span have also been noted. The microcomputer is proving a valuable addition to the clinician's therapeutic armamentarium.

Efficacy of aphasia treatment

The question of efficacy of speech and language treatment in the recovery from aphasia is an important issue in this era of limited resources, available personnel, and time constraints. A literature survey on efficacy reveals few adequately controlled studies focusing on the effects of speech and language treatment. Of the small group of studies whose major goal is the investigation of the effects of therapy, the methodologies, etiologies, severity of aphasia, and the nature of treatment being offered in each study have differed widely.

One such study was the report by Lincoln and co-workers[66] in 1984, which measured the effectiveness of speech treatment on patients with aphasia. The 191 subjects studied were divided into a treatment group and a no-treatment group. The investigators reported no significant differences in language performance when treated aphasic patients were compared with untreated patients and therefore surmised that treatment as currently practiced was not effective for most patients. However, their study appears to violate sound design principles for a controlled treatment task, including inadequate subject selection criteria, problematic statistical analysis, questionable randomized design, and variability of treatment offered. The treatment group subjects, for example, were to receive treatment up to 24 weeks two times a week; however, many subjects failed to receive all the treatment sessions.

In contrast, a few other studies are worth mentioning because they are recent, well designed, and present a controlled treatment trial. The Veterans Administration Cooperative Study[109] provided 8 hours of treatment each week for 48 weeks to a group of 67 aphasic subjects. The results indicated that both individually and group-treated patients made significant language gains during the treatment time. Furthermore, significant gains were observed in patients 26 to 48 weeks after onset, a period considered to be beyond the period of maximum spontaneous recovery. Sarno and Levita[90] in their 1979 study also noted substantial recovery 12 to 52 weeks after the stroke for global and fluent aphasic patients but reported no significant gains for the nonfluent aphasic subjects. Vignolo et al.[7] saw measurable gains with a minimum of three treatment sessions weekly but only in those patients who received at least 6 months of therapy.

A recent comprehensive study by Shewan and Kertesz[96] compared treated aphasic subjects with untreated aphasic subjects where the subjects were initially seen 2 to 4 weeks after stroke. The 100 subjects were studied for up to 1 year. The results showed that the treated aphasic subjects, regardless of type of treatment, improved and showed a significantly greater recovery in their language function than did the nontreated subjects. These data were similar to those

of Vignolo et al.,[7,105] who reported significant differences between treated and untreated aphasic patients. They found that treatment was most effective when initiated early and given for 6 or more months' duration.

The intensity and duration of treatment are often important factors in the aphasic patient's progress. With a motivated and neurologically stable patient, language intervention should be intensive—daily if possible—and should be available over a number of months if appropriate and measurable gains continue to be made. A study of 281 aphasic subjects revealed that treatment should be rendered for at least 3 hours each week for no less than 5 consecutive months.[105] As demonstrated by the Veterans Administration Cooperative Study, which provided 8 hours of therapy each week for 48 weeks, patients made significant improvement in language abilities when treatment was intense and continued over time.[109]

DYSARTHRIA

Another major communication disorder that is often confused with aphasia is the motor speech impairment known as *dysarthria*. Dysarthria is a speech disorder that has resulted from injury to the neural mechanisms that regulate speech movements.[77] Dysarthria does not refer to the symbolic, grammatical, or integrative language dysfunctions that result from aphasia, but rather to a disturbance in the neuromuscular production of speech. Defining dysarthria as a speech impairment also differentiates it from the cognitive-linguistic disorders seen in other impairments such as dementia. Including speech movement regulation in the definition distinguishes it from apraxia of speech, an articulation programming disorder involving damage to neural mechanisms that select and sequence speech.

Darley, Aronson, and Brown[21-23] view dysarthria as a group of speech disorders characterized by impairments in respiration, phonation, articulation, resonance, and prosody. The dysarthrias result from weakness, paresis, incoordination, and abnormal tone of the speech mechanism musculature.

Patients with dysarthria have retained the language symbols necessary for adequate communication, but when they speak they do so unclearly. Difficulty in mastication, swallowing, and controlling salivation is often observed. Darley and co-workers[23] have described six types of dysarthria associated with specific neuromuscular impairments. A summary of this classification schema is presented in Table 49-2.

The severity of the patient's speech impairment depends on the degree of neuromuscular involvement. The timing, force, strength, and coordination of speech movements are central to a patient's overall speech performance and intelligibility. Some individuals have slightly distorted speech, whereas others are more markedly impaired. Some patients have a speech system that is severely impaired with minimal

Table 49-2. Differential diagnostic patterns of dysarthria

Dysarthria types	Lesion site	Examples of medical diagnosis	Major neuromuscular symptoms	Predominant speech symptoms
Flaccid or bulbar palsy dysarthria	Lower motor neuron lesion; may affect selected cranial nerves, cranial nerve nuclei, or peripheral nerve fibers; occasionally impaired transmission across myoneural junction	Can occur with low brainstem stroke; poliomyelitis; myasthenia gravis	Flaccidity of musculature; hyporeflexia; muscular atrophy	Hypernasality; imprecise consonant production; breathy voice; monopitch; nasal emission; reduced speech loudness
Spastic or pseudobulbar palsy dysarthria	Upper motor neuron lesion; may involve damage to pyramidal system and/or extrapyramidal system	Multiple strokes; spastic cerebral palsy; multiple sclerosis; head trauma	Spasticity of musculature; hyperreflexia; paralysis or paresis; diffuse weakness	Imprecise consonant production; monopitch; strained-strangled voice quality; hypernasality; monoloudness
Ataxic or cerebellar dysarthria	Cerebellum	Multiple strokes; multiple sclerosis; head trauma; toxicity; tumor	Errors in timing, force, range, and direction of whole movements and of individual parts of movements; inaccurate movements; tremors often present	Imprecise consonants; excess and equal stress; irregular articulatory breakdown; vowels distorted; harsh voice; impaired loudness control
Hypokinetic dysarthria	Extrapyramidal system	Parkinson's disease	Alteration and reduction or paucity of movement; rigidity of muscle tone; rhythmic tremor at rest	Monopitch; reduced stress; monoloudness; imprecise consonants; inappropriate silences; short rushes of speech; harsh and breathy voice
Hyperkinetic dysarthria	Extrapyramidal motor system; may be lesion in subthalamic nucleus	Chorea; dystonia; drug toxicity; neurochemical disorders	Abnormal involuntary movements; excessive neuromotor activity; irregular and unpatterned movements; athetosis; dyskinesias	Imprecise consonants; prolongation of interword and/or intersyllable intervals; variable speaking rate; monopitch; harsh voice
Mixed or flaccid; spastic dysarthria	Degeneration of upper and lower motor neuron systems	Amyotrophic lateral sclerosis; multiple strokes	Pronounced weakness of the bulbar musculature; movements very slow; range of movement limited; spasticity usually present	Imprecise consonants; hypernasality; harsh voice; slow rate; monopitch and low pitch; short phrases

Modified from Darley, F, Aronson, AE, and Brown, JR: Motor speech disorders, Philadelphia, 1975, WB Saunders Co.

intelligible speech production, even on the single word level. If the person's speech production is so severely impaired that he or she cannot produce any intelligible words or even sounds, the disorder is termed *anarthria*. The person with anarthria is unable to use speech for daily functional communication owing to severe neuromuscular weakness, incoordination, or rigidity of the speech mechanism.

Diagnostic approaches

A thorough assessment of the dysarthrias involves reviewing the perceptual, physiologic, and acoustic aspects of speech production. The perceptual approach most commonly used in clinical practice is based on the Mayo Clinic perceptual classification system developed by Darley and colleagues.[21-23]

Thirty-eight speech and voice dimensions are rated by severity when the clinician subjectively evaluates the patient's speech. Dimensions such as vocal loudness level, imprecise consonant production, variable speaking rate, hypernasality, and vocal pitch level are included. The speech-language pathologist analyzes and rates the severity of the perceived speech characteristics with this classification system. The results of this perceptual feature analysis provide speech and voice symptom clusters that suggest the type of dysarthria and its possible neuromuscular basis. This evaluation is of course subjective and depends on the listening skills of each clinician.

The physiologic approach, which emerged at about the same time as the Mayo Clinic perceptual classification system, allows the clinician to obtain additional information during the dysarthria assessment. Proponents of this methodology view the dysarthrias as movement disorders rather than as speech disorders.[84] According to Netsell,[78] physiologic assessment emphasizes the evaluation of functional components of the patient's speech mechanism. Each vocal tract component is assessed to determine its severity and type of involvement following isolated and combined component testing during speech and nonspeech tasks. A patient may present perceptually with a breathy voice, monopitch, monoloudness, and imprecise consonant productions. The suspected physiologic components might include the larynx, velopharynx, tongue, jaw, and lips. It is only when objective data are obtained through instrumental measures such as radiographic, endoscopic, aerodynamic, and acoustic studies that a precise identification and localization of the breakdown can be realized. Such an evaluation provides a bridge between perceived symptoms and underlying pathophysiology.[84]

A third dimension in the evaluation of the dysarthrias is the inclusion of acoustic studies. Acoustic assessment allows for a more discrete interpretation of perceptual speech characteristics by employing precise measurements rather than by merely relying on clinician judgment. Voice characteristics such as vocal fundamental frequency (associated with pitch) and vocal intensity (associated with loudness)

can be easily measured in this manner along with temporal aspects of speech production. These data contribute to determining the location, severity, and type of impairments along the vocal tract.

Evaluation

Dysarthria assessment includes a perceptual evaluation of spontaneous speech, an examination of oral structures and their function, as well as the administration of formal tests and instrumental measures.

An oral examination requires direct observation of visible oral and pharyngeal structures. Any structural abnormality, such as increased tongue size, is noted. This portion of the assessment also includes oral, sensory, and motor testing, the latter focusing on muscle strength, range of motion, and coordination of movement. The data obtained from this testing provide information regarding the integrity of the cranial nerves innervating oral musculature.

In recent years attempts to formalize perceptual assessment have been made. Enderby's Frenchay Dysarthria Assessment (FDA)[30,31] and Yorkston and Beukelman's Assessment of Intelligibility of Dysarthric Speech (AIDS)[114] have expanded the clinician's evaluation tools. The FDA uses a nine-point scale to rate various behaviors and structures. The AIDS provides intelligibility ratings for the patient's single word and sentence length utterances and a measure of speaking rate. This is valuable for determining baseline performance and evaluating improvement after treatment. Both the FDA and the AIDS have recently been computerized for ease of data collection, scoring, and interpretation. Traditional articulation tests, such as the Templin-Darley Test of Articulation[103] and the Fisher-Logemann Test of Articulation Competence,[32] may be administered to determine the sound errors produced by the dysarthric speaker.

Investigation of the speech-acoustic signal using instrumental measurements includes oscillographic analysis, sound spectrography, and vocal fundamental frequency (pitch) and vocal intensity (loudness) measures of disordered speech and voice production. The oscilloscope is a piece of equipment that displays acoustic waveforms of speech signals on a screen. An oscillogram, the waveform display, can be used to measure parameters such as speech sound frequencies and speech segment duration. The spectrograph is a device that records acoustic speech signals, filters them, and then displays them on chemically treated paper or a videoscreen. The spectrogram, the filtered waveform display, also provides information on speech segment duration, fundamental frequency, voice onset time, glottal noise, and many other speech and voice characteristics. Pitch and loudness analyzers provide displays of specific voice parameters such as fundamental frequency and loudness. The Visi-Pitch, manufactured by Kay Elemetrics (Pinebrook, N.J.), is a device that displays frequency and intensity data on an oscilloscope screen; a digital readout of exact frequency

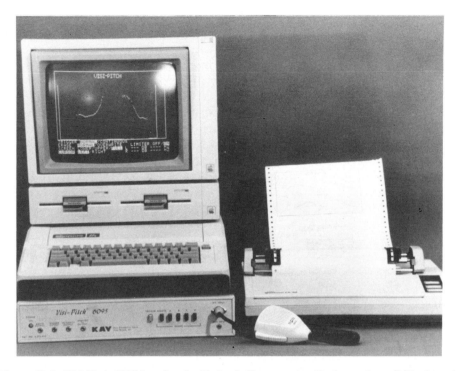

Figure 49-2. Visi Pitch 6095 interfaced with Apple IIe computer. Hard copy is available through attached printer.

measures is also available. Recent computerization of this instrument has increased its use for acoustic analysis of connected speech and ease of data tabulation and storage (Figure 49-2). These instruments validate the clinician's subjective perceptual evaluation. Instrumental measurements allow inferences to be made between perceived

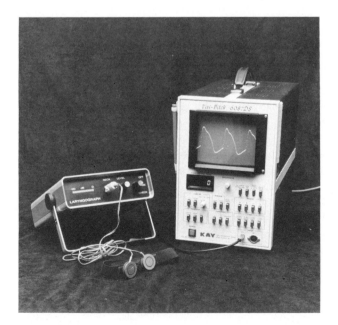

Figure 49-3. Laryngograph interfaced with Visi Pitch 6087 DS, which provides visual representation of vocal cord contact.

speech and voice characteristics and the physiologic dysfunction of vocal tract structures, especially of the laryngeal mechanism and its coordination with the respiratory mechanism.

Physiologic measurements, also using instrumental methods, include electromyography, electroglottography, fiberoptic endoscopy, videofluoroscopy, and aerodynamic assessment. Electromyography may be used to glean data regarding the muscle action potentials of the orofacial muscles.

Electroglottography is a method for assessing patterns of laryngeal fold contact by placing electrodes on the skin above the thyroid laminae. The Laryngograph, a simple electroglottograph offered by Larynograph, Ltd. (London, England) can be easily interfaced with the Kay Elemetric's Visi Pitch or an oscilloscope so that patterns of vocal fold contact can be visualized (Figure 49-3). Data obtained from this instrument may indicate aberrant vocal cord contact patterns associated with perceived voice parameters. For example, an electroglottographic waveform with a very long open phase may be indicative of decreased vocal fold contact and is often associated with a perceived breathy voice pattern.

Fiberoptic velopharyngeal and laryngeal endoscopy is an invasive technique that requires the passage of a small flexible fiberoptic scope transnasally for visualization of velopharyngeal and laryngeal structures and their functions. Endoscopy provides the speech-language pathologist and rehabilitation specialists with a dynamic picture of the speech musculature and structures during extended speech. The

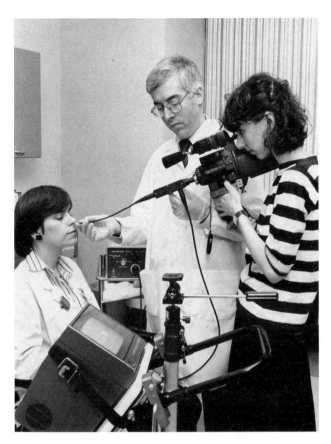

Figure 49-4. Fiberoptic velopharyngeal and laryngeal endoscopic evaluation is performed using endoscope, light source (behind examiner), video camera, screen, and tapedeck for permanent recording.

endoscope can easily be coupled with a video recorder and tape deck for permanent recording of the diagnostic information (Figure 49-4). This procedure has a distinct advantage over indirect laryngoscopy, which only allows for vocal cord visualization during the phonation of a single sound. When hypernasality is perceived, velopharyngeal incompetence is suspected. The use of endoscopy is one method for documenting velopharyngeal pathophysiology.

Videofluoroscopy is a radiographic assessment procedure for observing oral and velopharyngeal structures at rest, while moving, and during phonation. This unique ability to simultaneously view the physiology and hear the acoustic patterning of speech makes videofluoroscopy a valuable tool. During the procedure several drops of barium are inserted nasally to coat the nasopharynx and 1/3 teaspoon of barium is taken orally. Radiographic observation from a lateral position provides an excellent view of mandibular, labial, lingual, and velopharyngeal physiologic function during speech (see Figure 49-12). The anteroposterior view offers additional information regarding velopharyngeal phenomena.

Aerodynamic testing involves detailed measures of oral-

nasal air flow and pressure. A system containing a pneumotach and pressure transducers is used to determine the function of the respiratory system and of the larynx and velopharynx. These data can be easily visualized on an oscilloscope screen and photographed for documentation purposes. Subglottal air pressure is one parameter that can be evaluated using aerodynamic instrumentation. When aerodynamic testing reveals decreased subglottal air pressure in a dysarthric individual, for example, an associated decrease in vocal loudness is often the initial voice characteristic perceived.

Instrumental testing often reveals the underlying pathophysiology responsible for perceived speech and voice symptoms. Such assessment techniques are critical to the evaluation process, as their results provide objective data to verify the speech-language pathologist's subjective impressions. For additional information Baken[5] provided an extensive description of speech and voice measurement procedures and clinical instrumentation.

Treatment

The therapeutic management of the person with dysarthria concentrates on increasing effective communication (via speech or alternate systems) and improving speech intelligibility by either restoring function or using compensatory strategies to maximize residual function. Alternate and augmentative communication for severely dysarthric patients is discussed later in this chapter. Improving speech intelligibility can be accomplished using behavioral, instrumental, and prosthetic treatment approaches. These approaches overlap and are easily combined to restore functions and to compensate for decreased speech efficiency.

Traditional behavioral methods include oral motor exercises, speech sound production drills, vocal rate and loudness control, increasing speaking effort, and tactile monitoring of respiratory movements. Careful selection of the exercises and drill material, instruction to the patient, occasional direct manipulation of oral and respiratory structures, and clinician evaluation with patient self-evaluation are essential traditional treatment techniques. The reader is referred to Rosenbek and LaPointe[84] for a detailed description of traditional behavioral treatment methods.

Given the advent of new technology in recent years, the use of instrumental and microcomputer-based treatment techniques to effect changes in speech performance has rapidly increased. One such method involves administering visual biofeedback to the patient for single or multiple aspects of his or her speech behavior. This biofeedback is often paired with traditional behavioral techniques to obtain maximum gains. With continued treatment and progress toward criterion levels, the use of the visual biofeedback modality is gradually reduced. The result is improved speech production with the patient internalizing the feedback modality. Instrumental treatment also gives the dysarthric person knowledge of results following behaviorally oriented tasks.

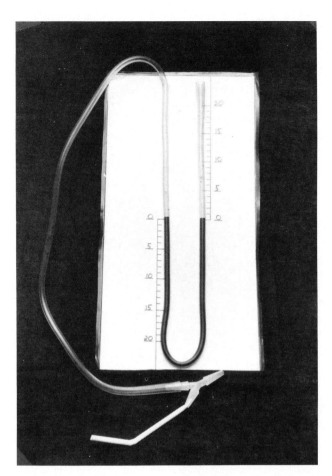

Figure 49-5. Fabricated U-tube oral manometer used in treatment to facilitate production of subglottal air pressure.

Instrumental remediation may be directed toward modification of respiratory behavior, specifically subglottal air pressure, which affects vocal loudness. Netsell and Hixon[79] have described the use of a simple modified oral manometer for the measurement of subglottal pressure. This device, a U-tube filled with colored water, is placed on a background of graph paper. The patient blows into the tube during nonspeech activities, displacing the water. Training increases the amount of generated subglottal pressure over longer periods of time, with eventual discontinuation of the use of the U-tube and replacement with traditional behavioral techniques (Figure 49-5). Similar training exercises can be accomplished with pressure-transducing devices. In addition, a portable microcomputer can be used during communication tasks to inform the wearer when his or her loudness falls below criterion levels. This device also indicates the accumulated time the speaker has spent above or at the appropriate loudness level.[86]

Instruments used for modifying laryngeal behavior include aerodynamic devices, the video fiberoptic scope, the electroglottograph, and acoustic analyzers. During speech activities there is potential for the use of the pneumotach-ograph to examine coordination of phonation and respiration.

Video fiberoptic feedback allows the patient to visualize the gross movements of the larynx during phonation. These techniques, when accompanied by vocal control therapy, can then aid in modifying laryngeal behavior. Similarly electroglottography, which provides the patient with biofeedback regarding vocal fold contact, can be paired with traditional behavioral methods to facilitate voice modification.[51] Acoustic analyzers, such as the Kay Elemetrics Visi-Pitch, are excellent devices for modifying pitch and loudness. This equipment allows the patient to compare his or her vocal performance against target models; such visual feedback helps the patient modify vocal production.

Measurements of nasal air flow and oral air pressure may be used in the modification of velopharyngeal valving. Air pressure and air flow readings are displayed on an oscilloscope screen so that patients receive feedback on the amount of air flowing through the nose and the air pressure in the oral cavity. For a patient with velopharyngeal incompetence this feedback can assist in decreasing perceived nasality and increasing speech intelligibility.[64] Feedback from video fiberoptic displays can indicate to the patient when velopharyngeal closure has been accomplished. This actual physiologic event can then be translated into a perceived "feeling" of closure. Eventually the patient may voluntarily perform required events with less reliance on instrumental feedback mechanisms.

To modify oral articulation, electromyography feedback has been successful. Facial muscle function and lip strength have been improved with this type of biofeedback. Concentration on muscle activity is directly related to speech production, and therefore, modification in muscle strength may result in a facilitation of speech production.

Microcomputer technology has also been incorporated into the dysarthria treatment regime. The use of voice recognition tasks (for example, Voice Interactive Learning, Voice Interactive Systems, Los Angeles) has also been employed to assist the patient with dysarthria attain intelligible speech productions. The patient is shown words or pictured stimuli on the computer screen and asked to produce his or her most intelligible production of that stimulus. This production is then coded into the computer's memory as a template of the patient's best production. Through practice, the patients' improved productions are continually recoded, requiring them to continue matching and superseding their own improved productions. These new applications offer additional areas for widespread use of microcomputers with the dysarthric population.

In some instances, therapeutic intervention produces only limited functional changes. Prosthetic management, which physically alters the musculoskeletal system, may become a viable alternative to achieve functional changes in speech production. Examples of prosthetic devices include the palatal lift speech prosthesis, the speech bulb obturator, the bite block, and various external supports for modifying posture, muscle tone, and strength of the orofacial and respiratory mechanisms.

The palatal lift provides partial or complete closure of the velopharyngeal port by elevating the soft palate upward and posteriorly toward the posterior pharyngeal wall (Figure 49-6). The speech bulb, sometimes used as an alternative to the palatal life, is constructed to fill the oronasopharyngeal lumen; both prosthetic devices improve the expiratory oral air flow and pressure. The optimal result is a reduced velopharyngeal opening with diminished nasal air flow and de-

creased perceived hypernasality. Additional effects include more precise consonant production and, at times, improved vocal loudness. These resultant changes facilitate overall speech intelligibility.

Successful treatment with the speech bulb obturator or palatal lift has been applied to patients with neurogenic velopharyngeal incompetence for over a decade.[4,55] The prosthesis is constructed following videofluoroscopic, fiberoptic, and aeorodynamic assessment, which documents the dimensions of the dysfunction.[78] In the actual construc-

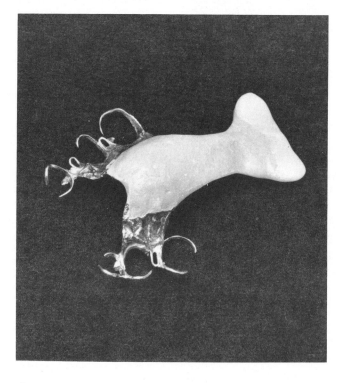

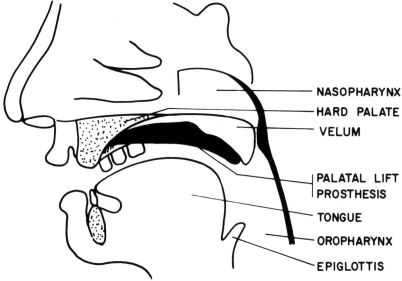

Figure 49-6. Palatal lift. Diagram shows its placement in oropharyngeal cavity.

tion, an initial impression is made of the maxillary area of the mouth and a stone cast is used to construct the prosthesis. Thermoplastic materials may be used to form the lift extension, which is then processed in acrylic resin. Retention may be obtained through stainless-steel clasps fitted around the teeth. For the edentulous patient, an attached acrylic lift can be connected to an upper denture.

The preferred conservative management for velopharyngeal incompetence with the neurogenically disordered adult has been the use of a speech prosthetic device. However, the pharyngeal flap procedure and Teflon injection, both surgical techniques, have also been widely used but with mixed results reported for the dysarthric population.[48]

Another prosthetic approach is the use of a bite block. The oral insertion of a bite block between the upper and lower molars to stabilize the jaw and to facilitate improved tongue movements may enhance some dysarthric speakers' facial movements. Additionally, the bite block may assist the speaker in inhibiting abnormal, involuntary movements. In some situations it may stabilize the jaw and allow the speaker to focus his or her energy during speech attempts on differentiated movements of the lips and tongue.[71] Bite blocks are also used in treatment with traditional oromotor exercises to improve labial and lingual function. Some patients who benefit from the stabilizing effects of the bite block during speech wear the block daily for improved speech sound production.

External modifications of posture, muscle tone, and strength can greatly influence speech performance. Neck braces, overhead slings, and simple changes in positioning (for example, placing the patient in supine position) may be used for the patient with movement disorders or weakened respiratory muscles. To provide more stable respiratory support for speech, for example, a patient may be asked to lean into a board fitted to body posture and fastened to the wheelchair.

Augmentative communication

Severely dysarthric individuals with poor or nonfunctional speech intelligibility may benefit from augmentative communication intervention as an immediate or long-term means of establishing communication between the patient, his or her family, and health care personnel. Augmentative communication is a specialized form of treatment involving the development of alternative systems of communication for the nonspeaking, severely physically handicapped individual whose linguistic and cognitive status remains largely intact. It is available to those individuals who have quadriplegia and severe motor speech impairment or anarthria as a result of congenital or acquired neurologic impairment. This population has little or no verbal, written, or gestural functional communication. The development of alternative systems of communication uses advanced technology in the form of electronic or portable microcomputer-based devices, as well as the person's residual vocal skills, facial expression, and gestures.

The focus of the augmentative treatment approach is on the establishment of effective and efficient communication between the nonspeaking individual and the listener. The communication system is tailored to meet the individual's

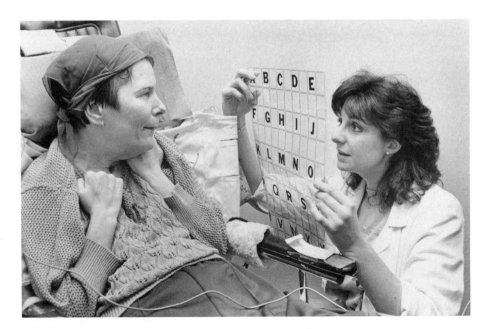

Figure 49-7. Patient interacting with clinician using Eye-Link, a direct selection, nonelectronic communicating system. Her medical diagnosis is bilateral strokes with resultant anarthria and quadriplegia.

needs by providing communication options such as synthesized speech, printed output, programmability, and portability. Although electronic devices may be used to promote more rapid and efficient one-to-one communication, simple nonelectronic systems may be implemented for individuals requiring more immediate reestablishment of communication (Figure 49-7).

For individuals whose motor speech disorder proves temporary or amenable to remediation, as in the case of Guillain-Barré syndrome, augmentative communication may optimize the effectiveness of message transmission until speech intelligibility improves. Often, however, augmentative intervention is the sole communication option open to those individuals whose severe dysarthria is permanent (for example, brainstem or bilateral stroke) or whose motor speech status is expected to deteriorate as a result of progressive, degenerative neuromuscular disease (for example, amyotrophic lateral sclerosis, multiple sclerosis, Parkinson's disease, muscular dystrophy). Many of these patients undergo tracheostomy or become ventilator dependent and have concomitant anarthria and severe physical disabilities. The patient's immobility as well as the inability to gesture or write to make his or her needs known results in communication isolation and environmental deprivation.

The specific motor impairments exhibited by the patient determine the method by which the message elements in the system are made accessible. Some quadriplegic individuals may have limited use of their hands or head as means of directly activating the communication device. This technique is known as direct selection. Individuals with more severe motor impairments such as ataxia may have only one reliable movement with which to activate a communication device. In this case the patient must wait until the message element or group of elements is displayed on the augmentative device. The patient in turn signals the listener by using his or her available motor movements, for example, by activating a switch or by using eye gaze, indicating that the desired message element has been reached. The technique, known as scanning, is a slower and less interactive method of access than is direct selection.

An awareness of the modes of access and the various electronic and nonelectronic treatment options available for this population enables the rehabilitation team to facilitate an effective communication avenue for the severely physically handicapped, nonspeaking person.

Evaluation

Augmentative communication intervention is conducted by a speech-language pathologist who performs a needs and communication abilities assessment to determine an individual's candidacy for a treatment regimen. An evaluation of the communicative environments and communication partners is a vital part of the appraisal protocol. Areas of cognitive and linguistic functioning, as well as motor speech and visual, hearing, and physical motor status, must also

be fully evaluated with the cooperation of the medical and interdisciplinary rehabilitation team. In addition, the patient's communication requirements must be identified; for example, the need for written output for correspondence and confidential messages or the need for vocal output through synthesized speech to alert a caregiver or to interact in a group situation must be considered. The individual's communication needs must be firmly established so the appropriate nonelectronic or electronic system may be prescribed.[10] Although a communication system may be designed for even the most severely physically disabled or sensory-impaired individual, the ideal augmentative communication candidate should have normal or nearly normal cognitive and linguistic functioning. In some circumstances, however, a simplified communication system may be provided for an individual whose cognitive and linguistic functioning is impaired.

Treatment

Most nonspeaking individuals seen in a rehabilitation environment benefit from a nonelectronic communication system in the form of a letter board, word board, or transparent eye-gaze system (Figure 49-7). This type of device often promotes rapid and efficient one-to-one communication between the patient and his or her family and with the health care support staff.[88] The diagnostic evaluation also guides the clinician in determining the necessity and appropriateness of electronic communication intervention, which may enable even the most severely disabled, nonspeaking individual to produce written and spoken output. The clinician is then faced with the task of integrating the patient's communication abilities, disabilities, and needs with available communication systems, whether they be nonelectronic or electronic communication aids or microcomputer-based systems.

The advent of electronic communication systems ushered in the use of dedicated communication devices that were designed mainly for communication purposes and intended specifically for the handicapped population.[87] These dedicated devices range from a direct-select, portable printout device such as the Cannon Communicator (Cannon USA, Lake Success, N.Y.) (Figure 49-8) to a more sophisticated and costly portable device with multiple access options, print capability, and vocal output as in the Light Talker (Prentke-Romich Co., Wooster, Ohio) (Figure 49-9). Although a complete description of all available devices is beyond the scope of this chapter, the reader may refer to Kraat and Sitver-Kogult[62] for a detailed listing and analysis of available systems.

Currently, the clinician may draw more recent advances in microcomputer technology in an effort to provide an electronic system of communication for the nonspeaking individual. In many cases the computer can mimic the function of a dedicated device at a lower cost. The clinician's decision then, to prescribe an electronic dedicated aid, a

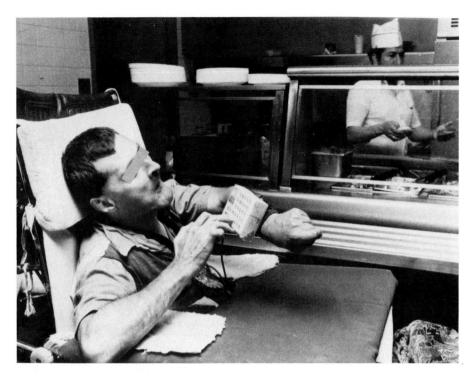

Figure 49-8. Patient using Cannon Communicator to order lunch at hospital canteen. Patient has dystonia muscularis deformans and anarthria.

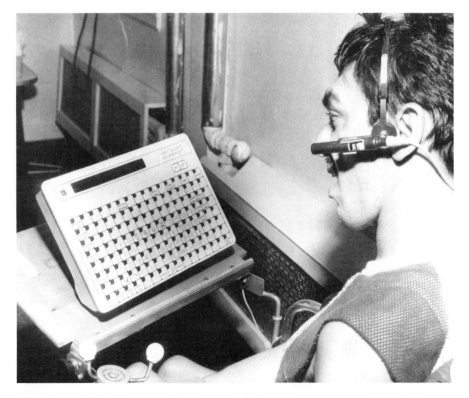

Figure 49-9. Patient with Light Talker uses infrared light pen to access individual letters.

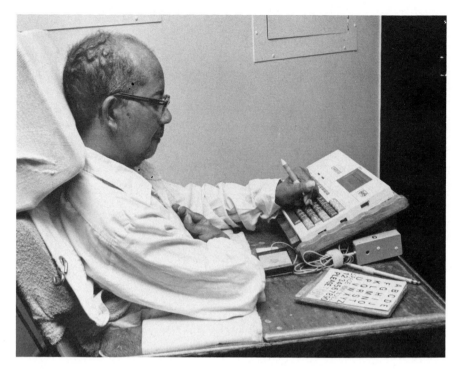

Figure 49-10. Patient with electronic Epson Speech PAC and nonelectronic letter board. This patient is quadriparetic and anarthric following bilateral strokes.

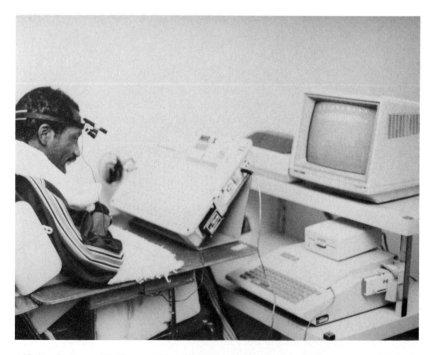

Figure 49-11. Patient with Express III, which is interfaced with Apple IIe computer. Adaptive firmware card (Adaptive Peripherals, Inc.) is used to operate computer through communication device. This elaborate system enables patient to write, produce synthesized speech, control his environment, and further his vocational goals by composing music. He is quadriplegic following viral encephalitis and is anarthric.

microcomputer-based device, or both, is based on the individual patient's needs as measured against the features inherent in various systems. Furthermore, a determination of selection techniques,[41,104] interfacing, system display, and modes of output[9,10] is central to the prescription of an appropriate device. The prescription of a device must also consider additional variables such as portability, independence, and speed of accessing the language output.

Finally, dedicated aids and microcomputers may be adapted to provide the features of written and spoken output for the handicapped population. Printed output can be accomplished with a liquid crystal display (LCD) and a built-in printer in the cases of dedicated aids, whereas a computer monitor and peripherally attached printer may serve to meet the same goal for a computer-based system (Figure 49-10). Similarly, both dedicated devices and microcomputers (stationary and portable) are capable of producing spoken output with speech synthesizers. Whereas some patients require only one type of output (spoken or written), other individuals have been noted to benefit from both types.

Technologic advances in the areas of dedicated communication aids and microcomputer-based systems have provided severely physically disabled individuals with a method for producing written and spoken output, thus enabling these individuals to realize their maximum communication and rehabilitation potentials (Figure 49-11). A speech-language pathologist trained in augmentative communication alternatives may creatively design a system, tailor it to meet individual communication needs, and provide intensive and individualized training with the system. The successful integration of an augmentative communication system therefore can improve the quality of life for the severely handicapped, nonspeaking individual. Augmentative communication intervention has proved itself to be a viable alternative for providing the severely motor and speech impaired population with an avenue for effective communication.

MANAGEMENT OF THE TRACHEOSTOMIZED, RESPIRATORILY IMPAIRED

In the respiratorily impaired population, maintaining a patent airway takes precedence over allowing active air flow through the vocal cords. Air is rerouted through the tracheostomy tube as opposed to passing through the vocal cords, resulting in a lack of air with which to phonate. This condition produces *aphonia,* or absence of voice. At times a fenestrated tracheostomy tube may be prescribed, which allows some air to leak into the upper airway and thereby permits voicing. However during periods of tracheostomy cuff inflation for purposes of airway protection, air passage through the folds is absent and as a result voicing is not feasible.

Patients who are ventilator dependent pose additional problems. If minimal cuff deflation is permitted, the patient needs instruction to coordinate phonation with ventilator breathing. In addition, ventilator modifications may also be explored to provide patients with increased air flow for speech purposes. When the rehabilitation plan includes weaning the patient from ventilator support or tracheostomy tube, a variation on the tracheostomy plug, called a speaking valve, may be appropriate. A Passy Muir Speaking Valve (Passy and Passy, Inc., Irving, Calif.) is an example of such a device. This device fits over the tracheostomy tube and acts as a one-way valve. It allows the passage of air into the trachea on inhalation, but automatically closes on exhalation, thereby shunting the air into the upper airway for speech.

When long-term aphonia is likely, due to the presence of a tracheostomy tube with an inflated cuff, a speaking tracheostomy tube may be appropriate (for example, the Communitrach I [Implant Technologies, Minneapolis], Portex Talking Tracheostomy Tube [Portex, Wilmington, Mass.], or the Pitt Tracheostomy Tube [American Hospital Supply, St. Louis]). These tubes allow the cuff to remain inflated to ensure airway protection. A small piece of tubing is connected to an outside compressed air source and channeled into the tracheal area above the level of the cuff. This air can then pass through the vocal folds to produce sound, which is later articulated into speech.

Tracheostomy tube modifications require good articulatory skills and are most appropriate for patients with high spinal cord injuries or static neurologic conditions (for example, poliomyelitis). Those patients with degenerative neuromuscular disease with a concomitant dysarthria usually exhibit compromised articulatory skills and are therefore best served using an alternative communication approach.

The absence of voice, coupled with the patient's apprehension concerning his or her respiratory status, makes immediate intervention on the part of the communication specialist mandatory. In such cases, a letter board can be provided to establish a means of immediate communication. Additionally, a standard hand-held electrolarynx or an electrolarynx that can be used intraorally or adapted for use with quadriplegic individuals can also be provided to allow communication access for the individual with aphonia.

DYSPHAGIA

Dysphagia is a swallowing disorder that may result from a variety of medical conditions. For discussion in this chapter, these include stroke, traumatic brain injury, progressive neurologic disease (for example, amyotrophic lateral sclerosis, muscular dystrophy, Parkinson's disease), and oropharyngeal carcinoma. Dysphagia may occur with a concomitant dysarthria or aphasia, depending on lesion site. The medullary reticular formation, located in the brainstem, is considered the swallowing "center" that organizes the information necessary for the swallow. Contributions of the cerebellum and cortex to the act of swallowing are less clearly defined.[68]

Deglutition is divided into four phases: the oral preparatory, or mastication phase; the oral phase, consisting of oral transit of the bolus; the pharyngeal phase, beginning when the swallow reflex initiates and the bolus is propelled through the pharynx; and the esophageal phase, when esophageal peristalsis pushes the bolus into the stomach.[27,68] The patient with dysphagia may have varying degrees of impairment in each phase. The speech-language pathologist is involved in managing impairment in the oral preparatory, oral, and pharyngeal stages. Esophageal problems usually require medical intervention.

The successful management of dysphagia involves a multidisciplinary team approach spearheaded by the swallowing therapist, usually a speech-language pathologist. The team includes the otolaryngologist, radiologist, dietician or nutritionist, physiatrist, nursing staff, and often the dentist or prosthodontist. Speech-language pathologists commonly assume the coordinating role in dysphagia management because of their expertise with oropharyngeal anatomy and normal and disordered deglutition, as well as their skills in administering direct dysphagia treatment.

Evaluation

The clinical evaluation often begins with a review of the onset, duration, and symptoms of the dysphagia. The clinician then performs an oromotor examination, relating the structure and function of the anatomy to oral and pharyngeal stage bolus control problems. Impaired tongue movement, for example, may cause decreased oral transit of the bolus and may impair timely initiation of the swallow reflex. If medically advisable, the speech-language pathologist may administer trial swallows of small amounts of liquid and semiliquid boluses to gain further information regarding oral stage problems and possible pharyngeal dysfunctions. The limitations of the clinical evaluation, usually conducted at bedside, are obvious. Definitive information is obtained *only* for oral stage functioning of the swallowing mechanism.

To obtain further objective information, the speech-language pathologist usually recommends that fiberoptic velopharyngeal and laryngeal endoscopy and radiographic videofluoroscopy be performed. Endoscopy provides a direct means of viewing the velopharynx, pharynx, and larynx during swallowing. This technique is valuable in delineating structural and functional impairments.[110,111] The instrument used for this procedure is the flexible fiberoptic endoscope and accompanying light source (usually halogen or xenon cool light system). Nasendoscopy is often performed by the otolaryngologist in cooperation with the speech-language pathologist. Relevant deficits identified during endoscopy include decreased velopharyngeal function, which may explain instances of nasal regurgitation, and incomplete vocal fold adduction, which suggests airway protection problems and a potential for aspiration.[52]

Videofluoroscopy is the procedure of choice in the eval-

uation of any dysphagic impairment that is not strictly limited to the oral phase. This radiographic assessment procedure, presently replacing cineradiography in many facilities, is the only technique available to image the deglutition process from the time the bolus is placed in the oral cavity to its passage into the esophagus.[67-69] Videofluoroscopy is usually performed by the radiologist in conjunction with the speech-language pathologist. The examination, also known as the modified barium swallow, consists of the administration of $\frac{1}{3}$ teaspoon barium liquid, $\frac{1}{3}$ teaspoon barium paste, and a one-quarter piece of graham cracker coated with barium during separate trials. The small quantities used decrease the danger of airway obstruction and limit the amount of material that can be aspirated. The patient is viewed from lateral and anteroposterior positions, each of which provides information on specific structural and functional disturbances (Figure 49-12).

Videofluoroscopy is the only method of documenting these functional and structural problems in the oral and pharyngeal stages of deglutition; however, since the entire swallowing tract, from mouth to stomach, functions as a whole, pharyngoesophageal interrelationships in deglutition must be considered. Esophageal disease often affects cricopharyngeal functioning and may thus interfere with aspects of the pharyngeal stage of swallowing.[28] In cases where esophageal dysfunction is suspected, an esophogram (barium swallow) follows the videofluoroscopy (modified barium swallow) to delineate a possible esophageal motility disorder. The two examinations provide different but integral information in the planning of a dysphagia treatment program.

Additional tests, such as the blue dye test, may be ordered as part of the total dysphagia protocol. This limited diagnostic procedure can only be used with the tracheostomized patient to identify gross aspiration.[11,17] Four drops of methylene blue dye are placed on the patient's tongue every 4 hours for 24 hours. In a variation, dye can be mixed with food or water and administered orally over three separate feedings. Blue dye obtained in suctioning is considered positive evidence of aspiration. The limitations of the blue dye test are that it can only be administered to patients with tracheostomy tubes, it only detects the presence (or absence) of significant aspiration, and it does not delineate between oral and pharyngeal stage swallowing problems.

Ultrasound, another dysphagia assessment tool that images the oral stage of swallowing, has the advantage of not exposing the patient to any radiation. However, this technique is restricted to oral phase evaluation only. Shawker and co-workers[94] and Stone and Shawker[101] described this procedure in more detail.

Treatment

Treatment for swallowing disorders includes indirect and direct intervention that is carried out by the speech-language pathologist following an extensive evaluation. Indirect treat-

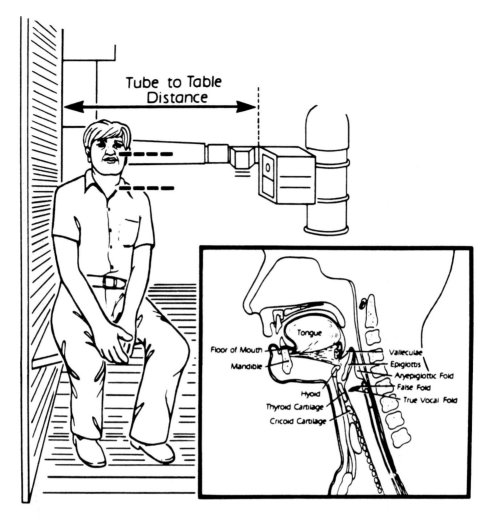

Figure 49-12. Patient seated on platform of radiographic table so oral cavity, pharynx, and cervical esophagus can be viewed in lateral plane. (From Logemann, J: Manual for the videofluorographic study of swallowing, Boston, 1986, College-Hill Press.)

ment is usually provided to the severely dysphagic patient who is unable to achieve sufficient nutrition and hydration orally or for whom oral intake is unsafe because of possible aspiration. Therapy may include oromotor strengthening exercises for labial, lingual, and mandibular weakness, which affects oral transit and bolus control, and thermal stimulation, a technique designed to facilitate a swallow. Direct dysphagia treatment involves the use of food and liquid in the therapy process. The speech-language pathologist often provides mealtime management strategies such as a postural modification. Additionally, airway protection techniques identified during videofluoroscopy might be prescribed. These may include the supraglottic swallow and the Mendelsohn maneuver, which facilitate opening of the upper esophageal sphincter. The treating clinician also recommends dietary changes to ensure the patient's safety during swallowing.

Recommendations for nutritional management are vital[37,68,70] and are usually provided by the dietary staff and nutritionist. Adequate nutritional intake and hydration are primary concerns. Suggestions for medical management are usually made in conjunction with the radiologist or otolaryngologist. Problems that arise medically, such as fistulas, cervical osteophytes, vocal fold paresis, and cricopharyngeal dysfunction, may warrant medical or surgical intervention.[27] Additionally, the patient's primary physician may be consulted on the need for alternate, nonoral feeding. Alternatives in these situations include nasogastric tube placement, pharyngostomy, esophagostomy, jejunostomy, or gastrostomy. Finally, the dental department may provide prosthetic management as needed. It can be surmised that team input is important to the successful management of the dysphagia disorder.

CLOSED HEAD INJURY

Closed head injury, a term referring to brain injury resulting from nonpenetrating head trauma, affects approximately 400,000 persons annually.[1] Many of those affected are adolescents and young adults under age 35, who are often involved in motor vehicle accidents. They face communication deficits caused by a complex interaction of cognitive and linguistic variables, which linger long after the acute onset of the damage. Generalized cognitive impairment, attentional, orientation, and memory deficits, and decreased speed of information processing are typical correlates of closed head injury. Although characteristic profiles of linguistic impairment are seen with focal lesions, diffuse lesions produce less predictable cognitive communication deficits. In addition, concomitant dysarthrias and dysphagias are often present.

Recent advances in the study of the neuropathology of closed head injury have helped define the types of lesions associated with particular injuries. Adamovich and coworkers[1] stated that there are two classes of lesions caused by varying injuries that can be differentiated. The first is direct impact injuries, such as a fall that causes focal cortical contusions found in the frontal and temporal lobe. The second type of lesion is from high acceleration injuries, such as motor vehicle accidents associated with diffuse axonal injury of the white matter and with focal lesions in the corpus callosum and the dorsolateral quadrant of the midbrain. The closed head injury patient also commonly faces cerebral edema, subdural or epidural hematomas, and hypoxia owing to cardiopulmonary arrest.

Evaluation

The assessment of the closed head injury patient is optimally an interdisciplinary approach, combining the expertise of the neuropsychologist, neurologist, speech-language pathologist, and occupational therapist. Team evaluation should delineate the impaired components of the cognitive-linguistic systems. The closed head injury patient presents with difficulties in organization, as well as in structuring and predication of thought, which leads to disorientation, confusion, reduced initiation, and reduced inhibition. Deficits in attention confound these difficulties, whereas higher-level deficits in "executive" functions can inhibit goal formation, selection, and ultimate achievement. Hagen[40] states that areas to be assessed therefore include attentional abilities (beginning with alerting and arousal), memory skills, and the ability to order sensory stimuli and internal thoughts.

Evaluation of these complex areas requires the administration of neuropsychologic batteries as well as more informal assessments. Ylvisaker and Holland[112] stressed the need to include tests of linguistic abilities and communicative functioning. Suggested standardized batteries include the Detroit Test of Learning Aptitude,[6] the Wechsler Memory Scale,[106] the Raven's Coloured Progressive Matrices,[82] the Boston Naming Testing,[53] and the Token Test.[72] These batteries address a range of cognitive and linguistic variables. More informal appraisal comprises evaluation of higher-level thought processing such as in metaphor and proverb interpretation, functional problem solving, and verbal absurdity analysis. Additionally, assessment of the patient's communicative functioning in terms of the pragmatics of language is generally required. Discourse skills and nonlinguistic skills such as eye contact and turn taking are also vital components to be evaluated.

Two well-known scales have proved valuable in providing information for treatment and in delineating prognostic indicators. They are the Rancho Los Amigos Scale of Cognitive Levels and Expected Behavior[40] and the Glasgow Coma Scale.[47] The former rates the head-injured patient by particular behaviors and places them within one of eight levels. The latter predicts recovery according to duration of coma after onset of closed head injury.

Treatment

Treatment of the closed head injury patient focuses on residual cognitive-linguistic skills. The speech-language pathologist provides treatment for those aspects of cognitive-linguistic dysfunction that affect functional communicative status with additional attention to any dysarthric or dysphagic component. One of the primary focuses of treatment is to develop in the patient the ability to practice, to learn from that practice, to use feedback purposefully, and to encourage relearning of daily skills, which will then enhance functional living.

Therapeutic intervention is also thought to be complementary to the natural recovery process following traumatic brain injury. Cognitive treatment programs are therefore hierarchic in overall structure and include careful ordering of abilities within that structure. For example, Adamovich and co-workers[1] suggested that treatment follow a three-stage hierarchy of arousal and alerting, operant retraining, and a community-oriented, self-reliant treatment program.

Therapy within this structure is also arranged in careful sequence. During an intermediate or goal-oriented phase, the clinician must select a task within the patient's ability and then increase complexity in gradual, controlled stages. For example, during a categorization activity, a patient would be first asked to sort objects into general categories, then after achieving this skill, to sort into more specific groupings. The goal of any treatment program is to increase the patient's functioning in the daily communicative environment. Other suggested treatment goals may include improving selective attention, developing vigilance for repetitive tasks, decreasing impulsivity in task initiation, increasing accuracy in repetitive tasks, initiating appropriate compensatory strategies, increasing awareness of deficit areas, and improving readiness and ability to modify behavior based on feedback.[29]

Treatment of the closed head injury patient can also be effectively delivered with a microcomputer. Parameters such as attention, perception, and visual tracking as well as language deficits can be addressed. Benefits of microcomputer intervention, as noted earlier, include the ability to provide a controlled, consistent presentation of task stimuli with objective feedback. A variety of cognitive rehabilitation software packages have been published to meet the needs of the patient with cognitive communication deficits.

Investigation and study findings of treatment efficacy with closed head injury populations have been cautiously optimistic[113] in recent years. Most favorable prognostic considerations are for younger patients, patients who spend less than 3 months in coma, and for those individuals who are highly goal oriented and motivated. Actual reported improvements in cognitive-linguistic performance are notable in interpersonal process recall (social-communicative performance[50]), effectiveness of strategy use,[26] and environmental enhancement.[38]

RIGHT HEMISPHERE DYSFUNCTION

The patient with right hemisphere dysfunction has impairments in overall communicative functioning secondary to nonlinguistic, extralinguistic, and, less significantly, linguistic deficits. The profile of the patient with right hemisphere dysfunction includes impaired attention and perception, pragmatic and prosodic disturbances, and usually mild linguistic deficits. The effect on communication is often profound: right hemisphere dysfunction patients demonstrate "linguistically adequate, but communicatively deficient output."[75]

Myers defined right hemisphere communication impairment as "an acquired disorder in the expression and reception of complex, contextually based communicative events resulting from a disturbance of the attentional and perceptual mechanisms underlying nonsymbolic, experiential processing."[75]

The role of the right hemisphere in communicative functioning has become clearer in recent years, partly because technologic advances have permitted delineation of the locus of right-sided lesions and their concomitant deficits. Evidence from split-brain studies has revealed differences in processing styles, with the left hemisphere dealing more effectively with descriptive systems, or "coded" behaviors, while the right is better suited for processing novel tasks, or experiences themselves.[35] Further disruptions in this experiential processing can cause lower-order perceptual deficits (for example, visuospatial impairment, neglect), prosodic and affective disturbances, linguistic disorders, and higher-order perceptual and cognitive problems.

Evaluation

The complexity of right hemisphere dysfunction necessitates an interdisciplinary management approach for expedient diagnosis and coordinated treatment. Neuropsychologists, neurologists, speech-language pathologists, and occupational therapists combine their areas of expertise to assess the functional ability of the right hemisphere dysfunction patient to interact within his or her environment. The speech-language pathologist, in order to assess those behaviors relevant to communicative functioning, must glean evaluative information from a variety of sources.

There are very few standardized batteries for the assessment of right hemisphere dysfunction. The RIC (Rehabilitation Institute of Chicago) Evaluation of Communication Problems in Right Hemisphere Dysfunction[15] is a recently published exception that provides standardized evaluation of right hemisphere correlates. Additional tests of visual perception, such as the Spatial Orientation Memory Test,[108] and assessment of higher level cognitive processes such as the Detroit Test of Learning Aptitude[6] may be administered. Linguistic assessment is usually performed using subtests of established aphasia batteries.

Pure linguistic diagnosis of the right hemisphere–impaired patient involves direct examination of receptive and expressive language modalities (comprehension of yes or no questions, following directions, discriminating verbal labels, naming, using grammatically complete utterances) as is typically conducted by the speech-language pathologist in aphasia remediation. Qualitatively different errors, however, are noted between aphasic patients and those exhibiting right hemisphere involvement. More directed attention in the linguistic modality is therefore necessary, especially for stimuli of increasing linguistic complexity. Higher linguistic functions such as comprehension of grammatically complex phrases was found to be significantly impaired for right hemisphere–involved patients as compared to control subjects in a study by McNeil and Prescott.[72]

Nonlinguistic disorders are also evidenced in the right hemisphere–involved patient. Specific attentional and perceptual deficits appear to confound the patient's ability to organize and sequence purposeful activities despite overall alertness and orientation to surroundings. Impaired facial recognition and geographic disorientation are common findings. Effects of these symptoms on communication can be dramatic and may isolate the patient from partaking communicatively and socially in daily activities.

Extralinguistic variables within right hemisphere dysfunction exceed the word-by-word comprehension of language utterances. It includes the ability to comprehend and express emotions and to use language in a pragmatic way, as in appreciating idiomatic expressions and humor. Both areas are a source of concern for clinicians working with the patient exhibiting right hemisphere involvement. The patient who demonstrates a deficit in these extralinguistic areas exhibits an overall hypoarousal in communicative performance that requires attention. Effect on performance can also be dramatic.

Treatment

Therapeutic remediation with the patient exhibiting right hemisphere impairments involves targeting a treatment program to meet the appropriate constellation of nonlinguistic, extralinguistic, and linguistic impairments. Pure linguistic impairments, as outlined previously, can be targeted with traditional aphasia treatment regimes if the impairment is not a part of a more encompassing perceptual or attentional disorder. Nonlinguistic and extralinguistic deficits, however, require an integrative and compensatory approach with overall communicative effectiveness as the final goal.

Nonlinguistic behaviors that affect communicative performances can be approached through counseling and through feedback paradigms. Compensatory strategies can be used to aid the patients in areas of orientation through visual mapping of the environment and more selective attention to tasks. Extralinguistic variables can also be included in treatment regimens through implementing goals designed to increase the patient's ability to distinguish critical from extraneous information. Cuing from the clinician can also be provided within treatment sessions to have the patient use facial expression and tone (pragmatic skills) within communicative endeavors. Additionally, the patient may capitalize on contextual cues from within his or her communicative environment to overcome perceptual difficulties and expand on visual and verbal strengths.

CONCLUSION

The ability to communicate with a variety of listeners in different environments through spoken, written, or gestural modalities is a unique skill available only to the human species. For this reason, speech-language pathologists and rehabilitation specialists must continue to integrate existing and new knowledge, technology, and creativity into the therapeutic process to help the communicatively impaired patient regain this precious ability. This chapter has provided basic knowledge on the diagnostic process, treatment alternatives, and prognostic considerations for the communicatively impaired, neurogenically disordered adult, while allowing the reader to appreciate the challenge that the physician and rehabilitation team face when working with these disordered individuals. It is hoped that concepts will be gleaned from this material and that sensitivity and skill will be shared with each communicatively impaired individual. Continued exploration into the field of communication and sciences and its disorders is encouraged and recommended.

ACKNOWLEDGMENT

I gratefully acknowledge the assistance of speech pathology staff from Goldwater Memorial Hospital, New York University Medical Center, and specifically, the contributions in the areas of emerging technology of Mark Leddy, Janet Cram, Karen Dikeman, Elizabeth Adams, and Cathy Salciccia.

REFERENCES

1. Adamovich, B, Henderson, JA, and Auerbach, S: Cognitive rehabilitation of closed head injured patients: a dynamic approach, San Diego, 1985, College-Hill Press.
2. Albert, M, Sparks, R, and Helm, N: Melodic intonation therapy for aphasia, Arch Neurol 29:130, 1973.
3. Alekoumbides, A: Hemispheric dominance for language: quantitative aspects, Acta Neurol Scand 57:97, 1978.
4. Aten, J: Efficacy of modified palatal lifts for improving resonance. In McNeil, MR, Rosenbek, JC, and Aronson, AE, editors: The dysarthrias: physiology, acoustics, perception and management, San Diego, 1984, College-Hill Press.
5. Baken, R: Clinical measurement of speech and voice, Boston, 1987, Little Brown & Co.
6. Baker, HJ, and Leland, AB: Detroit test of learning aptitude, New York, 1987, Bobbs-Merril Co.
7. Basso, A, Capitani, E, and Vignolo, LA: Influence of rehabilitation on language skills in aphasic patients, a controlled study, Arch Neurol 36:190, 1979.
8. Benson, DF: Aphasia, alexia, and agraphia, New York, 1979, Churchill-Livingston.
9. Beukelman, DR, Kraft, GH, and Freal, J: Expressive communication disorders in persons with multiple sclerosis: a survey, Arch Phys Med Rehabil 66:675, 1985.
10. Beukelman, DR, Yorkston, K, and Dowden, P: Communication augmentation: a casebook of clinical management, San Diego, 1985, College-Hill Press.
11. Bonanno, PC: Swallowing dysfunction after tracheostomy, Ann Surg 174:29, 1971.
12. Brown, JW: Aphasia, apraxia, and agnosia, Springfield, Ill, 1972, Charles C Thomas, Publisher.
13. Brown, JW, and Grober, E: Age, sex, and aphasia type, evidence for a regional cerebral growth process underlying lateralization, J Nerv Ment Dis 171:431, 1983.
14. Brown, JW, and Jaffe, J: Hypothesis on cerebral dominance, Neuropsychologia 13:107, 1975.
15. Burns, MS, Halper, AS, and Mogil, SI: RIC evaluation of communication problems in right hemisphere dysfunction, Gaithersburg, Md, 1985, Aspen Publishers.
16. Butfield, E, and Zangwill, DL: Re-education in aphasia: a review of 70 cases, J Neurol Neurosurg Psychiatry, 75:8, 1946.
17. Cameron, JL, and Zuidema, G: Aspiration in patients with tracheostomies, Surg Gynecol Obstet 136:68, 1978.
18. Collins, M: Diagnosis and treatment of global aphasia, San Diego, 1986, College-Hill Press.
19. Culton, GL: Spontaneous recovery from aphasia, J Speech Hearing Res 12:825, 1969.
20. Darley, F: Aphasia, Philadelphia, 1982, WB Saunders Co.
21. Darley, F, Aronson, AE, and Brown, JR: Differential diagnostic patterns of dysarthria, J Speech Hear Res 12:246, 1969.
22. Darley, F, Aronson, AE, and Brown, JR: Clusters of deviant speech dimensions in the dysarthrias, J Speech Hear Res 12:462, 1969.
23. Darley, F, Aronson, AE, and Brown, JR: Motor speech disorders, Philadelphia, 1975, WB Saunders Co.
24. Davis, GA, and Wilcox, MJ: Incorporating parameters of natural convention in aphasic treatment. In Chapey, R, editor: Language intervention strategies in adult aphasia, Baltimore, 1981, Williams & Wilkins Co.
25. Davis, GA, and Wilcox, MJ: Adult aphasia rehabilitation: applied pragmatics, San Diego, 1985, College-Hill Press.
26. Diller, L, and Gordon, W: Intervention for cognitive deficits in brain injured adults, J Consult Clin Psychol 49:822, 1981.
27. Donner, M, Bosma, J, and Robertson, D: Anatomy and physiology of the pharynx, Gastrointest Radiol 10:196, 1985.

28. Donner, MW, and Jones, B: The multidisciplinary approach to dysphagia, Gastrointest Radiol 10:193, 1985.

29. Dougherty, PM, and Radomski, MV: The cognitive rehabilitation workbook, Rockville, Md, 1987, Aspen Publishers, Inc.

30. Enderby, P: Frenchay dysarthria assessment, San Diego, 1983, College-Hill Press.

31. Enderby, P: The standardized assessment of dysarthria is possible. In Berry, W, editor: Clinical dysarthria, San Diego, 1983, College-Hill Press.

32. Fisher, H, and Logemann, J: The Fisher-Logemann test of articulation competence, Boston, 1971, Houghton-Mifflin.

33. Frydenberg, H, and Wheeler, D: Microcomputer assisted intervention for the speech and language impaired adult. In Grossfeld, M, and Grossfeld, C, editors: Microcomputer applications in the rehabilitation of communicative disorders, Rockville, Md, 1986, Aspen Publishers, Inc.

34. Geschwind, N: The apraxias: neural mechanisms of disorders of learned movement, Am Sci 63:188, 1975.

35. Goldberg, E, and Costa, L: Hemispheric differences in the acquisition and use of descriptive systems, Brain Lang 14:144, 1981.

36. Goodglass, H, and Kaplan, E: The assessment of aphasia and related disorders, Philadelphia, 1983, Lea & Febiger.

37. Groher, ME: Dysphagia: diagnosis and management, Stoneham, Mass, 1984, Butterworth Publishers.

38. Haarbauer-Krupa, J, et al: Cognitive rehabilitation therapy: late stages of recovery. In Ylvisaker, M, editor: Head injury rehabilitation: children and adolescents, San Diego, 1965, College-Hill Press.

39. Hagen, C: Language disorders in head trauma. In Holland, A, editor: Language disorders in adults: recent advances, San Diego, 1983, College-Hill Press.

40. Hagen, C, and Malkmus, D: Intervention strategies for language disorders secondary to head trauma, Atlanta, Ga, 1979, American Speech-Language-Hearing Association.

41. Harris, D, and Vanderheiden, GC: Augmentative communication techniques. In Schiefelbusch, RI, editor: Nonspeech language and communication analysis and intervention, Baltimore, 1980, University Park Press.

42. Helm-Estabrooks, N: Treatment of subcortical aphasia in language handicaps. In Perkins, WH, editor: Language handicaps in adults, Current therapy of communication disorders series, vol 3, New York, 1983, Thieme-Stratton, Inc.

43. Helm-Estabrooks, N, Fitzpatrick, PM, and Barresi, B: Visual action therapy for global aphasia, J Speech Hear Disord 47:385, 1982.

44. Hesselblad, J, Cram, JE, and Kerman-Lerner, P: Implementation and enhancements of a clinical microcomputer program. Presentation at Goldwater Memorial Hospital, New York University Medical Center, New York, 1987.

45. Holland, A: Case studies in aphasia rehabilitation using programmed instruction, J Speech Hear Disord 35:377, 1970.

46. Holland, A: Communicative abilities in daily living, Baltimore, 1980, University Park Press.

47. Jennett, B, et al: Disability after severe head injury: observations on the use of the Glasgow Outcome Scale, J Neurol Neurosurg Psychiatry 44:205, 1981.

48. Johns, DF: Surgical and prosthetic management of neurogenic velopharyngeal incompetency in dysarthria. In Johns, DF, editor: Clinical management of neurogenic communicative disorders, ed 2, Boston, 1985, Little Brown & Co.

49. Johns, DF, and Darley, FL: Phonemic variability in apraxia of speech, J Speech Hear Res 13:556, 1970.

50. Kagan, N: Interpersonal process recall, J Nerv Ment Dis 148:356, 1969.

51. Kapassakis, G, et al: Clinical instrumentation for the management of neurogenically-based speech and voice disorders, Paper presented at Goldwater Memorial Hospital, New York University Medical Center, New York, 1987.

52. Kapassakis, G, et al: Diagnosis and treatment of swallowing disorders, Paper presented at Goldwater Memorial Hospital, New York University Medical Center, New York, 1987.

53. Kaplan, E, Goodglass, H, and Weintraub, S: Boston naming test, Philadelphia, 1983, Lea & Febiger.

54. Katz, RC, and Nagy, VT: A computerized treatment system for chronic aphasic patients. In Brookshire, RH, editor: Clinical aphasiology: conference proceedings, Minneapolis, 1982, BRK Publishers.

55. Kerman, PC, Singer, L, and Davidoff, A: Palatal lift and speech therapy for velopharyngeal incompetance, Arch Phys Med Rehabil 54:271, 1973.

56. Kerman, PC, et al: Therapeutic strategies for language reacquisition in the severely expressively-impaired aphasic, Mini-seminar presented at American Speech and Hearing Association Annual Convention, Washington, DC, 1975.

57. Kerman-Lerner, P, et al: Efficacy of microcomputer treatment for reading disorders in aphasic adults, Paper presented at Annual Meeting of the American Congress of Rehabilitation Medicine, Baltimore, 1986.

58. Kertesz, A: Aphasia and associated disorders, New York, 1979, Grune & Stratton, Inc.

59. Kertesz, A: Western aphasia battery, New York, 1982, Grune & Stratton, Inc.

60. Kinsbourne, M: Hemi-neglect and hemisphere rivalry, Adv Neurol 18:41, 1977.

61. Kinsbourne, M, and Hiscock, M: Does cerebral dominance develop? In Segalowitz, S, and Gruber, F, editors: Language development and neurological theory, New York, 1977, Academic Press, Inc.

62. Kraat, AW, and Sitver-Kogult, M: Features of commercially available communication aids, Wooster, Mass, 1985, Prentke Romich Co.

63. LaPointe, LL: Base-10 programmed stimulation: task specification, scoring, and plotting performance in aphasia therapy, J Speech Hear Disord 42:90, 1977.

64. Leddy, M, et al: Clinical uses of instrumentation for dysarthria treatment: case studies, Paper presented at presentation at the New York State Speech-Language-Hearing Association Annual Convention, Kiamesha Lake, NY, 1987.

65. Lenneberg, EH: Biological foundations of language, Florida, 1984, Krieger.

66. Lincoln, NB, et al: Effectiveness of speech therapy for aphasic stroke patients: a randomized controlled trial, Lancet 2:1197, 1984.

67. Linden, P, and Siebens, A: Dysphagia: predicting laryngeal penetration, Arch Phys Med Rehabil 64:281, 1983.

68. Logemann, J: Evaluation and treatment of swallowing disorders, San Diego, 1983, College-Hill Press.

69. Logemann, J: Manual for the videofluorographic of swallowing, San Diego, 1986, College-Hill Press.

70. Logemann, J: Treatment for aspiration related to dysphagia: an overview, Dysphagia 1:34, 1986.

71. Lybolt, J, Netsell, R, and Farrage, J: A bite-block prosthesis in the treatment of dysarthria, Paper presented at the American Speech-Language-Hearing Association Convention, Toronto, 1982.

72. McNeil, MR, and Prescott, TE: The revised token test, Baltimore, 1978, University Park Press.

73. Mills, RH: Microcomputerized auditory comprehension training. In Brookshire RH, editor: Clinical aphasiology: conference proceedings, Minneapolis, 1982, BRK Publishers.

74. Minami, RT, et al: Velopharyngeal incompetency without overt cleft palate, a collective review with 98 patients, Plast Reconstr Surg 55:573, 1979.

75. Myers, PS: Right hemisphere communication impairment. In Chapey, R, editor: Language intervention strategies in adult aphasia, Baltimore, 1984, Williams & Wilkins.

76. Naeser, MA, et al: Aphasia with predominantly subcortical lesion sites: description of three capsular/putaminal aphasia syndromes, Arch Neurol 39:2, 1982.

76a. National Institutes of Health, National Institute of Neurological and Communicative Disorders and Stroke, Bethesda, Md, 1983, NIH Pub No 83-2222.

77. Netsell, R: A neurobiologic view of the dysarthrias. In McNeil, MR, Rosenbek, JC, and Aronson, AE, editors: The dysarthrias: physiology, acoustics, perception and management, San Diego, 1984, College-Hill Press.

78. Netsell, R: Neurobiological view of speech production and the dysarthrias, San Diego, 1986, College-Hill Press.

79. Netsell, R, and Hixon, TJ: A noninvasive method for clinically estimating subglottal air pressure, J Speech Hear Dis 43:326, 1978.

80. Obler, LK, et al: Aphasia type and aging, Brain Lang 6:318, 1978.

81. Porch, BE: Porch index of communicative ability, Palo Alto, 1983, Consult Psychologists Press.

82. Raven, JC: The coloured progressive matrices, London, 1963, HK Lewis & Co.

83. Rosenbek, JC: Treating apraxia of speech. In Johns, DF, editor: Clinical management of neurogenic communicative disorders, ed 2, New York, 1985, Little Brown & Company.

84. Rosenbek, JC, and LaPointe, LL: The dysarthrias: description, diagnosis, and treatment. In Johns, DF, editor: Clinical management of neurogenic communicative disorders, ed 2, Boston, 1985, Little, Brown & Co.

85. Rubens, AB: The role of changes within the central nervous system during recovery from aphasia. In Sullivan, M, and Kommers, M, editors: Rationale for adult aphasia therapy, Omaha, 1977, University of Nebraska Medical Center.

86. Rubow, R, and Swift, E: Microcomputer-based wearable biofeedback device to improve treatment carry over in parkinsonian dysarthria, J Speech Hear Disord 50:178, 1985.

87. Salciccia, CE: The microcomputer as an augmentative communication system In Grossfeld, M, and Grossfeld, C, editors: Microcomputer applications in the rehabilitation of communicative disorders, Rockville, Md, 1986, Aspen Publishers, Inc.

88. Salciccia, CE, Adams, E, and Christopher, F: Communication enhancement in groups with severely speech impaired persons, Paper presented at the New York State Speech-Language-Hearing Association Annual Convention, Kiamesha Lake, NY, 1987.

89. Sarno, MT: The functional communication profile manual of directions, Rehabilitation Monograph 42, New York, 1969, New York Institute of Rehabilitation Medicine, New York University Center.

90. Sarno, MT, and Levita, E: Recovery in treating aphasia in the first year, post stroke, Stroke 10:663, 1979.

91. Sarno, MT, Silverman, M, and Sands, E: Speech therapy and language recovery in severe aphasia, J Speech Hear Res 13:607, 1970.

92. Schuell, H: The Minnesota test for differential diagnosis of aphasia, Minneapolis, 1973, University of Minnesota Press.

93. Schuell, H, Jenkins, JJ, and Jiminez-Pabon, E: Aphasia in adults: diagnosis, prognosis and treatment, New York, 1975, Hoeber Medical Division, Harper & Row.

94. Shawker, T, Stone, M, and Sonies, B: Tongue pellet tracking by ultrasound: development of reverberation pellet, J Phonet 13:135, 1985.

95. Shewan, CM, and Bandur, DL: Treatment of aphasia: a language oriented approach, San Diego, 1986, College-Hill Press.

96. Shewan, CM, and Kertesz, A: Effects of speech and language treatment on recovery from aphasia, Brain Lang 23:272, 1984.

97. Smith, A: Objective indices of severity of chronic aphasia in stroke patients, J Speech Hear Disord 36:67, 1971.

98. Sparks, RW, Helm, N, and Albert, M: Aphasia rehabilitation resulting from melodic intonation therapy, Cortex 10:303, 1974.

99. Sparks, RW, and Holland, AL: Method: melodic intonation therapy for aphasia, J Speech Hear Disord 41:287, 1976.

100. Spreen, O, and Benton, AL: Neurosensory center comprehensive examination for aphasia, 1969, Neuropsychology laboratory, Development of Psychology, Victoria, BC, University of Victoria.

101. Stone, M, and Shawker, TH: An ultrasound examination of tongue movement during swallowing, Dysphagia 1:78, 1986.

102. Szekeres, SF, Ylivasaker, M, and Holland, AL: Cognitive rehabilitation therapy: early stages of recovery. In Ylvisaker, M, editor: Head injury rehabilitation: children and adolescents, San Diego, 1985, College-Hill Press.

103. Templin, M, and Darley, F: The Templin-Darley test of articulation, ed 2, Iowa City, 1970, University of Iowa Bureau of Educational Research and Service.

104. Vanderheiden, G, and Lloyd, L: Communication systems and their components. In Blackstone, S, editor: Augmentative communication: an introduction, Rockville, Md, 1986, American Speech and Hearing Association.

105. Vignolo, LA: Evaluation of aphasia and language rehabilitation: a retrospective exploratory study, Cortex 1:344, 1964.

106. Wechsler, D: Wechsler Adult Intelligence Scale—Revised, New York, 1981, American Psychological Association.

107. Wepman, JM: Recovery from aphasia, New York, 1951, Ronald Press Co.

108. Wepman, P, and Turaids, F: Spatial orientation memory test, Los Angeles, 1975, Western Psychological Services.

109. Wertz, RT, et al: Veterans Administration cooperative study on aphasia: a comparison of individual and group treatment, J Speech Hear Res 24:580, 1981.

110. Wilson, FB, Kudryk, WH, and Sych, JA: The development of flexible fiberoptic video nasendoscopy (FFVN): clinical-teaching-research applications, ASHA 28:25, 1986.

111. Yanagisawa, E: Office telescopic photography of the larynx, Ann Otol Rhinol Laryngol 91 (pt 1):354, 1982.

112. Ylvisaker, MS, and Holland, AL: Coaching, self-coaching, and rehabilitation of head injury. In Johns, DF, editor: Clinical management of neurogenic communicative disorders, Boston, 1985, Little, Brown & Co.

113. Ylvisaker, MS, and Szekeres, SF: Management of the patient with closed head injury. In Chapey, R, editor: Language intervention strategies in adult aphasia, Baltimore, 1986, Williams & Wilkins Co.

114. Yorkston, K, and Beukelman, D: Assessment of intelligibility of dysarthric speech, Tigard, Ore, 1981, CC Publications.

115. Zangwill, OL: Cerebral dominance and its relation to psychological functions, Edinburgh, 1960, Olvier & Boyd.

CHAPTER 50

Driver education for the physically disabled

JIRI C. SIPAJLO

Most members of our society take for granted the ability and the need to get around, "mobility." We especially take for granted driving a car. However, when one becomes physically disabled or in some way impaired and no longer can drive a car or use the public transportation system in the usual way, the need to maintain independence of movement becomes essential.

Although options to driving or using standard mass transportation do exist—public buses equipped with wheelchair lifts, special commercial ambulette transportation for the wheelchair-bound population, county or state "dial a ride" systems, and ramps and elevators to subways and trains—they all have drawbacks. Public buses and subways do not provide the much needed door-to-door transportation. Some are prohibitively expensive; the average wheelchair transportation in the New York City area costs approximately $80 per day, an unacceptable transportation cost for a person who has been vocationally retrained and is starting a new career with a salary to match. Some services must be reserved days in advance, making them inconvenient. Finally, for various reasons many of these transportation companies for the physically disabled eventually become tardy, resulting in unreliable transportation and an unreliable employee.

For the physically disabled, driver training and driver education programs of various degrees of sophistication can be found in commercial auto schools, high school driver education programs, universities that offer traffic safety and driver education programs, and Veterans Administration hospitals and as integral parts of rehabilitation departments that are usually associated with major medical centers.

ESTABLISHING DRIVER TRAINING PROGRAMS

When reliable, convenient, affordable mass transit and driver training programs are not available in the immediate area, one can take the following steps to establish driver training for the physically disabled. A staff member, an occupational therapist, or a physical therapist should be appointed to review existing possibilities in the community. The American Automobile Association publishes a handy booklet called *The Handicapped Driver's Mobility Guide,* which lists state-by-state facilities and agencies dealing with disabled drivers. These include the state motor vehicle department, local major automobile dealers, manufacturers of assistive devices, and modifiers of fully automatic vans that can be driven while sitting in a wheelchair. The nearest ongoing programs should be contacted, visited, and observed. Several days of observation of each program can provide a wealth of information about how to start a program and the kind of program that would be most suited for particular needs.

Using existing driver education programs

Many commercial auto school owners are unaware that able-bodied students can drive a training car equipped with basic assistive devices, such as hand controls, without any difficulty. Simple hand controls that operate the accelerator and the brake look like an additional directional signal lever and are usually found directly below the existing directional signal lever. The steering knob for left or right hand snaps in or out of the steering wheel in seconds; when the steering knob is not in use, the steering wheel is free for the hand-over-hand steering used by able-bodied students. In addition to the hand controls and the steering knob, a left accelerator pedal is mounted on the floor. With these devices a commercial auto school instructor can retrain most physically disabled individuals except for those so severely disabled that they would not be able to transfer into a car. Individuals who could benefit from the installation of these assistive devices in a commercial auto vehicle include those with weakness, paralysis, or absence of any one extremity or a combination involving two extremities, such as both lower extremities, both extremities on the left or the right side of the body, a combination of a left upper and right lower extremity, or right upper and left lower extremity.

Once owners or managers of a commercial auto school realize that the disabled student and the able-bodied students can drive the same car, they usually become interested in installing assistive devices, especially when they learn that installing hand controls usually does not require drilling holes. Placing an additional section of a carpet under the left gas pedal leaves no mark, and the car can be returned or sold unchanged.

After the car is equipped with the assistive device, the instructor should learn to use it, observe other programs, and be exposed to the problems of disabled individuals, such as the fundamentals of transfers from the wheelchair to the passenger seat of the car and then across to the driver's seat. The instructor should learn how to push and handle the wheelchair and how to fold it and dispose of it after the transfer.

An important difference exists between working with inpatients who have recently been injured and are in a hospital or rehabilitation setting and individuals who are congenitally disabled or have been discharged and have been living on the outside. Inpatients need and expect professional help from everyone they encounter while being rehabilitated, including, of course, the driving instructor. Outpatients who have been living on their own will be able to show the inexperienced instructor what to do and how to help if necessary. Therefore for safety reasons it is essential that during the interview the instructor learn the student's rehabilitation status, past experiences in transfers, and the presence of muscle spasms. Because some students lack sensation, the instructor must give particular attention to the student's sitting position to prevent pressure sores that could result from allowing any part of the affected body to press against hard objects or letting the feet slip under the pedals. In winter, care must be taken to avoid close proximity of a foot or a leg to the concentrated heat coming from a heater.

Once the program at a commercial auto school is established, the school can function as an independent outside agency to which the rehabilitation facility refers patients with no other responsibility of feedback. In other arrangements the medical facility cooperates with the commercial auto school by assisting the instructor at various levels, such as helping to transfer inpatients from their wheelchairs into the car and providing past medical history as it would pertain to driving and to the motor vehicle department's rules and regulations. The occupational therapist might be of help by modifying some devices, such as steering knobs or steering cuffs. In return, the commercial auto school could be expected to provide progress reports to the staff members at the rehabilitation facility.

Establishing an in-house driver education program

The hospital or rehabilitation center can establish its own in-house driver education program as an integral part of the physical rehabilitation process. An administrative staff consisting of the key members of the driver education department is established. This staff usually includes a physician, the coordinator, a psychologist, a supervisor in physical therapy or occupational therapy, a research associate, an administrative secretary, and a driver educator.

After the initial contacts and visits have been made by the institute's staff members to other ongoing programs, a day-long conference or a seminar on the subject of "driver education for the physically disabled" should be scheduled at the facility. The purpose is to demonstrate the need for a driver education program and the benefits it would provide to the disabled individual and the community at large. Some of the topics of discussion should include equipment, procurement of vehicles, assistive devices, simulators, the instructor staff, and the qualifications of the driving educator.

The panel members should include the staff of the driver education department and guest speakers from other ongoing programs. The other invited participants should include interested professionals from related fields, agencies, and associations including the motor vehicle department; insurance companies; major automobile dealers; the Office of Vocational Rehabilitation; American Automobile Association; manufacturers of assistive devices and equipment, such as hand controls; and companies that modify fully automatic vans for severely disabled drivers.

Part of the program should be set aside for an equipment display and demonstration of various vehicles equipped with different types of commercially available hand controls, such as the "push and pull," "push and right angle," and the "push and twist" principles. The vans should be equipped with the state-of-the-art operational systems and means of independent access, such as the different types of fully automatic lifts.

In the past, major U.S. automobile makers have annually loaned thousands of cars free to qualified driver education programs in the nation's high schools and universities. At times this practice has been extended to qualified nonprofit organizations and rehabilitation institutes that provide driver education for the physically disabled. Obviously, this is the most preferred arrangement, especially if the manufacturer allows the car to stay in the program for a whole year.

The advantages to this program are numerous. Aside from receiving a free car, the program is provided with a new car every year and therefore stays current with the automobile market. No maintenance or repair problems develop because the vehicles are under full new car warranty. In turn, the manufacturer and the local dealer gain visibility by having a driver education vehicle marked "courtesy of the local dealer" being driven throughout the community. Finally, after passing the road test, disabled students often purchase exactly the same type of car in which they were trained because they know they can drive that make and model. Thus the manufacturer often acquires a satisfied customer for life.

Sometimes manufacturers who will not lend a model to a driving program will offer a "favorable lease plan." Information on these plans can be obtained from the local participating dealer of each manufacturer.

Donated or purchased vehicles are not recommended. They tend to become out of date quickly and create cost problems after a few years of service.

Often the local representative of assistive devices, such as hand controls, will provide and install a demonstrator unit to a qualified program free of charge. Driving simulators are helpful but not essential when starting a program. Their big advantage is in regular driver education classes where there are 20 or more students for one instructor. In programs with one instructor for each student, as is the case with the disabled population, custom-designed simulators can be available.

Driving instructors and education

Driving instructors from commercial auto schools and driver educators at high school and university level programs provide professional driving instruction. Most states have specific rules and regulations pertaining to licensing and certification of instructors and programs.

The driver educators at high schools and universities must have academic and teaching credentials. Unless they have taught in an adult program, however, their experience consists of teaching high school–aged students, most of whom are well coordinated and are still in a continuous learning process. The commercial auto school's driving instructors are not required by law to have extensive academic training, but they do have experience teaching poorly coordinated students of all ages. Nonprofit organizations are often not subject to the rules and regulations governing the commercial or the high school and university level driver education programs.

Some universities and major medical centers, such as New York University, offer courses on a graduate and continuing education level to prepare the experienced driver educators or driving instructors to teach the physically disabled student how to drive safely. A typical course description is as follows:

This course presents the theory, principles, and practices of preparing the physically handicapped for their role as drivers; analyzing disabilities affecting driver performance; adapting the handicapped to the driving task through psychological evaluation and preparation. Automotive revision, neuromuscular skill training and/or utilization of prosthetic and assistive devices. This course also describes modification of vehicles to the needs of the handicapped.*

The person starting a program at a rehabilitation facility should thoroughly investigate the background of instructor candidates before hiring a driving instructor, driver educator, or other qualified individual with a valid driver's license.

Regardless of the rules and regulations, training a qualified driving instructor or driver educator to teach the physically disabled to drive seems to be more practical, economical, and expedient than training an experienced occupational therapist or a physical therapist to be a driving instructor. Any staff member being considered for the position of a driving instructor should begin by spending as much time as possible visiting other premises and observing high school or commercial auto school instructors teaching able-bodied students. Preferably they then serve in a part-time job in any kind of driver education program to get the benefit of maximum observation time and experience. They should attend courses in safety and driver education and finally become properly certified.

Individuals who are considering teaching the physically disabled to drive should enjoy driving and instructing and should expect to spend much of their working time in all kinds of traffic. The instructors should be enthusiastic about the work; relate easily with people and their problems; be optimistic, patient, diplomatic, and knowledgeable in the interpretation of the motor vehicle department's laws and regulations as they pertain to the physically disabled motorists; and above all, be strict about safety. The instructors should know their profession thoroughly, for they will be teaching students who are experts in their own field and who are now physically disabled. Students will come from all walks of life and may have very penetrating questions about any part of the program. In addition to expert manipulative skills, instructors should be thoroughly versed in defensive driving techniques.

Teaching the physically disabled to drive requires working with assistive devices; therefore the instructors should be inventive and imaginative and have the basic knowledge of the effects of physical laws, such as kinetic energy, gravity, centrifugal force, and body mechanics. To be able to adjust the hand controls in the car for the maximum benefit and comfort of each student, the instructor should understand the basic principles of leverage, fulcrum, and range of motion as they would apply to any student. Teaching the severely disabled students in a fully automatic van, the instructors should also be experienced in basic auto mechanics and systems, electrical wiring, and hydraulics.

Driving instructors as candidates for the in-house driver education program at a rehabilitation facility should be encouraged to take or monitor courses or lectures dealing with physical disability, attend staff meetings and patient's conferences, and observe patients being treated in various departments, such as occupational therapy or physical therapy and prosthetics. The candidates should be encouraged to become involved in patients' recreational activities to become acquainted with the various disability groups.

Throughout this introductory training and afterward, an occupational therapist or a physical therapist appointed

*Driver and traffic safety education for the physically handicapped, The Center for Safety, School of Education, New York University.

by the coordinator should closely supervise the driving instructor.

Length and number of lessons

Driving a motor vehicle safely on today's busy highways and congested streets is a complex task requiring creative participation on the part of the driver. The driving task consists of some of the following essential components: proper judgment and attitude (neither aggressive nor timid), adequate manipulative skills, defensive driving techniques, continuous environmental awareness and alertness, the ability to predict potential traffic hazards and deal with them in a safe manner, and the ability to drive and navigate day or night in various weather and road conditions.

To learn and master these skills takes time. The length and number of lessons vary from student to student and are adjusted according to the needs of each individual. Obviously, partial or total loss of a left leg will not affect the driving task greatly, especially if the individual had previously driven a vehicle with an automatic transmission. The evaluation would probably take two or three lessons to check for proper driving habits, build up confidence, and explain the rules and regulations of the motor vehicle department and insurance companies as they pertain to individuals with physical disabilities. Evaluating and instructing an individual who will require a left accelerator might take a little longer, depending usually on the driver's coordination and age. The length of training is usually not based on the complexity of the assistive device or system to be mastered but rather on the student's age, adaptability, and coordination. A 60-year-old who is "set in his ways" and undergoes right above-knee amputation might take longer to adjust to the left gas pedal extension than other students in the program who are more severely disabled. The motor vehicle department's recommendation of at least 25 lessons before undertaking a road test probably applies to the 16-year-old, well-coordinated high school student. The older the person is, the longer mastering a new task takes. The old rule of thumb to estimate the number of lessons required to learn a new skill is one lesson per year of the student's life.

Congenitally disabled students usually require the most extensive training. The congenitally disabled child misses out (when growing up) on the hand-eye coordination development that able-bodied children acquire by walking, running, riding a tricycle and bicycle, throwing and catching a ball, and playing in group games and scrimmages. For example, when a ball is thrown, the passer is predicting a collision course between the ball and the catcher. If children learn to predict the collision course, they can also learn to avoid it.

Children born into a wheelchair learn to steer it by manipulating the rear wheels, which they can propel independently or turn in the opposite direction, allowing them to achieve zero turning radius for their wheelchair. A car cannot do those things. The front wheels of a car are not casters as on the wheelchair; they are the steering wheels. Thus some congenitally disabled students have difficulty understanding the steering wheel's function.

Another phenomenon hampering the learning of driving skills in some individuals is their belief that they can drive because they have sat next to their parents all their lives and watched how "easy" driving is. They do not appreciate the required skills and knowledge until they are behind the wheel for the first time and are confronted with the task at hand.

Uncoordinated and inept students or individuals who feared driving or never wanted to learn to drive but now must develop new independence because of their disability will require extensive training. Sixty to 80 lessons are not uncommon.

BASIC DRIVER EDUCATION VEHICLE
Automobiles

The basic driver education vehicle is usually a two-door sedan of any size except compact. A two-door sedan offers the maximum door-opening space for a transfer from a wheelchair into the car and also allows easy placement of a wheelchair in the back of the passenger seat.

Storing a wheelchair in a medium-sized sedan might present a problem because of the recent manufacturing trend of making cars more compact. However, the new wheelchairs are made of much lighter material and are designed to be disassembled quickly and easily, not only the footrests and side arms but also the wheels. After the transfer of the driver from the wheelchair into the car is accomplished, the separate parts of the wheelchair can be easily stored in the back of the passenger seat piece by piece.

The two-door sedan should be power equipped with automatic transmission with the gear selector level on the steering column. (A gear selector on the floor interferes with, if not prohibits, transfers from the passenger's seat to the driver's seat.)

The vehicle should also have power steering, power brakes, adjustable steering wheel, air conditioning, and a power seat for the driver. The "60-40" power seat split is preferable (as compared to power bench seat) for the comfort of the student and the instructor. With this kind of seat the instructor can always sit in the same optimal position during the lesson, regardless of the body height of the student.

Preferably, the two-door sedan intended for a physically disabled individual should have a front-wheel drive that eliminates the transmission hump in the front compartment, easing the difficulty of transferring to the driver's seat. In addition, eliminating the hump helps in storing the wheelchair in the back of the passenger seat because it allows sufficient space to transfer the whole wheelchair.

As an alternative to storing the wheelchair inside the vehicle, devices are available that automatically fold and store a wheelchair inside a fiberglass storage box mounted on top of the car.

A simple directional signal lever is preferable to the complex directional signal lever that also operates high and low beams, windshield wipers, and the windshield washer. The simple directional signal is easily extended to the right side of the steering wheel for the disabled individual who has no use of the left arm. The complex directional signal arm usually has to be bypassed with separate electrical directional signals that are operated by fingers of a right hand while holding on to the steering knob.

The driver vehicle must be equipped with an instructor's separate rear view mirror, which is usually attached to the windshield next to the driver's rear view mirror by means of a suction cup, and a right-hand outside mirror.

The instructor's brake comes in several designs. The most preferable is the "steel rod" extension leading from the driver's brake to the passenger side. This system requires no maintenance after it is installed. The other designs are "cable and pulleys" and hydraulic systems. They require maintenance and tend to leave a mark on the floor carpet after they are removed.

The trunk of the car should be spacious enough to accept a standard-sized wheelchair. Leaving the student's wheelchair out of the car during a lesson is not recommended.

Vans

At least two fully automatic vans should be available in a driver education program. These vans should be of different makes, and they should be converted and modified by two different converting companies, locally located or at least having local representatives for routine maintenance and repairs.

The close proximity of a modifier is very important to the driver education program, not only for the maintenance of the driver education vehicles, but also for the convenience of the students. It is important to remember that each van is custom modified for each driver and every piece of equipment is new. Figure 50-1 is a sample of a typical van evaluation form. Invariably, after the students take possession of their vans, many trips back to the "shop" are needed for adjustments of various assistive devices and systems.

Both training vans should be converted and equipped with the following basic modifications: a raised roof (12-inch high), a raised sliding door, and a 6-inch power pan or a permanently lowered floor in the driver's area to accommodate a wheelchair. There are generally three types of raised roofs: the sport top, the 12-inch, and the 24-inch height. For a training vehicle, the 12-inch height seems most preferable. A vehicle with a 12-inch raised roof is relatively easy to work in for an average height instructor and comfortably accommodates most students. The sport top does not allow the door opening to be raised sufficiently, and the 24-inch raised roof is unnecessarily too high, creating a sway problem in a crosswind and in garaging of the vehicle.

Raised roofs should be insulated and reinforced with roll bars to provide protection in case of an accident.

Suggested items to order for a van for driver education programs include the following:

1. Chevrolet, Dodge, Ford van with a 138-inch wheel base
2. V-8 engine—302 or comparable engine
3. Automatic transmission
4. Heavy duty power brakes
5. Power steering
6. Heavy duty shock absorbers
7. Standard suspension
8. Stabilizer bar
9. Tilt steering wheel
10. Tinted windows (optional)
11. Additional courtesy lights
12. Low mount mirrors (western)
13. Seating arrangement—driver seat and a passenger seat
14. Heavy duty alternator (comes with A/C)
15. Heavy duty battery
16. Front air conditioning
17. Rear air conditioning (optional)
18. Rear heater (optional)
19. Rear window defogger (optional)
20. Auxiliary heater (optional)
21. Windows—all around (power)
22. Door-sliding
23. Steel-belted radial tires
24. Power door locks

One of the vans in the program should be a Ford because these vans have the roomiest interior in the driver's compartment and also the highest front windshield. This arrangement is very beneficial for individuals who are 6 feet tall and over and who intend to drive while sitting in their wheelchairs. Most likely they are also sitting on special cushions, which at times could add 2 or 3 inches to their height. Chevrolets are the second van choice and are preferable to Dodge vans, which have the least interior space in the driver's compartment to accommodate a wheelchair. Most foreign-made vans are designed so that the driver's seat is positioned directly above the fender of the front left wheel. This arrangement makes it impossible to fit a wheelchair in that space.

One van should be equipped with a "zero or no effort" steering system and "vacuum gas and brake" system (lateral or push and pull). Both systems, steering and the vacuum gas and brake, should have an automatic backup system that will supply power in case of an engine failure.

The other van should be equipped with a "low or reduced" effort steering system and a "low effort" brakes system. In addition to the 6-inch power pan, this van should be equipped with a removable six-way power seat for students who are able to transfer from their wheelchairs to the transfer seats. A transfer seat has a much sturdier construction than

```
                                    NAME:
                                    ADDRESS:
                                    TELEPHONE:
                                    DOB:
                                    CAUSE OF DISABILITY:
                                    DOCTOR:
                                    DX:
                                    ONSET:
```

DATE OF EVALUATION_____COUNSELOR_____

ROOM_____EXTENSION_____

The patient will be driving from_____manual wheelchair_____electric wheelchair

_____transfer seat   _____other

VEHICLE_____PASSENGER CAR_____ MINI VAN_____STANDARD VAN

1. EXTERIOR SWITCH BOX _____ regular key_____quad key_____keyless

_____ small toggles_____large toggles

2. AUTOMATIC DOOR OPENER_____Yes _____No

3. DOOR_____as is_____raised.

4. ROOF_____as is_____12"_____24"_____sport top.

5. LIFT_____automatic _____semi-automatic_____ fold-out_____rotary

_____side mount_____rear mount   _____ manual override.

6. FLOOR_____as is_____ wheelchair floor.

7. POWER PAN_____4"_____6"_____None.

8. SEAT_____transfer power   _____captain _____ swivel (manual or power).

9. DISCONNECT SEAT ON CASTERS_____Yes   _____No.

10. WHEELCHAIR LOCKDOWN_____driver position _____passenger position (manual)

_____transfer position

11. HARNESSING _____ chest restraint_____wheelchair seat belt

_____ regular seat belt (driver position)

_____ wall to floor shoulder harness (driver or passenger position)

_____ floor mounted seat belt (passenger position)

12. STEERING _____ factory power _____ reduced effort _____ 0 effort

_____ back-up system_____horizontal steering

_____vertical steering

13. TILT STEERING _____ Yes _____ No

14. STEERING POST EXTENSION _____ None_____ ".

15. DEEP DISH STEERING WHEEL_____ 8 1/2 X 6"   _____11 1/2 X 3 3/4"

_____13 1/2 X 2"   _____13 1/2 X 3 3/4"

_____15 X 4 1/8"   _____standard wheel

Figure 50-1. Sample van evaluation form used in prescribing systems and devices.

16. STEERING DEVICE _____ knob _____ bipin _____ tripin _____ cuff

_____ flat palm device _____ T bar _____ amputee ring

Position _____ .

17. HAND CONTROLS _____ right side mounted _____ left side mounted

_____ push-pull _____ push-right angle

_____ push-twist _____ quad adapter

_____ knee controls _____ reverse principle

_____ vacuum gas and brake (lateral or push and pull).

18. BRAKES _____ extremity _____ factory power brakes _____ low effort

_____ zero effort _____ back up system.

19. GEARSHIFT _____ as is _____ extension _____ crossover _____ remote.

20. IGNITION _____ as is _____ relocated _____ quad key _____ keyless.

21. PARKING BRAKE _____ as is _____ extension _____ remote.

22. DIRECTIONALS _____ as is _____ extension _____ remote _____ crossover.

23. WINDOWS _____ manual _____ power.

24. AIR CONDITIONING _____ front _____ rear.

25. HORN _____ as is _____ on hand controls _____ other _____ .

26. DIMMERS _____ as is _____ on hand controls _____ other _____ .

27. DASH BOARD EXTENSIONS _____ No _____ Yes

28. RELOCATED DASHBOARD AND POWER CONTROLS _____ on engine cover

_____ small or center quad console _____ small toggle switches

_____ large toggle switches _____ lights

_____ heater a/c fan _____ ignition _____ wipers _____ emergency brake

_____ power windows _____ door _____ lift _____ lift

_____ power pan _____ w/c lockdown if powered _____ remote gearshift.

29. CONTROLS RELOCATED TO DOOR _____ none _____ horn _____ wipers _____ dimmers

_____ windows _____ gearshift _____ ignition _____ emergency brake.

30. MIRRORS _____ right side view _____ full view _____ convex (right or left).

31. CB RADIO _____ No _____ Yes Comment _____ .

32. CRUISE CONTROL _____ Yes _____ Optional (order from factory).

33. DUAL BATTERY SYSTEM _____ Yes _____ No

34. TRAINING BRAKE _____ Yes _____ No

35. ONE ARM DEVICE _____ Mechanical _____ 0 effort _____ Other

BY _____

NOTE: If a rotary lift is ordered a sliding door must be ordered from the factory. Otherwise, either a double swing out door or the sliding door is okay.

Figure 50-1, cont'd. Sample van evaluation form used in prescribing systems and devices.

the wheelchair and, therefore, provides more protection in case of a collision.

These vans should be equipped with at least two different types of hand controls such as "push and pull," "push and twist," and "push right angle." In addition to the hand controls mounted on the left side of the steering wheel, there should be provision for hand controls that could be operated by a right hand.

Both vans should also be equipped with fully automatic lifts made by different manufacturers and based on different principles, such as an electric or hydraulic, rotary or fold-out.

If the student's van will be used primarily in a city, it is essential that the lift be mounted on the side of the van so the student will be able to exit and enter from the sidewalk. The rear door entry is preferred in rural areas where parking is predominantly end-in or at an angle, such as shopping malls, parking lots, and private driveways.

In addition to the two basic vans, it is recommended that an attempt should be made to secure periodic loan of specialized vehicles such as the "single lever system," "one arm driving system," "complete foot controls," and the converted mini vans.

Because of the extensive and permanent alteration of the vehicle (raised roof, raised door, and the power pan) one cannot expect to acquire the vans for the program on a free-loan basis from the manufacturers. Other than making an outright purchase, the program director should investigate and apply for grants or consider staging a campaign for donations.

Depending on the degree of use, the life expectancy of a training van is 4 to 5 years.

SUMMARY

The purpose of driver education programs for physically disabled individuals is to help them in their total rehabilitation. In addition to evaluating and training those who are able to learn, the professionals in these programs provide counseling to individuals who are not yet ready or who would not be able to drive because of their physical, visual, perceptual, or cognitive difficulties. However, for the majority of the disabled population, the ultimate goals are to increase mobility, independence, and a useful return to the community.

CHAPTER 51

General principles of orthotics and prosthetics

HANS RICHARD LEHNEIS

"Ortho" is a combining form derived from the Greek *orthos*, straight, normal, or true. The ending "tics" denotes a systematic pursuit of what the root of the words stands for. Orthotics then is the systematic pursuit of straightening or correcting. More specifically, orthotics deals with the application of exoskeletal devices to limit or assist motion of any given segment of the human body. Limitation of motion may mean immobilization (zero degrees of motion) to anything less than normal range of motion, whereas assistance of motion may mean motion throughout the normal range or through any specified range of motion. Applied for this purpose to patients suffering from neuromuscular or skeletal disorders, exoskeletal devices are called orthoses. This is a more inclusive term than brace or splint. The orthotist is a professional person who designs and, with the referring physician, helps prescribe orthoses based on proper patient evaluation.

The term "prosthetics" is derived from the Greek prefix *pros*, in addition to; *tithenai*, to put; and the ending *tics*. Thus prosthetics is the systematic pursuit of putting in addition to. Specifically, prosthetics deals with the addition or application of an artificial device called a prosthesis, to the body to replace partially or totally missing limbs or organs. The design and fitting of prostheses is performed by the prosthetist.

The terms "prosthetics" and "iso-organs" are distinguished semantically, "prosthetic" meaning adding to or supplementing.[3] If devices substitute for an organ or emulate

Table 51-1. Indications for ankle-foot orthoses*

Pathomechanical condition	Biomechanical device	Degree of spasticity	Sensory deficit
Weakness or absence of dorsiflexors	Posterior leaf-spring	None to mild	Reduced without mediolateral instability
Weakness or absence of dorsiflexors and plantar-flexors	Spiral	Mild to moderate	Reduced with valgus instability
Equinovarus with rotation of foot	Hemispiral	Moderate	Mild to moderate
Equinovarus without rotation of foot	Hemiposterior leafspring	Moderate	Mild to moderate
Other: pain, sensory deficit, structural	Solid ankle	Severe	Severe

From Lehneis, HR: Newsl Prosthet Orthot Clin 4:3, 1980.
*Criteria are based on musculoskeletal and neurological determinations rather than cause. Included are: (1) deformity, (2) joint mobility, (3) contractures, (4) motor power, (5) spasticity, (6) presence or absence of edema, and (7) sensory abnormalities, particularly proprioceptive.

its function, for example, an artificial pancreas or artificial heart, the organ replacement is isogenic. Isogenic devices require artificial logic and therefore biosensors to monitor input. The microprocessor makes possible iso-organs such as respirators, hemodialyzers, artificial endocrine systems, cardiac pacemakers, artificial hearts, verbal communicators for the nonvocal, artificial eyes, biofeedback devices, and artificial limbs.

Table 51-2. Functions of ankle-foot orthoses and contraindications

	Posterior leaf-spring	Hemiposterior leaf-spring	Spiral	Hemispiral	Posterior solid ankle
Biomechanical action	Prevents foot slap at heel strike; assists toe clearance in swing phase	Prevents foot slap at heel strike; assists toe clearance in swing phase with control of inversion	Prevents foot slap at heel strike; assists toe clearance in swing phase and push-off in stance phase with control of inversion and eversion; provides extension moment at knee to assist stability	Prevents foot slap at heel strike; assists toe clearance in swing phase with control of inversion; induces external torque on foot at heel strike	Immobilizes ankle in swing and stance phase
Indications	Motor weakness of ankle dorsiflexors	Motor weakness of ankle dorsiflexors and evertors with mild to moderate lateral instability and tendency toward varus (without foot internal rotation component)	Motor weakness of ankle dorsiflexors and/or plantar flexors with moderate mediolateral instability; mild motor weakness of knee extensors	Motor weakness of ankle dorsiflexors and evertors with moderate to severe lateral instability and/or strong tendency toward equinovarus; internal rotation of foot; moderate spasticity	Structural collapse of foot-ankle; pain caused by movement of ankle; severe spasticity with sustained clonus; severe sensory deficit
Contraindications					
Motor power	Moderate to severe weakness of ankle plantar flexors; inadequate knee strength; inadequate hip strength	Moderate to severe weakness of ankle plantar flexors; inadequate knee strength; inadequate hip strength	Pronounced imbalance of forces acting on ankle-foot complex; inadequate hip strength	Inadequate hip strength	Inadequate hip strength
Spasticity	Moderate to severe spasticity	Moderate to severe spasticity	Moderate to severe spasticity	Severe spasticity with sustained clonus	
Joint stability	Mediolateral ankle instability with marked varus/valgus	Valgus	Severe mediolateral ankle instability	Valgus	
Joint mobility	Ankle dorsiflexion limited to <90°; fixed deformity	Ankle dorsiflexion limited to <90°; fixed deformity	Ankle dorsiflexion limited to <90°; fixed deformity	Ankle dorsiflexion limited to <90°; fixed deformity	Significant functional movement of ankle during gait
Volume changes			Fluctuating edema	Fluctuating edema	Fluctuating edema

From Lehneis, HR: Newsl Prosthet Orthot Clin 4:3, 1980.

LOWER LIMB ORTHOTICS
Ankle-foot orthoses

Design and prescription of modern ankle-foot orthoses (AFOs) are based on the identification of a pathomechanical condition affecting the ankle-foot complex for the purpose of matching that condition with a biomechanical device (plastic AFO). Over the years this basic system has been improved to include modifying factors such as spasticity and sensory status (Table 51-1).[15]

Table 51-2 elaborates on the basic system by describing indications, contraindications, and biomechanical actions of each AFO.[15] Each of the AFOs described is shown in Figures 51-1 to 51-5.

Knee orthoses

There is an increasing number of knee orthotic designs available, most of which were designed for sports medicine applications. The major designs and the control they provide are summarized in Table 51-3.[4]

Supracondylar knee orthosis

The supracondylar knee (SK) orthosis[14] is designed to prevent genu recurvatum and to control genu varum or valgum. It must of course be appreciated that genu valgum or varum often cannot be reduced to a normal alignment with any device, including the supracondylar knee orthosis; however, further progression of the deformity can be prevented. Nevertheless, in most cases the degree of genu varum or valgum can be reduced in the SK orthosis. This is especially true in genu valgum because the orthosis applies forces in areas that not only are pressure tolerant, but where soft tissue is minimal. Therefore the effect of the orthosis on skeletal alignment is far greater than in genu varum.

The SK orthosis is a unitized plastic laminate structure that encases the knee mediolaterally and extends to a point approximately 4.5 cm proximal to the superior border of the patella. Distally it terminates approximately 7.5 cm above the malleoli. Posterior counterpressure to control genu recurvatum is applied in the popliteal area such that

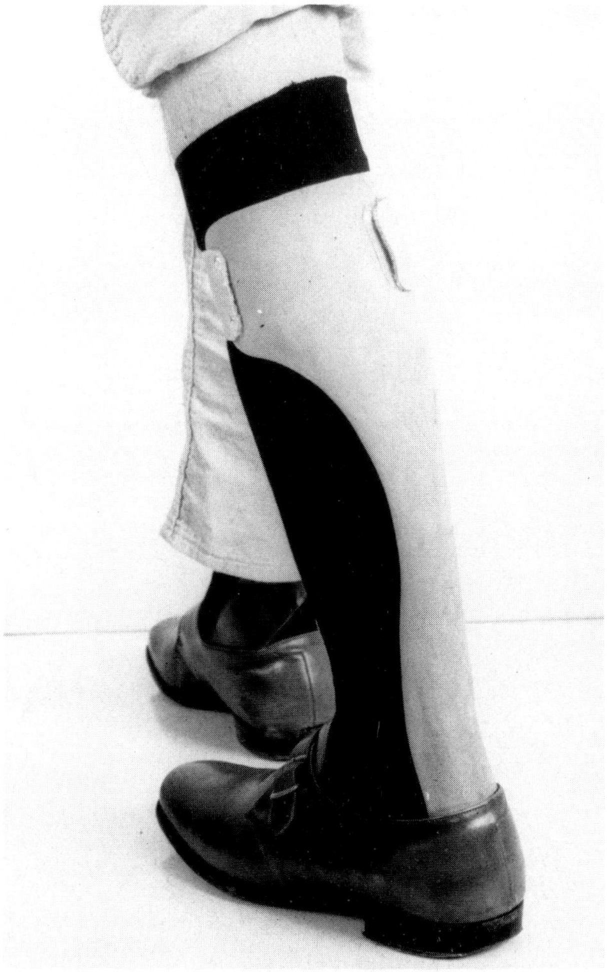

Figure 51-1. Posterior leaf-spring ankle-foot orthosis.

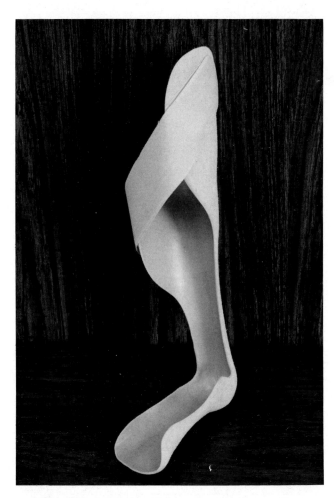

Figure 51-2. Hemiposterior leaf-spring ankle-foot orthosis.

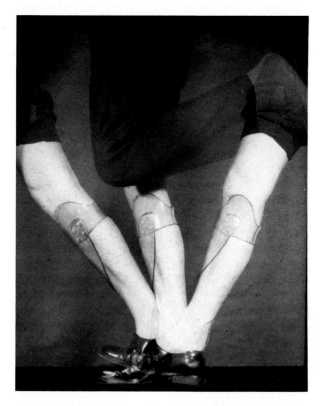

Figure 51-3. Spiral ankle-foot orthosis.

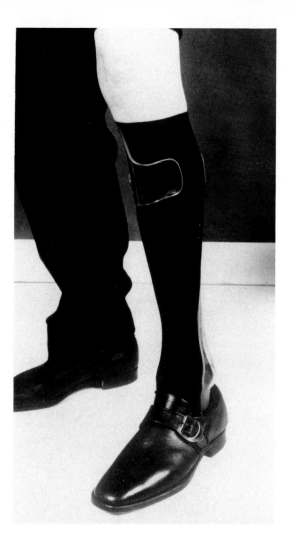

Figure 51-4. Hemispiral ankle-foot orthosis.

Table 51-3. Knee orthoses

	AP* control	ML† control	Collateral ligaments	Multiple ligaments	Rotary control	Recurva-tum	Patellar control	Postoperative	Varus/valgus control
Palumbo							X		
Marshall-PAC							X		
Teufel TKS		X				X			
Swedish Knee Cage						X			
Genucentric		X				X			
Lerman	X	X		X	X		X	X	
Lenox Hill		X		X	X				
External Cruciate Ligament	X	X		X	X				
TRIO	X	X		X	X			X	
Anderson Knee Stabilizer		X	X						
Iowa Knee Orthosis		X	X					X	
CARS—UBC		X							X
Generation II	X	X		X	X	X		X	
Can-Am	X	X			X				

From Beets, CL, et al: Orthot Prosthet 39:33, 1985.

* Anteroposterior.

† Mediolateral.

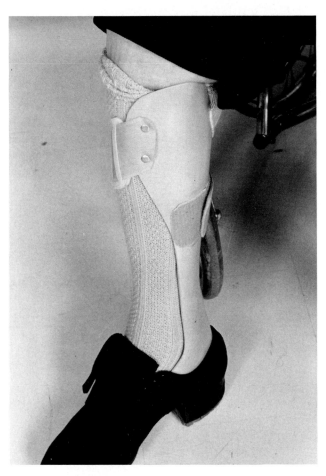

Figure 51-5. Posterior solid ankle-foot orthosis.

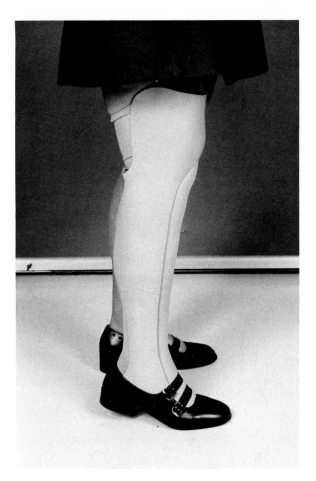

Figure 51-6. Supracondylar knee-ankle-foot orthosis.

knee flexion in the swing phase and for sitting is not restricted.

In contrast to the conventional knee cage, the SK orthosis does not possess a mechanical knee joint and thus is much lighter. Because of its light weight, the contoured fit provides adequate suspension, eliminating auxiliary suspension systems usually required with the conventional knee cage. Although the anterior brim protrudes when the wearer is sitting, patients do not find this objectionable. Rather, they are pleased with the cosmetic appearance of the orthosis because of the absence of straps, the flesh color of the plastic, and its close fit. The major functional advantage of the SK orthosis is its effectiveness in preventing genu recurvatum and in providing mediolateral stability.

Supracondylar knee-ankle orthosis

The supracondylar knee-ankle (SKA) orthosis[14] is indicated for patients who lack motor power in the knee extensors, as well as about the ankle. Prerequisites for successful use of this orthosis are good to normal hip extensors, absence of hip and knee flexion contractures, and absence of spasticity or only slight spasticity.

The SKA orthosis makes use of prosthetics technology in an orthotic application. Its design combines a modification of the protesi tibialis supracondylar (PTS) prosthesis and the SK orthosis with above-knee prosthetic alignment principles. This is achieved by immobilizing the ankel and foot in equinus in a plastic laminate (Figure 51-6). The equinus attitude results in alignment stability, producing a knee extension moment in the stance phase. Although the principle of placing the foot in equinus to achieve knee stability is not new and has been used in orthopedic surgery, it has not become a routine procedure. Patients thus treated may develop genu recurvatum or other structural changes in the knee joint over time. In the SKA, as in the SK orthosis, genu recurvatum is effectively controlled by the anterior extension of the brace above the knee, counteracted by a force applied in the popliteal area. Mediolateral stability of the knee is ensured by the supracondylar extensions.

Functionally, the absence of a mechanical knee joint with a lock in the SKA orthosis allows free knee flexion in the swing phase, which not only results in a more nearly normal gait pattern, but also conceivably reduces energy consumption. Another advantage is the light weight of the orthosis, which results in less patient fatigue. The flesh-colored, unitized structure is a closer-fitting and more cosmetically acceptable device. Like all plastic AFOs, the SKA orthosis fits inside the shoe. This feature, too, has been found more cosmetically pleasing and convenient.

Knee-ankle-foot orthoses

Virtually all AFOs in modern orthotics are plastic and do not incorporate stirrups and ankle joints. In plastic as well as conventional knee-ankle-foot orthoses (KAFOs), there are commonly stirrups attached to the shoe or a foot plate as well as ankle joints.

Stirrups

Stirrups may be attached either to the shoe or to a footplate, although plastic KAFOs are rarely if ever attached to a shoe. The solid stirrup, most commonly used, provides the most rigid and least bulky shoe attachment. The split stirrup allows the patient to transfer the brace to any shoe equipped with a flat caliper. The round caliper is indicated for patients who have a problem donning the brace and shoe, particularly children with cerebral palsy. With the round caliper the brace shoe and the brace itself can be donned separately and, once applied, can be interconnected. The solid stirrup may also be attached to a footplate made of metal or plastic, which allows the advantage of interchanging shoes.

Ankle joints

Ankle joints of most types may be used with the stirrups previously described, with the exception of the round caliper type. A limited-motion ankle joint is indicated for positive control of the plantar flexion or dorsiflexion angle to prevent contractures, to prevent excessive joint excursion when motor power about the ankle is inadequate, or to achieve control of a more proximal joint. For example, a plantar flexion stop can induce knee flexion, whereas a dorsiflexion stop produces a knee extension moment. A spring-loaded dorsiflexion assist is indicated when normal range of plantar flexion and dorsiflexion is permissible but the patient lacks adequate dorsiflexors.

Knee joints

Knee joints with a posterior offset are indicated when the patient has knee extensors but requires mediolateral control of the knee. The drop-ring lock is most commonly used when the patient lacks adequate knee extensors. A spring-loaded pull rod may be added to the drop-ring lock when the patient is unable to reach the knee. The spring load also provides automatic locking, rather than depending on gravity. The cam lock provides simultaneous locking and unlocking of the double-bar uprights and provides the greatest degree of rigidity. It is indicated primarily in weight-bearing braces or when semiautomatic unlocking is desired, by which the patient can use the edge of a chair to trigger the bail connecting the cam locks.

KAFOs may be of the conventional metal-leather design or may be plastic laminated (Figure 51-7) or vacuum molded from a thermoplastic sheet material.

The plastic KAFO may incorporate conventional ankle and knee components as described previously. Yet, improved fit, cosmesis, and reduction in weight can be achieved through the application of plastics and biomechanical principles to stabilize the knee more effectively than is possible with conventional brace bands and straps.[14] A suprapatellar shell eliminates the knee cap and controls the knee mediolaterally for proper alignment. The posterior thigh section aids in mediolateral control of the knee and acts anterioposteriorly to prevent genu recurvatum. The upper portion of the thigh section is quadrilaterally shaped to provide a comfortable fit and to control rotation. Rotational control may be augmented with a prosthetic suspension system such as a Silesian belt. The quadrilateral shape is also designed to provide ischial contact (not weight bearing, unless specifically indicated). This may be used to especially good advantage when hip extensors are weak. A high, well-

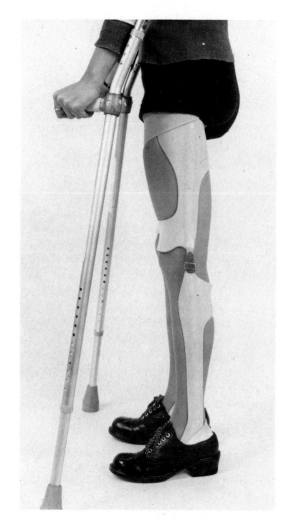

Figure 51-7. Knee-ankle-foot orthosis.

fitting, posterior thigh section will aid in creating a hip extension moment at heel strike when the knee is locked and a plantar flexion stop is used.

For paraplegic patients Craig-Scott orthoses[25] provide increased balance over conventional orthoses because of the rigid ankle unit and foot plate incorporated in the shoe sole. Double-action ankle joints, in which the springs are replaced with solid rods, permit alignment adjustability for optimum balance.

Hip-knee-ankle-foot orthoses

When a hip joint and pelvic belt or thoracic section is added to the KAFO, it becomes a hip-knee-foot orthosis (HKAFO). Hip joints may be used to control transverse rotation, increase lateral stability, substitute for hip flexion, and prevent hip flexion when a lock is used.

A free-motion hip joint is indicated for lateral stability and rotational control, although a Silesian belt may be adequate in certain cases. A posterior stop at the hip joint may be used not only to prevent hyperextension of the hip but to advance the braced leg forward. This can be done by using a posterior pelvic belt, which, through the pelvic band and posterior stop, advances the leg forward and thus substitutes for hip flexion to some degree.

The reciprocating gait orthosis (RGO)[23] (Figure 51-8) is increasingly used in paraplegic patients. It allows a reciprocal gait pattern, even though no active hip motors are present. This is accomplished by a cable control system connecting the mechanical hip joints. As one hip is flexed, the contralateral braced limb is extended. Hip flexion is accomplished by a combination of weight shift to the contralateral side and elbow extension on crutches or a walker.

In patients with high-level spina bifida, control of the pelvis has been typically problematic because of the imbalance of motor power around the hip joint. This can be readily appreciated when the differential innervation of the hip is considered. The hip flexors are at least partially innervated at the L2 and L3 level, whereas the hip extensors are innervated below the L3 level. Such imbalance at the L2 and L3 level of involvement causes the lordosis so often seen in these patients, often aggravated by hip flexion contractures. Control of the pelvis, and thus lordosis, has been difficult with conventional designs.

In analysis of the force system required to prevent hip flexion contracture, it becomes clear that the rigid portion of the pelvic band needs to be reversed from its conventional location[16] (Figure 51-9). This reversal consists of a plastic molded panel that extends superiorly to the level of the

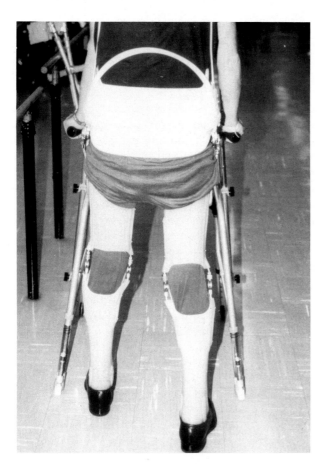

Figure 51-8. Reciprocating gait orthosis.

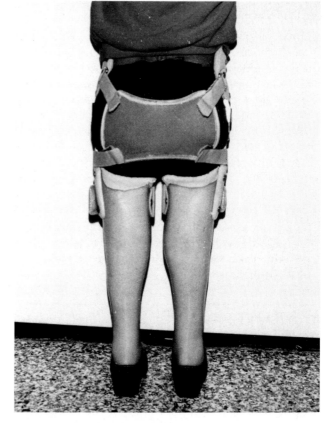

Figure 51-9. Orthotic pelvis control in spina bifida.

xiphoid process. The uprights of the hip joints are attached to the panel. An anteriorly directed force is provided by a leather hammock covering the buttocks. Straps attached on each of the four corners of the hammock run through D rings attached equidistant above and below the orthotic hip joint center. This system works quite effectively in controlling lordosis.

If the patient has a relatively severe hip flexion contracture, the hip joint uprights are attached to the panel by means of a single pivot placed approximately 5 cm below the lateral trim line of the panel. By gradual tightening of the straps of the buttock pad, some correction can often be achieved. The pivot allows the anterior panel to adapt to the changing angulation as correction is attempted.

It should also be noted that patients up to the age of approximately 6 years can be provided with solid ankles and knees because their legs are still short enough to sit without obstructing much of the space in front of the chair. Ths purpose of this is to provide the patient with maximum stability and lightweight orthoses. As the patient gains upper limb strength and mobility, knee joints with drop locks are added, usually of the lateral single-bar type. Double bars are used only when the patient is relatively heavy and there is a torsional problem. The ankle-foot portion of the orthosis remains of the solid ankle type. The solid ankle provides the largest possible base of support over which the patient's center of gravity can be maintained. This allows greater latitude than possible if orthotic ankle joints are used.

Fracture and weight-bearing orthoses

In recent years prefabricated fracture orthoses and components, that is, total contact shells, as well as plastic and adjustable metal knee and ankle joints, have become available to treat practically all levels of fracture of the limbs. Because these components are widely available commercially, they are not described here in detail.

Weight-bearing devices provide weight-bearing relief through the skeletal system. When relief below the knee is desired, a patellar tendon–bearing brace[1] is most commonly indicated. The weight-bearing characteristics of this brace are similar to those of a patellar tendon–bearing (PTB) prosthesis. For weight-bearing relief through the femur or for cases in which the PTB brace is inadequate (for example, tibial plateau fractures), ischial weight-bearing devices are indicated.[7] The quadrilateral socket, as used in prosthetics, offers optimal weight-bearing relief.

UPPER LIMB ORTHOTICS
Biomechanics

The shoulder, elbow, and hand are interdependent components that constitute a kinematic chain. Through the process of evolution, primates retained a more generalized structure of the forelimb than quadrupeds.[10] This is evi-

denced in increased movement in the shoulder joint, pronation and supination of the forearm, and increased range of motion of the digits. All primates evolved a forelimb, which became an ever more efficient prehensile organ. Primates developed greater pliability of the digits to adapt to varying sizes, shapes, and textures; an ever increasing cortical representation; and a highly developed sensory feedback system in the digits.[6]

In humans the vertebral border of the scapula is relatively long in proportion to any other border, typical of the family Hominidae. This is necessary to permit a greater degree of movement of the shoulder, and it provides a longer level arm for the serratus anterior and rhomboid muscles.

In the brachiators the thorax changes in cross-sectional shape. It becomes flatter ventrodorsally, placing the scapula more dorsally to allow better range of shoulder motion than the round cross section of the quadrupedal trunk, which primarily permits motion in one plane only.

The combination of a very well-developed S-shaped clavicle and a scapula that reaches its longest dimension at the vertebral border and that is placed dorsally makes possible powerful and great range of arm movement.[22]

In hominids (including *Homo sapiens*), the general proportion and shape of the shoulder, elbow, and forearm are similar. This is particularly true of the trochlea of the elbow joint, which is relatively broad, provides great lateral stability, and allows full extension of the forearm. Relative to other primates, there is a reduction in the length of the olecranon. This adaptation brings the attachment of the triceps tendon closer to the elbow's axis, thus increasing the angular velocity of the forearm when the triceps contracts.

The hand may be seen as a multifunctional organ.[9] It not only lends expression and feeling to our thoughts and speech, but can effectively substitute for other organ systems. It allows the blind to read and the dumb and deaf to speak and to hear. The functional value of the hand is related not only to its intrinsic characteristics, but to the mobility afforded by the proximal joints. The ever increasing range of motion permitted at the shoulder and the forearm rotation that developed in the course of evolution are necessary in manipulative activities.

In the higher primates opposition is greatly enhanced by a modification of the carpometacarpal joint.[26] Its articular surface is set oblique to the palm, providing a saddle joint that permits great mobility and universal motion. The human thumb is the longest of the digits. Because humans do not use the hand in locomotion, it has become a purely manipulative organ with greatly increased tactile function and enormous cortical representation.[28] It is this lack of specialization in human morphology that adapts us best to a given environment and circumstance.

Perhaps the most important factor in human's great dexterity is the retention of a long, movable thumb. This allows better opposition and permits larger objects to be grasped, and the flexor pollicis longus tendon provides powerful configurational adaptation.

Perhaps more important than musculoskeletal anatomy is the hand's sensory feedback and refined motor control. In the motor cortex the thumb alone occupies an area larger than the other four digits combined. The enhanced ability to oppose the thumb provides for a precision grip. Such dexterity is necessary when manipulating small objects and in performing certain activities of daily living. Simple things such as turning a doorknob, picking up a coin, holding a pen or pencil, and holding eating utensils require opposability of the thumb. The significance of this becomes quite clear when the ability to oppose the thumb is impaired, for example, in median nerve palsy or amputation of the thumb. In these cases many daily activities cannot be readily performed, if at all. In workmen's compensation cases it has been recognized that loss of the thumb accounts for greater than 50% dysfunction of the hand. In orthotic management of the impaired hand and prosthetic replacement of the thumb, the position of opposition is recognized and mechanically substituted for, greatly enhancing function.

General principles

Preservation of hand function, prevention of contractures, and replacement of lost hand function are the most important and difficult areas in orthotic management of upper limb disabilities.

Although it is impossible to include all the various designs of upper limb orthoses, those that represent the basic principles and are most commonly used are represented in this chapter. Nearly all orthoses are fabricated from aluminum, thermoplastic, or polyester laminates. Most orthoses are based on the principle of maintaining the thumb, if not

functionally then at least statically, in opposition to the index and middle fingers. The basic opponens orthosis illustrates this principle (Figure 51-10). Although it is most often used to prevent the first metacarpal from assuming a position parallel to the other metacarpals and to prevent web space contracture (for example, in a median nerve injury), it may serve a functional purpose simply by placing the hand in a functionally useful position.

Upper limb orthotic systems

A number of institutions have developed systems of upper limb orthotics, which in all cases are based on an opponens orthosis to which various components are added to ameliorate specific individual impairments.[13] All systems include various prehension orthoses, including externally energized systems for various levels of quadriplegia.[11,19]

These systems are best suited in the management of peripheral nerve injuries and other disease, for example, polio, Guillain-Barré syndrome, in which partial or complete recovery is anticipated, as well as for quadriplegic patients. The systems are applied not only to enhance function but also to protect the hand in a functional position and to prevent contracture while recovery takes place. Listed in chronologic order of development, the systems are:

1. Warm Springs System, developed at the Georgia Warm Springs Foundation
2. Rancho Los Amigos System, developed at the Rancho Los Amigos Hospital, Downey, California
3. Engen System, developed at the Texas Institute for Rehabilitation and Research, Houston
4. RIRM-NYU System, developed at the Rusk Institute of Rehabilitation Medicine, New York University Medical Center

Common to all systems is the principle of preserving the position of hand function, represented in the basic opponens orthosis. It serves as the basic module to which other components may be added, for example, forearm bar, metacarpophalangeal extension stop, or finger extension exist. The position of function is defined as the wrist extended 30 degrees, with the metacarpophalangeal joints flexed 30 degrees, interphalangeal joints extended, and the thumb placed in a position of abduction, opposite the index and middle finger. In the position of function, muscles and tendons crossing all joints are balanced and the likelihood of contractures is minimized. The purpose of orthotic management is to prevent contractures while maintaining the position of function. For a quadriplegic patient it is important to maintain this position in the early management, preferably as early as the day of injury. Thus the patient can ultimately be fitted with a functional prehension orthosis, which would not be accomplished if contractures were allowed to develop. Depending on the level of spinal cord injury, prehension orthoses may be driven by the finger or wrist or electrically driven (Figure 51-11).

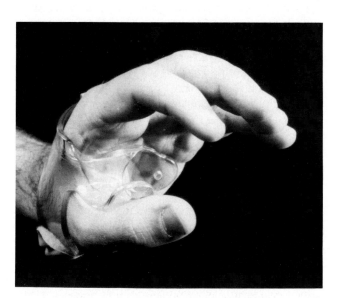

Figure 51-10. Basic opponens orthosis.

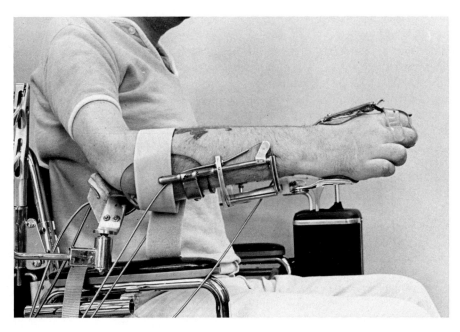

Figure 51-11. Electric arm orthosis.

Prefabricated splints

The prefabricated splints include ready-made splints, which are available from a number of manufacturers. This category includes Bunnell splints, various resting and positioning splints, and other devices for activities of daily living. Although some of these devices serve a very useful function (for example, adaptive devices for activities of daily living), some splints may be considered harmful because of improper positions imposed by certain designs. Prefabricated splints are used when the prognosis for patient recovery is good and short-term use of an orthosis is indicated, or in cases when the patient awaits the fitting of a more permanent orthosis.

Acute (temporary) splinting

Acute splints are applied in cases where immediate splinting is required (for example, soft tissue trauma or burns) or in cases where progressive changes in joint alignment are necessary. Most often this kind of splinting is provided by practitioners other than the orthopedic surgeon, that is, occupational or physical therapist, general practitioner, and nurse. Materials used for these purposes include the following:

1. Low-temperature thermoplastics. An increasing number of low-temperature thermoplastics has become available. In general they lend themselves well to this application, because they are easily handled and require a minimum amount of equipment. Each possesses unique physical characteristics such as color, stiffness, transparency, and temperature range.

2. Plaster of paris. Plaster casts are often applied as a temporary measure in an emergency setting to stabilize a joint or in progressive correction of contracted joints.

SPINAL ORTHOTICS

Although there is an abundance of spinal brace designs, only those most commonly used and presenting an example of motion control in various planes are described here.[12] The two-bar lumbar (sacroiliac or chairback) brace consists of a pelvic and a thoracic band and two paraspinal uprights. Its function is to control anteroposterior motion in the lumbar area. The pelvic band, as in all braces, should be placed as low as possible without interfering with sitting, at approximately the level of the coccyx. The thoracic band should extend to a point approximately 1.5 cm inferior to the inferior angles of the scapulae.

The four-bar lumbar (Knight) brace differs from the two-bar lumbar brace in the addition of lateral uprights connecting the pelvic and thoracic bands. Beyond controlling anteroposterior motion, it is designed to control mediolateral motion as well as to inhibit transverse rotation.

The two-bar thoracolumbar (Taylor) brace consists of a pelvic band and two paraspinal uprights extending to just below the spines of the scapulae. It is designed to control anteroposterior motion in the thoracic area. A thoracic band may be added when mediolateral motion control is desired.

The Williams flexion brace is designed to permit flexion of the lumbar spine but to resist extension. It also controls mediolateral motion.

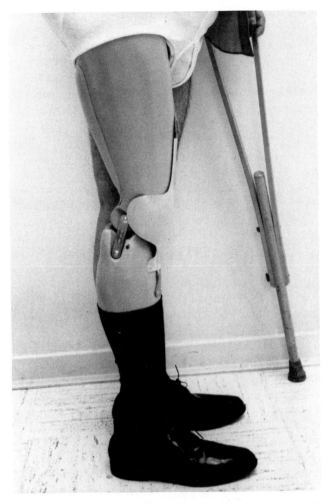

Figure 51-12. Exoskeletal above-knee prosthesis with polycentric knee joint.

In recent studies, corsets have been shown to be similar and sometimes superior in effectiveness to spinal braces. This may be explained by the fact that a well-fitted corset covers the entire abdominal area from the pubis to the xiphoid process, thereby creating a closed container. Thus an increase in intra-abdominal pressure can be effected, which to some extent relieves the spinal column.

Cervical orthoses reduce motion of the cervical spine and provide sensory feedback as a reminder to limit head and neck motions when so indicated. Soft collars are more effective in limiting flexion and extension than rotation and lateral tilting.

More rigid appliances such as the two- or four-poster cervical orthosis tend not to be any more effective than the soft collar, unless they extend inferiorly to the level of the xiphoid process. An example of such a device is the sterno-occipito-mandibular immobilizer (SOMI). This is often used after fracture or surgical intervention in the cervical spine and can be applied without moving the patient, for example,

in a postsurgical situation in the hospital. It is impossible to totally eliminate motion of the cervical spine, although the least motion can be obtained by the application of a plastic molded cervical-thoracic orthosis that includes stabilization of the forehead.[18] Without the forehead support the patient is still able to flex and rotate in the cervical spinal area. Such an orthosis is also referred to as a Minerva jacket. It must extend from the forehead over the occipital area and mandible inferiorly to the level of the floating ribs. However, maximal stabilization of the cervical spine can be achieved only with a halo-type orthosis, which includes skeletal fixation through pins that protrude into the skull from the halo ring. Lower levels of spinal instability that require mechanical support and fixation necessitate a bivalved plastic molded orthosis. Depending on the level of injury, such devices may extend caudally from the cervical spine to the pelvis and buttocks.

Hyperextension orthoses represent the three-point pressure system by applying pressure at the sternum, pubic, and lumbar areas. They are indicated in patients with fractures of the vertebral body. Through application of a hyperextension force, the superincumbent weight of the body is shifted to the posterior facets.

The cervico-thoraco-lumbo-sacral orthosis (CTLSO), also known as the Milwaukee brace, is used in controlling juvenile scoliosis and kyphosis. More recent designs, for example, the Boston scoliosis orthosis, eliminate the occipitomandibular support by providing a total-contact corrective force and are often used in lieu of the Milwaukee brace. Versions of the Boston brace are used in adults for low back pain and mechanical instability of the spinal column.

LOWER LIMB PROSTHETICS

The primary objectives of lower limb prosthetic design and component selection are to transfer body weight comfortably to the prosthetic socket, to achieve alignment stability, and to simulate normal locomotion. The degree to which these objectives can be realized depends greatly on the level of amputation. At any given level of amputation, however, there are significant variations from patient to patient. These relate to the patient's physical characteristics other than the amputation itself, the patient's age, and the patient's social and psychologic adjustment to amputation.

Prosthetics systems

There are two basic lower limb prosthetics systems for use above the level of Syme's amputation—the exoskeletal (Figure 51-12) and endoskeletal (Figure 51-13) types. Most commonly used is the exoskeletal, or crustacean, type in which the actual outer shape of the prosthesis also constitutes the supporting structure. The endoskeletal type, also referred to as the modular system, provides the supporting

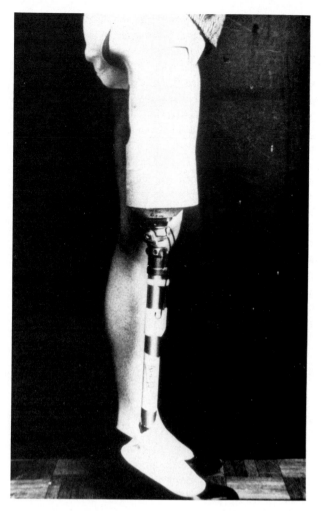

Figure 51-13. Endoskeletal above-knee prosthesis with flexible socket.

structure within the center of the prosthesis, that is, by means of a tubular system that interconnects the various components. One advantage of the endoskeletal-modular system is that components (for example, knee units) are interchangeable. They provide the clinician with greater latitude in exchanging modules—if one knee unit proves inadequate for a particular patient, it can be quickly interchanged, at least during the fitting stage. The foam body of the prosthesis is shaped to match the contralateral leg. The major problem with this system is the external cover of the foam body. Usually it is covered by a stocking and hose, which tend to tear easily. Nevertheless, especially for female amputees, it is the most cosmetic system, both visually and to the touch. Although some prosthetic skins are available, they tend to inhibit or influence knee motion in the above-knee prosthesis and are also likely to tear.

Prosthetic feet

Prosthetic feet are common to all amputation levels. The most commonly used prosthetic foot is the solid ankle cush-

ion heel (SACH) foot.[2] The SACH foot does not possess a mechanical ankle joint; rather it simulates plantar flexion by the compression of a soft rubber heel wedge that can be selected in various densities, depending on the patient's weight and gait pattern. With the exception of the hardwood or aluminum keel, the foot is made of flexible material that permits toe flexion and some adaptation to uneven terrain. While a modified version of the SACH foot is applicable to Syme's amputation prostheses, all other prosthetic foot-ankle components described in this section may be used in patients with a higher amputation level only.

More recent advances in prosthetic foot design are energy-storing feet, such as the Seattle Foot[5] and the Flex-Foot. These newer designs are distinguished from the SACH and other prosthetic feet by having a flexible component, that is, an energy-storing component, instead of a hardwood or aluminum keel. During weight bearing, energy is stored in the flexible material, for example, fiberglass laminate structure, or other plastic material, for example, Delrin. The stored energy is released at the time of heel-off and provides kinetic energy to propel the prosthesis forward, thus conserving energy.

The single-axis foot is rarely used today. It possesses a transverse mechanical ankle joint. Plantar flexion is controlled by a rubber bumper, which can be selected in various hardnesses. There is usually either a limited or rigid dorsiflexion stop to permit simulated push-off.

The multiaxis, or universal motion, foot (for example, Greisinger) is particularly useful in patients who have avocational interests, such as golf, in which transverse rotation as well as adaptation to uneven terrain is a necessity. However, most amputees who do not have such hobbies do not particularly gain from such a device because it is heavier and less cosmetic than any other type of prosthetic foot-ankle system. The universal ankle joint consists of a rubber block module interposed between the prosthetic foot and ankle unit and connected by a flexible connecting system.

Alternatively, rotator systems may be used with any foot component.[2] They consist of a disc with an elastomer control element to permit transverse rotation above the ankle or, in above-knee amputees, above the knee. All prosthetic feet or foot-ankle components can be used with any amputation level except Syme's level and below.

Prosthetic knee joints and controls

Although the physical construction of knee units differs between the two types of prosthetic systems, the actual functional capability is identical between exoskeletal and endoskeletal knee unit function. Prosthetic knee units may be distinguished on the basis of kinematics. There are two basic types: the single-axis knee and polycentric knee units of various types.[2] The latter include so-called physiologic knee joints, which are geometrically similar to the human knee joint. There are several other polycentric knee units whose shank and knee portions are connected by a linkage system in which the polycentric action is far exaggerated from that of the human knee. The purpose of such movement is to reduce the tendency toward buckling.

Prosthetic knee units may be provided with various control systems: stance phase control, swing phase control, or stance and swing phase control. Stance phase control may be provided in various ways. Alignment stability for stance phase control is described under above-knee amputation. Single-axis knees may be equipped with a manual locking mechanism, which can be engaged by the patient during ambulation for maximal safety and released when sitting.

Weight-actuated brake mechanisms apply body weight to tightly mate matching brake surfaces and prevent the knee from buckling of up to 15 degrees flexion.

The most sophisticated control is the Mauch swing and stance (SNS) hydraulic unit.[21] It includes a stumbling recovery that engages a mechanism to prevent buckling, yet allows the knee to be extended. In general, hydraulic mechanisms reduce the tendency toward buckling because of properties unique to hydraulic systems. Polycentric units inherently provide increased stance phase control, the degree of which depends on the linkage system or geometric configuration of the prosthetic knee.

Swing phase control may be provided by various means. In the single-axis knee a constant friction applied to the knee axis allows the patient to walk at a fixed cadence, which is selected by the patient and is dependent on the friction adjustment. If the patient changes cadences, for example, walks faster than the pace for which the friction control is set, the patient experiences excessive heel rise. Another swing phase control is a compression spring placed in the shank, which is progressively compressed as the knee is flexing in the swing phase. Once compressed, it aids in extending the knee at the end of the swing phase. Although pneumatic swing phase controls are available, they are less frequently used because they are more affected by temperature changes than are hydraulic units. Hydraulic units automatically adapt to varying cadences.

Toe prosthesis

Toe amputation usually requires nothing more than a shoe filler.

Lisfranc's prosthesis

Lisfranc's amputation prosthesis consists of a molded foot support encompassing as much of the dorsum of the foot as possible. A rigid anterior extension is added to the level of the normal toe break, and a toe filler is connected distally.

Chopart's prosthesis

Chopart's amputation and other partial foot amputations are highly undesirable from a prosthetic point of view. Although full end bearing is possible in most cases, an abnormal gait pattern results because of partial loss of the anterior lever arm during push-off. The prosthesis required

must often extend to the patellar tendon and immobilize the ankle joint to provide an anterior lever arm to achieve simulated push-off. Because plantar flexion is not possible, the gait remains somewhat abnormal. Furthermore, the prosthesis tends to be quite bulky and usually requires a larger shoe size. Cosmetically it is also undesirable, especially for female amputees.

Syme's prosthesis

Syme's amputation usually permits full weight bearing on the distal end. For female amputees, however, the Syme's prosthesis is cosmetically undesirable because it produces a bulbous end that cannot be cosmetically accommodated in the prosthesis. Syme's prosthesis must extend to the patellar tendon for leverage at heel-off and for partial weight bearing if full distal weight bearing cannot be tolerated. A medial opening in the distal one third of the prosthesis or an expandable inner socket is required to accommodate the bulbous end when donning the prosthesis. The socket consists of a plastic laminate attached to a modified SACH foot. Usually, there is no suspension required in Syme's prosthesis because the bulbous end serves that purpose.

Below-knee prosthesis

Below-knee amputation stumps above the level of Syme's amputation cannot tolerate any significant degree of distal weight bearing. Transfer of body weight therefore must occur in other pressure-tolerant areas. In the PTB prosthesis (Figure 51-14) a major portion of the body weight is distributed between the patellar tendon, counteracted by pressure in the popliteal area, and the medial tibial flare. The socket is intimately fitted to provide total contact over the entire stump area, including the distal end. A soft socket insert, although not absolutely necessary in all cases, is usually included. The socket is aligned with respect to the prosthetic foot in such a way as to provide mediolateral stability. In the sagittal plane it is aligned to produce knee flexion at heel strike, corresponding to a normal gait pattern, and to simulate push-off. Suspension of the PTB prosthesis is provided by either a suprapatellar cuff or an extension of the anterior socket brim over the patella, known as a suprapatellar or supracondylar prosthesis. Another method is to insert a supracondylar wedge between the medial portion of the socket and the medial femoral condyle. Although the PTB prosthesis provides a certain degree of mediolateral stability of the knee and is tolerated by most patients, a thigh corset and side bars may be added when additional knee stability is required or the surface area available in the PTB socket is insufficient to allow comfortable transfer of body weight to the prosthesis.

The conventional below-knee prosthesis with open-ended socket, thigh corset, and side joints is still indicated for a number of patients who cannot tolerate distal end contact and who must carry substantial weight in the thigh corset. Others for whom the conventional below-knee prosthesis is

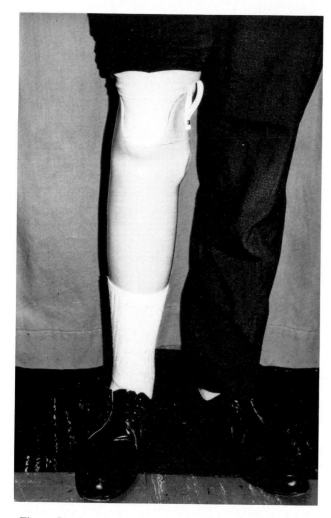

Figure 51-14. Patellar tendon–bearing below-knee prosthesis.

indicated are patients who are subject to fluctuations in stump size and new amputees who cannot readily obtain prosthetic services. Because the stump undergoes a number of changes during the first year following amputation, the new amputee can more readily maintain the fit of the prosthesis by adjusting the thigh lacer and adding stump socks.

Knee disarticulation prosthesis

In the past, surgeons were discouraged from performing disarticulations. Because of the length of the amputation, the prosthetic knee joints had to be placed on the outside of the prosthetic socket. This not only increased the bulk and worsened the appearance, but did not provide for adequate swing phase control, that is, controlling heel rise to adapt to varying cadences. This problem has been resolved with the development of the Orthopedic Hospital, Copenhagen (OHC) hydraulic swing phase control unit,[2] which allows the patient to walk with variable cadences and a more cosmetic prosthesis. The OHC unit is a four-bar polycentric knee mechanism and thus causes the shank to translate pos-

teriorly as the patient sits, eliminating any anterior protrusion. Knee disarticulation, whenever electively possible, is superior to an above-knee amputation because of the ability to yield end bearing and much improved proprioceptive feedback. It is also highly desirable from a surgical-medical point of view because of the reduced amputation trauma involved. It is not, however, recommended for female patients because of the bulk of the amputation itself with the addition of the prosthetic material surrounding the stump.

Because the knee disarticulation stump is bulbous distally, the prosthetic socket must either be fenestrated or contain a soft socket insert that is built up to provide a cylindric shape to insert the stump into the socket. The fenestration closure or soft socket insert is often sufficient to provide prosthetic suspension. Other suspension systems may be a suction socket design, which provides a valve distally so the socket is hermetically sealed once the stump is placed into the socket and the valve is sealed.

Gritti-Stokes prosthesis

Gritti-Stokes amputation and other supracondylar amputations result in reduced bulk and length and are partial or full end bearing. Either amputee type can achieve a very good gait, especially with hydraulic swing phase control mechanisms, other than the OHC knee unit.

Above-knee prosthesis

Above-knee amputation results in a stump that is unable to tolerate any appreciable end bearing. This stump is fitted with a quadrilateral socket that permits transfer of body weight through the ischial tuberosity. A total-contact socket provides optimal pressure distribution but is not indicated for all amputees. Contraindications are the same as those described for the PTB prosthesis in below-knee amputation. Recently the concept of the quadrilateral socket and ischial weight bearing has been challenged.[11] New socket configurations totally different from the quadrilateral socket are becoming increasingly popular.[21,24] Furthermore, the evolution of newer materials has made it possible to produce flexible sockets, that is, sockets that permit expansion of muscular tissue in selected areas while providing structural stability through a frame type of socket (Figure 51-15).[8] Obviously, such sockets are more comfortable, and they appear to have an advantage physiologically.

The alignment of the prosthesis in the sagittal plane must be such that knee stability is achieved. The simplest method is to place the axis of rotation of the mechanical knee somewhat behind the weight line. Additional stability is achieved from midstance to toe-off by minimizing or eliminating dorsiflexion. One must realize, however, that the farther the knee axis is placed posteriorly, the more difficult it is for the patient to initiate knee flexion. Alignment in the frontal plane should be such that the socket is adequately adducted to provide a supporting surface for the femur so the gluteus medius can stabilize the pelvis when the sound leg is in the

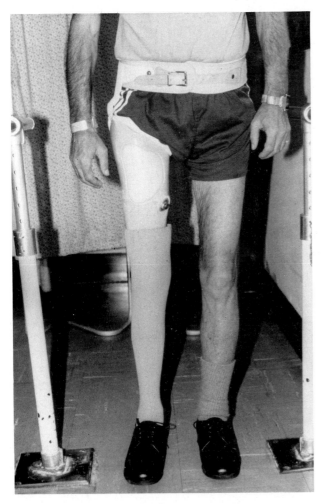

Figure 51-15. Above-knee prosthesis with flexible socket and hip joint and pelvic belt.

swing phase. The knee axis should be horizontal and the foot flat on the floor. A narrow base is desirable whenever possible to minimize the lateral excursion of the center of gravity.

In the past, single-axis knee joints with constant friction swing phase control were popular. However, they are rarely used today because of the aging patient population and the availability of improved control systems. Single-axis knee units with a manual knee lock are frequently prescribed for older patients to provide maximum safety. In patients who are weak or have poor stump conditions (for example, short stump), a weight-activated mechanism, or safety knee, is used. It provides safety on weight bearing, and on release of weight bearing the knee is free to swing. For younger patients, hydraulic or pneumatic control systems (Mauch SNS) are extremely useful in providing adaptation to varying cadences as well as stumble recovery. Less popular in the United States are polycentric knee units that simulate the kinematics of the normal anatomic knee joint and provide knee stability because of the geometric configuration. These

units tend to reduce energy consumption because of the relative shortening of the prosthesis in the swing phase and are best indicated for bilateral amputees.

The most sophisticated means of suspending the above-knee prosthesis is by negative pressure. This requires an accurate socket fit and maintenance of a suction seal in the proximal brim area. The patient must don the prosthesis by pulling the stump tissue into the socket by means of a stockinette. After the stockinette is removed, the suction valve is inserted and an airtight socket is created. The Silesian bandage is a flexible belt attached to the above-knee prosthesis, obliquely encircling the pelvis. It is an auxiliary to the suction suspension for extra security in short stumps. By its attachment points the Silesian bandage can control rotation and abduction-adduction. Suction suspension is contraindicated in patients whose stumps are subject to fluctuations in size, who perspire excessively, or who have very short stumps or deep scars in areas where a suction fit cannot be maintained. For these and patients who suffer from heart disease or are otherwise physically unable to exert themselves in the proper donning of the suction socket, a hip joint and pelvic band are indicated. In addition to suspending the prosthesis, the hip joint and pelvic band provide mediolateral and rotational stability. Ordinarily, stump socks are worn with this type of prosthesis. Any fluctuation in stump size can be accommodated by the addition or removal of stump socks.

Hip disarticulation prosthesis

The most common hip disarticulation prosthesis is the Canadian type. The unique location of the hip joint results in excellent alignment stability, yet permits the patient to walk with free-motion hip and knee joints. This is possible because the mechanical hip joint is purposely placed anterior and distal to the acetabulum. Thus the weight line passes behind the hip joint and produces hip extension. A control strap limits the degree of hip and knee flexion. A plastic laminated socket encircles the pelvis, terminating just above the crest of the ilium for suspension. More recently a hydropneumatic control system that coordinates knee flexion-extension and hip flexion-extension similar to that of a biarticular muscle has been developed to provide synergistic movement of the hip and knee joints.[20]

Hemipelvectomy prosthesis

The hemipelvectomy prosthesis is also of the Canadian type but has a socket that extends to that level of the xiphoid process to provide some weight bearing on the rib cage. Any of the knee or foot components previously described may be used with the Canadian hip disarticulation and hemipelvectomy prostheses.

Hemicorporectomy prosthesis

Hemicorporectomy prostheses of the most recent design include the alignment characteristics of the Canadian-type

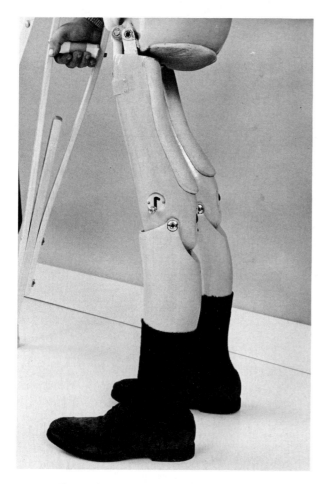

Figure 51-16. Hemicorporectomy prosthesis.

hip disarticulation prosthesis (Figure 51-16). The hip joint, however, is modified to incorporate a stride length control that allows the patient a reciprocal gait but requires mechanical locks at the knees. A shoulder control is used to unlock both hip joints to allow the patient to sit. The knee joints can be manually unlocked after the patient is seated.

UPPER LIMB PROSTHETICS

The objectives in upper limb prosthetics are quite different from those of lower limb prosthetics. Upper limb function is much more important in one's vocational and daily living activities than is lower limb function. Furthermore, an upper limb prosthesis is much less readily concealed than a lower limb prosthesis. The objectives, then, are replacement of function, especially prehension, and restoration of body image. Unfortunately, it is quite difficult to find both objectives effectively combined in the same terminal device.

Terminal devices

All terminal devices described here may be used for any level of amputation other than partial hand amputation. Ter-

minal devices are either voluntary opening or voluntary closing. Most common are voluntary-opening devices that are available in a functional hook or hand, as are the voluntary-closing devices. Rubber bands or spring loads are used to provide terminal device closing in voluntary-opening devices. Voluntary-closing devices include an alternating locking mechanism that allows the terminal device to be locked at any angle of opening; however, a second motion is required to unlock the terminal device. Either terminal device is interchangeable in the wrist unit, which may be friction controlled or may have a quick-change unit containing a rotation lock. Many patients find a hook considerably more functional than a hand because a hook is much lighter, less bulky, and more durable. Although prosthetic hands resemble the forms and colors of human hands, they are available in a limited number of sizes and therefore do not accurately match all individuals. The cosmetic glove covering the mechanical hand is susceptible to tearing and discoloration, which makes the prosthetic hand unsuitable for manual work. A prosthetic hook should be viewed as a tool rather than a hand replacement because it neither resembles the form and size of a hand nor functions in the same way. Just as tools are a necessary adjunct in the performance of certain activities of nonamputees, the function of a hook in such cases is far superior to that of a prosthetic hand.

Control systems

Harness control of terminal devices is through scapular abduction, shoulder flexion, or a combination of both. These motions are harnessed in a figure-of-8 or figure-of-9 harness and transmitted to the terminal device through a Bowden cable.

Myoelectric control uses EMG signals from residual muscles in the stump to switch on the actuator in a prosthetic hand, hook, or elbow. Electrical potentials generated when a muscle contracts to control an externally energized prosthesis do not require any shoulder harness to produce power to control the device. This eliminates the need for the various body movements needed in conventional operations. Electrodes built into the socket will, when the prosthesis is applied, pick up myopotentials when the muscle contracts. These signals are differentially amplified, rectified, and relayed for reliable control of the actuator. In below-elbow prostheses this is a very natural control, because one can use the residual extrinsic flexors and extensors of the hand and wrist. As little as 50 μV is sufficient to serve as a control signal.

Alternatively, electric switch control may be used with externally energized systems. A pull-switch may be incorporated into the harness system so that when the harness is stretched, the pull switch controls the actuator movement. A rocker or toggle switch may be placed such that rudimentary digits, for example, in phocomelia, can activate the controls. Yet the harnessing required in all but below-elbow prostheses is still the same as in conventionally con-

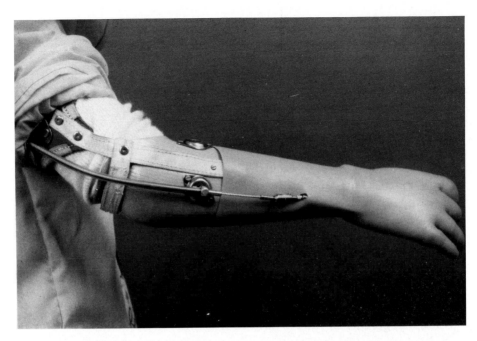

Figure 51-17. Wrist disarticulation prosthesis with triceps cuff.

trolled harness and cable control systems because of suspension needs. Patients must be properly selected for externally powered systems, because the electronic components are more susceptible to damage than conventional control systems.

Partial hand amputation

Partial hand amputees are rarely fitted with a functional prosthesis because of the technical difficulties involved. There is usually sufficient residual function and, most of all, sensibility that makes a functional prosthesis a poor trade-off. Instead, these patients can be provided with a cosmetic glove to replace missing portions of the hand.

Wrist disarticulation prosthesis

Wrist disarticulation is quite desirable from a functional point of view because the patient retains nearly full pronation-supination in the prosthesis.

The socket, as for all upper limb prostheses, is made of a plastic laminate and is shaped to permit maximal residual pronation and supination (Figure 51-17). A triceps cuff with flexible hinges serves as a reaction point for the control cable, as well as a link between the prosthesis and the front suspension strap of the harness.

Below-elbow prosthesis

Below-elbow amputees with long or medium-length stumps are fitted with the same prosthesis as wrist disarticulation amputees, with the exception of socket configuration. For the below-elbow amputee with a short stump, the Muenster-type prosthesis has achieved great popularity

(Figure 51-18). The socket extends posteriorly above the olecranon and intimately fits around the triceps tendon, thus suspending the prosthesis and eliminating the elbow hinges and triceps cuff. Although the Muenster-type prosthesis limits elbow flexion and extension, this has been found to be of little consequence in the unilateral amputee. Bilateral amputees, for whom maximum flexion-extension is a great necessity, may be fitted with a split socket.[2]

Elbow disarticulation prosthesis

Elbow disarticulation is desirable from a functional point of view. The patient retains nearly full range of internal and external rotation. Cosmetically it is undesirable for female amputees because of the bulk produced in the elbow area by the addition of outside-locking elbow hinges. The elbow unit contains an alternating locking mechanism, in which one control motion locks the elbow and the second control motion unlocks it. Terminal device control as well as elbow flexion is produced by the same motions discussed for wrist disarticulation. However, the housing is split in the elbow area so that elbow flexion occurs when the elbow is unlocked. When the elbow is locked, the same control motion operates the terminal device. The elbow lock is controlled by shoulder depression on the amputated side. The figure-of-8 harness includes a lateral and front suspension strap. The elbow lock control is attached to the front strap.

Above-elbow prosthesis

Prostheses for above-elbow amputees, with the exception of the elbow unit and the socket configuration, possess the same components as those described for elbow disarticu-

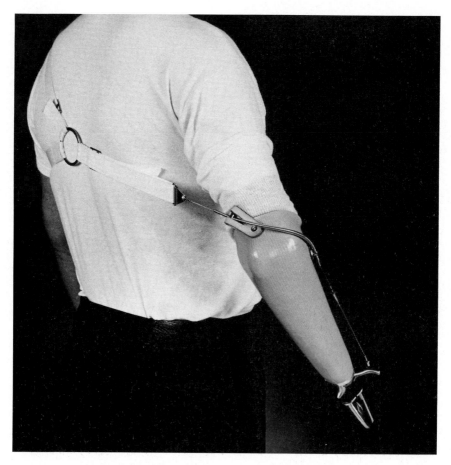

Figure 51-18. Below-elbow prosthesis with Muenster socket.

lation. The elbow unit contains an internal alternating locking system, as well as a turntable that permits passive control of internal and external rotation. Depending on the stump length, the proximal socket trim lines vary. For longer stumps, trim lines are identical to those for elbow disarticulation, but for a very short above-elbow stump they extend over the acromion and contain anterior and posterior wings to stabilize the arm against externally applied rotation forces.

Shoulder disarticulation prosthesis

Prostheses for shoulder disarticulation amputees require an extensive socket covering the scapula posteriorly and the pectoralis major anteriorly. Shoulder units vary from a free-motion abduction joint to friction-controlled shoulder flexion and abduction units. All other components are identical to those described for the above-elbow prosthesis. A chest strap harness with an elastic suspension strap serves to control the terminal device and elbow function. Because shoulder flexion is not available, the degree of residual scapular abduction is usually insufficient to provide full elbow flexion or terminal device operation unless an excursion amplifier is incorporated into the control system. Control of elbow

lock operation is obtained through shoulder elevation. The reaction point for the elbow lock cable is a waist band.

For this level of amputation, switch or myoelectric control (Figure 51-19) has advantages, as mentioned previously. Because shoulder flexion is not available, the patient is unable to obtain full range of elbow flexion and terminal device opening in a conventional system, except for the excursion amplifier. However, the excursion amplifier requires twice the force normally necessary to operate the harness control system.

Forequarter amputation prosthesis

The massive forequarter amputation and the absence of residual motor power often make a lightweight foam shoulder cap the device of choice to enable the patient to wear a shirt, blouse, or coat. Sometimes a passive cosmetic arm prosthesis, in which elbow flexion and locking are manually controlled, is indicated when improved appearance is desired.

With the advent of externally powered systems, and especially myoelectric control, some patients have been fitted with a semifunctional prosthesis. The terminal device is myoelectrically controlled from any available muscle from

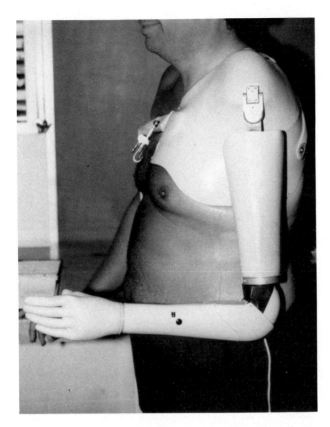

Figure 51-19. Shoulder disarticulation prosthesis with myoelectrically controlled elbow and hand.

the shoulder girdle, usually the upper trapezius. All other joint functions are friction or manually controlled.

REFERENCES

1. American Academy of Orthopaedic Surgeons: Atlas of orthotics, St. Louis, 1975, The CV Mosby Co.
2. American Academy of Orthopaedic Surgeons: Atlas of limb prosthetics: surgical and prosthetic principles, St. Louis, 1981, The CV Mosby Co.
3. Anbar, M: Computerized man: microprocessor-controlled prosthetics, Comput Med p 174, 1986.
4. Beets, CL, et al: Orthoses and the dynamic knee: a basic overview, Orthot Prosthet 39:33, 1985.
5. Burgess, EM, et al: Development and preliminary evaluation of the VA Seattle foot, J Rehab Res Dev 22:75, 1985.
6. Elliott, HC: The pyramidal system. In Textbook of neuroanatomy, Philadelphia, 1969, JB Lippincott Co.
7. Grynbaum, BB, Sokolow, J, and Lehneis, HR: Prosthetic principles in the management of fractures, J Chron Dis 23:201, 1970.
8. Jendrzejczyk, D: Flexible socket systems, Clin Prosthet Orthot 9:27, 1985.
9. Kaplan, EB: The hand as an organ. In Functional and surgical anatomy of the hand, Philadelphia, 1965, JB Lippincott Co.
10. LeGros Clark, WE: The evidence of limbs. In The antecedents of man New York, 1969, Harper & Row Publishers, Inc.
11. Lehneis, HR: Application of external power in orthotics. Orthot Prosthet 22:34, 1968.
12. Lehneis, HR: Principles of orthotics and prosthetics. In Rusk, HA: Rehabilitation medicine, ed 4, St. Louis, 1977, The CV Mosby Co.
13. Lehneis, HR: Upper-limb orthotics, Orthot Prosthet 31:14, 1977.
14. Lehneis, HR: Orthesenentwicklungen für die untere Extremitat aus der Sicht des Bioingenieurs, Orthopade 8:344, 1979.
15. Lehneis, HR: Plastic ankle-foot orthoses: Indications and functions, Newsl Prosthet Orthot Clin 4:3, 1980.
16. Lehneis, HR: Technical note: orthotic pelvis control in spina bifida, Clin Prosthet Orthot 8:26, 1984.
17. Lehneis, HR: Beyond the quadrilateral, Clin Prosthet Orthot 9:6, 1985.
18. Lehneis, HR, Chin, R, and Fornuff, D: Bivalved spinal orthoses for the structurally unstable spine, Clin Prosthet Orthot 7:9, 1983.
19. Lehneis, HR, and Wilson, RG: An electric arm orthosis, Bull Prosthet Res 10:4, 1972.
20. Lehneis, HR, et al: Advanced orthotics and prosthetics in cancer management: Rehabilitation monograph #63, New York, 1981, New York University Medical Center.
21. Long, IA: Normal shape–normal alignment (NSNA) above-knee prosthesis, Clin Prosthet Orthot 9:9, 1985.
22. Oxnard, CE: The functional morphology of the primate shoulder as revealed by comparative anatomical, osteometric and discriminate function techniques, Am Journal Phys Anthropol 26:219, 1967.
23. Personal communication, Durr-Fillauer Orthopedic, Orthopedic Division, Chattanooga, Tenn, 1985
24. Sabolich, J: Contoured adducted trochanteric-controlled alignment method (CAT-CAM): introduction and basic principles, Clin Prosthet Orthot 9:15, 1985.
25. Scott, BA: Engineering principles and fabricated techniques for Scott-Craig long leg brace for paraplegics, Orthot Prosthet J 25:14, 1971.
26. Tuttle, RH: Knuckle walking and the evolution of hominoid hands, Am J Phys Anthropol 26:171, 1967.
27. Tuttle, RH: Quantitative and functional studies on the hands of the anthropoidea, J Morphol 128:309, 1969.

CHAPTER 52 | Shoe correction and foot pathology

LAWRENCE I. KAPLAN

Although foot coverings were used as far back as 4 thousand years ago to prevent foot injuries, the shoe as we know it today probably began to develop in the early 1800s. Because the modern shoe is of such recent development, not surprisingly there is still some disagreement in methods of correcting the problem foot with shoe modifications.

Our knowledge of shoe correction is frequently based on trial and error. There has been little basic or clinical research compared to the research effort in prosthetic and orthotic areas since World War II. However, a significant amount of accumulated knowledge has become available that emphasizes the need for further research.

There are 26 bones in the foot, numerous ligamentous structures that connect one bone with another, and a number of extremely important muscles that can be primarily affected in foot disorders. Disorders of other structures of the lower extremities and the trunk also may contribute significantly to foot problems. For example, significant scoliosis of the trunk may result in one lower extremity being relatively longer than the other in the erect position, even though true lengths as measured from the anterosuperior iliac spines to the lower border of the medial malleoli may actually be equal. Such an extremity creates greater stress during the stance phase and has a tendency to strike the ground in a way that favors development of deformity as well as other disabilities such as splayed feet, dropped metatarsals, and claw and hammer toes. Furthermore, diseases of the nervous and the musculoskeletal system may be a major factor in producing foot disorders.

In genu varum, patients have a tendency to develop pes cavus, and in genu valgum, to develop pes planovalgus. For individuals with a paralysis secondary to poliomyelitis, resultant pathology may be the underlying factor in similar foot pathology. Weakness of the gastrocnemius soleus may result in dropfoot with contracture of the plantar fascia, and a cavus deformity may result. Weakness of the anterior tibial muscle may result in a planus foot. Thus it is evident that the whole patient must be examined even when the primary complaints concern the feet.

EXAMINATION OF THE FOOT

The foot should be examined with the patient in standing and reclining positions. With the patient standing, any abnormalities in appearance are noted. There should be a reasonably developed arch and a sustentaculum tali in its appropriate position on a medial aspect of the posterior portion of the foot. It should not be too low or too high.

Skin color should be evaluated. Hypertrophy may be present in the region of the fifth toe laterally or the first toe medially. Enlargements are usually found in the region of the metatarsophalangeal (MP) joint and tend to be reddened.

The angulation of the first and fifth toes is also important. They may be in an adducted position and may overlap the adjacent toes.

The appearance of a bunion in the region of the first toe is well recognized; however, much less is known about the tailor's bunion, which involves the fifth toe. This term is derived from the time when tailors commonly sat with their legs crossed and their fifth toes pressed against the hard floor. They also held their material against the lower sternum, which not infrequently caused an indentation on the lower aspect of that bone. Today the cause of tailor's bunion is the use of shoes that are too narrow and relatively sharply angulated.

On general examination one may notice a widening of the so-called transverse arch in the general region of the MP joints of the forefoot. This is referred to as a splayed foot.

With the patient in the erect position, it is possible to

note whether the longitudinal arch is too elevated, thus forming a cavus deformity, or too low, resulting in flatfoot, called pes planovalgus. The latter state may vary in degrees from minor flattening of the arch to the extreme change of a completely flat foot that is entirely in contact with the ground. The lateral aspect of the flat foot becomes projected to almost form a small ledge beyond the borders of the upper aspect of the foot.

Other observation requires notation of the presence or absence of deformed toes, to be described in a later section, and angulation of the heel that tends to be in the varus position with a cavus foot and inclines to a valgus position in a planus foot.

The examination proceeds with the patient walking the length of the examining room on the toes and then on the heels. The forefoot should clear the floor by at least an inch during this ambulation. The balance, stability, and phases of the gait of the individual are observed. For example, a patient with multiple sclerosis might have great difficulty in performing these movements, just as someone with weakness of the dorsiflexors or of the gastrocnemius and soleus might have difficulty in properly raising the heel to allow complete clearance in normal gait.

The patient should be asked to hold on to the examining table, leaving 15 to 18 inches between the body and table, and do knee flexion repetitions and again heel raises on each extremity separately. Further information is derived in this position regarding discomfort and malformation. This exercise allows the examiner to detect an otherwise unobservable varus or valgus position, metatarsal, or toe MP or IP incremented deformity or pain, calcaneal discomfort during heel raises, forefoot problems with pain of the metatarsals or toes during knee bends, presence of mild weakness of the gastrocnemius soleus, or weak anterior tibial musculature, and so on.

The patient then reclines on the table for further examination. Callosities may be present on the sole of the foot, especially in the region of the MP joints. Callosities tend to occur especially between the second and third toes and sometimes between the second, third, and fourth toes. They vary in thickness, depending on the undue pressure of the depressed arch. Callosities may also be noted along the medial border of the first toe, where there is otherwise no other disturbance of that toe, and on the lateral aspect of the fifth toe. Callus formation may relate to pes cavus, pes planovalgus, or shoes that are too narrow. Frequently callosities of the first and fifth toe are age related and are found in people who are in their forties or beyond.

The MP joints and the proximal IP joints and the middle and distal IP joints of the first to fourth toes should be tested separately. Significant tenderness of the MP joints on normal examination may indicate the presence of metatarsalgia, which is caused by compression of the joints against the floor and loss of the transverse arch. Tenderness in an IP joint may be caused by deformity in the claw or the hammer

position. In the clawed position the toes tend to maintain flexion at all levels, although they commonly can be straightened out with little difficulty. In hammer toe, the distal IP joint, instead of being flexed during standing, is held in an extended position, imparting the appearance of a hammer.

The first toe should be examined separately. The examiner should ask whether there is significant pain at rest, on ambulation, or both, especially on toe-off or shifting to the forefoot position during the stance phase. When there is pain on palpation, as well as limitation of active and passive range of motion at the MP joint and to some degree laterally of the first toe, the condition is called hallux rigidus.

In the congenital condition known as Morton's toe, the first toe may be shorter than the others. When the first toe is shorter, the second toe becomes the longest toe and must be considered in the proper fitting of shoes; the tip of the shoe must be related to the length of the second toe. There is also a condition in which the toes are separated from one another, in this area especially, which is known as metatarsus adductus.

NORMAL GAIT

The study of walking (gait) is necessary to understand the mechanics of foot disorders and the principles of treatment by shoe corrections and other means. During walking there is rapid movement from the calcaneus at heel strike along the lateral aspect of the foot across the metatarsals and phalanges to push-off on the big toe (Figure 52-1). The forces of the foot are dynamic.

Heel strike

As the foot hits the ground, the foot is in a varus position, or turned in, with the sole partially facing the opposite foot and only the lateral posterior portion of the heel in contact with the ground. This accounts for the greater wear of this portion of the heel in the normal well-shod foot. If the shoe is a flimsy slipper or sandal, it tends to slide laterally on the foot and wear occurs instead on the midposterior aspect of the heel.

Foot flat

Shortly after heel strike the sole of the foot moves to touch the ground. To arrive at this point—stance phase—the foot rotates in varus with the greater weight being taken along the lateral border of the sole until the foot is flat.

Midstance

In midstance the body weight is directly over the supporting extremity.

Push-off

Push-off is divided into heel-off and toe-off. In heel-off, as the heel of the supporting extremity rises from the ground, the ball of the foot and the toes are still in contact with the

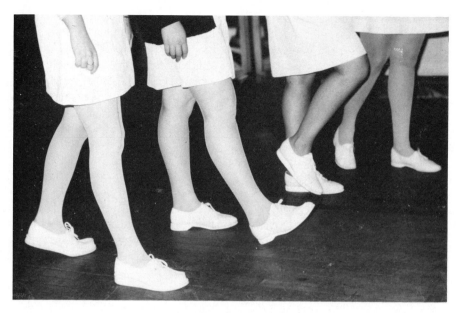

Figure 52-1. Phases of gait.

ground. Beyond this point, however, there is a roll-over across the ball of the foot from lateral to medial, with pressure being taken increasingly by the metatarsal region and the phalanges of the medial toes.

The push-off phase terminates in toe-off, when the entire foot rises from the gound and the extremity, then enters swing phase—forward propulsion of the leg.

At toe-off the normal big toe is in straight alignment with the rest of the foot. Meyers defined this line in stating that "the great toe must lie in such a position that its axis carried backward shall pass through the center of the heel." Greater weight is borne by the medial aspect of the first toe.

The foot is a second-class lever. A second-class lever can be thought of as a wheelbarrow in which the power is supplied through the handle bars by the individual who holds and pushes the wheelbarrow. The weight being carried is in the center, or container, section of the wheelbarrow, and the fulcrum is the wheel. In the foot the first toe is at the fulcrum. The weight is the body located between the first toe and the power source, which is the calf muscles acting at the heel. The center of gravity of the foot is located just anterior to the ankle joint during midstance.

An example of dysfunction occurs when the first toe is in some degree of valgus (turned out toward the little toe). This is common among wearers of pointed shoes, as well as in older persons who have gone barefoot during their lives. The lever is twisted at its fulcrum and creates inefficient movement in walking and running.

It has frequently been stated that shoes with pointed or cramped toe boxes are a major cause of hallux valgus. However, even in primitive populations, constant pressure against the medial aspect of the first toe during toe-off may account for the development of hallux valgus. MacLennan[1]

studied the prevalance of hallux valgus in an unshod neo-lithic New Guinea population. He found that it was frequently severe and increased with age, especially in women. Another study was done on the island of Tristan de Cunha. In the unshod population over 60 years of age, there was a greater tendency to hallux valgus, in men as well as women. The position of the foot during toe-off is probably critical with the increasing effect of pressure against the medial aspect of the first toe. In most instances in small children of this population, the alignment of the first toe seems to follow the axis line.

Full stance

Even when one is standing, there is still movement of the body (for example, swaying to balance), and the foot must constantly adjust to the changing position.

In full stance the concept of an anatomic metatarsal arch pertains with pressure on the first and fifth toes and on the calcaneus, the three points of contact when the foot is on the ground. One half of the load is found to be at the hind foot, and the other half is in the region of the forefoot. In the forefoot, one third of the load is borne by the big toe and two thirds by the other toes. Some studies report 50% of weight borne by the first toe in the forefoot and 50% by the other four toes.

NOMENCLATURE
Shoe (Figure 52-2)

The shoe consists of an upper part (or the upper), the sole, the heel, and the inner lining. The uppermost part of the posterior aspect of the shoe in the region of the heel, where the heel rests anatomically, is called the internal heel

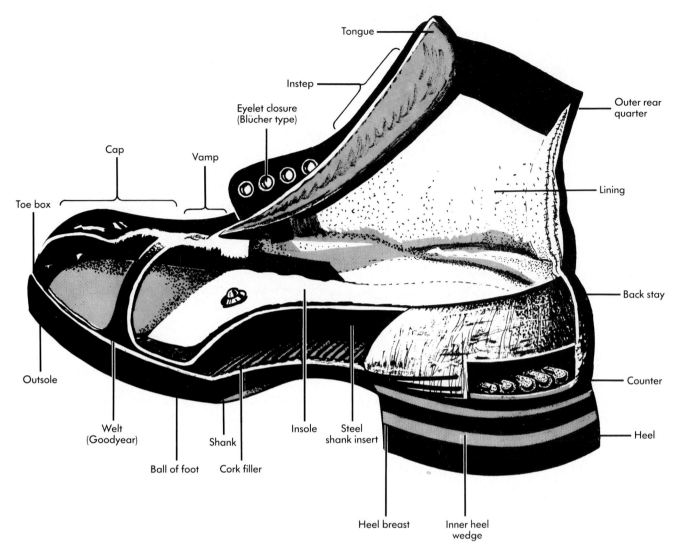

Figure 52-2. Anatomy of shoe.

seat. Below this is the base of the heel, where the heel is fastened. The heel proper is usually made out of leather or rubber; the anterior aspect is called the breast of the heel. The heel is also angled at its posterior to produce the pitch of the heel. The height of the heel is usually measured by manufacturers in eighths of an inch, for example, a three-eighths heel.

The sole consists of an anterior aspect called the ball of the shoe. Its widest part is located at the level of the metatarsal heads. The shank is the area between the anterior aspect of the heel and the ball of the sole. In orthopedic shoes there is often a piece of metal, the metal shank, which is placed between the layers of the sole. The anterior tip of the outer sole is spaced above the ground and is called the toe spring. The toe spring is the measured distance between the outer sole and the floor at the sole's tip. This allows the foot to rock through at push-off. The sole usually consists of at least two layers, the inner sole, seen on the inside of

the shoe, and the outer sole. The space between the insole and the outer sole is called the filler. This Goodyear welt construction is a feature of well-built shoes.

The upper part of the shoe has an anterior portion called the vamp. Attached to the vamp is the tongue of the shoe, which is the strip of leather lying under the laces. The anterior end of the tongue is called the throat, being the point at which the tongue is attached to the vamp, that is, the base of the tongue. Quarters consist of the posterior aspect of the upper, sometimes separated from the anterior aspect by a stitched line referred to as upper foxing. To prevent contact and abrasions in the region of the lateral malleolus, the lateral aspect is cut down lower than the medial.

The lace stay with its eyelets is the portion that contains the lace. The eyelets are usually ½ inch apart from one another, and there are usually four eyelets on each side of the lace stay. Several types of lace stays are in use. In the

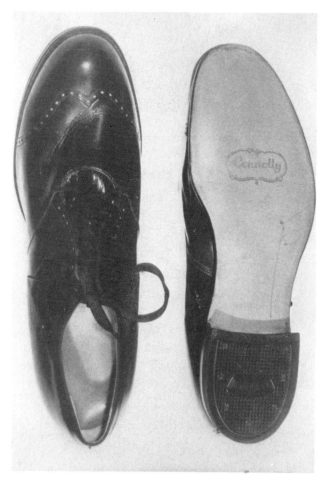

Figure 52-3. Blucher-type lace stay.

so-called Blucher type (Figure 52-3), the lace stay can be pulled apart one side from the other; the Blucher is part of the vamp. This allows for easy entry by separation of the two sides of the lace stay. The Balmoral type is usually part of the quarters and is connected at its distal anterior aspect in a V shape. The Balmoral, which is also laced, is difficult to open fully in the region of the vamp. People with problem feet find a Blucher type of opening easier to use than a Balmoral. The lining of the shoe should be perfectly smooth to prevent contact pressure against the foot.

The toe box, which is the very anterior part of the shoe, can be rigid and thus retain its shape and guard against injury to the toes, or can be soft, without any stiff material.

Most good shoes have a counter in their posterior quarter. The counter is usually made from a synthetic substance or ground leather, which is processed to become rigid and used to create a firm shape in the region of the heel. The counter usually extends to the heel breast, but special counters may extend medially or laterally farther forward as well as upward—over the malleoli, if necessary, for certain disabilities.

Foot

The foot is also described as having certain areas such as the ball that are identical to the ball of the shoe, being the region at the level of the metatarsal heads. The waist of the foot is between the calcaneal area and the metatarsal heads or ball; the instep, which is on the dorsum, is somewhat anterior to the waist of the foot and basically in the region of the lace stay of the shoe.

CORRECTIVE FOOTWEAR
Types of corrective footwear

The shoe with Goodyear welt construction is the most appropriate for adequate correction of foot disabilities, although other types may be sufficient. This type of shoe attaches the upper and lower parts; the upper is sewn to the welt and insole, and the lower portion or sole also is sewn to the welt. The space in between contains a filler material.

In the stitch-down type of shoe, another common variety, the upper is turned out and stitched down to the sole, and the cementing of a lining is cemented to the inner sole, the middle sole, and the insole; the outer sole is cemented to the middle sole. A small welt is added and stitched to all the layers.

Other styles of corrective shoes include those with the strap and buckle closure, in which the shoe can be closed by a simple strap laced through buckle. There is also a Velcro closure in which the Velcro passes through a wide buckle and is placed over the lace stay area (Figure 52-4). It is closed easily with one hand or simply by the palm of the hand pressing the Velcro sides together.

There is special footwear for those who experience difficulty in putting on shoes. The surgical or convalescent shoe is laced to the toe as in an athletic shoe. A shoe that has an opening in the back seam so that the foot is inserted from the rear of the shoe allows great ease of entry. The closure is lacing or Velcro (Figure 52-5). This is an excellent shoe for someone who cannot bend the hip, the knee, or back; the patient can simply place the shoe against a wall and slide the foot into it, closing it from behind. This shoe is also of value for someone with no ankle motion. Another shoe is made of elastic material (Goring) in which the lace stay area simply stretches open for easy entry.

Fitting corrective footwear

Proper prescription is a function of experience and is often more artful than scientific. I have patients bring the totally uncorrected shoe for my examination before corrective alterations. The planning of an effective prescription requires that the prescriber have expertise in the dynamics of muscle movement, knowledge of the pathomechanics of foot disabilities, a practical working knowledge of the construction and modification of shoes, and ingenuity and adaptability.

Professional responsibility requires the assurance that the shoe is the proper size before the shoe is changed. After

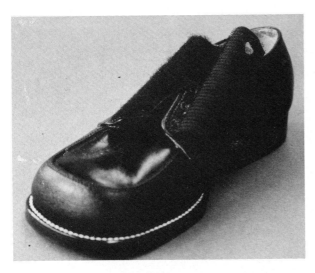

Figure 52-4. Velcro closure on corrective shoe.

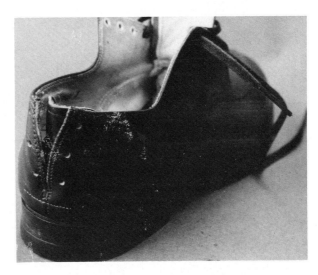

Figure 52-5. Corrective shoe with opening in back seam.

the corrections have been made, the patient wears the shoe for 1 week and then returns for final evaluation and corrections required.

Evaluation of the foot

The patient should disrobe except for underclothing so the entire alignment of the extremity can be evaluated. For example, patients with significant genu varum or genu valgum commonly have malalignment of the feet, pes planovalgus, or pes cavus because of the shape of the lower extremities. If there is a knee disability with one lower extremity in valgus, not infrequently both feet are totally different in appearance, one being in cavus and the other in planus. Careful observation must precede definitive corrective planning.

The patient should be observed while walking to see if there is eversion (toeing out) or inversion (toeing in). This is especially important in children. It is important to note the pattern of the movements and visualize corrections that might be needed, particularly in the presence of other types of disability from trauma of poliomyelitis. The patient should be examined while he or she is supine to determine the range of motion and malleability of the foot. Presence of callosities, corns, inappropriate positions of the toes such as hallux valgus, and spreading of the foot should be noted.

With the patient standing, the examiner should look for dropped metatarsals of the foot, toes spread out in the forward aspect (splaying), or the presence of claw toes or hammer toes. The foot should be grasped and moved throughout the normal range of motion to determine whether the heel cord is contracted, the foot is fixed in one position or another (as in eversion and inversion), there is loss of motor power and loss of active range in any of the ankle or foot directions, and the foot is rigid or normally loose. Finally, the presence of pain on manipulation of various

parts of the foot is noted. Included is pain of the toes on manipulation in flexion and extension, tenderness of an area such as the MP joints, pain over the ankle joint, medially or laterally, or pain on manipulation of the forefoot in relationship to the hind foot. There may be tenderness over the sole in the anterior aspect of the calcaneus and over the plantar fascia of the heel or other parts of the sole. Careful examination is crucial and is easily accomplished.

Evaluation of fit

The shoe must be the appropriate size for the patient. This is determined in the standing position. Any type of closure must be coapted or laced firmly. With laced shoes the eyelets must be parallel and the side of the closure separated by no less than ¼ to ½ inch. A gap at the top indicates that the shoe is too tight across the instep; a gap at the bottom reflects excessive wideness at the vamp.

The length of the shoe should be ½ to ¾ inch beyond the longest toe. In growing children a new shoe is required if there is less than ¼ inch of spacing left between the longest toe and the tip of the shoe. With a soft toe box, the examiner can feel the big toe up against the toe box and determine its distance from the toe tip. In the case of a rigid toe box in which the toes cannot be felt, the examiner measures the point of coincidence of the ball of the foot and the ball of the shoe. These should be equal from the heel-to-ball length. The MP joint, which juts out farthest medially, can be palpated along the ball of the shoe just beyond the beginning of the turn in the shank of the shoe.

When pinching the area of the vamp, just distal to the lace stay, the examiner should be able to grasp ¼ inch of leather between the fingers (Figure 52-6). Gapping at the sides of the shoe indicates incorrect fitting and probably means that the shoe is too narrow. There should also be a snug fit in the back seam area. When the patient walks,

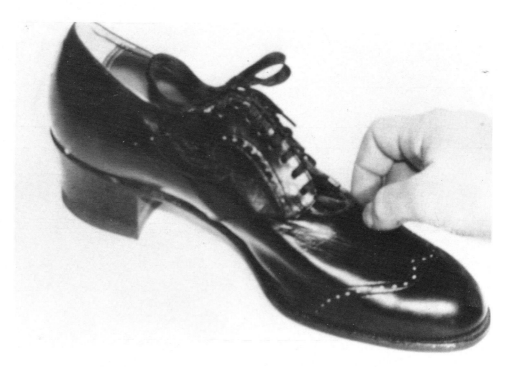

Figure 52-6. Evaluation of fit of shoe by pinching area of vamp.

there should be no piston action of the heel area in the shoe, although a small amount is permissible if the shoe is new and stiff. Whether the shoe has been worn properly can be determined by observing that the greatest degree of wear is at the outer aspect of the heel. There should also be a 1-inch band of wear under the MP joints across the sole of the shoe, especially under the first toe. In a child or an individual who runs, and in bicyclists, there may be greater wear under the toe tip region of the sole.

Goals of treatment

Based on the findings of the examination, a general course of action may be chosen: correction of the foot disabilities in alignment by the shoe or accommodation of disabilities by eliminating foot movement in the shoe through additions to the shoe. In the case of pain on movement or in the presence of a rigid foot structure, the option of choice is accommodation. This means making corrections to the shoe to substitute for the rigid or painful movement. The preferable alternative is to correct the position of the foot with the shoe to return the patient to a more normal gait. This can be done only if the foot is malleable and pain is not produced by the correction.

Pain relief

A dugout heel may relieve calcaneal discomfort caused by a calcaneal spur or inflammation of the fascial tissue (calcaneal fasciitis). The heel of the shoe can be dug out and the area filled with foam rubber and covered by a leather inner sole (Figure 52-7).

Prevention of progressive deformity

A platform or wedge type of shoe helps prevent descent of the medial-longitudinal arch from overweight or prolonged standing. This type of shoe provides extra support under the shank.

Mechanical substitution for loss of movement

A solid ankle cushion heel (SACH) and a rocker bar from shank to toe tip can be used to substitute for lost ankle or foot motion. The SACH is made of a rubber material that

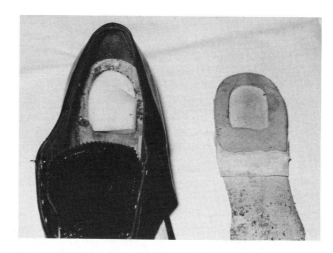

Figure 52-7. Dugout heel filled with foam rubber and covering insole.

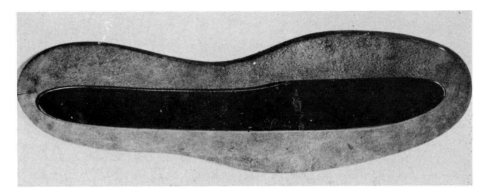

Figure 52-8. Steel insert used to eliminate motion through metatarsophalangeal joints.

comes in three densities to allow variable degrees of compression. It is used in artificial limbs when there is no ankle joint to permit the heel to compress and to allow the patient to be able to reach foot flat without excessive motion. This same rubber material can be used as an insert into the heel of a shoe. There are also several kinds of additions to the sole, such as the rocker and metatarsal bars. The rocker bar is rigid so that it may be "fixed" on certain lengths and apices; however, it can be adapted in many ways to permit efficient lifting of the heel from the ground, followed by toe-off. The rocker bar may be very small and found just posterior to the metatarsal heads, or it can be extended. The position of the bar can be varied in accordance with the patient's need. If the foot is very sensitive, the apex can be "skived"—a shoe term meaning to cut down the height of the correction. Thus a patient with a feeling of being elevated too high on an involved foot or both feet can be given a skived apex that can be made higher at some future date when the patient has accommodated to this type of correction.

A SACH can be used in combination with a rocker bar to permit the patient to descend to the sole and then to rock through the sole through the extended "shank to toe tip rocker bar." This substitutes for a rigid foot or lost ankle motion. This same type of dual correction can be used to eliminate painful motion and to allow the sole of the shoe to do the work.

Elimination of movement

Motion can be eliminated by using a semiflexible steel insert between the inner and outer sole or as part of a molded inner sole. Such a steel insert, which is used for many foot conditions, eliminates motion through the MP joints (Figure 52-8). It also accommodates a rigid deformity or a deformity that if corrected would produce pain.

Periodic reevaluation

Periodic reevaluations are an absolute necessity because, more than any other type of appliance, the shoe tends to wear and the distortion of weight bearing tends to produce changes in the correction. This is especially true with the growing foot that becomes bound in a smaller shoe with all the corrections in the wrong places. The problem is exacerbated when molded plates and arch supports are used.

Precautions

A prime principle is that it is a mistake to attempt to correct what cannot be corrected or what would become painful with shoe correction. Several other precautions must also be taken on prescribing and reevaluating a corrective shoe.

The additional weight of a corrected orthopedic shoe may be excessive to people who are markedly debilitated or have neurologic weaknesses of the lower extremities. The weight of the shoe may be so great that the patient may be unable to lift the lower extremity from the floor or it may cause easy and rapid fatigability and an inability to walk. This can be true in patients with paralytic poliomyelitis, peripheral neuropathy, or significant paresis. Under the circumstances it is important to compromise and to provide a light shoe with sufficiently designed corrections. Finally, the patient's reactions and use of the corrected shoe are critical. Sometimes what appear to be proper modifications leave the patient uncomfortable and in pain or unable to walk. The only course of action is to carefully restudy and remodify the shoes to overcome the patient's complaints and discomfort.

Physical laws of shoe correction

There are two important physical laws concerning shoe correction. The first is that pressure is inversely proportional to the square of the area. This is especially important to people with pain in the foot, as in the MP area, under the toes, in the region of the heel, or other locations. The guiding principle of modification is to spread the weight throughout the entire foot to lessen the pressure at any tender point. For example, if the patient has a cavus foot (high arch), undue pressure is present in the region of the heel, as well as over the MP joints. By filling in the longitudinal arch elevation with a scaphoid pad customized to match the arch height, the pressure will be extended along the midfoot, as well as to the heel and toe areas. Furthermore, by using a SACH or digging out under the metatarsal heads and filling this area with foam rubber, the pressure gradient is softened as well.

The second physical law involves the concept that each action involves an equal reaction. With regard to shoe modifications such as fillers, the harder the surface on contact, the harder the reactive effect against the foot. The softer the surface, the softer the reactive compression of the foot.

Correctional devices can be placed in one of three areas of the shoe:

1. As an insert on the inside of the shoe, called an inlay. These may be fixed or removable.
2. Sandwiched between the insole and the outsole. This can be done only on shoes such as the Goodyear welt, whose layers can be easily separated.

3. Modifications on the sole of the shoe. These are external and are referred to as overlays or onlays.

Inlays, especially if they are in the form of arch supports, either full length or three-quarter length, commonly require that shoe size be increased by one grade. However, they do not easily erode unless made of soft materials. In some instances when there is no good counter material in the shoe, the insert may deteriorate and flatten out. Sandwiches in the shoe do not erode because they do not contact the foot on the inside directly or the ground on the outside. External sole corrections do tend to wear, but they do not reduce the size of the shoe, nor do they distort its inner surface.

Materials

A number of materials are used to create the orthotic devices that are placed inside the shoe. SACH rubber is used frequently as an insert between the outer aspects and the base of the heel for creating a compressible heel.

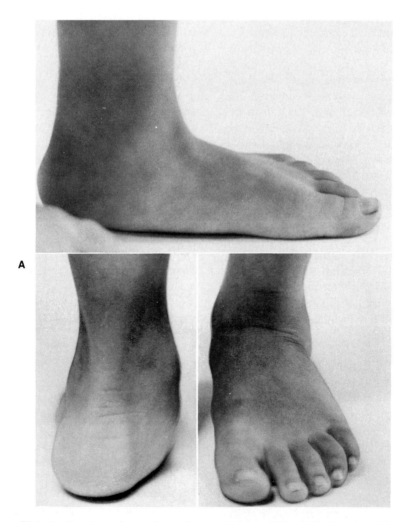

Figure 52-9. A, One type of pes planus. Note depression of longitudinal arch, without everted heel, abducted forefoot, or longitudinal rotation of metatarsals and phalanges.

Other materials include the following:

1. Plastizote, which comes in grades 1, 2, and 3 with different hardnesses known as durometer strength, from 20, 35, to 69 durometers of hardness (compressibility)
2. Aliplast, which comes in four degrees of rigidity known as 4E, 6A, 10, and XPE and from 23 to 68 durometers of hardness
3. Polyethylene foam (Pelite) from Japan, which also comes in a soft, medium, or firm density
4. Spenco, a nylon-covered rubber that has an excellent ability to cushion the foot and to absorb compression by the foot against it
5. Poron, a form of polyurethane foam that also takes compression rather well

All of these materials can be used to make the orthotic devices inside the shoe, whether removable or adherent to the inner aspect.

PATHOLOGIC CONDITIONS
Pes planovalgus

Pes planovalgus, or flatfoot, is an extremely common condition that is sometimes asymptomatic throughout a person's lifetime. In other cases it causes considerable difficulty. The condition varies in degree from a minimal lowering to complete collapse of the longitudinal arch (Figure 52-9). The foot becomes flattened on the ground with pronation of the hindfoot and abduction of the foot, which splays out laterally. The condition can be classified as first-, second-, third-, or fourth-degree pes planovalgus, depending on severity. Anatomically the condition is characterized by a descent of the navicular and the cuneiform bones, as well as a rotation of the talus downward and medially in relationship to the calcaneus. In the more serious cases the forefoot may be relatively internally rotated and abducted in relation to the midfoot and hindfoot.

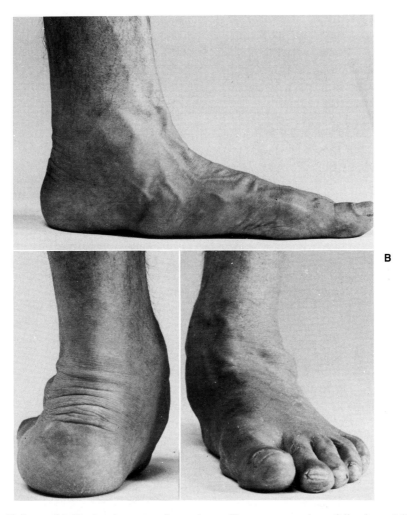

Figure 52-9, cont'd. B, Another type of pes planus. Foot appears to have fallen inward like a half-hemisphere. (From Mann, RA: Principles of examination of the foot and ankle. In Mann, RA, editor: Surgery of the foot, ed 5, St. Louis, 1986, The CV Mosby Co.)

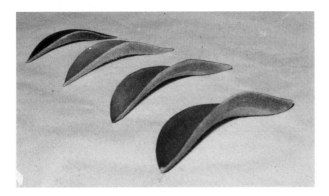

Figure 52-10. "Cookies" of various sizes.

Correction

The following are the objectives of corrections:
1. To elevate the medial aspect of the calcaneus in order to reverse the rotational component of the talus
2. To support and raise the longitudinal arch in order to relieve stress on the foot
3. In some cases, to derotate the forefoot into a degree of external rotation (pronation) relative to the hindfoot

A long medial counter is sometimes necessary to support the longitudinal arch. It should extend beyond the breast of the heel to the first cuneiform or, in extreme cases, even beyond, to provide greater support.

Scaphoid pads are placed under the medial longitudinal arch. They are usually made of a soft material such as rubber and covered with leather. Their height is determined by the severity of the planus deformity. A variation of the scaphoid pad is the "cookie," which is made of rigid leather for greater support (Figure 52-10). I recommend the use of the softer scaphoid pad, which causes less initial discomfort and has a similar function.

Wedges made of leather can be placed in the usual position as sandwiched material between the inner and outer sole (Figure 52-11), although in some types of shoes they can be glued as overlays under the sole. The wedges vary in thickness from 1/16 inch to approximately 1/4 inch, as required.

In children the correction is started with 1/16-inch thickness and built up as necessary, usually to no more than 1/8 inch. These wedges can also be placed under the base of the heel medially to bring the foot into greater supination at the heel in order to counter the pronation present. These "medial heel wedges" are sometimes described as medial "roof" wedges, meaning that they are above the heel rather than on the inferior surface. The heel of the shoe can also be extended medially to support the calcaneus, the scaphoid, and if necessary, the first cuneiform area. This is referred to as a Thomas heel (Figure 52-12). It ordinarily extends medially to the scaphoid bone only. Wedges can also be placed under the lateral sole of the shoe to combat the

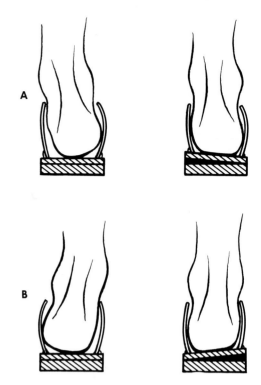

Figure 52-11. Heel lifts. **A,** Medial heel wedge for correction of valgus heel deformity. **B,** Lateral heel wedge for correction of varus heel deformity. (From Mann, RA: Conservative treatment and office procedures. In Mann, RA, editor: Surgery of the foot, ed 5, St. Louis, 1986, The CV Mosby Co.)

relative internal rotation of the forefoot (Figure 52-13). If this is done, the steel shank must be removed to permit torsion of the shoe. Steel wedges to supply a rigid shank are components of the manufacture of all orthopedic oxfords.

Orthopedic oxfords have a medial long counter, a straight inner shoe border, and a round toe box. This construction permits the first toe to remain in its normal position and prevents cramping of the toes. The wedge on a shoe usually extends to the midline of the sole, at which point it thins out to zero, a "feathering" of the wedge. This shoe suffices for the average patient. The prescription might read as follows: "Orthopedic oxford with long medial counter medial heel wedge of 1/16 or + thickness and Thomas heel with scaphoid pad" (Figure 52-14).

In more severe cases, such as those with painful metatarsals or plantar fasciitis, the entire anterior breast of the heel can be moved forward with expansion of the prescription to read, "Extended heel-breast anteriorly." This prescription improves the support to both the calcaneus and the longitudinal medial arch.

Another means of increasing the correction is to extend the medial path of the heel all the way forward to feather out in the region of the ball of the foot throughout the shank—a medial shank filler (Figure 52-15).

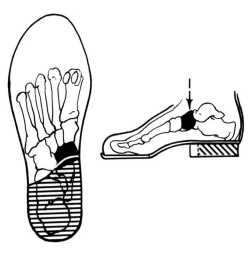

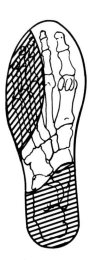

Figure 52-12. Thomas heel extends to midportion of navicular to provide support. (From Mann, RA: Conservative treatment and office procedures. In Mann, RA, editor: Surgery of the foot, ed 5, St. Louis, 1986, The CV Mosby Co.)

Figure 52-13. Combination of Thomas heel, which corrects heel valgus and supports navicular, and lateral sole lift, which corrects forefoot varus. This combination is used in treatment of flatfoot deformity. (From Mann, RA: Conservative treatment and office procedures. In Mann, RA, editor: Surgery of the foot, ed 5, St. Louis, 1986, The CV Mosby Co.)

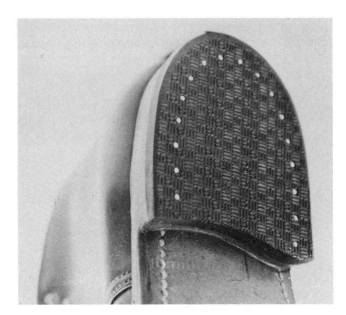

Figure 52-14. Thomas heel.

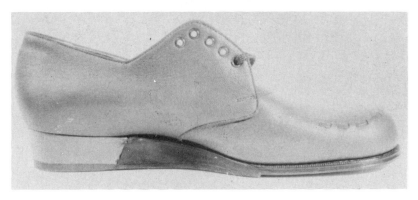

Figure 52-15. Medial shank filler.

Ordinarily, for pes planovalgus, the combination of Thomas heel, long medial counter, medial heel wedge, and scaphoid pad in an orthopedic oxford is sufficient. In some instances, when greater effect must be obtained, one can order a straight-last shoe in which an imaginary straight line drawn down the middle divides the shoe into two equal halves. A straight last removes the normal medial curve of the forefoot portion of the shoe. This allows for greater support of the forefoot in the shoe.

If the problem is even more severe and total support of the forefoot and the hindfoot is needed, a supinator "turned-in" last may be prescribed to produce a corrective shoe whose front aspect is deviated medially to varying degrees on the basis of the last used on the posterior aspect of the shoe. With a line drawn through the middle of the shoe, a greater part of the anterior aspect of the shoe would be located more medial to the line than ordinarily. This can also help to correct the abducted forefoot and to support the longitudinal arch. In a supinator-last shoe, one can still add corrections; in fact, the shoe ordinarily is constructed with a Thomas heel, a long medial counter, a medial heel wedge, as well as a scaphoid pad.

A child's foot must be evaluated on average every 3 months because of an interval of significant growth. Inserts such as arch supports are usually a poor idea in children, since even a small amount of growth places every point on the internal device in the wrong place in relation to the foot.

The corrections are better placed on the sole with the addition of a scaphoid pad, which can accommodate some degree of change in the size of the foot. In any case, especially in very active young children, the shoe will have worn out by the time it becomes too small.

Exercise for planus foot in the child

Exercise may be prescribed to strengthen the foot in young children. Some of these exercises are practicing walking forward and backward for several minutes every day on the lateral aspect of both feet with the feet turned in facing one another; stepping on a towel, grasping the cloth of the towel with the toes, and pushing it backward by flexing the toes toward the rear of the foot, which also helps to strengthen the arch; and using resistive exercises for the muscles of the sole of the foot, with special emphasis on the peroneus longus, which supports the arch, and the tibialis posterior.

The progressive resistive system is used starting with active exercises and building to maximum power for the muscle structures. However, with descent of the arch and malalignment of the bones, it is the ligamentous structures that normally keep the foot in proper alignment and these have been weakened and stretched. The ligaments cannot be tightened; however, strengthening the aforementioned two muscles in particular helps support the arch. Occasionally, an improvement of the arch by several degrees through the use of this exercise has been observed. However, the child must be old enough, usually 8 to 10 years of age,

before cooperation can be expected in performance of the exercises properly. Formal physical therapy control should be accompanied by a home exercise program.

Pes cavus

Pes cavus is as common a deformity as pes planovalgus. In pes cavus the medial longitudinal arch is curved higher than normal, forming a significantly high space between the walking surface or insole and the longitudinal arch. As a result, the plantar fascia eventually tightens in what is known as the windlass action. (A windlass is a handle that is turned to bring a pail of water to the surface of a well.) Because the fascia is inserted anteriorly over the superior surfaces of the proximal phalanges, the proximal phalanges are pulled downward, putting the MP joints into contact with the ground and destroying the transverse arch of the foot. As a result, the fat pads normally present under the MP joints thin out and become compressed against the bottom of the shoe, producing dropped metatarsals and, when pain occurs, metatarsalgia.

Because of the undue compression in the plantar area, the foot may develop an inflammatory process (plantar fasciitis) in the region of calcaneal plantar tissue and a calcaneal spur, which can be quite painful. The foot is in supination or turned so the sole tends to face inward to some degree. Simultaneously with dropped metatarsals there is a tendency for the ligaments to weaken in the foot and to cause spreading of the forefoot so the metatarsals are somewhat separated from one another more than is normal. This is referred to as a splayed foot.

As a result of the malalignment of the forefoot, calluses form underneath the sole in the region of the MP joints (Figure 52-16).

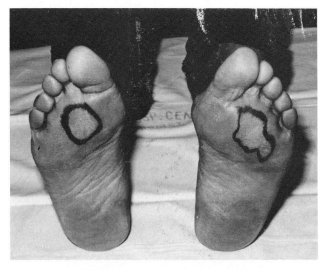

Figure 52-16. Callosities on sole of foot owing to malalignment of foot.

Corrections for pes cavus and its complications

There are several methods of treatment for pes cavus.

An orthopedic oxford with a long lateral counter rather than a medial counter supports the lateral aspect of the foot. This counteracts the development of undue pressure because of the high arch and supinated position.

The lateral aspect of the shoe can be flared by extending a wedged sole beyond the lateral borders. This may extend by ¼ to as much as ½ inch in severe cases. The wedge height is determined by the severity of the problem—from ⅛ to ¼ inch.

The arch can be filled in with a scaphoid pad of sufficient height to contact the medial sole in the region of the elevated longitudinal arch. It is sometimes beneficial to start with a lower support and over a period of time elevate the scaphoid pad to full correction as the patient can tolerate this change.

A reverse Thomas heel can be prescribed with the extension being on the lateral border of the shoe to the cuboid bone or beyond.

In less severe cases it may be sufficient to use an orthopedic oxford with a crepe sole, which softens the contact with the ground. The heel in this instance is replaced with a SACH insert to permit the foot to come into contact with the ground more easily. This is helpful because pes cavus tends to be a rigid deformity that is not aided by correction as much as by accommodation to the deformity.

A rocker bar from shank to toe tip with an apex posterior to the MP joints can be added. The insert of the shoe contains a scaphoid elevation to fill in the cavus deformity.

Splayed foot, dropped metatarsals, and claw or hammer toes may be present, as well as metatarsalgia, which can be determined by tenderness on palpation over the MP joints, particularly in the area of the second to fourth or fifth toes. This may be relieved by an inlay placed in the shoe with a scaphoid pad placed on top of this inlay. It will also be necessary to dig out the area of the inlay in the region of the MP joints so they are deeper than the rest of the support. If possible, the dugout area is filled with foam rubber covered with leather. This adjustment may be necessary under the toe tips, which may be pressing into the sole of the shoe.

When dropped metatarsals and claw and hammer toes are present, it is important to prescribe a high, wide, soft toe box with a straight inner border to permit the first toe to remain in normal position. A "deep shoe" is available that has extra room in the toe box and prevents development of corns and callosities over the upper surface of the toes, which in an ordinary shoe would be in contact with the toe box.

A quadrilateral pad (or dancer pad) is added to the shoe to take pressure off the metatarsal heads and elevate them. If the shoes are painful on manipulation, this correction may cause pain; therefore it should be omitted. A rocker bar on the sole of the deep shoe permits toe-off without pressure against the MP joints lying in a dugout repository. In most instances, however, it is possible to use metatarsal pads.

If there is undue pain at the calcaneal plantar surface, it is also possible to use a dugout heel as described earlier in the chapter. That, in combination with a SACH insert, is certain to relieve pain in the heel area. A rubber donut is sometimes used as a substitute for the dugout heel; however, in my experience it is totally inadequate.

When calcaneal fasciitis or a calcaneal spur is present, it is sometimes helpful to inject a combination of 3 to 4 ml of lidocaine 1% without epinephrine and 20 mg or 1 ml of dexamethasone into the midcalcaneal area or into the anterior border of the plantar surface of the calcaneus. This can significantly relieve the discomfort.

If the patient with claw toe or hammer toe deformity is not helped by the deep shoe or high, round, wide, soft toe box, the toe box of the shoe can be ballooned out by cutting out the leather on the upper surface and sewing a large elevated patch into the cutout area to eliminate any conceivable pressure against the toes. It is less cosmetic, and in my experience the deep shoe has been uniformly successful.

Pes equinus

Pes equinus can be an acquired or congenital deformity. It may occur as a result of weakness of the anterior tibial musculature in poliomyelitis or in multiple sclerosis from contracture of the forefoot and the inability to dorsiflex (Figure 52-17). The flexibility of the foot may remain complete, partial, or in a fixed deformity. This section addresses the more complicated rigid equinus deformity. The following are the correction objectives:

1. To compensate for the equinus position

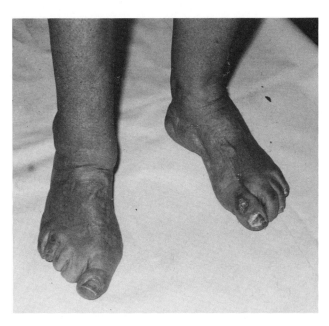

Figure 52-17. Pes equinus in polio.

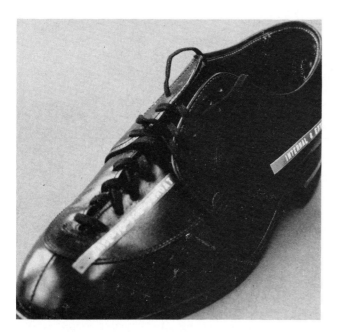

Figure 52-18. Shoe with lace stay extension to allow entry of foot into shoe.

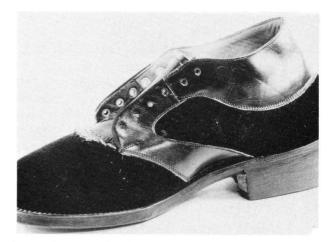

Figure 52-19. Addition of collar on shoe to help keep foot in shoe.

Table 52-1. Formula for placement of inlay in treating pes equinus

Heel height (inches)	Ball (inches)	Toe (inches)
½	½	¼
¾	½	¼
1	½	¼
1¼	¾	½
1½	¾	½
1¾	1	¾
2	1¼	¾
2¼	1½	1
2½	1¾	1
2¾	2	1
3	2¼	1¼
3¼	2½	1¼
3½	2¾	1¼
3¾	3	1½
4	3¼	1½
4¼	3½	1½
4½	3¾	1¾
4¾	4	1¾
5	4¼	1¾
5¼	4½	2
5½	4¾	2
5¾	5	2
6	5¼	2¼

2. To hold the foot in the shoe
3. To provide ease in putting the shoe on

The equinus position causes extensive pressure of the anterior aspect of the foot, which results in metatarsal compression on the plantar surface. If there is any flexibility in the position of the foot, this misfit should be corrected as much as possible.

Correction

In pes equinus of lesser severity a high-topped shoe is prescribed with a convalescent or surgical lacing to allow easy entry into the shoe (Figure 52-18). A regular shoe can sometimes be used with the addition of a "collar" that keeps the foot inside the shoe (Figure 52-19). Elevations on the inside of the shoe are prescribed to compensate for the necessity of increased heel height. The shoe may also be revised to permit an extension of the lace stay through the vamp and the addition of eyelets to lace the shoe to the toe box. This is sometimes referred to as a lace-to-toe throat.

Because the medial aspect of the foot is under stress and in the equinus position, another required modification is a medial longitudinal arch support.

There are several ways in which the heel can be elevated in the equinus foot. In the shoe with the collar, as much as ¾ inch can be added as part of a full-length inlay placed in the region of the heel and inclined toward the sole of the shoe using the formula shown in Table 52-1. In all instances the elevation must conform to the configuration of the equinus deformity.

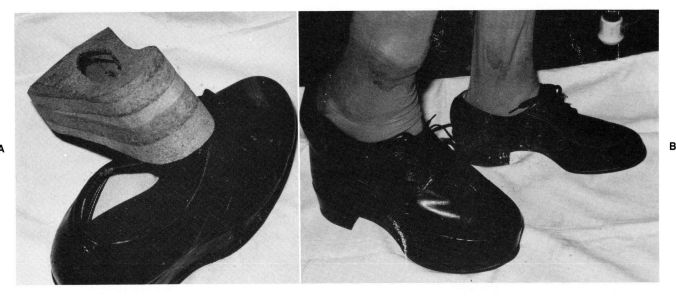

A

B

Figure 52-20. A, Hollowed-out cork used for elevation. **B,** Cork is sandwiched between inner and outer soles.

If the patient also has disability in the forefoot because of pressure against the metatarsals and metatarsalgia or dropped metatarsals, metatarsal pads or a rocker bar over the sole should be used.

When both lower extremities are of equal length, the heel and sole of the normal extremity must be raised to permit the patient to swing through freely. The adjustments of the shoe on the involved side cause it to be longer. The normal side must be made equal to permit proper gait.

Depending on the height of the required elevations, different substances may be used to make inlays and overlays. Cork or leather can be used, covered by an extra inlay of leather, if a full-length or three-fourths length arch support is used. Overlays on the sole up to approximately 1 inch can be made of leather; beyond this, cork is preferable because of its lighter weight. In cases where higher degrees of elevation are needed, hollowed-out cork is used for this specific reason. The cork is placed between the inner and outer soles; the latter is fabricated from leather of ¼ inch height (Figure 52-20).

Talipes equinovarus (equinovarus deformity)

In talipes equinovarus the same type of modifications are required as in equinus, with the addition of corrections for the varus position. Modifications can be added to bring the flexible foot into normal position, or accommodation can be made if the foot is in fixed position (Figure 52-21).

In talipes equinovarus it is also necessary to wedge the heel and sole on the medial aspect to position the foot flat on the floor. However, when the foot is flexible, the foot's position can be normalized by adding lateral heel and sole wedging and outflares (Figure 52-22). A lateral long counter must also be used to protect the outer aspect of the foot, which will be taking increased pressure as in pes cavus. Should there be excessive compression against the meta-

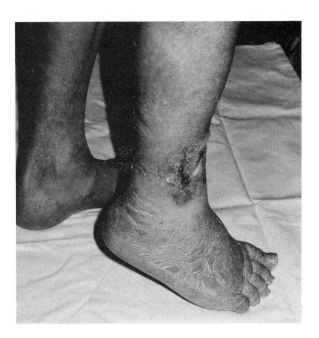

Figure 52-21. Equinovarus deformity.

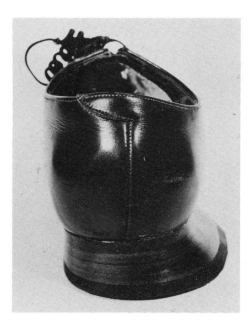

Figure 52-22. Shoe with outflare to help normalize position of foot with flexible varus deformity.

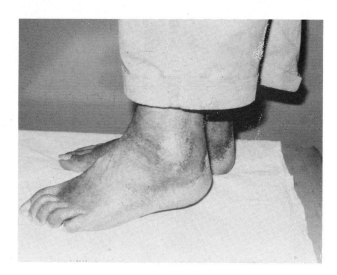

Figure 52-23. Feet of patient with chronic hemiplegia.

tarsals, especially on the lateral aspect of the foot, insoles with dugout areas filled with foam rubber in this area must be used.

The degree of flaring can vary up to more than ½ inch. If there is still undue pressure, especially with a high-topped shoe, the lateral counters can be made higher, up to and including the malleolus and sometimes almost to the top of the shoe. This gives added support to the lateral aspect of the ankle. If the high counter causes pressure, it can be ballooned out to some degree to prevent pressure at any particular point, much as one does with splinting or prosthetic devices.

Short leg

Short lower extremities caused by a genetic or growth-related defect, such as fracture in a growing site before full growth is achieved or early poliomyelitis, require elevations of the shoe. The same principles and numeric formulas for shoe elevations in pes equinus are applicable here as well (Table 52-1).

If the length disparity is less than ½ inch, elevation is not recommended except for certain instances involving the equinus position. I do not add the sole elevation for cosmetic reasons. For example, if a ¾-inch adjustment is required, ½ inch may be added to the heel in several ways, one of them being to place a heel cushion (hard rubber) as an inlay glued to the heel area. The other ¼ inch can be obtained by cutting the height of the opposite heel by that amount or elevating the heel on the involved side by a ¼-inch addition.

Hemiplegia

The foot problem in hemiplegia is usually a flexible or fixed equinus deformity, frequently with some degree of varus. The first toe usually becomes hyperextended and is clearly identified only if the patient is examined without shoes (Figure 52-23).

The varus deformity is easily perceived. The toe problem is treated by prescription of a high, deep, soft, wide toe box that prevents excessive pressure against the digit.

The patient may be given a short metal leg brace that must be attached to the shoe. An alternative is a polypropylene brace that may be inserted into the shoe.

The shoe must have the following characteristics:
1. It must be an orthopedic shoe and in some cases a "high" shoe to prevent pumping of the foot in the shoe.
2. It must have a rigid shank and a ¼-inch leather sole.
3. The lace stay must be of the Blucher type, preferably with some type of special closure such as Velcro, straps, or buckles, especially if the patient also has an upper extremity disability.

The steel shank should be reinforced with a tongue to permit connection to the stirrup, which is the attachment of the sole for the brace. Figure 52-23 shows a patient with hemiplegia with contracture of the ankle, fixed in plantar flexion. The treatment consists of elevating the heel, usually by adding a heel cushion glued as an inlay in the shoe, with or without the addition of a heel lift.

If the foot is in varus and flexible, slight lateral heel and sole wedges may be used to bring the foot into proper alignment during stance phase. If the position is fixed, me-

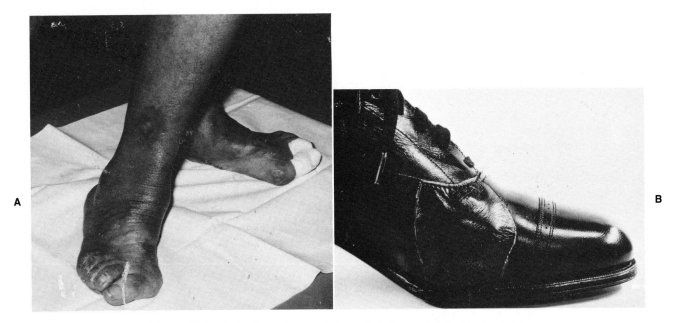

Figure 52-24. A, Hallux valgus. **B,** Shoe with balloon patch for hallux valgus.

dial heel and sole wedges are used to accommodate the contractures.

Gastrocnemius-soleus paralysis

Paralysis of the gastrocnemius-soleus muscles is commonly seen in poliomyelitis and peripheral neuropathy. As a result of the weakness of the gastrocnemius muscle, the calcaneus tends to be pulled forward and the plantar fascia tends to contract and become stressed by this position. The peroneal muscles, in attempting to plantar flex the foot, increase the cavus deformity, resulting in pes cavus. The patient ends up with toes in the claw and hammer position and metatarsalgia with dropped metatarsals.

Treatment for this condition, which is usually a fixed deformity, is to accommodate as with fixed pes cavus. The longitudinal arch area is filled with scaphoid elevations, with a dugout area under the MP joints and also under the toe tips to protect them. The preferable filler is foam rubber. The shoe should have a high, soft, wide, round toe box with a straight inner border. The shoe must also have a long lateral counter to protect the lateral aspect of the foot.

Conditions of the forefoot
Hallux valgus (bunion)

Hallux valgus is usually an acquired condition with varied etiologies. It is much more common in females than in males and in the shod population, especially these who wear pointed or tight shoes with high heels. However, it is also seen as a result of certain congenital defects such as metatarsus varus or adductus, a condition in which the first toe

is considerably separated from the second and consequently tends to be pushed toward the second toe, creating a valgus deformity. It can also be present with Morton's toe, a congenital short first metatarsal.

The degree of valgus tends to increase as the patient ages. Not uncommonly the first toe overlaps the second toe or forces the second toe to overlap the third toe. Consequently, an exostosis forms over the MP joint on the medial aspect of the first toe, and there is also an inflammatory and chronic thickening of the connective tissue in the area superficial to the exostosis. The MP joint is narrowed, with destruction of the joint region of the bunion. It can be treated by ballooning out a patch of similar leather to give adequate room for the bunion. Figure 52-24 shows a typical hallus valgus deformity, as well as a shoe with a ballooned-out patch.

Tailor's bunion can be caused by pressure on the lateral aspect of the fifth toes. It occurs in a pes cavus deformity where there is undue pressure along the lateral aspect of the foot and in splayed feet with a spread forefoot, as in pes planovalgus, as well as pes cavus. It is also seen in those who wear ill-fitting shoes. The condition is an exostosis of the lateral MP joint with an inflammatory process similar to that seen in hallux valgus.

The treatment is usually relatively simple. The shoe should have a wide, round, soft toe box with a lateral sole wedge of ⅛ inch thickness to move the center of gravity more toward the medial side of the foot. If other disabilities accompany the tailor's bunion, they must be corrected. The objective of treatment in this condition is usually to accommodate rather than to correct the position of the toes, but frequently it is possible to support the flattened transverse arch, which is commonly flexible and pain free. If there is marked tenderness of the MP joints on palpation, as well as significant pain in passive flexion and extension of these joints, accommodation rather than correction is made.

Claw toes

Claw and hammer toes are quite different. In the former the MP joint is quite extended and the proximal and distal interphalangeal joints are in flexion. In hammer toes the MP joint is extended, the proximal IP joint is flexed, and the distal IP joints are in extension with significant painful compression of these toes against the inner sole of the shoe.

Because of the position of the toes there is a tendency to develop corns, especially over the proximal IP joints, as well as callosities under the MP joints. This is most common in the area of the second to the fifth toes, particularly the second, third, and fourth toes.

Correction, when feasible, involves the placement of a metatarsal pad, either triangular or quadrilateral, to elevate the transverse arch (Figure 52-25). Several types of correction may be added to the sole of the shoe, including a metatarsal bar. This is a bar with abrupt edges, both anteriorly and posteriorly, just posterior to the MP joints, used as an onlay on the sole of the shoe. I believe that it is much more helpful to use the Denver bar (Figure 52-26), which supports the entire metatarsal area, instead of supporting only the distal aspect of the metatarsal. The bar consists of a leather extension on the sole. This is narrowed in front of the posterior aspect of the MP joints and widened to accommodate to the foot's flat position, passing backward along the metatarsal length. The anterior aspect can be slightly abrupt or, as I prefer, feathered at its anterior end, that is, completely confluent with the sole.

In the presence of significant pain or rigid deformity, accommodation must be made. An orthopedic oxford with a high, soft side, deep toe box, straight inner border, and preferably with a ¼-inch-thick crepe sole of hard rubber can be used. Placement of a semiflexible steel shank from the calcaneus to the toe tip between the inner and outer soles is necessary to allow for rigidity of the shoe so it does not flex at toe-off during the late aspect of stance phase. A SACH insert and a rocker bar, placed from shank to toe tip, are used to allow the patient to pass through stance phase

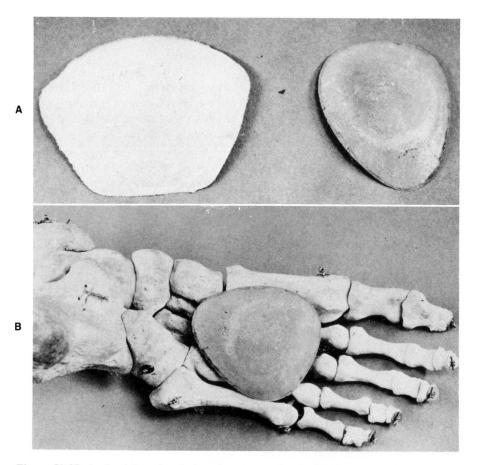

Figure 52-25. A, Quadrilateral and triangular metatarsal pads. **B,** Metatarsal balloon placement.

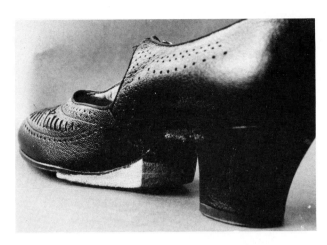

Figure 52-26. Denver bar.

easily with significant toe spring (Figure 52-27). It is usually necessary to employ an insert, either of leather with Neoprene material or Plastizote. This permits digging out of the insole under the metatarsophalangeal joints and the toe tips to allow for pain relief in these areas during gait. This type of shoe is extremely comfortable and eliminates discomfort and disability. Occasionally a patient requires a balloon patch to be placed over the toe box to make extra room for the toes; however, with the deep shoe, this is rarely necessary.

In addition to acquiring modified shoes, the patient is advised to bathe the feet in warm water for about 20 minutes in the bathtub, sitting on a stool outside of the tub. The bath is followed by use of a No. 1 fine emery cloth, obtained in a hardware store, to gently brush away only the easily removable parts of the callus. This regimen, twice a week over a period of a few months along with the shoe corrections, should cause the callus to disappear. Corn pads can be stuck to the corn areas to prevent contact with the top of the shoe and to allow healing.

Hallux rigidus

Hallux rigidus, caused by osteoarthritis or rheumatoid arthritis of the first MP joint, involves painful, marked re-

striction without the valgus deformity. It is treated by completely eliminating all motion at the MP level.

The shoe must have a straight inner border and a wide, round, soft toe box. The shoe is made rigid by placing a semiflexible steel shank straight through from the calcaneus to the toe, beyond the MP joint, and using a SACH and a rocker bar from shank to toe tip, skived, because a large toe spring is usually not necessary. There should also be a long medial counter and a scaphoid pad to prevent undue pressure on the first toe.

Another recommended treatment uses a three-quarter-length arch support with a Morton's toe extension. This is a soft leather extension under the first MP joint that provides a degree of immobility to the toe (Figure 52-28). It is helpful in milder cases but is ineffective in more severe ones.

Morton's toe

The first metatarsal is congenitally short, resulting in inappropriate toe-off and eventual disability in the area of the first and second toes. Because the first toe is inadequate for toe-off, the second toe, which is longer, is forced to take a greater amount of weight. This results frequently in a thickening of the second metatarsal shaft.

The treatment for this condition is the same as for hallux rigidus. One may use a semiflexible steel insert placed through the sole, the rocker bar, and SACH or an arch support with Morton's toe extension, depending on the severity of the disability.

Morton's neuroma

Morton's neuroma is a common condition in which undue compression between the third and the fourth toes causes formation of a neuroma on the digital nerves passing through the toe web, between the third and fourth anterior aspects of the metatarsal shafts. On palpation the area is very tender. The patient complains of burning and tenderness in this region while walking.

The mild neuroma usually responds to injections of lidocaine and dexamethasone, plus a long-acting steroid of the triamcinolone type. I use 2 ml of lidocaine 1% without epinephrine and 0.5 ml each of dexamethasone solution and

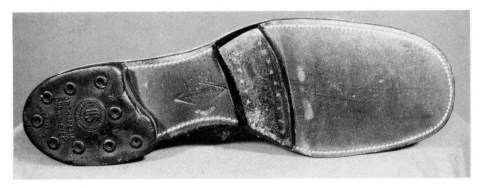

Figure 52-27. Rocker bar.

triamcinolone suspension. This is injected into the toe web area of greatest tenderness between the third and the fourth toes. One may also use anti-inflammatory agents such as indomethacin or ibuprofen for a short period of time. Physical therapy is often helpful; the prescribed sequence is a whirlpool for 20 minutes, dipping of the foot in paraffin for 15 minutes, followed by lidocaine 1% without epinephrine, combined with hydrocortisone and iontophoresis, 5 to 15 mA, for a period of 10 to 15 minutes.

The shoe corrections consist simply of a lowered heel,

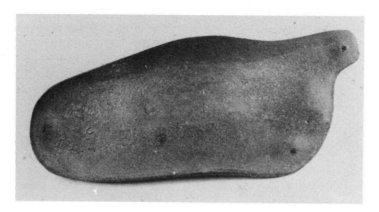

Figure 52-28. Morton's toe extension.

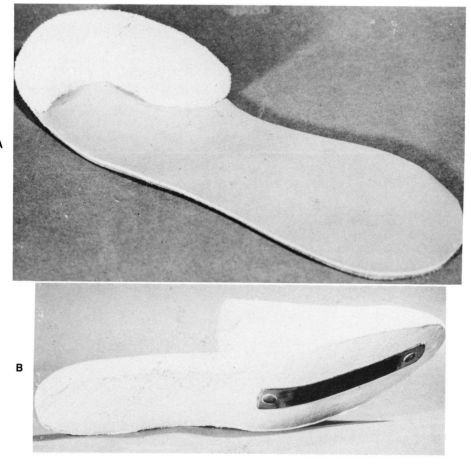

Figure 52-29. A, Foam rubber forefoot filler. **B,** Forefoot filler with steel bar.

usually of the SACH type, and a rocker bar from shank to toe tip plus a scaphoid pad to distribute the pressure along the sole and make toe-off easy without much pressure over the neuroma. A quadrilateral metatarsal pad is placed as an inlay. Further, a lateral ⅛-inch sole wedge to move gravity toward the medial foot may help. If these measures do not bring relief within a reasonable amount of time, I recommend surgical excision.

Amputation of the forefoot

In cases of amputation of the toes, an ordinary shoe, possibly with a rigid steel shank and a rocker bar, allows for easy toe-off. Some patients can walk in an ordinary oxford with little problem; however, in amputations farther posterior on the foot, such as through the midtarsal area, an appropriate filler is necessary. Shoes for patients with amputations at this level should include a semiflexible steel shank through the sole, as well as a rocker bar and, preferably, a SACH. The forefoot filler, made of foam rubber on an inlay inserted into the shoe, may also have a semiflexible steel bar inserted onto the inlay itself (Figure 52-29). If the steel addition is added to the inlay, the long steel shank is unnecessary. The foam rubber filler must have a perfectly smooth posterior edge to prevent pressure against the stump. A leather liner on the stump end of the filler is helpful. It too should be absolutely smooth and wrinkle free.

Fractures of the phalanges or the metatarsals

Simple fractures of the phalanges require little support except during the first 1 or 2 weeks, when they may be quite painful. I have found it helpful to use a rigid shoe when the patient can afford to purchase it. The shoe, containing a semiflexible insert to the sole and a rocker bar from shank to toe tip, eliminates all motion. In my opinion the technique of binding the fractured phalanx to the contiguous phalanx increases the pain by permitting the normal toe to tug on the fractured toe, causing a greater problem than originally existed.

Greater immobilization is indicated for a metatarsal fracture. A full-length arch support, incorporating a semiflexible steel bar and a rocker bar on the sole of the shoe, full length from shank to toe tip, helps considerably in diminishing the discomfort and allowing for healing.

CONCLUSION

Some cases are so complicated because of massive disability that only custom shoes or loose-fitting, simple coverings may be used. Generally, with problems of lesser magnitude, the goals of relieving pain and making the patient more comfortable can be accomplished in a number of ways. More complicated cases such as old severe poliomyelitis with distortion of the foot, peripheral vascular disease with partial amputations, and complete distortion, swelling, and malalignment of the foot from various severe ailments require custom shoes or loose-fitting foot coverings. It is necessary for the prescriber to be familiar with the underlying disability and the available methods of treatment for correction or accommodation to obtain proper results.

REFERENCE

1. MacLennan, R: Prevalance of hallux valgus in a neolithic New Guinea population, Lancet 1:1398, 1966.

ADDITIONAL READINGS

American Academy of Orthopaedic Surgeons: Orthopedic appliance atlas, vol I, Ann Arbor, Mich, 1952, JW Edwards.

Ball, Richard D: Current concepts in shoes and foot orthosis, Boston, 1984.

Bull Prosthet Res Dept. of Medicine and Surgery, Veterans Administration, 10-2, Fall 1964.

Dickson and Diveley, RL: Functional disorders of the foot, Philadelphia, 1953, JB Lippincott Co.

Gamble, FO, and Yale, I: Clinical foot roentgenology, Baltimore, 1966, Williams & Wilkins Co.

Hauser, ED: Diseases of the foot, Philadelphia, 1950, WB Saunders Co.

Hauser, ED: Congenital clubfoot, Philadelphia, 1966, WB Saunders Co.

Human locomotion and body form, Morton, 1952.

Kaplan, L: Shoes and the foot. In Ruskin, A: Current therapy in physiatry, Philadelphia, 1984, WB Saunders Co.

Kelikian, H: Hallux valgus: allied deformities of the forefoot and metatarsalgia, Philadelphia, 1967, WB Saunders Co.

Licht, S: Orthotics, Physical Medicine Library, vol. 9, 1966.

Shoes for all people by prescription, Med Times, June 1914.

CHAPTER 53 ‖ Wheelchairs

COLIN A. McLAURIN

To most people the word "wheelchair" conjures an image of an invalid who has been cast aside from life's mainstream and just sits and waits for an attendant to wheel him for a short walk. Fortunately, thanks largely to the exceptional athletes who have refused to be bound by a wheelchair, this attitude is changing. Also changing is the design of the wheelchair itself, to reflect an image of mobility, comfort, and style. Like automobiles, wheelchairs are not only essential items of modern living for over 1 million people, but also an expression of one's self-image. Most recent changes have been toward the sporty style brought on by the athletes and favored by young wheelchair users. Whatever the style of wheelchair, some basic principles can enhance mobility, comfort, and general utility. An understanding of these principles can aid in the selection of a wheelchair for an individual patient.

HUMAN FACTORS AND PROPULSION

If mobility is considered as ease of propulsion, the principles can be examined in two categories—those attributed to the user and those attributed to the wheelchair. A good prescription includes correct matching of these attributes.

Human factors

Several studies have been undertaken to determine the metabolic cost and efficiency of wheelchairs using hand rims, cranks, and levers. Engel[5] and Brattgard[2] are among the pioneers in this work. They have shown that levers and cranks provide nearly double the efficiency of hand rims. Hildebrandt and Seeliger (Figure 53-4, *B*) have developed a sophisticated lever drive system that is being readied for the market. In the United States most of the work has been done by two investigators, Glaser,[7] who has studied extensively the physiologic effects of wheelchair propulsion, and

Brubaker,[3] whose work is of particular importance because it included factors that affect the design of the wheelchair.

According to Brubaker, three major factors contribute to efficient use of the muscles: seat position, type of propulsion (lever or hand rims), and mechanical advantage. These have been studied on a specially built dynamometer, shown in Figure 53-1. This piece of equipment allows seat adjustment in the vertical, fore, and aft directions, as well as load and speed adjustment, independent for the left and right sides. In addition, instantaneous torque, arm motion, metabolic cost, and heart rate can be monitored, with information recorded by computer with available printout. Figure 53-2 illustrates the effect of seat position using hand rims and single-acting levers. From this illustration it is apparent that the levers are approximately 50% more efficient, and seat position has a significant effect on rim propulsion but minimal effect on levers within the range tested.

The effect of mechanical advantage for hand rims is shown in Figure 53-3. An increase of about 50% in efficiency is realized by using a 2:1 ratio at a typical level terrain workload. As the workload increases, this advantage is lost, and for ascending hills a gearing-down rather than gearing-up could be preferable. Two-speed gearing with hand rims has been demonstrated in prototypes, but it does add cost, weight, and complexity because some switching lever is required. With levers the selection of one suitable ratio is easier to obtain if the levers are connected to the drivewheels with a chain or belt. With several obvious advantages to lever drive, it is surprising that it is not more popular. The most common form has been in use in Europe for many years for outside use. It uses a connecting rod from the lever to the drivewheel (Figure 53-4, *A*). Steering is accomplished by twisting a handle on top of a lever connected to the casters. In spite of excellent performance

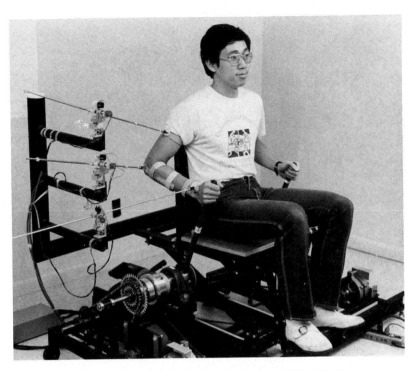

Figure 53-1. Wheelchair dynamometer developed at University of Virginia. Dynamometer records speed, work, instantaneous torque, and arm position. When it is used with breath analyzer, efficiency is easily computed.

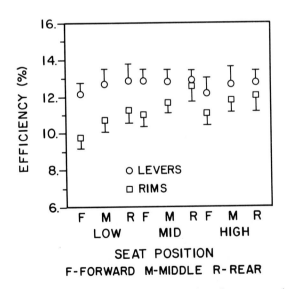

Figure 53-2. Propulsion efficiency plotted against seat position for hand rims and single-acting levers. (From Brubaker, CE, McClay, IS, and McLaurin, CA: Effect of seat position on wheelchair propulsion efficiency. In Proceedings of the Second International Conference on Rehabilitation Engineering, Washington, DC, 1984, Rehabilitation Engineering Society of North America.)

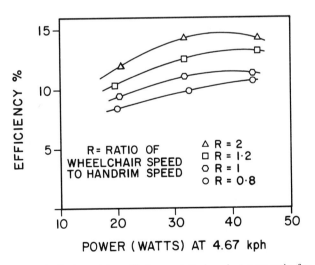

Figure 53-3. Propulsion efficiency plotted against gear ratio for hand rims at various workloads. (From Brubaker, CE, McClay, IS, and McLaurin, CA: Effect of seat position on wheelchair propulsion efficiency. In Proceedings of the Second International Conference on Rehabilitation Engineering, Washington, DC, 1984, Rehabilitation Engineering Society of North America.)

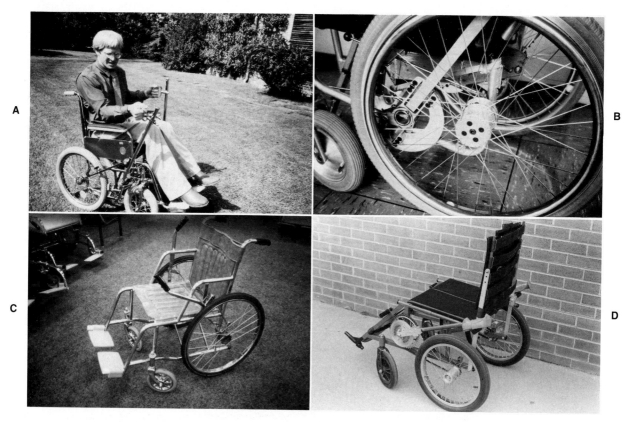

Figure 53-4. Examples of lever-drive wheelchairs. **A,** Ortopedia (commercially available). **B,** Seeliger (prototype). **C,** Matsunaga (commercially available). **D,** University of Virginia (prototype).

for street use, two difficulties are presented—loss of maneuverability in close quarters and inability to relax the arms and coast between strokes. Subsequent systems have overcome this latter disadvantage. The Poirier has a silent ratchet in the drive linkage but requires an extra control to reverse. The Matsunaga (Figure 53-4, *C*) also uses silent ratchets, and reverse is obtained by stroking backward from a neutral position. This limits the effective stroke length. Performance is further reduced because the pivot position is located near the elbow, thus using elbow extension rather than shoulder and elbow motion, with subsequent early fatigue. Herron[8] has developed a ratcheting lever drive that can be fitted to a conventional wheelchair. Bicycle-type brakes with the controls on the levers allow steering in the conventional manner, but the drive must be disconnected for reverse, using hand rims. Seeliger has developed an elegant double-acting lever system that provides a neutral gear, reverse, hill gear, hill holder, drum brake, and steering. Hand rims are still used indoors.

Brubaker, McClay, and McLaurin have attempted to provide the advantages of levers with the versatility and use of hand rims. In their model (Figure 53-4, *D*) the lever is connected to the drive chain through a clutch that is engaged by moving the levers inward; thus forward, reverse, or braking is instantly available. Propulsion is similar to the motion of rowing, with the clutch engaged and disengaged at the beginning and end of each stroke. "Wheelies" and all other functions have been well demonstrated by new users after a brief learning period in this wheelchair. In spite of these many advances, the simple hand rim will probably remain as the drive system of choice for many years.

Farey[6] introduced a hand rim with a cross section considerably larger and somewhat egg shaped. This has an instant appeal and should be more popular in the future. Vinyl and other coatings improve the force that can be applied with a weak grip but introduce problems of skin trauma in braking. A recent survey of Paralyzed Veterans of America members[14] indicated that 85% would welcome some type of dynamic braking, which has been available in Europe for some time. Brakes operating on the tire are simple but lose effectiveness if the tire is underinflated or wet. Drum brakes as used on bicycles are effective but add to the weight and cost. However, it seems likely that some type of dynamic brake will be in common use in the near future.

DESIGN CONSIDERATIONS

Several factors in wheelchair design affect ease of propulsion and mobility. On a hard, level surface, tires have a prominent role. Tests at the University of Virginia Rehabilitation Engineering Center on a specially built treadmill have shown that high-pressure pneumatic tires have only one fourth of the rolling resistance of conventional hard gray rubber. Lower pressures and some of the newer synthetic airless tires fall somewhere between these two values. The pneumatic tires have a further advantage in that they provide a comfortable ride and lessen the stresses on the wheelchair frame. Properly designed synthetic tires approach the pneumatics in efficiency, and the advantages of long wear and flat-free performance combined with some type of springs may result in the ideal tire for the future. Carpet can increase the rolling resistance by a factor of 4 or more. For off-pavement use, larger pneumatic tires offer advantages, although no data are available for the rolling resistance on grass, gravel, or sand. The rolling resistance is also a factor of wheel diameter. The small caster wheels have much greater drag for a given load; therefore it is advantageous to keep most of the weight on the main wheels. It is interesting to note that the force necessary to overcome the rolling resistance is directly proportional to weight but largely independent of speed.

Casters

Casters can affect performance in other ways. Wheelchairs with front casters tend to turn downhill on a side slope; with rear casters the tendency is to turn uphill. The mechanical effort required to overcome this turn is a function of the angle of the slope and the distance of the center of gravity from the main axles. In a typical situation, a 2-degree slope requires double the mechanical effort. However, the metabolic cost may not be as great because only one arm may be in motion, with the other used only for braking. The rear-castered wheelchair, because the center of gravity is behind the main axles, is directionally unstable. Any disturbance that initiates a change in direction results in the mass of the wheelchair and rider forcing the main wheels further into the turn. The rider is constantly correcting for this factor at all but the lowest speeds.

Whether front or rear, caster shimmy is a common and dangerous phenomenon. This rapid oscillation of the caster increases the rolling resistance by a factor of 6 or more, which is similar to applying a brake, and this can and does cause the rider to be thrown out of the wheelchair. Road irregularities such as gravel can initiate flutter, but for any caster assembly there is a critical speed at which flutter will continue once it has started. Formulas have been developed to predict this critical speed, which can be increased by increasing the trail, decreasing the weight or flywheel effect, using a dual-tread caster tire, or introducing friction to the caster stem. A simple friction damper has recently been developed, consisting of a set of conical wedges and a spring mounted inside the caster stem tube. The spring forces the wedges to grip the stem and automatically adjusts for any wear. Depending on the strength of the spring, the friction

force can be preset to prevent flutter for speeds of 6 mph or more without increasing turning resistance significantly.

Weight

Weight is perhaps the most common consideration in today's wheelchair. The typical wheelchair of a few years ago weighed about 50 pounds. Sports wheelchairs weigh about half that much, but the recent trend to the use of swing-away footrests, removable armrests, and full-height back supports has brought a modern lightweight wheelchair into the 30- to 35-pound range. This weight reduction is quite significant when loading the wheelchair into an automobile but has little effect on rolling resistance on level terrain. When a rider is propelling the wheelchair up a hill, every pound counts. Pushing a wheelchair up a 1 in 12 ramp (approximately 5-degree incline) at 1 mph with a total weight of 200 pounds requires about 33 watts. The highest work output using hand rims recorded at the University of Virginia was 125 watts—by a world-class athlete.

There are several ways to reduce weight in a wheelchair. The most common is use of high-strength, lightweight materials. Conventional frames have been made from mild steel tubing or stainless steel. More recently, chromium molybdenum steel, aluminum alloy, graphite, and titanium have been used. All these materials exhibit a much greater ratio of strength to weight, but all have some drawbacks that could lead to early failure. Mild steel is very forgiving and yields on impact to absorb the energy without fracturing. The high-strength steels must be thinner to save weight, which increases problems with welding. Also, internal stresses must be relieved through heat treatment to obtain maximum frame strength. Aluminum alloys are more difficult to weld and are more subject to fatigue failure caused by repeated high stresses. Titanium is light, strong, and corrosion resistant but is also very expensive and difficult to work and weld. Graphite epoxy tubing offers the best

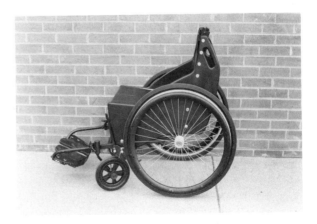

Figure 53-5. Composite wheelchair prototype designed and fabricated by NASA at Langley Air Force Base and University of Virginia. Panels have foam core with skins of Kevlar and graphite.

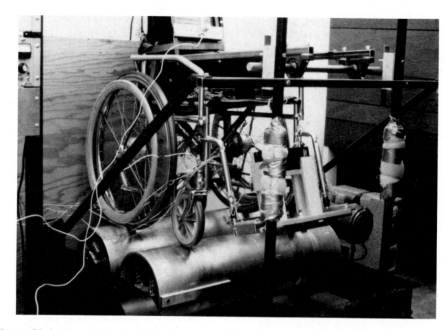

Figure 53-6. Wheelchair on double-drum tester. Tester simulates driving over slats and uneven terrain, and strain gauges monitor effects on frame. (Courtesy University of Virginia.)

strength-to-weight ratio; it is used extensively in modern aircraft. However, fittings for the joints pose a problem, and when graphite fractures it shatters somewhat like glass, resulting in a catastrophic failure. Attempts have been made to use composite plastics, particularly for seats, side panels, and wheels (Figure 53-5). These panels may be made with a foam core and skins of graphite and Kevlar that provide toughness and strength. Injection-molded plastics have been standard for caster wheels for some time and are used for main wheels. The material may find its way into other components such as footplates, but the high cost of molds and the relatively low strength-to-weight ratio have restricted its use to date.

Another method for reducing weight is by more efficient design. Strain gauges located at various points on the wheelchair frame indicate that some members are very highly stressed, while others are only lightly stressed. Before the use of computer analysis there was no way of correctly estimating the stresses in a closed loop structure such as a side frame of a wheelchair. In recent years software has become available for such an analysis using a personal computer. Kauzlarich and co-workers[9] have refined a program specifically for wheelchair side frames, and this allows an engineer to readily determine the frame stresses at any point in response to a given load condition. Thacker, Kauzlarich, and Todd[16] have used more complex software and larger computers to analyze more complex wheelchair structures, including composite panel assemblies. Thacker and Kauzlarich have further studied the forces on a wheelchair caused by various static and dynamic loading conditions (Figure 53-6). The load conditions include dropping off a curb and rolling over a standard ½-inch by 1½-inch slat at different speeds. The frame stresses can be affected by tires and springs, which are included in the investigation.

Sitting comfort

Tires and springs can also affect sitting comfort, which is perhaps the area in which the most improvement can be expected in the future. Choices in wheelchair seating have traditionally been limited to seat width. More recently a choice of back heights has become available, with some models featuring adjustable heights (Figure 53-7). The use of quick-disconnect main wheels with a choice of axle positions allows some adjustment in seat angle. Reclining backs have been available for many years, but any variation from these few choices would necessitate custom design or the use of seat inserts, which could be either off-the-shelf items or custom fitted for the individual. Most people readily agree that standard wheelchair seating leaves a great deal to be desired, but information regarding correct seating is difficult to obtain. Nwaobi, Hobson, and Trefler[13] have been investigating the effect of posture on spasticity and arm function for patients with cerebral palsy. Preliminary analysis indicates that 90% hip flexion and a near-vertical back support may be optimal. Hobson and Reger[9] have been gathering anthropometric information for several disability groups among wheelchair users. A report of this information is available from the University of Virginia or Memphis Rehabilitation Engineering Center.[1a] Chung[4] has been recording contour shapes and seat pressure patterns for a number of spinal cord–injured subjects at different seat and back angles (Figure 53-8). A 10-degree change in angle can make

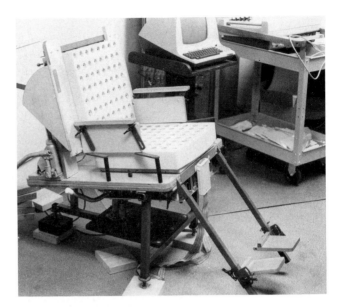

Figure 53-8. Fitting seat with adjustable back and seat angles. Cushions are instrumented to record seat and back contours. (Courtesy University of Virginia.)

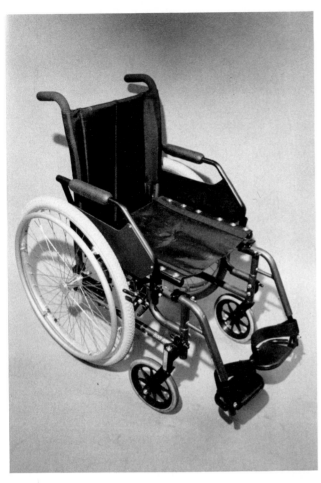

Figure 53-7. Typical modern wheelchair with adjustable back height, wheel position, and footrests (Invacare Rolls 500 ATS).

a significant difference in the pressure patterns on the four different cushion types investigated. It is too early to predict the best postural and shape configurations for individual prescriptions, but it is becoming apparent that a thorough assessment using an adjustable seat may soon become a routine prerequisite to prescription.

SPECIAL WHEELCHAIR DESIGNS

The typical modern wheelchair is a useful mobility aid but has many limitations. To overcome these shortcomings, special-purpose wheelchairs have been and will continue to be developed. However, there appears to be a limited market for these designs (Figure 53-9). The array of special designs includes sports models for road racing and basketball, all-terrain models for trail and beach, indoor models for the office or home, models that allow standing or seat elevation, stairclimbers, and wheelchairs for traveling in aircraft, public transport, or automobiles. Sports wheelchairs are typically lightweight and nonfolding, and they are often custom built. Road racers have large steerable caster wheels for

easy rolling, and basketball wheelchairs have small casters for flutter-free maneuverability. All-terrain wheelchairs typically have large pneumatic tires and possibly four-wheel drive. The Staircat, a prototype manual stairclimber, actually worked quite well, but it was heavy and expensive and presented a liability problem for the manufacturer. A powered model such as the Access (Figure 53-12, *E*) has a better chance of survival because it weighs less and the mechanism is simpler. Stand-up wheelchairs are available with battery-powered lifting or spring assist. Seat and knee restraints are needed for most users to maintain the standing position. Travel wheelchairs include those stowed on board airliners for access to the lavatory while in flight, narrow models for access to hotel bathrooms, and wheelchairs designed or modified for use in private autos. The use of wheelchairs in autos presents problems for storage or securement if they will be occupied in transit. The stowage problem has been addressed by a committee of the Society of Automotive Engineers,[15] which has a computer register of some 150 automobiles describing the space behind the seat and in the trunk. The proposed ANSI/RESNA Wheelchair Standards include the corresponding dimensions of the folded wheelchair so stowage can be assessed. The securement of a wheelchair with user in a van or bus is a serious problem that has been inadequately addressed. Crash studies at the University of Michigan have shown that riding sideways is a very dangerous practice. Perhaps the simplest and most adaptable method of securement is the use of four cargo straps, one from each corner of the wheelchair to a ring attached to the frame or reinforced floor of the vehicle. The Q-Straint (Figure 53-10) is an example. Most wheelchairs are not strong enough to withstand the stresses of a collision and may need to be reinforced.

POWERED WHEELCHAIRS

Powered wheelchairs had their start by the addition of batteries, motors, and controllers to standard wheelchairs. The first practical design was developed in the early 1950s by Klein[12] at the National Research Council in Ottawa, Canada, based on a homemade conversion in Pennsylvania by an unknown inventor. The Klein design (Figure 53-11) would not look out of place today, and for many years it was the basis for commercial models. The first significant change was from friction drive to belt drive, and the second from on-off switches to variable speed control. Heavier extended frames and 20-inch wheels were also introduced, but it was not until a few years ago that they came into common use. Perhaps the first commercial model that was built from scratch, rather than using conventional wheelchair design, was the Swedish Permobile.

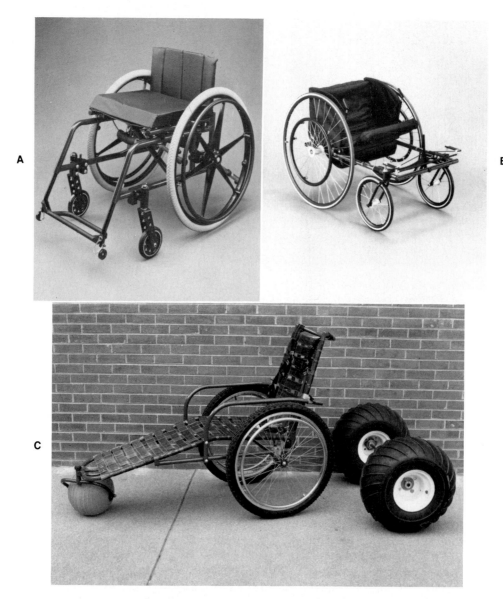

Figure 53-9. Some special-purpose wheelchairs. **A,** Basketball and court sports. **B,** Road racer. **C,** All-terrain wheelchair. Large wheels can be replaced with low-pressure all-terrain tires for use on beach. **D,** Stand-up wheelchair. **E,** Staircat—manual stairclimbing wheelchair. **F,** Stowaway— designed for use on airliners. (**A** and **B** courtesy Invacare Corp.; **C** and **F** courtesy University of Virginia; **D** courtesy Imex Medical, Inc.)

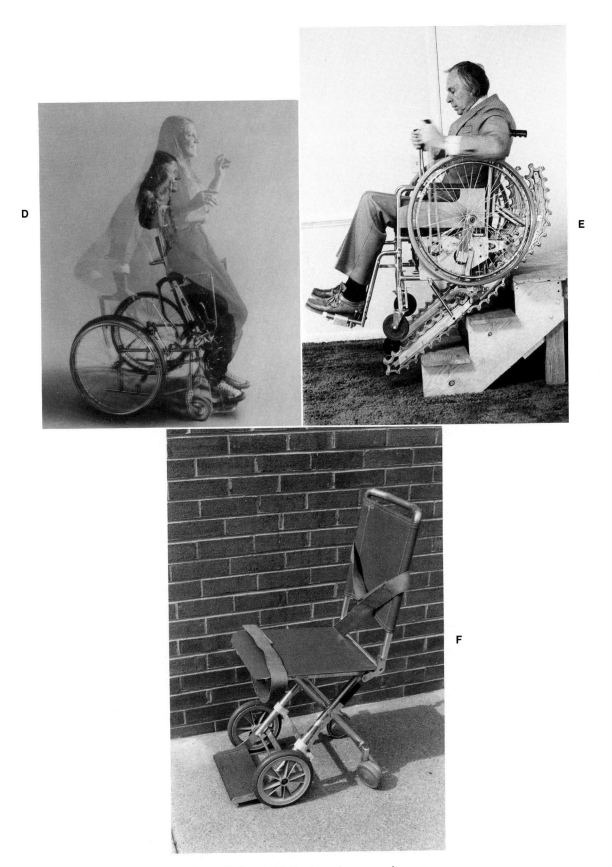

Figure 53-9, cont'd. For legend see opposite page.

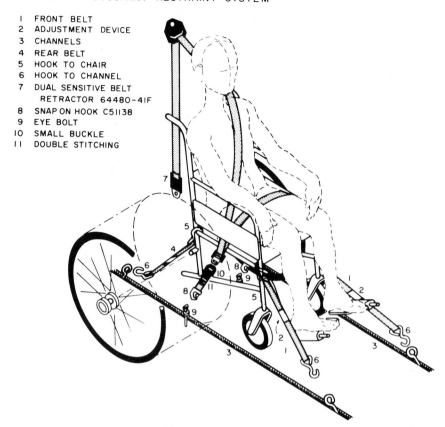

WHEELCHAIR OCCUPANT RESTRAINT SYSTEM

1 FRONT BELT
2 ADJUSTMENT DEVICE
3 CHANNELS
4 REAR BELT
5 HOOK TO CHAIR
6 HOOK TO CHANNEL
7 DUAL SENSITIVE BELT
   RETRACTOR 64480-41F
8 SNAP ON HOOK C51138
9 EYE BOLT
10 SMALL BUCKLE
11 DOUBLE STITCHING

Figure 53-10. Q-Straint. Method for restraining wheelchair occupant developed at Queens University at Kingston, Ontario, Canada. (Courtesy G.A.B. Saunders.)

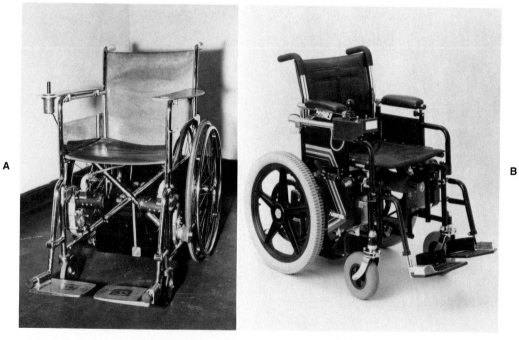

Figure 53-11. A, First practical electric wheelchair, designed by G.L. Klein in early 1950s. **B,** Modern equivalent. (Courtesy Invacare Corp.)

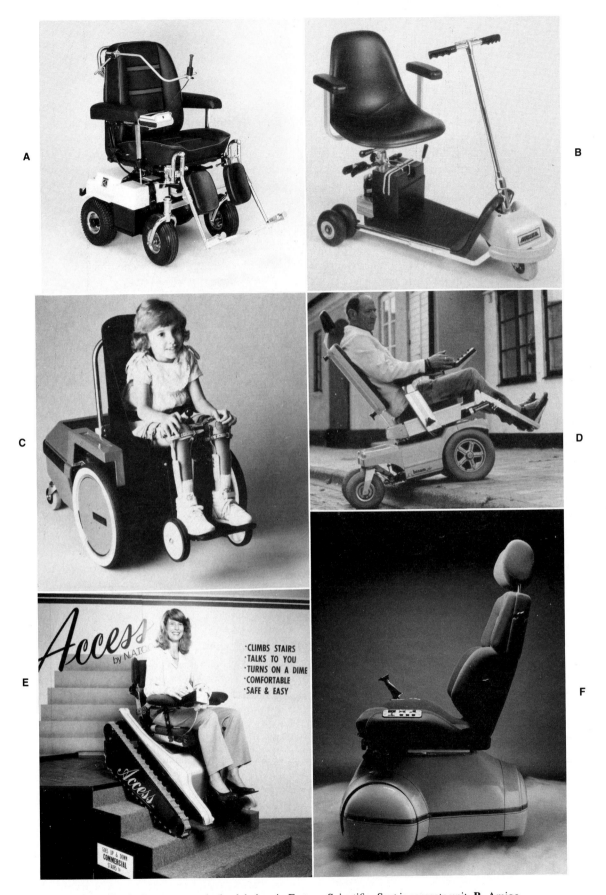

Figure 53-12. Some powered wheelchairs. **A,** Fortress Scientific. Seat is separate unit. **B,** Amigo—three wheelers. **C,** Turbo—features elevating seat for children. **D,** Besam. Swedish design with optional powered back rest and leg rests. **E,** Access. Stair-climbing model. **F,** Alexa—with sportscar seat and omnidirectional wheels. (**B** Courtesy Amigo Sales, Inc.; **C** courtesy Invacare Corporation; **D** courtesy Besam, Landskrona; **F** courtesy Rehabilitative Engineering Research and Developmental Center, Stanford University.)

A conference titled "Wheelchair III,"[18] held in San Diego in 1982, marked a turning point. At this conference it was stated that the ideal powered wheelchair should have a powered base or chassis on which a standard or special seat can be fastened. An example of this concept is the Fortress Scientific (Figure 53-12, *A*). The typical design has evolved into a low-profile power unit with smaller-diameter drive wheels and larger, more rugged casters, both with wide-tread pneumatic tires. One of the main advantages of this design is that custom seating can become a practical reality. Many standard support sections are now available for fabricating a seat for an individual. Multiadjusting car seats may be used if desired.

Performance testing of several powered wheelchairs at the University of Virginia[17] showed that at normal speeds on hard level surface, efficiency was on the order of 25%. The losses occur throughout the power train, motor, controller, transmission, and tires, with most attributed to the motor and controller. Much of the problem lies with the necessity for a motor with sufficient power to climb ramps with a heavy rider, which means that operation is not the most efficient when driving level. The problem could be solved in part with an automatic transmission but not without increasing cost and complexity.

The technical design of the power systems has undergone some changes, although lead acid batteries and permanent magnet motors are still universal. Geared drives have replaced belts in many instances, with greater reliability. Controllers nearly always use pulse width modulation (PWM), which chops the flow of electricity from the battery into short bursts of energy. The duration of each burst determines the power available to the motors. The controller is an expensive, heavy, power-consuming component that still presents some problems in reliability and requires further research. One feature found in some models is velocity control, which means that the speed remains constant despite changes in terrain. This ensures straight travel on sloping surfaces, limits speed on a downhill slope, and also prevents fishtailing if the wheelchair has casters in the rear. This wheel configuration is inherently unstable in a powered or manual wheelchair. The center of mass is behind the fixed wheels and, once disturbed from its neutral position by a change in direction of the main wheels, tends to drive them further into a turn.

Batteries are often considered to be the biggest problem for powered wheelchair users. The deep discharge lead acid battery is the standard, with a gel type used wherever air travel is a necessity. In both of these batteries charging is as important as discharging in prolonging the life of the battery. The chargers should be shut off when full capacity has been reached, and most new chargers do this automatically. The charging cycle for the liquid batteries is somewhat different from that for gel cells, and it is important to ensure that the charger has been designed for the battery in question.

Much research has been done in recent years to develop batteries with greater energy capacity for the same size and weight, but so far there is no practical alternative to lead acid batteries. However, there is a very significant difference between types of lead acid battery. Batteries with tubular positive plates have been shown to have a life span of three or four times the conventional flat-plate designs. If these can be made available in a size suitable for wheelchairs, the national savings could be several million dollars per year.

Powered wheelchairs have appeared in much greater variety than manual wheelchairs, no doubt because propulsion is not limited by arm motion. The first major change was embodied in the Amigo (Figure 53-12, *B*), a simple three-wheeler that has since spawned many competing alternatives. Typically these three-wheelers are used by persons who have some ability to stand and walk short distances. In general they exemplify a trend toward a personal mobility vehicle that will probably find an increasing market among elderly and moderately disabled individuals. Other wheelchairs of interest are the Turbo for children (Figure 53-12, *C*); the Besam, a Swedish design with powered seat and leg adjustments (Figure 53-12, *D*); the Access, which can climb steps up to 30 degrees (Figure 53-12, *E*); and the Alexa, which is omnidirectional (Figure 53-12, *F*).

WHEELCHAIR STANDARDS

With so much happening in wheelchair design and so many features and options becoming available, it is difficult for a purchaser or a user to decide on the most appropriate model. Although cost and esthetics are important factors, performance and fit should be foremost in the decision process. Both these factors are addressed in the new wheelchair standards published by the American National Standards Institute and the International Organization for Standardization[10] in 1987. Twelve standards will be published describing the dimensions and performance of the wheelchair, as will a further standard that explains the use of these standards in choosing a wheelchair.

The main value of the standards is to ensure safety and to inform the purchaser or user. Five of the standards apply to all types of wheelchairs and deal with strength, burning behavior, brakes, and dimensions. The strength tests include fatigue cycling as well as static and impact loads. Every wheelchair must pass these tests, which are graded according to the weight category of the user—25, 50, 75, or 100 kg. Each wheelchair must also pass the burning tests, which guard against inflammability from cigarettes. Dimensions, folded and unfolded, include mass and turning space. One standard addresses seating dimensions, recording 21 measurements that can be related to the corresponding measurements of the user. The standard specifies the method of measurement and does not restrict the actual dimensions. Similarly, the brake test records the angle of incline on which the parking brakes will hold and, in the case of a powered wheelchair, the stopping distance from full speed.

For manual wheelchairs one additional test provides information on the tipping angle in all directions. For powered wheelchairs, six additional tests are required to provide information on dynamic stability, energy consumption, speed, acceleration, and obstacle climbing. Powered wheelchairs must also pass tests of operation in conditions of heat, cold, and rain and safety aspects of the power and control system.

The best guarantee for excellence in any product is an informed consumer. The introduction of these standards should do much to achieve that purpose.

REFERENCES

1. American National Standards Institute, Committee Z360: Wheelchair Standards, Washington, DC, 1987, Rehabilitation Institute of North America.
1a. Anthropometry for the physically disabled, Vol 1. Cerebral palsy, 1987, University of Tennessee Rehabilitation Engineering Center.
2. Brattgard, SO, Grimby, G, and Hook, O: Energy expenditure and heart rate in driving a wheelchair ergometer, Scand J Rehabil Med 2:143, 1970.
3. Brubaker, CE, McClay, IS, and McLaurin, CA: Effect of seat position on wheelchair propulsion efficiency. In Proceedings of Second International Conference on Rehabilitation Engineering, Ottawa, Canada, June 17-22, 1984.
4. Chung, K-C: Tissue contour and interface pressure on wheelchair cushions, doctoral dissertation, Charlottesville, 1987, University of Virginia.
5. Engel, P, and Hildebrandt, G: Wheelchair design—technological and physiological aspects, Proc R Soc Med 67:409, 1974.
6. Farey, A: Personal communication, 1981.
7. Glaser, RM, et al: Metabolic and cardiopulmonary response to wheelchair and bicycle ergometry, Proc Am Physiolog Soc 1066, 1979.
8. Herran, M: Personal communication, 1985.
9. Hobson, D, and Reger, SI: Seat design factors for wheelchairs: Task 9, wheelchair mobility. In University of Virginia Annual report, Charlottesville, 1986.
10. International Organization for Standardization Technical Committee ISO/TC 173, ISCI.
11. Kauzlarich, JJ, et al: Computer aided design (CAD) of wheelchair sideframes, Tech Rep, Charlottesville, 1987, University of Virginia Rehabilitation Engineering Center.
12. Klein, GL: A wheelchair electric drive designed for the use of quadriplegics, Rep MM234, Dec 1953, National Research Council of Canada.
13. Nwaobi, O, Hobson, D, and Trefler, E: Hip angle and upper extremity movement time in children with cerebral palsy, Proceedings of the RESNA Conference, Memphis, June 24-28, 1985.
14. Paralyzed Veterans of America: Adult wheelchair users survey, Washington, DC, 1982.
15. Society of Automotive Engineers, Adaptive Devices Subcommittee of the SAE Human Factors Engineering Committee.
16. Thacker, JG, Kauzlarish, JJ, and Todd, BA: Frame design, Task 13, Charlottesville, 1986, University of Virginia Rehabilitation Engineering Center.
17. University of Virginia Charlottesville Rehabilitation Engineering Center: Wheelchair Mobility, 1976-1981. Charlottesville.
18. Wheelchair III—Report of a workshop on specially adapted wheelchairs and sports wheelchairs, San Diego, 1982, RESNA.

CHAPTER 54

Technology in rehabilitation

AN ORDERLY APPROACH TO ENGINEERING DESIGN

ARTHUR EBERSTEIN

The development of devices to aid the handicapped is not a new concept in rehabilitation but is as old as the cane or crutch. What is new is that the rehabilitation specialist has recognized the complexities of modern science and engineering and the need for specialized knowledge to effect solutions for the problems of handicapped persons. Dramatic and varied accomplishments in science and engineering during the 1980s have mandated the inclusion in the rehabilitation team of a technical specialist with particular knowledge and training. "If we can put a man on the moon, we should be able to build a better wheelchair or prosthesis" is an often repeated petition that the advanced level of technical progress used in space research be applied to rehabilitation needs.

Rehabilitation engineering is a relatively new specialty that is characterized more easily by what it involves in practice than by any formal engineering training. The engineer working in rehabilitation medicine uses engineering principles and procedures to ameliorate the handicaps of disabled people. Because of the varied nature of impairments, the applied principles may be derived from electrical, chemical, mechanical, or material engineering. The competent rehabilitation engineer not only has knowledge of all these specialties but is also well versed in the unique and multiple problems of the handicapped population.

PRINCIPLES OF DESIGN AND DEVELOPMENT

Solutions to rehabilitation engineering problems are not accomplished by trial and error but by a step-by-step approach that encompasses the entire design process, from identification of the problem to development and manufacture of the final product. The main phases involved in planning are described in this section and can be applied to any project, whether developing a new device or improving an old one.

Definition of the problem

The process of product design starts with identification and formulation of the problem. In most instances the problem is identified by the patient through requests for specific aids or for improvement of devices already in use. Problems may also be identified by a generalized review or assessment of patient needs performed by the rehabilitation team. For a clear understanding of the problem, good communication must exist among all members of the rehabilitation team and the patient. After the problem has been identified, one should be able to determine whether it is unique or widespread and to estimate the number of potential users of the solution.

Literature review

Once the problem has been formulated, the next step, which is very important but unfortunately overlooked in many laboratories, is review of the literature. The importance of a thorough review of the literature cannot be overemphasized. A literature review is performed to determine, first of all, if a solution to the problem already exists. Second, a literature review can determine whether state-of-the-art technology can be applied directly for a solution or new technology needs to be developed. Excellent sources for literature review are *Cumulative Index Medicus,* the National Library of Medicine's monthly bibliography of biomedicine literature, and *Excerpta Medica,* which publishes abstracts in *Rehabilitation and Physical Medicine.*

Problem solutions and design

Once past accomplishments and current possibilities are understood, creative and innovative ideas may be generated. This phase of the design process may be approached in different ways. Some engineers recommend the checklist approach for generating ideas, especially where the objective is modification of existing solutions. Checklists may give questions directed toward reviewing the technical base of ideas and developing new ideas, or they may list the key elements and features of each idea. The designers then systematically modify or eliminate each item.

Another approach, useful for new problems that require innovative solutions, is brainstorming. The objective of a brainstorming session is to generate as many solutions for a given problem as possible without regard to their attributes or eventual applicability. The session includes all members of the rehabilitation team, such as medical engineering, allied health, and technical professionals, as well as, if possible, the consumers of the eventual product. The active participation of a patient can stimulate creativity and permit consideration of aspects of the problem that would be missed otherwise.

After all suggested solutions have been compiled, the best is chosen by painstaking review and discussion. The benefit of team participation becomes evident in this step. In rehabilitation engineering, the most effective solution to a problem is not always determined by considering only the technical aspects; there are social and psychologic considerations as well. A patient may be fitted with the most advanced and efficient prosthesis but refuse to wear it because of its color or shape. There are variables in every design that the engineer could know of only through consultation with patients or allied health professionals.

After formulation of the solution, the role of the rehabilitation engineer is to design and construct the first prototype.

Evaluation

All devices must undergo thorough evaluation to ensure that all functional and technical requirements are met, including reliability and safety. Frequently, problems do not surface until the device is clinically tested with a patient. The process of product evaluation can be divided into two steps: internal clinical evaluation and external clinical evaluation.

Testing the first prototype in the clinic will verify the design specifications and provide data regarding its technical performance, quality assurance, and safety factors. At this stage any problems with the use of the device by the patient will become obvious and should be scrutinized carefully by the engineer. Inevitably, redesign, redevelopment, and reevaluation will be required. It may be necessary to repeat this cycle many times until the performance goals defined by the rehabilitation team and the consumer are finally met. It must be emphasized again that human acceptance is an important factor in rehabilitation engineering; it should not be minimized.

When the prototype is acceptable, a number of other prototypes can be made and tested to gain further experience. Additional data can be collected regarding acceptability and durability.

External clinical evaluation involves making the device available to other clinics for field evaluation. This is an important step if the device is to be submitted to a manufacturer and recognized by the Food and Drug Administration. Field evaluation is one of the most efficient ways to measure the performance and the likely success of a new device.

TECHNOLOGY FOR THE HANDICAPPED

Rehabilitation engineering is widely diverse in its applications and accomplishments: from wheelchairs to hydraulic knee controls and from house modifications to functional electrical stimulation of paralyzed muscles. The rehabilitation engineer is concerned with research and development and with the delivery of services to the disabled. Recognizing this diversity, it is helpful to outline the various activities in terms of general functional categories of need:

I. Function and physical restoration
   A. Prostheses
      1. Upper extremity
         a. Above elbow, below elbow, and shoulder disarticulation
         b. Body-powered prosthesis
         c. Myoelectric hand and arm
      2. Lower extremity
         a. Above knee, below knee, and hip disarticulation
         b. Passive swing
         c. Stance control
   B. Orthoses
      1. Braces, casts, splints, orthopedic shoes
      2. Nonpowered orthoses—articulation braces, hand splints, mobile arm supports
      3. Powered orthoses—upper and lower extremities
      4. Functional electrical stimulation—upper and lower extremities
   C. Joint replacement—hip, knee, ankle, shoulder, elbow, wrist, finger
II. Activities of daily living
   A. Self-care aids
   B. Home aids: lifts, transfer devices, feeding, hygiene, access modifications
   C. Environmental control systems
   D. Robotic aids
III. Mobility
   A. Wheelchairs—motorized, nonpowered, sport, stairclimbing, reclining
   B. Licensed vehicles—driver control, modified for wheelchairs
   C. Public transit—modified for wheelchairs
IV. Accessibility—architectural barrier removal
V. Communication
   A. Systems for neurologically and speech impaired
   B. Computer access

VI. Employment
    A. Job station modifications—machine tools and office equipment adaptations
    B. Specialized assistive devices for job performance
VII. Body function assistive devices
    A. Respiratory assistive devices
    B. Micturition and defecation control
    C. Copulation aids

Although this outline is long, it could be much expanded, for example, by including aids for the hearing and visually impaired. It is difficult to describe the state of the art of such widely varied programs; however, advances in technology for the handicapped have been made in almost all categories. For example, a curb-climbing wheelchair has been constructed. This wheelchair has portable ramps attached to the side, leaving enough room to pass through standard doors. The ramps are lowered by the paraplegic to ascend normal curbs. Another example is a nonverbal communication aid, inexpensive and portable, that produces voice or printed messages. Messages are entered into the device with a keyboard, and each character is displayed as it is entered. When complete, the message can be spoken or saved for later use.[3]

Sometimes the solution to a problem may be simple but very significant. The modification of an electric wheelchair to permit control by foot movement[2] exemplifies the almost daily problem-solving tasks confronted by the engineer. Another example of this is the modification devised for a patient with C7 quadriplegia to meet an ambulation goal. An ordinary walker was modified by fabricating polyvinyl chloride–acrylic alloy guards lined with foam to reduce palmar pressure. This permitted the patient to use wrist and finger extension during walker advancement and to walk 300 meters with a Craig-Scott orthosis.[5]

Besides the development of new devices, considerable research is going on in all phases of rehabilitation engineering. One example is a study to investigate the load on the shoulder joint and muscles in adults during the lifting of burdens from floor to table level. The procedure employed recording surface electromyography and the calculation of loading movements of force using a static biomechanical model.[1]

Application of electrostimulation to men to achieve erection, semen release, or both is an example of a more difficult problem solved by long-term research. This system used constant-current rectal probe stimulation.[4] Also developed were catheter techniques for antegrade collection of the semen, uncontaminated by urine.

A high priority in rehabilitation engineering is the need to quantify the effects of various therapeutic treatments and devices on the handicapped. In most cases the outcome of treatment is evaluated by professionals on the basis of subjective analysis. Current technologic expertise should provide accurate and quantifiable measures of progress in a therapeutic program or in the application of new devices.

REFERENCES

1. Arborelius, UP, Ekholm, J, and Memeth, G: Shoulder joint load and muscular activity during lifting, Scand J Rehabil Med 18:71, 1986.
2. Harrison, E, Jr, and Vise, GT, Jr: Simple devices for the physically disabled, Paraplegia 22:182, 1984.
3. Trimble, J, and Kampschoer, C: Portable communication aid with synthetic speech, J Rehab Res Dev 22:323, 1985.
4. Warner, H, et al: Electrostimulation of erection and ejaculation and collection of semen in spinal cord injured humans, J Rehab Res Dev 23:21, 1986.
5. Yarkony, GM: Jones-Hedman walker modification for C7 quadriplegic patient, Arch Phys Med Rehabil 67:54, 1986.

CHAPTER 55

Computers in rehabilitative medicine

ROBERT L. MAGNUSON AND JEROME STENEHJEM

The introduction of computers to rehabilitation medicine has caused excitement, promise, and hope for the disabled.[17,53] Although the implementation of computers in rehabilitation has been slow, their impact is now being felt by patients. Therapeutic devices with on-board microprocessors are being used in the treatment of paralysis to collect electromyographic (EMG) data and change treatment parameters.[49] Interactive computer systems are being used in cognitive training for the brain injured.[1,9] Speech and language systems have begun using sophisticated voice recognition methods for monitoring and correcting articulation, rate, and syntax.[16,27] For those without speech, alternative communication has become richer (Figure 55-1).[15,47,58] The affordability and dependability of computer systems have contributed to their proliferation in rehabilitation medicine.

Computer systems provide the unique ability to examine large amounts of information in ways not previously possible. This allows the computer to assist in professional communication, training of rehabilitation professionals, decision making, practice management, accounting, and research. As technology continues to expand the options, applications will be restricted by only ingenuity.

THERAPEUTIC TOOLS

Many experts in rehabilitation and computers have foreseen the use of microprocessors to help patients directly. The increasing capabilities and decreasing costs of computers have allowed many developments. Teaching is a basic process in rehabilitation. Improved awareness of behaviors often increases rehabilitation's success in improving human function.

Behavior monitoring

Computers can monitor behavior that may cause pressure ulcers to develop in spinal cord–injured patients. Seating pressures can be measured and stored in a microprocessor system attached to a wheelchair.[3,22] Figure 55-2 illustrates the basic components. Besides providing an audible cue to remind the patient, this monitor stores duration of shifts and the interval since the last shift for later transmittal to a computer system for tabular or graphic display. Figure 55-3 displays one day of data on each line. The frequent upward spikes represent pressure relief events, and long uninterrupted declines represent prolonged sitting. Without such monitoring the rehabilitation team could not know about pressure relief behavior patterns.[22] Newer versions of these systems provide the option of visual or audible cues to the patient. The cost of the monitoring system is projected at a small fraction of the surgical care costs for treating a pressure ulcer.

Physiologic monitoring

Monitoring of electrophysiologic data is another area in which computers have assisted rehabilitation. Since the early 1970s ambulatory electrocardiographic data (Holter monitoring) has been analyzed automatically by analog-to-digital conversion and computer analysis of waveforms and events. Stenehjem and Swenson[52] are analyzing ambulatory EMG data to assess spasticity in complete spinal cord injury. Analog-to-digital conversion allows manipulation of data to assess the number and severity of spastic motor contractions as well as daily variations in muscle spasm activity. Quantitative measurement over time enhances evaluation of the best approaches to reduce spasticity.

Memory assistance

Brain-injured patients with impaired memory can benefit from programmable wristwatches, which can store and display up to 99 events per day, addresses, telephone numbers, and other useful information. The watches can be programmed by a family member using a personal computer.

```
U R HOLDING IN UR HAND A          NALS 2 SELECT FORM A MAT
MINOR MIRACLE----FOR IN           RIX----IE
NO OTHER WAY COULD I COM          ROW 3 COLUMN 2 ON CARD 4
MUNICATE                           SELECTS A PARTICULAR PH
2 U WITH THE SAME DEGREE          RASE
 OF PRECISION AND ECONOM          I WOULD HAVE A FEW PHRAS
Y                                 ES SPELLED OUT AND HANDY
WHAT'S LEFT OF MY ORAL S          IN THE COMPUTER
PEECH IS VERY SEVERLY CO          RIGHT NOW I'M BLAZING AW
MPROMIZED ----4 EXAMPLE           AY ON SPEED SETTING 4 BE
I WOULDN'T EVEN TRY 2 SA          CAUSE OF TWO FACTORS----
Y                                 1----THE PIECE OF WOOD W
THE PREVIOUS PHRASE----'          ITH THE SWITCHES TAPED O
VERY HARD' IS PROBABLY T          N AND
HE MOST THAT I WOULD ATT          2----THE FACT THAT I CUR
EMPT                              RENTLY HAVE THE ABILITY
SO 3 CHEERS 4 THIS TOOL-          2 TWITCH MY MUSCLES IN M
---WITH IT I CAN CONTINU          Y FINGERS AND WRIST
E 2 HAVE FULL COMMAND OF          PERHAPS  IF THE SWITCHES
 THE PRICELESS RESOURCE            WERE BETTER ARRANGED I
OF LANGUAGE                       COULD GO FASTER ----
HOWEVER IT IS NOT THE TO          THEN AGAIN IF I LOSE THI
OL 4 MAKING A SNAPPY RES          S SET OF MUSCLES I WILL
PONSE----                         HAVE 2 HOPE THAT I CAN F
IT TAKES TIME FOR ME 2 G          IND ANOTHER EQUALLY EFFI
ET RIGGED UP AND READY 2          CIENT INTERFACE
 OPERATE                          GIVEN THE COURSE OF ALS
I THINK THER R SIMPLER W          IT WILL CONTINUE 2 B ANO
AYS FOR DEALING WITH THE          THER IN A LONG SERIES OF
NEED 4 'CANNED' PHRASES            EVERCHANGING EVERCHALLE
PERHAPS BY USING EYE SIG          NGING REALITIES
```

Figure 55-1. Patient's words.

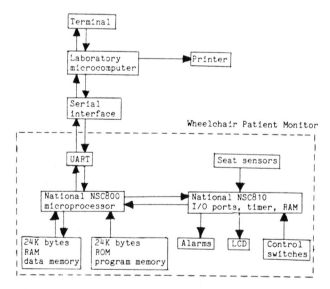

Figure 55-2. Block diagram of wheelchair patient monitor. Seat sensors detect weight shifts, which are monitored by microprocessor. Stored data are relayed via the serial interface to laboratory computer for analysis and display. (From Cummings, WT, et al: Arch Phys Med Rehabil 67:172, 1986.)

They have a four-line, 40-character display that prompts the wearer with the purpose of each scheduled alarm to sequence their daily activities.

Cognitive rehabilitation

Interactive computer programs can direct cognitively impaired patients in learning lost skills by reiterative processes performed at an optimal pace. Cognitive retraining programs have been developed for use on inexpensive personal computers. There are various programs for cognitive retraining. Some commercial games, instructional programs, and word-processing programs have been useful without modification. In the early 1980s Gianutsos[13] introduced special computer programs for cognitive rehabilitation to improve perception, response speed, recall, and memory span. Additional programs have been developed by psychologists, occupational therapists, speech pathologists, and family members to address the cognitive problems from different perspectives.[13,30] Games are incorporated in programs written by Lambert[30] and others to maintain the patient's participation for longer periods. Therapy goals are defined, and when performance approaches the goal behavior, positive feedback is provided through scoring. Programs with the therapeutic goals of

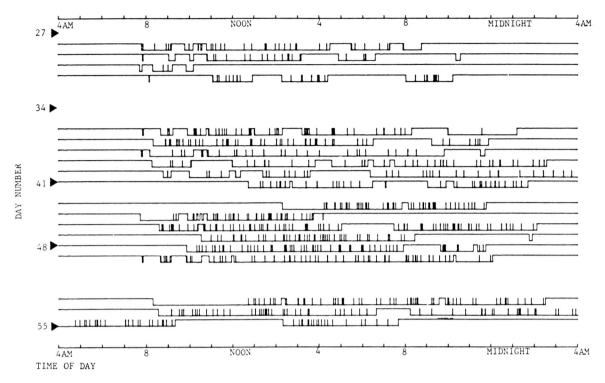

Figure 55-3. Each line represents one day of monthly log from wheelchair pressure monitor, with each spike representing pressure relief maneuver. When baseline stayed down, as in the period 8 AM to noon near bottom of chart, patient failed to perform lift-offs. When patient is out of chair, baseline is up. Day numbers on left side are Sundays. (From Grip, JC, and Merbitz, CT: Comput Meth Prog Biomed 22:137, 1986.)

symbolic processing (Figure 55-4, *A*), shape recognition (Figure 55-4, *B*), sequencing tasks, recall with interrupting tasks simulating real world challenges, money management skills, and so on are available for head injury patients. The carryover of computer-trained skills to daily functioning requires further documentation, but traditional therapeutic goals of right-left discrimination, body scheme, spatial relations, form constancy, figure-ground discrimination, tracking, eye-hand coordination, sequencing, response rate, time concepts, bilateral skills, attention span, memory, mathematics skills, organization and categorization, problem solving, and living skills can be logically pursued with computer technology.

Communication disorders

In communication disorders the microcomputer has begun to assist in evaluation of problems, instructional sessions, and direct communication efforts.[16,27] Testing and teaching strategies for word finding and comprehension have often been direct conversions of methods used by speech pathologists. But the addition of voice recognition input devices allows the computer to hear and respond to the patient's attempts to phonate and articulate sounds. When the speech

product meets the pattern recognition specifications, the system can provide rewarding output for the user. Fried-Oken[10] reported improvement in articulatory precision by a brain-injured patient. Conversely, the computer itself determines normal sounds of words; it only compares the pattern with its templates. If the phonation is consistent, it is accepted as a match. Group discussion has taken place through computer conferencing. Remarkably open self-help group interactions have taken place through computers, and this may expand opportunities for the disabled to share their strengths.[45]

ASSISTIVE DEVICES
Environmental control

Environmental control for the severely disabled has been improved significantly through the use of desktop computers. The first environmental control devices were too large and limited in choice of devices. Commercially available devices can now interface with Apple or IBM desktop computers. The computers provide virtually unlimited expansion, control of remote devices through home power lines, time delay, and remote access through off-site tele-

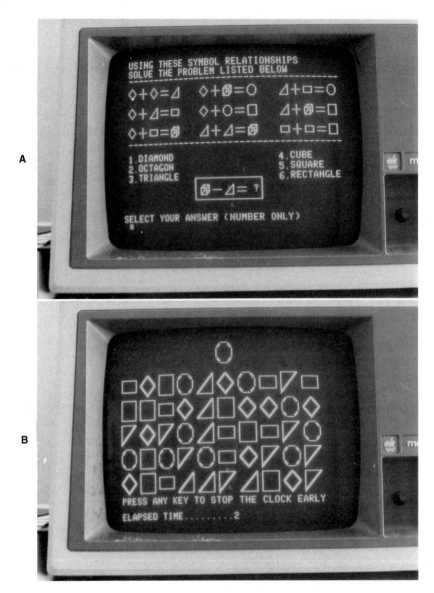

Figure 55-4. A, Apple computer screen from "Math with Shapes," symbolic problem game. **B,** "Find the Shape," timed shape recognition game that requires visual monitoring of both sides of computer screen. (Courtesy Karen Lambert Foundation.)

phones.[32,48] Many of the newer devices are relatively inexpensive because they have been designed and marketed for general use.

Prosthetics and orthotics

The use of computers in prosthetics and orthotics has been limited, except for research applications. The Utah Artificial Arm, developed at the University of Utah Center for Biomechanical Design,[24] uses a hybrid system that incorporates digital and analog systems to control the motion of the device. This device has been successfully commercialized. The need for extreme ruggedness to give adequate reliability and the relatively small market size have slowed

development of more advanced systems. Research developments continue in the areas of bracing, incorporating functional electrical stimulation,[28,37,42] robot controllers as assistive devices,[46] and other microprocessor-based systems.

Speech synthesis

Speech synthesis has been progressing rapidly because of technologic advances in inexpensive memory and faster computer clock rates. Combinations of phonetic and word recognition techniques with artificial phrasing, accenting, and end-of-sentence recognition are improving the quality of synthesized speech.[48,53,58] Text readers are now readily available. These devices have been of major benefit to the visually impaired. The vocally impaired have not benefited as greatly because of the lack of data input methods that can approximate normal speech rates. Programmed statements, phrases, or words have minimally increased telephone access for the vocally impaired.

Employment opportunities

Computers offer a unique employment opportunity for the physically disabled.[32,56] Electronic transfer of digital information allows opportunities for home-based employment. The absence of need for mobility enhances the suitability of such employment. However, computer programming and related fields require high cognitive function combined with discipline and creativity. The percentage of able-bodied individuals who successfully meet these criteria is small. This also holds true for the disabled, but it is an arena in which they can compete equally.

Interfaces with users

Adaptation of computer systems for the severely disabled has yielded ingenious solutions. A Morse code interface converts on-off signals to ASCII character input.[47] Although the data input rates are initially slow, time can improve data entry rates to a practical level. Voice recognition techniques are advancing rapidly.[15] This allows hands-free input at the computer terminal and may provide additional employment opportunities for patients with high-level spinal cord injury. Most systems require a voice signature learning routine to define the characteristics of each person's voice for adequate discrimination.

PATIENT CARE MANAGEMENT
Records

Word processing has been a major use of computers in the office setting. The word processor is frequently used as an advanced typewriter with document storage, retrieval, and rewrite capabilities. This is appropriate but does not begin to use the potential of the more advanced systems. Storage and quick retrieval of common phrases, diagnoses, headings, treatment plans, and so on should be routine. Referral acknowledgments, team conference report cover letters, and other routine and periodic correspondence can be automatically generated by merging standard statements and lists of referring physicians. Team conference reports can be created in individualized narrative form, stored, and retrieved with a minimum of keystrokes (macros). Automatic spelling correction, custom glossaries, and other proofing techniques are common. Tutorial programs can teach the operator how to run specific software programs quickly and easily.

Free-form text

Some computer programs sort through free-form text to find, extract, and manipulate some data. These programs require many cycles of the computer's central processing unit (CPU) resulting in slow response, even with high-speed processors. A problem with the free-form text approach is lack of consistency and completeness of the dictated data.

Programmed text

To improve the completeness of data and to electronically retrieve frequently used terms, Granger and Delabarre[18] adapted the Programmed History and Physical for rehabilitation patients in 1972. This approach used automatic typewriters and mixed selected prerecorded keystrokes with free-form narrative. It employed worksheets for recording the data and encouraged completeness and standard terminology. It also allowed branching of data collection with optional sheets for brain injury and spinal cord injury patients.

Frequently encountered data can be programmed to build a useful database of information. Standardization enhances the comparison of patients and allows reduction in storage requirements. If the data are organized in the same sequence, high-speed sorting is possible. The same information can be used in reports for different purposes without reentry of repetitive data. The deliberate intermingling of free-form text with programmed text restores eloquent opportunities for describing the uncommon. The tremendous value of structured data collection has been recognized by others involved in the production of computerized medical records.[25,26]

Educating the clinician in the importance of systematic medical record keeping is a critical step in developing a database from admission records. Such a database could allow a quantum leap in the rehabilitation sciences' base of information.

Patient assessment

The computer participates in all areas of patient assessment. It can record performance in eye-hand coordination with video game–style testing. It can also measure gait,[50,57] quantify the function of balance, or extract small-amplitude signals for multimodality evoked-potential measurements.[38] New radiologic capabilities for imaging the brain and other body parts have also evolved. As the physician collects this information and it is combined with data from the history and physical examination and from other members of the rehabilitation team, a state of information overload can impair effectiveness in dealing with the patient's need. Lehmann and associates[31] and Brown[2] have developed programs to assist in case management.

Consultation reporting

In 1986 Stineman and co-workers[55] reported the use of the "Cardiac Physiatric Consultation Software," which was designed to create clearly typed reports for hospital charts without transcription delays. It encouraged high-quality, uniform patient evaluations by various physicians seeing cardiac rehabilitation patients in consultation. The system

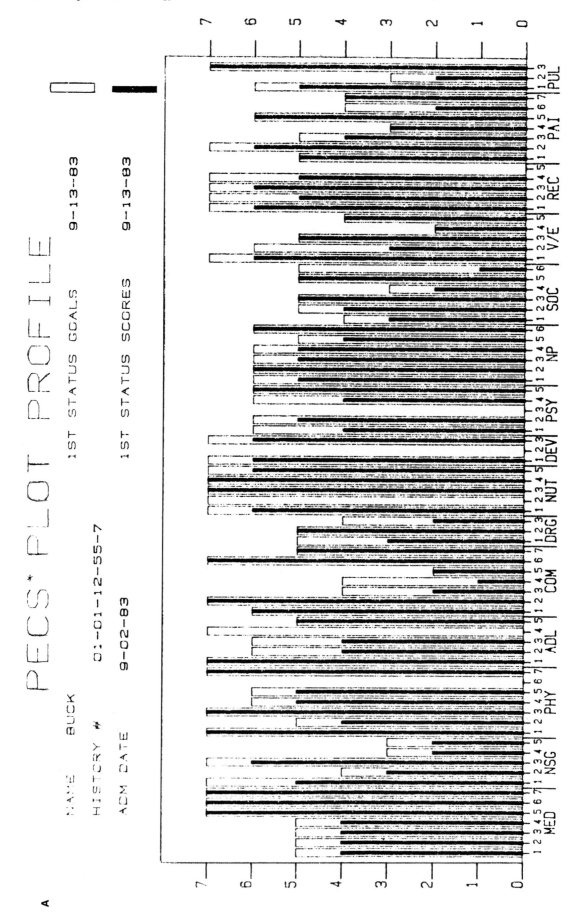

Figure 55-5. A, Sample of PECS functional graphing of team conference data. Original computer printed graph was two colored.

Continued.

allows infinite variations in describing the patient's historical and physical findings. The program produces a one- or two-page narrative form document in 13 sections. Descriptions of cardiac activity protocols are available. The data are also used to prepare a "Consultation Service Patient Summary Sheet," which is referenced for team rounds and rotating staff physicians.

Electrodiagnostic reports

Reporting of electromyographic and electrodiagnostic studies can be enhanced by computer. The format adapted by Granger and Delabarre[18] for programmed history and physical examination is easily used for collecting the patient history. The report is verified and amplified with free-form narrative. Selected parts of the neurologic examination and manual muscle strength testing can be rapidly recorded in tabular format. Nerve conduction studies are usually standardized and can be modified for the circumstances. Velocities can be calculated from input data. "Boiler-plate" storage of all the electromyographically accessible muscles with their root and peripheral innervation allows rapid and accurate assembly of reports.

Because the computer always spells the text as it was stored, review is reduced to verification of the facts, not proofreading. Most word processing programs have optional spelling verification functions to check the free-form text. This approach allows preparation of the final electrodiagnostic report within 20 minutes of the completion of the

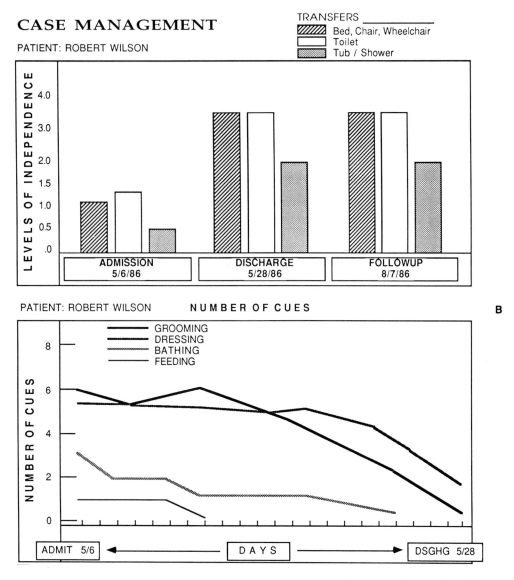

Figure 55-5, cont'd. B, Sample of R/COM functional graphing of team conference data. (**A** courtesy Harvey and Jellinek. **B** courtesy C. Gerald Warren and Associates.)

studies. In this way the patient can take the completed report back to the referring physician. Use of the computer's information-processing ability in electrodiagnosis is addressed in the section on decision support.

Functional assessment

Functional assessment is a natural extension of the history and physical examination. Rating scales have been developed for different types of disabilities.[8,19-21] The Long-Range Evaluation System (LRES) is a computerized assessment method of tracking patients with physical deficits.[19]

The arduous process of defining the functional skills to be measured and tracked has been begun on a national level by the joint task force of the American Academy of Physical Medicine and Rehabilitation and the American Congress of Rehabilitation Medicine. The information gathered in the functional assessment process has different uses. The members of the rehabilitation team need to document progress to third-party payors so the patient may continue to receive rehabilitative services.

A sensitive scale is needed to discriminate small gains in function. The difference between minimal assistance and moderate assistance in transferring from a bed to a wheelchair may not be important to a program reviewer who sees that at both levels the patient will need assistance from someone. The computer can take data recorded on one scale and convert them to corresponding points on another scale if common definitions have been planned. In this way the needs of differing perspectives are met.

Problem-oriented progress notes

Problem-oriented records were first used at the University of Vermont to improve the organization of medical care, using a systematic approach developed by Weed.[59] This was adapted to rehabilitation by Dinsdale and co-workers[6] in 1969. Programmed progress notes have not yet been reported in the rehabilitation literature. Psychiatric occupational therapy notes were programmed successfully at the Naval Regional Medical Center, San Diego, and used from 1975 until 1981. They established the SOAP note format, which decreased the time spent in note writing and increased completeness and legibility of the data. General nursing notes have been developed on database software. As more computer technology becomes available for input by rehabilitation therapists, nurses, and physicians, these important sequential data entries can be expected to save time and enhance care of the patient through improved communication. The free-form narrative will be needed for special situations but need not be stored or retrieved for statistical purposes.

Team conferences

Rehabilitation team conference summaries can be approached with a structured format to reduce dictation time and increase reliable collection of information. This format

can simultaneously generate data for program assessment. Information can be contributed by each of the rehabilitation team members. Commercial programs, such as Patient Evaluation Conference System (PECS), developed by Harvey and Jellinek, and R/COM developed by Warren (Figure 55-6), allow various other functions and are in use in several rehabilitation centers. When combined with the entry history and physical examination, medications, laboratory findings, and final diagnoses, these data can be restructured into a discharge summary report.[54] This automated summary saves staff time because only review and verifying signature is needed. The report can be ready to accompany the patient leaving the rehabilitation care unit to return to the referring physician.

DECISION SUPPORT

With the ability to collect, store, retrieve, and manipulate large amounts of data in controlled processes, the computer has some of the capabilities of the human brain. Although it is not capable of many human thought processes, the computer can perform specific tasks at near-perfect levels, repeatedly and without tiring.

Decision responsibility

The computer can present data in a manner that allows decisions to be made with clearer understanding. Some systems collect data, make decisions, and take action without human intervention. Because of the potential for harm, these systems are closely controlled by the Food and Drug Administration. Those systems that reach decisions but require human intervention for action are not as closely controlled. When accountants review the accuracy of simple spreadsheet programs marketed for business purposes, they often find serious errors in their data.[7] Therefore the use of all computer programs in medicine requires careful monitoring for accuracy and proper performance by the user.

Artificial intelligence

Since the early 1970s serious work has been done in medical computing to develop artificial intelligence programs that approach specific problems in ways that would simulate the thought processes of a good clinician. Miller[36] looked at several of these programs to see if they uncover new design problems, offer new solutions to help deal with problems, develop new tools to help handle similar problems, and make illustrative mistakes that can point to new constructive directions. One of these systems was AI/RHEUM, developed at the University of Missouri to perform rheumatologic diagnosis. The system was able to diagnose diseases with high accuracy in patients whose diagnoses were known to the computer. When 11 patients with diagnoses not known to the computer were presented, seven were given incorrect diagnoses and four did not receive diagnoses.[29] Thus it may fail to recognize when the correct diagnosis is beyond its capability.

Researchers at the University of Maryland developed the TIA system to help assess transient ischemic attacks and to recommend therapy.[36] The system's localization of the brain lesion had better agreement with an "expert" than the specialists caring for the patients. Recommending appropriate therapy for a medical problem for which there was no consensus of treatment among neurologists produced considerable disageement. With the lack of consensus, the computer system will not likely be accepted by potential physician-users.

Electrodiagnosis

With the integration of computers and electromyographic instruments, the primary goals have been signal processing and easier setting of parameters for various neurophysiologic studies. The quantification of potentials and the use of averaging techniques to reduce random noise is opening new areas of electrodiagnosis, as discussed in other areas of this book. However, there would appear to be even more promise in the use of the computer's information management powers.

In 1976 Magnuson and Friedman[11,34] reported the development of a software prototype for computer-assisted electrodiagnostic data acquisition. The basic program ran on a minicomputer and allowed an electromyographer without computer-programming skills to enter an anatomic model of the peripheral nervous system's connection to each accessible muscle and a branching logic tree by responding to system prompts. When the system's data solicitation processor was employed by the examiner, it sequenced the requests for data depending on the logic tree being used and the examination results at any point. This system allowed the examiner to collect unsolicited data, to skip entry of solicited data, to edit entered data, and to modify the programmed interpretations before the report was generated. The system terminated data solicitation and gave no interpretation when its knowledge base limits were exceeded.

At the Medical College of Georgia, Rivner and Swift[44] are proceeding with development of MYAL, a computerized electromyographic data management system, which collects electrodiagnostic data on a desktop personal computer. This system uses a rule-based diagnostic system for data collection and knowledge base development. It can generate a report without producing diagnostic assistance. Both systems have potential for training of electromyographers.

Requirements for system success

For the computer to be used successfully for decision support in health care, it must do several things.[36] It must produce alterations in the care provided, and these changes must be improvements, such as fewer diagnostic or management errors. The results of these alterations should be shown to improve the health and functioning of patients and the overall health care delivery process so the computer system is cost effective. Its users must be willing to use it. If physicians do not think it is useful and choose not to use

it, the system will have a short history. A system is dependent on all its parts: hardware, programming, medical knowledge, costs, and perceived rewards. Sometimes the difference between acceptance and rejection depends on the speed of the computer's processor and disk drive retrieval time. These are technologic factors that can advance dramatically in brief intervals and give new promise to a marginally functioning system.

DATA ANALYSIS

Data analysis is performed on a daily basis by every clinician. Information is collected through chart review, patient interview and examination, and other sources before decisions are made and acted on. When information is entered into some type of storage device that allows it to be handled as discrete data, the data can be manipulated to provide additional information. Data can be displayed in several formats, such as graphic, spreadsheet, list, and text. Each of these formats has specific advantages in presenting information. Data that are not reviewed and used in decision making reflect wasted time and money. Data that are presented so trends and correlations can be seen and comparisons made will justify the cost.

Database terms

Database nomenclature has been standardized to improve communication. The essential elements include characters, fields, records, and files. A group of characters comprising numbers or words may occupy a field. (For example, "123 Elm Street" may be the data occupying the field named "Address.") Additional fields such as name and telephone number could be grouped as a record of an individual patient. A group of records could be assembled to represent a mailing address file. The American Rheumatism Association has developed a large data bank for long-term storage of multipurpose data to track the complexities of chronic disease.[12] On this very large system or on the smaller personal computer database, the records or data can be displayed by a variety of formats including list, spreadsheet, graphic display, flowsheet, or text.

Lists

List formats are the first step in data collection and entry. The list is one of the easier ways to collect and enter data. The list typically includes all of the needed information for decision making. However, because of their cumbersome nature, lists are not conducive to analysis.

The list can be created using computer prompts that ask for specific information in a specific order to ensure completeness. Many commercially available databases have custom-designed screens that the user creates to suit his or her needs. An example of a simple list format is shown in Figure 55-7, *A*.

List formats can be restructured into various formats, including charts and spreadsheets. The chart format takes

```
        name:      ABLE              name:      SMITH
         age:        79               age:         32
        diag:      L HEMI            diag:      SCI C6
         adm:    03-Mar-87            adm:    18-Mar-87
         dis:    27-Mar-87            dis:    06-May-87
        cost:     $20,000            cost:     $20,000


A       name:      JONES             name:      LINCOLN
         age:        79               age:         20
        diag:      R HEMI            diag:         HT
         adm:    20-Feb-87            adm:    31-Dec-86
         dis:    29-Apr-87            dis:    20-Apr-87
        cost:     $20,000            cost:     $65,000
```

```
       name    age      diag        adm          dis        cost
       ABLE     65    L HEMI     03-Mar-87    27-Mar-87    $20,000
B      JONES    79    R HEMI     20-Feb-87    29-Apr-87    $20,000
      SMITH     32    SCI C6     18-Mar-87    06-May-87    $20,000
    LINCOLN     20        HT     31-Dec-86    20-Apr-87    $65,000
```

Figure 55-6. A, List format of data for six fields of four records from one file. This format is frequently used during data entry. **B,** Simple chart format example from **A** with spreadsheet program. May also be described as "view" format.

the list data and creates rows or columns of similar fields (Figure 55-7, *B*).

Spreadsheets

The spreadsheet is perhaps the most versatile method of data display for numeric manipulation. It is a chart format with improved versatility. The values of a single record can occupy one row, and additional records can be added vertically to form columns. Cell values may be words (text or labels), numbers, or logical characters. Cells, rows, or columns may be added to the spreadsheet by computing values derived from other cells or groups of cells within the spreadsheet.

Columns or portions of columns can be totaled. Rows or selected cells from rows may be added or subtracted. Any mathematic operation dealing in real numbers may be performed on any combination of cells. A simple example would be to compute length of stay from admission and discharge dates. Figure 55-8 is a display of the data in Figure 55-7, with derived average and difference values. The last column is calculated from the difference of the admitting and discharge dates. The cost/day is calculated by dividing the days spent in the hospital into the total bill to derive the cost per day. One of the important uses of spreadsheets is in modeling known situations and then inserting hypothetic values to predict results. Spreadsheets can allow up to hundreds of columns and thousands of rows. Although many of the sophisticated database programs can perform some of these operations during the report-writing phase, they have not yet replaced the power of the spreadsheet.

Flowsheets

The flowsheet is used to depict values that lie along a continuum, such as time. Flowsheets can be particularly useful in determining the critical path a project may take on the basis of limited time and resources. As resources continue to dwindle and acuity increases, flowsheets for improving rate of rehabilitation without sacrificing quality may be more widely used.

Graphic display

Graphic display of data typically compares a variable over time or some other parameter. The value, for example, bed census, is depicted on the *y* axis (ordinate) over its range, for example, time, along the *x* axis (abscissa). If a relationship exists between the two values, it may be seen graphically. This process typically yields points distributed across the *x-y* coordinates. If one of the values is formed from discrete steps, such as the months of the year or days of the week, this value can be placed on the abscissa (horizontal axis), and a bar graph may be drawn. When parts of a whole are depicted as a percentage of the whole, a pie chart can

name	age	diag	adm	dis	cost	hos days
ABLE	65	L HEMI	03-Mar-87	27-Mar-87	$20,000	24
JONES	79	R HEMI	20-Feb-87	29-Apr-87	$54,000	68
SMITH	32	SCI C6	18-Mar-87	06-May-87	$56,000	49
LINCOLN	20	HT	31-Dec-86	20-Apr-87	$65,000	110
AVE AGE	49			TOTALS	$195,000	251
				AVE STAY		62.75
				COST/DAY	$777	

Figure 55-7. Spreadsheet created from data shown in Figure 55-6 combines data display and manipulation.

be drawn. Frequently two columns from a spreadsheet will be graphed to illustrate a relationship.

Text

Data can and have been effectively presented in a text format. Text is still the most frequently used method for transferring data from one physician to another, as in daily notes, conference reports, and hospital summaries. Text is frequently the final common pathway for the vast amounts of data that are distilled to make a decision. This is the method of order writing and documenting completion of orders. The computer has improved methods for handling text through databases and word processing. Frequently used names, diagnoses, and phrases can be stored for rapid retrieval. Documents can be searched for specified words and phrases. Text is not regularly handled as data. However, text may be converted to database formats in the future with the advancement of artificial intelligence, improved processing speeds, and algorithms.

EDUCATION
Graduate training

Medical education with computers has become widely used.[33,51] The instructor needs to anticipate many aspects of the lesson that usually would be spontaneously handled during a lecture, in interaction between teacher and students. Multiple-choice responses have fewer options to consider than natural language approaches and are easier to program. It takes 40 to 150 hours to prepare a 1-hour computer lesson.

Several areas relevant to rehabilitation have begun to develop. A program on anatomy of the forearm, using a computer model generated from frozen sections and combining videodisc media, opens new options for visually exploring spatial relationships of nerves, muscles, bones, and vessels.[35] The program allows rotation of the image, making structures just under the viewed layer partially visible, removing layers sequentially, or presenting only specific structures, such as peripheral nerves. A program to develop the diagnostic skills needed to assess neuromuscular dysfunc-

tion in infants suspected of having cerebral palsy is already commercially available. This program uses a desktop computer with laser videodisc. A growing list of computer-assisted learning programs of interest to physiatrists appear in medical computer journals. Several rehabilitation training programs are exploring development of computer lessons specifically for physiatry.

Continuing medical education

Training programs developed for graduate education that will run on widely available hardware systems may be disseminated to practicing physiatrists. Several commercially available programs to update drug interactions and to help evaluate and manage dementia and other subjects are also of interest. The use of computers to access computerized information services, such as MEDLINE (see below), is now common even in the smallest hospital medical libraries. Introduction of computerized patient files in hospitals and physiatrists' practices will facilitate new possibilities for analysis of practice problems and identification of learning needs based on the individual physician's practice profile. The American Academy of Physical Medicine has formed a task group to explore enhancement of the availability of computer-assisted continuing medical education in rehabilitation.

Patient education

Patient-oriented programs for instruction are available for diabetes, sexual dysfunction, and heart attack. It is anticipated that the technology developed for these programs can be used in training patients and their caregivers in various areas of rehabilitation.

MEDICAL INFORMATION RETRIEVAL SYSTEMS

Articles appearing in most major journals, such as the *Archives of Physical Medicine and Rehabilitation,* are indexed on several computerized database information systems. This allows rapid, on-line searching of the current literature by subject and author. The use of MEDLINE and other systems that offer structured queries may require knowledge in their use to get the listing the physician desires. Medical librarians are frequently willing to instruct groups of physicians who want to perform their MEDLINE searches personally. Some cross-indexed filing systems, such as Orthobase, can also retrieve abstracts and full text. Some systems include only textbooks, some only journals. Illustrations pose a challenge and are not available through these services. With the development of affordable telefacsimile boards for desktop computers to allow transmission of graphic data via the computer's modem and printer, more electronic medical journals are anticipated.

Computer bulletin boards can be integrated with medical databases, as in the American Medical Association's MINET. The physician-subscriber can access these services with almost any small computer system using communication software and a modem to modulate and demodulate the digital data. Electronic mail can be sent and received with these systems. Some practices use these or voice mail services that record the digitized spoken message and repeat it when requested. Smaller versions in hospitals can allow access to patient's radiologic and other data. In some hospitals, interpretations awaiting transcription may be accessed via a touch-tone phone, as with voice mail.

RESEARCH

Research applications for computers in rehabilitation medicine are vast and continuing to grow rapidly. The computer can collect large amounts of data, then process, analyze, make decisions, and implement actions quickly. Rehabilitation medicine deals with physical impairments. These impairments are represented as paralysis, loss of speech, loss of limb, and so on. The computer promises to bridge the gap for patients with impaired motor or cognitive systems and thereby improve or restore function. Computer models of human functions are being used to explore theories of language and cognitive processes.[14,43]

Research in prosthetics for upper extremity amputees has demonstrated the power of the computer in above-elbow amputation prosthesis control. Jacobsen[23] demonstrated effective three-degree-of-freedom control by simultaneously monitoring up to 12 torso and stump electromyographic sites. These electromyographic data are processed, and humeral rotation, elbow flexion, and wrist rotation torques are computed. Control signals are sent to servomotors in the artificial arm, which effect the desired motion. A unique concept that postulates the use of torso reactive forces as a signal source allows the computer to determine where the arm should be in space during a given reactive force. Three-degree-of-freedom control is accomplished without the need for extensive training or complicated maneuvers by the patient.

Research in functional electrical stimulation (FES) is being advanced through the use of computers to assess limb position, monitor multiple parameters, and vary stimulation current according to selected algorithms.[49] In the early 1980s research in computer-controlled FES bicycle ergometry that could sense leg position and stimulate the quadriceps muscle during the appropriate phase of the cycle stroke became widespread.[39,41] FES devices are now commercially available for home and hospital use.

Muscle retraining

The computer has expanded the role of FES in the treatment of various forms of paralysis.[40] The simplest FES devices produce on-off cycles of electrical current to simulate repetitive motor activity. The computer has allowed control over all stimulation parameters, including waveform, frequency, cycle on-off times, treatment times, and storage of treatment parameters on removable storage devices or random access memory. Patient use records are also kept with some home units, allowing monitoring of compliance in home treatment programs. The addition of biofeedback in later FES units requires computing ability to determine whether the criteria for stimulation are met. When the computer has determined that the monitored surface electromyographic signal has reached an appropriate amplitude, the stimulation is triggered. Although these biofeedback and FES devices are available, their efficacy has been demonstrated in only a few studies.

REFERENCES

1. Bracy, OL: Cognitive rehabilitation: a process approach, Cognitive Rehabil 4:10, 1986.
2. Brown, M: Computerized approach to case management and outcome measurement in medical rehabilitation, paper presented at National Association of Research and Training Centers Conference, Washington, DC, May 6-8, 1985.
3. Cummings, WT, et al: Microprocessor-based weight shift monitors for paraplegic patients, Arch Phys Med Rehabil 67:172, 1986.
4. De Luca CJ: Decomposition of the EMG signal and analysis of the motor unit action potential trains, personal communication, 1985.
5. Desmedt, JE: Computer-aided electromyography, Basel, 1983, S.J. Karger.
6. Dinsdale, SM, et al: The problem-oriented medical record in rehabilitation, Arch Phys Med Rehabil 51:488, 1970.
7. Ditlea, S: Spreadsheets can be hazardous to your health, Personal Computing, January, 1987, p 60.
8. Feinstein, AR, et al: Scientific and clinical problems in indexes of functional disability, Ann Intern Med 105:413, 1986.
9. Fisher, L, et al: Computerized cognitive rehabilitation for the rural head injury patient, International Conference on Rural Rehabilitation Technologies, Grand Forks, ND, October 1984.
10. Fried-Oken, M: Voice recognition device as a computer interface for motor and speech impaired people, Arch Phys Med Rehabil 66:678, 1985.
11. Friedman, LA: Software design specifications for an interactive fault location-diagnosis system, Spec Rep 7-11, San Diego, June 1977, Navy Personnel Research and Development Center.
12. Fries, JF, and McShane, DJ: ARAMIS (the American Rheumatism Association Medical Information System)—a prototype system, West J Med 145:798, 1986.

13. Gianutsos, R: Using computer-based therapies to ameliorate hemiplegic deficits, paper presented at National Association of Rehabilitation Research and Training Centers Conference, Washington, DC, May 6-8, 1985.

14. Gigley, HM: Studies in artificial aphasia: experiments in processing change, Comput Meth Prog Biomed 22:43, 1986.

15. Glenn, JW, and Miller, KH: Voice terminal may offer opportunities for employment to the disabled, Am J Occup Ther 30:309, 1976.

16. Goldman, R, and Dahle, AJ: Current and emerging applications of microcomputer technology in communication disorders, Top Lang Disorders 6:11, 1985.

17. Gordon, WA, et al: Improving rehabilitation outcomes in persons who have experienced stroke or traumatic brain damage, National Association of Rehabilitation Research and Training Centers Conference, Washington, DC, May 6-8, 1985.

18. Granger, CV, and Delabarre, EM: Programmed examination formats: use in rehabilitation medicine, Arch Phys Med Rehabil 55:235, 1974.

19. Granger, CV, and Gresham, GE, editors: Functional assessment in rehabilitation medicine, Baltimore, 1984, Williams & Wilkins Co.

20. Granger, CV, Sherwood, CC, and Greer, DS: Functional status measures in a comprehensive stroke care program, Arch Phys Med Rehabil, 18:555, 1977.

21. Granger, CV, et al: Stroke rehabilitation: analysis of repeated Barthel Index measures, Arch Phys Med Rehabil 60:14, 1979.

22. Grip, JC, and Merbitz, CT: Wheelchair-based mobile measurement of behavior for pressure sore monitoring, Comput Meth Prog Biomed 22:137, 1986.

23. Jacobsen, SC: Control systems for artificial arms, doctoral thesis, Cambridge, 1973, Massachusetts Institute of Technology.

24. Jacobsen, SC, Knutti, DF, and Sears, HH: Development of the Utah artificial arm, IEEE Trans Biomed Eng BME 29:249, 1982.

25. Kanner, IF: Programmed medical history-taking with or without computer, JAMA 207:317, 1969.

26. Kanner, IF: Programmed physical examination with or without computer, JAMA 215:1281, 1971.

27. Katz, RC: Using microcomputers in the diagnosis and treatment of chronic aphasic adults, Semin Speech Lang 5:11, 1984.

28. Keith, MW, et al: Strategies for improved manipulation and grasp in the tetraplegic upper extremity using functional neuromuscular stimulation, Arch Phys Med Rehabil 67:628, 1986.

29. Kingsland, L, et al: Testing a criteria-based consultant system in rheumatology. In Proceedings of MEDINFO-83, Amsterdam, 1983.

30. Lambert, C: Perspectives of a programmer/consumer. Presented at the 60th Annual Session of the American Congress of Rehabilitation Medicine, Los Angeles, November 8, 1983.

31. Lehmann, JF, et al: Computerized data management as an aid to clinical decision-making in rehabilitation medicine, Arch Phys Med Rehabil 65:260, 1984.

32. Littman, J: Open doors, PC World, March, 1984.

33. Llaurado, JG: Commentary: how to write computer lessons, Int J Biomed Comput 18:71, 1986.

34. Magnuson, RL, and Friedman, LA: Development of software package for computer-assisted electrodiagnostic data acquisition, paper presented at 38th Annual Assembly of the American Academy of Physical Medicine and Rehabilitation, San Diego, Nov 9, 1976.

35. Meals, RA, and Kabo, JM: Computerized anatomy instruction, MD Comput 3:30, 1986.

36. Miller, PL: The evaluation of artificial intelligence systems in medicine, Comput Meth Prog Biomed 22:5, 1986.

37. Nathan, RH: The development of a computerized upper limb electrical stimulation system, Orthopedics 7:1170, 1984.

38. Pavot, AP, et al: Diagnostic value of multimodality evoked potentials in cerebrovascular accidents, Bull Am Soc Clin Evoked Potentials 4:16, 1986.

39. Petrofsky, JS, and Phillips, CA: The use of functional electrical stimulation for rehabilitation of spinal cord injured patients, Cent Nerv Syst Trauma 1:57, 1984.

40. Petrofsky, JS, Phillips, CA, and Petrofsky, SH: Electronic physicians' prescription system for functional electrical stimulation (FES) patients, J Neurol Orthop Med Surg 6:239, 1985.

41. Petrofsky, JS, et al: Aerobic trainer with physiological monitoring for exercise in paraplegia and quadriplegic patients, J Clin Eng, 10:307, 1985.

42. Petrofsky, JS, et al: Computer synthesized walking: An application of orthosis and functional electrical stimulation (FES), J Neurol Orthop Med Surg 6:219, 1985.

43. Reggia, JA, and Berndt, RS: Modelling reading aloud and its relevance to acquired dyslexia, Comput Meth Prog Biomed 22:13, 1986.

44. Rivner, MH, and Swift, TR: A computerized EMG data management system, personal communication, 1986.

45. Schneider, SJ, and Tooley, J: Self-help computer conferencing, Comput Biomed Res 19:274, 1986.

46. Seamone, W, and Schmeisser, G: Early clinical evaluation of a robot arm/worktable system for spinal cord injured persons, J Rehabil Res Dev 22:38, 1985.

47. Shannon, DA, et al: Morse code controlled computer aid for the nonvocal quadriplegic, Med Instrum 15:341, 1981.

48. Smith, C, editor: Discovery 84: technology for disabled persons, conference papers, Chicago, 1984.

49. Solomonow, M, et al: External control of rate, recruitment, synergy and feedback in paralyzed extremities, Orthopedics 7:1161, 1984.

50. Stanic, U, et al: Standardization of kinematic gait measurements and automatic pathological gait pattern diagnostics, Scand J Rehabil Med 9:95, 1977.

51. Starkweather, JA: The computer as a tool for learning, West J Med 145:864, 1986.

52. Stenehjem, JC, and Swenson, JR: Spasticity monitoring using long-term EMG, Arch Phys Med Rehabil 67:679, 1986.

53. Stern, PH, and Ollayos, CW: Personal computer-based programs for the handicapped, Prosthet Orthot Int 8:82, 1984.

54. Stern, PH, and Rubin, EH: Computerized discharge summaries, Arch Phys Med Rehabil 60:25, 1979.

55. Stineman, MG, et al: Cardiac physiatric consultation software. Proceedings of the AAMSI Congress, Anaheim, Calif, May 8-10, 1986.

56. Stride, BD: Computer vocations for severely physically disabled persons: survey results, Arch Phys Med Rehabil 66:505, 1985.

57. Takebe, K, and Basmajian, JV: Gait analysis in stroke patients to assess treatments of foot drops, Arch Phys Med Rehabil 57:305, 1976.

58. Veterans Administration Rehabilitative Engineering Research and Development Service Programs. Part II, Bull Prosthet Res 18:62, 1981.

59. Weed, LL: Medical records, medical education, patient care, Chicago, 1970, Yearbook Medical Publishers.

PART VIII | **PSYCHOSOCIAL AND ECONOMIC ASPECTS OF REHABILITATION**

CHAPTER 56

Psychiatry and rehabilitation

SAUL H. FISHER

Since rehabilitation began as a serious endeavor in medicine, it has been recognized that emotional and mental attitudes can exert a decisive effect on the outcome of the process.[9]

Patients may be considered for referral to a psychiatrist or psychologist for the following reasons: behavioral disturbances caused by organic brain damage; overt psychopathology in the form of neurotic, psychotic, or sociopathic behavior, including addiction, alcoholism, and sexual disturbances; emotional problems such as severe anxiety, depression, or hostility; suicidal ideas or acts; bizarre physical symptoms and signs that do not conform to a known organic pattern or are exaggerated beyond what can be explained pathologically; and lack of improvement in rehabilitation without obvious physical or psychologic reasons.

There have been a number of major advances in psychiatry relevant to rehabilitation medicine: revised classification of psychiatric disorders by the American Psychiatric Association based on more objective criteria,[17] expansion of liaison-consultation psychiatry,[13] advances in basic neurosciences such as receptor sites and neurotransmitters,[4] advances in psychopharmacology,[3] increased use of behavioral therapy,[16] retraining techniques,[5,8] and short-term group and family therapies.[20] In this limited space, some are mentioned in discussion of specific problems.

DENIAL OF DISABILITY

First described by von Monakow[18] in 1885 in a blind patient, the phenomenon of denial of disability was observed in 1896 by Anton.[1] In 1914 Babinski[2] applied the term "anosognosia" to patients with left hemiplegia who completely denied or were unaware of their paralysis. Although denial is more common in patients with brain damage, more so in the acute phase, it has been observed in patients without brain damage, including paraplegics and amputees.

Weinstein and Kahn,[19] in a study of 104 brain-damaged patients, classified denial according to explicit expression in verbal terms ("I am not paralyzed, the person in the next bed is.") and implicit expression in terms of feeling or behavior (unrealistic goals, such as a quadriplegic patient rejoining his basketball team). The mood of patients with explicit verbal denial is usually bland and affable during interviews but may be depressed and perplexed outside of interviews. Euphoric and hypomanic or paranoid and depressed attitudes are more prominent in the group showing implicit denial. The patient's mood may change many times in the course of a day.

Denial is an important defense of the ego, permitting individuals to act as if they were not disabled. It can serve as an excuse for refusing help and aids patients to overcome overwhelming feelings of inferiority and helplessness. In some individuals, when this defense is unwittingly pierced (for example, seeing oneself in a mirror in the ambulation room), the result may be a severe agitated depression.[6]

In cases of complete denial, attempts at suggestion or logical argument are futile. Rather than attempt to deal directly with the denial, the clinician should work around it. Every effort should be made to engage the patient in rehabilitation procedures, which should be introduced gently and over time. Time and the therapeutic milieu are effective in most cases. When denial is implicit and there is considerable emotional lability, transquilizers such as the diazepene compounds or haloperidol may be given with supportive psychotherapy. Antidepressants such as the tricyclic compounds may also be used.

BRAIN-DAMAGED PATIENT

In a rehabilitation program, brain-damaged patients constitute a large percentage of the patient population. Most of their injuries are caused by cerebrovascular disease and cerebral palsy, but head trauma, postoperative brain tumor, and multiple sclerosis cause a fair number. They often pose special problems, not only in presenting symptoms but also in management.

In a sense the term "brain-damaged patient" is a misnomer, because in behavior and mental function, brain-damaged persons may differ as much from each other as they do from patients without brain damage. The fact of brain injury is not sufficient to determine how a person thinks or experiences the world. It is difficult to generalize, but from a psychiatric point of view the management of a brain-damaged person requires inquiry into four overlapping areas: nature of the brain injury, mental makeup and behavior of the person, services that a rehabilitation program can offer, and the social environment the person must face.

Concerning the brain injury itself, the following prognostic factors have been noted:

1. Age at which injury occurred. If the injury occurs early in life, as in cerebral palsy, habit patterns to cope with the defects are difficult to change.
2. Site of the lesion. For example, temporal lobe lesions tend to be more disruptive than lesions elsewhere in the brain.
3. Size of the lesion. This is often misleading. A very small lesion in a setting of generalized disease (for example, cerebrovascular disease) can be very serious. On the other hand, some patients with hemispherectomy show no striking impairment of ability.
4. Nature of damage. A clean gunshot wound may leave virtually no sequelae, whereas a stroke may produce gross changes in behavior.
5. Length of time since damage occurred. Many World War II brain-injury patients were able to function at their preinjury level when reexamined 10 years later, despite extensive brain wounds.

The knowledge provided by these facts may be insufficient to plan a treatment program. Knowledge of the patient's premorbid life history may be of crucial importance. For example, a successful, hard-driving business person may be depressed not as a direct consequence of brain damage but by loss of independence. Similarly, a person who has been independent all his life may show the same attitude toward the rehabilitation challenge.

Intimate knowledge of the rehabilitation program is necessary, including skills that can be taught, personnel involved in teaching, and other patients in the program. In addition, knowledge of the meaningful environment alternatives that confront the patient on discharge is important.

As stated previously, behavioral reactions to brain damage are varied. From the rehabilitation viewpoint, patients may be divided into two groups: those who show limited, specific, or no deficits ("nonorganic" mental syndrome) and those who demonstrate profound global impairment ("organic" mental syndrome).

"Nonorganic" mental syndrome

The "nonorganic" mental syndrome group consists of those with limited impairment of sensory or motor modal-

ities, but with essentially intact structure of the mental apparatus. Patients in this group may be depressed, show exaggerated dependency reactions, or exhibit any of the gamut of behavioral disturbances. However, when these disturbances occur, they generally are not the result of brain damage per se but reactions to internal and external stresses.

"Organic" mental syndrome

The "organic" mental syndrome group usually demonstrates profound behavioral disturbance, anxiety, and disorders in mentation, characterized by perceptual insecurity and distortions, thought disorders, regression, and disorders of body image.

Perceptual insecurity

Perceptual insecurity refers to the profound difficulties that some brain-damaged patients have in apprehending and integrating their experience. Although perceptual insecurity might be associated with or caused by sensory deficits, the two are not identical. At times the perceptual difficulty may be manifested in such diverse phenomena as visual inattention or fluctuation in memory, orientation, and concentration. Perceptual anomalies such as displacement and projection of sensations, reversals of commonly perceived shapes, and denial of experiences are reported.

Thinking disturbances

Thinking disturbances are lost powers to properly categorize experiences. Patients with thinking disturbances can no longer grasp essential similarities in their surroundings; that is, they cannot think abstractly but can reason concretely. Logical relationships either are difficult to establish or are based on irrelevant aspects of stimuli. For example, an object may be identified by its use and not its more general connotation. The patient may refer to an apple as something you eat and not as a fruit, or a chair as something you sit on and not as a piece of furniture.

Regression

Childlike responses characterize regression. Patients are profoundly dependent and tend to see the world according to their needs, wishes, and fears. They have a low tolerance for frustration. Psychologic tests and overt behavior are childlike in some respects but may show evidence of mature functioning. Children who sustained injuries at birth or early in life do not show regression as often as they show uneven development of skills and aptitudes.

Body image disturbance

Body image disturbance is one of the signal characteristics of brain damage. This finding may be elicited by a variety of neurologic and psychologic tests.

• • •

These four characteristics generally overlap and are seldom found to exist independently. They are associated with states of acute and profound anxiety, low frustration tolerance, stereotyped thinking, impulse disorders, fluctuating attention span, or extreme, debilitating loss of energy and lack of motivation.

Management of brain-damaged patients depends on evaluation. Patients who belong to the "nonorganic" category are treated like any other patient in the service. Untoward emotional reactions can be helped by insight and supportive psychotherapy. Psychoactive drugs in small doses may be necessary during periods of stress or crisis.

Patients with "organic" brain damage require special management. The rehabilitation program and goals are usually limited. Few activities are prescribed, and special efforts are made to keep the patient's environment constant so therapists and classes remain stable. Repetition and drill in teaching are emphasized. Many trials are needed to attain mastery in a skill, and these trials are spaced rather than massed together. Staff members are encouraged to build warm, personal relationships with the patients and not to react personally to aggressive and abusive behavior directed at them. Gentleness and firmness are the rule. A firm therapist presents a fixed, predictable figure in a world that has become otherwise disordered.

Recent research has suggested specific techniques for treatment of the perceptual and cognitive impairments resulting from brain damage.[5,8]

Psychotherapy for patients with organic brain damage is usually limited to support and is reality oriented. Psychoactive medications such as tranquilizers, antidepressants, hypnotics, and stimulants may be used, but with caution. Dosage is usually smaller than usual, and the potential for side effects and interactions must be kept in mind.

ANXIETY

Every patient who suffers physical disability probably experiences anxiety. Anxiety is a condition of heightened and often disruptive tension accompanied by a vague and disquieting feeling of prospective harm or distress. Through its effect on the autonomic nervous system, anxiety is likely to disrupt physiologic functions. Acute anxiety may produce generalized visceral tension, with spasms of the cardiac and pyloric ends of the stomach, intestinal symptoms, palpitation, tachycardia, extrasystole, and vasomotor flushing or blanching. The patient may assume a tense posture, show excessive vigilance, and have an uneven or strained voice and widely dilated pupils.

When anxiety is intolerable or unacceptable, a variety of defenses are brought into play to minimize painful feelings. These defenses often present themselves as symptoms and determine the diagnosis attached to the anxiety. Thus anxiety may be repressed from conscious awareness. It may be displaced onto an object or a situation to produce a phobia. It may be converted into a hysteric symptom. It may be controlled and walled off by means of obsessions or compulsions. Behavioral symptoms such as apathy, boredom,

and hyperactivity may appear. Anxiety may lead to psychosomatic disorders or hypochondriasis.

Depending on the qualitative and quantitative aspects of anxiety and on its defenses, it is called reactive (realistic) or neurotic. (Present-day DSM-III-R classification uses the diagnosis Adjustment Disorder or Anxiety State.[11,17]) In the reactive patient the anxiety is considered to be appropriate to the situation. In the neurotic patient the anxiety is greater than called for, or defenses are expressed in neurotic symptoms such as phobias or hysteria.

Most patients with physical disability manifest realistic or mildly neurotic anxiety that does not interfere significantly with rehabilitation. Such patients respond well to support, a sympathetic milieu, and rehabilitation procedures. In some patients anxiety interferes with rehabilitation because motor, perceptual, or cognitive performance becomes either disorganized and fragmented or rigid and inhibited. Supportive and insight therapy can be effective, aided by tranquilizers such as the benzodiazepine compounds. On occasion panic disorder with or without agoraphobia is observed; in this case the tricyclic antidepressants as well as behavioral therapy can be effective.

DEPRESSION

All patients with physical disability experience depression, just as they do anxiety. Depression may vary from mild sadness to the extremes of suicide and psychotic delusions. The degree of depression is determined less by the nature of the disability than by the individual who suffers it and its meaning to that person.

Depression may present itself in a variety of ways. Patients with the milder forms of depression are quiet, inhibited, unhappy, discouraged, and uninterested in their surroundings. In more severe states there is a constant unpleasant tension. These patients' interests are limited and always melancholy. Conversation is difficult, and patients are dejected and hopeless. They are so preoccupied with depressive rumination that attention, concentration, and memory are impaired. Insomnia, especially in the form of early awakening, is common. Vegetative symptoms such as constipation, anorexia, fatigue, and headaches are frequent complaints. Delusions may appear, and patients usually express ideas of guilt, unworthiness, and impoverishment. When elements of anxiety and anger are present, patients may become agitated. (These types of depression are classified in DSM-III-R as Adjustment Disorder with Depressed Mood; Dysthymic Disorder or Depressive Neurosis; Major Affective Disorder, Bipolar with Depression and Mania; or Major Depressive Disorder.[12])

Patients may defend themselves against depression by acting cheerful, even euphoric. In rare instances this may progress to states of hypomania or mania. Cheerful patients are often deceptive, because the observer admires them and reacts to them positively. However, there is always some element of depression that may reveal itself during an interview.

Guilt may be part of the depression. Guilt may be felt for real or imagined faults, and patients dredge up all kinds of experiences from the past to explain the accident or illness and heap blame on themselves.

Depression is also caused by loss of mastery resulting from the disability. The loss is related to mourning or grief and to a loss of self-esteem. Much of our self-esteem is derived from accomplishments that have social value. In the maturing process we learn to walk, talk, control our bladders and bowels, dress ourselves, wash ourselves, and perform a host of other activities. When a physical disability strikes, many of these skills are lost, some permanently. The patient is projected back into a childlike, helpless state, and this leads to depression.

Fortunately, a patient with mild depression does not often present a management problem. Usually, the therapeutic milieu, personnel, and activity provide sufficient support and outlets that the rehabilitation process is not disturbed. Patients with more severe depression usually reveal inhibited activity. Because the rehabilitation process is impaired, in these cases the depression is more likely to be recognized. Supportive psychotherapy is indicated.

When depression is severe, and particularly when the patient expresses suicidal thoughts, psychiatric consultation should be sought. Pharmacotherapy with antidepressive medication is used. This includes the tricyclic antidepressants such as imipramine and amitryptiline and perhaps some of the newer second-generation groups. On occasion monoamine oxidase inhibitors or lithium may be used. Attention must be paid to medication side effects, such as hypotension and anticholinergic actions, interactions with other medications, and pharmacodynamics in general. Most severely depressed patients respond well to such therapy.[12,14]

SUICIDE

Psychiatric problems pose few threats to patients' lives. Suicide is the most prominent problem, and proper evaluation of a suicidal threat demands experience and judgment.[15]

Patients often make remarks such as "I wish I were dead" or "I'm too much of a burden." The clinician should listen respectfully and carefully and reflect the patient's feeling tone as accurately as possible in terms of both quality and intensity. There is a difference, for example, between sadness and despair.

Some situations must be taken more seriously: depression of a neurotic or psychotic character; history of a past suicide attempt by the patient or a family member or friend or a history of a major affective disorder; persistent threats of suicide; anorexia, severe weight loss, insomnia, listlessness, apathy, hopelessness, continuous weeping, and general motor retardation that cannot be explained on the basis of the patient's disease or disability; dreams of death, mutilation, funerals, rejoining departed close persons; and loneliness or alienation.

Several specific comments are in order concerning suicide:

1. Although grossly disturbed psychotic patients are not usually accepted in a rehabilitation service, some psychotic patients may be. Some may have survived a suicide attempt that led to the physical disability.
2. Rehabilitation services see a large number of elderly patients. Suicide rates rise with increasing age in the general population. This has not been observed in patients on the rehabilitation service. However, the risk may increase after the patients have been discharged.
3. Sociologic studies have indicated a correlation between incidence of suicide and social disintegration and isolation. It may be that a rehabilitation setting provides even the most deprived patient with social support. This is a potent antidote to the isolation that is apparently a predisposing factor in suicide.

When suicidal threat is considered serious, or there is doubt, psychiatric consultation is necessary. Treatment is instituted, which may be instruction regarding management, continued psychotherapy, antidepressive medication, or, on rare occasions, electroconvulsive shock therapy. Despite present-day opposition to this therapy, it can be very effective in selected cases and may be lifesaving.

AGGRESSION AND HOSTILITY

The third of the triad of basic emotions (anxiety and depression being the others) is hostility or anger. Anger is most difficult to manage because it is socially the least acceptable. It also produces angry reactions in others and may be threatening to a patient dependent on others.

A hostile, aggressive patient may be exhibiting a reaction to the disability, seeing it as an unfair act of fate. The patient's anger may simply reflect a need to strike back at an unknown force that has so changed life. The patient may displace and project anger at physicians, nurses, other staff members, or patients.

Management can be a sorely trying experience. The initial impulse on the part of the staff is to react in kind, which only aggravates the situation. The best way is to be patient and attempt to understand the forces driving the patient. This is not always easy, especially when the welfare of other patients is concerned. Psychotherapy over time is helpful, as is behavioral therapy. At times, use of tranquilizers, mainly the benzodiazepine compounds, may be necessary.

In patients who have a personality disorder, management is more difficult. Therapy must be intensive and may require group therapy.

DEPENDENCY

Among the characteristics that differentiate humans from lower organisms is the long period of dependency they require for maturation. This dependency is physical, emotional, and social. Under normal, healthy circumstances, and barring obstacles to growth and maturation, the child gives up many dependencies and becomes an independent and mature adult, able to depend on others when in need and to be socially interdependent.

However, some individuals fail to grow in this way. They remain dependent and helpless, using a variety of conscious and unconscious adaptations to cope with stressful situations. They may repress earlier experiences and feelings and proceed to maturation, while unconsciously struggling to repair injuries suffered in earlier development.

Physical disability deprives patients of their mature skills and projects them into a state of actual dependency. Because the goals of rehabilitation often contradict those of dependent reactions, the very outcome of rehabilitation may rest on the management of dependency needs, based on an understanding of the dynamics behind them. A reasonably mature and well-integrated person may bend in the face of the acute problems created by the disability and may fall back for purposes of security. Dependency in such a patient is a reaction to anxiety and helplessness and serves as a psychologic crutch. Such dependency needs should be satisfied by means of support, sympathy, and warm acceptance. In time the patient usually gives up the dependency and makes progress in the rehabilitation program. In this case dependency is a temporary adaptation, and under favorable circumstances the patient's basic health and maturity will reemerge. (This assumes the absence of extensive brain damage or overwhelming disability.)

Where dependency behavior has played an important role in the patient's life and has become a basic part of his character structure (Dependent Personality Disorder), management is much more difficult. The disability fits into the patient's immature outlook on life and is used not only as a crutch to relieve anxiety but also as a pattern for an entire way of life. To attempt to satisfy the demands of such patients is futile, because they are insatiable. To deny the demands leads to bitter complaints and overt hostility. In general, the attitude of the staff should not be overtly hostile, but it must be reasonable and firm. At best, even in patients without disability, personality disorders are difficult to treat. It may be necessary to set partial and limited goals that are oriented to the rehabilitation process.

PAIN

Pain is a frequent accompaniment of physical disability. Although the source of pain is often tangible, determined by anatomy and pathology, on occasion it is not. Similarly, even though the source is tangible, the nature and degree may not seem consistent with the disease. This finding has led to a separation of pain into organic and psychogenic. This categorization may be convenient, but it often leads to errors in management.

In the final analysis all pain is a psychic phenomenon.

Consciousness of the sensation is dependent on the higher nervous centers and is subjective in nature. Unless this fact is emphasized, a dichotomy in thinking and practice may result—a tendency to treat the pain rather than the patient. Because pain can inhibit rehabilitation and lead to interpersonal difficulties, its proper management may spell the success or failure of the rehabilitation.

Pain produces emotional changes even in well-adjusted individuals. It increases dependency needs, self-centeredness, and irritability. Environmental factors also play a role. Pain tends to appear worse at night because of anxiety, isolation, and absence of external interests and diversions.

Patients vary in their threshold to painful stimuli. Tolerance may be constitutionally determined, but personality differences can be observed. The dependent, immature patient and the anxiety-ridden patient are more reactive to pain. The detached, emotionally controlled patient shows a higher tolerance. Hysteric patients may show conversion phenomena via pain, paresthesia, or anesthesia, with or without organic disease.

Successful management of pain stems from a thorough medical and psychosocial evaluation. This approach forms the basis for the numerous pain centers and clinics that have developed in the 1980s. All means of relieving the pain should be exhausted. Adjustments in the patient's life should be part of the therapeutic plan. Decrease in physical activity, use of rest periods, simplification of or decrease in responsibilities, and exhaustive inquiry as to possible sources of painful feelings in the environment—past, present and future—should be considered.

Psychotherapy and physical therapy, behavioral therapy including relaxation techniques and hypnosis, and analgesic medications have been used effectively.[7] Addiction to and dependency on narcotic and nonnarcotic drugs are dangers. Because tolerance usually precedes either physical or psychologic dependence, special attention should be given to it. Tolerance probably depends more on frequency of dose than size, so careful choice of drug and dose is necessary. Intermittent pain requires a short-acting drug such as meperidine (Demerol), although continuous pain requires longer-acting drugs such as levorphanol tartrate (Levo-Dromoran) or methadone. Codeine can be used freely with discretion, because it is rarely addictive. All narcotic drugs produce cross-addiction, and tolerance to one results in increased tolerance to all.

Finally, in recent years, psychoactive drugs such as tricyclic antidepressant drugs (imipramine, amitryptiline) have been found to be effective in the treatment of pain, particularly pain of neurologic origin. Where anxiety plays a role in pain, the benzodiazepine drugs may be used.

CONVERSION REACTION

Some individuals cope with anxiety or conflict by developing a physical impairment unrelated to the real underlying pathology. Disturbances of sensation and motion are the most common. The former include anesthesia, paresthesia, and pain. Superficial or deep sensation may be affected. Disturbances of motion include paralyses, usually of limbs, digits, or speech mechanisms, and uncontrolled movements such as tics or convulsions.

Because many of the phenomena of conversion simulate the syndromes seen in rehabilitation medicine, differential diagnosis is of the utmost importance, although at times very difficult. The patient with conversion usually demonstrates the following characteristics:

1. The neurologic signs follow the patient's idea of anatomic distribution, such as in stocking and glove anesthesia. Inconsistent and physiologically impossible combinations are seen, such as hysteric paraplegia without loss of bowel and bladder control or without expected atrophy of muscles.
2. The conversion symptoms have a symbolic meaning and are related to unconscious conflict or to the precipitation situation.
3. The patient reveals far less anxiety than organic illness of the same degree would be expected to show—*la belle indifference*.
4. Patients display features of a neurotic personality. They are suggestible and prone to therapeutic suggestion such as faith cures and placebos.

Treatment includes suggestion, hypnosis, and occasionally more intensive psychotherapy. It must be emphasized that conversion reactions are not deliberate and thus differ fundamentally from malingering.

SEXUAL PROBLEMS

Of all the problems confronting the disabled patient, probably least has been written about problems with sexual function. The disabled patient seldom ventures to discuss them, and the examiner often fails to question the patient. Both are anxious, both are protective. The disability is often so overwhelming and the problems so difficult that discussion of sexual problems seems of low priority. Discussing the problem may carry the feeling that one is adding insult to injury.

Sexual behavior is dependent on both biologic and psychologic factors. Biologic, neurologic, and endocrinologic factors are necessary for adequate physiologic sexual functioning. Behaviorally, early psychosocial development, along with numerous social and cultural experiences, leads to conscious and unconscious attitudes that affect sexual fantasies and impulses. Sex in human beings is more than a biologic phenomenon. It is a profoundly emotional experience, carrying a host of emotional attitudes, both positive and negative, and often reflecting the deepest sources of self-esteem and satisfaction.

In physically disabled persons sexual function may be interfered with in two ways: anatomic injury to the genitalia or spinal cord, which may make some forms of sexual

function impossible, and psychologic changes resulting from a disability, such as doubts about adequacy, attractiveness, and potency.[10]

Problems of the male are different than those in the female. In the male, cord injury leads to partial or complete impotence. Paraplegic males who are impotent are more depressed, withdrawn, and emotionally overwhelmed than those who are potent. They regard their bodies as useless and present more difficulties in constructively dealing with readjustment and rehabilitation. Many are apprehensive at the thought of returning home to their wives and families.

In the female, problems include not only attractiveness and acceptability problems but also the ability to bear children. Anatomically and physiologically, physical disability does not impair sexual receptivity in females. Because of sensory difficulties, vaginal and clitoral orgasm may be impaired. However, as with the male, this lack does not preclude sexual satisfaction. Nor is fertility always impaired in females. (See Chapter 62 for further discussion of sexual problems.)

Sexual activity also induces fear other than those mentioned: fear of recurrence of the disease and physical disability, for example, stroke or heart attack. Studies indicate that normal sexual activity does not increase the chances of recurrence.

REFERENCES

1. Anton, G: Blindheit nach beiderseitiger Gehirnerkrankung mit Verlust der Orientierung in Raume, Mittherlungen des Vereines der Ärzte in Steiermark 33:41, 1896.
2. Babinski, J: Contribution à l'etude des troubles mentaux dans l'hemiplégie organique cérébrale (anosognosie), Rev Neurol 27:845, 1914.
3. Baldessarini, RJ: Chemotherapy in psychiatry, ed 2, Cambridge, Mass, 1985, Harvard University Press.
4. Coyle, JT: Introduction to the world of neurotransmitters and neuroreceptors, APA Psychiatry Update Ann Rev 4:3, 1985.
5. Diller, L, and Gordon, WA: Interventions for cognitive deficits in brain injured adults, J Consult Clin Psychol 49:822, 1981.
6. Fisher, SH: Mechanism of denial in physical disabilities, Arch Neurol Psychiatry 80:782, 1958.
7. Fordyce, WE, et al: Some implications of learning in problems of chronic pain, J Chronic Dis 21:179, 1968.
8. Gordon, WA, et al: Perceptual remediation in patients with right brain damage—a comprehensive program, Arch Phys Med Rehabil 66:353, 1985.
9. Grayson, M, Levy, J, and Powers, A: Psychiatric aspects of rehabilitation. Rehabilitation Monographs 2, New York, 1952, Institute of Physical Medicine and Rehabilitation, New York University Medical Center.
10. Held, JP, et al: Sexual attitude reassessment workshop: effect on spinal cord injured adults, their partners, and rehabilitation professionals, Arch Phys Med Rehabil 56:14, 1975.
11. Klein, DF: The anxiety disorders, APA Psychiatry Update 3:390, 1984.
12. Klerman, GL: Depressive disorders, APA Psychiatry Update 2:354, 1983.
13. Lipowski, ZJ: Consultation-liaison psychiatry, APA Psychiatry Update 3:177, 1984.
14. Robinson, RG, Lipsey, JR, and Price, TR: Diagnosis and clinical management of post-stroke depression, Psychosomatics 26:769, 1985.

15. Roy, A, editor: Suicide, Baltimore, 1986, Williams & Wilkins Co.

16. Spiegel, D, and Agros, WS: Psychiatric contributions to medical care, APA Psychiatry Update Ann Rev 5:526, 1986.

17. Spitzer, RL, editor: Diagnostic and statistical manual of mental disorders, ed 3-R, Washington, DC, 1987, American Psychiatric Association.

18. Von Monakow, C: Experimentelle und pathologisch-anatomische Untersuchungen über die Beziehungen der sogenannten Sehsphare zu den infrakortikalen Opticuscentren und zum N. opticus, Arch Psychiatry 16:151, 1885.

19. Weinstein, EA, and Kahn, R: Denial of illness: symbolic and psychologic aspects, Springfield, Ill, 1955, Charles C Thomas, Publisher.

20. Yalom, ID, et al: Group psychotherapy, APA Psychiatry Update Ann Rev 5:655, 1986.

ADDITIONAL READINGS

APA Psychiatry Update Annu Rev 1-7, 1982–88.

Drugs for psychiatric disorders, Med Lett 28:99, 1986.

Drugs that cause psychiatric symptoms, Med Lett 28:81, 1986.

Goldstein, G, and Ruthven, L: Rehabilitation of the brain-damaged adult, New York, 1983, Plenum Press.

Kaplan, HI, and Sadock, BJ: Comprehensive textbook of psychiatry, ed 4, Baltimore, 1985, Williams & Wilkins Co.

Rizack, MA, and Hillman, CDM: The Medical Letter handbook of adverse drug interactions, New Rochelle, 1985, The Medical Letter.

Yodofsky, SC, et al: Neuropsychiatry, APA Psychiatry Update Ann Rev 4:101, 1985.

CHAPTER 57

Psychologic services in medical rehabilitation

LEONARD DILLER

A psychologic service is concerned with two overlapping dimensions—facilitating patient rehabilitation fit and assessing and managing patients with psychologic difficulties. Patient rehabilitation fit involves identifying patients who can profit from rehabilitation services, what goals can be reasonably set for a given individual if accepted for a rehabilitation program, how the tasks can be brought into harmony with the needs of a given person, and what strategies should be pursued to facilitate the rehabilitation process. In a sense the psychologist serves as a consultant to a team of skilled professionals who conduct assessments and therapies. The second dimension of concern focuses on the person with psychologic problems. In this case the role of the psychologist is closer to that of the traditional clinician, who assesses psychopathologic conditions and treats people with psychologic problems. In either case an effective psychologic service requires that the psychologist be routinely available and be a team member in the overall medical rehabilitation service system.[19]

The effectiveness of a psychologic service is closely related not only to the technical skills of the psychologist, but also to the application of those skills to help solve problems as they unfold. Effectiveness, then, depends on timeliness of consultations and interventions and ease of communication between the psychologist and the other members of the team.

Although the psychologist as diagnostician and psychotherapist applies the traditional skills of a clinician to rehabilitation patients, the psychologist as consultant to the rehabilitation team must draw on a set of skills beyond individual psychologic diagnosis or therapy. These skills require knowledge of disease and disability characteristics, and of rehabilitation services. This knowledge includes the dynamics involved in the interactions between people emerging from severe trauma or illness and a team of professionals, who may be eager to restore and rehabilitate their patients as quickly as possible.

PSYCHOLOGIC RESPONSES IN MEDICAL REHABILITATION

Individual patients entering a medical rehabilitation program are usually emerging from the stress of acute trauma or illness. They may be facing the permanent loss of a body part or loss of vital skills or bodily functions. In addition to anxiety related to uncertainty over the future, a threat exists to the body image and the integrity of the entire individual, including a sense of continuity and self-esteem. The patient's values and energies become focused on grappling with loss and with survival as an impaired or disabled individual.

Anxiety is accompanied by a narrowing of perspective; the individual may focus only on the present and have a difficult time in projecting expectations. Future planning is difficult. During this period the individual may hover between feelings that complete recovery or restitution of function will occur (denial) and feelings that no further recovery or restitution of functions can take place and that life is over (depression). In this frame of mind individuals may set arbitrary periods for recovery. When the magic date, for example, 6 months, passes without recovery taking place, the patient sets another date. Patients will often seek confirmation of signs of recovery by hyperalertness to their own body sensations and functions; to the comments of other patients, particularly those with similar conditions; and to the comments and attitudes expressed by members of the rehabilitation team. The patients reinforce this selective attention to signs of recovery by defense mechanisms, translated into statements such as "I'm different," "It's not really happening," or "There will be a cure for me." Most observers regard denial and depression as inevitable with some individual differences in their timing and duration. In one form or another, individuals go through stages in adaptation to loss, similar to those seen in mourning.[21] These stages or steps involve refusal to believe the loss is real, continued search to try to recover the loss, realization that life will continue, and acceptance of the fact that life can be lived despite the loss. Manifestations of these phases may include shock, denial, anger, guilt, bargaining, somatization, and depression.[32] It is critical to note that negative emotions are common and not exceptional in rehabilitation settings. Although these stages have been observed most frequently in settings where people are admitted soon after onset, they may also appear at further points in time, such as in the case of parents of children with developmental disabilities who may go through chronic mourning. Some observers have argued against the inevitability of going through these stages before accepting disability.[33] Others have noted that, while stages in acceptance may be normal, clinical problems may occur when the negative emotions (anger, depression, anxiety) become fixated to the point that they interfere with the patient's maximum use of the program. The patient's premorbid personality is often a factor, not only in defining a context within which a disability is perceived, but also because some disabilities may arise as a result of imprudent or impulsive behavior, suicidal gestures, or engagement in high-risk sports.[12]

Life circumstances, including age, sex, and vocational and family status, also constrain the way patients perceive the disability, their support systems, and available opportunities. For example, middle-class people have better outcomes than lower-class people.

The 1980s have seen an expanding body of knowledge in the emerging field of health psychology. This field, closely allied to behavioral medicine, is of interest to physiatrists. Whereas earlier work in psychosomatic medicine focused on psychic factors as causes of physiologic changes and physical symptoms, and somatopsychology has focused on the idea that disability and personality structure are basically unrelated,[31] health psychology is concerned with psychologic factors as adaptation to specific illnesses. Although no compelling evidence exists that specific personality traits are associated with specific populations, certain issues have received more attention in certain disability groups and may highlight what is common in all disability groups. Examples include sexual function in the paraplegic,[33] faith in the medical diagnosis in the multiple sclerosis patient,[29] fear of activity in the cardiac patient,[3,20] breakdown in communication between patient and family or between patient and physician in the cancer patient,[23] and compliance with therapy in the pain patient.[4] More detailed discussion of specific diseases and disabilities may be found in *Coping with Chronic Disease* by Burish and Bradley.[5]

REHABILITATION SETTINGS—SOME PSYCHOLOGIC IMPLICATIONS

Rehabilitation medicine settings may be generally considered as places in which diagnostic and therapeutic services are organized to meet the needs of patients with impairments or disabilities associated with combinations of physical, psychologic, social, and vocational disturbances resulting from disease or trauma. In inpatient settings as well as in some outpatient programs, much time is spent in attending classes, in which patients acquire skills to function more independently. Staff members devote a great deal of energy to these educational efforts. Bleiberg and Merbitz[2] examined close to 9000 chart entries for a group of spinal cord injury patients and found that 65% of the notes were concerned with statements that reflected teaching and learning and attempts to accelerate or decelerate specific behaviors.

In a sense one might argue that rehabilitation presents a patient with a series of tasks that must be mastered. Rehabilitation is unique in the scope and organization of its tasks, which include many quality of life issues beyond those normally considered in medical settings. Further reflection suggests that the tasks pose different kinds of demands. These demands can be rank ordered into a hierarchy of preference or difficulty. Consider the sample of inpatients who were interviewed when entering a comprehensive medical inpatient program. Although almost every patient wanted complete recovery, 80% wanted improvement in aspects of activities of daily living (ADL), 40% wanted help in social and vocational domains, and only 10% wanted help for psychologic problems. The goals are hierarchic in the sense that those who wanted recovery or even recovery and improvement in ADL did not necessarily want improvement in the psychosocial areas. Those who wanted improvement in the less frequently mentioned domains always wanted improvement in the more frequently mentioned domains. The fact that only 10% wanted to achieve psychologic goals of greater self-confidence and reduction in fear and anxiety is puzzling; objective estimates of psychologic disturbance in inpatient settings are said to be close to 50%,[1] and clinical estimates may be higher. The reason for the rank order of preferences may be that people tend to be more focused on physical recovery when entering a rehabilitation program. The tasks in physical restoration activities address the immediate physical demands. The tasks in the psychologic, social, and vocational areas focus on the future and are more complex. ADL skills are learned in childhood. Social and vocational skills are learned through adolescence and adulthood. They are more difficult to deal with than task demands in physical and occupational therapy.[8]

Indeed, the individual's ability to use all of the therapeutic modalities available in a rehabilitation setting may be a mark of ego strength. Paradoxically, people who are most depressed and most somatically preoccupied and seemingly in greatest need of psychologic therapy may be most reluctant to participate in a talking therapy or plan for the future.

Some of the problems of noncompliance with rehabilitation programs that have been traditionally described as problems in motivation may therefore be regarded from a different perspective. The task demands of the program may not be congruent with the patient's abilities at a given time. The rehabilitation staff must reexamine the goals it has set for the patient and ask itself two questions: What tasks can the individual perform within the structure of the program? What conditions should be altered to facilitate enhanced performance? This line of reasoning conforms with three views. Shontz[31] argued that as rehabilitation workers have grown increasingly sophisticated, there has been a shift in attributing motivational problems from the intrapsychic exclusively to problems related to pressures and obstacles in the environment as well. Based on experimental demonstration, Wool, Sigel, and Fine[37] hypothesized that exposing spinal cord injury patients to experiences of success helps to immunize them against feelings of learned helplessness. Fordyce's more radical statement argued that the control of response contingencies by manipulating reinforcement properties of environments can alter learning in important ways.[11] Thus "pain behaviors" (inactivity, complaints) can be reduced by reinforcing the nonpain behaviors (being active and not speaking of the pain).

Fordyce's example points to an additional aspect of rehabilitation and the role of the psychologist. Psychologic treatment can often be delivered by the psychologist collaborating intensively with another member of the team who may actually conduct the treatment. For example, Varni and associates[34] used social rewards and manipulation of task performance to help diminish crying in a 3-year-old girl with severe burns who would not comply with occupational therapy. Redd[30] used principles of behavior modification to establish self-feeding behavior in a child in a pediatric rehabilitation unit. Applications to physical therapy appear particularly useful. Thus Klein, Kewman, and Sayoma[18] used behavior modification successfully to address the complaints of a woman with a 16-year history of gait problem and multiple somatic complaints. Gouvier and colleagues[15] used reward and desensitization procedures for two patients who resisted the use of orthopedic devices.

PSYCHOLOGIC EVALUATION

Psychologic assessments may be divided into two major categories, each of which has different purposes and consumes different amounts of time and energy.

Psychologic screening

Psychologic screenings are generally brief, ranging from 15 minutes to 60 minutes, and are applied routinely to as many patients as possible on entry or just before entry to a program. The aims of the screening are to help determine patient program fit, define major needs of the patient in the psychologic sphere, set goals for a patient, anticipate problems in working with a patient or in implementing goals, and delineate the personal resources a patient can draw on to make maximal use of the program. Psychologic screenings may rely on interviews or brief samples of standard tests. They serve to provide useful information to other members of the team, to make the patient known to the psychologist, make the psychologist known to the patient in the event that problems occur in the course of the program, and to identify patients who may need more intensive assessment and interventions by the psychologist.

Psychologic examinations

More intensive psychologic evaluations are often used for assessment in the following populations or situations in rehabilitation[16]:

1. The weight and role of functional versus organic elements in understanding and managing a symptom complex or behavioral pattern
2. Patients with histories of suspected or actual personality disturbances
3. Patients with problems in educational or vocational planning
4. Patients with known or suspected brain damage
5. Patients who pose management problems for the rehabilitation team

In all of these instances, the written referral to the psychologist should contain specific questions or issues that prompted the referral. The more specific the question, the more focused the assessment and report can be.

In considering psychologic reports, several models might be noted. First, psychologic assessments may be viewed as x-ray studies that provide a picture of an underlying psychic structure, whether one is regarding the structure of personality or mental abilities. From the underlying structure, one makes a deduction about the nature and extent of a problem. From this viewpoint psychologic tests have the virtue of yielding objective scores based on standardized methods of administration, which can be compared against normative groups. For certain diagnostic issues, such data are invaluable. However, for certain issues the questions behind the referral are narrower and more immediate. Should a patient be discharged or continued on the program? How serious is the presenting problem? For example, a patient may speak of depression and hint at self-destructive behavior. How much attention should be paid to the comments? Is the patient's complaint of pain merely an excuse for not cooperating on a program? Is the patient playing staff members against each other? Should one confront or go along with the patient? The physician can expect a direct correlation between the specificity of the question and the specificity of the recommendations.

In working with populations of disabled people, experienced psychologists recognize that some patients may fail for reasons that are irrelevent to competence. These include the following:

1. Sensory limitations, for example, vision or hearing loss, may diminish adequacy of response.
2. Motor impairments, for example, paralyses, may limit ability to perform manual tasks.
3. Cultural impoverishment. For example, children with congenital disabilities may not have the advantage of normal environmental stimulations or may have distorted histories of social reinforcement.
4. Many items on behavioral or personality questionnaires that might indicate a pathologic psychic disturbance could be explained by other factors. For example, difficulty in falling asleep, usually attributed to anxiety, may occur because the patient is being tested in an inpatient hospital setting, where sleeplessness is common. "I feel depressed" might be a common response for a person emerging from severe trauma. Traditional notions of psychopathology may not apply in settings where anxiety and depression occur with such frequency.
5. Adequate norms. Test standards are usually compiled from samples of people who are physically able, with none of the limitations listed here.

To obviate some of these difficulties, psychologists have developed tests that bypass impairments. An individual who cannot speak or write might be presented with the tests in a multiple-choice format. Some psychologists have developed norms based on large numbers of subjects with the same disability to indicate how a particular patient compares with other patients in the same setting.[14] In some instances where neither of the above options apply, it is helpful to suspend normal criteria such as time limits. Providing cues might also be useful. Although the use of standard norms in this situation may or may not be appropriate, because standard conditions of test administration were not maintained, any change in test conditions should be acknowledged in the report.

Although the choice of specific tests to evaluate a patient might be left to the psychologist, the following may be noted.

Personality tests

Personality tests may be divided into projective and objective tests. Projective tests such as the Rorschach Test and the Thematic Appreciation Test use deliberately ambiguous stimuli so that the way the person responds reflects the person's attitudes, affect, style, thought processes, and needs rather than being intrinsic to the stimulus. Projective tests are most useful for the study of idiosyncratic features of personality and psychodynamics. Because they are difficult to reduce to quantitative dimensions with norms, they are seldom used in research.

Objective tests use unambiguous stimuli and elicit responses that can be scored and compared against norms.

Objective tests of personality may yield multidimensional, broad-ranging profiles such as the Minnesota Multiphasic Personality Inventory (MMPI) or the Millon Behavioral Health Inventory.[27] However, some objective tests may be narrower in scope and targeted for specific dimensions, such as affect (for example, Multiple Affect Adjective Check List), attribution of responsibility (for example, locus of control), or behavior pattern.[17] Because objective tests do not require as much clinical skill in their administration, they can be self-administered or administered by a less well-trained person.

Cognitive tests

The most popular tests of intelligence in current use are the Wechsler Intelligence Scales,[35] which have versions for adults and children. The Wechsler Scales view intelligence as an average of a sampling of 11 abilities in different areas. In addition to the average score and separate verbal and performance scores, clinicians have used profiles of scores as valuable clues to differential impairments in mental abilities that point to psychopathology or brain damage. Thus two people with the same intelligence may have different profiles of abilities, which are more important diagnostically than the overall intelligence level. For use when time does not permit a full-scale assessment, shortened versions of the Wechsler Scales have been developed. In addition, brief mental status examinations can be used for screening purposes and might be incorporated as part of clinical examinations. These include the Mini Mental State,[9] which has been used for stroke patients, and the Dementia Rating Scale,[26] which has been used to assess orientation and memory loss in elderly and dementia patients. Test batteries designed for specific populations, such as quadriplegics suspected of having brain damage, are useful.[37] A detailed discussion of test batteries used in clinical neuropsychology may be found in *Neuropsychological Assessment* by Lezak.[24] Caplan discussed their application in a rehabilitation setting.[6] Finally, it should be noted that patients who need to be assessed for educational or vocational purposes may require extensive batteries of cognitive assessments.

Other tests

Interests, vocational aptitudes, and educational attainments may also be incorporated into test batteries. Thus a full-scale workup may last from 3 to 10 hours.

PSYCHOLOGIC INTERVENTIONS

Psychologic interventions are usually equated with counseling and psychotherapy. In nonrehabilitation settings psychotherapy is usually identified with the treatment of symptoms and conflicts related to intrapsychic problems that have a long history. In rehabilitation, individuals who present such problems constitute a minority of patients requiring interventions. The primary problems deal with the psychology of loss and dependency in a stressful context of having to learn new skills. Psychologic interventions aim to (1) support and facilitate the resolution of emotional conflicts and disturbing negative affects, (2) enhance compliance with the task demands of a rehabilitation setting, (3) reduce emotional distress, and (4) improve cognitive or behavioral disturbances following brain damage (see Chapter 9). A survey of types of psychotherapy in an inpatient setting indicates that psychologic support, to reinforce the individual's assets and resources to cope with problems, is the most frequent type of psychotherapy. Providing information in the context of a good emotional relationship, dealing with issues of planning, and working with negative reactions and conflicts occur about equally often.[7,8]

In addition to individual psychotherapy, group therapy is also useful. Group psychotherapy in rehabilitation settings is usually time limited. It may vary in degree of emphasis from a given structured topic, such as assertiveness training, to open ended. In general, experience suggests that groups that are focused and have informational components such as lectures are more successful than open-ended groups that feature only discussions of emotions. Groups may often be helpful if there is co-leadership, with psychologists leading groups together with a physician or other health professionals.

Active, ongoing consultation is an important component of a psychologic service program. Patients may sometimes place rehabilitation team members under stress because of their demands. Gans[13] has noted instances of anger on the part of rehabilitation team members in a stroke unit who felt powerless to deal with patients who were uncooperative or denied the presence of a disability. Therapists often have to deal with anxious and depressed patients. An important point to note is that the misjudging of patients may occur in both directions—the staff may think some patients are anxious when they are not, or they may overlook patients who are anxious. Lawson[22] has tracked significant events in a group of spinal cord injury patients while undergoing rehabilitation. These events included sickness, physician's prognosis, personal events, and last 5 days in the hospital. All of these serve to heighten depression or elation, which spill over into performance on the program and may require consultation.

ROLE ISSUES

Counseling and mental health consultation touch on the competencies of a number of related fields, including social work, psychiatry, and rehabilitation counseling. Palmer and co-workers[28] reported an interdisciplinary team approach to help obviate role confusion, overlapping efforts, and discontinuity of care. Among the considerations are definition of the goals of the intervention and the specific needs of the population, the skills and duties basic to the training of each discipline, areas of overlap and exclusiveness, tasks

Table 57-1. Task assignments to psychosocial team members

Task	Social work	Psychology	Psychiatry
		Psychosocial discipline	
Psychosocial screening	X		
Discharge planning	X		
Community service liaison	X		
Problem-focused counseling	X		
Cognitive evaluation		X	
Personality evaluation		X	
Behavioral change programs		X	
Psychotherapy		X	X
Differential diagnosis			X
Management of dangerous and psychotic patients			X
Treatment of alcohol and drug addiction			X
Monitoring psychotropic medication			X
Collaborating with rehabilitation team	X	X	X
Family conferences	X	X	X
Group therapy	X	X	X
Pain management	X	X	X
Sex counseling	X	X	X

From Palmer, S, et al: Arch Phys Med Rehabil 66:690, 1985.

performed by each discipline, available resources in terms of time and personnel, and integration of efforts of the team members. Table 57-1 presents an approach to these issues.

Specialty and subspecialty groups within psychology have mushroomed in recent years. It is therefore important for the physiatrist to be aware of some distinctions to achieve the kind of service being sought. Although space does not permit detailed considerations, the following may be noted. Within the last two decades there has been a division of the American Psychological Association, whose nearly 1000 members are considered rehabilitation psychologists. Not all of these psychologists engage in clinical work, but all are involved in rehabilitation and are familiar with issues in disability and rehabilitation. This group arose because it was recognized that the main emphasis in training and interests in clinical psychology has been in mental health and psychiatric settings. The clinical populations and treatment aims in such settings overlap those of a rehabilitation setting, but they are not the same. Two other specialty groups have evolved as needs in the field have become more differentiated. Health psychology is concerned with the issues of maintenance of health and prevention and adaptation to disease, and clinical neuropsychology is concerned with identifying the presence of brain damage and its consequences for behavior. These subfields are closely allied to rehabilitation psychology and have common interests. They have developed a growing body of data and techniques of interest to rehabilitation professionals.

REFERENCES

1. Berven, NL, Habeck, RV, and Malec, JF: Predominant MMPI: 168 profile clusters in a rehabilitation medicine sample, Rehabil Psychol 30:209, 1985.
2. Bleiberg, J, and Merbitz, C: Learning goals during initial rehabilitation hospitalization, Arch Phys Med Rehabil 64:448, 1984.
3. Bloom, LJ: Psychology and cardiology collaboration in coronary treatment and prevention, Prof Psychol 10:485, 1979.
4. Bradley, LD: Coping with pain. In Burish, TG, and Bradley, LD, editors: Coping with chronic disease. New York, 1983, Academic Press, Inc.
5. Burish, TG, and Bradley, LD, editors: Coping with chronic disease, New York, 1983, Academic Press, Inc.
6. Caplan, B: Neuropsychology in rehabilitation: its role in evaluation and intervention, Arch Phys Med Rehabil 63:362, 1982.
7. Diller, L: Psychological theory in rehabilitation counseling, J Couns Psychol 6(3):61, 1959.
8. Diller, L: Client-counselor relationships to counseling in rehabilitation process. In Jacobs, A, Jordan, J, and DiMichael, S, editors: Client counselor relationships in vocational rehabilitation, New York, 1961, Bureau of Publishers, Teachers College, Columbia University.
9. Folstein, MD, Folstein, SE, and McHugh, PR: Mini-mental state, J Psychiatr Res 12:189, 1975.
10. Fordyce, WE: Personality characteristics in men with spinal cord injury as related to manner of onset of disability, Arch Phys Med Rehabil 45:541, 1964.
11. Fordyce, WE: Behavioral methods for chronic pain and illness, St Louis, 1976, The CV Mosby Co.
12. Fordyce, WE: Interdisciplinary process: implications for rehabilitation psychology, Rehabil Psychol 27:5, 1982.
13. Gans, J: Hate in the rehabilitation setting, Arch Phys Med Rehabil 64:176, 1983.
14. Gordon, WA, et al: The evaluation of deficits associated with right brain damage: Normative Data on the Institute of Rehabilitation Medicine test battery. New York, 1980, New York University Medical Center, Research and Training Center on Head Trauma and Stroke.
15. Gouvier, WD, et al: Behavior modification in physical therapy, Arch Phys Med Rehabil 66:113, 1985.
16. Grzesiak, RC: Psychological services in rehabilitation medicine: clinical aspects of rehabilitation psychology, Prof Psychol 10:511, 1979.
17. Jenkins, CD, Zyzanski, SJ, and Rosenman, RH: Jenkins Activity Survey Manual, New York, 1979, The Psychological Corp.
18. Klein, Kewan, and Sayoma.
19. Koocher, GP, Sourkes, BM, and Keane, WM: Pediatric oncology consultations: a generalizable model for medical settings, Prof Psychol 10:475, 1979.
20. Krantz, D, and Deckel, AW: Coping with coronary heart disease and stroke. In Burish, TG, and Bradley, LA, editors: Coping with chronic disease, New York, 1983, Academic Press, Inc.
21. Kübler-Ross, E: Questions and answers on death and dying, New York, 1974, Macmillan, Inc.
22. Lawson, NC: Significant events in rehabilitation process: patient's point of view, Arch Phys Med Rehabil 59:573, 1978.
23. Levy, SM: The process of death and dying: Behavioral and social factors. In Burish, TG, and Bradley, LA, editors: Coping with chronic disease, New York, 1983, Academic Press, Inc.
24. Lezak, MD: Neuropsychological assessment, ed. 2, New York, 1983, Oxford University Press.
25. Lifshitz, K: Problems in the quantitative evaluation of the psychoses of the senium, J Psychol 19:295, 1960.
26. Mattis, S: Mental status examination for organic mental syndrome for the elderly patient. In Bellak, L, and Karasau, TB, editors: Geriatric psychiatry, New York, 1976, Grune & Stratton, Inc.
27. Millon, T, Green, CJ, and Meagher, RB: The MBHI: a new inventory for psychodiagnostian in medical settings, Prof Psychol 10:25, 1979.
28. Palmer, S, et al: Psychosocial success in rehabilitation, Arch Phys Med Rehabil 66:690, 1985.
29. Pavlou, M, et al: A program of psychologic service delivery in a multiple sclerosis center, Prof Psychol 10:563, 1979.
30. Redd, WH: Treatment of excessive coping in a terminal cancer patient: a time series analyses, J Behav Med 2:81, 1979.
31. Shontz, FA: Psychological adjustment to disability, Arch Phys Med Rehabil 59:251, 1978.
32. Stewart, T, and Shields, CR: Grief in chronic illness: assessment and management, Arch Phys Med Rehabil 66:447, 1985.
33. Trieschmann, R: The psychological social and vocational adjustment to spinal cord injury: a strategy for future research, Rep 13 P 159011-9-01, Washington, DC, April, 1978, Rehabilitation Services Administration.
34. Varni, J, et al: Behavioral management of chronic pain in children care study, Arch Phys Med Rehabil 61:375, 1980.
35. Wechsler, D: The measurement of adult intelligence, ed 3, Baltimore, 1944, Williams & Wilkins Co.
36. Wilmot, CB, et al: Occult head injury: its evidence in spinal cord injury, Arch Phys Med Rehabil 66:227, 1985.
37. Wool, RN, Siegel, D, and Fine, PR: Task performance in spinal cord injury: effect of helplessness in training, Arch Phys Med Rehabil 61:321, 1980.

CHAPTER 58

Vocational rehabilitation counseling services

PATRICIA DVONCH

In attempting to discuss the state of the art of vocational rehabilitation counseling services, one must first define what vocational rehabilitation counseling is and describe its current place in rehabilitation. Defining vocational rehabilitation counseling is no easy task, for its unique niche is not readily apparent. As a counseling specialty, it overlaps extensively with general psychologic counseling, social work practice, and what is currently called community counseling. Yet the strength and influence of the discipline of vocational rehabilitation counseling, with interpersonal counseling skills central to the process, can be traced to World War I, when disabled veterans required job placement.

After World War II rehabilitation in general and vocational rehabilitation counseling in particular experienced its greatest growth. Factors that contributed to this included federal monetary support to provide training for professionals in all areas of rehabilitation and health and human services personnel who were positioned to take advantage of federal grants. Vocational rehabilitation counselors, because of their specialized training, consistently have been found to possess the very specific skills necessary to coordinate, plan, and promote a safe and timely return to work for clients with disabling conditions.

By the 1960s the number of graduate programs in rehabilitation counseling had grown to more than 55. Today there are 84 such programs, located in universities as separate departments or as leading programs in departments of allied health services, counseling psychology, special education, and educational psychology.

Vocational counseling services in the rehabilitation process have been changing, yet in some ways have remained the same since 1920, when Congress voted into law vocational rehabilitation services for World War I disabled veterans and injured industrial workers. Changes include the shorter length of time available for evaluation and vocational planning; the shorter stay for a client in a rehabilitation hospital; and the serving of clients as outpatients in a comprehensive not-for-profit rehabilitation center rather than in a hospital. Perhaps the strongest evidence of change resides in a word—"optimum" has replaced "maximum" as the goal of state and federal vocational rehabilitation services.

Change has also occurred in types of disabling conditions. Although persons with amputations and spinal cord injuries remain a significant percentage of the vocational service population, persons with diagnoses of traumatic brain injury (TBI), developmental disabilities, and severe mental and emotional retardation now tend to be the clients who require long-term planning and creative, innovative vocational evaluation techniques.

In many respects the task of the vocational rehabilitation counselor is similar to what it was in the 1920s: 3 weeks to 6 months is considered an end point for physical restoration; education and previous work evaluation are the principal determinants in establishing job potential; labor market needs are considered; and the attitudes and fears that many employers have about an employee's chance of further disability are still obstacles. The Great Depression heavily influenced types of services provided, even as today, when a tight job market and dramatically changing technology determine the services needed.

These changes contribute to a renewed vitality and create an arena for creativity and innovation for the vocational rehabilitation counselor in planning and implementing services for the disabled client. The following pages define the role of the vocational rehabilitation counselor and discuss current practice, history, evolution, and selected legislation that has molded the professional and the profession. Attention is also given to how, what, and to whom services are provided; the impact of improved medical technology and consequent changes in groups served; the kind and severity of disabling conditions encountered today; and future trends.

VOCATIONAL REHABILITATION COUNSELOR

The professional rehabilitation counselor works with people who have physical, mental, and social disabilities to help them understand their capabilities and limitations and use this knowledge to build vocationally and socially productive lives. In addition to conducting individual and group counseling sessions, vocational rehabilitation counselors may perform a variety of other tasks, depending on their employment setting. Counselors collect and analyze occupational, educational, social, psychologic, and medical data to form a basis for understanding the client's current problems and concerns. Counselors administer tests, collate data, and interpret the results to help clients develop appropriate vocational plans and secure employment. Counselors also work with employers to develop job opportunities when clients have disabilities that prevent their return to their former jobs. Vocational rehabilitation counselors assist clients to find appropriate services provided by other professionals or agencies. To determine if the methods and techniques used to accomplish these tasks are effective, counselors conduct follow-up studies and engage in other methods of evaluation and research.

Vocational rehabilitation counselors also serve as advocates for persons with disabilities to raise public awareness and acceptance of clients' needs, rights, and abilities. Counselors promote the development of service programs and support new or revised legislation to meet these needs.

HISTORY

The vocational rehabilitation counselor (originally called the placement worker) came early to rehabilitation, as the need for employment for returning disabled World War I veterans became clear. These disabled veterans were provided with rehabilitation services and were readily assimilated into the work force during the boom years of the 1920s; 97% were placed between 1918 and 1928.[7]

The United States Employment Service, established in 1917 through the Smith-Hughes Act, included a section for handicapped civilians. In 1920 legislation mandated "vocational rehabilitation of persons disabled in industry or otherwise" and their return to employment (66th Congress, H.R. 4438). Evaluation of education and previous work were the principal means of establishing the job potential of a client. The job market conditions in a client's community determined successful placement. After the stock market crash of 1929 lack of jobs made the situation bleak. For many disabled veterans, industrial workers, and miners, becoming disabled meant unemployment and forced retire-

ment from social and community life. Few had pensions, and most subsisted on government welfare.

It soon became apparent that physical restoration or stability alone was insufficient. When the patient returned home, he or she faced new problems in coping with activities of daily living. Thus rehabilitation staff directed their attention to the disabled client in the home, providing training and techniques to move the client toward independence. With successful transition to home and community, a new hurdle was faced: finding appropriate employment. Job placement then became a primary task for rehabilitation professionals.[5]

The first sign of government responsibility toward injured workers was the establishment of workmen's (now worker's) compensation. This concept was first accepted in Europe around the turn of the century. Remuneration of an injured worker was made the concern of the state and payable by industry. In 1911 New Jersey became the first state in the United States to provide such financial compensation to injured workers. Not until 1918 to 1919 was rehabilitation included in similar legislation in Massachusetts, Minnesota, and Wisconsin, when these states provided for "replacement" of the injured worker. This marked the beginning of the state-federal program of rehabilitation that included vocational provisions.[7,14]

When rehabilitation began, as a helping discipline, it focused on physical restoration. The holistic concept—viewing the client as a social being—came much later. In a 1927 review of rehabilitation practices in 12 New York City agencies,[10] the employment department at the International Center for the Disabled (ICD; at that time called the Institute for the Crippled and Disabled) determined that properly evaluating the client's potential and skill and gaining the cooperation of industry were two requisites of the placement worker. Thus training in case management, psychologic counseling, the industrial process, and labor market trends was necessary. In other words, the placement worker had to be a "world of work" specialist as well as prepared in psychologic theory and interpersonal counseling skills. The ICD study also revealed that canvassing employers was the most productive method of finding job openings. Numbers of classified advertisements in the newspapers were used as the basis for determining labor market needs and trends.

At that time some professionals had college training and some even had knowledge of the industrial process, but they made up a small percentage of the total providing services to place disabled workers. The lack of analysis of and information on the qualities and qualifications needed by placement workers was apparent.

The client's attitude and motivation to work were vital factors in securing employment. Other obstacles encountered were lack of vocational training facilities and the attitudes of employers who saw the disabled person as not competitive. Clients, on average, made one visit to the New

York State Bureau for Rehabilitation (Division of Vocational Rehabilitation), the number of client contacts at other agencies in this study varied. ICD had the most frequent contact—they required clients to come in every day until they were placed.

A Montreal International Labour Office report in 1945 assessed the training and employment of disabled persons around the world.[10] The study credited voluntary agencies with the thrust to facilitate the "occupational reestablishment of disabled persons." At that time a disabled person was defined as "any person who by reason of a physical defect . . . whether congenital or acquired by accident, injury or disease, is or may be expected to be totally or partially incapacitated for remunerative occupation." Rehabilitation was defined as "the rendering of a disabled person fit to engage in a remunerative occupation."[8] Vocational rehabilitation was seen as a continuous process, one that needed integration and coordination of services for success. The criteria were (and still are in the U.S. state-federal system): a disability likely to remain for at least 12 months, financial need for (a majority of) services provided, and the potential for employment.

Between World War I and World War II the Veterans Administration developed a separate program for disabled soldiers. The state-federal offices of vocational rehabilitation were established nationally, and the employment services division took over the placement function with a special program called Selective Placement of the Handicapped. Until recently clients who completed their rehabilitation programs through the DVR offices were referred for placement to the selective placement counselor of the state employment offices. Thus, inadvertently, the basis on which our profession came into existence—placement—was for practical purposes removed from the roster of required services provided by the state rehabilitation counselor.

In 1942 Dr. Howard A. Rusk (then a major in the U.S. Army) organized a small program in rehabilitation at the Missouri Army/Air Forces Convalescent Center. The patients included large numbers of veterans with spinal cord injuries with resulting paraplegia and quadriplegia. For the first time in history these veterans were surviving the initial trauma.[2]

At the same time Dr. Henry Kessler, returning from the South Pacific, had established a major amputation center at Mare's Island Naval Hospital in California. Rusk and Kessler, leaders in the rehabilitation movement, met in New York City and asked ICD to provide vocational rehabilitation programs for their patients who were convalescing in hospitals in the area. ICD's excellent faculty and well-trained staff, with their wealth of clinically interesting materials, made this agency a national clearing house for the newest technology and training. From this collaboration a chain of Spinal Cord Injury (SCI) centers was established in 1945. Dr. James Garrett was recruited from ICD by the federal government to head the vocational rehabilitation and em-

ployment services special counseling unit for disabled veterans. Vocational counseling was the mainspring of the entire program, running through each stage of recovery. There was to be systematic and adequately supervised case counseling from inception to completion, based on the fundamental principle that *ability* rather than *disability* would be the focus.[8]

These actions led to the establishment of a series of rehabilitation centers to provide physical and occupational therapy; develop physical and work tolerance; offer trade and occupational trial periods; and give medical, psychologic, and vocational counseling services to realize the goals and potentials of each client. These centers had medical and orthopedic specialists and vocational specialists to provide transitional vocational instruction, job analysis, career information, and general education services to the client.

At about this same time the U.S. Office of Vocational Rehabilitation took direct action. A statement prepared for committee hearings in the House of Representatives emphasized the following points: "Because of the individualized nature of analysis and advisement . . . it [vocational counseling] represents the heart of the program . . . the future welfare of not only disabled persons but also their dependents is contingent upon the quality of this service."[8] Training needs for these specialists were listed and included the ability to interpret medical reports; the ability to distinguish between clinical counseling and placement counseling; familiarity with the world of work, the risks of work in industry, and many different occupations; skill in the use of psychologic tests and measurements; and knowledge of psychiatry without being a psychiatrist or a psychologist. In sum this specialist had to objectively recognize and interpret essential facts that enabled the disabled individual to share fully in determining and carrying out a plan to capitalize assets and minimize liabilities. This specialist had to integrate and coordinate the medical and vocational services of rehabilition step by step from the disparate diagnoses of many specialists from the beginning of medical treatment to placement and employment.[2] Civil service certification and later master's degrees in psychology, education, or personnel administration and, finally, rehabilitation counseling gradually came to be the basic educational requirements to practice as a vocational rehabilitation counselor. As early as 1918, however, these required skills had already become the core of a 1-week orientation program held at ICD. Twenty-five members of the helping professions attended. Until the 1940s ICD provided training and internships to professionals in rehabilitation and to students in medicine, physical and occupational therapies, psychology, social work, vocational advisement, and education.

The first master of arts degree program in vocational rehabilitation was established in 1941 at New York University, when Roland H. Spaulding, an aeronautic engineer, hung a sign on his office door that read, "Vocational Rehabilitation Counseling." He was named director of ICD's vocational rehabilitation services in 1942. These events formally established the extensive activities of vocational rehabilitation as a separate profession and paved the way for effective coordination with other established disciplines in ICD and agencies throughout the United States. An emerging concept crucial to success was that one person acting as a skilled rehabilitation coordinator should give focus to the findings of the professionals involved (the team) and make rehabilitation for the client a unified experience.[14]

A limitation in our federal rehabilitation legislation is that rehabilitation evaluation and planning for disabled persons is voluntary. No special arrangement or process has been instituted to induce employers, physicians, or insurers to train or retrain (either themselves or through referral) disabled workers, patients, or claimants. Employers are rarely required to hire or rehire a reasonable number of persons with disabilities (quota system). Other countries, such as Australia, Brazil, France, Great Britain, New Zealand, Japan, South Africa, and the U.S.S.R., have at one time instituted quota systems, whereby disabled workers must make up a certain percentage (often 3% to 6%) of the total work force of any one employer. Businesses in many democratic, entrepreneurial societies object to this, as it sets one group in competition with others. Also, many employers fear the risk and costs of further illness or accident. However, the Second Injury clause, established in the United States in 1945 and made a part of the workers' compensation law, has helped ease the resistance of employers.

Individual states (Michigan, California, and recently Massachusetts) and several other countries have made rehabilitation services a part of the workers' compensation program. The manner in which such mandates were carried out, however, could be problematic. For instance, some countries relied wholly on retraining to restore disabled workers to their job and overlooked the wide variety of needs that had to be met. By 1945 greater emphasis was placed on using a gamut of services, and retraining became viewed as only one phase in the total integrated plan. Linking one process to the others became the key to a total plan.[8]

Employers' acceptance of disabled persons as workers has always been an obstacle to placement. To remedy this, the Veteran's Preference Act of 1944 reserved certain federal jobs, such as guard, elevator operator, and custodial and messenger positions, for disabled veterans. Vendor positions in newsstands in all U.S. government buildings were to be reserved for persons with visual impairments.

As commissioner of the Office of Vocational Rehabilitation in the 1950s, Mary Switzer developed and promoted effective and landmark legislation. After her era, during the halcyon days of the Great Society (1960 to 1968), rehabilitation as a basic individual right grew, and medical research promised many technologic breakthroughs. These developments have enabled persons with a broader array of disabling conditions to be rehabilitated into the community and work force today.

The year 1954 is often cited as the starting date of the discipline known as vocational rehabilitation counseling. In actuality the vocational rehabilitation counselor was "becoming" since the first placement officer or employment counselor attempted to place the World War I disabled veteran in 1918. It has been an evolutionary process that culminated in a distinct profession in 1954, when the federal government enacted Public Law 93.143 and substantially increased funding for client services, research, and training of professional personnel. The need, then and now, is for "properly trained personnel who invest in themselves scientific training, tolerant understanding, and warm compassion."[15]

CURRENT PRACTICE

The following case is presented to illustrate changes that have occurred in the last 5 to 10 years in comprehensive rehabilitation center practice. In 1961 a typical patient referral from a private hospital to a comprehensive rehabilitation hospital center might have been Peter Grant, an 18-year-old spinal cord–injured motorcycle accident victim with a diagnosis of quadriplegia at the C4 to C5 level. This hypothetical patient had a middle-class background and a supportive family and had anticipated attending college. The prognosis for return of physical and sensory function below the level of injury was guarded. His stay at the center was expected to be between 10 and 16 months. He had no loss of intellectual function. A thorough, exhaustive evaluation began on day 1 with a comprehensive medical examination by a physiatrist, functional capacity assessments by physical and occupational therapists, and an intensive social and family history taken by a social worker. In the first week the patient was also interviewed by a psychologist and a vocational counselor. Other specialists would see him as the need arose (for example, an orthotist for bracing and a psychiatrist, if indicated).

A case conference with these specialists was held at the end of the first week. All presented their findings, and a tentative rehabilitation plan was drawn up with the physiatrist in charge, assuming prime responsibility for monitoring the progress of the plan. The patient then entered the conference to learn of the findings and to discuss and modify or agree to the plan.

In the following months the patient had a rigorous schedule of medical monitoring, physical exercise, evaluation of functional capacities, and practice in activities of daily living. He explored his vocational interests and abilities and planned career goals. For this client goals included contacts with colleges and universities to find one that was accessible to students in wheelchairs. In the early 1960s only two or three colleges nationwide were wheelchair accessible. Scheduled sessions with the psychologist were necessary to assist this young, formerly active and independent man to confront his emotions and reactions to sudden trauma and loss, which are manifest in numerous and different ways for each individual. Meetings with the social worker were productive in working toward resolution of some of the familial, social, and financial concerns that confront newly disabled patients.

As early as feasible, Peter was encouraged to participate in social and recreational activities at the center, including trips to local restaurants, theaters, and sporting events, which provided opportunities to test his physical strength and to encounter social situations in his new capacity. Weekends at home helped him to experience and begin to resolve changed feelings in family relationships and friendships, to learn about his functional capacity to care for himself, and to accept his new dependency on others.

All of these activities are part of a complex psychologic-behavioral phenomenon that the vocational counselor sees in occupational adjustment and affect the eventual success of a placement plan. To take an active role in vocational services, to select a vocational goal, to seriously plan and have the capacity to pursue a college program, to get and hold a job—all of these are influenced by the client's feelings and values, by family relationships, experiences with peers and social situations, and attitudes of employers and fellow employees.[17] As his rehabilitation program at the center concluded, 18 months after his admission, Peter Grant traveled to a university in the midwest with his vocational counselor. Their goals were to assess living accommodations, campus accessibility, and attitudes of faculty and students to his disabled status and to complete his matriculation. During the next 4 years the counselor continued regular contacts and vocational counseling sessions with him, working with him and his family to explore and help resolve academic, medical, and social relationship issues that had the potential to interfere with his vocational goals.

Job placement activities began early in his senior year. The counselor and client worked together to identify available jobs in the client's home area, to check the accessibility of the workplace, and to determine employer response to job and environmental accommodation that would be needed. Follow-up services would be available until Peter Grant and the employer had reached an agreement that satisfactory adjustment had occurred. All the foregoing were and are recognized as integral elements in a comprehensive rehabilitation plan.

Today, this plan differs in several crucial ways. The patient is admitted, according to the new diagnostic related grouping (DRG) method, for a 3-week stay in a comprehensive rehabilitation center. He or she is interviewed by similar specialists, and a plan is drawn up. Because of the time limit, the major services provided are medical stabilization and care, intensive physical therapy sessions for muscle strengthening and instruction in home exercises, occupational therapy, evaluation and instruction in activities of daily living, and provision of necessary splints and other assistive devices. Discharge planning with the social worker and family is then done. This plan also includes a 2-day live-in experience with a family member in the center's apartment to acquaint and instruct both in necessary changes at home. Vocational counseling may be done but generally centers on current physical problems, as it is usually still early in the recovery process. Vocational rehabilitation assessment and program planning are carried out on an outpatient basis. This necessitates transportation planning and family cooperation. Commonly, the client is referred for sponsorship of services to outside rehabilitation agencies, such as the Office of Vocational Rehabilitation or private (profit or not-for-profit) rehabilitation agencies, that are closer to the client's home and community.[11] Many factors have contributed to the development of this new approach. The field must wait for longitudinal assessment of outcomes before one can support or decry the new regulations.

In the 1970s vocational counselors experienced a gradual change in their case loads. Fewer clients had spinal cord injuries, amputations, and other orthopedic injuries, and more clients had diagnoses of mental illness, mental retardation, and developmental disabilities. The Rehabilitation Service Administration (RSA) had stated that mental illness and mental retardation had priority for services among the severe disabilities listed in the 1973 Vocational Rehabilitation Act.

These new mandates brought many changes in the provision of services by state and federal OVR agencies and private not-for-profit rehabilitation agencies and centers in type of clients seen, length of client stay, and cost of programs. For example, in 1965, of 300 sheltered workshops that offered any service to patients discharged from mental hospitals, only 47 described themselves as specialized in serving the mentally ill. By 1984 nearly 800 agencies offered special work programs for this population.[1] Black states:

A separation between work and therapy programs does persist [even to the present], losing the advantage of tangible information in vocational activities; e.g., patient adjustment to independent living, to achievement of self-esteem, and even as a tangible gauge to effects of medication, seen to be viewed as alien to psychotherapy.*

Mental retardation and developmental disabilities have also received tremendous government support. New treatment modalities continue to be developed and assessed through implementation to ameliorate the devastating effects of these congenital and acquired deficits. The effects touch the lives of individuals, family, and society at tremendous monetary and psychologic cost.

---

*Black, BJ, editor: Work as therapy and rehabilitation for the mentally ill, Professional Monograph Series, vol 1, Altro Institute for Rehabilitation for the Mentally Ill.

Today we hear phrases such as "supported employment," "consortium-based transition," and "community-based work adjustment." Supported employment is paid work for persons with severe disabilities who require ongoing support to remain employed. Clients are placed on the job first and are then trained by an agency job coach. To bridge the gap from school to work for school-age youth with special needs, consortium-based transition services are provided at the work site by school or agency personnel. The goal is to obtain earned income; the program is work focused. The Vocational Rehabilitation Act (1986) calls for "school and rehabilitation counselors to work closely together to help high school students with disabilities to enter the work world."[6] Community-based work adjustment programs are distinguished from traditional work adjustment programs by their location in community businesses and industry as service agency-supervised, time-limited experiences.[9] All these programs call for high-level professional skills, including knowledge of employer psychodynamics and sensitivity to verbal and nonverbal communication. Reluctant employers are just as challenging as reluctant (and compliant) clients.[19]

Today closed head injuries occupy vocational counselors and work evaluators in hospital rehabilitation units and comprehensive rehabilitation centers. An estimated 800 per 100,000 people suffer brain injury from head trauma. Most head injuries result from incidents involving falls, beatings, stabbings, motor vehicles, and hand guns. Recent research shows that some regeneration, albeit haphazard, is possible in patients with head and spinal cord injuries.[16]

In Israel, where coma victims are taken to coma rehabilitation hospitals, 60% are ambulatory or able to walk in 6 months. In the United States, however, less than one coma patient in 10 is transferred to a rehabilitation facility. A move toward regional rehabilitation hospitals specializing in treating head trauma is evident. Research continues to identify cognitive predictors of long-term outcome and factors contributing to rehabilitation program success. Training task performance outcomes tend to differentiate between patients with good outcomes and those with less than desired outcomes. Training tasks include formulating goals and intention planning, carrying out plans, monitoring performance, and making appropriate adjustments.[4]

Patients with intact verbal skills, abstract reasoning, and insight often do not function well in their daily activities. Musante states that one in 200 persons requires care after closed head injuries each year, with a cost to the public of 2 billion per year.[12] Increases in motor vehicle accidents and decreases in mortality because of improved acute care of head-injured patients have presented a serious challenge to medical and rehabilitation practitioners. Government figures show that these patients are predominantly male, between the ages of 15 and 24 years, and adults with minimal work history and very often naive conceptions of the demands of society and the world of work.[18] The complexity

and chronic nature of the limitations that patients have and their lack of response to traditional evaluation methods increase the challenge.

Unlike the localized insult of a stroke or tumor, which yield predictable patterns, TBI produces mixed behavior patterns and diffuse generalized damage, especially in cognition and behavior. Often it is only when a patient is referred for vocational evaluation and job exploration that the extent of the damage and greater understanding of specific deficits emerge. For example, one young man who was able to score above average on most paper-and-pencil aptitude tests, to articulate a realistic and organized plan of action for himself, and to demonstrate insight into his problems convinced his counselor of his readiness to attend college. However, his daily functioning level was so poor that he required supervised living arrangements. He was unsuccessful in completing a college course because he frequently forgot to attend class, indicating a lack of orientation to time. Although his test scores had shown retention of past learning, new learning did not carry over.

Conversely, it is easy to underestimate a client's abilities if he or she has unintelligible speech and severe perceptual and physical limitations. Some individuals have the ability to compensate to the degree that they can live independently and obtain employment. Specialized approaches in evaluation, training, and placement are required. As an example, a young man with global aphasia, right-sided sensory loss, and little use of his right hand performed well below average on all standardized work samples and was unable to read or write. He had, however, excellent problem-solving skills and was able to devise techniques to perform two-handed tasks. Over time and with an individualized training and job placement program, he obtained summer employment in a large corporate mailroom at a level competitive with non-disabled employees.[12]

Since new learning may be affected by memory deficits as well as language, assessment of learning potential for brain-injured clients is crucial. Because of the stigma attached to brain damage and cognitive malfunction, the affected individual and the family commonly focus on the less stressful area of physical functioning, totally overlooking cognitive deficits. Fear of discovering limitations and unavailability of a cognitive and perceptual retraining program have delayed or prevented opportunities for rehabilitation and return to community and employment.

Musante recommends that assessment programs done by a trained psychologist or speech-language therapist be carried out before or during the work evaluation. The combination and degree of cognitive deficits and psychologic trauma can be confusing to both client and professionals. Restructuring and modification of evaluation and testing procedures are essential, calling for keen observation, problem-solving skills, specificity of recommendations for remediation, training and job restructuring, and creativity.

TRENDS

Vocational rehabilitation counseling was the first profession to provide services focusing on return to work—on employment, not employability.[3] Optimizing human potential is recognized as the common goal of the total rehabilitation process. The philosophy of rehabilitation rests on a humanistic, holistic approach. Recognition of the uniqueness and diversity of the individual operates from a realistic theory of the nature of human beings. To carry out this philosophy, many services must be provided by professionals from a variety of disciplines. Each professional must possess expertise in that discipline and, in the process, seek to provide continuity and collaboration—concepts inherent in rehabilitation. This requires special characteristics in the practitioner. For the vocational rehabilitation counselor these include awareness, acceptance, sensitivity, flexibility, and resourcefulness.[13]

Essentially, the vocational rehabilitation counselor is and always has been a placement professional, helping to move and motivate the client to deal with the psychologic trauma resulting from the physical or sensory insult dealt by accident, war, disease, or birth and to realize the ultimate goal of holding a job. Still, it has come as something of a surprise to many vocational rehabilitation counselors and to rehabilitation counselor educators that as professional practitioners they are expected to be leaders in meeting the nation's need to return disabled individuals to work.

Vandergoot points out that research outcomes indicate "on-the-job training, as in supported work programs, and individualized placement planning, produce more favorable outcomes than pre-placement training or counseling alone. Active counselor involvement [is a key ingredient] to monitor the plan."[20] Further, Vandergoot notes, "of all rehabilitation services offered to clients, from intake to post-placement, significant outcomes lie in their contribution to placement."[20]

The number of rehabilitation counselors engaged in placement activities for their clients has grown tremendously in the past 10 years. This trend stems partially from federal mandates for placement, from supportive work projects, from the independent living movement, and from civil rights legislation (1973) for the handicapped. Zadny and James note that studies have repeatedly shown that counselors spend relatively little time on placement.[22] In response to this, placement specialists have been trained and used as alternative providers of direct job placement services. However, it has been suggested that their efficiency or effectiveness may be suspect.[20] More recently, as insurers of major corporations and industry have come to grips with escalating insurance and health costs, they are discovering that rehabilitation counselors can be instrumental in the safe and timely return to work of their injured and ill employees.

Most vocational rehabilitation counselor graduates of 2-year master's degree programs still choose to initially work for state and federal vocational rehabilitation agencies or not-for-profit comprehensive rehabilitation centers. A small number of graduates may wish to go directly into private rehabilitation practice, but generally, agency experience under supervision is desired to become proficient and ready for the more autonomous work of the private practitioner. Work-injured clients seen by skilled, experienced counselors in private rehabilitation are generally more receptive to the concentrated coordination of services that leads to return to work than is the problematic client population that most vocational rehabilitation counselors see in the public and not-for-profit sector.

A reason for the increasing number of vocational rehabilitation counselors entering private practice is simply supply and demand. An increase in the number of disabled workers because of work or accident injuries and the concomitant increased insurance costs have made it imperative for the corporate sector to look for effective, timely solutions. In response to this need private rehabilitation agencies have emerged as an alternative to the long-established federally funded public and not-for-profit agencies. At the same time there has been a notable growth in the number of workers' compensation and disability management programs in public and not-for-profit agencies. The impetus to establish such separate programs hinges on the need to shorten the time from onset of injury to return to work for the disabled worker if job placement is to be effected.

A number of states (California, Minnesota, Michigan, and Massachusetts) have mandated vocational rehabilitation services as a benefit and requirement for all recipients of workers' compensation. The implementation of this implies that there will be a better understanding by the claimant of benefits derived from workers' compensation, of his or her responsibilities to work toward a safe but timely return to work, and of how decisions are made for a cash settlement or continued monthly payments to age 65 years.

Corporate interest and the need for timely, high-quality services and return to work have clearly effected changes in program planning, types of services, and focus of goals for clients in traditional rehabilitation agencies.

FUTURE TRENDS

Rising medical costs have caused industry and insurance companies to take an active role in countering the tremendous increase in payments to employees who have been disabled. The unique skills of the vocational rehabilitation counselor are proving to be of greater use and value, especially in coordinating the various services and in the range and quality of direct services provided to the disabled worker and in cost containment to the insurer and employer.

Exorbitant medical, hospital, and insurance costs have been decisive factors in the establishment of the new guidelines for hospital admission and care. Experience and new data show that monetary disincentives and the distancing from work that time imposes erode the disabled employees' motivation to return to work in a timely fashion.

These are hotly debated issues and will continue to ignite the imagination, the sensitivity, and the professionalism of rehabilitation practitioners in the next decade. Private practice rehabilitation and supported work concepts have contributed to an accelerated change in providing services. Working with clients as co-managers is necessary to ensure real progress and positive long-term outcomes. Clients must be engaged in every aspect of their rehabilitation, and matters should be discussed realistically, hopefully, and with full respect for the client. Clients need to contribute, to help evaluate data, and to work toward solutions. Wright calls this the principle of co-management, stating, "involvement enhances motivation to make the plan work; the potential for learning is greatly increased when one is actively guiding one's own behavior."[21]

Courage, pride, and honor are words brought to life through the rehabilitation process by clients. Client and counselor take justifiable satisfaction in the client's growth, independence, and achievement, which are the goals of the vocational rehabilitation process.

REFERENCES

1. Black, BJ, editor: Work as therapy and rehabilitation for the mentally ill, Professional Monograph Series, vol 1, New York, 1986, ALTRO Rehabilitation Services.
2. Dean, RJN: New life for millions: rehabilitation for America's disabled, New York, 1972, Hastings House Publishing.
3. Deneen, LJ, and Hessellund, TA: Counseling the able disabled: rehabilitation consulting in disability compensation systems, San Francisco, 1986, Rehabilitation Publications.
4. Fryer, J: Identifying cognitive predictors of long-term outcome, Boston, 1986, New Medico Head Injury Systems.
5. Gellman, W: In Marinelli, RP, and Dell Orto, AE: The psychological and social impact of physical disability, New York, 1977, Springer Publishing Co, Inc.
6. Guidepost: American Association for Counseling and Development, Nov 26, 1986.
7. Hinshaw, D: Take up thy bed and walk, New York, 1948, GP Putnam & Son.
8. International Labour Office: Training and employment of disabled persons: a preliminary report, Montreal, 1945, International Labour Office.
9. JM Foundation: Search for excellence, New York, 1987, JM Foundation.
10. LeDame, M: Securing employment for the handicapped: a study of placement agencies in New York City, New York, 1927, Department of Industrial Studies, Russell Sage Foundation.
11. Mesch-Spinello, J: Personal communication, November 1986.
12. Musante, SE: Issues relevant to the vocational evaluation of the traumatically head injured client, Vocational Eval Work Adjustment Bull Spring 45, 1983.
13. Payne, JS, et al: Rehabilitation techniques: vocational adjustment for the handicapped, New York, 1984, Human Sciences Press, Inc.
14. Robinault, IP: ICD experience, 1917-1981, New York, 1981, International Center for the Disabled.
15. Rusalem, H, and Malikin, D: Contemporary vocational rehabilitation, New York, 1976, New York University Press.
16. Shea, JF: A neurosurgeon looks at TBI and rehabilitation, Boston, 1986, New Medico Head Injury Systems.
17. Siegel, MS: Principles in management of vocational problems. In Rusk, HA, editor: Rehabilitation medicine, ed 4, St Louis, 1977, The CV Mosby Co.
18. The silent epidemic: rehabilitation of people with traumatic brain injury, Rehabilitation brief, vol 9, no 4, Washington DC, NIHR.
19. Sinick, D: The job placement process. In Rusalum and Malikin, editors: Contemporary vocational rehabilitation, New York, 1976, New York University Press.
20. Vandergoot, D: Review of placement research literature: implications for research and practice, Rehabil Counsel Bull 20:243, 1987.
21. Wright, BA: Physical disability: a psychological approach, ed 2, New York, 1983, Harper & Row.
22. Zadny, JJ, and James, LFL: Time spent on placement, Rehabil Counsel Bull 21:31, 1977.

CHAPTER 59

Therapeutic recreation

CLAUDETTE LeFEBVRE AND DORIS BERRYMAN

Rehabilitation has aptly been described as a distinctly human enterprise[22] whose ultimate aim is to assist disabled individuals to attain or regain those rights, roles, and responsibilities that effectively define life in their surrounding communities.[8] Truly integrated community living, however, encompasses all dimensions of life, and it is increasingly evident that for disabled individuals:

Living and working in the community is not enough! Participating in the community means having leisure choices and using a variety of community resources, whether they be walking in the park, taking evening courses, or going out with friends. Leisure means having these opportunities for self-development and personal-social fulfillment.*

Illness, stress, and trauma are conditions that, by the imposition of temporary or prolonged limitations, have concomitant impacts on individuals, families, and the community at large. Limitations may be considered functional or handicapping when, at any point in the life cycle, they act to impede, disrupt, or interfere with the effectiveness of outcomes between individuals and their physical or social environments. Functional effectiveness is broadly reflected and measured across the life span in individual competence (or the lack thereof) in such behavioral arenas as mastery of developmental tasks and functions, assumption of increased responsibility for meeting one's own needs, ability to carry out routine activities of daily living, assumption of a diversity of situationally and contextually appropriate social roles and repertoires, and achievement of a personally satisfying and fulfilling life-style, including the play, recreation, and leisure domains.

---

*Hutchinson, P, and Lord, J: Recreation integration: issues and alternatives in leisure services and community involvement, Ottawa, 1979, Leisurability Publications, Inc.

Leisure functioning is increasingly recognized as an integral component in the quality of life and in the maintenance of a satisfying and rewarding life-style. Leisure effectiveness is reflected and measured across the life cycle in relation to the development of age-appropriate play behaviors and repertoires, the scope and depth of participation in culturally normative recreation activities and experiences, and the realization of leisure interests, preferences, values, and resourcefulness.

Disabled individuals have the same basic needs for satisfying play, recreation, and leisure experiences as do their nonimpaired peers upon which are superimposed actual or presumed limitations associated with impairment and with a diversity of physical, social, or attitudinal barriers extant in the environment. The need to integrate therapeutic recreation services in the medical treatment of patients has been apparent for some time.[6] As Vash notes, "Rehabilitation centers and hospitals have long included recreation programs for their patients, but their character has made a significant change in recent years."[24]

During the early era of the rehabilitation movement (when the overall focus was on the medical treatment of impairment and vocational training)[7] recreation services were primarily viewed as passive entertainment or diversion, largely designed to "fill evening or weekend hours not taken up by medical, nursing, or therapy activities."[24] As rehabilitation services have broadened in scope and holistic foci, so has therapeutic recreation been more clearly defined in its professional mission. Therapeutic recreation services are ultimately designed and implemented "to facilitate the development, maintenance, and expression of an appropriate leisure life-style for individuals with physical, mental, social or emotional limitations."[18] As integral members of the comprehensive rehabilitation treatment team, therapeutic recreation specialists are concerned with enhancing patients' leisure functioning and effectiveness in a diversity of settings and with "facilitating patients' adaptation to the community."[11] Accordingly, "by now, most programs have evolved into recreation preparation, emphasizing exposure to feasible alternatives and training in the constructive use of leisure time *after* returning to the community."[24] Therapeutic recreation processes, as those of rehabilitation, can be viewed from a dual perspective—as a learning process for individuals with congenital impairments or developmental disabilities and as a process of readjustment to community living in instances of trauma, illness, or acquired disorders.[8]

HISTORICAL OVERVIEW

Recreation and play activities of one type or another have for centuries been used in the treatment of various illnesses and disabilities. Organized programs of recreation activities in health care settings, however, first emerged during World War I. Moderate expansion of these services continued throughout the 1920s and 1930s, particularly in institutions serving mentally retarded and emotionally disturbed persons. World War II brought a great acceleration to the hospital recreation movement and increased recognition of the value of professionally planned and supervised recreation programs in the total treatment of patients. After that war there was continued expansion of hospital recreation services in military, veterans', and other public, private, and voluntary institutions throughout the United States. During this time a variety of terms, such as "hospital recreation," "medical recreation," "recreational therapy," and "recreation for the ill and handicapped," were used to describe the services provided. A number of colleges and universities began to offer graduate degree programs, usually called hospital recreation or recreation for the ill and handicapped. Job titles used included recreation worker, recreation specialist, and recreation therapist. These titles, along with therapeutic recreation specialist, are still used today.

During the 1960s the term "therapeutic recreation" was brought into general use, and professionals involved in this facet of the total recreation movement expanded their conceptual base and programmatic thrust. The profession moved from a narrow identification with institutional settings and specific disabled groups toward identification with a humanistically oriented process or service and concern for all ill, disabled, or handicapped persons, including such special population groups as the aged, disadvantaged, and delinquent in both institutional and community settings. Also during this period colleges and universities began changing the names of their degree programs to therapeutic recreation, and the profession developed and implemented a voluntary registration plan for professionals in the field. In 1969 a group of leading professionals in the field formulated a statement of definition that for the next 10 years

was the definition most often used by the profession. Therapeutic recreation was defined as "a process which utilizes recreation services for purposive intervention in some physical, emotional, and/or social behavior to bring about a desired change in that behavior and to promote the growth and development of the individual."[12] Although this definition provided some guidance to the field, its focus proved to be too broad. Peterson and Gunn state, "The resulting impact of this definition was the continued programming for patients based on the individual practitioner's or agency's interpretation of the definition. Client need could be viewed as almost anything that the therapeutic recreation specialist wished to address."[18]

The 1970s generated many creative and innovative programs for special populations in a variety of settings, and some of them brought new insights for alternative perspectives from which the field might be viewed. From 1970 to 1986 the field expanded considerably in number of practitioners with professional training, number of agencies adding therapeutic recreation services, and in efforts to make service delivery and research more professional and sophisticated. Accreditation of undergraduate and graduate programs in therapeutic recreation was established, and the voluntary registration plan evolved into a voluntary certification plan that is recognized by many state and local civil service agencies and numerous institutions and organizations. Philosophy became a critical issue as the profession became increasingly aware that a clear and concise definition was essential to its immediate existence and future expansion.

After several years of study and discussion the National Therapeutic Recreation Society in 1981 adopted the "leisure ability" philosophy and model as its official position. This provided the field with a philosophical basis with well-defined direction for the conceptualization and delivery of therapeutic recreation services and definite implications for research and content of preservice and inservice training programs. This philosophy states that the purpose of therapeutic recreation is "to facilitate the development, maintenance, and expression of an appropriate leisure life-style for individuals with physical, mental, social or emotional limitations."[18] The process of achieving this goal involves the selection, development, implementation, and evaluation of goal-oriented services based on individual assessment and program referral procedures in three areas of professional service: therapy (treatment), leisure education, and recreation participation.

The concept of leisure life-style that is central to this statement of purpose has been defined by Peterson and Gunn as "the day-to-day behavioral expression of one's leisure-related attitudes, awareness, and activities revealed within the context and composite of the total life experience."[18] One's leisure life-style interacts with all other aspects of one's life, and although its quality and nature may vary, it is nevertheless true that each person has one. Viewed from this perspective, it is apparent that therapeutic recreation is much more complex than the simple provision of enjoyable activity or delivery of an isolated "therapy" using activity as the medium.

Figure 59-1 portrays the leisure ability approach to therapeutic recreation service developed by Peterson and Gunn.[18] The nature and purposes of interventions and services, roles of the therapeutic recreation specialist, and the concept of levels or degrees of freedom for clients' participation are shown. The model also illustrates the "concept of a continuum, implying movement through the various service components."[18] The three areas of service, the concomitant roles of the specialist, and the nature of interventions used usually overlap or occur simultaneously. That is, a given client, based on assessment results, might be involved in one activity to improve a specific functional ability and in another to acquire particular leisure knowledge or recreation skill.

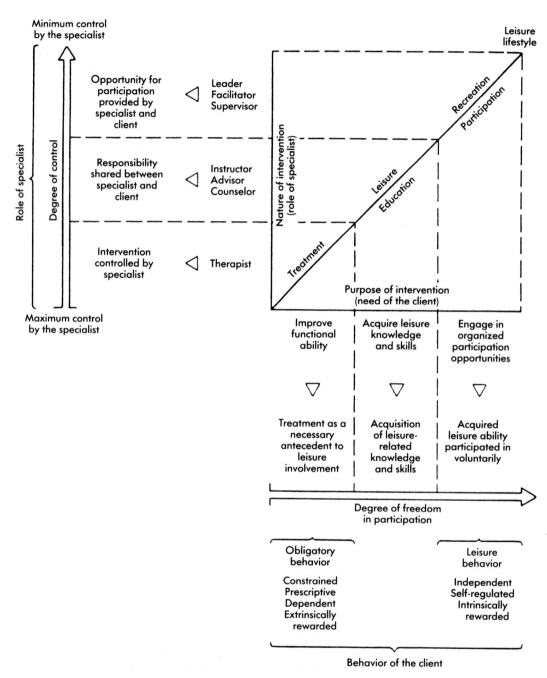

Figure 59-1. Therapeutic recreation service model. (From Peterson, CA, and Gunn, SL: Therapeutic recreation program design: principles and procedures, ed 2, Englewood Cliffs, NJ, 1984, Prentice-Hall, Inc. Reprinted by permission of Prentice-Hall, Inc.)

This model of therapeutic recreation service is based on three principles:

1. Play, participation in recreation, and positive attitudes toward leisure are essential to the growth and development of the child and to balanced living and stress reduction for the adult.
2. Individuals who are limited by impairment, disability, or social condition have the same rights to and need for play, recreation, and leisure involvement.
3. Sound, comprehensive therapeutic recreation service is client oriented and based on behavioral assessment, identified treatment and learning goals, program referral procedures, and appropriate evaluation procedures.

Individual assessment and treatment planning serve as the basis for selection and implementation of appropriate activities, content, and intervention strategies in the professional areas of recreation therapy, leisure education, and recreation participation. These processes are described in the following sections.

ASSESSMENT AND DOCUMENTATION

Halpern and Fuhrer have defined functional assessment in rehabilitation as "the measurement of purposeful behavior in interaction with the environment, which is interpreted according to the assessment's intended uses."[8] The term "assessment" usually refers to employing various methods (for example, tests, questionnaires, observations, ratings, and interviews) of gathering pertinent information on behavioral variables that are relevant to a particular decision-making process. Ideally, in rehabilitation information is gathered on physical, mental, emotional, social, and vocational functional abilities and typical behaviors. Results of these appraisals are then used to determine treatment and service plans and to provide a baseline of data needed for evaluating client progress and service effectiveness.

The therapeutic recreation specialist gathers assessment information on the client's physical, mental, emotional, and social abilities and behaviors in relation to the behavioral and skill requirements of recreation and play activities and the activity preferences, recreation participation patterns, and leisure awareness, attitudes, and satisfactions of the individual. This information, shared with the client, is used to identify treatment or learning goals related to the play, recreation, and leisure aspects of the client's life that are compatible with the overall rehabilitation or habilitation goals established for the client; to develop a treatment program plan for achieving the identified goals; to assist in identifying environmental factors that may need to be modified; and to serve as baseline data for evaluating client progress and service effectiveness. Cohen and Anthony suggest that there should also be a resource assessment to identify "those *environmental* strengths and deficits that are related to achieving the overall rehabilitation

goal."[4] They feel such an assessment is essential because "factors outside the client's capacities and outside the client's control are critical in the client's attainment of his or her rehabilitation goal."[4]

Specific assessment instruments and techniques employed will depend on the nature of the client's impairment and extent of disability, overall rehabilitation goals, and pertinent assessment information obtained by other members of the rehabilitation team. For example, assessment of an individual who has had a traumatic leg amputation would focus on identifying the client's recreation interests, participation patterns, perceived future activity participation, and leisure awareness, attitudes, and satisfactions. Assessment of an individual who has suffered a cerebrovascular accident would include, in addition to that given above, information on physical (including speech), mental, emotional, and social abilities and deficits. Sufficient information on the client's performance in some of these behavior domains may already be available from assessments done by other rehabilitation team members. The therapeutic recreation specialist would do only those additional assessments necessary for obtaining information needed to develop an appropriate therapeutic recreation plan with the client.

Currently, only a few published instruments are available to assess behaviors, awareness, attitudes, activity preferences, and interests related to play, recreation, and leisure. The Leisure Diagnostic Battery by Witt and Ellis[25] consists of seven separate scales. Five of these assess various aspects of the construct of perceived freedom: Perceived Leisure Competence Scale, Perceived Leisure Control Scale, Leisure Needs Scale, Depth of Involvement in Leisure Scale, and Playfulness Scale. The other two scales are Barriers to Leisure Opportunities and Knowledge of Leisure Opportunities. The battery was designed for children and adolescents but has been used for assessing adults in psychiatric, hospital, and nursing home settings. The Leisure Activities Blank by McKechnie[14] is a list of 120 activities for which the respondent indicates past and present participation and intended future participation. Through factor analysis the author has clustered the activities for the Past Scale (which includes present) into six activity categories and the Future Scale into eight activity categories. The Recreation Behavior Inventory (RBI) by Berryman and Lefebvre[3] is a criterion-referenced instrument that assesses levels of performance in 92 behaviors under the broad categories of sensory (14), cognitive (25), and perceptual motor (53) domains. The behaviors included in the RBI are either important developmental milestones or are frequently required for participation in various play and recreation activities. The behaviors are assessed by a three-point rating scale of clients' actual behaviors as they participate in 20 specially designed activities. Each activity is designed to elicit one to 10 behaviors. Although the instrument was designed for disabled children and adolescents, it has been used by therapeutic recreation specialists for assessing adults in psychiatric, developmental disabilities, rehabilitation, and nursing home settings.

In addition to these three instruments, several other instruments have been published in professional journals and conference proceedings. Permission for their use may be obtained by writing to the authors of the instruments. Some of these instruments, described briefly below, have been designed for general use in the field; others, although designed for a particular agency, could be effectively used in a variety of other settings.

Edwards' Constructive Leisure Activities Survey[5] is an interview schedule designed to determine the client's past, present, and future leisure activities, interest, needs, and preferences. The survey includes five categories: physical and outdoor activities, social activities, arts and crafts, learning, general welfare, and personal satisfaction. The State Technical Institute Leisure Activities Project (STILAP) developed by Navar[16] is a self-report checklist of 123 leisure and recreation activities for which the client indicates frequency of participation or interest in learning. The 123 activities are organized into 14 categories of participation patterns and include physical, mental, social, and creative activities. The Comprehensive Evaluation in Recreational Therapy (CERT) Scale, developed by Parker and associates,[17] is a criterion-referenced observational rating form that assesses and monitors 25 behaviors commonly displayed in recreation activities. It was designed for adolescents and adults in short-term psychiatric settings but is usable in other treatment settings. Beard and Ragheb's Leisure Satisfaction Scale[1] consists of 51 closed-ended questions and uses a five-point Likert scale for responses. This scale assesses satisfaction in six subscales developed through factor analysis: psychological, physiological, educational, social, relaxational, and environmental and esthetic. A 24-item short form is also available. The Leisure Attitude Scale developed by Ragheb and Beard[19] is a 36 closed-ended item questionnaire, using a seven-point Likert-type scale for responses. There are 12 items in each of three attitude categories: cognitive, affective, and behavioral. All of these instruments are examples of available assessment tools that are useful in assessing various aspects of recreation activity and leisure interests, preferences, participation patterns, attitudes, and satisfactions.

Another important method for obtaining pertinent information about clients is behavioral observation recording. Observation techniques are particularly appropriate for assessing play behaviors, social skill acquisition, behavior modification, environmental modification, and perceptual-motor skill development. Levy, in describing such techniques as continuous recording, frequency count or event recording, duration recording, latency recording, and interval recording, states:

Observation is becoming one of the more salient methods of gathering social data. Like all other scientific methods of knowing about human behavior, it has to be carried out systematically, based within a theoretical-conceptual framework, and must contain appropriate checks and controls to establish its reliability and validity.*

As stated earlier, assessment results are used to determine client treatment goals and service plans and to provide baseline information for evaluating client progress and service effectiveness. One method for ensuring that these goals are met is Goal Attainment Scaling (GAS). In describing its application to therapeutic recreation, Touchstone states:

GAS is a personalized client goal planning and evaluation method that is not influenced by setting or diagnosis . . . Originally developed as a program evaluation approach for community mental health, GAS has since been applied to goal setting for both individuals and organizations across a wide spectrum of human and rehabilitation services.†

GAS is a systematic process with three basic phases: specifying the most significant behaviors or problem areas that need clinical intervention, based on available assessment data; scaling and weighting the identified behaviors or problem areas; and scoring the outcome of the interventions used in implementing the treatment or rehabilitation plan. For GAS to be effective the therapeutic recreation specialist must obtain behavioral assessment data; be able to analyze recreation and play activities; carry out sequential or developmental task analysis; and translate the activity and task analysis information into specific behavioral descriptions that accurately describe expected results of clinical interventions.[23]

Another system often used in hospitals is Problem-Oriented Medical Records (POMR). POMR applies the same basic concept of using systematic client data input for client goal planning, treatment, and evaluation but does not require the quantified scaling, weighting, and scoring procedures used in GAS. The POMR format includes five components: database or initial assessment, problem list, initial plan, progress notes, and discharge summary. In institutions or clinical agencies using either GAS or POMR the client record or chart is organized according to client problems rather than by each professional discipline, which is the more traditional method used in hospitals.

Regardless of the documentation system employed by the rehabilitation service, the therapeutic recreation specialist should determine an appropriate method of providing input to the client's treatment and rehabilitation plan. Navar[15] has provided the therapeutic recreation specialist with an excellent discussion on this subject, which includes problem identification, initial treatment plan, progress notes, and discharge summary using the POMR system; the procedures involved in writing a therapeutic recreation treatment plan, and instructive examples. The procedures include obtaining

---

*Levy, J: Ther Rec J 16:25, 1982.
†Touchstone, WA: Ther Rec J 18:24, 1984.

assessment information, referral information, and specification of treatment and rehabilitation goals, programs in which the client will be involved, frequency and duration of participation, staff and client responsibilities, facilitation styles and approaches, and schedule for reevaluation. She also describes the content and procedures for maintaining progress notes and methods of recording observations of client behaviors. She discusses physical fitness, gross motor development, cognitive development, social skills, emotional functioning, and independent functioning as problem areas that can be addressed by therapeutic recreation. She also discusses leisure attitudes, leisure and recreation activity skills, leisure resources, social skills, and recreation participation.

The therapeutic recreation treatment plan should also provide for working with the client to plan his or her recreation participation and leisure involvement after discharge from the rehabilitation service. The client's needs, interests, abilities, limitations, and future residence should be considered. Peterson and Gunn state, "Master planning enables appropriate identification of client needs and selection of program components from all levels of the Therapeutic Recreation Service Model to meet the identified needs."[18] Client needs in leisure involvement, identified through the assessment process, ultimately determine the nature, form, and content of therapeutic recreation plans designed for and with individuals in rehabilitation treatment programs and settings. At various stages in their rehabilitation experience clients may be engaged sequentially or concurrently in one or more of the three distinct professional areas of service (recreation therapy, leisure education, and recreation participation) that comprise the therapeutic recreation continuum.

RECREATION THERAPY

Recreation therapy focuses not on the treatment of initial pathologic conditions but on the functional deficiencies or limitations imposed by pathologic conditions. Program approaches and strategies in the recreation therapy mode are both process and content oriented, as they focus on the enhancement of "functional behavior areas that are considered to be prerequisites to, or a necessary part of, leisure involvement and life-style."[18] Recreation treatment plans are designed and implemented to enhance functional play; physical, social, mental, emotional, and social behaviors; and skills considered essential for participation in normalized recreation and leisure experiences. Improved functional ability is the specific predetermined outcome. Services in the treatment mode generally adhere to a medical model format: individual or small group recreation therapy programs are most commonly provided on a prescriptive or program-referral basis after comprehensive assessment of client limitations, needs, interests, priorities, and abilities. Recreation therapy modalities focus on individuals and the manner in which they adjust to, cope with, or compensate

for illness or disability. Although specific programs are often conducted with groups of clients with similar diagnoses or impairments, individual assessment and treatment planning *always* serve as the basis for recreation therapy services. Disability is a distinctly personal experience. As Stolov notes, "There is no one-to-one correlation between a disease [or injury] and the spectrum of associated disability problems. The same disease [or traumatizing condition] can produce separate sets of disability problems in different individuals."[21] Clients' responses to the primary disability (expressed in such forms as withdrawal, isolation, antisocial or regressed behaviors, excessive dependency, inappropriate emotional affect, and so on) may serve as the basis for the development of secondary handicaps or disabilities. Peterson and Gunn note, "Because the secondary disabilities are often in the social and emotional areas, they are very amenable to therapeutic recreation treatment-oriented services."[18] Effective individual or group treatment plans (often referred to as program protocols) include specification of objectives, performance measures, designated staff intervention approaches, and activities that are carefully selected to be compatible with client needs, overall program content, and specific treatment objectives. Selection of activities for inclusion in recreation therapy programs is most appropriately made on the basis of activity analysis—a systematic process designed to identify the unique potentials of each activity that elicits or requires specific behaviors and skills leading to achievement of established treatment goals and objectives. Peterson and Gunn state, "In the treatment mode, activities are used not for their recreation or leisure potential but rather for their specific inherent contribution to behavioral change."[18]

In summary, process- and content-oriented programs and interventions in the recreation therapy mode always have specific predetermined outcomes for improved functional ability, with activities and experiences designed and implemented to enhance individuals' behaviors and skills in the play, physical, mental, emotional, and social domains; determine the need for or appropriateness of modified or adapted recreation activities, experiences, and equipment; counteract the potential secondary handicapping effects of stress, hospitalization or institutionalization, and learned helplessness; and enhance clients' active involvement and participation in the total rehabilitation process.

LEISURE EDUCATION

Establishment and expression of an appropriate and personally satisfying leisure life-style ultimately depends on the individual's acquisition and enhancement of diverse leisure-related knowledge, skills, and attitudes. Despite the severity of initial limitations and handicaps, all individuals have the right to participate in a diversity of meaningful and personally satisfying leisure experiences, and personal leisure effectiveness can be enhanced "as the individual acquires new knowledge, skills, attitudes, and abilities."[18]

Although services in the therapy mode adhere to a medical model format, program content and strategies in leisure education more typically approximate those of educational and counseling model formats. Many content areas in the leisure education mode are appropriate to small group education settings and experiences, but individual or small group counseling experiences should be considered when dealing with highly specific or unique client problems or issues. Regardless of the specific format adopted, however, it is essential that leisure education programs, content, and intervention strategies conform to normalization principles and practices and that the client be viewed as an active participant in the process, sharing responsibility with the therapeutic recreation specialist for attainment of mutually predetermined outcomes. Predetermined outcomes in the leisure education mode should enhance cognitive understanding and personal appreciation of leisure in its diverse forms; identify individuals' leisure interests, preferences, and attitudes; clarify individuals' leisure values; provide realistic appraisals of actual or presumed limitations resulting from disability that may hinder involvement in leisure experiences; develop or reestablish appropriate social interaction and friendship patterns; and enhance leisure resourcefulness. Resourcefulness refers to the individual's "capacity to develop interests which have meaning in themselves as well as expressing underlying preoccupations"[20] and to the "ability to carry through the interests to realization"[20] in a diversity of settings.

Leisure can be viewed from two viewpoints. Objectively, leisure is the amount of free, unobligated, or discretionary time left over after the demands of work (or school) and the daily requirements of subsistence have been met. Subjectively, leisure is a state of mind experienced by individuals as they engage in activities during free hours. Regardless of one's preferred definition, however, there appears to be a general consensus that leisure experiences are "at their best when free-time activities are freely chosen and intrinsically motivated."[10]

A major focus of leisure education is to develop a repertoire of effective recreation interests and skills. Recreation skills are an integral component of each individual's unique life-style. Selection of appropriate activities for inclusion in leisure education programs should be made on the basis of the following criteria:

1. The overall program provides a diversity of opportunities for participation in individual or group recreation experiences at various levels of specialization in the physical, social, cognitive, creative, and cultural arenas.
2. Activities are within the functional ability and behavior limitations of participating clients.
3. Activities are age appropriate and culturally normative.
4. Opportunities are provided for clients to participate in a variety of activities in the community.
5. Activities are compatible with clients' overall life situations and personal resources, whether the client is at home or in an institution.
6. Activities offered provide opportunities for continued development and involvement in later life.
7. The client is involved in the selection process.

It should be noted that "the issue is not simply one of acquiring as many leisure skills as possible. It is more important to assist the individual in selecting and developing adequate skills in a number of activities that will potentially be a source of enjoyment and personal satisfaction for the individual."[18]

RECREATION PARTICIPATION

The recreation therapy and leisure education components of the therapeutic recreation services continuum are developmental prerequisites to the establishment of an effective leisure life-style; the recreation participation mode is an integral part of the expression of an individual leisure life-style:

Recreation in varying forms, amounts, and quality is a life-continuous form of experience and expression. It is integrally related to all other facets of life's circumstances and experiences, either as the receptor or reflector of such influences or as their shaper or molder. Thus recreation may be seen both as being integrated with total life patterns and as being in itself one of life's integrating forces.*

Recreation participation programs are conducted on the premise that clients have developed the activity skills and preparatory abilities necessary for satisfying, enjoyable involvement. Outcomes for this mode are broadly stated in terms of clients' expressed enjoyment, self-expression, and satisfaction from participation in diverse, self-selected activities that closely approximate community-based recreation and leisure experiences.

Recreation participation programs in rehabilitation settings can also be viewed as a "living laboratory," providing clients with an appropriate arena for testing and practicing skills being developed in related therapy modalities. Recreation provides a unique setting for observation of what the client *does do* as opposed to what the client *can do*. Both the rehabilitation center and available community facilities, services, and situations can be used as social testing grounds for client performance. When appropriate, recreation programs also serve as a social forum in which clients and significant others can renew previously established patterns of recreation involvement or develop new family and

---

*Frye, V, and Peters, M: Therapeutic recreation: its theory, philosophy, and practice, Harrisburg, Penn, 1972, Stackpole Books.

friendship networks. The scope of potential activities and experiences that can be offered is limited only by the resources of the facility and the creativity of facilitators.

As indicated earlier, an essential aspect of comprehensive therapeutic recreation service is planning with the client for his or her recreation participation and leisure involvement after discharge from the rehabilitation service. This plan would include information on the various leisure resources available in the community or treatment setting in which the client will live. The therapeutic recreation specialist should contact these resources and make arrangements for referral of the client to them.

Rapoport and Rapoport describe the resourceful person as one who "can take the intelligence he has, the competence he is able to develop, and within the framework of his material means and social values apply them to weave a life that is satisfying."[20] It is appropriate that rehabilitation agencies and therapeutic recreation programs have increasingly moved toward models of service that emphasize participant self-determination; facilitate individual potentialities; allow individuals to find their own life solutions in work and leisure; and foster spontaneity, autonomy, and synergistic recreation.[2]

REFERENCES

1. Beard, JG, and Ragheb, MG: Measuring leisure satisfaction, J Leis Res 12:20, 1980.
2. Berryman, DL, and Borris, ER: Leisure and recreation services. In Valletutti, PJ, and Christoplos, R, editors: Preventing physical and mental disabilities: multidisciplinary approaches, Baltimore, 1984, Paul H Brookes Publishing Co.
3. Berryman, DL, and Lefebvre, CB: Recreation behavior inventory, ed 2, Denton, Tex, 1984, Leisure Learning Systems.
4. Cohen, BF, and Anthony, WA: Functional assessment in psychiatric rehabilitation. In Halpern, AS, and Fuhrer, MJ, editors: Functional assessment in rehabilitation, Baltimore, 1984, Paul H Brookes Publishing Co.
5. Edwards, PB, and Boland, PA: Leisure counseling and consultation, Pers Guid J 58:435, 1980.
6. Frye, V, and Peters, M: Therapeutic recreation: its theory, philosophy, and practice, Harrisburg, Penn, 1972, Stackpole Books.
7. Goldenson, RM: Dimensions of the field. In Goldenson, RM, editor: Disability and rehabilitation handbook, New York, 1978, McGraw-Hill Book Co.
8. Halpern, AS, and Fuhrer, MJ, editors: Functional assessment in rehabilitation, Baltimore, 1984, Paul H Brookes Publishing Co.
9. Hutchinson, P, and Lord, J: Recreation integration: issues and alternatives in leisure services and community involvement, Ottawa, 1979, Leisurability Publications, Inc.
10. Iso-Ahola, SE: The social psychology of leisure and recreation, Dubuque, 1980, Wm C Brown Co.
11. Kaplan, PE: Physical medicine and rehabilitation. In Valletutti, PJ, and Christoplos, F, editors: Preventing physical and mental disabilities: multidisciplinary approaches, Baltimore, 1979, University Park Press.
12. Kraus, R: Therapeutic recreation service: principles and practices, ed 2, Philadelphia, 1978, WB Saunders.
13. Levy, J: Behavioral observation techniques in assessing change in therapeutic recreation/play settings, Ther Rec J 16:25, 1982.
14. McKechnie, GE: Manual for the leisure activities blank, Palo Alto, 1975, Consulting Psychology Press, Inc.
15. Navar, N: Documentation in therapeutic recreation. In Peterson, CA, and Gunn, SL: Therapeutic recreation program design: principles and procedures, ed 2, Englewood Cliffs, NJ, 1984, Prentice-Hall, Inc.
16. Navar, N: Leisure skill assessment process in leisure counseling. In Szmanski, DJ, and Hitzhusen, GL, editors: Expanding horizons in therapeutic recreation VI, Columbia, Mo, 1979, Technical Education Services, University of Missouri.
17. Parker, RA, et al: Comprehensive evaluation in recreation therapy scale: a tool for patient evaluation, Ther Rec J 9:143, 1975.
18. Peterson, CA, and Gunn, SL: Therapeutic recreation program design: principles and procedures, ed 2, Englewood Cliffs, NJ, 1984, Prentice-Hall, Inc.
19. Ragheb, MG, and Beard, JG: Measuring leisure attitudes, J Leis Res 14:155, 1982.
20. Rapoport, R, and Rapoport, RN: Leisure and the family life cycle, London, 1975, Routledge & Kegan Paul.
21. Stolov, WC: Introduction. In Stolov, WC, and Clowers, MR: Handbook of severe disability, Washington DC, 1981, US Department of Education, Rehabilitation Services Administration.
22. Stubbins, J, editor: Social and psychological aspects of disability: a handbook for practitioners, Austin, 1977, Proed.
23. Touchstone, WA: A personalized approach to goal planning and evaluation, Ther Rec J 18:24, 1984.
24. Vash, CL: The psychology of disability, New York, 1981, Springer Publishing Co.
25. Witt, PA, and Ellis, G: The measurement of perceived freedom in leisure, J Leis Res 16:110, 1984.

CHAPTER 60

Americans with severe disabilities

VICTIMS OF OUTMODED POLICIES

RONALD W. CONLEY AND JOHN H. NOBLE, JR.

In this chapter we examine the ways in which public policy at the federal, state, and local levels interferes with the optimal social adjustment of persons with severe disabilities. This is a topic that, for two reasons, is both timely and important. First, the role of government in the provision of income support and services to persons who have disabilities has become large and complex. Government programs are often the primary resource available to disabled persons. In consequence, the requirements determining eligibility for the receipt of income support and services often dominate how persons with severe disabilities conduct their lives. Second, our expectations as to what severely disabled persons can and should achieve have changed in revolutionary ways in recent years. For example, it is increasingly accepted that persons who would formerly have been placed in institutional care for their protection and well-being can live in community-based residences and participate in community activities. In addition, it is now becoming apparent that many people who were formerly placed in sheltered workshops, work activity centers, or day care can be employed as members of an integrated work force in regular employment sites.

These facts raise the obvious question of whether the programs that were created in earlier years to serve persons with severe disabilities are consistent with current treatment philosophies. As this chapter demonstrates, many of the current programs are outmoded. We hasten to add, however, that this is not the fault of the legislators who enacted the laws that created the programs. In general, the programs were based on the available knowledge about how to improve the lives of persons with severe disabilities. The ex-

isting problems result from the failure of the programs to evolve as rapidly as the technology of providing care is changing.

This chapter discusses the problems of persons with severe disabilities and the problems of persons with severe mental retardation. The term "persons with severe disabilities" encompasses persons with all kinds of severe, disabling conditions, including mental retardation. An in-depth analysis of issues related to severely mentally retarded persons is presented to highlight problems generally applicable to a much wider range of persons with severe disabilities.

DEFINITIONS AND PREVALENCE

The term "disability" is defined in different ways for different purposes. Unfortunately, these different definitions have led to serious misunderstandings about the extent of disability and the capabilities of persons who have disabilities. In consequence, we begin by defining disability and other important terms used throughout the chapter.

We define a person as disabled if that person has functional limitations that result from one or more chronic physical or mental impairments. The loss of a limb (or loss of or restriction of its use), for example, is considered an impairment. If the impairment causes an inability (or reduction in ability) to walk, climb, lift, bend, or reach, the person with the impairment is considered disabled. As another example, brain damage—an impairment—often leads to reduced capacity to reason—a disability. The conceptual distinction between impairments and functional limitations or disabilities is consistent with the usage of Nagi[27] and the World Health Organization (WHO).[33] Although the term "handicap" is not used here, many of the problems that we describe as arising from society's adverse judgments

This paper was written by the authors in their private capacity. No official support or endorsement by the U.S. Department of Health and Human Services is intended or should be inferred.

or behaviors toward disabled persons fall within the meaning of the WHO definition of handicap, that is, the disadvantages experienced by individuals with impairments and disabilities as they interact with their physical and social surroundings.

Functional limitations or disabilities (we use the terms interchangeably) in turn often affect the way individuals carry out or respond to social expectations and roles. Such limitations also affect the way society responds to disabled individuals. For want of a better term, we refer to these consequences of functional limitations as the "ultimate effects" of chronic conditions or impairments (these terms may also be used interchangeably). These ultimate effects are numerous and have substantial effects on the well-being of an individual, his or her family, and society.

Many examples of types of ultimate effects can be given. The affected individual usually experiences psychic distress. Often there is a loss of or reduction in the capacity to engage in paid work. This loss of work capacity may extend to productive activities for which pay is not usually received, such as housework, child care, and home maintenance. The individual who has a functional limitation may also experience reduced ability to engage in nonwork activities that are considered normal for a person's age and sex, including visiting friends and relatives, driving a car, participating in sports, and so on. The ability to form personal relationships, such as having close friends, marrying, and having children, may be diminished. A parent may have to forego work to provide child care. Parents may have fewer children. Siblings may have to limit their education because of reduced family financial resources. And society often has to respond by providing special services, such as residential care, special education, extra medical care, respite care, and counseling.

Obviously, the number of the ultimate effects becomes enormous as the results of disabling conditions ripple through society. Reduced income and increased treatment costs, for example, probably lead to a lower rate of capital formation than would have otherwise occurred, slowing future economic growth.

Most people who hear and use the term "disability" generally think of persons with severe chronic impairments, such as the absence of a limb, mental retardation, and so on, and assume that these impairments cause functional limitations. This common definition of the term "disability" permeates both the professional and lay literature. Unfortunately, disability is often defined in technical ways that are inconsistent with the way most people use the term. The difference between popular and technical meanings of the term has led to frequent misunderstandings among those who use it and to differences of opinion about the implications of existing data on disabled persons.

As a specific illustration, most disability surveys do not consider a person with a chronic condition to be disabled unless he or she is unable to work. The survey reports often describe the population on which they are collecting information as "work disabled." This causes many functionally impaired persons who are working, including some persons who are severely impaired, not to be counted. Because of this technical definition of disability, we often come across reports that stress the finding that most disabled persons do not work, seemingly oblivious to the fact that the finding is an artifact of the definition. This technical survey definition has led to widespread failure to appreciate the fact that many severely impaired Americans are productively employed. Furthermore, this misunderstanding of the data has caused the term "disability" to become synonymous in some people's minds with failure—an inference that has profound negative consequences for disabled people who seek to live normal lives.

The importance of these observations is underscored by the fact that at least 18.5 million Americans, aged 17 to 64 years, were limited in their activities because of a chronic physical or mental condition in 1979.[23] More than one fourth of these people, however, were not limited in their ability to perform their major activity, generally working or keeping house. Almost one half were limited but not totally prevented from doing their major activity. Only about one fifth were totally unable to perform their major activity.

These statistics might appear to differentiate among those in the United States who are severely, moderately, or mildly disabled. Reliance on such data, however, would be simplistic and misleading. Among persons who report partial or even no limitation in work activity are some who, by the common definition, would be considered severely disabled—persons with multiple amputations, with IQs below 50, and so on. And if persons who report great difficulty in working are closely examined, we find some who, by the common definition, do not have severe disabilities.

The policy implications of these data are clear. Whether Americans with disabilities secure and retain substantial work depends not only on their disabling condition and its severity, but also on many other variables, such as their attitudes toward work; the vigor of the economy; and the service system that provides income support, medical care, and vocational and other services. We believe that widely prevailing attitudes toward persons labeled as "disabled" and the misguided policies that have sprung from these attitudes account for much of the dependency and economic idleness of the affected individuals.

NORMALIZATION AND THE FEDERAL ROLE

To highlight the policy issues and stakes further, we focus on persons who are moderately, severely, or profoundly mentally retarded or who are mildly mentally retarded and physically or emotionally impaired. Collectively, this group can be considered to have severe mental retardation. They often have IQs of 55 or less. More often than not, they also have other impairments, such as cerebral palsy, epilepsy, heart disease, and psychiatric disorders. Estimates vary, but we believe that there are about 400,000 adults in the United States with IQs below 50.[7]

A great deal has been learned about the adaptive capacity of persons with severe mental retardation in the last 25 years. Twenty-five years ago, the advice most often given to a family with a severely mentally retarded infant was to place the infant in an institution so that he or she might receive adequate lifelong care and the parents might save themselves the embarrassment and encumbrance of such a child. Today, however, such an infant usually remains with the natural family during childhood. As a child, the severely mentally retarded individual generally receives special education and in some cases regular schooling to develop productive capabilities and skills. As an adult, that individual may live in the community, in a group home or in an independent residence; participate in community activities; and engage in meaningful, substantial work.

Recognition that persons with severe mental retardation are capable of much more than living out their lives in an institution has created the ideology of normalization. The goal of normalization is to assist Americans with all kinds of severe disabilities to live as nearly normal a life as possible. In this regard we are still learning just how normal a life a severely disabled person can lead.

In the past the capacity of persons with severe mental retardation to learn, to live in the community, and to work has been greatly underestimated. At present, public programs are in the throes of changing to reflect our better understanding of the capacity of these individuals to live outside of institutions and to take part in community life.

The federal government has often provided leadership in changing or creating programs to promote normalized living for people with severe disabilities. The U.S. Congress has enacted a number of major laws that have dramatically changed expectations and the types of services provided to people with severe disabilities.

In 1971 the Intermediate Care Facilities for Mentally Retarded (ICF/MR) Persons program was enacted, primarily to improve the quality of care provided in state institutions. Almost from the beginning, however, the program was used to support some community residential programs.

The Rehabilitation Act of 1973 directed state vocational rehabilitation agencies to give priority to serving "those individuals with the most severe handicaps."

In 1975 the Education for all Handicapped Children Act was passed. It required participating states to provide all disabled children, regardless of the degree of their disability, with a free, appropriate public education. Today few children with disabilities in the United States lack access to educational services.

In 1976 the Social Security Act was amended to permit Supplemental Security Income (SSI) to be paid to residents in public residential facilities with 16 or fewer residents.

Previously, SSI payments could not be made to residents in public facilities.

In 1981 Title XIX of the Social Security Act was amended to allow the secretary of the Department of Health and Human Services to grant waivers to states to use Medicaid funds for nonmedical services to persons who are elderly or have disabilities and would otherwise require institutional care. The Home and Community-Based Services Waivers Program was explicitly designed to promote the development and provision of community-based care and to avoid needless institutionalization.

The Developmental Disabilities Act of 1984 established "employment-related activities" as one of four priority services to be provided under the basic support grant program. This act defines a developmental disability as one that begins before age 22 years and substantially limits an individual's functioning in three of seven major life activities.

Despite these positive actions by the federal government, there remain numerous impediments in the service system to the attainment of a normal life and maximum independence by severely disabled Americans.

MISCONCEPTIONS ABOUT WORKERS WITH SEVERE DISABILITIES

There are three common misconceptions about mentally retarded persons that are largely applicable to persons with other forms of severe disability. The first is that persons with mental retardation are unable to work. This is clearly untrue of persons with IQs from 55 to 70. Follow-up studies have shown that the percentage of persons in this IQ range who are employed is only slightly below the percentage employed among the general population.[7] Persons with IQs below 55 are usually either not employed or employed in work activity centers. There is rapidly accumulating evidence, however, that even persons in this low IQ range can do substantial jobs if placed in suitable work settings and given appropriate support.[4,19,25,29-32] Persons with severe mental retardation are increasingly employed as dishwashers, bus persons, janitors, and horticultural workers and in a wide variety of other jobs.[19]

The second misconception is that even if persons with severe mental retardation are employed, their earnings will necessarily be low. This reflects the fallacious belief that earnings vary directly with intelligence and represents a fundamental misunderstanding about the nature of the job market. There are a large number of different types of jobs in the economy, each requiring different combinations of reasoning ability, strength, dexterity, experience, training, and other traits. Many of these jobs can be effectively done by persons with limited intelligence. The productivity of workers with mental retardation on these jobs is sometimes as high as or even higher than the productivity of much brighter persons would be if placed in the same job. Place a learned professor on a job requiring a pick and shovel, and his productivity will often be far below the norm.

The key to productivity, of course, is proper placement and motivation. On most jobs, because of the division of labor, productivity must be measured for a group of workers rather than for a single worker. Alternatively stated, the absence of a single worker often greatly affects the productivity of co-workers. How many businesses, for example, would continue to produce effectively without janitorial staff? In consequence, the wages paid to individual workers reflect the relative bargaining power of persons in a producing enterprise, rather than what the esoteric concept of individual "marginal productivity" would imply. What advantages do persons who are not mentally retarded have over persons who are? First and most obvious, non–mentally retarded persons can acquire skills that command a higher rate of pay than those to which mentally retarded persons can aspire. Second, non–mentally retarded persons can perform a wider variety of existing jobs, which eases their job search. Third, non–mentally retarded persons have superior ability to shop around, try different jobs, and eventually find one that is personally satisfying. In contrast, persons with mental retardation often require assistance and support to locate and retain work of any kind.

The third misconception is that the intellectual limitation is primarily at fault when work cannot be found by a mentally retarded person. However, many factors affect the prospects of mentally retarded persons searching for work, including the existence of other physical and emotional disorders; attitudes toward work; personal habits, such as punctuality, neatness of dress, and ability to use public transportation; job discrimination; and the availability of appropriate training and assistance in locating and retaining work. Although the intellectual limitation may be one impeding factor, it usually takes more than the intellectual limitation to prevent a person from working; in fact, the intellectual limitation is often the least important factor in causing job failure.

FEDERAL ROLE

Persons with mental retardation have the same basic needs and are subject to the same kinds of problems as everybody else in the population. In consequence, persons with mental retardation and other disabling conditions make use of most of the public programs that are generally available to other Americans, as well as some programs specifically designed to serve them. Among the most important of these programs are income support provided by the SSI or the Social Security Disability Insurance (SSDI) programs, including the Childhood Disability Beneficiary (CDB) component of the SSDI program; medical care provided by Medicaid or Medicare; social services provided through the social service block grant; education in either regular or special education classes; and vocational services provided by the state-federal vocational rehabilitation program or the state employment services.

Many additional programs provide benefits to persons with severe disabilities. Income support may also come through civil service, railroad retirement, and private pension plans. Some persons receiving income support are eligible for food stamps. In addition to public programs, there are many private organizations that provide social and vocational services.

Most persons with severe mental retardation or other severe disabilities need more than one of these services. It is quite possible, for example, for some beneficiaries of the SSDI/CDB program to also receive a supplement from the SSI program and food stamps. In addition, these beneficiaries are also usually eligible for Medicare, Medicaid, or both. In some cases these same people also receive vocational and social services.

This leads us to a critical observation. To determine the impact of public programs on individuals, we must examine the combined effect of all programs; one program cannot meaningfully be evaluated in isolation. The full range of programs must be regarded as providing a system of services for severely disabled persons. Thus, when employment programs fail to assist persons with severe disabilities to return to work, it may be the result of the work disincentives existing in other programs, rather than the fault of the employment program. Although the need to take a holistic approach in evaluating programs for severely disabled persons may appear obvious, the sad fact is that programs are usually assessed and modified as though their effects occur in isolation.

LIFE CYCLE TRANSITIONAL PERSPECTIVE

To understand the needs of persons with severe mental retardation or other childhood disabilities and of their families, it is necessary to consider the whole life cycle and ask, "What are the major transitions through which they must pass, and what are their needs at each transition point?" This will assist in assessing the strengths and weaknesses of the existing service system.

The birth of a child with a severe disability, such as mental retardation, leads to a fairly predictable sequence of life events and transitions until the end of life is reached.[28] The first major transition is from hospital to home. The parents of the child must accept and understand the disabling condition if they are to undertake the difficult task of caring for their child. In additon to meeting the child's physical care needs, the parents must provide the stimulation and environment needed to foster the child's development to the limits of his or her capacity.

The second major transition takes place when the child reaches preschool age. Preschool nursery and Head Start programs help the child in social training and stimulation, while offering needed respite to parents.

The third transition occurs when the child enters school. At this time the school and parents must develop an individualized education plan that seeks to optimize the child's capacity for learning and social maturation. During this extended period the child should learn how to care for himself or herself, and acquire prevocational and vocational skills within the limits of his or her capacity.

As with people without disabilities, when the late adolescent or young adult leaves school between the ages of 18 and 22 years, transition to adult life, employment, and independent living should occur. For a young adult with a disability this is a critical transition, the success of which requires the support of family, friends, peers, and employers. Families often need help in accepting and promoting their child's departure from home to live as independently as possible. For the severely disabled "independent living" often means sharing a supervised apartment or other congregate living arrangement and taking up supported employment or sheltered work in the community in which they grew up.

Finally, severely disabled persons who work can at some point expect to retire. Such persons, like those without disabilities, may need help in adjusting to a life-style of greater leisure and opportunities for more social and recreational activities.

PROBLEMS IN EVALUATING PROGRAMS

In conducting studies on disability, economists use three basic tools. The first is cost-of-condition analysis—the cost of mental retardation, the cost of all disabling conditions, and so on. The social cost of a disabling condition is usually defined as the total sum of the costs of all of the ultimate effects caused by that condition, plus the cost of efforts to prevent the condition such as vaccinating children against rubella.[6] The social cost includes the loss of productivity among persons in the defined group; the value of the loss of homemaking services and other unpaid work; the value of the possible loss of family stability; the value of treatment services, such as special education and residential care, that can be ascribed to the condition; and so on. Cost-of-condition analyses may cover a single year for all of the persons with that condition or may span the lifetime of persons born with the condition during a given year.

The second economic tool is cost-benefit analysis. Cost-benefit analysis has a direct relationship to cost-of-condition analysis. Suppose a program is established or expanded to prevent, treat, or rehabilitate a person with mental retardation or some other disabling condition. Some of the ultimate effects measured under cost-of-condition analysis increase as a result of the program. These are the costs in the cost-benefit calculation. Other ultimate effects decrease. These are the benefits. A comparison of these two types of

changes in the components of the cost of a condition constitute cost-benefit analysis.

The third economic tool is cost-effectiveness analysis, which establishes a goal that is usually measured in nonmonetary terms, such as reducing institutional populations by a given number, and then compares the relative costs of the various ways of attaining this goal. When it can be used, cost-effectiveness analysis is usually much simpler than cost-benefit analysis.

Unfortunately, many empiric and conceptual problems are involved in implementing and interpreting all of these forms of economic analysis.

There are problems of missing data. Obviously, disabling conditions have many effects. At best we measure only a few of these effects, such as the loss of earnings of people with disabilities, the increase in their earnings after rehabilitation, and the costs of treatment and rehabilitation. Effects on the earnings of other family members are usually mentioned but rarely quantified. Effects on the work efforts of siblings or their future college achievements are rarely even mentioned, although they are obviously relevant in discussing the effects of disability. Even for obvious variables, such as the earnings of disabled persons, we rarely have sufficient data to estimate the *increase* in earnings that can be ascribed to rehabilitation without making a number of very judgmental assumptions.

There are also problems of imputing a monetary or market value to many of the effects of disabling conditions. This is obviously true for psychic costs and for losses in the ability to carry on such normal activities as riding the bus, going shopping, and so on. It is even true for such activities as homemaking.

There are problems with the different weighing of costs and benefits. Although economists are concerned primarily with easily measured variables, such as earnings and treatment costs, other people, such as parents, may attach much less importance to these variables and place much greater emphasis on psychic costs and family stability.

There are also problems of distribution. The costs of programs are usually borne by taxpayers, and the benefits are largely received by persons who are handicapped. Technically, one cannot compare costs borne by one group and benefits received by another. Although such information may be useful in deciding whether a program should be funded, it will require a judgment on the desirability of redistributing income in addition to a comparison of benefits and costs.

There are problems in defining the appropriate decision units. Although economists stress the importance of conducting cost-benefit analyses based on marginal changes in the program (that is, changes in a part of the program that is realistically subject to a funding decision), it is next to impossible to determine the benefits that result from changing only a small part of the program. Who can say which persons in a vocational rehabilitation program would not have been served if the program had not expanded?

There are also problems of discounting. Obviously, much of the benefits and some of the costs in rehabilitation programs will not occur until future years and must be discounted to present value. Although this is one of the most significant variables affecting the results of cost-benefit analysis, there is little consensus, either empirically or conceptually, about what constitutes the appropriate discount rate. Using two rates, as is sometimes done, merely doubles the number of calculations. And telling policy makers that the best measure of benefits probably lies between the two sets of calculations greatly increases the likelihood of instant dismissal of the results.

There are many additional technical problems in conducting economic analyses; the problems cited are only the most important ones. However, one should not conclude from this enumeration of the problems that economic studies have little value. On the contrary, analyses that identify and refine cost and benefit information are of immense value to decision makers. It is essential, however, to be aware of the limitations of cost-benefit analyses and to recognize that, although these analyses can assist in decision making, they are not substitutes for the ultimate value judgments that must be made.

The problems that arise in conducting economic studies have contributed to a major evolutionary change in the way cost-benefit and cost-effectiveness analyses are generally carried out. Because it is impossible in cost-benefit analysis to place monetary values on many important benefits, such analysis has been modified to allow the benefits of various programs to be identified and measured but when appropriate left in nonmonetary terms. In the case of deinstitutionalization, for example, one would array a range of benefits that would include increased earnings, increased ability to perform activities of daily living, increased use of community resources, and so on. When conducted in this fashion, such analyses have commonly been referred to as program evaluation. Actually, "program evaluation" is a general term that includes as a special case the form of cost-benefit analysis in which all benefits are measured in monetary terms.

A basic problem with cost-effectiveness analysis is that it assumes that the benefits being sought can be held constant across different ways of providing services. In fact, it is usually the differences in benefits among alternative ways of providing services and not the differences in costs that are the determining factor in choosing which program should be adopted. As examples, supported work is preferred over adult day care because of the superior benefits it provides to persons with severe mental retardation. Community-based residences are preferred over institutional care because of the obvious benefits to persons who require some form of supervised care. Even a choice among different ways of providing community-based residential care is often based

as much on differences in the way the alternatives affect the well-being of residents as on differences in costs.

Therefore, in comparing alternative means of providing services, we increasingly examine *both* the benefits and costs of the alternatives and, when appropriate, the benefits are left in nonmonetary form. As in the case of cost-benefit analyses, cost-effectiveness analyses are a special case of a generalized program evaluation approach in which the benefits can be assumed to remain constant over the various alternatives.

Although it is not generally done, cost-of-condition analyses could also be as easily done by leaving some of the ultimate effects of nonmonetary form, so that cost of condition analyses would be modified to conform to the realities of our knowledge of the ultimate effects of conditions in the same way that cost-benefit analyses and cost-effectiveness analyses have been modified.

The next logical step in the evolution of methods to evaluate programs is still in its initial stages. This next step is to evaluate the benefits and costs of the programs in the service system as a whole, rather than program by program.

PROBLEMS IN THE SERVICE SYSTEM

The current U.S. system that provides income support and services to severely disabled persons has a number of flaws that cause it to fail to achieve socially desirable goals in many cases.[8] Some of the more important of the obstacles to the desired goal attainment are described below.

Coordination problems

Despite our earlier observation that the different programs serving persons with disabilities collectively comprise a system of services and should be conceptualized and evaluated as such, a lack of coordination and integration among the various programs has been frequently identified as a major problem in the provision of services. In general, the various programs do not operate as a cohesive system but as a loose aggregation of independently functioning units that on occasion clash and interfere with one another's operations. There are a number of reasons for this. Legislative consideration is rarely given to how these programs interact when they are being considered for modification or renewal. In addition, coordination problems are exacerbated because the programs are sometimes managed at the federal level (for example, income support programs), sometimes at the state level (for example, Medicaid and vocational rehabilitation), and sometimes at the local level (for example, public housing and transportation).

Disparate program goals and motivations

In our view the most important reason for the lack of coordination is a lack of common objectives among programs. The income support and medical care programs were not designed to encourage employment but to support persons unable to work. As another example, social workers, lawyers, family members, group home operators, and others are usually more concerned with ensuring that severely disabled persons have a secure income than with returning them to work.

Work disincentives

The existing system of services, particularly the income support and health care programs, contain major work disincentives for individuals receiving benefits. These work disincentives take several forms. First, there is often a strong effect on the net gain from work such that a beneficiary returning to work either receives a small net increase in income or suffers an actual decrease in disposable income. In considering the effects of a return to work, the total benefit package must be considered—loss of income support, loss of medical care coverage, and loss of social services.

The potential income loss is particularly striking in the SSDI program, including the CDB component. Beneficiaries who return to work and earn the substantial gainful activity (SGA) wage of $300 per month or more—about three fifths of the minimum wage for a full-time worker—are allowed a 9-month trial work period. At the end of the trial work period, they are reevaluated. If thought capable of earning more than $300 per month, they are terminated from SSDI. Since benefits are usually higher than $300 per month (the average SSDI benefit is half again this high) the reward for returning to work is a loss of income more often than not. In addition, taxes and normal work-related expenses have to be paid out of this income.

Before 1981 an SSI recipient who began to work was also placed on a trial work period. At the end of 9 months the recipient was reevaluated and terminated from SSI if considered capable of earning over the SGA level per month. Since the SGA level is currently $300 per month and at that time was close to the SSI payment rate for individuals and considerably below the payment rate for couples, and since taxes and normal work expenses would have to be paid out of earnings, there was substantial disincentive for SSI recipients to accept employment paying over the SGA amount, unless they were capable of earning significantly more than the SSI monthly payment. In 1988 the SSI payment was $354 per month for individuals and $532 per month for couples. The SGA level has remained unchanged

To reduce these work disincentives, Congress approved two special 3-year demonstrations beginning in 1981. One demonstration, incorporated as Section 1619(a) of the Social Security Act, authorized special cash benefits to be paid to working SSI recipients as long as their earnings were below the federal break-even point. This special demonstration project was extended in 1984 and then made permanent in 1986 in the Employment Opportunities for Disabled Americans Act (P.L. 99-643).

Under the Section 1619(a) program, after an initial $85 is disregarded, the payments to SSI recipients are reduced by $1 for every $2 of earnings. In 1988 all SSI payments did not terminate until the break-even points of $793 per month for an individual and $1149 per month for a couple. This program greatly reduces but does not eliminate the work disincentives in the SSI program.

Continuation of health benefits is often as important, if not more important, to persons with severe disabilities as receipt of ongoing income support payments. Before 1981 SSDI/CDB beneficiaries who lost their entitlement to cash benefits would also lose their entitlement to Medicare benefits. However, in 1980 Congress passed legislation that extended Medicare benefits for 36 months after the termination of cash benefits for SSDI/CDB beneficiaries who returned to work. This also reduced but did not eliminate this source of work disincentive.

Before 1981 SSI recipients who lost their entitlement to cash benefits usually lost their entitlement to Medicaid. To address this disincentive, Congress passed a special 3-year demonstration, incorporated as Section 1619(b) of the Social Security Act, that continued Medicaid coverage to some SSI recipients who returned to work and whose SSI was terminated because their earnings exceeded the break-even point. Medicaid protection is continued if recipients (1) continue to qualify on the basis of limited assets, (2) would not be able to pay for medical benefits equivalent to Medicaid, and (3) would have difficulty maintaining their employment without such coverage. This special demonstration was extended in 1984 and then made permanent in the Employment Opportunities for Disabled Americans Act of 1986.

A second type of work disincentive arises because of the effect of public programs on the security of income. Most people, whether or not they have a disability, are as much concerned about the security of their income as they are about the amount. They will sometimes forego higher paying jobs in favor of those that are protected by seniority, tenure, civil service, or some other means. Similarly, it is reasonable to expect that recipients of public support would feel little incentive to exchange a secure source of monthly income for employment that adds little to net income and sometimes even decreases it. These recipients are no less concerned about income security than anyone else.

In 1980 Congress attempted to reduce the fear of loss of income among recipients of disability income by providing a 15-month reentitlement period following the trial work period for both the SSDI/CDB and SSI programs. In 1986, as part of the Employment Opportunities for Disabled Americans Act, Congress repealed the use of time-limited trial work and extended reentitlement periods, which had become obsolete and confusing under the now permanent provisions of Sections 1619(a) and 1619(b), for disabled SSI recipients.

A third way in which public programs create work disincentives is by fostering defeatist attitudes toward work. To qualify for SSDI/CDB or SSI, applicants must prove that they are unable to work at the SGA level. For persons who have not worked since their injury or the onset of their disease or at any time during their lives, this may consist of demonstrating that they have one of a long list of conditions that are presumed to show inability to earn at a substantial gainful activity level. Persons who have a work history or whose conditions are not listed must prove inability to earn at the SGA level through the use of medical and other evidence. It is likely to take between 2 months and 1 year to document inability to earn at this level to the satisfaction of the Social Security Administration. During this time the applicant, his or her family, lawyer, and others are busily engaged in proving that the applicant cannot work. This process often has destructive effects on the applicant's morale and willingness to even try to return to work.

The extent of work disincentives in the SSDI/CDB, SSI, Medicare, and Medicaid programs has been substantially reduced since 1980. Of particular importance is the Employment Opportunities for Disabled Americans Act of 1986, which not only made permanent the Section 1619(a) and 1619(b) demonstration programs for disabled SSI recipients who return to work, but also simplified the administration of these programs and reduced much of the capriciousness that existed in these programs. As mentioned previously, the 1986 act eliminated the time-limited trial work and reentitlement periods because they were no longer needed. In addition, program participants can now move freely between the regular SSI, the Section 1619(a), and the Section 1619(b) programs. Before the 1986 act there were circumstances under which it was possible for a disabled SSI recipient to forfeit all claim to continuing Section 1619(a) payments if, for any reason, the recipient lost entitlement to SSI payments for a single month (for example, earnings may have been too high because of holiday overtime, a year-end bonus, or a gift).

Despite the reduction in work disincentives since 1980, major work disincentives still remain in the service system. These remaining disincentives partly explain why there has been no great rush of recipients to return to work. Remaining disincentives include the following:

1. The SSDI/CDB still makes no provision for reducing benefits gradually as earnings rise, and as a result, many SSDI/CDB beneficiaries who return to work face a substantial income loss.

2. Although the Section 1619(a) and 1619(b) programs have been made permanent, continuing disability reviews are required within 12 months of an SSI recipient's entry into the Section 1619(a) program. It is unclear as to the extent to which high earnings will trigger or incline the persons making the disability evaluation toward a finding that the recipient is not sufficiently disabled to qualify for continuing SSI payments.

3. Persons applying for SSI must still prove inability to work at the SGA level of $300 per month, a requirement that places the qualifying conditions for SSI in direct opposition to the intent and purposes of the Section 1619(a) and 1619(b) programs, which permit SSI recipients to have earnings up to the federal breakeven point before losing entitlement to SSI payments and even higher earnings before losing entitlement to Medicaid.

4. Persons receiving extended Medicaid benefits under the Section 1619(b) program still must fall below an annual income threshold to maintain eligibility for the program. This has allegedly caused some SSI recipients to refuse promotions and to reduce hours of work. This is a particularly important consideration, given that some SSI recipients are uninsurable under private plans.

5. This same lack of insurability may cause some SSDI/CDB beneficiaries to be concerned about the loss of Medicare benefits that will occur 3 years after they lose entitlement to cash benefits.

6. The different rules governing the payment of benefits under the SSDI/CDB and SSI programs may also cause serious work disincentives among persons who are eligible for both programs.

More elaborate descriptions of these and other work disincentives may be found in Conley, Noble, and Elder.[8]

We believe that current and previous work disincentives are an unintended consequence of a basic fallacy that underlies these income support and health care financing programs. The legislative mandate of these programs is to provide basic income support and health care financing only if program participants are unable to engage in work at a substantial gainful activity wage level. This assumes that the world can be divided into persons who are capable of this level of work and those who are not. Work capacity, however, depends on a great many variables in addition to the disabling condition (for example, age, education, motivation, and work experience). The way that these variables interact and affect work capacity is imperfectly understood. Predictions of work capacity are highly subjective and often are disputed, as evidenced by the extensive litigation among permanent disability cases in workers' compensation (which, by the way, is a system that was originally designed to avoid litigation).

We do not believe that existing methods of assessing work capacity are adequate.[24] For SSDI/CDB and SSI programs the initial determination of work disability is made by the disability determination service, usually located in the state vocational rehabilitation agency. Forms and medical reports from the Social Security Administration are the basis of decisions. As patently flawed as this process is, we know of no other process that would be better, largely because we believe that the process is based on a flawed premise.

We believe that most severely disabled persons can work if placed in a suitable job and given appropriate services and support. Unfortunately, by rewarding people for convincing the Social Security Administration that they cannot work, the existing system makes it unlikely that these individuals will ever attempt to return to work.

In this regard, it is worth emphasizing that the importance of making the provisions of the Section 1619(a) and 1619(b) programs permanent lies not only in reducing the work disincentives inherent in the SSI program, but also in creating a fundamental change in the public's perception of disabled persons receiving public support. No longer are disabled SSI recipients to be regarded as inherently unable to work. Instead, they will henceforth be considered persons who may be helped to return to substantial employment. The inconsistencies between the treatment of persons receiving SSI payments and SSDI/CDB benefits and between persons already receiving benefits and those applying for benefits for the first time cannot possibly go unnoticed. These inconsistencies highlight inequities and stimulate continuing efforts by the U.S. Congress to further reduce the remaining work disincentives.

Creation and perpetuation of poverty

To become eligible for SSI and in most cases Medicaid in 1987, individual applicants could have no more than $1800 in countable assets, and couples could have no more than $2700 in countable assets. In determining countable assets, SSI applicants are entitled to disregard the value of their home and, with some limitations, their car, as well as some insurance, personal effects, and a burial plot. Each year about 20% of the applicants for SSI are turned down because of excess assets. Some SSI recipients are terminated for this reason. Thus some people must spend their life savings before they can qualify for SSI and Medicaid.

This stringent asset limitation has several harmful effects on both the individual and the society. First, not only does it cause some people to spend themselves into poverty, but the lack of resources for emergencies may itself act as a deterrent against SSI and Medicaid recipients taking a chance to reestablish their independence. Moreover, the asset restriction creates a clear disincentive to save. This reduces capital formation, encourages unnecessary consumption, and may create habits that are counter to the American work ethic. In any event discouraging people from saving for future needs is clearly nonnormalizing. Although few SSI recipients have income sufficient to enable them to save any significant sums, the ability and desire of SSI recipients to save may become increasingly important as rising numbers of people with disabilities return to work under the Section 1619(b) program. In many cases eligibility for extended Medicaid benefits under the 1619(b) program will continue, even though earnings may exceed $20,000 per year.

Problems have also arisen for severely disabled persons in residential care. In some cases these institutionalized persons have managed to save a substantial amount of the small sums of earnings or income support benefits they are allowed to keep. Social workers and group home managers have learned to caution these residents against being too frugal.

Even the SSDI/CDB program has features that create poverty. One such feature is the 2-year hiatus between the time of being declared eligible for SSDI/CDB benefits and the time at which these beneficiaries become eligible for Medicare benefits. During this time they must spend their own funds for medical services or apply for Medicaid benefits. The 2-year waiting period causes Medicare benefits to be denied to a group that is likely to have above average need for medical services and limited likelihood of being able to obtain or afford insurance protection for medical needs. In addition, there is a 6-month wait between the time of becoming disabled and the earliest time at which individuals can receive SSDI/CDB benefits.

Institutional bias of programs

The Title XIX ICF/MR program is the major federal source of funding for both institutional and community care of persons with mental retardation and developmental disabilities. In fiscal year 1985 it accounted for 34.2% of a total of $7.773 billion in federal spending for persons with mental retardation and developmental disabilities.[5] To gain perspective on the significance of this source of revenue, it is useful to reflect that federal expenditures for SSI payments constituted 19.7% of total federal spending for mentally retarded and developmentally disabled persons in fiscal year 1985; SSDI, 16.4%; noninstitutional Medicaid, 3.1%; Title XX social services, 2.8%; vocational rehabilitation state grants, 1.7%; and 43 other federal programs, 4.7%.

The growth of federal reimbursements for institutional care of persons with mental retardation and developmental disabilities since 1977 has been explosive. The federal share of expenditures for state institutional services has increased from 23% to 45%, rising from $570 million in 1977 to $1.91 billion in 1984. In contrast, the federal share of expenditures for community services increased from 6% to 21%, rising from $45 million in 1977 to $663 million in 1984. Total spending for community care of persons with mental retardation and developmental disabilities has grown from $745 million in 1977 to $3.1 billion in 1984, an increase of 316%. State general funds account for 70% of total community services spending for mentally retarded and developmentally disabled persons.

During a time of rapid growth in both institutional and community spending the Title XIX ICF/MR program, because of its institutional bias, has acted as a drag on the development of needed community services for persons with mental retardation and developmental disabilities and has reduced their prospects for employment. The explanation for this lies in the history, basic philosophy, and assumptions of the program.

Federal ICF/MR funds were used by the states to finance state-operated institutions for mentally retarded persons.

When the ICF/MR program was instituted in 1971, the states had to spend substantial sums of state money to upgrade staff, plant, and equipment to meet the higher federal "active treatment" and fire and life-safety standards. The institutions thus represent a "sunk cost" that the states are reluctant to abandon for a number of reasons. First, the only way in which states can recoup these "sunk costs" is through continued occupancy of the Medicaid certified institutions, so that depreciation on these buildings can be included in Medicaid charges. Second, the capital cost of developing community residential facilities that are not certified as ICF/MR facilities by Medicaid must be entirely financed by state and local funds. Third, the states (and local governments) must pay a large share of the costs of operating community residential facilities if they are not certified as ICF/MR facilities, since the primary source of funds other than state revenues is from residents who receive SSI or who have some earnings. Finally, the ICF/MR program simplifies administration by placing all authority for decisions about individual services into the hands of a single authority, adopting a medical model that assumes that residents require 24-hour supervised care. Given this requirement, residents could hardly be encouraged to engage in substantial work.

The open-ended character of the ICF/MR program makes it easy for the states to pass along to the federal government a substantial portion of the wage and benefit increases that are demanded by often unionized state employees. Buttressed by the unions and the families of institutionalized residents, the states have sought to hang onto their ICF/MR-funded institutions, despite the rising tide of opinion that community-based residences are superior to institutions.

The bias toward institutional care is sometimes further reinforced by funding arrangements between state and local governments. Where local governments do not share in the cost of institutional care but must pay some portion of the cost of community-based services, as in Virginia, there is a strong incentive to avoid development of community alternatives to institutional care of the mentally retarded and developmentally disabled. In fiscal year 1984, for example, the federal government through Medicaid and Medicare contributed almost half (49.03%) of Virginia's expenditure of $98,294,000 for the care of persons with mental retardation and developmental disabilities in state institutions. The share of the federal government in the provision of community care for mentally retarded citizens was much smaller; thus the share of the Virginia state government was correspondingly much larger. Moreover, the share of the total cost of community care that must be borne by the states is increasing because of declining local and federal government support and a static contribution from families and philanthropic organizations. Under these financial circumstances, it is not surprising that Virginia has not taken more aggressive steps to reduce the size of its ICF/MR-funded institutional pro-

grams for mentally retarded and developmentally disabled persons. To do so would require substantially greater state tax effort in the face of predictable taxpayer resistance.

The Home and Community-Based Services Waivers program, enacted in 1981, represented the first weakening of the institutional bias of the ICF/MR program. It lessened the bias toward institutionalization for persons who are aged, mentally ill, or mentally ill and are eligible for Medicaid support. (Persons in institutions for the mentally ill cannot qualify for Medicaid unless they are under age 22 years or over age 64 years.) This program permitted states to purchase nonmedical services for persons in the community who would otherwise be institutionalized. Two restrictions on this program were that the cost had to be less than the corresponding cost of institutional care and that there had to be evidence that these persons would in fact be in institutions in the absence of these services. The latter restriction in particular has limited the use of this program. To show that persons served under a waiver could have been institutionalized, states had to establish that there were beds available in an institution for these persons, that an institution would otherwise be built, or by some other means. For these and other reasons states have not rushed to take advantage of this program.

Lack of family support

Lack of community services influences many families to institutionalize their child. Families with a severely disabled child at home often sustain an extraordinary burden beyond the initial sense of shock, denial, grief, shame, guilt, and depression that typically accompanies the discovery. These burdens include social isolation from stigma or rejection by kin or neighbors; financial and opportunity costs; excessive amounts of time required to provide personal care; difficulty with physical management; difficulty in ordinary family routines, such as shopping, house cleaning, and finding ample recreational outlets; the acquisition of special parenting skills to cope with medical emergencies and promote the child's adaptive behavior; stress that often results in poor physical health; and strained family relationships between siblings and parents.[17] In the absence of community support families of lower socioeconomic status with few resources tend to seek out-of-home placement of their severely disabled child. Many studies indicate that the lack of community services often precipitates a family's decision to institutionalize their child.[1,11-13,18,22]

Although most states offer some form of family support as a means of encouraging families to maintain their severely disabled member at home, there is great variation in the type and amount of services provided. Many states offer only limited case management and respite care—two of the most critically needed services. State funding support is extremely limited. In the early 1980s it ranged from $3.6 million annually in Pennsylvania for supportive services for

11,548 persons to $23,000 in Connecticut for cash subsidies for 15 families.[17] Federal support for family support services is extremely limited and thus places most of the fiscal burden for such services on state or local revenues.

Limited funds for long-term vocational support

The rapidly developing emphasis on providing supported work to persons with severe disabilities who cannot maintain employment with traditional vocational rehabilitation services alone has generated a need for the provision of supported work services (for example, long-term supervision, transportation to work, a job coach, and so on). Unfortunately, there are severe limitations on the funds available for these purposes.

Obviously, persons in ICF/MR facilities are prime candidates for the provision of such services. Until recently, however, Medicaid had a flat prohibition against the provision of vocational services of any type. Efforts by the states to provide such services resulted in a spate of audit exceptions involving the use of ICF/MR funds to pay for prevocational and vocational services. Instead of promoting the "helplessness" of ICF/MR residents, it would be consistent with the intent of the ICF/MR program to take every means of encouraging their higher level of functioning. Ironically, rigid ICF/MR funding regulations are motivating the states to withhold community care and employment options from people with severe disabilities. In places where the ICF/MR funds are used to pay for supported employment services, the program operators run the risk of an audit exception and liability for paying back to the federal government many thousands of dollars. The prohibition against the use of Medicaid funds to pay for vocational services is a major reason why most persons in ICF/MR facilities are placed in adult day care programs rather than work programs.

Changes in the service system that will expand the provision of long-term vocational services are beginning to be made. The Consolidated Omnibus Budget Reconciliation Act of 1985 specifically authorized the use of Medicaid funds for the provision of prevocational and supported employment services for persons leaving institutional care under a Home and Community-Based Services Waiver. Although this change is a major step in the right direction, it has two significant limitations. These services are authorized for only a small number of persons with severe disabilities who are eligible for Medicaid, and the failure to explicitly include vocational services as authorized services creates ambiguity as to the range of employment services that can be provided.

In addition, the 1986 Amendments to the Rehabilitation Act of 1973 (P.L. 99-506) created a new formula grant to the states for the purpose of providing supported work services. The 1987 budget, however, was small—only $27 million.

State and local government conservatism

It is no secret among state and local government fiscal officers that the relationship between reimbursement charges and *actual* costs of providing the reimbursable service is weak. In the face of pressures to minimize state or local government program expenditures, fiscal officers are constantly on the lookout for cross-subsidy opportunities; that is, opportunities to spread the cost of nonreimbursable services over reimbursable service sectors. The underlying principle is, "Whenever possible, spend the other fellow's dollar before your own." Thus support staff who provide both reimbursable and nonreimbursable services are often charged to the reimbursable cost center. Similarly, there are substantial opportunities to collect reimbursement for nonexistent employees by delaying prompt replacement of employees who leave.

When a cross-subsidy strategy is discovered and implemented, one level of government succeeds in shifting to another level a portion of the legitimate costs of providing services to its citizens. Clearly, any change in the reimbursement or funding rules by the level of government to which costs are shifted threatens the cross-subsidy strategy and could force painful readjustments in the budget of the government unit taking advantage of cost-shifting possibilities. For this reason, among others, state and local governments often seek to maintain the status quo. Unless the federal government can be induced to pick up the costs, state and local governments, while vociferous in complaints about perceived program inadequacies or inequities, generally follow rather than take the lead in making needed program changes.

The twisting of state programs to optimize the yield of federal funds creates a dilemma for federal policy makers. Although federal policy dictates much of what states will ostensibly do in a given program sector, there is no assurance that federal program standards will be fully implemented. Lynn[21] explains that "elected state officials have on the whole a greater sense of responsibility toward economy and efficiency in governmental operations than they do toward the effectiveness of coverage of human services." Thus, to the extent that state officials see opportunities to balance the state budget by shaving the cost of care in the human services sector or by shifting costs to the federal government, they may be perceived by taxpayers as securing apparent "economies and efficiencies."

Federal funds as free goods

State and local governments sometimes perceive and use federal funds as a "free good" rather than as a scarce resource to be carefully husbanded. Thus a program arrangement that is more expensive than some other alternative in total program costs may be perpetuated because the state or local government share of the total costs of the more expensive arrangement is less than it would be in the alternative. This phenomenon, more than anything else, explains why local governments, which often do not share in the cost of institutional care, are willing to see the state and federal governments pay institutional costs running to $60,000 or more per year. Similarly, it is financially and politically cheaper for state governments to sustain these very high costs when the federal government is paying the lion's share.

Problems of federal oversight

The inconsistent and sporadic oversight of federally funded programs is one of the major causes of program quality erosion that occurs over time. This phenomenon is undoubtedly related to the short "shelf life" of federal appointed officials and the time it takes for them to gain understanding of the statutory, regulatory, and technologic foundations of the programs they administer.[16] Federal oversight policies invite diverse interpretations of acceptable practice among the states and periodic confrontation between the federal government and the states. For example, Martha Derthick's[10] revelations about the use of federal funds by the states to pay for a wide variety of goods and services in the guise of social services led to the capping of social service expenditures and, ultimately, to the Social Services Block Grant. This happened after the U.S. Congress, in reaction to strong state pressure and numerous suits against the federal government, passed legislation to pay for most of the Title XX expenditures that the federal auditors disallowed.

Political versus economic perspectives

Perhaps the greatest obstacle to economic rationality is the political perspective of public officials that tends to brush aside information and analyses that do not satisfy the dominant power interests at hand.[3] It is not that the political perspective ignores economic considerations; rather, it selects the economic argument most consistent with the decision that is going to be made to satisfy the dominant political interests.

Societal stereotyping is a factor that weighs heavily in the decisions of government officials. Negative stereotypes about the functional capacities of severely handicapped persons crowd out information and analysis that would suggest that these stereotypes are inaccurate. When economic arguments for providing certain kinds of services run counter to the negative stereotypes, the arguments tend to be ignored. When the economic arguments support these negative stereotypes, these arguments are eagerly grasped and used to buttress the decision that will be made to satisfy the dominant power interest in any event.

Unfortunately, the conclusions reached by some economic studies can easily be misinterpreted as supporting negative societal stereotypes about the capacities of disabled people and provide ammunition for those who stress dependency rather than substantial work for persons with dis-

abilities. These studies have usually concluded that limitations in physical and mental fitness are closely related to diminished ability to produce on the job or that employers prefer nondisabled workers, even if educationally or culturally disadvantaged, to workers with disabilities.[2,14,15,20] These interpretations of the data stress the "apparent" effects of the disabling condition rather than the combined and interacting effects of other employment impediments (such as age and limited education), the effects of work disincentives, the effects of discrimination by employers, or the potential of new vocational techniques and careful job placement to enable workers with severe disabilities to engage in substantial employment. Unfortunately, these studies perpetuate the misleading presumption that the term "disability" is synonymous with failure.

It is no wonder that those who do not accept these negative stereotypes have resorted to litigation to force an impartial and comprehensive sifting of the evidence and consideration of the human capacities and constitutional rights of persons with severe disabilities. It is extremely important to weigh carefully the empiric evidence for and against theories that are inherently prejudicial to the best interests of classes of people who are negatively stereotyped by the dominant society.

Such careful sifting of available evidence and knowledge is particularly important in the case of supported work when data on its effectiveness are limited.[27] Conventional attitudes may quickly lead to the conclusion that the benefits of supported work will fall short of its costs. In fact, before such conclusions can be reached, we face a long period of increasing the amount and improving the quality of the data that are collected, improving the methods used to provide supported work, and improving the techniques used to evaluate supported work. We believe that subsequent studies of supported work will not support earlier studies that concluded that earnings among severely disabled persons will tend to result in costs to society that exceed the value of the benefits.[14]

Bureaucratic insensitivity

Bureaucratic insensitivity to the needs of handicapped persons is an endemic problem. It is epitomized by the way the Social Security Administration implemented the continuing disability investigations required by Section 221(i) of the Disability Amendments of 1980. Thousands of people who had not worked for years were cut off from the SSDI or SSI rolls without regard for the fact that their lack of recent labor force experience made them hard to employ. No attempt was made to ease them back into the labor force through the provision of rehabilitation services. As a result of the inept handling of the continuing disability reviews and termination of benefits, a number of people, in despair, committed suicide. Gordon D. of Eugene, Oregon, a childhood polio victim diagnosed as paranoid schizophrenic, was one such individual.[26] After the Social Security Administration dropped him from the disability rolls, he committed suicide, leaving a note to his family that read, "I no longer have any income whatsoever and there is no way I can work. . . . I have no life any more. . . . I can't afford to eat. . . . I don't feel like a man any more."

These problems develop because people making programmatic decisions are insensitive to or unaware of the limitations, needs, and adjustment problems of persons with disabilities. Such problems also arise if administrators and bureaucrats are concerned only about the operation of their small part of the service system and do not consider the effects of their actions on the individual. Finally, such problems arise because of the failure of administrators and bureaucrats to see the complicated interrelationships or lack thereof among the various programs in the services system and the ways in which the service system will respond to their actions. To the extent that educational and training programs in the area of disability fail to sensitize future practitioners to the issues and to instill in them the philosophy and practices of normalization, these workers will continue to have a limited vision of how their practice adds to or detracts from the normalization of the lives of the severely disabled. In consequence, they will be less likely to lobby for incorporating the principles of normalization into public policy,[3] and bureaucratic insensitivity will continue to create problems for the effectiveness and humane functioning of the service system.

Conflict of interest

Related to the weakness of federal oversight is the conflict of interest that comes from the delegation of responsibility in the ICF/MR program to the state Medicaid agency to monitor the operations of other state agencies that receive Medicaid reimbursement for the services they provide. To expect one state agency to disallow reimbursements for substandard practices and thereby increase total program costs to the state is naive. As a matter of principle, it is important to avoid policies that create a conflict of interest for the parties involved. To partly counter this problem, Congress has authorized funds for federal "look-behind" audits to ensure that persons in Medicaid-certified institutions receive care in accordance with federal regulations.

Special interest groups

The strong economic interests and political power of state employees and the communities that contain the large institutions must be reckoned with. Usually, the majority of the members of these constituencies wish to see that the institutions are maintained to protect jobs and businesses. A a bloc, state employees, whether or not unionized, have considerable influence with legislators. Political parties are sometimes quick to exploit the discontent that arises when an institution or part of an institution is threatened with closure. "Internal" agency discussions about closing down

a building or ward, not to mention a whole facility, are often quickly made public.

Even national politicians are not immune from these pressures. For example, federal legislation has urged the states to look after the economic interests of state employees in the course of deinstitutionalization. Caught between federal and local pressures, the states sometimes simply continue institutional care rather than deal with the profoundly disruptive effects that large scale layoffs create in the state civil service system and in the communities in which the large institutions are located.

Thus, even when the benefits appear to be greater than the costs of community care,[9] strong countervailing political arguments and pressures exerted by employee groups and the communities to keep an institution open may prevail.

POSSIBLE SOLUTIONS

We believe that the present system of services for persons with mental retardation and other severe disabilities is in need of further major reappraisal and restructuring so that it supports rather than hinders the attainment of normalized living. More important, we believe that the country is on the verge of making needed major changes in the service system. The old conventional wisdom that stressed dependency and the development of programs oriented primarily toward helpless Americans is being replaced by a new wisdom that stresses the potential for independent living among Americans with severe disabilities. The goals of community-based living and employment in integrated settings for severely disabled persons are endorsed by almost all Americans. The U.S. Congress, state legislatures, and local governments have been changing laws and restructuring the service system to make these goals an actuality for increasing numbers of Americans with severe disabilities.

Although this chapter focuses primarily on changes in federal laws, it is worth noting that virtually all the states are currently engaged in a reappraisal of their day programs for persons with severe disabilities, particularly those who are severely mentally retarded, with a view to moving persons in adult day care to employment-oriented activities, especially supported employment in integrated work settings.

We believe the following types of changes are currently and urgently needed. This list of needed changes is not exhaustive, and many variations in ways of making these changes are possible.

Establishing uniform national objectives

The lack of uniform and consistent goals for the different programs comprising the service system is a major impediment to program coordination and program efficiency. Uniform national objectives should be established. Among the potential national objectives (which would also become objectives for each program) are employment for disabled persons; income support and medical coverage when needed; residential placement in the most appropriate and least restrictive care setting; and participation in community activities appropriate to the individual's age, sex, and education (for example, use of public transportation and eating in restaurants). Each program in the service system should be evaluated according to the extent to which it assists disabled Americans to attain those goals. More important, it is the service system as a whole that should be evaluated and altered when necessary to enhance the attainment of the goals.

Changing eligibility requirements

The emphasis on demonstrating inability to work as the condition of eligibility for program benefits should be eliminated. Given the unreliability of the judgmental predictions involved and the harmful effects of the process, it is more sensible to require only that applicants prove that they would have substantial difficulty in locating work by virtue of their functional limitations. Benefits could then be granted with the expectation and on the condition that the individual would accept services that are designed to assist them to return to work. This would not be a particularly great departure from current practice. Often applicants for SSDI/CDB or SSI are declared eligible for benefits on the basis of their medical condition alone.

Ensuring income increases for return to work

Individuals who return to work should always significantly increase their income. One important step has already been taken. The Section 1619(a) and 1619(b) programs of the Social Security Act that authorize continuing cash benefits and Medicaid coverage to working SSI recipients has been made permanent. This eliminated the great uncertainty that formerly surrounded the continuation of these programs.

Additional steps could be taken. First, the formula for determining SSDI benefits could be revised to reduce benefits as earnings increase. This will probably require a two-stage reduction formula. The first part would cover earnings up to the federal SSI break-even point and would apply the same formula for reducing benefits as is used for SSI recipients. The second part would involve greater reductions in benefits for each dollar of earnings; for example, benefits might be reduced by $3 for each $4 of earnings to prevent the federal break-even point for SSDI from reaching levels that are too high to be socially acceptable. One would also need to consider whether the earnings disregarded should be limited to $85, as is currently the practice for SSI recipients, or be increased. At present, the first $300 of earnings are effectively disregarded for SSDI/CDB beneficiaries.

Second, Medicare and Medicaid coverage could be made permanent for SSDI and SSI beneficiaries, regardless of their current income or assets, who cannot obtain health insurance from their employer or privately because of their disabling condition. This provision need not be totally financed by tax funds, since employers could be required to pay an amount equivalent to what they pay for health benefits for other workers. In addition, beneficiaries could be required to contribute to the costs of these programs on a sliding scale based on their income.

Providing lifetime security for the severely disabled

Lifetime income security should be provided for persons with severe disabilities. To encourage persons with severe disabilities to work, they could be made permanently eligible for income support and health care coverage. Thus, if they lost their jobs, they would be immediately reentitled to needed benefits. Given the severity of the disabilities of these persons, one can anticipate that some will experience a lifelong pattern of interspersed work and public benefits. We believe, however, that this is preferable to the exclusive receipt of public benefits.

Providing lifelong eligibility for income support and health care would remove one problem that may undermine the effectiveness of the Section 1916(a) and 1619(b) programs. Currently, periodic case reevaluation can conclude that the SSI recipient who earns above the SGA wage level is not disabled and therefore no longer eligible for SSI payments. Lifelong eligibility would enable severely disabled persons to establish or reestablish entitlement for SSDI and SSI if they are not working; they are not eligible for other benefits, such as unemployment compensation; and they are seeking work, engaged in a program designed to help them find work, or assessed as unemployable. Similarly, severely disabled persons will be able to establish or reestablish entitlement for health care support if private insurance is not available at a reasonable price (for example, if they change jobs and their new employer does not provide medical insurance as a fringe benefit).

Improving service coordination

The coordination of the services used by persons with severe disabilities should be improved. Identification of the major transition points in the lives of people with severe disabilities (such as from school to adult life) should be given particular attention. Improving service coordination is critical to the cost-effective use of society's resources. There is great waste in the way program resources are fragmented in their application to individual clients.

There are several ways of improving program linkages. First, the eligibility determinations for SSDI/CDB, SSI, and the federal-state vocational rehabilitation programs could be unified. Sometimes a person is declared unfeasible for vocational rehabilitation by a state agency and is also refused SSDI or SSI on the grounds that he or she is not sufficiently disabled to qualify. In addition, the Social Security Administration often terminates persons from the SSDI or SSI rolls on the grounds that they have "medically recovered" without consideration for the fact that these persons have not worked for some time and cannot easily find employment. To resolve these problems, disabled persons who apply to these programs could be assured eligibility for one or the other. Furthermore, SSDI or SSI program participants who recover medically could be maintained on the rolls until after they have received adequate services to enable them to return to work.

Second, the individual service plans of state special education, vocational rehabilitation, adult social services, and health care programs could be integrated into a single unified plan for each client. Ideally, this unified plan would specify a common set of independent living goals, the specific client attainments expected at the points of major life transitions, and the phased and linked inputs of all relevant agencies. In developing the individual service plans and the unified plan, a life cycle perspective should be taken. Stress should be placed on identifying interagency linkages and ensuring that the different agencies comply with their part of the unified plan. A unified plan should be made a condition for receipt of federal funds by the relevant state and local agencies.

Third, federal income support and health care programs should participate in the development of a service plan for persons with severe disabilities. In many states joint planning among state and local agencies already exists, and a plan is not valid until approved by the representatives of the different agencies. We are proposing that the representatives of federal agencies become part of the team that develops a service plan and become signatories to that plan. At present, the lack of participation by representatives of the federal income support programs, such as SSDI/CDB and SSI, and the health care financing programs, such as Medicare and Medicaid, as well as other programs, limits the planning perspective and truncates the range of service options that might be pursued. At times the lack of federal participation causes the federal agencies to work at cross purposes with state and local agencies.

Without assurance of income support and health care coverage for given individuals, it is difficult to develop a long-term plan that will lead, for example, to placement in a supervised apartment and a job in a regular or supported work environment. Above all, coordination activities among federal and state agencies should have the pivotal goal of enhancing the individual's independence of functioning. Thus the decision to apply for SSDI/CDB or SSI should be an interim step on the way to vocational rehabilitation and eventual placement in some kind of remunerative employment that permits at least partial reduction of the individual's dependency on these payments for income.

Finally, one agency should be designated as the "lead" agency for given clients, with case management responsibility and a case services budget to immediately pay for an urgently needed service when it cannot be obtained in any other way. In this manner delays can be avoided in providing immediately needed services (for example, for vocational training that would otherwise be delayed because the state rehabilitation agency has exhausted its annual budget or for respite or attendant care when a caregiving family member gets sick). A single agency need not be the lead agency for all disabled persons. Instead, separate agencies could be designated to be lead agencies for persons with mental retardation, blindness, hearing impairments, and so on. The designated lead agency would also be responsible for providing vigorous oversight of the implementation of the individual service plans by other responsible agencies.

National data system

A national uniform data system should be developed for persons who are disabled. This data system should identify the extent to which disabled persons achieve social goals, the types of programs that are provided, the costs of these programs, and other information. This would require consolidation and coordination of the data systems of different programs providing services to disabled persons as well as additional information beyond that collected by the individual agencies. All income support and human services agencies responsible for implementing an individual service plan could be required to participate in the uniform information system.

Such a data system would become the basic tool with which to evaluate the success of the service system and to identify areas in which the service system is not effectively achieving social goals. Equally important, because of the many variations in ways of providing services, it would be the basis for beginning to understand which types of services are most effective in achieving social goals and minimizing costs and which groups of people with disabilities are most effectively served by the different services. There is, for example, still much to be learned about the most effective mechanisms of providing community-based residential housing and supported work.

A national data system would create a basic force driving the service system to increasingly greater levels of effectiveness. Part of the reason for the slow progress that has been made in such areas as deinstitutionalization, despite widespread acceptance of the general concept for at least 25 years, is that the rudimentary information available on the implementation of deinstitutionalization concealed the failures and inadequacies of the system and did not identify which types of community housing were most effective for which groups of disabled people. An information system that exposed these problems would lead to political demands that the system improve performance.

Removing program bias

The institutional bias inherent in the ICF/MR program needs to be removed. In fact, there are two issues that must be dealt with. One is to remove the often described institutional bias in the ICF/MR program, and the other is to encourage the states to undertake the administratively more difficult task of placing persons with severe disabilities in community-based residences. Even if federal funding was made neutral in the type of housing that could be paid for with federal dollars, it is likely that some states would still be reluctant to move residents from large institutions to the community.

Senator John Chaffee has introduced several bills (for example, S. 2053) that would address these issues. The bills would not only permit states to use ICF/MR funding to move residents of large Medicaid certified ICF/MR institutions to small community-based residents, but would require the states to move the great majority of current residents of large institutions in a 10-year period as a condition of continued Medicaid funding. There are two separate, distinct options inherent in the Chaffee bills—one to create more flexibility in the use of funds, and the other to require states to move in the direction of greater reliance on community-based care.

A major concern with creating greater flexibility in the ICF/MR program is that, because it is open ended, there would be an increase in the number of people served and much greater costs. This leads to the next option, which is to put a cap on the amount of federal funds that could be used to support community-based housing for persons with mental retardation and developmental disabilities. If combined with greater flexibility in the use of funds, this would have the effect of converting the ICF/MR program into a block grant program. Such a block grant should probably be extended to encompass the provision of support and services to families providing care to their children with severe disabilities and thus not be limited to funding community residential programs. This option could be extended to require states to emphasize family support programs and community residences, as is done in the Chaffee bills.

Some persons oppose creating a block grant out of the ICF/MR program. They fear that it would become an easy target for subsequent budget cuts. Another concern is that, because states vary widely in the extent of the use of the ICF/MR program, it would be difficult to protect the funding of high-use states while allocating funds to other states without greatly expanding the budget. To gain support for the creation of a block grant, some increase in current expenditures would probably have to be accepted and assurances given that future funding would at least keep pace with inflation.

The Home and Community-Based Services Waivers program was another approach to increasing the flexibility of the use of federal funds for residential support while assuring that there would not be a significant increase in the federal budget. Since the program is restricted to persons who would have needed to be institutionalized in the absence of the program and actually could have been (as demonstrated by empty institutional beds or some other means), it is usually regarded as too restrictive for optimal state development of community services. Nevertheless, it is clearly a step in the right direction and does give rise to another option that could easily be implemented at no federal costs. That option is to convert the waivers program into an optional service, so that the states do not have to keep returning for federal approval of waivers for services that are intended to be permanent when instituted.

One way to induce states to redirect resources from institutions to community-based care is to make this a condition of the receipt of federal funds. Another less intrusive option would be to use different cost-sharing ratios for community versus institutional care. This could be done in the context of the current ICF/MR program, any modification of that program, or the development of a block grant.

A major problem in the change from institutional care to community-based residential care is the lack of federal "up-front," or initial, funds to pay the capital and conversion costs. This lack of funds often results in the strong opposition of state and local governments to significant reductions in institutional populations, since they must rely on depreciation through subsequent Medicaid reimbursement to recoup these funds (if the facilities are certified as ICF/MR). One advantage of converting to a block grant lies in the ability to structure it so that states have more leeway to use these funds for the initial costs of developing community-based facilities. In any event, any federal reform effort should consider methods of providing initial funds for the development of community-based facilities. The states are more likely to go along with needed reforms if they do not have to bear the cost of conversion by themselves.

These options have the common thrust of moving away from the requirement of the current ICF/MR program that residents be in need of 24-hour care that induces many state and local governments to deny many people with severe disabilities access to less restrictive care environments.

Increasing funding for long-term vocational programs

Funding should be increased for long-term vocational support. As large numbers of severely disabled persons are moved into integrated employment, the need for long-term vocational support to assist these individuals to retain their employment will rise substantially. The following are ways of providing this support:

1. Increase the amount available for supported work under the 1986 Amendments to the Rehabilitation Act of 1973.
2. Permit Medicaid funds now used to support day activities to be applied instead to supported employment, thereby not only providing needed funds but also eliminating an overwhelming work disincentive inherent in the Medicaid program.

Decreasing program-created poverty

The procedures of public programs that push people into poverty need to be reduced. There is little reason to impose a 6-month waiting period on applicants who obviously meet the medical criteria for eligibility for SSDI/CDB or to impose a 2-year waiting period before entitlement to Medicare. A stronger emphasis on assisting these beneficiaries to return to work might be more cost effective.

Consideration might also be given to eliminating the asset test for persons applying for SSI, Medicaid, or both. Another alternative would be to calculate the actual or imputed income on countable assets over the permitted level and reduce the SSI payment according to some formula (for example, by the entire amount, by the same $1 for $2 reduction factor as is currently used, or by some intermediate formula). Similarly, if co-payment provisions are established for recipients of Medicaid, this return on assets could be added to the recipient's income, which would presumably be the basis for determining the level of co-payment required.

CONCLUSION

Many people will regard these options as radical and expensive. These views are shortsighted. Indeed, it is possible that these reforms would result in lower, not higher, costs. Obviously, it is difficult to predict the net effect on costs of changes as substantial as those that we have proposed. Nonetheless, there are several reasons to believe that costs will not rise substantially and may even fall.

To begin with, the changes discussed will not only greatly improve the services provided to severely disabled Americans, but in many cases may be funded by shifting resources from inappropriate services to appropriate services. Obvious examples of such fund shifting possibilities are moving clients from institutions to community-based rsidential care and moving clients from adult day care to integrated work. In addition, there will be cost savings as people with severe disabilities are moved, partially or totally, from dependency on SSDI/CDB and SSI for income to gainful employment. Further, the services that they receive will not only often be more appropriate, but also less expensive than the ones now provided. Community residences are generally less expensive than institutional care, and supported work costs less than adult day care.

It must be granted that some additional number of Americans with severe disabilities may receive services under a more flexible service system than are now served under the current system. But it should also be noted that they will probably receive lower cost services and that these costs may well be offset by the savings that we have described. Moreover, one should anticipate that there will be continued pressure to provide services to persons who are not now being served, so that improvements to the service system can forestall inappropriate and expensive future expansion of the current system with all its built-in sources of inefficiency.

We do not regard the aforementioned options as radical. In fact, they are simply projections of trends that are currently in place and gaining momentum. In any event, the inertia and inefficiency of the current system of services must somehow be overcome. Adopting these options for change would promote attainment of the social goal of independence for Americans with severe disabilities. Cries of "administrative infeasibility" must be countered with the reminder that programs are funded with hard-earned taxpayer money to achieve the social goals set forth by legislation. The limitations of existing programs should not be allowed to rationalize curtailment of these goals.

We believe the yield in increased independence of functioning among Americans with severe disabilities would be substantial if the federal government were to leverage in the ways that we have suggested the billions of dollars that it now spends yearly for income support and services to the nation's estimated 2 million institutionalized persons and the 3.7% to 7.2% of the noninstitutionalized population who are severely limited in their activities.[23] We also believe that such federal action is the only way to overcome the inherent conservatism of state and local governments.

REFERENCES

1. Allen, MK: Persistent factors leading to application for admission to a residential institution, Ment Retard 10:25, 1972.
2. Berkowitz, M, Fenn, P, and Lambrinos, J: The optimal stock of health with endogenous wages, J Health Economics 2:139, 1983.
3. Bevilacqua, JJ, and Noble, JH, Jr: Chronic mental illness: a problem in politics, Paper presented at the National Conference on the Chronic Mental Patient, Kansas City, August 13, 1984.
4. Boles, S, et al: Specialized training program: the structured employment model. In Pain, S, Bellamy, G, and Wilcox, B, editors: Human services that work: from innovation to practice, Baltimore, 1984, Paul H Brookes Publishing Co.
5. Braddock, D, Hemp, R, and Howes, R: Public expenditures for mental retardation and developmental disabilities in the United States, Chicago, 1985, The University of Illinois at Chicago.
6. Conley, RW: Down syndrome: economic burdens and benefits of prevention. In Dellarco, VL, Voytek, PE, and Hollaender, A, editors: Aneuploidy, etiology and mechanisms, New York, 1985, Plenum Press.
7. Conley, RW: The economics of mental retardation, Baltimore, 1973, The Johns Hopkins Press.
8. Conley, RW, Noble, JH, Jr, and Elder, J: Problems with the service system. In Kiernan, W, and Stark, J, editors: Pathways to employment for adults with developmental disabilities, Baltimore, 1986, Paul H Brookes Publishing Co.
9. Conroy, JW, and Bradlay, VJ: The Pennhurst longitudinal study: a report of five years of research and analysis, Philadelphia, 1985, Temple University Developmental Disabilities Center.
10. Derthick, M: Uncontrolled spending for social services grants, Washington DC, 1975, The Brookings Institution.
11. Downey, KJ: Parents' reasons for institutionalizing severely mentally retarded children, J Health Hum Behavior 6:163, 1965.
12. Eyman, K, Dingman, F, and Sabagh, G: Association of characteristics of retarded patients and their families to speed of institutionalization, Am J Mental Deficiency 71:93, 1966.
13. Graliker, BV, and Koch, R: A study of factors influencing placement

of retarded children in a state residential institution, Am J Ment Defic 69:553, 1965.

14. Haveman, RH: A benefit-cost and policy analysis of the Netherlands social employment program, Leiden, 1977, University of Leiden.

15. Haveman, RH, Halberstadt, V, and Burkhauser, RV: Public policy toward disabled workers, Ithaca, NY, 1984, Cornell University Press.

16. Heclo, H: A government of strangers: executive politics in Washington, Washington DC, 1977, The Brookings Institution.

17. Human Services Research Institute: Supporting families with developmentally disabled members: review of the literature and results of a national survey, Draft report to the Office of Human Development Services, Boston, 1984, US Department of Health and Human Services.

18. Justice, RS, Bradley, J, and O'Connor, G: Foster family care for the retarded: concerns of the caretaker, Ment Retard 9:12, 1971.

19. Kiernan, WE, McGaughey, MJ, and Schalock, RL: Employment survey for adults with developmental disabilities, Boston, 1986, The Developmental Evaluation Clinic, Children's Hospital.

20. Levitan, S, and Taggart, R: Jobs for the disabled, Baltimore, 1979, The Johns Hopkins Press.

21. Lynn, LE, Jr: The state and human services, Cambridge, Mass, 1980, The MIT Press.

22. Maney, AC, Pace, R, and Morrison, DF: A factor analytic study of the need for institutionalization: problems and populations for program development, Am J Ment Defic 69:372, 1964.

23. Mathematica Policy Research, Inc: Digest of data on persons with disabilities, Washington, DC, 1984, Mathematica Policy Research, Inc.

24. McCrary, P, and Blakemore, T: A guide to learning curve technology to enhance performance prediction in vocational evaluation, Menomonie, 1985, University of Wisconsin, Stout Vocational Rehabilitation Institute.

25. McLeod, B: Real work for real pay, Psychology Today 19:42, 1985.

26. Mental Health Law Project: Letter from Norman S. Rosenberg, Washington DC, 1983, Mental Health Law Project.

27. Nagi, SZ: Disability and rehabilitation: legal, clinical and self-concepts and measurement, Columbus, 1969, Ohio State University.

28. Noble, MA: Nursing's concern for the mentally retarded is overdue, Nurs Forum 9:192, 1970.

29. Noble, JH, Jr, and Conley, RW: Accumulating evidence on the benefits and costs of supported and transitional work for persons with severe disabilities, Paper presented at the Annual TASH Conference, San Francisco, November 7, 1986.

30. Poole, D: Supported work services employment project, Grant No 90-DD-0065, Richmond, 1985, Virginia Commonwealth University School of Social Work.

31. Rhodes, L, Ramsing, K, and Valenta, L: An economic evaluation of supported employment within one manufacturing company, Paper presented at the Annual TASH Conference, San Francisco, November 7, 1985.

32. Wehman, P: Competitive employment: new horizons for severely disabled individuals, Baltimore, 1981, Paul H Brookes Publishing Co.

33. World Health Organization: International classification of impairments, disabilities, and handicaps, Geneva, 1980, World Health Organization.

CHAPTER 61

Clinical social work

MAURICE V. RUSSELL

As an intrinsic part of the rehabilitation process, the clinical social worker has a unique role, not only as a member of a distinct discipline, but also as a member of the rehabilitation team. It is the combined functions of the rehabilitation team that deal with diagnosis, treatment plan, and follow-up care of the disabled patient. Depending on the nature of the diagnosis and its origin and severity, the treatment plan must always extend into the community, particularly with the involvement of family members and significant others who may have a relationship with the patient.

The developmental stage of the patient (infancy, childhood, adolescence, young adulthood, and old age) greatly influences the prognosis of the disability and governs the determination of suitable or adequate capacity for adaptation and adjustment to the diagnosis. Implicit in this process is the initial assessment of the problem, the patient's reaction to the disorder, the reaction of the family or spouse to the presenting problem, and the availability of resources—financial, emotional, public, or private agencies and services—all of which contribute to the total helping process and the ultimate maximum adjustment to the rehabilitation effort. Beyond the specific physical situation, in other words, there are a host of significant components that must combine in some orderly and systematic fashion if the patient is to receive maximum benefit.

Although social workers have specific training in a variety of helping methods—casework, group work, community activity, and advocacy—the critical element must be an understanding of the clinical problem. All planning and subsequent interventions must be based on a clear clinical understanding of the problem. In addition, the social worker should recognize that all patients are different and cannot be treated routinely if their total treatment plan is to produce successful results. Without individuation of each patient, the treatment effort will be mechanical and guaranteed to create resistance in the patient. Although institutional structures have routine procedures for assessment and standardized approaches to specific diagnoses, they also must identify individual factors such as the critical question of patient and family motivation for adaptation and change, adjustment to rehabilitation methodology, and capacity for dealing with mandatory management expectations.

DEFINITIONS

The words "impairment," "disability," and "handicap" are often used interchangeably and convey different meanings to the speaker and the listener. It would be helpful to clarify these terms in order to clarify different aspects of the rehabilitation process and goals. *Impairment* is a more generic word that literally means to worsen, so it might be applied to stages of disability or handicap or, in a larger sense, to quality of life.

Disability is a loss in personal coping and adaptation ability that causes limitations in daily living. It may include disturbances of the adaptive and adjustment mechanisms that ordinarily permit a relatively stable and healthy reaction of a person to the psychosocial, economic, and physical demands of life.

Handicap is a general term meaning a limitation of bodily motion or circumstances in daily living that prevents or makes a physical activity impossible (for example, missing arm.) Some professionals examine other aspects of handicap such as economic, sociocultural, and vocational factors. These are more sociologic than physical but contribute to total view of person as they contribute to basic phyical limitations. In the diagnostic assessment and establishment of realistic goals for a handicapped person, these additional "social" factors cannot be ignored. For example, it may be assumed that a handicapped young black adolescent coming from a poorly educated, financially marginal household will have additional handicaps beyond actual physical limitations. These are the areas in which the expertise and competence of the clinical social worker come sharply into focus.

Having established one of the goals of rehabilitation as restoration of maximal healthful living, it would be helpful to refine the definition of health as mutually understood by members of the rehabilitation team. In the simplest biologic sense, at all stages of normal development health involves a minimum of three essential ingredients:

1. Functional capacity, or the ongoing management of physiologic capacities and adequate psychologic and social behavior, determines the estimated goals or limitations in which the behavior takes place. With aging, psychologic and social behavior are important in helping individuals cope with bodily changes and tolerate mechanical devices and other altering circumstances in the human organism.

2. Adaptive capacity is the capacity to achieve stability or develop compensatory defenses when there are upsetting changes in the physical self or the external environment. It is critical in assessing motivation for rehabilitation efforts. The basic adaptive capacity is the most difficult or resistant to change.

3. Organizing capacity reflects the highest order of human expression in regard to optimizing adjustment. It is the effort or ability to match physical conditions or limitation with environmental and social aspirations and expectations. It is this area of activity that most deeply reflects education, culture, family tradition, and a host of nonbiologic or social elements. An area for the expertise of clinical social work is the preparation of a psychosocial history and analysis to help the rehabilitation team develop realistic treatment goals based on past history and family ego strengths, cohesion, and supportive elements available in forms of community resources. (For example, deeply religious families have often found considerable strength and capacity for adaptation through their religious convictions and beliefs.)

EPIDEMIOLOGY

Although exact numbers of handicapped persons cannot be determined because of differences in terms and methodology, much has been written about the large number of handicapped persons, both nationally and internationally. As far back as the 1970 census, the President's Committee on the Employment of the Handicapped concluded that one in 11 adults under age 65 had a handicap that affected employability. The census showed a total of 121 million persons in the United States in the typically employable age range of 16 to 64 years of age. (The military service and institutions were not included.) Of this number, 11,265,000 persons had handicaps that had existed for 6 months or

longer. Thus over 9%, or 1 in every 11 Americans under 65, were handicapped.[8] The survey examined four demographic characteristics: years of school completed, income in 1969, poverty status, and labor force status. The findings were that the handicapped had less schooling and lower earnings than the nonhandicapped; the proportion of handicapped in poverty status was twice that of the general population. The committee also noted that handicapped adults who were not working or looking for work thought job opportunities did not exist. This factor may help explain the fact that a disproportionate number of handicapped persons were unemployed.[8]

The Bureau of Education for the Handicapped estimated there were 3,103,000 physically handicapped children through age 19 in the United States from 1974 to 1975. Of these, 2,293,000 were speech impaired, 328,000 were crippled and otherwise health impaired, 49,000 were deaf, 228,000 were hard of hearing, 66,000 were visually handicapped, and 40,000 were deaf and blind or otherwise multihandicapped. A 1971 Department of Health, Education and Welfare study of the prevalence of "10 impairment groups" estimated there were 9,760,000 persons aged 65 or over with one or more of impairments.[9] All study findings indicated their figures were conservative; however, even using conservative figures and continuing to omit the military and persons in institutions, the total number of handicapped persons is in excess of 25 million.

The growing and increasing number of severely handicapped persons is attributed to the following causes:

1. The incredible advances in medical care, both technically and in quality, as well as mechanical substitutes to perform vital bodily functions or substitutes for parts of the body. Earlier and more effective intervention in life-threatening medical complications has enabled an increasingly larger number of extensively handicapped persons to survive.

2. The increased environmental risks of urban and rural life caused by industrialization and mechanization. With increased use of technical equipment, the growth of industry, and so on, there are increased opportunities for accidents by automobiles, farm equipment, and industrial plants. Air pollutants further increase risks, particularly in chronic pulmonary obstructive disease.

3. A rapidly aging population that is vulnerable to all the natural handicapping conditions of age (stroke, atherosclerosis, diabetes). Ironically, persons live longer as a result of advances such as antibiotic drugs and tranquilizers but then develop the usual disabilities of old age, making them vulnerable to conditions requiring rehabilitation intervention or referral to nursing homes or specialized care, all of which prolong life.

4. Increasing and more sophisticated institutional arrangements for children and adults with birth defects.

Formerly fatal conditions such as cystic fibrosis and neuromuscular, renal, and cardiopulmonary diseases have now contributed to an increase in the number of aged persons. (Note the development of hemodialysis alone and the impact on renal disease survival.)

REHABILITATION PROCESS

The goal in rehabilitating the handicapped is to reverse or control handicapping problems. Unlike the medical model, which assumes specific treatment, rehabilitation is predicated on a set of factors—adaptation, coping, and adjustment—rather than cure. Poor health, injury, and illness become more critical when cure is impossible, as is often true with rehabilitation patients. This set of circumstances can be approached only through the rehabilitation process, which requires a problem-solving, goal-focused, and coordinated approach to improving the condition of the patient. The process also requires the patient to change his or her life-style, react to the problem, and change his or her physical environment. The team must address the optimal possible adjustment through counseling, concrete resources, medical care, orthotic adaptations, and modifications. The social workers' responsibilities include being familiar with the availability of community resources, offering counseling to patients and significant others about the presenting problem, and explaining the rehabilitation process. The following are specific areas with which social work must be involved (always in conjunction with the relevant team members):

1. Early assessment of the medical, psychosocial, and educational impairment and initial management of conditions that led to the handicap.

2. Assessment of the actual and potential capabilities of the patient and of the team members serving him or her in a responsive, coordinated psychosocial system that includes the patient as part of the planning. Planning focuses on the reduction of social and physical barriers and enabling the patient to participate as fully as possible in appropriate community activities.

3. Involvement in a dynamic plan of care that includes evaluation, diagnosis, prognosis, and ultimate discharge. The plan should also include guidelines for achieving goals.

4. Inclusion of patient and significant others throughout the entire plan of care with arrangements for follow-up as indicated or referral to another facility, for example, one nearer the patient's home.

5. Helping the patient move from dependent to more independent functioning, particularly with respect to goals for education, training, social adjustment, and interpersonal relationships.

Rehabilitation services are being increasingly developed (see "Quality Assurance and Evaluation") through careful planning. The initial process of diagnosis involves identifying specific functional problems (how feasible or desirable is their resolution) and the ultimate prognosis that accounts for temporary, chronic, or unchangeable impairments and complications. The social worker's assessment of strengths of the patient and significant others is a serious component of this prognosis. Careful and sensitive analysis of these data helps to justify the goals of care and to determine priorities and, above all, assists in establishing realistic expectations so neither the patient nor the team members become frustrated, angry, disappointed, and bitter about the experience.

REHABILITATION TEAM

The rehabilitation team is the core of the diagnosis, treatment, and follow-up care for the patient who is disabled or handicapped. The elusive quality of team interaction must be blended with the individual professional expertise of the clinical social worker to work out the best possible outcomes for the patient and for family members, especially the spouse and parents. The social worker must be able to approach the team with a sense of competence while contributing toward the combined competence of all team members involved. This is not an easy task for a variety of reasons.

The team notion is not new in medical treatment or health care. There has always been a commitment to team process, but it does not always work smoothly. Mental health models in psychiatry are perhaps the most notable in their clinical combination of psychiatrist, psychologist, psychiatric nurse, and social worker. It is, incidentally, this model that led to the development of the early child guidance movement for the treatment of childhood schizophrenia and behavior disorders. This resulted in the formation of the American Orthopsychiatric Association in 1923, which was the first to give equal status to each of the disciplines involved. Decision making and the allocation of tasks were shared or divided among the various disciplines. For legal and credentialing reasons, the psychiatrists assumed the major decision making and discharge planning responsibility concerning matters such as the readiness of the psychiatric patient to move back into the community without harm to himself or the community. With the development of the community mental health movement in the 1960s (stimulated by the Kennedy family's interest in mental health and mental retardation) there were a variety of innovative approaches such as rotating various team members as team leaders. Of all team members, social workers were the most knowledgeable about the family-parental-community role and the availability of community resources for follow-up. This was further enhanced by their work with self-help and other groups.

The rehabilitation team is larger and more complex than the psychiatric model because the rehabilitation process, which follows acute care intervention, of necessity must use all the various skills of care. The emphasis shifts according to the nature of the problem and what aspects of treatment are indicated on an individual basis. The development of the "therapeutic milieu" for treating psychiatric patients, as expounded by Maxwell Jones in his classic development of the therapeutic community as a treatment model, was a significant innovation that pointed out that the roles of team members varied; for example, primary therapists were designated according to which person on the team had the most effective relationship with the patient, not according to professional status. The responsibility for the family has always been the major assignment of the clinical social worker, since this responsibility requires knowledge of community resources that assist families. Public and private agencies are available and needed for after-hospital assistance.

As is evident from the earlier discussion, the smooth working of the rehabilitation team is critical if treatment goals are to be attained. Issues of competition, status, and seniority are inevitable at local patient evaluation conferences, as well as at senior department heads meetings. Departments must vie for space, personnel, equipment, and budget flexibility; competition automatically ensues. Administration has a responsibility to help resolve these issues in an equitable fashion, and to develop an objective approach to its policy and decision making because it affects the growth or limitations of the disciplines comprising the rehabilitation team. Many of the roles overlap, and the relationships must permit an opportunity to discuss mutual roles and the appropriate allocation of tasks to various patients. This overlapping is strikingly apparent in the psychosocial issues, specifically between social work and psychology.

Palmer[6] discussed role confusion, overlap, and duplication of effort in rehabilitation medicine. She presents a team as a method for identifying service goals, differentiating roles, coordinating goals, and educating staff on the expertise and use of various disciplines. Falck[3] similarly discussed interdisciplinary collaboration with regard to social work activity. He proposed the team process as "a form of behavior that must be learned and involves people who make mutual adaptations to each other's differences such as profession, method, use of knowledge, skill and professional goal. The effective collaborative behavior he suggested includes the following qualities:

1. Thorough commitment to the profession's values and ethics and belief in the usefulness of one's profession
2. Belief in a holistic approach to the client's problems
3. Recognition of the interdependency of practice
4. Recognition of the expertise of colleagues and others

Team success as well as team failure must be equally shared. Mature professionals are aware of their own knowledge, values, and skills yet are able to recognize, appreciate, and accept those of their colleagues on the team.

REHABILITATION SOCIAL WORKER

By its very nature, the rehabilitation setting and process, whether in an acute care setting or a separate rehabilitation facility, exacts a heavy toll on social workers emotionally and professionally. The ethical dilemmas and values of the worker must be enmeshed with those of the team and the philosophy of the setting. They must face their own philosophy of life regarding: What is optimal quality of life? What is possible, desirable, and realistic? In what manner can or should we expect people to function? The severity of the disability and the coping capacity exacted from some patients, spouses, parents is frequently overwhelming. Social workers' maximum effective functioning is impaired if their values conflict with those of the team. This process also involves priority setting. It is not easy to face the parents of a promising young athletic adolescent who has suffered spinal cord injury and will never be able to walk again. The constant pressure of high expectations and limited outcomes creates sources of personal pain and conflict for social work staff. In large complex medical centers, it is possible to transfer and shift workers when they start to evidence and verbalize feelings of "burnout" and lack of effectiveness.

The staff requires the energy to be patient, creative, and resourceful. Overidentification with the presenting problem and family and social situation can interfere with objective professional functioning. Workers require constant support from their supervisors and administrators.

They must be able to work comfortably as team members with specific knowledge—frequently without intensive supervision. Their initial diagnostic psychosocial evaluations are critically important to the initial team conference and to generating a realistic plan of care. There will be moments of feeling inadequate and helpless, particularly with patients who do not respond to the process and who must be discharged to home with supports or to another facility.

Medical information (at least the implications of the diagnosis) must be understood, especially to help patients anticipate and plan with physicians and other team members in carrying out their role with families and community agencies. As the major liaison with families, social workers must have the ability to convey the team's thinking about future objectives to the patients and families.

There is no single social work strategy that embodies all modes of intervention: casework, group work, advocacy, education, and consultation. It becomes the social workers' responsibility to report to the team what resources are available and accessible; this information can greatly effect team planning, particularly if treatment goals are not being realized. The team needs to know other options exist for this patient. The social worker's experience with the community is important to the patient and family because community resources change constantly; even more important, eligibility for outside services is a complex and confusing issue. Most families cannot afford the extra items required for patients such as wheelchairs, prostheses, or home care attendants and are not knowledgeable about access to free building modifications to accommodate to the handicap. Many patients and their families must move to other housing if their own housing is crowded, inaccessible, or otherwise not appropriate. This of course is determined by the situation of the patient. One of the most complex and haunting questions is when, if, and how a patient can live independently in the community. This becomes a treatment goal if the patient wants to assume independent functioning apart from the family.

The social worker's role in group education cannot be underestimated. Groups of all kinds—patients, families, children, other professionals—offer considerable support and direct information sharing. During group activity, other team members should be encouraged to contribute information from their own disciplines. Groups of patients with similar diagnoses can be encouraged to work together on creative solutions and mutual understanding. The more aggressive and resilient patients and families are helpful to patients who are frightened and immobilized by the realities of their goals and living patterns. The tendency of social workers to find their reward in effecting rapid change stems from the psychiatric model that is part of social work training in psychosocial assessment and counseling. Because rehabilitation is gradual and often lasts a lifetime, it can be frustrating because the gains are slow and gratification is delayed, if it comes at all.

As with other patients, the rehabilitation patient's condition changes over time (especially with the aging process), and the worker must adjust to these changes with new approaches and creative ideas to meet the changing condition. Sooner or later, despite the advantages of independent living, independence may no longer be feasible or practical. Healthy adults also have problems with aging, but the process is even more complicated for the disabled person. With patients requiring skilled nursing home care, complications caused by their disability may create a need for more care than the nursing home can provide. One of the most exciting new developments is the movement of handicapped groups to create advocacy programs for improved services from publicly supported programs such as housing. Most of the larger urban areas have local offices of the handicapped to offer services to these patients and to address their problems in adjusting and surviving in the community.

The team must consider issues such as timing and the patient's readiness for more complex rehabilitation tasks. While treating the patient, the social worker must also consider the community as part of his or her treatment responsibility so that the community can get ready to receive the patient back into its midst. Former routines and activities (such as attending church) must be considered, since the patient may not be as mobile as formerly.

For those patients returning to communities without resources for the disabled, the social worker must use creativity and imagination. One young woman patient was going blind as a result of juvenile diabetes. Her husband worked all night as a truck driver, and they were the parents of newborn twins. They lived in a trailer camp in a very depressed community, and there were no established home care agencies in their community. The social worker, with the patient's permission, suggested placing an advertisement in the local newspaper, and they were subsequently able to get several volunteers locally who came to help the couple.

One of the social worker's special contributions to the team should be assessing the impact of the patient's psychosocial situation. Some of the most commonly identified psychosocial considerations in regard to disability are similar to those of nonhandicapped persons. The difference is that the health care experience is much longer in rehabilitation than in care for the acutely ill. The most frequently expressed psychosocial concerns focus on the following:

1. Health-care procedures, tests, treatment procedures, length of hospitalization, and sources of financing
2. Loss of status in household or community (the wage earner who can no longer support his or her family) and life-style and financial adjustments
3. The ability to respond to the needs and demands of others, being dependent on family or others, and becoming a burden on society
4. Initial concerns about ultimate outcome: fear of pain, prolonged discomfort, and of the unknown (death, loss of all functions)
5. Sexuality: loss of sensation, inability to perform sexually and its impact on spouse or partner
6. What to do after leaving the hospital—about managing alone or about remaining in the family if unable to contribute in any way
7. Past interpersonal and family problems, previous occupational problems, and related financial stresses and how these relate to current situation
8. Family members' attitudes toward the patient—expectations and plans or goals for the patient and themselves; the need to examine role readjustments and the ability to create new family systems relationships, power relationships, and decision-making processes
9. What is available in the community for support services: educational, vocational, social, ongoing future health care needs
10. Responses of those who must provide care; conflicts between patients and the health-care team regarding planning

PERSONNEL NEEDS

As mentioned earlier, the rehabilitation process is an amalgam of types of services and forms of assistance. The objective becomes directed toward an adaptive process in which the patient is the major focus. At the same time, another objective becomes the patient's independence from the services of others, which means that the patient and family must become actively involved and develop maximum understanding of the process and the goals. One of the greatest problems in the rehabilitation process is the difficulty frequently created by the patient's and family's denial of the seriousness of the disability or the unlikelihood of total recovery. A great effort must be made to cultivate the patient and family as fully as possible. Since each patient has a special set of problems (both physically and emotionally), efforts must be made to construct appropriate special plans based on knowledge derived from the intake study (derived from a variety of information sources) but stressing the psychosocial background of patient and family.

The personnel involved in rehabilitation include a broad range of specialists in rehabilitation medicine, physical and occupational therapists, orthotists, nursing specialists, audiologists, rehabilitation counselors, speech pathologists, psychologists, and clinical social workers. These personnel are augmented by an array of supportive personnel such as recreational specialists and volunteers. Staff shortages and competition between settings is one of the serious problems in providing rehabilitation services. One of the greatest shortages is in medical specialists in rehabilitation. In 1972, when it was estimated that there was a national need for 3500 to 6200 medical rehabilitation specialists, there were an estimated 1600 to 1800 available. Accordingly, if the annual population growth rate of 3.5% to 5.5% continues, the shortage will last through the 1980s.[5]

A study done by the Council on Social Work Education estimated that in 1970 approximately 17% of social workers were in the health field. It was further estimated that there would be a minimum of 199,000 social work openings requiring higher education (preferably at the master's degree level). If the distribution remains the same as in 1970, about 31,000 of these openings would be in the health field.[10] As with the physicians in rehabilitation, the traditional shortage of social workers in rehabilitation will become increasingly critical as competition for trained personnel develops in the health field. For years, the U.S. Social and Rehabilitation Service (SRS) had been placing grants in social work training to prepare students for working with handicapped people and to include material about disability and rehabilitation in curriculum for all social work students. These grants have been discontinued by the current federal administration, further reducing the ability of potential social workers—especially those from minority and economically limited backgrounds—to become trained, since the costs of education have radically increased.

DEVELOPMENTAL STAGES: PSYCHOSOCIAL IMPLICATIONS

Considerable emphasis has been placed on the social worker's special competence in the area of psychosocial diagnosis of the handicapped patient. Part of that diagnosis concerns the effect of specific phases of the life cycle on the patient and his or her situation.

A handicapped child in a household and community poses special problems such as schooling, peer relationships, and family reactions. On a physical level, depending on the nature of the problem, the child will not be able to go through the normal developmental tasks of children such as talking, walking, and eating. If diagnosis and treatment involve frequent trips to institutions (clinics) or agencies, such trips may be frightening; the child may feel deprived and see the process as a further indication of difference from siblings. The nature and varieties of discipline become problematic when a parent is feeling guilty or overprotective of the child. Some handicapped children respond to their condition by excessive aggression and determination. Within the proper context, this may be appropriate for the coping task, yet it can have unpleasant consequences in interpersonal or peer relationships. Much work has been done about the personality of handicapped people in relation to their adaptation to the problem. Frequently, other children in the school or community will taunt or ridicule a handicapped child. Unless there is parental agreement about handling the child throughout the growing years, there is constant friction and conflict, particularly if the parents are giving major attention to the child.

Adolescence is in and of itself a highly problematic life stage. The emergence of sexuality and sexual feelings creates enormous anxiety in the nonhandicapped child. When there is loss of body part or body function, the teenager may withdraw and become depressed, especially since peer approval is critical at this time. The various forms of acting out by the handicapped youngster can be self-destructive and cause regression to earlier stages of dependency. The role and place of authority becomes highlighted at this age, and testing out can be expected to take place, as when the teenager pushes his parents to see if they really love him.

Disabilities occurring in the young adult stage may be extremely traumatic, since this is a time of early marriage, child rearing, and beginning financial struggles. Accidents occurring at this stage are severely disruptive to the young person or couple. The various role functions (whether male or female) will be thrown into disarray if the disability results in a serious change in life-style and functioning. Partners must take on new and different roles to accommodate the other's handicap. The impact on young children of a parent's sudden disability can have serious effects on the child's developing personality.

Children born with genetic defects or missing limbs are understandably shocking to the young couple. Parents react in a variety of ways: some mothers shudder with repugnance and are unable to nurture a deformed child. Depending on the extent of the deformity, some parents will decide not to take a child home but have it placed in an institution. All of these decisions give rise to tremendous amounts of guilt, particularly if the condition is experienced as genetically transmitted from one spouse or other. This often leads to conflict between the couple and decisions to separate or divorce. The physician and social worker must quickly move into such situations to help sort out the complicated feelings of both parents and to help them move toward a solution. Some parents, on the other hand, exert enormous dedication to the handicapped child, to the extent of personal sacrifice. This may lead to neglect of other siblings in the home or the spouse. At another level, parents may deny the responsibility for the child or deny the child's special needs.

In middle and old age, there are special considerations concerning the onset of disability or disabling disease process. Again, marital status and children's reactions come into focus. Children may resent having to care for a disabled parent when they are trying to make their own family and marriage adjustments. The elderly pose particular problems because of their fragility and the questionable prognosis. This is usually compounded by other complaints such as failing eyesight and arthritis, which make independent living highly problematic.

The social worker has a special role to play in all these life situations by providing counseling or making available educational groups for patients of comparable age or with comparable diagnoses.[5] Supportive or self-help groups can be very enabling to the handicapped at all stages of their lives.

DISCHARGE PLANNING

Discharge planning is the complex collaborative process by which patients are discharged from hospitals to their homes with an array of home health care services or to an institution (health-related, skilled nursing, or hospice). In the acute care setting most patients return home with minimum difficulty, since their condition is usually transitory or episodic (minor surgeries, orthopedic problems, gastrointestinal disorders). With supportive families, the patient's return should be relatively uncomplicated.

The situations of those patients who require considerable care upon discharge, however, become complicated. Every rehabilitation patient has some kind of discharge problem. If a wheelchair is required, for example, the living quarters must permit passage of a wheelchair. Obviously a patient living alone will have problems if his home care needs (such as wound dressing) require the services of another person. Even when there are family members, their availability is not guaranteed, because the spouse may be employed and the elderly spouse may be too fragile to lift a heavy patient or push a wheelchair. The need for a nursing home or some other specialized program requires immediate attention to financing, transportation, special equipment, and the availability of needed resources. With a shortage of nursing homes and mandatory state health department regulations, planning can take a long time and become an involved process. New York University Medical Center has addressed this problem over a period of time and has developed a

model discharge planning unit (DPU) by which all complex placement problems are routed through their range of services by the social worker involved with the case.[4]

Since the Director of Social Service at New York University Medical Center was assigned the title Coordinator of Discharge Planning (as mandated by Professional Standards Review Organization legislation), the DPU is placed within the Social Service Department and because of its high priority, complexity, and impact on hospital planning. It is administered by the Assistant Director of Social Service. The unit consists of an MSW social worker, a BSW social worker, two registered nurses, and a clerk. These functions are combined with those of a transportation coordinator, an equipment coordinator, and a medicaid representative. To plan for complex discharges, all personnel must cooperate to ensure timeliness, financial eligibility, necessary equipment, method of transportation, and other essential factors. In reviewing the recent and pending legislation of the New York State Hospital Association in March 1987, we listed the implications for social service and the DPU. Some of the recently devised forms include a PRI (patient review instrument) to be requested by the social worker and prepared by the nurse in the DPU. This will require an evaluation of the patient's condition and care needs at time of discharge: ability to feed self, mobility, extra care needs, additional equipment, and so on. (Patients requiring respirator help, for example, are extremely complex cases, since the average nursing home cannot monitor such specialized care.)

Documentation becomes the most critical aspect of this planning. Reimbursement rates depend on the level of care required and the demonstrated documentation of efforts at discharge. This is predicated on patient reaching ALOC (alternate level of care status), which means the patient is ready to go to another facility. Other problems of implementation occur: patients must be ready and informed; families who must be involved often "disappear" or conceal or transfer assets; patients with psychiatric or substance abuse problems are difficult to place; patients' rights must be observed. These are only a few of the possible problems in discharge encountered by the social worker and the discharge planning unit.

Admissions must be considered in this discussion, since discharge planning should begin even before admission. For example, we know an elderly woman coming in for hip replacement must have some assistance when returning home. Since this is an elective admission, arrangements for after-hospital care should be made before the inpatient surgery. Correct information at the point of entry in the system is vitally important such as details of insurance coverage, amount of time, and so on. Family cooperation should be stressed and encouraged, since their cooperation, especially at time of discharge, is particularly critical for rehabilitation patients. As much psychosocial information as possible not only enables the team to plan treatment but also to arrange an effective and appropriate discharge.

QUALITY ASSURANCE AND PROGRAM EVALUATION

For a long time, rehabilitation lacked quality control regulations, particularly for patient outcomes. The development of voluntary accreditation of rehabilitation facilities developed by the Commission on Accreditation of Rehabilitation Facilities (CARF) is a beginning step toward this effort. Just as the Joint Commission for Accrediting Hospitals has defined specific standards for rehabilitation programs, so has CARF. Starting with the earlier Professional Standards Review Organization (PSRO) legislation, a series of methods to examine health care practice has evolved; these include peer review, medical audit, and quality assurance. Similarly, the National Association of Social Workers (NASW) has identified needs for quality of care and competence. A joint committee representing the Social Work Section of the American Public Health Association and Health Quality Standards Committee of NASW compiled a policy statement (1981) entitled NASW standards for social work in health care settings.[6] It is significant that they listed 11 standards that describe the director's responsibilities, program structure and functions, policies and procedures, budget, space and equipment, and documentation. The last standard requires review and evaluation of social work services, at least yearly, with written records and pre-established criteria and standards. The standards indicate feedback mechanisms and implementation for corrective measures.

The AHA *Joint Commission Manual* is specific about rehabilitation services; it indicates individual criteria for each discipline and interdisciplinary collaboration.[1] For social work the manual indicates assessment and intervention relative to psychosocial factors and the social context of the disabled patient; the scope of patient's coping history and current psychosocial adaptation to the disability; assessment of immediate and extended family members; assessment of housing and living arrangements, and source of income. It also includes casework counseling, education groups, and community linkages. The monitoring of goals relevant to discharge planning is stressed.

It is clear that a major effort is being directed toward eliminating duplication of services and achieving efficient care and competent standards of practice for all health-care practitioners, not just social workers. The threat of loss of accreditation has caused institutions offering all forms of health care to be vigilant and concerned about defining and meeting the highest-quality standards by which services can be measured and evaluated.

FUTURE IMPLICATIONS

Within health-care systems, there are mounting pressures to deal with the increasing costs of care through cost-containment measures and quality assurance standards. At the same time, other changes are taking place in the form and structure of health-care organization. Above all, the notion of "for profit" is entering the health-care scene. Hospitals are buying hotels, health spas, restaurants, and shopping centers; the intent is to acquire income-producing services that will return funds to the institution. Mount Sinai Hospital in New York City has recently mounted an aggressive public relations marketing campaign to advertise its services through the media at a cost of approximately $3 million. It stresses quality of care at the hospital and pushes for higher census rates (maximal bed utilization). There is also a trend toward hospital mergers, which would consolidate resources and diversity of services. The impact of diagnostic related groups (DRGs) has led to increasing use of home health-care services in a variety of forms.

Most social workers are not familiar with the determination of costs in the hospital setting. Currently social workers are a component of the per diem rate for almost all third party payers. Ambulatory care social services are not covered except as a portion of Medicare and Medicaid physician visits. Thus all ambulatory care programs impose a deficit on their institutions. If fee-for-service continues as major source of health care payments, social workers will have to modify their "philanthropic" philosophy to a more realistic appraisal of their value and what to charge reimbursement agents. Possible solutions have been suggested by the passage in 1977 of the third-party payments law, which recognizes qualified social workers as vendors of services to patients who are insured for mental health services, just as with psychologists and psychiatrists. There must be certification and licenses to ensure social work competence, which has been defined by NASW at different levels of performance.

As with the acute care patients, it appears that disabled patients will be receiving increasing amounts of care in their home rather than in institutional settings. Technologic advances and computer systems have enabled severely handicapped persons to function remarkably well as homemakers, office workers, and in all types of occupations that were impossible in the past. These changes may create other kinds of problems as the number of elderly persons increases and as more persons with disabilities are sustained with devices that prolong life and maximize social functioning. Social workers must adapt their own skills, values, and roles to meet these rapid changes in the health-care field.

REFERENCES

1. American Hospital Association: Accreditation manual for hospitals, Chicago, 1987, The Association.
2. Bureau of Education for the Handicapped: Estimated number of handicapped children served and unserved by type of handicap, Washington, DC, 1976, US Office of Education. (Mimeo.)
3. Falck, Hans: Interdisciplinary education and implications for social work practice, J Educ Social Work 13:30, 1977.
4. Foster, A, and Brown, DG: The social work role in hospital discharge planning: and administrative case history, Social Work Health Care 4:55, 1978.
5. Lowin, A, and Sanderregger, L: Rehabilitation medicine: need, supply, demand, 1972-87, Minneapolis, Minn, 1974, Commission on Rehabilitation Medicine.

6. NASW: Standards for social work in health care settings, Washington, DC, 1981, National Association of Social Workers.

7. Pendarvis, JF, and Grinnell, RM: The use of a rehabilitation team for stroke patients, Social Work Health Care 6:77, 1980.

8. President's Committee on Employment of the Handicapped: One in eleven handicapped adults in America: a survey based on 1970 U.S. census data, Washington, DC, US Government Printing Office. (No date.)

9. Public Health Service, Health Resources Administration: Prevalence of selected impairments: United States 1971, Series 10, No. 99, Washington, DC, 1973, US Department of Health, Education and Welfare.

10. Siegel, Sheldon: Social service needs: an overview to 1980, New York, 1975, Council on Social Work Education.

ADDITIONAL READINGS

Colachis, SC, Jr: New directions in health care, Arch Phys Med Rehabil 65:291, 1984.

Cramand, D, and Titus, LM: Discharge to independent living for the chronically ill patient: a case study, Social Work Health Care 10:123, 1985.

Miller, RS, and Rehr, H: Social work issues in health care, Englewood Cliffs, NJ, 1983, Prentice-Hall, Inc.

Palmer, S, et al: Psychosocial services in rehabilitation medicine: an interdisciplinary approach, Arch Phys Med Rehabil 66:690, 1985.

Snyder, B, and Keefe, K: The unmet needs of family caregivers for frail and disabled adults, Social Work Health Care 10:123, 1985.

Stoller, EP: Sources of support for the elderly during illness, Health Social Work 7:111, 1982.

CHAPTER 62

Psychosexual issues in rehabilitation

FRANCES SOMMER ANDERSON

In the last two decades knowledge of human sexuality has markedly increased, perhaps as a result of an atmosphere in which sexuality is acknowledged as a vital aspect of human identity. In 1975 the World Health Organization called attention to the importance of sexual health, challenging health-care professionals to integrate the somatic, emotional, intellectual, and social aspects of sexual being to enhance and enrich personality and quality of life.[100] Many believe that a feeling of sexual adequacy is at the core of our identity.[31] Professionals in rehabilitation medicine agree that interpersonal, psychosocial, and psychosexual needs, as well as physical and medical problems, are important concerns in rehabilitation.[31,85,93] Much has been written advocating evaluation of sexual functioning, sex education, and sexual rehabilitation[4,27,38,86] to ensure comprehensive rehabilitation. The negative impact of impaired sexual functioning on medical, psychologic, and vocational rehabilitation of the chronically ill and physically disabled has been documented.[74,122] Shrey and co-workers[94] found an increase in depression, anxiety, and feelings of being overwhelmed by the rehabilitation program in clients with sexual dysfunction.

Studies of the health-care professional's role in rehabilitation have found that physicians, psychologists, social workers, and other professionals are often ignorant and ambivalent about their roles in the sexual rehabilitation of their clients.[30,93,94] This can lead to role ambiguity and overlap. Health-care professionals have tended to ascribe the responsibility for sexual rehabilitation to other professionals on the rehabilitation team.[85] Obstacles for all who attempt to help the client with sexual concerns are cultural taboos, personal discomfort, and inadequate educational preparation for the task.[30,32,33] Counselors' apprehension and uneasiness have been traced to embarrassment, confusion, lack of knowledge, moral and religious convications, and discomfort with their own sexuality.[34]

This chapter addresses fundamental aspects of sexual rehabilitation. First, a database is provided for health-care professionals to use as a component of a comprehensive sexual rehabilitation program. This review of the sexual problems and concerns of individuals with spinal cord injury, stroke, multiple sclerosis, and neuromuscular disease is followed by an overview of the social and personal implications of physical disability, since sexual rehabilitation efforts must occur in this context. Approaches to staff training and methods of integrating sexuality into the rehabilitation program are also discussed.

IMPACT OF PHYSICAL DISABILITY ON SEXUAL FUNCTIONING
Spinal cord injury

According to Trieschmann,[114] more than 60% of spinal cord injuries occur in people aged 15 to 29 years. Motor vehicle accidents are the most common cause. Sports injuries, such as those from diving, surfing, and skiing, result in quadriplegia more often than paraplegia. In this group 82% are male, and 18% are female. Among those aged 60 years and older, falls are the primary cause of spinal cord injury.

Men with spinal cord injuries

The long-range impact of spinal cord injury on sexual functioning cannot be predicted in the first several weeks after the trauma because of "spinal shock"—the suppression of reflex activity below the level of the injury.[1] During this period there may also be atonic paralysis of the bladder and rectal sphincters, as well as sensory loss. Priapism may occur in some men because of venous stasis. Amelar and Dubin[1] stated that deficits lasting 6 months or more are likely to be permanent. Erection, ejaculation, and fertility are affected.

Erectile functioning. In general, sexual sequelae are determined by the level of the lesion. Incomplete lesions are associated with a better prognosis. Complete upper motor neuron lesions are associated with a higher rate of erections but less frequent ejaculation and orgasm.[15,109] Until recently the majority of investigations of sexual functioning after spinal cord injury have used retrospective data obtained through interviews and psychologic screening.[10,15,29,54] Objective evaluations of the erectile capability of spinal cord–injured patients can be done using a nocturnal penile tumescence monitor, described by Karacan and co-workers[61-63] and Leyson and Powell.[72]

Lamid[69] measured changes in penile tumescence related to the level of spinal cord injury, completeness of lesion, and presence of the bulbocavernous reflex. The subject population was 12 quadriplegics and 12 paraplegics, ranging in age from 20 to 57 years (mean, 31.4 years). The postinjury period lasted from 0.6 to more than 12 months. All subjects were interviewed for preinjury and postinjury sexual histories, and all received complete physical, neurologic, and urologic examinations. There was no control for current medications. The mean duration of an erectile episode during sleep was greater for quadriplegics than for paraplegics ($p < .01$). Similarly, the mean increase in penile circumference was greater for the quadriplegic ($p < .01$). There were more quadriplegics with full erections and more paraplegics with no erections. These three findings were consistent with previous studies.[15,29] Subjects with incomplete lesions had a greater expansion, but this difference was not statistically significant, unlike the results of studies by Comarr and Vigue[29] and Bors and Comarr.[15] The nocturnal penile tumescence was not affected by type of urinary drainage used nor related to the presence of sex dreams and reflexogenic erections. Further, the bulbocavernous reflex was not associated with increased penile tumescence, in agreement with Karacan and associates.[61]

A number of researchers have reported that erections sufficient for intercourse are found in less than 25% of spinal cord–injured men.[59,90,109,124] Techniques for triggering reflexogenic erections and prolonging the erection have been described by various authors.[19,92]

The use of penile prostheses—silicone rod implants and inflatable penile prostheses—has been discouraged by Amelar and Dubin.[1] Problems such as infection, tissue breakdown, and extrusion of the prosthesis can occur. The caution necessary in evaluating the suitability of these devices in the context of a couple's relationship has been stressed by Stewart and Gerson.[104]

More recently Green and Sloan[46] reported the use of penile prosthesis in 40 spinal cord–injured patients since 1981. They combined early sexual counseling in the acute phase of injury and implantation no less than 9 to 12 months after injury. Early counseling involved private and group sessions focused on reassessing body image as it relates to sexuality and the level of injury. These sessions included a partner

when possible. The emotional aspects of sexuality were elaborated in addition to the sexual alternatives to penovaginal intercourse. The penile prosthesis was mentioned as an option. Further counseling after discharge was offered. The experience of previous investigators was used to avoid the high probability of complications.[89,118] Suitable surgical candidates were identified as those who had stable bladder programs, a recent urologic radiography evaluation, sterile urine at implantation, and absence of open skin lesions. The 40 subjects included 28 paraplegics and 12 quadriplegics, with a mean age of 33 years (range, 21 to 60 years). Thirty-one subjects had complete lesions. Candidates with high self-esteem, motivation, and general care of activities of daily living were selected. Of 36 patients followed up in 1985, 31 had intercourse regularly and were pleased with the prosthesis. Four complained that the semirigid rod was not rigid enough for vaginal intercourse.

Ejaculatory functioning. Ejaculatory functioning in men with spinal cord injuries is variously reported as severely limited. In 1976 Sandowski[92] observed that only a few men who have erections can ejaculate. Amelar and Dubin[1] stated that less than 10% of men with spinal cord injury are able to ejaculate. Of course, these figures are averages across all levels of spinal cord injury and are not based on detailed, controlled studies of sexual functioning in spinal cord–injured men. More recently, Larsen and Hejgaard[70] in Denmark and Sjogren and Egberg[98] in Sweden reported greater sexuality and fertility in younger than in older men, regardless of the severity of the deficits. Sjogren and Egberg[98] studied 21 Swedish men (mean age, 27 ± 4 years) with completely transected cords (determined clinically) at least 1 year after the trauma. The significance of sexuality was unaltered for the majority. Most men had continued to have intercourse, and one half reported feeling orgasmic. The greater capability for penetration and ejaculation found in this study may be due to the younger age of the subjects, cultural differences in attitudes toward sexuality, and the fact that the interview used four graded scales in assessing sexual functioning. Further, the authors suggested that changes in sexual functioning may be easier to cope with earlier in life, when gender roles and sexual identity are in the process of being established.

In both of these studies the major obstacles to sexual fulfillment were not directly related to sexual functioning per se. Larsen and Hejgaard[70] reported that bladder dysfunction led to a fear of involuntary urination and that the use of the catheter, diaper, or drainage bag contributed to negative feelings about sexual activity. Sjogren and Egberg[98] found that locomotor impairment and autonomous dysreflexia (excessive activation of the autonomic nervous system) were more frequently cited as causes of sexual displeasure than were sexual dysfunctions per se. For those with lesions above T4 autonomic dysreflexia was common, characterized by a sudden pounding headache from increased blood pressure,[90] flushing, sweating, and cardiac arrhythmias because of elevated catecholamine levels.[1] Subjects with midcervical lesions were less satisfied than those with low cervical or high thoracic injuries. Although subjects had the same genital physiologic impairments, those with midcervical lesions had more motility and activity restrictions and less input from generalized erogenous skin areas than did those with other levels of lesion.

Fertility. Infertility in spinal cord–injured men may be due to an inability to ejaculate or to retrograde ejaculation.[5,81] Retrograde ejaculation is more common if the lesion is in the upper lumbar segments and is rare otherwise.[19] Retrograde ejaculation can result from neurologic disturbances, transurethral resection of the bladder neck to improve micturition, or both.[14,37,58,111] Brindley[19] recommended the implantation of a sacral anterior root stimulator instead of bladder neck resection if fertility is at issue. Prolonged intermittent or continuous catheterization can lead to prostatitis, epididymitis, and epididymo-orchitis, which can produce obstructive ductal lesions and testicular damage.[14] Sandowski[92] noted that testicular atrophy is more common when the lesion is below D11. Spermatogenesis may be severely impaired[82] because of denervation of lumbar spinal nerves passing through the sympathetic trunk in the L3 to L6 area. Further, damage to the thermoregulatory centers in the T10 to T12 region may result in elevated testicular temperatures. There have been conflicting reports on serum levels of luteinizing hormone (LH), follicle-stimulating hormone (FSH), testosterone, and estradiol in men with spinal cord injuries. Bors[16] and Kikuchi[66] and their co-workers found these levels to be normal, but Hayes[51] and Mizutani[80] and their associates found elevated LH and FSH with normal prolactin and testosterone levels in 30% to 50% of paraplegic men.

Even when ejaculation is possible, aspermia may result from neurogenic causes, such as the failure of ductal sperm conduction because of interference with the innervation of the epididymitis, vasa deferentia, and seminal vesicles.[1] David and co-workers[36] found normal hormonal and sperm metabolic values but severe disturbances in spermatogenesis and spermiogenesis, their causes unclear. Brindley[19] believes that deficient semen results from a combination of nondrainage, chronic infection, and raised scrotal temperature.

Despite frequently documented problems with erection and fertility, some investigators continue to pursue methods to stimulate an ejaculation to produce sperm for insemination. In general, these techniques should be tried as soon as possible after injury, because semen quality and fertility decline rapidly after injury. Electrical stimulation was described by Horne and co-workers[55] and used by Thomas[112] and Francois[43] and their co-workers. Brindley[20,21,22] described two methods—electroejaculation and the use of vibrators—to improve the prospects for obtaining semen. Electroejaculation, described in detail by Brindley,[20] is induction of seminal emission using electrical stimulation produced by electrodes inserted in the rectum. It has been used

in animals since 1938; the first human pregnancy resulting from this technique was documented by Thomas and associates[112] in 1975. The first live births were noted by Francois and co-workers[43] and Brindley.[22] Vibratory stimulation has also been described by Comarr[28] and used by Francois and co-workers[42] and Brindley.[21]

In a study of 81 men with predominantly complete spinal injuries of more than 6 months' duration, Brindley[19] reported that 59% had an ejaculation using vibratory stimulation. Vibratory stimulation was successful in 75% of cases when injury was sustained more than 6 months earlier and when a hip flexion was obtained in response to scratching the soles of the feet (indicating that L2 to S1 are intact, enabling a reflex ejaculation). The vibratory stimulation yielded better semen than electroejaculation because the semen was free from urine contamination. With successive use of either technique, however, the quality of the semen improved. Electroejaculation was as successful in the first 6 months after injury as later, whereas vibratory stimulation was rarely successful before 6 months from the time of injury. Eleven pregnancies were achieved in this study: three by electroejaculation, seven by vibratory stimulation, and one by masturbation.

Brindley[19] reached the following conclusions based on this and other studies. He estimated that for those with complete cord lesions, using both electroejaculation and vibratory stimulation, semen should be obtained in 51% of the cases, with 23% fertile. He pointed out that this projection is only for those who do not have damaged intermediate horn cells in segments T11 to L2, inclusive. If these segments are spared, the two techniques described should yield semen. Ejaculation and impregnation in coitus for those with incomplete lesions is possible, because T12 to L2 segments are accessible to reflexive and psychologic influences mediating ejaculation. If the damage is complete and below T12, ejaculation is psychogenic, whereas complete lesions above T12 result in reflex ejaculations.

A third method being used to produce sperm for fertilization is the use of intrathecal injections of neostigmine (Prostigmin), introduced by Guttmann[48,49] in 1949. Variable results have been reported by Spira,[102] Piera,[84] Chapelle and co-workers,[23] and Iwatsubo and co-workers.[57] The mechanism of ejaculation after intrathecal injection of neostigmine is twofold[15,49,110]: direct stimulation of spinal sexual centers by neostigmine and the removal of skeletal muscle reflexes that may inhibit sexual function. The spinal sexual centers are divided into two parts: seminal emission mediated by the sympathetic center linked to the hypogastric nerves in segments T11 to L2 and ejaculation proper mediated by the somatic center associated with pudendal nerves in segments S2, S3, and S4.

The major problem associated with this technique is the possibility of autonomic hyperreflexia[52] provoked by the contraction of seminal vesicles and bulbocavernous muscles during ejaculation, usually in lesions above T5.[49] This potential can be controlled by intravenous injections of atropine or pentolinium.[49] Additional precautions are described by Otani and co-workers[83]: nothing by mouth should be allowed for several hours before the injection, an intravenous line should be secured, atrophine and a ganglionic blocking agent should be readily available, and blood pressure and pulse rate should be monitored for several hours after the injection. Chapelle and associates[24] reported a successful pregnancy using this method with a man who had damage from T7-T8 to T11-T12 7 years earlier. Otani and co-workers[84] described a 33-year-old man who sustained a compression fracture of T6 in a fall, resulting in complete paralysis below T9, who later fathered a child after an intrathecal injection of neostigmine. This was the fourth successful case using this method.

Women with spinal cord injuries

Less research has been published on the sexual problems of spinal cord–injured women[41,113] perhaps because the number of spinal cord–injured men far exceeds that of women. Also, the mechanics of sexual intercourse seem to require fewer adjustments for women.[8] Vaginal lubrication continues, and some women report experiencing orgasms.[87] Fertility is unaffected—menstrual periods and ovulation continue.[116] Menstrual cramps and labor pains are no longer felt. Finding suitable birth control may be difficult, however. Birth control pills are not recommended because of the associated risk of blood clotting. The diaphragm can be mechanically difficult to use. Intrauterine devices and condoms are better choices, and sterilization may be an option.

In a recent study of pregnancy and delivery Verduyn[120] described 33 spinal cord–injured women who had a total of 50 deliveries. Potential problems for these women were early labor, hyperreflexia, urinary tract infection, and spinal cord injury care. The results of a mail survey indicated that 22 of 27 women with injury at T6 or above had experienced hyperreflexia during delivery. Seven of these had had cesarean sections. Hyperreflexia was a more serious threat for this group than for those with lower lesions. Postpartum complications included dehiscence of the episiotomy, thrombophlebitis, pulmonary emboli, and urinary tract infections. The author strongly recommended relying on the spinal cord–injured woman's experience in managing skin care, hyperreflexia, and other aspects of her treatment. In addition, the obstetrician should consult a spinal cord specialist to prepare for the complications that may arise.

Stroke

There are far fewer investigations of sexual functioning in patients after stroke than after spinal cord injury. Sjogren and Fugl-Meyer[100] pointed out that difficulty determining the site and size of the lesion, varying degrees of cognitive and perceptual impairment, dysphasia, impaired judgment, and motoric dysfunction (with or without spasticity) contribute to the problems of designing controlled studies and obtaining valid and reliable input from victims of stroke.

In four studies that assessed changes in sexual functioning after stroke, all reported a significant negative impact of hemiplegia and hemiparesis. Kalliomaki and co-workers[60] found that 70% of men and 44% of women reported a decrease in the frequency of intercourse after stroke. One third of the subjects reported decreased libido, the reduction being more common in right than in left hemiplegia. Leshner, Fine, and Goldman,[71] studying a group 50 to 70 years old, also found a significant decrease in the frequency of intercourse; 45% had ceased intercourse.

Fugl-Meyer and Jaasko[44] evaluated sexual activity in 23 women and 62 men, aged 57.5 ± 9 years, who had had one stroke either 6 years or 1 year before the study. These investigators did not control for locus of damage. Before the stroke 83% of the patients had been sexually active. After the stroke 36% reported the same frequency of intercourse, 33% reported a decreased frequency, and 31% ceased having intercourse. These results are consistent with those of Kalliomaki and associates.[60] The poststroke interval was not significant. The degree of motor deficit was not related to change in frequency of intercourse. An important factor was impaired sensation in one half of the body. Those in the decreased frequency and cessation groups were more likely to experience impaired sensation. Further, an increase in custodial attitudes of the nondisabled partner was positively related to a decrease in frequency of intercourse. The authors stressed that sexual maladjustment is part of general psychologic maladjustment. After the stroke the "sexual ego" is put under stress by the spouse's attitudes, traditional sex role definitions, stigmatization of the disability, regressive dependency, and fear of loss of attractiveness. Further, the temporal relation of sexual activity to the onset of stroke can cause fear and guilt.

Sjogren and Fugl-Meyer[100] assessed specific changes in coital habits and the prevalence of erectile and orgasmic dysfunction in 51 subjects, sexually active before stroke, whose mean age at stroke was 53 ± 8 years. The stroke-to-study interval and the side of hemiplegia were not controlled for. Similar to the preceding studies, there was a significant reduction of coital frequency and an increase in levels of sexual problems, more for men than for women. Forty-six percent of men and women ceased or reduced the duration of foreplay, although less change occurred for women than men. The majority reported having been relatively satisfied with the frequency and duration of sexual activity before stroke. After the stroke men were greatly dissatisfied with the frequency of intercourse, duration of foreplay, and total time for sex play. In contrast, women were much less dissatisfied, possibly because they had accepted a less active sexual style or had less pleasure from intercourse before the stroke. The incidence of excitatory erectile dysfunction was three times more common after than before the stroke. Orgasmic dysfunction was reported by 84% of men after stroke. Erectile dysfunction was the main complaint for men, compared with general fatigue for women. In general, the higher the level of prestroke sexual dysfunction, the less change after stroke, leading to lower sexual frustration and dysfunction compared with prestroke levels.

Sjogren and Fugl-Meyer[99] studied the extent to which the degree of physical disability and daily dependency affect sex and leisure and assessed the temporal factor. Using an interview, they assessed motor performance, cutaneous sensitivity, and activities of daily living status in a group of 110 subjects who were less than 66 years at stroke (71% men, 29% women). They also found a decrease in the frequency of intercourse and leisure in approximately 75% of the subjects. These changes were directly related to the degree of physical impairment and levels of dependency in daily living. Changes in the frequency of intercourse were independent of the stroke-to-study interval. Changes in frequency of intercourse were directly related to impaired cutaneous sensitivity.

Sjogren and associates[97] assessed parameters of sexual behavior in 22 right hemisphere–damaged and 29 left hemisphere–damaged patients after stroke: frequency and duration of intercourse, incidence of erectile and orgastic dysfunction, and sex partner's drive. For men and women the frequency and duration of foreplay and intercourse was markedly reduced. Erectile problems, rare before stroke, were reported by the majority of the 39 men after stroke. Orgastic dysfunction was fairly common for women but not men before the stroke. After the stroke, 75% of the women and 64% of the men had orgastic dysfunction and reported a decrease in the partner's sex drive. The reported increase in duration of foreplay in men was related to an attempt to overcome erectile dysfunction. The side of the hemiplegia was not significantly correlated with a change in any of the parameters studied. This finding is in contrast to other studies, which have concluded that aphasic patients have particular sexual difficulties, perhaps because of the negative impact of impaired communication on the relationship with the partner.[25] Kinsella and Duffy[67] reported that 83% of the aphasic patients in their study sample ceased having sexual relations after the stroke.

Sjogren[96] conducted a more focused study of sexual function, fulfillment, and partner responsiveness before and after stroke in the population described in the preceding study. The findings were related to the prevalence of "performance-orientated" attitudes toward sexual activity and to sexually stigmatic tendencies. Like the results of the study by Sjogren and co-workers,[97] 15% of the men reported retarded ejaculation after stroke, compared with no problems before stroke. Erectile problems were cited as the primary reason for a decline in sexual enjoyment, followed by fatigue, fear of relapse, reduced sensation, and orgastic problems. Women cited fatigue as the primary reason for decrease in enjoyment, as they did in the Sjogren and Fugl-meyer[100] study. The tendency to "observe" one's sexual perfor-

mance—"spectatoring"—increased significantly for men after stroke. Sixty percent of women reported such tendencies before stroke, with an insignificant change after stroke.

After the stroke women and men experienced a decrease in verbal and nonverbal partner responsiveness. Fifty percent of the group felt that they themselves were less responsive. Fifty percent of the men and 33% of the women felt that their partners were less responsive. Overall fulfillment was markedly decreased for men and somewhat decreased for women. This reduction was associated with changes in sexual function and partner responsiveness. In a sample of 39 of the 51 subjects, a performance orientation during sexual activity was common, and there was a general tendency toward stigmatization. Sexual stigmatization was associated with a decline in general sexual satisfaction, dissatisfaction with the frequency of intercourse, a decrease in one's own responsiveness to the partner's initiative, and an increase in the frequency of erectile spectatoring.

As Fugl-Meyer and Jaasko[44] noted, the neurophysiologic substrates of sexual function require further investigation to clarify whether the reported erectile dysfunction and apparently decreased libido after stroke are centrally mediated. They further question the possibility of negative effects of antihypertensive drugs on erectile function.[53] Sjogren et al.[97] addressed both of these issues. In a detailed evaluation of 15 men they found that serum levels of FSH, LH, and prolactin were within the normal range. The response to human chorionic gonadotropin (HCG) was normal. The levels of hormones were not associated with reported changes in sexual function or with sexual function per se. They concluded that hormonal factors were not responsible for the sexual dysfunctions found in their study group; that is, vascular brain lesions did not appear to impair the pituitary-gonadal axis in men. Further, they failed to find an association between erectile dysfunction and the use of antihypertensive drugs.

The consensus of these investigators is that the negative impact of a stroke on the individual's sex life is due primarily to the individual's style of coping with the disability rather than to physiologic deficits brought about by the cerebral damage. For example, Sjogren and Fugl-Meyer[99] concluded that the marked changes in sexual intercourse observed in their study were a function of maladaptive coping with disease-related, intrapersonal, and interpersonal factors. Disease-related factors identified were movement restrictions, sensation deficits, impaired cerebral integration, and problems with energy production. These obstacles in and of themselves do not prevent sexual activity and intercourse. Specifically, the authors pointed out that the loss of exteroception of one half of the penis need not adversely affect intercourse.[47] Intrapersonal factors, such as the individual's reaction to and assessment of the meaning of the sequelae of the stroke, are particularly important. Reactive depression, anxiety, fear of relapse, lack of information, regressive dependency, and feelings of stigmatization are significant obstacles to adaptive coping. The performance orientation described by Sjogren,[96] for example, may be a general orientation to life and can result in a drastic loss of self-esteem when the individual cannot measure up to personal expectations. For people who have valued intellectual ability and occupational success, the reduced somatic and mental capacity, loss of occupation, and fear of relapse can lead to fixation in a dependent role. Interpersonal factors then come into play. The dependency of one partner may produce a shift in roles, and the able-bodied partner may become an authoritarian, parental custodian. Each partner's role expectations come into focus, and the possible amibivalence about the new roles can easily affect the sexual relationship. Indeed, Sjogren and associates[97] documented that the increased custodial attitude of the partner was associated with a decrease in the frequency of intercourse. An increase in dependency in self-care had the same effect.

Multiple sclerosis

Little has been published on the sexual problems of people with multiple sclerosis (MS), even though sexual disturbances have been cited by Minderhoud and co-workers[79] to be an important feature of the disease that can appear early.[73] One of the earliest studies of the relationship between sexual functioning and MS was reported by Ivers and Goldstein[56] in 1963. These researchers evaluated 144 patients (37% male). Twenty-six percent of the men were impotent; for 3% impotence was the main symptom of the disease. Miller and co-workers[78] reportred that 60% of the men in that study sample experienced erectile dysfunction and that emotional factors played a primary role in one third of this group. Vas[119] found that 47% of a sample of 37 men reported some degree of erectile dysfunction, despite absence of marked neurologic disability. He hypothesized that the dysfunction was caused by a lesion of the spinal cord in its lateral horn or in connecting pathways in the dorsolumbar area. He also noted that the patients reporting impotence had a lower than average level of circulating testosterone.

In a questionnaire survey of 302 people with MS, Lilius and associates[73] found that 91% of the men and 72% of the women reported a change in their sex life. Approximately half of the group were dissatisfied with their sex life or had ceased to have sexual activity. Sixty-two percent of men cited disturbances in erection as the major problem; only 20% of the men had normal erections. Women reported loss of orgasm (33%), loss of libido (27%), and spasticity (12%) as major problems. The duration of the MS was not related to the incidence of sexual disturbances.

A survey of 100 MS patients reported by Szasz and co-workers[107] revealed that almost 50% were less sexually active or no longer active after the onset of MS. Fifty percent were concerned about the change. In a subsequent investigation Szasz and co-workers[106,107] used a five-point Sexual Functioning Scale with 73 MS patients to clarify the natural history of sexual problems in MS patients. They found that 45% were less sexually active or inactive after the onset of the MS, and 27% were concerned about this change. Difficulties with toilet transfer and bladder functioning distinguished this group from a group that was as active after the onset of MS as before. The authors suggested that the changes in sexual activity were not related to demographic variables. Rather, they concluded that impairments related to the course of MS were responsible for the changes in sexual practices. They suggested that the impact of problems with ambulation and difficulties in maintaining preillness financial standards could have a psychologic impact with negative implications for sex role definitions.

Valleroy and Kraft[117] used a questionnaire with 217 patients to evaluate the extent and types of sexual dysfunction in MS patients. This group was experiencing minor mobility limitations—75% did not use a wheelchair, and more than one half were ambulatory without assistive devices. In general, the finding was that sexual dysfunction can be expected in at least 50% of women and 75% of men with MS, regardless of mobility level, mildness of symptoms, and lack of spasticity and bladder dysfunction. Spasticity and bladder dysfunction were associated with sexual dysfunction, whereas loss of mobility, weakness, and depression were not. Even when spasticity and bladder dysfunction were absent, 50% of cases reported sexual dysfunction. Overall, 56% of women and 75% of men complained of sexual difficulties. For women sexual complaints (in order of decreasing frequency) were fatigue, decreased sensation, decreased libido, decreased frequency or loss of orgasm, and difficulty with arousal. Erectile dysfunction was the most common problem cited by men, with decreased sensation, fatigue, decreased libido, and orgasmic dysfunction following.

Minderhoud and associates[79] used a questionnaire to evaluate the frequency and nature of sexual dysfunctions among MS patients with mild mobility impairment. A control group of neurologic outpatients was chosen to match the MS patients in age and sex. Their data are consistent with earlier reports of the high incidence of sexual dysfunction in the MS population. Seventy-one percent of men and 74% of women reported sexual dysfunction, compared with 19% of the control group. There was a significant correlation of serious sexual dysfunction with disturbances of bladder and anal sphincter function. They suggested that separate damage in the lower part of the spinal cord is responsible for the sexual dysfunctions and the bladder and sphincter disturbances.

Neuromuscular disease

Investigations of sexual functioning in individuals with neuromuscular disease have been reported by Anderson and Bardach[3]; Anderson, Bardach, and Goodgold[4]; and Anderson.[2] These investigators were the first to systematically assess the impact of neuromuscular disease on sexual functioning and psychosexual adjustment. One earlier investigator had noted abnormally small testes, underdeveloped genitalia, and gynecomastia in males with Duchenne type muscular dystrophy.[75] Lundberg[75] also observed testicular atrophy in males with myotonic dystrophy and ocular myopathy.

Anderson and Bardach[3] published a pilot study in which they assessed sexual functioning in 20 subjects with early onset of symptoms of neuromuscular disease and a relatively rapid rate of progression and in 20 subjects with neuromuscular disease characterized by a relatively slower rate of progression. Using a structured interview, they failed to find any evidence of impairment of physiologic sexual functioning. Rather, the impact of the disease in both groups had its most adverse effects on the psychosexual aspect of sexual functioning. Specifically, in the group with early onset and rapid progression, physical limitations had interfered with psychosocial and psychosexual development, resulting in extremely limited sociosexual contacts. The subjects reported great dissatisfaction with their severely restricted range of sexual experiences and with the many environmental and attitudinal obstacles to socialization. Autoerotic activities, such as masturbation and sexual fantasizing, were frequently relied on as sexual outlets in this group. Although mobility and movement limitations were present because of muscle weakness, muscle atrophy, contractions, and respiratory constraints, these variables were not critical when compared with the psychosocial variable.

In the group of subjects with relatively slow progression of neuromuscular disease the emotional impact of the progression of the disease was a more critical determinant of sexual practices than the degree of physical limitations per se. Loss of self-esteem, depression, and anxiety were common reactions to changes in vocational status. Additional stresses were changes in physical attractiveness and in sexual practices necessitated by physical limitations imposed by the disease. In this group the focus of rehabilitation efforts was on expanding sex role definitions and on effecting attitudinal changes to increase the range of acceptable sexual activities for each partner.

PSYCHOSOCIAL AND PSYCHOSEXUAL IMPLICATIONS OF DISABILITY

Conine[30] has identified three obstacles to sexual readjustment for the physically disabled individual: psychologic reactions, communication dysfunctions, and physical limitations. Similarly, Ray and West,[87] in discussing rehabilitation of the paraplegic patient, delineated the social, sexual, and personal implications of the disability. Clearly, interventions to facilitate sexual rehabilitation must be tailored to the individual in an atmosphere of acceptance and trust,[11] taking into consideration the multiple factors noted previously. The psychologic impact of the disability on the person's self-image, feelings of worth and self-respect, and happiness may be negative and thus may generalize to a person's image of sexual attractiveness. Expectations about one's body are drastically altered, often leading to shame and self-doubt over loss of control, especially during sexual activity.[12,18,108] Depression from frustration over motoric slowness and clumsiness and people's reactions to them are common.[87] Thus one's self-image can be adversely affected in one's own eyes, as well as in the eyes of others.

In our culture physical disability is seen as a stigma or marker of difference from others, leading to discredit and disqualification from ordinary participation in society.[45,64] Sjogren and Fugl-Meyer[100] noted that changes in sex life with a partner after a stroke were positively related to increased feelings of stigmatization. Stigmatization can lead to social exclusion and rejection.[91] As Siller[95] demonstrated, attitudes toward the disabled are multidimensional. Clearly, positive attitudes toward disabled individuals can be seen in people's tendencies to be helpful and considerate.[68] However, many can be distressed and embarrassed in the presence of a disabled person and try to avoid contact.[68,101,115]

Multiple variables affect the emotional adjustment and, consequently, the psychosexual adjustment of the disabled individual. For example, premorbid intellectual ability, personality characteristics, family relationships, life-style, and values are important.[17,35,40] "Physique as a prime mover" in contemporary American society has been identified by Wright[123] as a major contributor to the negative impact of physical disability. For the individual who has valued physical appearance and prowess, mobility limitations may be especially devastating. In another vein, for the person who has valued intellectual achievements, awareness of the cognitive deficits after a stroke can be traumatic. In addition, the general meaning of the injury to the individual is important. For example, Katz and associates[65] found that disabled war veterans had a more positive self-image than people who had accidents at work.

Verwoerdt[121] identified three groups of factors that affect an individual's response to acute illness. Related to the illness itself, severity of symptoms, degree of disability, perceived threat to life, duration and rate of progression of illness, and the particular body part affected are important variables. The patient's age, sex, body image, and premorbid personality and coping mechanisms are patient variables. Social variables, such as family, social, and employment environment, must also be considered.

Engel[39] hypothesized that the stress of illness must be defined to account for intrapsychic factors as well as the external effects of the illness. The individual's intrapsychic experience is determined by past experiences and stresses, especially by unresolved intrapsychic conflicts. Engel has cited loss or threat of loss of psychic objects, injury or threat of injury, and frustration of drives as intrapsychic sources of stress. Some of the real or fantasized potential losses for the physically disabled person are loss of part of the body; loss of body function; loss of status in the family, social, and professional group; loss of future plans, home, finances, job, profession, and so on. Other stressors may be a threat to narcissistic integrity—fear of loss of love and approval; fear of loss of control of developmentally achieved functions (for example, bowel and bladder control); the reactivation of feelings of guilt and shame; and fear of retaliation for past transgressions.[105]

Mobility limitations result in physical and practical problems of meeting people by restricting one's ability to circulate in a social situation. This constriction of social sphere can lead to a lack of confidence in dealing with people's ignorance and rudeness. Thus the physically disabled person must contend with the physical disability *and* society's attitudes toward it. Friendships are often affected by the disability through people's anticipation that greater damands will be placed on them by their disabled friend. Further, friends' emotional response to the disability may make them reluctant to engage as they did before. These factors can lead to a change in one's circle of friends. Some find it easier to talk with other disabled persons, for example.[87]

Sandowski[92] stated that fear and lack of knowledge are the main psychologic factors that prevent realization of full sexual potential for the spinal cord–injured person. Indeed, David, Gur, and Razin,[35] in a study of male paraplegics who married nondisabled women after the injury, found that the women lacked knowledge about their husband's sexual capacities and the effect of the injury on the men's fertility. The wives were more dissatisfied with their inability to become pregnant and bear children than with the lack of sexual relations. Self-doubt about one's attractiveness as a sexual partner can have a negative impact on performance in a sexual situation that has been complicated by a spinal cord injury or other physical disability. Obviously, knowledge of alternative techniques, practice, and perseverance, together with an understanding partner and a sense of humor, can help surmount obstacles.[85]

Some investigators have reported that a return to preinjury sexual functioning is more important for many paraplegics and quadriplegics than a return to walking.[13,27,29] More recently researchers have looked at the relative value of sexual loss in relation to other functional losses for spinal cord–injured men, who suffer the most drastic physical limitations as a result of spinal cord damage. For example, Hanson and Franklin[50] found that rehabilitation staff overemphasize the relative importance of "normal" genital functioning when compared with the paraplegics' and quadriplegics' ratings of the relative importance of functional losses. These authors stressed that rehabilitation staff should carefully assess the relative importance of sexual loss for each patient to avoid the danger of conveying the message that intact genitals are essential to one's masculine identity. They also noted that dealing with sexual issues with patients can be exciting and stimulating and thus can meet needs of the staff as much as the needs of the patient. In a study of 11 male and 11 female paraplegics, aged 20 to 40 years, Ray and West[87] found that most had some sexual difficulties, but that these were not of greater importance than the social and personal implications of the disability.

DEVELOPING A PROGRAM FOR SEXUAL REHABILITATION

Many approaches to sexual counseling and rehabilitation have been described in the last decade.* In making recommendations for an approach to integrating sexual counseling into a rehabilitation program for individuals with neuromuscular disease, Anderson, Bardach, and Goodgold[4] addressed the fundamentals of sexual counseling: attitudes, knowledge, and skills. An assessment of the health care professional's *attitudes* toward all aspects of sexuality is considered a prerequisite by most researchers who have developed sexual rehabilitation programs. Cole, Chilgren, and Rosenberg's[27] model has been particularly successful in raising the participants' awareness of their *attitudes* and feelings about their own and others' sexuality, including the sexuality of physically disabled people. Their Sexual Attitude Reassessment seminars, called SARs, have been adapted for use in many settings. They were recently recommended by Madorsky and Dixon[76] as an important component of the sexual rehabilitation program at Casa Colina Hospital for Rehabilitation Medicine in Pomona, California. A primary goal is to reduce anxiety about sexual matters, using desensitization techniques, thereby enabling the professional to respond to clients' questions comfortably and without censure.

A second fundamental of sexual counseling—*knowledge*—is more easily achieved. Mastery of the basic information about the anatomy and physiology of sexual functioning, along with the most recent research data on the specific impact of disability on sexual functioning, is important. Each health care professional can then focus on the particular domain of rehabilitation that he or she is best equipped to explore with the client. For example, the physical therapist can be particularly helpful in recommending positions for sexual activity to overcome balance problems and so on. The rehabilitation nurse often has pertinent information about management of bowel and bladder incontinence, which can be an obstacle to sexual enjoyment.

The basic counseling *skills*—the ability to listen and communicate—are particularly important in assessing and treating sexual problems. Clients are often embarrassed and anxious, and many disguise their concerns. The creation of an atmosphere of acceptance of the clients' sexuality is essential. Careful and thorough exploration of clients' questions and concerns, using knowledge of potential obstacles, is necessary before problems can be resolved.

Madorsky and Dixon[76] have described a model for the integration of modern sex education, counseling, and therapy into the *initial* comprehensive rehabilitation plan for

---

*References 3, 4, 6-8, 26, 27, 38, 77, 88, 103.

spinal cord–injured individuals. Obviously, it can be modified to address the concerns of the majority of rehabilitation clients. The program is based on three assumptions: that sexual functioning is a legitimate, important concern of rehabilitation, that early intervention maximizes function and minimizes secondary complications, and that the opportunity for involvement of all rehabilitation staff and clients is important.

Madorsky and Dixon[76] use the PLISSIT model of sex therapy, developed by Annon.[6,7] The model provides a vertical emphasis in sex therapy, beginning with *permission*. An atmosphere of permission is achieved by using the physician as the authority figure to introduce the topic of sexuality during the admission interview and examination. The physician assesses sexual functioning and makes recommendations for further exploration in other areas of the rehabilitation program. *Limited information* is provided by each member of the rehabilitation team as it relates to his or her area of responsibility and expertise. *Specific suggestions* are given when indicated by a detailed evaluation of the client's personal strengths, level of adjustment to the disability, and current sexual relationship. *Intensive therapy* is provided by the psychologist and physician, based on an assessment of the individual's needs. Couple exercises, sensate-focus exercises, and social skills training are some of the recommendations that may be given. This program maximizes the involvement of the staff and the client.

Bardach and Anderson[8] and Anderson, Bardach, and Goodgold[4] have described a problem-oriented, or functional, approach to assessing and treating some of the obstacles to sexual activity that arise because of physical limitations. Bardach and Anderson,[8] for example, identify such problems as bladder incontinence, bowel incontinence, spasticity, arousal and sensation, motor losses, and positioning and make recommendations for surmounting these obstacles. Anderson, Bardach, and Goodgold[4] provide a manual for health care professionals to use in sexual rehabilitation of individuals with neuromuscular diseases. One section of this manual identifies functional limitations, such as loss of mobility, contractures, problems with balance and coordination, and low endurance, and suggests methods of overcoming these difficulties. Bardach and Padrone[9] have produced a two-part film, "Choices: In Sexuality with Physical Disability,"* that uses a problem-oriented approach in which disabled persons and their partners relate and discuss their experiences. Part 1 explores such concerns as one's perception of self as sexual, fears of rejection, establishing relationships, and so on. In part 2 specific problems, such as incontinence, lost and diminished sensation, arousal, positioning, and communication, are presented explicitly, with possible solutions offered.

---

*This product is available as a 16 mm film and in ¾- and ½-inch Beta or VHS videocassettes from Mercury Productions, 17 West 45th Street, New York, NY 10036.

REFERENCES

1. Amelar, RD, and Dubin, L: Sexual function and fertility in paraplegic males, Urology 20:62, 1982.
2. Anderson, FS: Sexual problems of patients with neuromuscular diseases, Med Aspects Hum Sexuality, 18:82, 1984.
3. Anderson, F, and Bardach, JL: Sexuality and neuromuscular disease: a pilot study, Int Rehabil Med 5:21, 1983.
4. Anderson, F, Bardach, JL, and Goodgold, J: Sexuality and neuromuscular disease, Rehabilitation Monograph, No 56, New York, 1979, Rusk Institute of Rehabilitation Medicine.
5. Anderson, TP, and Cole, TM: Sexual counseling of the physically disabled, Postgrad Med 58:117, 1975.
6. Annon, J: The behavioral treatment of sexual problems, vol 2, Intensive therapy, Honolulu, 1976, Enabling Systems.
7. Annon, J: The behavioral treatment of sexual problems, vol 1, Intensive therapy, Honolulu, 1974, Kapiolani Health Services.
8. Bardach, JL, and Anderson, F: Sexual therapy in rehabilitation. In Murray, R, and Kijek, JC, editors: Current perspectives in rehabilitation nursing, vol 1, St Louis, 1979, The CV Mosby Co.
9. Bardach, JL, and Padrone, F: Choices: in sexuality with physical disability (filmstrip), New York, 1982, Mercury Productions.
10. Berkman, AH, Weismann, R, and Frielich, MH: Sexual adjustment of spinal cord injured veterans living in the community, Arch Phys Med Rehabil 59:29, 1978.
11. Blanchard, MG: Sex education for spinal cord injured patients and their nurses. In Krueger, DW, editor: Rehabilitation psychology: a comprehensive textbook, Rockville, Md, 1984, Aspen Systems Corp.
12. Blanchard, MG: Sex education for spinal cord injured patients and their nurses, Paraplegia News 29:30, 1976.
13. Bloom, DS: Sexual aspects of physical disability, Am Arch Rehabil Ther 22:32, 1974.
14. Bors, E, and Comarr, AE: Neurological urology, Baltimore, 1971, University Park Press.
15. Bors, E, and Comarr, AE: Neurological disturbances of sexual function with special reference to 529 patients with spinal cord injury, Urol Surgery 10:191, 1960.
16. Bors, E, et al: Fertility in paraplegic males: a preliminary report of endocrine studies, J Clin Endocrinol 10:381, 1950.
17. Braakman, R, Orbaan, IJC, and Blauw-van Dishoeck, M: Information in the early stages after spinal cord injury, Paraplegia 14:95, 1976.
18. Bregman, S: Sexuality and the spinal cord injured woman, Minneapolis, 1975, Sister Kenny Publishers.
19. Brindley, GS: The fertility of men with spinal injuries, Paraplegia 22:337, 1984.
20. Brindley, GS: Electroejaculation: its technique, neurological implications and uses, J Neurol Neurosurg Psychiatry 44:9, 1981.
21. Brindley, GS: Reflex ejaculation under vibratory stimulation in paraplegic men, Paraplegia 19:299, 1981.
22. Brindley, GS: Electroejaculation and the fertility of paraplegic men, Sexuality Disability 3:223, 1980.
23. Chapelle, PA, Gaussel, JJ, and Grossiord, A: Reflexions concernant les problemes genito-sexuales des paraplegiques, Ann Med Physique 12:1, 1974.
24. Chapelle, PA, et al: Pregnancy of the wife of a complete paraplegic by homologeous insemination after an intrathecal injection of neostigmine, Paraplegia 14:173, 1976.
25. Charatan, FB, and Fisk, A: Mental and emotional results of strokes, NY State J Med 7:1403, 1978.
26. Chipouras, S: Ten sexuality programmes for spinal cord injured persons, Sexuality Disability 2:301, 1979.
27. Cole, TM, Chilgren, R, and Rosenberg, P: New program of sex education and counselling for spinal cord injured adults and health care professional, Intern J Paraplegia 11:111, 1973.

28. Comarr, AE: Sexual function among patients with spinal cord injury, Urologica Internationalis 23:134, 1970.

29. Comarr, EA, and Vigue, MS: Sexual counseling among male and female patients with spinal cord and/or cauda equina injury, part 1, Am J Physical Med 57:107, 1978.

30. Comfort, A, editor: Sexual consequences of disability, Philadelphia, 1978, George F. Stickley Co.

31. Conine, TA: Sexual rehabilitation: the roles of allied health professionals. In Krueger, DW, editor: Rehabilitation psychology: a comprehensive textbook, Rockville, Md, 1984, Aspen System Corp.

32. Conine, TA, and Evans, JH: Sexual adjustment in chronic obstructive pulmonary disease, Respir Care 26:871, 1981.

33. Conine, TA, et al: Sexual rehabilitation of the handicapped: the roles and attitudes of health professionals, J Allied Health 9:260, 1980.

34. Cressy, JM, Comar, A, and Estin, MD: Sexuality and spinal cord injury, Spinal Cord Injury Digest 3:23, 1981.

35. David, A, Gur, S, and Rozin, R: Survival in marriage in the paraplegic couple, Paraplegia 15:198, 1978.

36. David, A, Ohry, A, and Rozin, R: Spinal cord injuries: male infertility aspects, Paraplegia 15:11, 1977.

37. Dollfus, P, et al: Impairment of erection after external sphincter resection, Paraplegia 13:290, 1976.

38. Eisenberg, MG, and Rustad, LC: Sex education and counselling program on spinal cord injury service, Arch Phys Med Rehabil 57:135, 1976.

39. Engel, GL: Psychological development in health and disease, Philadelphia, 1962, WB Saunders Co.

40. Feinblatt, A, Anderson, FS, and Gordon, W: Psychosocial and vocational considerations. In Leek, JC, Gershwin, ME, and Fowler, WM, editors: Principles of physical medicine and rehabilitation in the musculoskeletal diseases, Orlando, Fla, 1986, Grune & Statton, Inc.

41. Forner, JV: The female paraplegic in Spain: preliminary report, Paraplegia 21:176, 1983.

42. Francois, N, et al: L'ejaculation par le vibromassage chez le paraplegique a propos de 50 cas avec 7 grossesses, Ann Med Physique 23:24, 1980.

43. Francois, N, et al: Electroejaculation of a complete paraplegic followed by pregnancy, Paraplegia 16:248, 1978.

44. Fugl-Meyer, AR, and Jaasko, LJ: Post stroke hemiplegia and sexual intercourse, Scand J Rehabil Med 12(suppl 7):158, 1980.

45. Goffman, E: Stigma, Englewood Cliffs, NJ, 1963, Prentice-Hall, Inc.

46. Green, BG, and Sloan, SL: Penile prostheses in spinal cord injured patients: combined psychosexual counselling and surgical regimen, Paraplegia 24:167, 1986.

47. Gunterberg, B, and Petersen, J: Sexual function after major resections of the sacrum with bilateral or unilateral sacrifice of sacral nerves, Fertil Steril 27:1146, 1976.

48. Guttmann, L: The effect of Prostigmin on the reproductive function in the spinal man, Proceedings of the Fourth International Neurological Congress, vol 2, Paris, 1949, Masson.

49. Guttmann, L, and Walsh, JJ: Prostigmin assessment of fertility in spinal man, Paraplegia 9:39, 1971.

50. Hanson, RW, and Franklin, MR: Sexual loss in relation to other functional losses for spinal cord injured males, Arch Phys Med Rehabil 57:291, 1976.

51. Hayes, PJ, et al: Testicular endocrine function in paraplegic men, Clin Endocrinol 11:549, 1979.

52. Head, H, and Riddoch, G: The automatic bladder, excessive sweating and some other reflex conditions in gross injuries of the spinal cord, Brain 40:188, 1917.

53. Hogan, MJ, Wallin, JD, and Baer, RM: Antihypertensive therapy and male sexual dysfunction, Psychosomatics 21:234, 1980.

54. Hohmann, GW: Consideration in management of psychosexual adjustment in spinal cord injured males, Rehabil Psychol 19:50, 1972.

55. Horne, HH, Paull, DP, and Munro, D: Fertility studies in the human male with traumatic injuries of the spinal cord and cauda equina, N Engl J Med 239:959, 1948.

56. Ivers, RR, and Goldstein, NP: Multiple sclerosis: a current appraisal of symptoms and signs, Proc Mayo Clinic 38:457, 1963.

57. Iwatsubo, E, Imamura, A, and Hoshino, O: Reevaluation of prostigmine test for male paraplegics, Orthopaed Traumatol Surgery 27:1163, 1984.

58. Jameson, RM: The long term results of transurethral division of the external urethral sphincter in the neuropathic urethra with reference to potency, Paraplegia 20:299, 1982.

59. Jochheim, KA, and Wahle, H: A study of sexual function in 56 male patients with complete irreversible lesions of the spinal cord and cauda equina, Paraplegia 8:166, 1970.

60. Kalliomaki, JL, Markanen, TK, and Mustonen, VA: Sexual behavior after cerebral vascular accident, Fertil Steril 12:156, 1961.

61. Karacan, I, et al: Nocturnal penile tumescence and diagnosis in diabetic impotence, Am J Psychiatry 135:191, 1978.

62. Karacan, I, Williams, RL, and Thornby, JI: Sleep related penile tumescence as a function of age, Am J Psychiatry 132:932, 1975.

63. Karacan, I, et al: Some characteristics of nocturnal penile tumescence in young adults, Arch Gen Psychiatry 26:315, 1972.

64. Katz, K: Stigma: a social psychological analysis, Hillsdale, NJ, 1981, Lawrence Erlbaum Associates, Publishers.

65. Katz, S, Shurka, E, and Florian, V: The relationship between physical disability, social perceptions and psychological stress, Scand J Rehabil Med 10:109, 1978.

66. Kikuchi, TA, et al: The pituitary-gonadal axis in spinal cord injury, Fertil Steril 27:1142, 1976.

67. Kinsella, GJ, and Duffy, FD: Psychosocial readjustment in the spouses of aphasic patients, Scand J Rehabil Med 11:129, 1979.

68. Kleck, R: Physical stigma and nonverbal cues emitted in face to face interaction, Hum Relations 21:19-28, 1968.

69. Lamid, S: Nocturnal penile tumescence studies in spinal cord injured males, Paraplegia 23:26, 1985.

70. Larsen, E, and Hejgaard, N: Sexual dysfunction after spinal cord or cauda equina lesions, Paraplegia 22:66, 1984.

71. Leshner, M, Fine, HL, and Goldman, A: Sexual activity in older stroke patients, Proceedings of the 51st Annual Session of the ACRM, 1974, Arch Phys Med Rehabil 55:578, 1974.

72. Leyson, JFJ, and Powell, RB: Comparative study of 2 nocturnal penile tumescence monitors in the diagnosis of impotence, J Med Soc NJ 79:647, 1982.

73. Lilius, HG, Valtonen, EJ, and Wikstrom, J: Sexual problems in patients suffering from multiple sclerosis, J Chron Dis 29:643, 1976.

74. Linder, H: Perceptual sensitization to sexual phenomena in the chronic physically handicapped, J Clin Psychol 9:67, 1953.

75. Lundberg, PO: Observations in endocrine function in ocular myopathy, Acta Neurol Scand 42:39, 1966.

76. Madorsky, JG, and Dixon, TP: Rehabilitation aspects of human sexuality, West J Med 139:174, 1983.

77. Melnyk, R, and Montgomery, R: Attitude changes following a sexual counselling program for spinal cord injured persons, Arch Phys Med Rehabil 60:601, 1979.

78. Miller, H, Simpson, CA, and Yeates, WK: Bladder dysfunction in multiple sclerosis, Br Med J 1:1265, 1965.

79. Minderhoud, JM, et al: Sexual disturbances arising from multiple sclerosis, Acta Neurol Scand 70:299, 1984.

80. Mizutani, S, et al: Plasma testosterone concentration in paraplegic men, J Endocrinol 54:363, 1972.

81. Mooney, TO, Cole, TM, and Chilgren, RA: Sexual options for paraplegics and quadraplegics, Boston, 1974, Little Brown & Co.

82. Morales, PA, and Harden, J: Scrotal and testicular temperature studies in paraplegics, J Urol 79:972, 1958.

83. Otani, T, Kondo, A, and Takita, T: A paraplegic fathering a child after an intrathecal injection of neostigmine: case report, Paraplegia 24:32, 1985.

84. Piera, JB: The establishment of a prognosis for genitosexual function in the paraplegic and tetraplegic male, Paraplegia 10:271, 1973.

85. Quastel, LN: Sexual rehabilitation of the physically disabled and chronically ill. In Freeman, DS, and Trute, B, editors: Treating families with special needs, Ottawa, Candada, 1981, Canadian Association of Social Workers.

86. Ray, C, and West, J: Coping with spinal cord injury, Paraplegia 22:249, 1984.

87. Ray, C, and West, J: Social, sexual and personal implications of paraplegia, Paraplegia 22:75, 1984.

88. Romano, M, and Lassiter, R: Sexual counseling with the spinal-cord injured, Arch Phys Med 53:568, 1972.

89. Rossier, A, and Fam, BA: Indication and results of semi-rigid penile prostheses in spinal cord injury patients: long term followup, J Urol 131:59, 1981.

90. Rossier, A, et al: Sexual function and dysreflexia, Paraplegia 9:51, 1971.

91. Rubington, E, and Weinberg, MS, editors: Deviance: the interactionist perspective, New York, 1973, Macmillan Publishing Co.

92. Sandowski, CL: Sexuality and the paraplegic, Rehabil Lit 37:322, 1976.

93. Sha'ked, A, and Flynn, RJ: Normative sex behavior and the person with a disability: training of rehabilitation personnel, J Rehabil 44:30, 1978.

94. Shrey, DE, Kiefer, JS, and Anthony, WA: Sexual adjustment counseling for persons with severe disabilities: a skill-based approach for rehabilitation professionals, J Rehabil 45:28, 1979.

95. Siller, J: The measurement of attitudes toward physically disabled persons. In Herman, CP, Zanna, MP, and Higgins, ET, editors: Physical appearance, stigma, and social behavior: the Ontario symposium, vol 3, Hillsdale, NJ, 1986, Lawrence Erlbaum Associates, Publishers.

96. Sjogren, K: Sexuality after stroke with hemiplegia. II. With special regard to partnership and adjustment and to fulfillment, Scand J Rehabil Med 15:63, 1983.

97. Sjogren, K, Damber, JE, and Liliequist, B: Sexuality after stroke with hemiplegia. I. Aspects of sexual function, Scand J Rehabil Med 15:55, 1983.

98. Sjogren, K, and Egberg, K: The sexual experience in younger males with complete spinal cord injury, Scand J Rehabil Med (suppl) 9:189, 1983.

99. Sjogren, K, and Fugl-Meyer, AR: Adjustment to life after stroke with special reference to sexual intercourse and leisure, J Psychosom Res 26:409, 1982.

100. Sjogren, K, and Fugl-Meyer, AR: Sexual problems in hemiplegia, Int Rehabil Med 3:26, 1981.

101. Snyder, ML, et al: Avoidance of the handicapped: an attributional analysis, J Personal Soc Psychol 37:2297, 1979.

102. Spira, R: Artificial insemination after intrathecal injection of neostigmine in a paraplegic, Lancet 270:670, 1956.

103. Steger, JC, and Brockway, JA: Sexual enhancement in spinal cord injured patients: behavioral group treatment, Sexuality Disability 3:84, 1980.

104. Stewart, TD, and Gerson, SN: Penile prosthesis: psychologic factors, Urology 7:400, 1976.

105. Strain, JH, and Gross, S: Psychological care of the medically ill: a primer in the liaison psychiatry, New York, 1975, Appleton-Century-Crofts.

106. Szasz, G, Paty, D, and Maurice, WL: Sexual dysfunctions in multiple sclerosis, Ann NY Acad Sci 436:443, 1984.

107. Szasz, G, et al: A sexual functioning scale in multiple sclerosis, Acta Neurol Scand (suppl) 101:37, 1984.

108. Taggie, JM, and Manley, MS: A handbook on sexuality after spinal cord injury, Englewood, Colo, 1978, M Scott Manley, Publisher.

109. Talbot, HS: The sexual function in paraplegics, J Urol 73:91, 1975.

110. Tarabulcy, E: Sexual function in the normal and in paraplegia, Paraplegia 10:210, 1972.

111. Thomas, DG: The effect of trans-urethral surgery on penile erections in spinal cord injury patients, Paraplegia 13:286, 1976.

112. Thomas, JS, Mcleish, G, and McDonald, IA: Electroejaculation of the paraplegic male followed by pregnancy, Med J Austr 2:798, 1975.

113. Thornton, CE: Sexuality counselling of women with spinal cord injuries, Sexuality Disability 4:276, 1979.

114. Trieschmann, RB: Spinal cord injuries: psychological, social and vocational adjustment, New York, 1980, Pergamon Press.

115. Tringo, JL: The hierarchy of preference toward disability groups, J Special Ed 4:295, 1970.

116. Turk, R, Turk, M, and Assejev, V: The female paraplegic and mother-child relations, Paraplegia 21:186, 1983.

117. Valleroy, ML, and Kraft, GH: Sexual dysfunction in multiple sclerosis, Arch Phys Med Rehabil 65:125, 1984.

118. Van Arsdalen, KN, et al: Penile implants in spinal cord injury patients for maintaining external appliances, J Urol 126:331, 1981.

119. Vas, CJ: Sexual impotence and some autonomic disturbances in men with multiple sclerosis, Acta Neurol Scand 45:166, 1969.

120. Verduyn, WH: Spinal cord injured women, pregnancy and delivery, Paraplegia 24:231, 1986.

121. Verwoerdt, A: Psychopathological responses to the stress of physical illness. In Lipowski, ZJ, editor: Psychosocial aspects of physical illness, vol 8. Advances in psychosomatic medicine series, Basel, 1972, S Krager.

122. Weiss, AJ, and Diamond, MD: Sexual adjustment, identification and attitudes of patients with myelopathy, Arch Phys Med Rehabil 47:245, 1966.

123. Wright, BA: Physical disability: a psychosocial approach, ed 2, New York, 1983, Harper & Row, Publishers.

124. Zeitlin, AB, Cottrell, TL, and Floyd, FA: Sexology of the paraplegic male, Fertil Steril 8:337, 1957.

Index

Italicized page numbers indicate illustration; t indicates table.